Tucson, Arizona

Dear Readers:

We are proud to present the 11th annual edition of the **COMPLETE GUIDE TO PRESCRIPTION & NON-PRESCRIPTION DRUGS.** Each new edition provides information regarding drugs newly approved by the U.S. Food and Drug Administration as well as added information about established drugs.

The members of the large team that works together to make this book possible include the publishers, The Body Press/Perigee Books of the Putnam Publishing Group; my wife, Jo Alyce Griffith, who contributed in many ways; and Randy Summerlin as editor. These and more played big roles in this updated version for 1994. As always, I am also grateful to the host of scientists and workers in the fields of pharmacology, organic chemistry and pharmacy for discovering the facts and principles published here. We are fortunate to live when there are so many effective and safe medications for so many human illnesses. I am grateful, too, for the many of you who read and use this book. Your health is important to all of us.

I view my job as that of a translator, reporter and organizer of the opinions of the majority of experts. I have attempted to reduce technical writing to a readily understandable level and format so you can easily use the information for better health for yourself or for those to whom you may provide care.

In addition to being healing, curative, or life-saving, many drugs can also cause new symptoms, unnecessary pain, prolonged hospital stays, or unfortunate new illnesses. To prevent or minimize these adverse effects, wise use of all drugs requires the full cooperation of doctors, nurses, pharmacists, manufacturers and patients.

I challenge each of you to be fully informed before you take any medicine, including those you prescribe for yourselves. There are many reasons why medication errors occur. You can prevent most of those errors yourself by being fully informed about the medicines you take and by constantly reviewing and acting upon this knowledge.

You are the most important member of your own health-care team.

Sincerely yours,

H. Winter Griffith, M.D.

H. Winter Griffith, M.D.

COMPLETE GUIDE TO PRESCRIPTION & NON-PRESCRIPTION

DRUGS

By H. WINTER GRIFFITH, M.D.

Technical consultants:
John D. Palmer, M.D., Ph.D.
William N. Jones, B.S., M.S.

NEW!
Revised for 1994
Over 5000 Brand Names
Over 700 Generic Names

THE BODY PRESS/PERIGEE

Notice: The information in this book is true and complete to the best of our knowledge. The book is intended only as a guide to drugs used for medical treatment. It is not intended as a replacement for sound medical advice from a doctor. Only a doctor can include the variables of an individual's age, sex and past medical history needed for wise drug prescription. This book does not contain every possible side effect, adverse reaction or interaction with other drugs or substances. Final decision about a drug's safety or effectiveness must be made by the individual and his doctor. All recommendations herein are made without guarantees on the part of the author or the publisher. The author and publisher disclaim all liability in connection with the use of this information.

The Body Press/Perigee Books
are published by
The Putnam Publishing Group
200 Madison Avenue
New York, NY 10016

Library of Congress Cataloging-in-Publication Data

Griffith, H. Winter (Henry Winter).
    Complete guide to prescription & non-prescription drugs / by H. Winter Griffith;
technical consultants, John D. Palmer, William N. Jones.—Rev. for 1994.
      p. cm.
    Includes index.
    ISBN 0-399-51835-5
    1. Drugs—Popular works. 2. Drugs, Non-prescription—Popular works.
I. Title. II. Title: Complete guide to prescription and non-prescription drugs.
    [DNLM: 1. Drugs—handbooks. 2. Drugs—popular works. 3. Drugs,
Non-prescription—handbooks. 4. Drugs, Non-prescription—popular works.
QV 39 G854c 1994]
RM301.15.G75 1994   93-30019 CIP
615'.1—dc20
DNLM/DLC
for Library of Congress

Printed in the United States of America

1 2 3 4 5 6 7 8 9 10

CONTENTS

ABOUT THE AUTHOR

H. Winter Griffith, M.D., has authored 25 medical books, including the *Complete Guide to Symptoms, Illness & Surgery; Complete Guide to Pediatric Symptoms, Illness & Medications;* and *Complete Guide to Sports Injuries,* each now published by The Body Press/Perigee Books. Others include *Instructions for Patients; Drug Information for Patients; Instructions for Dental Patients; Information and Instructions for Pediatric Patients; Vitamins, Minerals and Supplements;* and *Medical Tests—Doctor Ordered and Do-It-Yourself.* Dr. Griffith received his medical degree from Emory University in 1953. After 20 years in private practice, he established and was the first director of a basic medical-science program at Florida State University. He then became an associate professor of family and community medicine at the University of Arizona College of Medicine.

Technical Consultants

John D. Palmer, M.D., Ph.D.
  Associate professor of pharmacology, University of Arizona College of Medicine
  Associate professor of medicine (clinical pharmacology), University of Arizona
    College of Medicine

William N. Jones, Pharmacist, B.S., M.S.
  Clinical pharmacy coordinator, Veterans Administration Medical Center, Tucson,
    Arizona
  Adjunct assistant professor, Department of Pharmacy Practice, College of
    Pharmacy, University of Arizona

DRUGS AND YOU

My first day of pharmacology class in medical school started with a jolt. The professor began by writing on the blackboard, "Drugs are poisons."

I thought the statement was extreme. New drug discoveries promised to solve medical problems that had baffled men for centuries. The medical community was intrigued with new possibilities for drugs.

In the 30 years since then, many drug "miracles" have lived up to those early expectations. But the years have also shown the damage drugs can cause when they are misused or not fully understood. As a family doctor and teacher, I have developed a healthy respect for what drugs can and can't do. I appreciate my professor's warning more than ever.

A drug cannot "cure." It aids the body's natural defenses to promote recovery. Likewise, a manufacturer or doctor cannot guarantee a drug will be useful for everyone. The complexity of the human body, individual responses in different people and in the same person under different circumstances, past and present health, age and sex influence how well a drug works.

All effective drugs produce desirable changes in the body, but a drug can also cause undesirable adverse reactions or side effects in some people. Despite uncertainties, the drug discoveries of the last 40 years have given us tools to save lives and reduce discomfort. Before you decide whether to take a drug, you or your doctor must ask, "Will the benefits outweigh the risks?"

The purpose of this book is to give you enough information about the most widely used drugs so you can make a wise decision. The information will alert you to potential or preventable problems. You can learn what to do if problems arise.

The information is derived from many authoritative sources and represents the consensus of many experts. Every effort has been made to ensure accuracy and completeness. Where information from different sources conflicts, I have used the majority's opinion, coupled with my clinical judgment and that of my technical consultants. Drug information changes with continuing observations by clinicians and users.

Information in this book applies to generic drugs in both the United States and Canada. Generic names do not vary in these countries, but brand names do.

BE SAFE! TELL YOUR DOCTOR

Some suggestions for wise drug use apply to all drugs. Always give your doctor or dentist complete information about the drugs you take, including your medical history, your medical plans and your progress while under medication.

MEDICAL HISTORY

Tell the important facts of your medical history including illness and previous experience with drugs. Include allergic or adverse reactions you have had to any medicine in the past. Describe the allergic symptoms you have, such as hay fever, asthma, eye watering and itching, throat irritation and reactions to food. People who have allergies to common substances are more likely to develop drug allergies.

List all drugs you take. Don't forget vitamin and mineral supplements; skin, rectal or vaginal medicines; eyedrops and eardrops; antacids; antihistamines; cold and cough remedies;

inhalers and nasal sprays; aspirin, aspirin combinations or other pain relievers; motion sickness remedies; weight-loss aids; salt and sugar substitutes; caffeine; oral contraceptives; sleeping pills or "tonics."

FUTURE MEDICAL PLANS

Discuss plans for elective surgery, pregnancy and breast-feeding. These conditions may require discontinuing or modifying the dosages of medicines you may be taking.

QUESTIONS

Don't hesitate to ask questions about a drug. Your doctor, nurse or pharmacist will be able to provide more information if they are familiar with you and your medical history.

YOUR ROLE

Learn the generic names and brand names of all your medicines. Write them down to help you remember. If a drug is a mixture, learn the names of its generic ingredients.

TAKING A DRUG

Never take medicine in the dark! Recheck the label before each use. You could be taking the *wrong* drug! Tell your doctor about any unexpected new symptoms you have while taking medicine. You may need to change medicines or have a dose adjustment.

STORAGE

Keep all medicines out of children's reach. Store drugs in a cool, dry place, such as a kitchen cabinet or bedroom. Avoid medicine cabinets in bathrooms. They get too moist and warm at times.

Keep medicine in its original container, tightly closed. Don't remove the label! If directions call for refrigeration, keep the medicine cool, but don't freeze it.

DISCARDING

Don't save leftover medicine to use later. Discard it before the expiration date shown on the container. Dispose safely to protect children and pets.

REFILLS

All refills must be ordered by your doctor or dentist, either in the first prescription or later. Only the pharmacy that originally filled the prescription can refill it without checking with your doctor or previous pharmacy. If you go to a *new* pharmacy, you must have a new prescription, or the new pharmacist must call your doctor or original pharmacy to see if a refill is authorized. Pharmacies don't usually transfer prescriptions.

If you need a refill, call your pharmacist and order your refill by number and name.

Use one pharmacy for the whole family if you can. The pharmacist then has a record of all of your drugs and can communicate effectively with your doctor, you and your family.

LEARN ABOUT DRUGS

Study the information in this book's charts regarding your medications. Read each chart completely. Because of space limitations, most information that fits more than one category appears only once.

Take care of yourself. You are the most important member of your health-care team.

GUIDE TO DRUG CHARTS

The drug information in this book is organized in condensed, easy-to-read charts. Each drug is described in a two-page format, as shown in the sample chart below and opposite. Charts are arranged alphabetically by drug generic names, and in a few instances, such as *ADRENOCORTICOIDS, TOPICAL*, by drug-class name.

A *generic name* is the official chemical name for a drug. A *brand name* is a drug manufacturer's registered trademark for a generic drug. Brand names listed on the charts

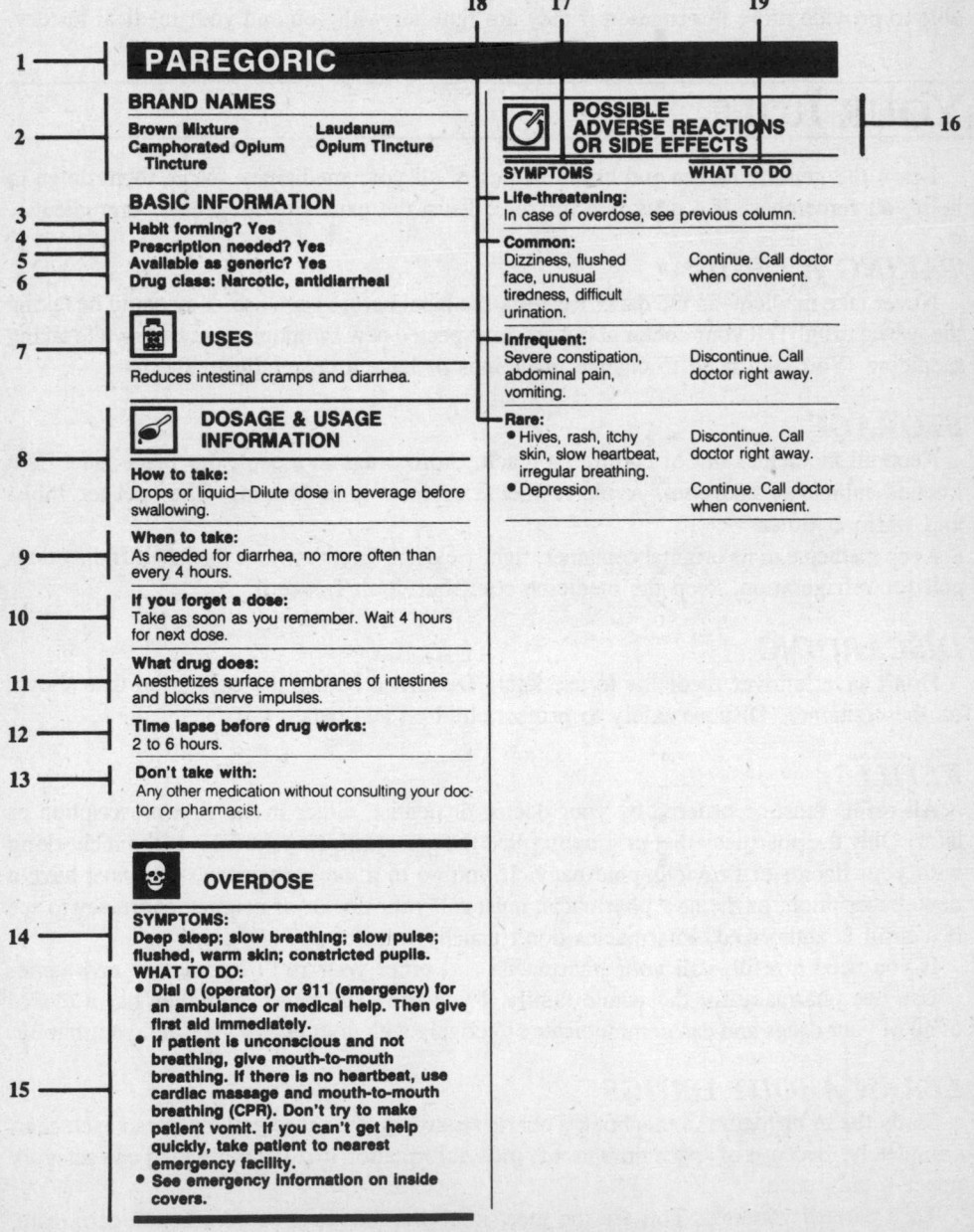

PAREGORIC

BRAND NAMES

Brown Mixture
Camphorated Opium
  Tincture

Laudanum
Opium Tincture

BASIC INFORMATION

Habit forming? Yes
Prescription needed? Yes
Available as generic? Yes
Drug class: Narcotic, antidiarrheal

USES

Reduces intestinal cramps and diarrhea.

DOSAGE & USAGE INFORMATION

How to take:
Drops or liquid—Dilute dose in beverage before swallowing.

When to take:
As needed for diarrhea, no more often than every 4 hours.

If you forget a dose:
Take as soon as you remember. Wait 4 hours for next dose.

What drug does:
Anesthetizes surface membranes of intestines and blocks nerve impulses.

Time lapse before drug works:
2 to 6 hours.

Don't take with:
Any other medication without consulting your doctor or pharmacist.

OVERDOSE

SYMPTOMS:
Deep sleep; slow breathing; slow pulse; flushed, warm skin; constricted pupils.
WHAT TO DO:
- Dial 0 (operator) or 911 (emergency) for an ambulance or medical help. Then give first aid immediately.
- If patient is unconscious and not breathing, give mouth-to-mouth breathing. If there is no heartbeat, use cardiac massage and mouth-to-mouth breathing (CPR). Don't try to make patient vomit. If you can't get help quickly, take patient to nearest emergency facility.
- See emergency information on inside covers.

POSSIBLE ADVERSE REACTIONS OR SIDE EFFECTS

SYMPTOMS	WHAT TO DO
Life-threatening:	
In case of overdose, see previous column.	
Common:	
Dizziness, flushed face, unusual tiredness, difficult urination.	Continue. Call doctor when convenient.
Infrequent:	
Severe constipation, abdominal pain, vomiting.	Discontinue. Call doctor right away.
Rare:	
• Hives, rash, itchy skin, slow heartbeat, irregular breathing.	Discontinue. Call doctor right away.
• Depression.	Continue. Call doctor when convenient.

include those from the United States and Canada. A generic drug may have one or ma[...]
brand names.

To find information about a generic drug, look it up in the alphabetical charts. To lea[...]
about a brand name, check the index first, where brand names are followed by their gener[...]
ingredients and chart page numbers.

The chart design is the same for every drug. When you are familiar with the chart, yo[...]
can quickly find information you want to know about a drug.

On the next few pages, each of the numbered chart sections below is explained. Thi[...]
information will guide you in reading and understanding the charts that begin on page 2[...]

PAREGORIC

20 — 👉 **WARNINGS & PRECAUTIONS**

21 — **Don't take if:**
You are allergic to any narcotic.

22 — **Before you start, consult your doctor:**
If you have impaired liver or kidney function.

23 — **Over age 60:**
More likely to be drowsy, dizzy, unsteady or constipated.

24 — **Pregnancy:**
No proven harm to unborn child. Avoid if possible.

25 — **Breast-feeding:**
Drug filters into milk. May depress infant. Avoid.

26 — **Infants & children:**
Use only under medical supervision.

27 — **Prolonged use:**
Causes psychological and physical dependence.

28 — **Skin & sunlight:**
No problems expected.

29 — **Driving, piloting or hazardous work:**
Don't drive or pilot aircraft until you learn how medicine affects you. Don't work around dangerous machinery. Don't climb ladders or work in high places. Danger increases if you drink alcohol or take medicine affecting alertness and reflexes, such as antihistamines, tranquilizers, sedatives, pain medicine, narcotics and mind-altering drugs.

30 — **Discontinuing:**
May be unnecessary to finish medicine. Follow doctor's instructions.

31 — **Others:**
Great potential for abuse.

🔲 **POSSIBLE INTERACTION WITH OTHER DRUGS**

GENERIC NAME OR DRUG CLASS	COMBINED EFFECT
Analgesics*	Increased analgesic effect.
Antidepressants*	Increased sedation.
Antihistamines*	Increased sedation.
Carteolol	Increased narcotic effect. Dangerous sedation.
Central nervous system (CNS) depressants*	Increased central nerve system depression.

32 — (bracket for POSSIBLE INTERACTION WITH OTHER DRUGS table)

Clozapine	Toxic effect on the central nervous system.
Ethinamate	Dangerous increased effects of ethinamate. Avoid combining.
Fluoxetine	Increased depressant effects of both drugs.
Guanfacine	May increase depressant effects of either medicine.
Leucovorin	High alcohol content of leucovorin may cause adverse effects.
Methyprylon	May increase sedative effect to dangerous level. Avoid.
Mind-altering drugs*	Increased sedation.
Nabilone	Greater depression of central nervous system.
Narcotics, other*	Increased narcotic effect.
Phenothiazines*	Increased sedative effect of paregoric.
Sedatives*	Excessive sedation.
Sleep inducers*	Increased effect of sleep inducers.
Sotalol	Increased narcotic effect. Dangerous sedation.
Tranquilizers*	Increased tranquilizer effect.

32 (right bracket)

🔲 **POSSIBLE INTERACTION WITH OTHER SUBSTANCES**

INTERACTS WITH	COMBINED EFFECT
Alcohol:	Increases alcohol's intoxicating effect. Avoid.
Beverages:	None expected.
Cocaine:	None expected.
Foods:	None expected.
Marijuana:	Impairs physical and mental performance.
Tobacco:	None expected.

33 (bracket for POSSIBLE INTERACTION WITH OTHER SUBSTANCES)

*See Glossary

1—GENERIC NAME

Each drug chart is titled by generic name, or in a few instances, by the name of the drug class, such as *DIGITALIS PREPARATIONS.*

Sometimes a drug is known by more than one generic name. The chart is titled by the most common one. Less-common generic names appear in parentheses following the first. For example, vitamin C is also known as ascorbic acid. Its chart title is *VITAMIN C (Ascorbic Acid).* The index will include a reference for each name.

Your drug container may show a generic name, a brand name or both. If you have only a brand name, use the index to find the drug's generic name and chart.

If your drug container shows no name, ask your doctor or pharmacist for the name and record it on the container.

2—BRAND NAMES

A brand name is usually shorter and easier to remember than the generic name.

The brand names listed for each generic drug in this book may not include all brands available in the United States and Canada. The most-common ones are listed. New brands appear on the market, and brands are sometimes removed from the market. No list can reflect every change. In the few instances in which the drug chart is titled with a drug-class name instead of a generic name, the generic and brand names all appear under the heading *BRAND AND GENERIC NAMES.* The *BRAND NAMES* are in lower case letters, and *GENERIC NAMES* are in capital letters.

Inclusion of a brand name does not imply recommendation or endorsement. Exclusion does not imply that a missing brand name is less effective or less safe than the ones listed. Some generic drugs have too many brand names to list on one chart. The most common brand names appear, or a complete list of common brand names for those drugs is on the page indicated on the chart.

Lists of brand names don't differentiate between prescription and non-prescription drugs. The active ingredients are the same.

If you buy a non-prescription drug, look for generic names of the active ingredients on the container. Common non-prescription drugs are described in this book under their generic components. They are also indexed by brand name.

Most drugs contain *inert,* or inactive, ingredients that are *fillers, dyes* or *solvents* for active ingredients. Manufacturers choose inert ingredients that preserve the drug without interfering with the action of the active ingredients.

Inert substances are listed on labels of non-prescription drugs. They do not appear on prescription drugs. Your pharmacist can tell you all active and inert ingredients in a prescription drug.

Occasionally, a tablet, capsule or liquid may contain small amounts of sodium, sugar or potassium. If you are on a diet that severely restricts any of these, ask your pharmacist or doctor to suggest another form.

BASIC INFORMATION

3—HABIT FORMING

A drug habit can be physical or psychological. A drug that produces physical dependence leads to addiction. It causes painful and sometimes dangerous effects when withdrawn.

Psychological dependence does not cause dangerous withdrawal effects. It may cause stress and unwanted behavior changes until the habit is broken.

4—PRESCRIPTION NEEDED?

"Yes" means a doctor must prescribe the drug for you. "No" means you can buy this drug without prescription. Sometimes low strengths of a drug are available without prescription, while high strengths require prescription.

The information about the generic drug applies whether it requires prescription or not. If the generic ingredients are the same, non-prescription drugs have the same dangers, warnings, precautions and interactions as prescribed drugs. The information and warnings on containers for non-prescription drugs may not be as complete as the information in this book. Check both sources.

5—AVAILABLE AS GENERIC?

Some generic drugs have patent restrictions that protect the manufacturer or distributor of that drug. These drugs may be purchased only by brand name.

In recent years, drug manufacturers have marketed more drugs under generic names. Drugs purchased by generic name sometimes are less expensive than brand names.

Some states allow pharmacists to fill prescriptions by brand names or generic names. This allows patients to buy the least expensive form of a drug.

A doctor may specify a brand name because he or she trusts a known source more than an unknown manufacturer of generic drugs. You and your doctor should decide together whether you should buy a medicine by generic or brand name.

Generic drugs manufactured in other countries are not subject to regulation by the U.S. Food and Drug Administration. Drugs manufactured in the United States are subject to regulation.

6—DRUG CLASS

Drugs that possess similar chemical structure and similar therapeutic effects are grouped into classes. Most drugs within a class produce similar benefits, side effects, adverse reactions and interactions with other drugs and substances. For example, all the generic drugs in the narcotic drug class will have similar effects on the body.

Some information on the charts applies to all drugs in a class. For example, a reference may be made to narcotics. The index lists the class—narcotics—and lists drugs in that class.

The names for classes of drugs are not standardized, so classes listed in other references may vary from the classes in this book.

7—USES

This section lists the disease or disorder for which a drug is prescribed.

Most uses listed are approved by the U.S. Food and Drug Administration. Some uses are listed if experiments and clinical trials indicate effectiveness and safety. Still, other uses are included that may not be officially sanctioned, but for which doctors commonly prescribe the drug.

The use for which your doctor prescribes the drug may not appear. You and your doctor should discuss the reason for any prescription medicine you take. You alone will probably decide whether to take a non-prescription drug. This section may help you make a wise decision.

DOSAGE & USAGE INFORMATION

8—HOW TO TAKE

Drugs are available in tablets, capsules, liquids, suppositories, injections, transdermal patches (See Glossary), aerosol inhalers and topical forms such as drops, sprays, creams, ointments and lotions. This section gives general instructions for taking each form.

This information supplements drug-label information. If your doctor's instructions differ from the suggestions, follow your *doctor's* instructions.

Instructions are left out for how *much* to take. Dose amounts can't be generalized. Dosages of prescription drugs must be individualized for you by your doctor. Non-prescription drugs have instructions on the label regarding how much to take.

9—WHEN TO TAKE

Dose schedules vary for medicines and for patients.

Drugs prescribed on a schedule should usually be taken at approximately the same times each day. Some *must* be taken at regular intervals to maintain a steady level of the drug in the body. If the schedule interferes with your sleep, consult with your doctor.

Instructions to take on an empty stomach mean the drug is absorbed best in your body this way. Many drugs must be taken with liquid or food because they irritate the stomach.

Instructions for other dose schedules are usually on the label. Variations in standard dose schedules may apply because some medicines interact with others if you take them at the same time.

10—IF YOU FORGET A DOSE

Suggestions in this section vary from drug to drug. Most tell you when to resume taking the medicine if you forget a scheduled dose.

Establish habits so you won't forget doses. Forgotten doses decrease a drug's therapeutic effect.

11—WHAT DRUG DOES

This is a simple description of the drug's action in the body. The wording is generalized and may not be a complete explanation of the complex chemical process that takes place.

12—TIME LAPSE BEFORE DRUG WORKS

The times given are approximations. Times vary a great deal from person to person, and from time to time in the same person. The figures give you some idea of when to expect improvement or side effects.

13—DON'T TAKE WITH

Some drugs create problems when taken in combination with other substances. Most problems are detailed in the Interaction column of each chart. This section mentions substances that don't appear in the Interaction column.

Occasionally, an interaction is singled out if the combination is particularly harmful.

OVERDOSE

14—SYMPTOMS

The symptoms listed are most likely to develop with accidental or purposeful overdose. Overdosage may not cause all symptoms listed. Sometimes symptoms are identical to ones listed as side effects. The difference is intensity and severity. You will have to judge. Consult a doctor or poison-control center if you have any doubt.

15—WHAT TO DO

If you suspect an overdose, whether symptoms are apparent or not, follow instructions in this section. Expanded instructions for emergency treatment for overdose are on the inside cover.

16—POSSIBLE ADVERSE REACTIONS OR SIDE EFFECTS

Adverse reactions or side effects are symptoms that may occur when you take a drug. They are effects on the body other than the desired therapeutic effect.

The term *side effect* implies expected and usually unavoidable effects of a drug. Side effects have nothing to do with the drug's intended use.

For example, the generic drug paregoric reduces intestinal cramps and vomiting. It also often causes a flushed face. The flushing is a side effect that is harmless and does not affect the drug's therapeutic potential.

The term *adverse reaction* is more significant. For example, paregoric can cause serious adverse allergic reaction in some people. This reaction can include hives, rash and severe itch.

Some adverse reactions can be prevented, which is one reason this information is included in the book. Most adverse reactions are minor and last only a short time. With many drugs, adverse reactions that might occur will frequently diminish in intensity as time passes.

The majority of drugs used properly for valid reasons offer benefits that outweigh potential hazards.

17—SYMPTOMS

Symptoms are grouped by various body systems. Symptoms that don't naturally apply to these body systems or which overlap systems are listed under "Others."

18—FREQUENCY

This is an estimation of how often symptoms occur in persons who take the drug. The four most common categories of frequency can be found under the **SYMPTOMS** heading and are as follows. **Life-threatening** means exactly what it says: Seek emergency treatment immediately. **Common** means these symptoms are expected and sometimes inevitable. **Infrequent** means the symptoms occur in approximately 1% to 10% of patients. **Rare** means symptoms occur in fewer than 1%.

19—WHAT TO DO

Carefully follow the instructions provided opposite the symptoms that apply to you.

20—WARNINGS AND PRECAUTIONS

Read these entries to determine special information that applies to you.

21—DON'T TAKE IF

This section lists circumstances when drug use is not safe. On some drug labels and in formal medical literature, these circumstances are called *contraindications*.

22—BEFORE YOU START, CONSULT YOUR DOCTOR

This section lists conditions under which a drug should be used only with caution and supervision.

23—OVER AGE 60

As a person ages, physical changes occur that require special considerations. Liver and kidney functions decrease, metabolism slows and the prostate gland enlarges in men.

Most drugs are metabolized or excreted at a rate dependent on kidney and liver functions. Small doses or longer intervals between doses may be necessary to prevent unhealthy concentration of a drug. Toxic effects and adverse reactions occur more frequently and cause more serious problems in older people.

24—PREGNANCY

The best rule to follow during pregnancy is to avoid all drugs, including tobacco and alcohol. Any medicine—prescription or non-prescription—requires medical advice and supervision.

This section will alert you if there is evidence that a drug harms the unborn child. Lack of evidence does not guarantee a drug's safety.

25—BREAST-FEEDING

Many drugs filter into a mother's milk. Some drugs have dangerous or unwanted effects on the nursing infant. This section suggests ways to minimize harm to the child.

26—INFANTS & CHILDREN

Many drugs carry special warnings and precautions for children because of a child's size and immaturity. In medical terminology, *newborns* are babies up to 2 weeks old, *infants* are 2 weeks to 1 year, and *children* are 1 to 12 years.

27—PROLONGED USE

With the exception of immediate allergic reactions, most drugs produce no ill effects during short periods of treatment. However, relatively safe drugs taken for long periods may produce unwanted effects. These are listed. Drugs should be taken in the smallest dose and for the shortest time possible. Nevertheless, some diseases and conditions require an indefinite period of treatment. Your doctor may want to change drugs occasionally or alter your treatment regimen to minimize problems.

The words "functional dependence" sometimes appear in this section. This does not mean *physical* or *psychological addiction*. Sometimes a body function ceases to work naturally because it has been replaced or interfered with by the drug. The body then becomes dependent on the drug to continue the function.

28—SKIN & SUNLIGHT

Many drugs cause *photosensitivity*, which means increased skin sensitivity to ultraviolet rays from sunlight or artificial rays from a sunlamp. This section will alert you to this potential problem.

29—DRIVING, PILOTING OR HAZARDOUS WORK

Any drug that alters moods or that decreases alertness, muscular coordination or reflexes may make these activities particularly hazardous. The effects may not appear in all people, or they may disappear after a short exposure to the drug. If this section contains a warning, use caution until you determine how a new drug affects you.

30—DISCONTINUING

Some patients stop taking a drug when symptoms begin to go away, although complete recovery may require longer treatment.

Other patients continue taking a drug when it is no longer needed. This section gives warnings about prematurely discontinuing. Some drugs cause symptoms days or weeks after they have been discontinued.

31—OTHERS

Warnings and precautions appear here if they don't fit into the other categories. This section includes storage instructions; how to dispose of outdated drugs; changes in blood, urine and other laboratory tests; warnings to persons with chronic illness and other information.

32—POSSIBLE INTERACTION WITH OTHER DRUGS

Drugs interact in your body with other drugs, whether prescription or non-prescription. Interactions affect absorption, elimination or distribution of either drug. The chart lists interactions by generic name or drug class. An asterisk (*) beside drug-class names in this column reminds you to "See Glossary" in the back of the book, where that drug class is described and where generic drug names for that class are listed.

If a drug class appears, the generic drug interacts with any drug in that class. Drugs in each class that are included in the book are listed in the index. Occasionally drugs that are not included in this book appear in the Interaction column.

Interactions are sometimes beneficial. You may not be able to determine from the chart which interactions are good and which are bad. Don't guess. Consult your doctor if you take drugs that interact. Some combinations are fatal.

Some drugs have too many interactions to list on one chart. The additional interactions appear on the continuation page indicated at the bottom of the list.

33—POSSIBLE INTERACTION WITH OTHER SUBSTANCES

The substances listed here are repeated on every drug chart. All people eat food and drink beverages. Many adults consume alcohol. Many people use cocaine and smoke tobacco or marijuana. This section shows possible interactions between these substances and each drug.

DRUGS OF ABUSE

Each of the drug charts beginning on page 2 contains a section listing the interactions of alcohol, marijuana and cocaine with the therapeutic drug in the bloodstream. These three drugs are singled out because of their widespread use and abuse. The information is factual, not judgmental.

The long-term effects of alcohol and tobacco abuse are numerous. They have been well publicized and information is provided here as a reminder of the inherent dangers of these drugs.

Drugs of potential abuse include those that are addictive and harmful. They usually produce a temporary, false sense of well-being. The long-term effects, however, are harmful and can be devastating to the body and psyche of the addict.

Refresh your memory frequently about the potential harm from prolonged use of *any* drugs or substances you take. Avoid unwise use of habit-forming drugs.

These are the most common drugs of abuse:

TOBACCO (NICOTINE)

What it does: Tobacco smoke contains noxious and cancer-producing ingredients. They include nicotine, carbon monoxide, ammonia, and a variety of harmful tars. Carcinogens in smoke probably come from the tars. Most are present in chewing tobacco and snuff as well as smoke from cigarettes, cigars, and pipes. Tobacco smoke interferes with the immune mechanisms of the body.

Short-term effects of average amount: Relaxation of mood if you are a steady smoker. Constriction of blood vessels.

Short-term effects of large amount inhaled: Headache, appetite loss, nausea.

Long-term effects: Greatly enhanced chances of developing lung cancer. Impaired breathing and chronic lung disease (asthma, emphysema, bronchiectasis, lung abscess and others) much more likely. Heart and blood vessel disease more frequent and more severe when they happen. These include myocardial infarction (heart attack), coronary artery disease, heart beat irregularities, generalized atherosclerosis (hardening of the arteries making brain, heart, and kidney more vulnerable to disease), peripheral vascular disease such as intermittent claudication, Buerger's disease and others. Tobacco and nicotine lead to an increased incidence of abortion and significantly reduce the birth weight of children brought to term and delivered of women who smoke during pregnancy. Tobacco smoking causes higher frequency not only of lung cancer, but also increases the likelihood of developing cancer of the throat, larynx, mouth, esophagus, bladder, and pancreas.

Cigarette smoking has been linked to this many deaths per year in the U.S. alone:
    80,000 lung cancer
    22,000 other cancer
    15,000 chronic lung disease
    225,000 cardiovascular disease
346,000 TOTAL

ALCOHOL

What it does:

• Central Nervous System

Depresses, does *not* stimulate, the action of all parts of the central nervous system. It depresses normal mental activity and normal muscle function. Short-term effects of an average amount: relaxation, breakdown of inhibitions, euphoria, decreased alertness. Short-term effects of large amounts: nausea, stupor, hangover, unconsciousness, even death.

• Gastrointestinal System

Increases stomach acid, poisons liver function. Chronic alcoholism frequently leads to permanent damage to the liver.

• Heart and Blood Vessels

Decreased normal function, leading to heart diseases such as cardiomyopathy and disorders of the blood vessels and kidney, such as high blood pressure. Bleeding from the esophagus and stomach frequently accompany liver disease caused by chronic alcoholism.

• Unborn Fetus (teratogenicity)

Alcoholism in the mother carrying a fetus causes *fetal alcohol syndrome (FAS),* which includes the production of mental deficiency, facial abnormalities, slow growth and other major and minor malformations in the newborn.

Signs of Use:

Early signs: Prominent smell of alcohol on the breath, behavior changes (aggressive; passive; sexually uninhibited; poor judgment; outbursts of uncontrolled emotion, such as rage or tearfulness).

Intoxication signs: Unsteady gait, slurred speech, poor performance of any brain or muscle function, stupor or coma in *severe* alcoholic intoxication with slow, noisy breathing, cold and clammy skin, heartbeat faster than usual.

Long-term effects:

Addiction: Compulsive use of alcohol. Persons addicted to alcohol have severe withdrawal symptoms when alcohol is unavailable. Even with successful treatment, addiction to alcohol (and other drugs that cause addiction) has a high tendency to relapse. (Memory of euphoric feelings plus family, social, emotional, psychological, and genetic factors probably are all important factors in producing the addiction.)

Liver disease: Usually cirrhosis; also, deleterious effects on the unborn child of an alcoholic mother.

Loss of sexual function: Impotence, erectile dysfunction, loss of libido.

Increased incidence of cancer: Mouth, pharynx, larynx, esophagus, liver, and lung.

Changes in blood: Makes clotting less efficient.

Heart disease: Decreased normal function leading to possible damage and disease.

Stomach and intestinal problems: Increased production of stomach acid.

Interference with expected or normal actions of many medications: Detailed on every chart in this book, drugs such as sedatives, pain killers, narcotics, antihistamines, anticonvulsants, anticoagulants, and others.

MARIJUANA (CANNABIS, HASHISH)

What they do: Heighten perception, cause mood swings, relax mind and body.
Signs of use: Red eyes, lethargy, uncoordinated body movements.
Long-term effects: Decreased motivation. Possible brain, heart, lung and reproductive system damage.

AMPHETAMINES

What they do: Speed up physical and mental processes to cause a false sense of energy and excitement. The moods are temporary and unreal.
Signs of use: Dilated pupils, insomnia, trembling.
Long-term effects: Violent behavior, paranoia, possible death from overdose.

BARBITURATES

What they do: Produce drowsiness and lethargy.
Signs of use: Confused speech, lack of coordination and balance.
Long-term effects: Disrupts normal sleep pattern. Possible death from overdose, especially in combination with alcohol.

COCAINE

What it does: Stimulates the nervous system, heightens sensations and may produce hallucinations.

Signs of use: Trembling, intoxication, dilated pupils, constant sniffling.

Long-term effects: Ulceration of nasal passages where sniffed. Itching all over body, sometimes with open sores. Possible brain damage. Possible death from overdose.

OPIATES (CODEINE, HEROIN, METHADONE, MORPHINE, OPIUM)

What they do: Relieve pain, create temporary and false sense of well-being.

Signs of use: Constricted pupils, mood swings, slurred speech, sore eyes, lethargy, weight loss, sweating.

Long-term effects: Malnutrition, extreme susceptibility to infection, the need to increase drug amount to produce the same effects. Possible death from overdose.

PSYCHEDELIC DRUGS (LSD, MESCALINE)

What they do: Produce hallucinations, either pleasant or frightening.

Signs of use: Dilated pupils, sweating, trembling, fever, chills.

Long-term effects: Lack of motivation, unpredictable behavior, narcissism, recurrent hallucinations without drug use ("flashbacks"). Possible death from overdose.

VOLATILE SUBSTANCES (GLUE, SOLVENTS)

What they do: Produce hallucinations, temporary, false sense of well-being and possible unconsciousness.

Signs of use: Dilated pupils, flushed face, confusion.

Long-term effects: Permanent brain, liver, kidney damage. Possible death from overdose.

CHECKLIST FOR SAFER DRUG USE

- Tell your doctor about *any* drug you take (even aspirin, allergy pills, cough and cold preparations, antacids, laxatives, vitamins, etc.) *before* you take *any* new drug.

- Learn all you can about drugs you may take *before* you take them. Information sources are your doctor, your nurse, your pharmacist, this book and other books in your public library.

- Don't take drugs prescribed for someone else—even if your symptoms are the same.

- Keep your prescription drugs to yourself. Your drugs may be harmful to someone else.

- Tell your doctor about any symptoms you believe are caused by a drug—prescription or non-prescription—that you take.

- Take only medicines that are *necessary*. Avoid taking non-prescription drugs while taking prescription drugs for a medical problem.

- Before your doctor prescribes for you, tell him about your previous experiences with any drug—beneficial results, side effects, adverse reactions or allergies.

- Take medicine in good light after you have identified it. If you wear glasses to read, put them on to check drug labels. It is easy to take the wrong drug at the wrong time.

- Don't keep any drugs that change mood, alertness or judgment—such as sedatives, narcotics or tranquilizers—by your bedside. These cause many accidental deaths by overdose. You may unknowingly repeat a dose when you are half asleep or confused.

- Know the names of your medicines. These include the generic name, the brand name and the generic names of all ingredients in a drug mixture. Your doctor, nurse or pharmacist can give you this information.

- Study the labels on all non-prescription drugs. If the information is incomplete or if you have questions, ask the pharmacist for more details.

- If you must deviate from your prescribed dose schedule, tell your doctor.

- Shake liquid medicines before taking.

- Store all medicines away from moisture and heat. Bathroom medicine cabinets are usually unsuitable.

- If a drug needs refrigeration, don't freeze.

- Obtain a standard measuring spoon from your pharmacy for liquid medicines. Kitchen teaspoons and tablespoons are not accurate enough.

- Follow diet instructions when you take medicines. Some work better on a full stomach, others on an empty stomach. Some drugs are more useful with special diets. For example, medicine for high blood pressure is more effective if accompanied by a sodium-restricted diet.

- Tell your doctor about any allergies you have. A previous allergy to a drug may make it dangerous to prescribe again. People with other allergies, such as eczema, hay fever, asthma, bronchitis and food allergies, are more likely to be allergic to drugs.

- Prior to surgery, tell your doctor, anesthesiologist or dentist about any drug you have taken in the past few weeks. Advise them of any cortisone drugs you have taken within two years.

- If you become pregnant while taking any medicine, including birth-control pills, tell your doctor immediately.

- Avoid *all* drugs while you are pregnant, if possible. If you must take drugs during pregnancy, record names, amounts, dates and reasons.

- If you see more than one doctor, tell each one about drugs others have prescribed.

- When you use non-prescription drugs, report it so the information is on your medical record.

- Store all drugs away from the reach of children.

- Note the expiration date on each drug label. Discard outdated ones safely. If no expiration date appears and it has been at least one year since taking the medication, it may be best to discard it.

- Pay attention to the information in the charts about safety while driving, piloting or working in dangerous places.

- Alcohol, cocaine, marijuana or other mood-altering drugs as well as tobacco—mixed with some drugs—can cause a life-threatening interaction, prevent your medicine from being effective or delay your return to health. Common sense dictates that you avoid them during illness.

COUGH AND COLD MEDICINES

Coughs and colds are among humans' most common ailments, and the commercial medicines available for treatment are numerous.

There are over 350 brands of medicines (each with a registered name) designed to relieve symptoms caused by the common cold, influenza and other minor respiratory illnesses. Most of these medications are over-the-counter (OTC) medicines and can be purchased without a prescription.

Although these drugs may be safe when taken alone, interactions between these medicines and other non-prescription or prescription drugs, when taken together, may produce undesirable or unsafe results. So, for your own safety, you should study the information in this book with regard to the ingredients of each brand name cough or cold medicine you are taking. Follow these steps to learn about the safety of your drug:

1. Determine the brand name of your drug.

2. Look on the label for the generic ingredients that are used in your brand of medicine.

3. For each generic ingredient, consult the index or look up each generic drug in the alphabetized drug charts. Read the information about how to use the drug safely, especially regarding its use (interaction) with other drugs you may be taking simultaneously.

The generic ingredients of cough and cold medicines fall into several drug classes:

Antihistamines control allergy symptoms. All antihistamines may cause drowsiness, decreased reflexes and decreased ability to concentrate. Therefore, don't drive vehicles or pilot aircraft until you learn how this medicine affects you. Don't work around dangerous machinery. Don't climb ladders or work in high places. The danger increases if you drink alcohol or take other medicines that affect alertness and reflexes, such as other antihistamines, tranquilizers, sedatives, pain medicines, narcotics and mind-altering drugs. They all may cause other side effects or adverse reactions.

Decongestants relieve symptoms of nasal or bronchial congestion. All decongestants may cause nervousness, irregular heartbeats in some people, dizziness, confusion and other side effects. Conduct your daily activities with these effects in mind.

Antitussives reduce frequency and severity of cough. These may be either *narcotic* (codeine and hydrocodone) or *non-narcotic* (dextromethorphan). Narcotic cough suppressants are habit-forming and may cause some of the same mental changes that can take place with antihistamines. The most common non-narcotic antitussive medicine, dextromethorphan, is not habit-forming but has other side effects.

Expectorants loosen secretions to make them easier to cough up. The most common expectorant is guaifenesin, which has very few side effects but doesn't loosen secretions very efficiently.

Analgesics relieve aches and pains. The most common analgesics in cough and cold medicines are aspirin and acetaminophen.

To learn the details about any cough or cold remedy you may take, look up the brand names in the index of this book. Then consult the generic drug charts listed for each brand name.

DRUG CHARTS

ACETAMINOPHEN

BRAND NAMES

See complete list of brand names in the *Brand Name Directory*, page 904.

BASIC INFORMATION

Habit forming? No
Prescription needed? No
Available as generic? Yes
Drug class: Analgesic, fever-reducer

 USES

Treatment of mild to moderate pain and fever. Acetaminophen does not relieve redness, stiffness or swelling of joints or tissue inflammation. Use aspirin or other drugs for inflammation.

 DOSAGE & USAGE INFORMATION

How to take:
- Tablet or capsule—Swallow with liquid.
- Effervescent granules—Dissolve granules in 4 oz. of cool water. Drink all the water.
- Elixir—Swallow with liquid.
- Suppositories—Remove wrapper and moisten suppository with water. Gently insert larger end into rectum. Push well into rectum with finger.
- Powder—Sprinkle over liquid, then swallow.

When to take:
As needed, no more often than every 3 hours.

If you forget a dose:
Take as soon as you remember. Wait 3 hours for next dose.

What drug does:
May affect hypothalamus—part of brain that helps regulate body heat and receives body's pain messages.

Time lapse before drug works:
15 to 30 minutes. May last 4 hours.

Continued next column

 OVERDOSE

SYMPTOMS:
Stomach upset, irritability, sweating, diarrhea, loss of appetite, abdominal cramps, convulsions, coma.
WHAT TO DO:
- **Call your doctor or poison-control center for advice if you suspect overdose, even if not sure. Symptoms may not appear until damage has occurred.**
- **See emergency information on inside covers.**

Don't take with:
- Other drugs with acetaminophen. Too much acetaminophen can damage liver and kidneys.
- Any other medicine without consulting your doctor or pharmacist.

 POSSIBLE ADVERSE REACTIONS OR SIDE EFFECTS

SYMPTOMS	WHAT TO DO
Life-threatening:	
In case of overdose, see previous column.	
Common:	
Lightheadedness.	Continue. Call doctor when convenient.
Infrequent:	
• Trembling.	Continue. Call doctor when convenient.
• Pain in lower back or side.	Discontinue call doctor right away.
Rare:	
• Extreme fatigue; rash, itch, hives; sore throat and fever after taking regularly a few days; unexplained bleeding or bruising; blood in urine; painful or frequent urination; jaundice; anemia.	Discontinue. Call doctor right away.
• Decreased volume of urine output.	Continue. Call doctor when convenient.

ACETAMINOPHEN

WARNINGS & PRECAUTIONS

Don't take if:
- You are allergic to acetaminophen.
- Your symptoms don't improve after 2 days use. Call your doctor.

Before you start, consult your doctor:
If you have kidney disease or liver damage.

Over age 60:
Don't exceed recommended dose. You can't eliminate drug as efficiently as younger persons.

Pregnancy:
No proven harm to unborn child. Avoid if possible.

Breast-feeding:
No proven harm to nursing Infant.

Infants & children:
Use only under medical supervision.

Prolonged use:
- May affect blood system and cause anemia. Limit use to 5 days for children 12 and under, and 10 days for adults.
- Talk to your doctor about the need for follow-up medical examinations or laboratory studies to check liver function, kidney function.

Skin & sunlight:
No problems expected.

Driving, piloting or hazardous work:
Avoid if you feel drowsy. Otherwise, no restrictions.

Discontinuing:
Discontinue in 2 days if symptoms don't improve.

Others:
May interfere with the accuracy of some medical tests.

POSSIBLE INTERACTION WITH OTHER DRUGS

GENERIC NAME OR DRUG CLASS	COMBINED EFFECT
Anticoagulants, oral*	May increase anticoagulant effect. If combined frequently, prothrombin time should be monitored.
Isoniazid	Increased risk of liver damage.
Nicotine	Increased effect of acetaminophen.

POSSIBLE INTERACTION WITH OTHER SUBSTANCES

INTERACTS WITH	COMBINED EFFECT
Alcohol:	Drowsiness, long-term use may cause toxic effect in liver.
Beverages:	None expected.
Cocaine:	None expected. However, cocaine may slow body's recovery. Avoid.
Foods:	None expected.
Marijuana:	Increased pain relief. However, marijuana may slow body's recovery. Avoid.
Tobacco:	None expected.

*See Glossary

3

ACETAMINOPHEN & SALICYLATES

BRAND NAMES

See complete list of brand names in the *Brand Name Directory,* page 905.

BASIC INFORMATION

Habit forming? No
Prescription needed?
  High strength: Yes
  Low strength: No
  Yes, for some combinations
Available as generic? No
Drug class: Analgesic, fever-reducer, anti-inflammatory (non-steroidal)

 ## USES

- Treatment of mild pain and fever.
- Salicylates are useful in the treatment of inflammatory conditions such as stiffness, swelling, joint pain of arthritis or rheumatism. For long term use for inflammatory problems, separate drugs instead of this combination may be safer and more effective.

 ## DOSAGE & USAGE INFORMATION

How to take:
- Tablet or capsule—swallow with liquid.
- Effervescent granules—dissolve granules in 4 oz. of cool water.

When to take:
As needed, no more often than every 3 hours or as prescribed by your doctor.

If you forget a dose:
Take as soon as you remember. Wait 3 hours for next dose.

Continued next column

 ## OVERDOSE

SYMPTOMS:
Ringing in ears; nausea; vomiting; diarrhea; dizziness; fever; deep, rapid breathing; hallucinations; coma; unusual sweating; blood in urine; thirst; vision problems; nervousness.
WHAT TO DO:
- **Dial 0 (operator) or 911 (emergency) for an ambulance or medical help. Then give first aid immediately.**
- **See emergency information on inside covers.**

What drug does:
- May affect hypothalamus, the part of the brain that helps regulate body heat and receives body's pain messages.
- May affect production of prostaglandins to reduce inflammation.

Time lapse before drug works:
15 to 30 minutes. May last 4 hours.

Don't take with:
- Other drugs with acetaminophen or aspirin or other salicylates. Too much can cause damage to liver, kidneys and peripheral nerves.
- Any laxative containing cellulose.
- If medicine you take has a buffering agent added, don't take with tetracyclines.
- Any other medicine without consulting your doctor or pharmacist.

 ## POSSIBLE ADVERSE REACTIONS OR SIDE EFFECTS

SYMPTOMS	WHAT TO DO
Life-threatening:	
In case of overdose, see previous column.	
Common:	
• Jaundice, vomiting blood, black stools, cloudy urine, nausea and vomiting, unexplained tiredness, discomfort on urinating.	Discontinue. Call doctor right away.
• Indigestion or heartburn.	Continue. Call doctor when convenient.
Infrequent:	
Shortness of breath; wheezing (for medicines containing aspirin); decreased urine volume; feet swelling; black or tarry stools; pain on urinating; nausea and vomiting; skin rash, hives; sore throat, fever; easy bruising.	Discontinue. Call doctor right away.
Rare:	
• While taking medicine: Sudden decrease in urine volume.	Discontinue. Call doctor right away.
• After discontinuing medicine: Swelling of feet; rapid weight gain; bloating or puffiness; any urinary problems, such as painful, cloudy or bloody urine.	Check with doctor immediately.

ACETAMINOPHEN & SALICYLATES

WARNINGS & PRECAUTIONS

Don't take if:
- You are allergic to acetaminophen or any salicylates. *
- Your symptoms don't improve after 3 days use.
- You take a buffered form and need to restrict sodium in your diet.
- You have a peptic ulcer.
- You have a bleeding disorder.

Before you start, consult your doctor:
- If you have ever had peptic ulcers.
- If you have had gout.
- If you have asthma or nasal polyps.
- If you have kidney disease or liver damage.

Over age 60:
Don't exceed recommended dose. More likely to be harmful to kidney and liver or cause hidden bleeding in stomach or intestines. Watch for black stools or decreased urine output.

Pregnancy:
Risk to unborn child outweighs drug benefits. Don't use.

Breast-feeding:
Drug passes into milk. Avoid drug or discontinue nursing until you finish medicine. Consult doctor on maintaining milk supply.

Infants & children:
Overdose frequent and severe. Keep bottles out of children's reach. Consult doctor before giving to persons under age 18 who have fever and discomfort of viral illness, especially chicken pox and influenza. Probably increases risk of Reye's syndrome *.

Prolonged use:
- High doses for severe inflammatory conditions taken for long periods may increase likelihood of kidney damage.
- Talk to your doctor about the need for follow-up medical examinations or laboratory studies to check liver function, kidney function.

Skin & sunlight:
Aspirin combined with sunscreen may decrease sunburn.

Driving, piloting or hazardous work:
No problems expected unless you feel drowsy.

Discontinuing:
No problems expected.

Others:
- Children up to 12 years—Don't take more than 5 doses per day for more than 5 consecutive days.
- Adults—Don't take for more than 10 consecutive days.
- Urine test for sugar may be inaccurate.
- Don't take if container has a strong vinegar-like odor.
- May interfere with the accuracy of some medical tests.

*See Glossary

POSSIBLE INTERACTION WITH OTHER DRUGS

GENERIC NAME OR DRUG CLASS	COMBINED EFFECT
Antacids*	Decreased aceta-minophen and salicylates effect.
Anticoagulants*	Increased anticoagulant effect. Abnormal bleeding.
Antidiabetics, oral*	Low blood sugar.
Aspirin and other salicylates*	Likely toxicity.
Barbiturates*	Increased liver toxicity.
Carbamazepine	Increased liver toxicity.
Carteolol	Decreased antihypertensive effect of carteolol.
Cortisone drugs*	Increased cortisone effect. Risk of ulcers and stomach bleeding.
Furosemide	Possible salicylate toxicity, decreased furosemide effect.
Hepatotoxic drugs*	Increased liver toxicity.
Indomethacin	Risk of stomach bleeding and ulcers.

Continued page 932

POSSIBLE INTERACTION WITH OTHER SUBSTANCES

INTERACTS WITH	COMBINED EFFECT
Alcohol:	Increased chance of stomach irritation and bleeding.
Beverages:	None expected.
Cocaine:	None expected. However, cocaine may deter body's recovery. Avoid.
Foods:	None expected.
Marijuana:	Possible increased pain relief, but marijuana may deter body's recovery. Avoid.
Tobacco:	None expected.

5

ACETOHYDROXAMIC ACID (AHA)

BRAND NAMES

Lithostat

BASIC INFORMATION

Habit forming? No
Prescription needed? Yes
Available as generic? No
Drug class: Antibacterial, antiurolithic

 USES

- Treatment for chronic urinary-tract infections.
- Prevents formation of urinary-tract stones. Will not dissolve stones already present.

 DOSAGE & USAGE INFORMATION

How to take:
Tablet—Swallow with liquid. If you can't swallow whole, crumble tablet and take with liquid or food.

When to take:
At the same time each day, according to instructions on prescription label.

If you forget a dose:
Take as soon as you remember up to 2 hours late. If more than 2 hours, wait for next scheduled dose (don't double this dose).

What drug does:
Stops enzyme action that makes urine too alkaline. Alkaline urine favors bacterial growth and stone formation and growth.

Time lapse before drug works:
1 to 3 weeks.

Don't take with:
- Alcohol or iron.
- Any other medicine without consulting your doctor or pharmacist.

 OVERDOSE

SYMPTOMS:
Loss of appetite, tremor, nausea, vomiting.
WHAT TO DO:
Overdose unlikely to threaten life. If person takes much larger amount than prescribed, call doctor, poison-control center or hospital emergency room for instructions.

 POSSIBLE ADVERSE REACTIONS OR SIDE EFFECTS

SYMPTOMS	WHAT TO DO
Life-threatening:	
In case of overdose, see previous column.	
Common:	
• Appetite loss, nausea, vomiting.	Discontinue. Seek emergency treatment.
• Anxiety, depression, mild headache, unusual tiredness	Continue. Call doctor when convenient.
Infrequent:	
• Loss of coordination, slurred speech, severe headache, sudden change in vision, shortness of breath, clot or pain over a blood vessel, sudden chest pain, leg pain in calf (deep vein blood clot).	Discontinue. Seek emergency treatment.
• Rash on arms and face.	Discontinue. Call doctor right away.
Rare:	
• Sore throat, fever, unusual bleeding, bruising.	Discontinue. Call right away.
• Hair loss.	Continue. Call doctor when convenient.

ACETOHYDROXAMIC ACID (AHA)

WARNINGS & PRECAUTIONS

Don't take if:
You have severe chronic kidney disease.

Before you start, consult your doctor:
- If you are anemic.
- If you have or have had phlebitis or thrombophlebitis.

Over age 60:
Adverse reactions and side effects may be more frequent and severe than in younger persons.

Pregnancy:
Studies inconclusive on harm to unborn child. Animal studies show fetal abnormalities. Decide with your doctor whether drug benefits justify risk to unborn child.

Breast-feeding:
No proven problems. Avoid if possible.

Infants & children:
Not recommended. Safety and dosage have not been established.

Prolonged use:
Talk to your doctor about the need for follow-up medical examinations or laboratory studies to check blood pressure, liver function, kidney function, urinary pH.

Skin & sunlight:
No problems expected.

Driving, piloting or hazardous work:
Don't drive or pilot aircraft until you learn how medicine affects you. Don't work around dangerous machinery. Don't climb ladders or work in high places. Danger increases if you drink alcohol or take medicine affecting alertness and reflexes, such as antihistamines, tranquilizers, sedatives, pain medicines, narcotics and mind-altering drugs.

Discontinuing:
Don't discontinue without consulting doctor. Dose may require gradual reduction if you have taken drug for a long time. Doses of other drugs may also require adjustment.

Others:
No problems expected.

POSSIBLE INTERACTION WITH OTHER DRUGS

GENERIC NAME OR DRUG CLASS	COMBINED EFFECT
Dapsone	Increased risk of adverse effect on blood cells.
Iron	Decreased effects of both drugs.

POSSIBLE INTERACTION WITH OTHER SUBSTANCES

INTERACTS WITH	COMBINED EFFECT
Alcohol:	Severe skin rash common in many patients within 30 to 45 minutes after drinking alcohol.
Beverages:	None expected.
Cocaine:	None expected.
Foods:	None expected.
Marijuana:	None expected.
Tobacco:	None expected.

ACRISORCIN (Topical)

BRAND NAMES

Acrisorcin Cream

BASIC INFORMATION

Habit forming? No
Prescription needed? Yes
Available as generic? No
Drug class: Antifungal (topical)

 USES

- Used on skin to treat tinea versicolor, a yeast infection that changes the color of skin it affects. Sometimes called "sun fungus," it's more common in adolescents and adults and more likely to occur with exposure to heat and high humidity.
- Acrisorcin is not useful for other fungus or yeast skin infections.

 DOSAGE & USAGE INFORMATION

How to use:
- Cream, lotion, ointment—Bathe and dry area before use. Apply small amount and rub gently.
- After using, wash hands with soap to prevent medicine from getting in eyes.

When to use:
Apply at night.

If you forget a dose:
Take as soon as you remember.

What drug does:
Unknown. Probably removes outer layer of skin to remove the infecting fungus.

Time lapse before drug works:
2 to 3 weeks.

Don't use with:
Any other medicine without consulting your doctor or pharmacist.

 OVERDOSE

SYMPTOMS:
None expected.
WHAT TO DO:
Not for internal use. If child accidentally swallows, call poison-control center.

 POSSIBLE ADVERSE REACTIONS OR SIDE EFFECTS

SYMPTOMS	WHAT TO DO
Life-threatening:	
None expected.	
Common:	
None expected.	
Infrequent:	
Redness, itching, blistering, hives, new skin rash.	Discontinue. Call doctor right away.
Rare:	
None expected.	

WARNINGS & PRECAUTIONS

Don't use if:
You are allergic to acrisorcin.

Before you start, consult your doctor:
If you are allergic to any substance such as dyes or preservatives.

Over age 60:
No problems expected.

Pregnancy:
No problems expected, but check with doctor.

Breast-feeding:
No problems expected.

Infants & children:
Use only under close medical supervision.

Prolonged use:
May lead to skin sensitivity.

Skin & sunlight:
May cause itching.

Driving, piloting or hazardous work:
No problems expected.

Discontinuing:
No problems expected.

Others:
- Check with doctor if no improvement in 6 weeks.
- Do not apply plastic wraps over treated skin.

 ## POSSIBLE INTERACTION WITH OTHER DRUGS

GENERIC NAME OR DRUG CLASS	COMBINED EFFECT
None expected.	

 ## POSSIBLE INTERACTION WITH OTHER SUBSTANCES

INTERACTS WITH	COMBINED EFFECT
Alcohol:	None expected.
Beverages:	None expected.
Cocaine:	None expected.
Foods:	None expected.
Marijuana:	None expected.
Tobacco:	None expected.

ACYCLOVIR (Oral & Topical)

BRAND NAMES

Zovirax   Zovirax Ointment

BASIC INFORMATION

Habit forming? No
Prescription needed? Yes
Available as generic? No
Drug class: Antiviral

 USES

- Treatment and prevention of severe herpes infections of genitals occurring for first time in special cases.
- Treatment of severe herpes infections on mucous membrane of mouth and lips in special cases.
- Used for shingles (herpes zoster) and chicken pox (varicella) in special cases.

 DOSAGE & USAGE INFORMATION

How to take:
- Capsule—Swallow with liquid. If you can't swallow whole, open capsule and take with liquid or food.
- Tablet—Swallow with liquid. If you can't swallow whole, crumble tablet and take with liquid or food.
- Suspension—Swallow with liquid.
- Ointment—Apply to skin and mucous membranes every 3 hours (6 times a day) for 7 days. Use rubber glove when applying. Apply 1/2-inch strip to each sore or blister. Wash before using.

When to use:
As directed on label.

Continued next column

 OVERDOSE

SYMPTOMS:
Hallucinations, seizures, kidney shutdown.
WHAT TO DO:
- Dial 0 (operator) or 911 (emergency) for an ambulance or medical help. Then give first aid immediately.
- See emergency information on inside covers.

If you forget a dose:
- Oral—Take as soon as you remember up to 2 hours late. If more than 2 hours, wait for next scheduled dose (don't double this dose).
- Ointment—Apply as soon as you remember.

What drug does:
- Inhibits reproduction of virus in cells without killing normal cells.
- Does not cure. Herpes may recur.

Time lapse before drug works:
2 hours.

Don't take with:
Any other medicine without consulting your doctor or pharmacist.

 POSSIBLE ADVERSE REACTIONS OR SIDE EFFECTS

SYMPTOMS	WHAT TO DO
Life-threatening:	
In case of overdose, see previous column.	
Common:	
Rash, hives, itch, mild pain, burning or stinging of skin, lightheadedness, headache, joint pain, diarrhea.	Continue. Call doctor when convenient.
Infrequent:	
Confusion, hallucinations, trembling, dizziness.	Discontinue. Call doctor right away.
Rare:	
Abdominal pain, decreased appetite, nausea, vomiting, breathing difficulty, blood in urine, decreased urine volume, acne, insomnia.	Discontinue. Call doctor right away.

10

WARNINGS & PRECAUTIONS

Don't take if:
You are allergic to acyclovir.

Before you start, consult your doctor:
- If pregnant or plan pregnancy.
- If breast-feeding.
- If you have kidney disease.
- If you have any nerve disorder.

Over age 60:
Adverse reactions and side effects may be more frequent and severe than in younger persons.

Pregnancy:
Risk to unborn child outweighs drug benefits. Don't use.

Breast-feeding:
- Oral—Drug passes into milk. Avoid drug or discontinue nursing until you finish medicine. Consult doctor for advice on maintaining milk supply.
- Ointment—No special problems expected. Consult doctor.

Infants & children:
Use only under special medical supervision by experienced clinician.

Prolonged use:
- Don't use longer than prescribed time.
- Talk to your doctor about the need for follow-up medical examinations or laboratory studies to check pap smear, kidney function.

Skin & sunlight:
No problems expected.

Driving, piloting or hazardous work:
No problems expected.

Discontinuing:
May be unnecessary to finish medicine. Follow doctor's instructions.

Others:
- Women: Get Pap smear every 6 months because those with herpes infections are more likely to develop cancer of the cervix. Avoid sexual activity until all blisters or sores heal.
- Don't get medicine in eyes.
- Protect from freezing.
- Check with doctor if no improvement in 1 week.
- May interfere with the accuracy of some medical tests.

POSSIBLE INTERACTION WITH OTHER DRUGS

GENERIC NAME OR DRUG CLASS	COMBINED EFFECT
Other medications that can cause toxic effects on kidneys, such as amikacin amphotericin B capreomycin colistimethate colistin cyclosporine gentamycin kanamycin neomycin netilmicin polymixin B probenecid streptomycin tiopronin tobramycin vancomycin	Possible increased kidney toxicity.
Zidovudine	Increased risk of nerve damage.

POSSIBLE INTERACTION WITH OTHER SUBSTANCES

INTERACTS WITH	COMBINED EFFECT
Alcohol:	No problems expected.
Beverages:	No problems expected.
Cocaine:	Increased chance of brain and nervous system adverse reaction. Avoid.
Foods:	No problems expected.
Marijuana:	Increased chance of brain and nervous system adverse reaction. Avoid.
Tobacco:	No problems expected.

*See Glossary

ADRENOCORTICOIDS (Nasal)

BRAND AND GENERIC NAMES

BECLOMETHASONE
(Nasal)
Beconase
Beconase AQ
Decadron Turbinaire
DEXAMETHASONE
(Nasal)
FLUNISOLIDE (Nasal)

Nasacort
Nasalide
Rhinalar
TRIAMCINOLONE
(Nasal)
Vancenase
Vancenase AQ

BASIC INFORMATION

Habit forming? No
Prescription needed? Yes
Available as generic? No
Drug class: Adrenocorticoid (nasal);
anti-inflammatory (steroidal), nasal

 USES

- Treats nasal allergy.
- Treats nasal polyps.
- Treats non-infectious inflammatory nasal conditions.

 DOSAGE & USAGE INFORMATION

How to take:
- Read patient instruction sheet supplied with your prescription. Usually 1 or 2 sprays into each nostril every 12 hours.
- Save container for possible refills.

When to take:
At the same time each day, according to instructions on prescription label.

If you forget a dose:
Use as soon as you remember up to an hour late. If you remember more than an hour late, skip this dose. Don't double the next dose.

Continued next column

 OVERDOSE

SYMPTOMS:
None expected.
WHAT TO DO:
Overdose unlikely to threaten life. If person takes much larger amount than prescribed, call doctor, poison-control center or hospital emergency room for instructions.

What drug does:
- Subdues inflammation by decreasing secretion of prostaglandins in cells of the lining of the nose and by inhibiting release of histamine.
- Very little, if any, of the nasal adrenocorticoid gets absorbed into the bloodstream.

Time lapse before drug works:
Usually 5 to 7 days, but may be as long as 2 to 3 weeks.

Don't take with:
Any other medicine without consulting your doctor or pharmacist.

 POSSIBLE ADVERSE REACTIONS OR SIDE EFFECTS

SYMPTOMS	WHAT TO DO
Life-threatening:	
None expected.	
Common:	
Burning or dryness of nose, sneezing.	Continue. Call doctor when convenient.
Infrequent:	
Crusting inside the nose, nosebleed, sore throat, ulcers in nose, cough, dizziness, headache, hoarseness, nausea, runny nose.	Discontinue. Call doctor right away.
Rare:	
• White patches in nose or throat.	Discontinue. Call doctor right away.
• Eye pain, wheezing respiration.	Discontinue. Seek emergency treatment.

WARNINGS & PRECAUTIONS

Don't take if:
You are allergic to cortisone or any cortisone-like medication.

Before you start, consult your doctor:
If you know you are allergic to any of the propellants in the spray. These include benzalkonium chloride, disodium acetate, phenylethanol, fluorocarbons, propylene glycol.

Over age 60:
No special problems expected.

Pregnancy:
Probably safe, but check with doctor.

Breast-feeding:
Probably safe, but check with doctor.

Infants & children:
Probably safe, but check with doctor.

Prolonged use:
Not recommended.

Skin & sunlight:
No special problems expected.

Driving, piloting or hazardous work:
Don't drive or pilot aircraft until you learn how medicine affects you. Don't work around dangerous machinery. Don't climb ladders or work in high places.
Danger increases if you drink alcohol or take medicine affecting alertness and reflexes.

Discontinuing:
No special problems expected.

Others:
No special problems expected.

 ## POSSIBLE INTERACTION WITH OTHER DRUGS

GENERIC NAME OR DRUG CLASS	COMBINED EFFECT
None expected.	

 ## POSSIBLE INTERACTION WITH OTHER SUBSTANCES

INTERACTS WITH	COMBINED EFFECT
Alcohol:	None expected.
Beverages:	None expected.
Cocaine:	None expected.
Foods:	None expected.
Marijuana:	None expected.
Tobacco:	None expected.

ADRENOCORTICOIDS (Topical)

BRAND AND GENERIC NAMES

See complete list of brand and generic names in the *Brand Name Directory,* page 905.

BASIC INFORMATION

Habit forming? No
Prescription needed? For some
Available as generic? Yes
Drug class: Adrenocorticoid (topical)

 ## USES

Relieves redness, swelling, itching, skin discomfort of hemorrhoids; insect bites; poison ivy, oak, sumac; soaps, cosmetics; jewelry; burns; sunburn; numerous skin rashes; eczema; discoid lupus erythematosus; swimmers' ear; sun poisoning; hair loss; scars; penphigus; psoriasis; pityriasis rosea.

 ## DOSAGE & USAGE INFORMATION

How to use:
• Cream, lotion, ointment, gel—Apply small amount and rub in gently.
• Topical aerosol—Follow directions on container. Don't breathe vapors.
• Other forms—Follow directions on container.

When to use:
When needed or as directed. Don't use more often than directions allow.

If you forget an application:
Use as soon as you remember.

What drug does:
Reduces inflammation by affecting enzymes that produce inflammation.

Time lapse before drug works:
15 to 20 minutes.

Don't use with:
Any other medicine without consulting your doctor or pharmacist.

 ## OVERDOSE

SYMPTOMS:
None expected.
WHAT TO DO:
If person swallows or inhales drug, call doctor, poison-control center or hospital emergency room for instructions.

 ## POSSIBLE ADVERSE REACTIONS OR SIDE EFFECTS

SYMPTOMS	WHAT TO DO
Life-threatening: None expected.	
Common: None expected.	
Infrequent: Infection on skin with pain, redness, blisters, pus; skin irritation with burning, itching, blistering or peeling; acne-like skin eruptions.	Continue. Call doctor when convenient.
Rare: None expected.	

Note: Side effects are unlikely if topical adrenocorticoids are used in low doses for short periods of time. High doses for long periods can possibly cause the adverse reactions of cortisone (see CORTISONE).

ADRENOCORTICOIDS (Topical)

WARNINGS & PRECAUTIONS

Don't take if:
You are allergic to any topical adrenocorticoid (cortisone) preparation.

Before you start, consult your doctor:
- If you plan pregnancy within medication period.
- If you have diabetes.
- If you have infection at treatment site.
- If you have stomach ulcer.
- If you have tuberculosis.

Over age 60:
Adverse reactions and side effects may be more frequent and severe than in younger persons, especially thinning of the skin.

Pregnancy:
Risk to unborn child outweighs drug benefits. Don't use.

Breast-feeding:
No problems expected.

Infants & children:
- Use only under medical supervision. Too much for too long can be absorbed into bloodstream through skin and retard growth.
- For infants in diapers, avoid plastic pants or tight diapers.

Prolonged use:
- Increases chance of absorption into bloodstream to cause side effects of oral cortisone drugs.
- May thin skin where used.
- Talk to your doctor about the need for follow-up medical examinations or laboratory studies to check complete blood counts (white blood cell count, platelet count, red blood cell count, hemoglobin, hematocrit), adrenal function.

Skin & sunlight:
No problems expected.

Driving, piloting or hazardous work:
No problems expected.

Discontinuing:
May be unnecessary to finish medicine. Follow doctor's instructions.

Others:
- Don't use a plastic dressing longer than 2 weeks.
- Aerosol spray—Store in cool place. Don't use near heat or open flame or while smoking. Don't puncture, break or burn container.
- Don't use for acne or gingivitis.

POSSIBLE INTERACTION WITH OTHER DRUGS

GENERIC NAME OR DRUG CLASS	COMBINED EFFECT
Antibiotics* (topical)	Decreased antibiotic effects.
Antifungals* (topical)	Decreased antifungal effect.

POSSIBLE INTERACTION WITH OTHER SUBSTANCES

INTERACTS WITH	COMBINED EFFECT
Alcohol:	None expected.
Beverages:	None expected.
Cocaine:	None expected.
Foods:	None expected.
Marijuana:	None expected.
Tobacco:	None expected.

*See Glossary

ALLOPURINOL

BRAND NAMES

Alloprin	Purinol
Apo-Allopurinol	Zurinol
Lopurin	Zyloprim
Novopural	

BASIC INFORMATION

Habit forming? No
Prescription needed? Yes
Available as generic? Yes
Drug class: Antigout

 ## USES

- Treatment for chronic gout.
- Prevention of kidney stones caused by uric acid.

 ## DOSAGE & USAGE INFORMATION

How to take:
Tablet—Swallow with liquid or food to lessen stomach irritation.

When to take:
At the same times each day.

If you forget a dose:
- 1 dose per day—Take as soon as you remember up to 6 hours late. If more than 6 hours, wait for next scheduled dose (don't double this dose).
- More than 1 dose per day—Take as soon as you remember up to 3 hours late. If more than 3 hours, wait for next scheduled dose (don't double this dose).

What drug does:
Slows formation of uric acid by inhibiting enzyme (xanthine oxidase) activity.

Time lapse before drug works:
Reduces blood uric acid in 1 to 3 weeks. May require 6 months to prevent acute gout attacks.

Don't take with:
Any other medicine without consulting your doctor or pharmacist.

 ## OVERDOSE

SYMPTOMS:
None expected.
WHAT TO DO:
Overdose unlikely to threaten life. If person takes much larger amount than prescribed, call doctor, poison-control center or hospital emergency room for instructions.

 ## POSSIBLE ADVERSE REACTIONS OR SIDE EFFECTS

SYMPTOMS	WHAT TO DO
Life-threatening: None expected.	
Common: Rash, hives, itch.	Discontinue. Call doctor right away.
Infrequent: • Jaundice (yellow skin or eyes.)	Discontinue. Call doctor right away.
• Drowsiness, diarrhea, stomach pain, nausea or vomiting without other symptoms, headache.	Continue. Call doctor when convenient.
Rare: • Sore throat, fever, unusual bleeding or bruising.	Discontinue. Call doctor right away.
• Numbness, tingling, pain in hands or feet.	Continue. Call doctor when convenient.

 ## WARNINGS & PRECAUTIONS

Don't take if:
You are allergic to allopurinol.

Before you start, consult your doctor:
If you have had liver or kidney problems.

Over age 60:
Adverse reactions and side effects may be more frequent and severe than in younger persons.

Pregnancy:
Studies inconclusive on harm to unborn child. Animal studies show fetal abnormalities. Decide with your doctor whether drug benefits justify risk to unborn child.

Breast-feeding:
Drug passes into milk. Avoid drug or discontinue nursing.

Infants & children:
Not recommended.

Prolonged use:
Talk to your doctor about the need for follow-up medical examinations or laboratory studies to check liver function, kidney function, complete blood counts (white blood cell count, platelet count, red blood cell count, hemoglobin, hematocrit), and serum uric-acid determinations.

Skin & sunlight:
No problems expected.

Driving, piloting or hazardous work:
Avoid if you feel drowsy. Use may disqualify you for piloting aircraft.

Discontinuing:
Don't discontinue without doctor's advice until you complete prescribed dose, even though symptoms diminish or disappear.

Others:
Acute gout attacks may increase during first weeks of use. If so, consult doctor about additional medicine.

POSSIBLE INTERACTION WITH OTHER DRUGS

GENERIC NAME OR DRUG CLASS	COMBINED EFFECT
Ampicillin	Likely skin rash.
Anticoagulants, oral*	May increase anticoagulant effect.
Antidiabetics, oral*	Increased uric-acid elimination.
Azathioprine	Greatly increased azathioprine effect.
Chlorpropamide	May increase chlorpropamide effect.
Chlorthalidone	Decreased allopurinol effect.
Cyclophosphamide	Increased cyclophosphamide toxicity.
Diuretics, loop*	Decreased allopurinol effect.
Diuretics, thiazide*	Decreased allopurinol effect.
Ethacrynic acid	Decreased allopurinol effect.
Furosemide	Decreased allopurinol effect.
Indapamide	Decreased allopurinol effect.
Iron supplements*	Excessive accumulation of iron in tissues.
Mercaptopurine	Increased mercaptopurine effect.
Metolazone	Decreased allopurinol effect.
Probenecid	Increased allopurinol effect.
Theophylline	May increase theophylline effect.

POSSIBLE INTERACTION WITH OTHER SUBSTANCES

INTERACTS WITH	COMBINED EFFECT
Alcohol:	None expected, but may impair management of gout.
Beverages:	Caffeine drinks. Decreased allopurinol effect.
Cocaine:	Decreased allopurinol effect. Avoid.
Foods:	None expected. Low-purine diet* recommended.
Marijuana:	Occasional use— None expected. Daily use—Possible increase in uric-acid level.
Tobacco:	None expected.

*See Glossary

AMANTADINE

BRAND NAMES

Symadine   Symmetrel

BASIC INFORMATION

Habit forming? No
Prescription needed? Yes
Available as generic? Yes
Drug class: Antiviral, antiparkinsonism

USES

- Prevention and treatment for Type-A flu infections.
- Relief for symptoms of Parkinson's disease.

DOSAGE & USAGE INFORMATION

How to take:
- Capsule—Swallow with liquid or food to lessen stomach irritation.
- Syrup—Dilute dose in beverage before swallowing.

When to take:
At the same times each day. For Type-A flu it is especially important to take regular doses as prescribed.

If you forget a dose:
Take as soon as you remember. Wait 4 hours for next dose. Return to schedule.

What drug does:
- Type-A flu—May block penetration of tissue cells by infectious material from virus cells.
- Parkinson's disease and drug-induced extrapyramidal* reactions—Improves muscular condition and coordination.

Time lapse before drug works:
- Type-A flu—48 hours.
- Parkinson's disease—2 days to 2 weeks.

Continued next column

OVERDOSE

SYMPTOMS:
Heart-rhythm disturbances, blood-pressure drop, convulsions, toxic psychosis, confusion, slurred speech, rolling eyes.
WHAT TO DO:
- Dial 0 (operator) or 911 (emergency) for an ambulance or medical help. Then give first aid immediately.
- See emergency information on inside covers.

Don't take with:
- Alcohol
- Any other medicine without consulting your doctor or pharmacist.

POSSIBLE ADVERSE REACTIONS OR SIDE EFFECTS

SYMPTOMS	WHAT TO DO
Life-threatening:	
In case of overdose, see previous column.	
Common:	
• Hallucinations, confusion, lightheadedness.	Continue. Call doctor when convenient.
• Dizziness, headache, purple blotches, appetite loss, nausea.	Continue. Tell doctor at next visit.
• Dry mouth.	No action necessary.
Infrequent:	
• Fainting, slurred speech.	Discontinue. Call doctor right away.
• Difficult or painful urination.	Continue. Call doctor when convenient.
Rare:	
• Rash, uncontrollable rolling of eyes, irregular heartbeats, blurred vision, sore throat, fever, vomiting.	Discontinue. Call doctor right away.
• Constipation.	Continue. Tell doctor at next visit.

WARNINGS & PRECAUTIONS

Don't take if:
You are allergic to amantadine.

Before you start, consult your doctor:
- If you have had epilepsy or other seizures.
- If you have had heart disease or heart failure.
- If you have had liver or kidney disease.
- If you have had peptic ulcers.
- If you have had eczema or skin rashes.
- If you have had emotional or mental disorders or taken drugs for them.

Over age 60:
Adverse reactions and side effects may be more frequent and severe than in younger persons.

Pregnancy:
Studies inconclusive on harm to unborn child. Animal studies show fetal abnormalities. Decide with your doctor whether benefits justify risk to unborn child.

Breast-feeding:
Drug passes into milk. Avoid drug or discontinue nursing until you finish medicine. Consult doctor for advice on maintaining milk supply.

Infants & children:
Use only under medical supervision.

Prolonged use:
Skin splotches, feet swelling, rapid weight gain, shortness of breath. Consult doctor.

Skin & sunlight:
No problems expected.

Driving, piloting or hazardous work:
Don't drive or pilot aircraft until you learn how medicine affects you. Don't work around dangerous machinery. Don't climb ladders or work in high places. Danger increases if you drink alcohol or take medicine affecting alertness and reflexes.

Discontinuing:
- Parkinson's disease—Don't discontinue without doctor's advice until you complete prescribed dose, even though symptoms diminish or disappear.
- Type-A flu—Discontinue 48 hours after symptoms disappear.

Others:
- Parkinson's disease—May lose effectiveness in 3 to 6 months. Consult doctor.
- Amantadine may increase susceptibility to German measles.

POSSIBLE INTERACTION WITH OTHER DRUGS

GENERIC NAME OR DRUG CLASS	COMBINED EFFECT
Amphetamines*	Increased amantadine effect. Possible excessive stimulation and agitation.
Anticholinergics*	Increased benefit, but excessive anti-cholinergic dose produces mental confusion, hallucinations, delirium.
Antidyskinetics*	Confusion, hallucinations, nightmares.
Antihistamines*	Confusion, hallucinations, nightmares.
Appetite suppressants*	Increased amantadine effect. Possible excessive stimulation and agitation.
Levodopa	Increased benefit of levodopa. Can cause agitation.
Phenothiazines*	Confusion, hallucinations, nightmares.
Sympathomimetics*	Increased amantadine effect. Possible excessive stimulation and agitation.
Tricyclic Antidepressants	Confusion, hallucinations, nightmares.

POSSIBLE INTERACTION WITH OTHER SUBSTANCES

INTERACTS WITH	COMBINED EFFECT
Alcohol:	Increased alcohol effect. Possible fainting.
Beverages:	None expected.
Cocaine:	Dangerous overstimulation.
Foods:	None expected.
Marijuana:	None expected.
Tobacco:	None expected.

*See Glossary

AMBENONIUM

BRAND NAMES

Mytelase

BASIC INFORMATION

Habit forming? No
Prescription needed? Yes
Available as generic? No
Drug class: Cholinergic, antimyasthenic

 USES

- Diagnosis and treatment of myasthenia gravis.
- Treatment of urinary retention and abdominal distention.

 DOSAGE & USAGE INFORMATION

How to take:
- Tablet—Swallow with liquid or food to lessen stomach irritation.
- Extended-release capsules and tablets— Swallow each dose whole with liquid; do not crush.

When to take:
As directed, usually 3 or 4 times a day.

If you forget a dose:
Take as soon as you remember up to 2 hours late. If more than 2 hours, wait for next scheduled dose (don't double this dose).

What drug does:
Inhibits the chemical activity of an enzyme (cholinesterase) so nerve impulses can cross the junction of nerves and muscles.

Time lapse before drug works:
3 hours.

Don't take with:
Any other medicine without consulting your doctor or pharmacist.

 OVERDOSE

SYMPTOMS:
Muscle weakness or paralysis, cramps, twitching or clumsiness; severe diarrhea, nausea, vomiting, stomach cramps or pain; breathing difficulty; confusion, irritability, nervousness, restlessness, fear; unusually slow heartbeat; seizures, blurred vision, extreme fatigue.
WHAT TO DO:
- Dial 0 (operator) or 911 (emergency) for an ambulance or medical help. Then give first aid immediately.
- See emergency information on inside covers.

 POSSIBLE ADVERSE REACTIONS OR SIDE EFFECTS

SYMPTOMS	WHAT TO DO
Life-threatening:	
In case of overdose, see previous column.	
Common:	
• Mild diarrhea, nausea, vomiting, stomach cramps or pain.	Discontinue. Call doctor right away.
• Excess saliva, unusual sweating.	Continue. Call doctor when convenient.
Infrequent:	
• Confusion, irritability.	Discontinue. Seek emergency treatment.
• Constricted pupils, watery eyes, lung congestion, urgent or frequent urination.	Continue. Call doctor when convenient.
Rare:	
None expected.	

WARNINGS & PRECAUTIONS

Don't take if:
- You are allergic to any cholinergic or bromide.
- You take mecamylamine.

Before you start, consult your doctor:
- If you plan to become pregnant within medication period.
- If you have bronchial asthma.
- If you have heartbeat irregularities.
- If you have urinary obstruction or urinary-tract infection.

Over age 60:
Adverse reactions and side effects may be more frequent and severe than in younger persons.

Pregnancy:
No proven harm to unborn child. Avoid if possible. May increase contractions of the womb close to time of delivery.

Breast-feeding:
No problems expected, but consult doctor.

Infants & children:
Not recommended.

Prolonged use:
Medication may lose effectiveness. Discontinuing for a few days may restore effect.

Skin & sunlight:
No problems expected.

Driving, piloting or hazardous work:
Don't drive or pilot aircraft until you learn how medicine affects you. Don't work around dangerous machinery. Don't climb ladders or work in high places. Danger increases if you drink alcohol or take medicine affecting alertness and reflexes, such as antihistamines, tranquilizers, sedatives, pain medicine, narcotics and mind-altering drugs.

Discontinuing:
Don't discontinue without doctor's advice until you complete prescribed dose, even though symptoms diminish or disappear.

Others:
No problems expected.

POSSIBLE INTERACTION WITH OTHER DRUGS

GENERIC NAME OR DRUG CLASS	COMBINED EFFECT
Anesthetics, local or general*	Decreased ambenonium effect.
Antiarrhythmics*	Decreased ambenonium effect.
Antibiotics*	Decreased ambenonium effect.
Anticholinergics*	Decreased ambenonium effect. May mask severe side effects.
Cholinergics, other*	Reduced intestinal-tract function. Possible brain and nervous-system toxicity.
Guanadrel	Decreased ambenonium effect.
Guanethidine	Decreased ambenonium effect.
Mecamylamine	Decreased ambenonium effect.
Nitrates*	Decreased ambenonium effect.
Procainamide	Decreased ambenonium effect.
Quinidine	Decreased ambenonium effect.
Tiremethaphan	Decreased ambenonium effect.

POSSIBLE INTERACTION WITH OTHER SUBSTANCES

INTERACTS WITH	COMBINED EFFECT
Alcohol:	No proven problems with small doses.
Beverages:	None expected.
Cocaine:	Decreased ambenonium effect. Avoid.
Foods:	None expected.
Marijuana:	No proven problems.
Tobacco:	No proven problems.

AMILORIDE

BRAND NAMES

Midamor

BASIC INFORMATION

Habit forming? No
Prescription needed? Yes
Available as generic? Yes
Drug class: Diuretic

 USES

Treatment for high blood pressure and congestive heart failure. Decreases fluid retention and prevents potassium loss.

 DOSAGE & USAGE INFORMATION

How to take:
- Tablet—Swallow with liquid.
- Capsule—Swallow with liquid. If you can't swallow whole, open capsule and take with liquid or food. Instructions to take on empty stomach mean 1 hour before or 2 hours after eating.

When to take:
At the same time each day, preferably in the morning. May interfere with sleep if taken after 6 p.m.

If you forget a dose:
Take as soon as you remember up to 8 hours late. If more than 8 hours, wait for next scheduled dose (don't double this dose).

What drug does:
Blocks exchange of certain chemicals in the kidney so sodium is excreted. Conserves potassium.

Continued next column

 OVERDOSE

SYMPTOMS:
Rapid, irregular heartbeat; confusion; shortness of breath; nervousness; extreme weakness.
WHAT TO DO:
- Dial 0 (operator) or 911 (emergency) for an ambulance or medical help. Then give first aid immediately.
- If patient is unconscious and not breathing, give mouth-to-mouth breathing. If there is no heartbeat, use cardiac massage and mouth-to-mouth breathing (CPR). Don't try to make patient vomit. If you can't get help quickly, take patient to nearest emergency facility.
- See emergency information on inside covers.

Time lapse before drug works:
2 hours.

Don't take with:
Any other medicine without consulting your doctor or pharmacist.

 POSSIBLE ADVERSE REACTIONS OR SIDE EFFECTS

SYMPTOMS	WHAT TO DO
Life-threatening:	
In case of overdose, see previous column.	
Common:	
Headache, nausea, appetite loss, vomiting, mild diarrhea, constipation, decreased interest in sex.	Continue. Call doctor when convenient.
Infrequent:	
• Shortness of breath, fever, chills, unusual tiredness or weakness, confusion.	Discontinue. Call doctor right away.
• Dizziness, bloating, muscle cramps, dry mouth.	Continue. Call doctor when convenient.
Rare:	
None expected.	

 WARNINGS & PRECAUTIONS

Don't take if:
- You are allergic to amiloride.
- Your serum potassium level is high.

Before you start, consult your doctor:
- If you plan to become pregnant within medication period.
- If you have diabetes.
- If you have heart disease.
- If you have kidney or liver disease.

Over age 60:
Adverse reactions and side effects may be more frequent and severe than in younger persons. More likely to exceed safe potassium blood levels.

Pregnancy:
No proven harm to unborn child. Avoid if possible.

Breast-feeding:
No problems expected, but consult doctor.

Infants & children:
Not recommended.

AMILORIDE

Prolonged use:
Talk to your doctor about the need for follow-up medical examinations or laboratory studies to check blood pressure, kidney function, ECG* and serum electrolytes.

Skin & sunlight:
Increased sensitivity to sunlight.

Driving, piloting or hazardous work:
Don't drive or pilot aircraft until you learn how medicine affects you. Don't work around dangerous machinery. Don't climb ladders or work in high places. Danger increases if you drink alcohol or take medicine affecting alertness and reflexes, such as antihistamines, tranquilizers, sedatives, pain medicine, narcotics and mind-altering drugs.

Discontinuing:
Don't discontinue without doctor's advice until you complete prescribed dose, even though symptoms diminish or disappear.

Others:
Periodic physical checkups and potassium-level tests recommended.

POSSIBLE INTERACTION WITH OTHER DRUGS

GENERIC NAME OR DRUG CLASS	COMBINED EFFECT
Acebutolol	Increased antihypertensive effect. Dosages may require adjustment.
ACE inhibitors*: captopril, enalapril, lisinopril	Possible excessive potassium in blood.
Amiodarone	Increased risk of heartbeat irregularity due to low potassium.
Antihypertensives*	Increased effect of both drugs.
Blood-bank blood	Increased potassium levels.
Calcium supplements*	Increased calcium in blood.
Diuretics, other*	Increased effect of both drugs.
Lithium	Possible lithium toxicity.
Nicardipine	Dangerous blood pressure drop. Dosages may require adjustment.
Nimodipine	Dangerous blood pressure drop.
Nitrates*	Excessive blood pressure drop.
Potassium supplements*	Increased potassium levels.
Sodium bicarbonate	Decreased potassium levels.

POSSIBLE INTERACTION WITH OTHER SUBSTANCES

INTERACTS WITH	COMBINED EFFECT
Alcohol:	Increased blood pressure drop. Avoid.
Beverages: Low-salt milk.	Possible excess potassium levels. Low-salt milk has extra potassium.
Cocaine:	Blood pressure rise. Avoid.
Foods: Salt substitutes.	Possible excess potassium levels.
Marijuana:	None expected.
Tobacco:	None expected.

*See Glossary

23

AMILORIDE & HYDROCHLOROTHIAZIDE

BRAND NAMES

Moduret   Moduretic

BASIC INFORMATION

Habit forming? No
Prescription needed? Yes
Available as generic? Yes
Drug class: Diuretic (thiazide),
  antihypertensive

USES

- Controls, but doesn't cure, high blood pressure.
- Reduces fluid retention (edema), decreasing likelihood of congestive heart failure.

DOSAGE & USAGE INFORMATION

How to take:
Tablet—Swallow with liquid. If you can't swallow whole, crumble tablet and take with liquid or food.

When to take:
At the same time each day, no later than 6 p.m.

If you forget a dose:
Take as soon as you remember up to 2 hours late. If more than 2 hours, wait for next scheduled dose (don't double this dose).

What drug does:
- Forces sodium and water excretion, conserves potassium, reducing body fluid.
- Relaxes muscle cells of small arteries.
- Reduced body fluid and relaxed arteries lower blood pressure.

Time lapse before drug works:
2-6 hours. May require several weeks to lower blood pressure.

Continued next column

OVERDOSE

SYMPTOMS:
Cramps, weakness, drowsiness, weak
pulse, coma, rapid, irregular heartbeat.
WHAT TO DO:
- **Dial 0 (operator) or 911 (emergency) for an ambulance or medical help. Then give first aid immediately.**
- **See emergency information on inside covers.**

Don't take with:
- Any other medicine without consulting your doctor or pharmacist.
- Non-prescription drugs without consulting doctor.

POSSIBLE ADVERSE REACTIONS OR SIDE EFFECTS

SYMPTOMS	WHAT TO DO
Life-threatening:	
In case of overdose, see previous column.	
Common:	
• Increased thirst, irregular heartbeat, cramps in muscles, numbness and tingling in hands and feet, thready pulse, shortness of breath.	Discontinue. Call doctor right away.
• Tiredness, weakness, diarrhea, headache, appetite loss, nausea, constipation, decreased interest in sex.	Continue. Call doctor when convenient.
Infrequent:	
• Mood changes, dizziness, lightheadedness.	Continue. Call doctor when convenient.
• Fever and chills, red tongue, cracked mouth corners, black stools, dry mouth.	Discontinue. Call doctor right away.
Rare:	
Jaundice; unusual bleeding or bruising; abdominal pain with vomiting; sore throat, sores in mouth; hives; skin rash; joint pain.	Discontinue. Seek emergency treatment.

AMILORIDE & HYDROCHLOROTHIAZIDE

WARNINGS & PRECAUTIONS

Don't take if:
You are allergic to amiloride or any thiazide diuretic drug.

Before you start, consult your doctor:
• If you are allergic to any sulfa drug.
• If you have gout, diabetes, heart disease.
• If you have liver, pancreas or kidney disorder.

Over age 60:
Adverse reactions and side effects may be more frequent and severe than in younger persons, especially dizziness and excessive potassium loss.

Pregnancy:
Risk to unborn child outweighs drug benefits. Don't use.

Breast-feeding:
Drug passes into milk. Avoid drug or discontinue nursing until you finish medicine.

Infants & children:
Not recommended unless closely supervised.

Prolonged use:
• You may need medicine to treat high blood pressure for the rest of your life.
• Talk to your doctor about the need for follow-up medical examinations or laboratory studies to check blood pressure, kidney function, electrocardiogram and serum electrolytes.

Skin & sunlight:
May cause rash or intensify sunburn in areas exposed to sun or sunlamp. Avoid overexposure.

Driving, piloting or hazardous work:
Don't drive or pilot aircraft until you learn how medicine affects you. Don't work around dangerous machinery. Don't climb ladders or work in high places. Danger increases if you drink alcohol or take medicine affecting alertness and reflexes, such as antihistamines, tranquilizers, sedatives, pain medicine, narcotics and mind-altering drugs.

Discontinuing:
Don't discontinue without medical advice.

Others:
• Hot weather and fever may cause dehydration and drop in blood pressure. Dose may require temporary adjustment. Weigh daily and report any unexpected weight decreases to your doctor.
• May cause rise in uric acid, leading to gout.
• May cause blood-sugar rise in diabetics.
• Get periodic check-ups and potassium-level laboratory tests.

POSSIBLE INTERACTION WITH OTHER DRUGS

GENERIC NAME OR DRUG CLASS	COMBINED EFFECT
Allopurinol	Decreased allopurinol effect.
Antidepressants, tricyclic (TCA)*	Dangerous drop in blood pressure. Avoid combination unless under medical supervision.
Antihypertensives, other*	Increased effect of both drugs.
Barbiturates*	Increased hydrochlorothiazide effect.
Beta-adrenergic blockers*	Increased antihypertensive effect. Dosages of both drugs may require adjustments.
Blood-bank blood	Increased potassium levels.
Carteolol	Increased antihypertensive effect.
Cortisone drugs*	Excessive potassium loss that causes dangerous heart rhythms.
Cyclosporine	Increased potassium levels.

Continued page 932

POSSIBLE INTERACTION WITH OTHER SUBSTANCES

INTERACTS WITH	COMBINED EFFECT
Alcohol:	Dangerous blood pressure drop.
Beverages: Low-salt milk.	Possible excess potassium levels. Low-salt milk has extra potassium.
Cocaine:	Increased risk of heart block and high blood pressure.
Foods: Salt substitutes.	Possible excess potassium levels.
Marijuana:	May increase blood pressure.
Tobacco:	None expected.

*See Glossary

AMINOBENZOATE POTASSIUM

BRAND NAMES

KPAB
Potaba
Potassium
  Aminobenzoate

Potassium
Para-
  aminobenzoate

BASIC INFORMATION

Habit forming? No
Prescription needed? Yes
Available as generic? No
Drug class: Antifibrosis

 ## USES

Reduces inflammation and relieves contractions in tissues lying under the skin that have become tight from such disorders as dermatomyositis, Peyronie's disease, scleroderma, pemphigus, morphea.

 ## DOSAGE & USAGE INFORMATION

How to take:
- Tablets—Dissolve in liquid or take with food to prevent stomach upset.
- Capsules—Take with full glass of liquid.
- Oral solution—Swallow with liquid to lessen stomach upset.
- Powder—Mix with liquid.

When to take:
At the same times each day, according to instructions on prescription label. Usually taken with meals and at bedtime with a snack.

If you forget a dose:
Take as soon as you remember up to 2 hours late. If more than 2 hours, wait for next scheduled dose (don't double this dose).

What drug does:
May increase ability of diseased tissues to use oxygen.

Time lapse before drug works:
May require 3 to 10 months for improvement to begin.

Continued next column

 ## OVERDOSE

SYMPTOMS:
Nausea, vomiting.
WHAT TO DO:
Overdose unlikely to threaten life. If person takes much larger amount than prescribed, call doctor, poison-control center or hospital emergency room for instructions.

Don't take with:
Any other medicine without consulting your doctor or pharmacist.

 ## POSSIBLE ADVERSE REACTIONS OR SIDE EFFECTS

SYMPTOMS	WHAT TO DO
Life-threatening: None expected.	
Common: Appetite loss, nausea, rash, fever.	Continue. Call doctor when convenient.
Infrequent: • Low blood sugar (hunger, anxiety, cold sweats, rapid pulse).	Discontinue. Seek emergency treatment. (Note: Take sugar or honey on the way to emergency room.)
• Sore throat.	Discontinue. Call doctor right away.
Rare: None expected.	

AMINOBENZOATE POTASSIUM

 WARNINGS &
PRECAUTIONS

Don't take if:
You are allergic to aminobenzoate potassium or aminobenzoic acid (PABA).

Before you start, consult your doctor:
- If you have low blood sugar.
- If you have diabetes mellitus.
- If you have kidney disease.

Over age 60:
Adverse reactions and side effects may be more frequent and severe than in younger persons, particularly low blood sugar.

Pregnancy:
Safety not established.

Breast-feeding:
Drug passes into milk. Avoid drug or discontinue nursing.

Infants & children:
Not recommended. Safety and dosage have not been established.

Prolonged use:
Talk to your doctor about the need for follow-up medical examinations or laboratory studies to check complete blood counts (white blood cell count, platelet count, red blood cell count, hemoglobin, hematocrit).

Skin & sunlight:
No problems expected.

Driving, piloting or hazardous work:
No problems expected.

Discontinuing:
No problems expected.

Others:
If you become acutely ill and cannot eat well for even a short while, tell your doctor. These circumstances can lead to low blood sugar, and dosage may need adjustment.

 POSSIBLE INTERACTION
WITH OTHER DRUGS

GENERIC NAME OR DRUG CLASS	COMBINED EFFECT
Dapsone	Decreased dapsone effect.
Methotrexate	Increased methotrexate effect and toxicity.
Salicylates*	May increase salicylate blood level.
Sulfa drugs* (sulfonamides)	Decreased sulfa effect.

 POSSIBLE INTERACTION
WITH OTHER SUBSTANCES

INTERACTS WITH	COMBINED EFFECT
Alcohol:	None expected.
Beverages:	None expected.
Cocaine:	None expected.
Foods:	None expected.
Marijuana:	None expected.
Tobacco:	None expected.

AMINOGLUTETHIMIDE

BRAND NAMES

Cytadren

BASIC INFORMATION

Habit forming? No
Prescription needed? Yes
Available as generic? No
Drug class: Antiadrenal, antineoplastic

USES

- Treats Cushing's syndrome.
- Treats breast malignancies.

DOSAGE & USAGE INFORMATION

How to take:
Tablets—Swallow with liquid. If you can't swallow whole, crumble tablet and take with liquid or food. Instructions to take on empty stomach mean 1 hour before or 2 hours after eating.

When to take:
Follow doctor's instructions exactly.

If you forget a dose:
Take as soon as you remember up to 2 hours late. If more than 2 hours, wait for next scheduled dose (don't double this dose).

What drug does:
Suppresses adrenal cortex.

Time lapse before drug works:
1 to 2 hours.

Don't take with:
Any other medicines (including over-the-counter drugs such as cough and cold medicines, laxatives, antacids, diet pills, caffeine, nose drops or vitamins) without consulting your doctor.

OVERDOSE

SYMPTOMS:
None expected.
WHAT TO DO:
Overdose unlikely to threaten life. If person takes much larger amount than prescribed, call doctor, poison-control center or hospital emergency room for instructions.

POSSIBLE ADVERSE REACTIONS OR SIDE EFFECTS

SYMPTOMS	WHAT TO DO
Life-threatening:	
None expected.	
Common:	
Skin rash on face and hands.	Continue. Tell doctor at next visit.
Infrequent:	
• Dizziness, drowsiness, unexplained fatigue, low back pain, pain on urinating, clumsiness, unusual eye movements, appetite loss.	Discontinue. Call doctor right away.
• Vomiting, skin darkening, depression, headache, muscle pain.	Continue. Call doctor when convenient.
Rare:	
Unusual bleeding or bruising.	Discontinue. Call doctor right away.

WARNINGS & PRECAUTIONS

Don't take if:
- You have recently been exposed to chicken pox.
- You have shingles (herpes zoster).

Before you start, consult your doctor:
- If you have decreased thyroid function (hypothyroidism).
- If you have any form of infection.

Over age 60:
Adverse reactions and side effects may be more frequent and severe than in younger persons. You may need smaller doses for shorter periods of time.

Pregnancy:
May cause birth defects. Avoid if possible.

Breast-feeding:
Effect not documented. Consult your doctor.

Infants & children:
Effect not documented. Consult your pediatrician.

Prolonged use:
Talk to your doctor about the need for follow-up medical examinations or laboratory studies to check thyroid function, liver function, serum electrolytes (sodium potassium, chloride) and blood pressure.

Skin & sunlight:
No problems expected.

Driving, piloting or hazardous work:
No problems expected.

Discontinuing:
No special problems expected.

Others:
- Advise any doctor or dentist whom you consult that you take this medicine.
- May affect results in some medical tests.
- May cause decreased thyroid function.

 ## POSSIBLE INTERACTION WITH OTHER DRUGS

GENERIC NAME OR DRUG CLASS	COMBINED EFFECT
Anticoagulants*	Decreased anticoagulant effect.
Clozapine	Toxic effect on the central nervous system.
Cortisone-like drugs*	Decreased cortisone effects.
Dexamethasone	Dexamethasone effect decreased by half.
Phenprocoumon	Decreased anticoagulant effect.
Sertraline	Increased depressive effects of both dugs.
Trilostane	Too much decrease in adrenal function.

 ## POSSIBLE INTERACTION WITH OTHER SUBSTANCES

INTERACTS WITH	COMBINED EFFECT
Alcohol:	Increased stomach irritation.
Beverages: Coffee, tea, cocoa.	Increased stomach irritation.
Cocaine:	No proven problems.
Foods:	No proven problems.
Marijuana:	No proven problems.
Tobacco:	No proven problems.

*See Glossary

AMIODARONE

BRAND NAMES

Cordarone

BASIC INFORMATION

Habit forming? No
Prescription needed? Yes
Available as generic? No
Drug class: Antiarrhythmic

 USES

Prevents and treats life-threatening heartbeat irregularities involving both the large chambers of the heart (auricles and ventricles).

 DOSAGE & USAGE INFORMATION

How to take:
Tablets—Swallow whole with liquid or food to lessen stomach irritation. If you can't swallow whole, crumble tablet and take with liquid or food.

When to take:
According to prescription instructions.

If you forget a dose:
Skip this dose and resume regular schedule. Do not double the next dose. If you forget 2 doses or more, consult your doctor.

What drug does:
- Slows nerve impulses in the heart.
- Makes heart muscle fibers less responsive to abnormal electrical impulses arising in the electrical regulatory system of the heart.

Continued next column

 OVERDOSE

SYMPTOMS:
Irregular heartbeat, loss of consciousness, seizures.
WHAT TO DO:
- **Dial 0 (operator) or 911 (emergency) for an ambulance or medical help. Then give first aid immediately.**
- **If patient is unconscious and not breathing, give mouth-to-mouth breathing. If there is no heartbeat, use cardiac massage and mouth-to-mouth breathing (CPR). Don't try to make patient vomit. If you can't get help quickly, take patient to nearest emergency facility.**
- **See emergency information on inside covers.**

Time lapse before drug works:
2 to 3 days to 2 to 3 months.

Don't take with:
Any other medicine without consulting your doctor or pharmacist.

 POSSIBLE ADVERSE REACTIONS OR SIDE EFFECTS

SYMPTOMS	WHAT TO DO
Life-threatening:	
Shortness of breath, difficulty breathing, cough.	Discontinue. Seek emergency treatment.
Common:	
• Walking difficulty, fever, numbness or tingling in hands or feet, shakiness, weakness in arms and legs.	Discontinue. Call doctor right away.
• Constipation, headache, appetite loss, nausea, vomiting.	Continue. Call doctor when convenient.
Infrequent:	
• Skin color change to blue-gray, blurred vision, cold feeling, dry eyes, nervousness, scrotum swelling or pain, insomnia, swollen feet and ankles, fast or slow heartbeat, eyes hurt in light, weight gain or loss, sweating.	Discontinue. Call doctor right away.
• Bitter or metallic taste, diminished sex drive, dizziness, flushed face, coldness and unusual tiredness.	Continue. Call doctor when convenient.
Rare:	
Jaundice, skin rash.	Discontinue. Call doctor right away.

 WARNINGS & PRECAUTIONS

Don't take if:
You are allergic to amiodarone.

Before you start, consult your doctor:
- If you have liver, kidney or thyroid disease.
- If you have heart disease other than coronary artery disease.

Over age 60:
- Adverse reactions and side effects may be more frequent and severe than in younger persons. Ask about smaller doses.
- Pain in legs (while walking) considerably more likely.

Pregnancy:
Safety to unborn child unestablished. Thyroid abnormalities possible in fetus. Avoid if possible.

Breast-feeding:
Drug passes into milk. Avoid drug or discontinue nursing until you finish medicine. Consult doctor for advice on maintaining milk supply.

Infants & children:
Safety not established. Use only under close medical supervision.

Prolonged use:
- Blue-gray discoloration of skin may appear.
- Don't discontinue without consulting doctor. Dose may require gradual reduction if you have taken drug for a long time. Doses of other drugs may also require adjustment.
- Talk to your doctor about the need for follow-up medical examinations or laboratory studies to check ECG*, SGPT*, serum alkaline phosphatase, SGOT*, thyroid function.

Skin & sunlight:
May cause rash or intensify sunburn in areas exposed to sun or sunlamp. Avoid undue exposure, use sunscreens.

Driving, piloting or hazardous work:
Avoid if you feel dizzy or lightheaded. Otherwise, no problems expected.

Discontinuing:
- Don't discontinue without consulting doctor. Dose may require gradual reduction if you have taken drug for a long time. Doses of other drugs may also require adjustment.
- Notify doctor if cough, fever, breathing difficulty or shortness of breath occur after discontinuing medicine.

Others:
- Learn to check your own pulse. If it drops to lower than 50 or rises to higher than 100 beats per minute, don't take amiodarone until you consult your doctor.
- May interfere with the accuracy of some medical tests.

 POSSIBLE INTERACTION WITH OTHER DRUGS

GENERIC NAME OR DRUG CLASS	COMBINED EFFECT
Antiarrhythmics, other*	Increased likelihood of heartbeat irregularity.
Anticoagulants*	Increased anticoagulant effect.
Beta-adrenergic blockers*	Increased likelihood of slow heartbeat.
Calcium channel blockers*	Possible heart block.
Cholestyramine	May decrease amiodarone blood levels.
Digitalis	Increased digitalis effect.
Diltiazem	Increased likelihood of slow heartbeat.
Diuretics*	Increased risk of heartbeat irregularity due to low potassium level.
Encainide	Increased effect of toxicity on the heart muscle.
Flecainide	Increased flecainide effect.
Isoniazid	Increased risk of liver damage.
Nicardipine	Possible increased effect and toxicity of each drug.
Nifedipine	Increased likelihood of slow heartbeat.
Phenytoin	Increased effect of phenytoin.
Procainamide	Increased procainamide effect.
Propafenone	Increased effect of both drugs and increased risk of toxicity.
Quinidine	Increased quinidine effect.
Verapamil	Increased likelihood of slow heartbeat.

 POSSIBLE INTERACTION WITH OTHER SUBSTANCES

INTERACTS WITH	COMBINED EFFECT
Alcohol:	Increased risk of heartbeat irregularity. Avoid.
Beverages:	None expected.
Cocaine:	Increased risk of heartbeat irregularity. Avoid.
Foods:	None expected.
Marijuana:	Possible irregular heartbeat. Avoid.
Tobacco:	Possible irregular heartbeat. Avoid.

*See Glossary

AMOXICILLIN

BRAND NAMES

Amoxil	Novamoxin
Apo-Amoxi	Polymox
Augmentin	Trimox
Clavulin	Wymox

BASIC INFORMATION

Habit forming? No
Prescription needed? Yes
Available as generic? Yes
Drug class: Antibiotic (penicillin)

 ## USES

Treatment of bacterial infections that are susceptible to amoxicillin.

 ## DOSAGE & USAGE INFORMATION

How to take:
- Tablet or capsule—Swallow with liquid on an empty stomach 1 hour before or 2 hours after eating.
- Chewable tablets—Chew well before swallowing.
- Liquid—Take with cold beverage. Liquid form is perishable and effective for only 7 days at room temperature. Effective for 14 days if stored in refrigerator. Don't freeze.

When to take:
Follow instructions on prescription label or side of package. Doses should be evenly spaced. For example, 4 times a day means before meals and bedtime.

If you forget a dose:
Take as soon as you remember. Continue regular schedule.

What drug does:
Destroys susceptible bacteria. Does not kill viruses.

Continued next column

 ## OVERDOSE

SYMPTOMS:
Severe diarrhea, nausea or vomiting.
WHAT TO DO:
Overdose unlikely to threaten life. If person takes much larger amount than prescribed, call doctor, poison-control center or hospital emergency room for instructions.

Time lapse before drug works:
May be several days before medicine affects infection.

Don't take with:
Any other medicine without consulting your doctor or pharmacist.

 ## POSSIBLE ADVERSE REACTIONS OR SIDE EFFECTS

SYMPTOMS	WHAT TO DO
Life-threatening:	
Hives, rash, intense itching, faintness soon after a dose (anaphylaxis); difficulty breathing.	Seek emergency treatment immediately.
Common:	
Dark or discolored tongue.	Continue. Tell doctor at next visit.
Infrequent:	
• Mild nausea, vomiting, diarrhea.	Continue. Call doctor when convenient.
• Bloody urine, face and ankle swelling.	Discontinue. Call doctor right away.
Rare:	
Unexplained bleeding or bruising, weakness, sore throat, fever, abdominal cramps, convulsions.	Discontinue. Call doctor right away.

WARNINGS & PRECAUTIONS

Don't take if:
You are allergic to amoxicillin, cephalosporin antibiotics, other penicillins. Life-threatening reaction may occur.

Before you start, consult your doctor:
- If you are allergic to any substance or drug.
- If you take birth control pills.

Over age 60:
You may have skin reactions, particularly around genitals and anus.

Pregnancy:
Studies inconclusive on harm to unborn child. Animal studies show fetal abnormalities. Decide with your doctor whether drug benefits justify risk to unborn child.

Breast-feeding:
Drug passes into milk. Child may become sensitive to penicillins and have allergic reactions to penicillin drugs. Avoid amoxicillin or discontinue nursing until you finish medicine. Consult doctor for advice on maintaining milk supply.

Infants & children:
No problems expected.

Prolonged use:
- You may become more susceptible to infections caused by germs not responsive to amoxicillin. Super infection also a potential.
- Talk to your doctor about the need for follow-up medical examinations or laboratory studies to check SGPT*, SGOT*.

Skin & sunlight:
No problems expected.

Driving, piloting or hazardous work:
Usually not dangerous. Most hazardous reactions likely to occur a few minutes after taking amoxicillin.

Discontinuing:
Don't discontinue without doctor's advice until you complete prescribed dose, even though symptoms diminish or disappear.

Others:
- May interfere with the accuracy of some medical tests.
- Birth control pills may not be effective. Use additional birth-control measures.

POSSIBLE INTERACTION WITH OTHER DRUGS

GENERIC NAME OR DRUG CLASS	COMBINED EFFECT
Beta-adrenergic blockers*	Increased chance of anaphylaxis (see emergency information on inside front cover).
Birth control pills	Impaired contraceptive efficiency.
Chloramphenicol	Decreased effect of both drugs.
Erythromycins*	Decreased effect of both drugs.
Loperamide	Decreased amoxicillin effect.
Paromomycin	Decreased effect of both drugs.
Probenecid	Increased effect of all penicillins.
Sodium benzoate & sodium phenylacetate	May reduce effect of sodium benzoate & sodium phenylacetate.
Tetracyclines*	Decreased effect of both drugs.
Troleandomycin	Decreased effect of both drugs.

POSSIBLE INTERACTION WITH OTHER SUBSTANCES

INTERACTS WITH	COMBINED EFFECT
Alcohol:	Occasional stomach irritation.
Beverages:	None expected.
Cocaine:	No proven problems.
Foods: Acidic fruits or juices, aged cheeses, wines, syrups (if taken with).	Decreased antibiotic effect.
Marijuana:	No proven problems.
Tobacco:	None expected.

*See Glossary

AMPHETAMINES

BRAND AND GENERIC NAMES

Amfetamine
AMPHETAMINE
AMPHETAMINE
  SULFATE
Biphetamine 12½
Biphetamine 20
Desoxyn Gradumet

Dexedrine
Dexedrine Spansule
DEXTROAMPHETA-
  MINE
METHAMPHETAMINE
Oxydess
Spancap

BASIC INFORMATION

Habit forming? Yes
Prescription needed? Yes
Available as generic? Yes
Drug class: Central nervous system
  stimulant

 ## USES

- Prevents narcolepsy (attacks of uncontrollable sleepiness).
- Controls hyperactivity in children under special circumstances.

 ## DOSAGE & USAGE INFORMATION

How to take:
- Tablet—Swallow with liquid.
- Extended-release capsules and tablets—Swallow each dose whole with liquid; do not crush.

When to take:
- At the same times each day.
- Short-acting form—Don't take later than 6 hours before bedtime.
- Long-acting form—Take on awakening.

If you forget a dose:
- Short-acting form—Take up to 2 hours late. If more than 2 hours, wait for next dose (don't double this dose).
- Long-acting form—Take as soon as you remember. Wait 20 hours for next dose.

Continued next column

 ## OVERDOSE

SYMPTOMS:
Rapid heartbeat, hyperactivity, high fever, hallucinations, suicidal or homicidal feelings, convulsions, coma.
WHAT TO DO:
- Dial 0 (operator) or 911 (emergency) for an ambulance or medical help. Then give first aid immediately.
- See emergency information on inside covers.

Time lapse before drug works:
15 to 30 minutes.

Don't take with:
Any other medicine without consulting your doctor or pharmacist.

 ## POSSIBLE ADVERSE REACTIONS OR SIDE EFFECTS

SYMPTOMS	WHAT TO DO
Life-threatening:	
In case of overdose, see previous column.	
Common:	
• Irritability, nervousness, insomnia, euphoria.	Continue. Call doctor when convenient.
• Dry mouth.	Continue. Tell doctor at next visit.
• Fast, pounding heartbeat.	Discontinue. Call doctor right away.
Infrequent:	
• Dizziness; reduced alertness; blurred vision; unusual sweating.	Discontinue. Call doctor right away.
• Headache.	Continue. Call doctor when convenient.
• Diarrhea or constipation, appetite loss, stomach pain, nausea, vomiting, weight loss, diminished sex drive, impotence.	Continue. Tell doctor at next visit.
Rare:	
• Rash, hives; chest pain or irregular heartbeat; uncontrollable movements of head, neck, arms, legs.	Discontinue. Call doctor right away.
• Mood changes, swollen breasts.	Continue. Call doctor when convenient.

 ## WARNINGS & PRECAUTIONS

Don't take if:
- You are allergic to any amphetamine.
- You will have surgery within 2 months, including dental surgery, requiring general or spinal anesthesia.

Before you start, consult your doctor:
- If you plan to become pregnant within medication period.
- If you have glaucoma.
- If you have heart or blood vessel disease or high blood pressure.
- If you have overactive thyroid, anxiety or tension.
- If you have a severe mental illness (especially children).

AMPHETAMINES

Over age 60:
Adverse reactions and side effects may be more frequent and severe than in younger persons.

Pregnancy:
Risk to unborn child outweighs benefits of drug. Don't use.

Breast-feeding:
Drug passes into milk. Avoid drug or discontinue nursing.

Infants & children:
Not recommended for children under 12.

Prolonged use:
- Habit forming.
- Talk to your doctor about the need for follow-up medical examinations or laboratory studies to check blood pressure, growth charts in children, reassessment of need for continued treatment.

Skin & sunlight:
No problems expected.

Driving, piloting or hazardous work:
Don't drive or pilot aircraft until you learn how medicine affects you. Don't work around dangerous machinery. Don't climb ladders or work in high places. Danger increases if you drink alcohol or take medicine affecting alertness and reflexes.

Discontinuing:
May be unnecessary to finish medicine. Follow doctor's instructions.

Others:
- This is a dangerous drug and must be closely supervised. Don't use for appetite control or depression. Potential for damage and abuse.
- During withdrawal phase, may cause prolonged sleep of several days.
- Don't use for fatigue or to replace rest.

POSSIBLE INTERACTION WITH OTHER DRUGS

GENERIC NAME OR DRUG CLASS	COMBINED EFFECT
Anesthesias, general*	Irregular heartbeat.
Antidepressants, tricyclic (TCA)*	Decreased amphetamine effect.
Antihypertensives*	Decreased antihypertensive effect.
Beta blockers*	High blood pressure, slow heartbeat.
Carbonic anhydrase inhibitors*	Increased amphetamine effect.
Doxazosin	Decreased doxazosin effect.
Furazolidine	Sudden and severe high blood pressure.
Haloperidol	Decreased amphetamine effect.
MAO inhibitors*	May severely increase blood pressure.
Nabilone	Greater depression of the central nervous system.
Phenothiazines*	Decreased amphetamine effect.
Prazosin	Decreased prazosin effect.
Sodium bicarbonate	Increased amphetamine effect.
Sympathomimetics*	Seizures.
Thyroid hormones*	Heartbeat irregularities.

POSSIBLE INTERACTION WITH OTHER SUBSTANCES

INTERACTS WITH	COMBINED EFFECT
Alcohol:	Decreased amphetamine effect. Avoid.
Beverages: Caffeine drinks.	Overstimulation. Avoid.
Cocaine:	Dangerous stimulation of nervous system. Avoid.
Foods:	None expected.
Marijuana:	Frequent use— Severely impaired mental function.
Tobacco:	None expected.

*See Glossary

35

AMPICILLIN

BRAND NAMES

Amcill	Penbritin
Ampicin	Polycillin
Ampilean	Polycillin-N
Apo-Ampi	Prinicipen
Novo-Ampicillin	Totacillin
Omnipen	Totacillin-N
Omnipen-N	

BASIC INFORMATION

Habit forming? No
Prescription needed? Yes
Available as generic? Yes
Drug class: Antibiotic (penicillin)

USES

Treatment of bacterial infections that are susceptible to ampicillin.

DOSAGE & USAGE INFORMATION

How to take:
- Capsules—Swallow with liquid on an empty stomach 1 hour before or 2 hours after eating.
- Chewable tablets—Chew well before swallowing.
- Liquid—Take with cold beverage. Liquid form is perishable and effective for only 7 days at room temperature. Effective for 14 days if stored in refrigerator. Don't freeze.

When to take:
Follow instructions on prescription label or side of package. Doses should be evenly spaced. For example, 4 times a day means before meals and at bedtime.

If you forget a dose:
Take as soon as you remember. Continue regular schedule.

Continued next column

OVERDOSE

SYMPTOMS:
Severe diarrhea, nausea or vomiting.
WHAT TO DO:
Overdose unlikely to threaten life. If person takes much larger amount than prescribed, call doctor, poison-control center or hospital emergency room for instructions.

What drug does:
Destroys susceptible bacteria. Does not kill viruses.

Time lapse before drug works:
May be several days before medicine affects infection.

Don't take with:
Any other medicine without consulting your doctor or pharmacist.

POSSIBLE ADVERSE REACTIONS OR SIDE EFFECTS

SYMPTOMS	WHAT TO DO
Life-threatening:	
Hives, rash, intense itching, faintness soon after a dose (anaphylaxis); difficulty breathing.	Seek emergency treatment immediately.
Common:	
Dark or discolored tongue.	Continue. Tell doctor at next visit.
Infrequent:	
• Mild nausea, vomiting, diarrhea.	Continue. Call doctor when convenient.
• Bloody urine, face and ankle swelling.	Discontinue. Call doctor right away.
Rare:	
Unexplained bleeding or bruising, weakness, sore throat, fever, abdominal cramps, convulsions.	Discontinue. Call doctor right away.

WARNINGS & PRECAUTIONS

Don't take if:
You are allergic to ampicillin, cephalosporin antibiotics, other penicillins. Life-threatening reaction may occur.

Before you start, consult your doctor:
- If you are allergic to any substance or drug.
- If you take birth control pills.

Over age 60:
You may have skin reactions, particularly around genitals and anus.

Pregnancy:
Studies inconclusive on harm to unborn child. Animal studies show fetal abnormalities. Decide with your doctor whether drug benefits justify risk to unborn child.

Breast-feeding:
Drug passes into milk. Child may become sensitive to penicillins and have allergic reactions to penicillin drugs. Avoid ampicillin or discontinue nursing until you finish medicine. Consult doctor for advice on maintaining milk supply.

Infants & children:
No problems expected.

Prolonged use:
- You may become more susceptible to infections caused by germs not responsive to ampicillin. Super-infection also a potential.
- Talk to your doctor about the need for follow-up medical examinations or laboratory studies to check SGPT*, SGOT*.

Skin & sunlight:
No problems expected.

Driving, piloting or hazardous work:
Usually not dangerous. Most hazardous reactions likely to occur a few minutes after taking ampicillin.

Discontinuing:
Don't discontinue without doctor's advice until you complete prescribed dose, even though symptoms diminish or disappear.

Others:
- Urine sugar test for diabetes may show false positive result.
- Birth control pills may not be effective. Use additional birth-control methods.

POSSIBLE INTERACTION WITH OTHER DRUGS

GENERIC NAME OR DRUG CLASS	COMBINED EFFECT
Beta-adrenergic blockers*	Increased chance of anaphylaxis (see emergency information on inside front cover).
Birth control pills	Impaired contraceptive efficiency.
Chloramphenicol	Decreased effect of both drugs.
Erythromycins*	Decreased effect of both drugs.
Loperamide	Decreased ampicillin effect.
Probenecid	Increased effect of all penicillins.
Paromomycin	Decreased effect of both drugs.
Sodium benzoate & sodium phenylacetate	May reduce effect of sodium benzoate & sodium phenylacetate.
Tetracyclines*	Decreased effect of both drugs.
Troleandomycin	Decreased effect of both drugs.

POSSIBLE INTERACTION WITH OTHER SUBSTANCES

INTERACTS WITH	COMBINED EFFECT
Alcohol:	Occasional stomach irritation.
Beverages:	None expected.
Cocaine:	No proven problems.
Foods: Acidic fruits or juices, aged cheese, wines, syrups (if taken with).	Decreased antibiotic effect.
Marijuana:	No proven problems.
Tobacco:	None expected.

*See Glossary

AMYL·NITRITE INHALANT

BRAND NAMES

Amyl Nitrate Inhalant

BASIC INFORMATION

Habit forming? No
Prescription needed? Yes
Available as generic? Yes
Drug class: Coronary vasodilator

 ## USES

Treats angina pectoris attacks. *Note:* Don't use amyl nitrite expecting a "high" or as an aphrodisiac. Serious, harmful side effects may occur when amyl nitrate is abused.

 ## DOSAGE & USAGE INFORMATION

How to take:
Cover the glass capsule with a protective cloth and then crush between your fingers. Inhale 1 to 6 times. Remain seated while you inhale. Repeat dose in 5 minutes if needed.

When to take:
Only when chest pain occurs. If relief doesn't occur with first capsule within 5 minutes, crush another. If inhaling 2 capsules in 10 minutes doesn't bring relief, go to emergency room.

If you forget a dose:
No set dosage schedule. Use only when needed.

What drug does:
Relaxes coronary arteries that supply blood to the heart muscle.

Time lapse before drug works:
1 to 5 minutes.

Don't take with:
Any other medicine without consulting your doctor or pharmacist.

 ## OVERDOSE

SYMPTOMS:
Blue lips, fingernails; dizziness, fainting, head pressure, shortness of breath, fast heartbeat.
WHAT TO DO:
- **Dial 0 (operator) or 911 (emergency) for an ambulance or medical help. Then give first aid immediately.**
- **See emergency information on inside covers.**

 ## POSSIBLE ADVERSE REACTIONS OR SIDE EFFECTS

SYMPTOMS	WHAT TO DO
Life-threatening:	
In case of overdose, see previous column.	
Common:	
Continuing fast heartbeat, pulse; headache, restlessness.	Discontinue. Call doctor right away.
Infrequent:	
Dizziness, lightheadedness.	Discontinue. Call doctor right away.
Rare:	
Continuing dizziness.	Discontinue. Call doctor right away.

WARNINGS & PRECAUTIONS

Don't take if:
You have had a recent head injury.

Before you start, consult your doctor:
- If you are anemic.
- If you have glaucoma.
- If you have overactive thyroid.
- If you have had a recent myocardial infarction.

Over age 60:
Adverse reactions and side effects may be more frequent and severe than in younger persons. You may need smaller doses for shorter periods of time.

Pregnancy:
Risk to unborn child outweighs drug benefits. Don't use.

Breast-feeding:
No documented problems. Best to avoid.

Infants & children:
Effect not documented. Consult your pediatrician.

Prolonged use:
Request follow-up studies to check liver function, kidney function, blood counts, platelet counts, heart function and blood pressure.

Skin & sunlight:
No problems expected.

Driving, piloting or hazardous work:
Avoid if you feel confused, drowsy or dizzy.

Discontinuing:
None expected.

Others:
- Advise any doctor or dentist whom you consult that you take this medicine.
- May affect results in some medical tests.

POSSIBLE INTERACTION WITH OTHER DRUGS

GENERIC NAME OR DRUG CLASS	COMBINED EFFECT
Antihypertensives*	Increased side effects of fainting and dizziness.
Sympathomimetics*	Reduces amyl nitrite effects.

POSSIBLE INTERACTION WITH OTHER SUBSTANCES

INTERACTS WITH	COMBINED EFFECT
Alcohol:	Excess lightheadedness.
Beverages: Coffee, tea, cocoa.	Reduces amyl nitrite effects.
Cocaine:	Central nervous system toxicity. Avoid.
Foods:	None expected.
Marijuana:	Excess central nervous system stimulation. Avoid.
Tobacco:	No special problems expected.

ANALGESICS (Topical-Otic)

BRAND AND GENERIC NAMES

ANTIPYRINE AND
BENZOCAINE
Aurafair
Auralgan
Aurodex
Auromid
Oto

BASIC INFORMATION

Habit forming? No
Prescription needed? Yes
Available as generic? No
Drug class: Analgesic (otic), anesthetic

 USES

Relieves pain of middle ear infections (otitis media). It does not treat the infection itself.

 DOSAGE & USAGE INFORMATION

How to use:
- Warm ear drops under running water around the unopened bottle.
- Lie down with affected ear up.
- Adults—Pull ear lobe back and up.
- Children—Pull ear lobe down and back.
- Drop medicine into ear canal until canal is full.
- Stay lying down for 2 minutes.
- Gently insert cotton plug into ear to prevent leaking.

When to use:
Every 1 to 2 hours for 4 hours, then 4 times a day when needed for pain.

If you forget a dose:
Use as soon as you remember.

What drug does:
Functions as a topical anesthetic/analgesic on the eardrum.

Time lapse before drug works:
10 minutes.

Don't use with:
Any other medicine without consulting your doctor or pharmacist.

 OVERDOSE

SYMPTOMS:
None expected.
WHAT TO DO:
Not intended for internal use. If child accidentally swallows, call poison-control center.

 POSSIBLE ADVERSE REACTIONS OR SIDE EFFECTS

SYMPTOMS	WHAT TO DO
Life-threatening: None expected.	
Common: None expected.	
Infrequent: Itching or burning in ear (probably represents allergic reaction).	Discontinue. Call doctor right away.
Rare: None expected.	

WARNINGS & PRECAUTIONS

Don't use if:
You are allergic to any local anesthetic (name usually ends with 'caine').

Before you start, consult your doctor:
If eardrum is ruptured.

Over age 60:
No problems expected.

Pregnancy:
No problems expected.

Breast-feeding:
No problems expected.

Infants & children:
No problems expected.

Prolonged use:
Not intended for prolonged use.

Skin & sunlight:
No problems expected.

Driving, piloting or hazardous work:
No problems expected.

Discontinuing:
No problems expected.

Others:
- Keep cool, but don't freeze.
- Don't touch tip of dropper to any other surface.
- Don't rinse the dropper, wipe with clean cloth and close tightly.

POSSIBLE INTERACTION WITH OTHER DRUGS

GENERIC NAME OR DRUG CLASS	COMBINED EFFECT
None expected.	

POSSIBLE INTERACTION WITH OTHER SUBSTANCES

INTERACTS WITH	COMBINED EFFECT
Alcohol:	None expected.
Beverages:	None expected.
Cocaine:	None expected.
Foods:	None expected.
Marijuana:	None expected.
Tobacco:	None expected.

ANDROGENS

BRAND AND GENERIC NAMES

See complete list of brand and generic names in the *Brand Name Directory*, page 906.

BASIC INFORMATION

Habit forming? No
Prescription needed? Yes
Available as generic? Yes
Drug class: Androgen

 USES

- Corrects male hormone deficiency.
- Reduces "male menopause" symptoms (loss of sex drive, depression, anxiety).
- Decreases calcium loss of osteoporosis (softened bones).
- Blocks growth of breast-cancer cells in females.
- Corrects undescended testicles in male children.
- Reduces breast pain and fullness following childbirth.
- Augments treatment of aplastic anemia.
- Stimulates weight gain after illness, injury or for chronically underweight persons.
- Stimulates growth in treatment of dwarfism.

 DOSAGE & USAGE INFORMATION

How to take:
- Tablets or capsules—With food to lessen stomach irritation.
- Injection—Once or twice a month.

When to take:
At the same time each day.

If you forget a dose:
Take as soon as you remember up to 2 hours late. If more than 2 hours, wait for next scheduled dose (don't double this dose).

Continued next column

 OVERDOSE

SYMPTOMS:
None expected.
WHAT TO DO:
Overdose unlikely to threaten life. If person takes much larger amount than prescribed, call doctor, poison-control center or hospital emergency room for instructions.

What drug does:
- Stimulates cells that produce male sex characteristics.
- Replaces hormone deficiencies.
- Stimulates red-blood-cell production.
- Suppresses production of estrogen (female sex hormone).

Time lapse before drug works:
Varies with problems treated. May require 2 or 3 months of regular use for desired effects.

Don't take with:
Any other medicine without consulting your doctor or pharmacist.

 POSSIBLE ADVERSE REACTIONS OR SIDE EFFECTS

SYMPTOMS	WHAT TO DO
Life-threatening:	
Intense itching, weakness, loss of consciousness.	Seek emergency treatment immediately.
Common:	
• Acne or oily skin, deep voice, enlarged clitoris in females; frequent erections, swollen breasts in men.	Continue. Call doctor when convenient.
• Sore mouth; higher sex drive, decreased testicle size, impotence in men.	Continue. Tell doctor at next visit.
Infrequent:	
• Yellow skin or eyes.	Discontinue. Seek emergency treatment.
• Depression or confusion, flushed face, rash or itch, nausea, vomiting, diarrhea, swollen feet or legs, headache, shortness of breath, rapid weight gain, chills, difficult urination; vaginal bleeding in women; scrotum pain in men.	Discontinue. Call doctor right away.
Rare:	
• Hives, black stool.	Discontinue. Seek emergency treatment.
• Sore throat, fever, abdominal pain.	Discontinue. Call doctor right away.
• Appetite loss, halitosis.	Continue. Call doctor when convenient.

ANDROGENS

WARNINGS & PRECAUTIONS

Don't take if:
You are allergic to any male hormone.

Before you start, consult your doctor:
- If you might be pregnant.
- If you have cancer of prostate.
- If you have heart disease or arteriosclerosis.
- If you have kidney or liver disease.
- If you have breast cancer (males).
- If you have high blood pressure.
- If you have migraine attacks.
- If you have high level of blood calcium.
- If you have epilepsy.

Over age 60:
- May stimulate sexual activity.
- Can make high blood pressure or heart disease worse.
- Can enlarge prostate and cause urinary retention.

Pregnancy:
Risk to unborn child outweighs drug benefits. Don't use.

Breast-feeding:
Drug passes into milk. Avoid drug or discontinue nursing until you finish medicine. Consult doctor for advice on maintaining milk supply.

Infants & children:
Don't give to children younger than 2. Use with older children only under medical supervision.

Prolonged use:
- Reduces sperm count and volume of semen.
- Possible kidney stones.
- Unnatural hair growth and deep voice in women.
- Talk to your doctor about the need for follow-up medical examinations or laboratory studies to check complete blood counts (white blood cell count, platelet count, red blood cell count, hemoglobin, hematocrit).

Skin & sunlight:
No problems expected.

Driving, piloting or hazardous work:
No problems expected.

Discontinuing:
No problems expected.

Others:
- May cause atrophy of testicles.
- Will not increase strength in athletes.
- May cause liver cancer.
- In women, may cause male-like changes such as deepened voice, increased hair growth.

POSSIBLE INTERACTION WITH OTHER DRUGS

GENERIC NAME OR DRUG CLASS	COMBINED EFFECT
Anticoagulants*	Increased anticoagulant effect.
Antidiabetics, oral*	Increased antidiabetic effect.
Chlorzoxazone	Decreased androgen effect.
Hepatotoxic drugs* (other)	Increased liver toxicity.
Insulin	Increased antidiabetic effect.
Oxyphenbutazone	Decreased androgen effect.
Phenobarbital	Decreased androgen effect.
Phenylbutazone	Decreased androgen effect.

POSSIBLE INTERACTION WITH OTHER SUBSTANCES

INTERACTS WITH	COMBINED EFFECT
Alcohol:	None expected.
Beverages:	None expected.
Cocaine:	No proven problems.
Foods: Salt.	Excessive fluid retention (edema). Decrease salt intake while taking male hormones.
Marijuana:	Decreased blood levels of androgens.
Tobacco:	No proven problems.

*See Glossary

BRAND AND GENERIC NAMES

Americaine
BENZOCAINE
DIBUCAINE
Ethyl Aminobenzoate
Fleet Relief
Nupercainal
PRAMOXINE
Pontocaine Cream

Pontocaine Ointment
Preparation "H"
Proctofoam
TETRACAINE
TETRACAINE
  AND MENTHOL
Tronolane
Tronothane

BASIC INFORMATION

Habit forming? No
Prescription needed? Yes, for some.
Available as generic? Yes, Dibucaine. No
  others, but most brands are available
  without prescription.
Drug class: Anesthetic (rectal)

USES

- Relieves pain, itching and swelling of hemorrhoids (piles).
- Relieves pain of rectal fissures (breaks in lining membrane of the anus).

DOSAGE & USAGE INFORMATION

How to use:
- Rectal cream or ointment—Apply to surface of rectum with fingers. Insert applicator into rectum no farther than 1/2 and apply inside. Wash applicator with warm soapy water or discard.
- Aerosol foam—Read patient instructions. Don't insert into rectum. Use the special applicator and wash carefully after using.
- Suppository—Remove wrapper and moisten with water. Lie on side. Push blunt end of suppository into rectum with finger. If suppository is too soft, run cold water over wrapper or put in refrigerator for 15 to 45 minutes before using.

When to use:
As directed.

Continued next column

OVERDOSE

SYMPTOMS:
None expected.
WHAT TO DO:
Not intended for internal use. If child accidentally swallows, call poison-control center.

If you forget a dose:
Use as soon as you remember.

What drug does:
Deadens nerve endings to pain and touch.

Time lapse before drug works:
5 to 15 minutes.

Don't use with:
Any other medicine without consulting your doctor or pharmacist.

POSSIBLE ADVERSE REACTIONS OR SIDE EFFECTS

SYMPTOMS	WHAT TO DO
Life-threatening: None expected.	
Common: None expected.	
Infrequent:	
• Nervousness, trembling, hives, rash, itch, inflammation or tenderness not present before application, slow heartbeat.	Discontinue. Call doctor right away.
• Dizziness, blurred vision, swollen feet.	Continue. Call doctor when convenient.
Rare:	
• Blood in urine.	Discontinue. Call doctor right away.
• Increased or painful urination.	Continue. Call doctor when convenient.

ANESTHETICS (Rectal)

WARNINGS & PRECAUTIONS

Don't use if:
You are allergic to any topical anesthetic.

Before you start, consult your doctor:
• If you have skin infection at site of treatment.
• If you have had severe or extensive skin disorders such as eczema or psoriasis.
• If you have bleeding hemorrhoids.

Over age 60:
Adverse reactions and side effects may be more frequent and severe than in younger persons.

Pregnancy:
No proven harm to unborn child. Avoid if possible.

Breast-feeding:
No problems expected.

Infants & children:
Use caution. More likely to be absorbed through skin and cause adverse reactions.

Prolonged use:
Possible excess absorption. Don't use longer than 3 days for any one problem.

Skin & sunlight:
No problems expected.

Driving, piloting or hazardous work:
No problems expected.

Discontinuing:
May be unnecessary to finish medicine. Follow doctor's instructions.

Others:
• Report any rectal bleeding to your doctor.
• Keep cool, but don't freeze.

POSSIBLE INTERACTION WITH OTHER DRUGS

GENERIC NAME OR DRUG CLASS	COMBINED EFFECT
Sulfa drugs*	Decreased anti-infective effect of sulfa drugs.

POSSIBLE INTERACTION WITH OTHER SUBSTANCES

INTERACTS WITH	COMBINED EFFECT
Alcohol:	None expected.
Beverages:	None expected.
Cocaine:	Possible nervous-system toxicity. Avoid.
Foods:	None expected.
Marijuana:	None expected.
Tobacco:	None expected.

ANESTHETICS (Topical)

BRAND NAMES

See complete list of brand names in the *Brand Name Directory*, page 906.

BASIC INFORMATION

Habit forming? No
Prescription needed?
  High strength: Yes
  Low strength: No
Available as generic? Yes
Drug class: Anesthetic (topical)

 ## USES

- Relieves pain and itch of sunburn, insect bites, scratches and other minor skin irritations.
- Relieves discomfort and itch of hemorrhoids and other disorders of anus and rectum.

 ## DOSAGE & USAGE INFORMATION

How to use:
- Suppositories—Remove wrapper and moisten suppository with water. Gently insert larger end into rectum. Push well into rectum with finger.
- All other forms—Use only enough to cover irritated area. Follow instructions on label.

When to use:
When needed for discomfort, no more often than every hour.

If you forget an application:
Use as needed.

What drug does:
Blocks pain impulses from skin to brain.

Time lapse before drug works:
3 to 15 minutes.

Don't take with:
Any other medicine without consulting your doctor or pharmacist.

 ## OVERDOSE

SYMPTOMS:
If swallowed or inhaled—Dizziness, nervousness, trembling, seizures.
WHAT TO DO:
- Dial 0 (operator) or 911 (emergency) for an ambulance or medical help. Then give first aid immediately.
- See emergency information on inside covers.

 ## POSSIBLE ADVERSE REACTIONS OR SIDE EFFECTS

SYMPTOMS	WHAT TO DO
Life-threatening:	
None expected.	
Common:	
None expected.	
Infrequent:	
• Nervousness; trembling; hives, rash, itch; inflammation or tenderness not present before application; slow heartbeat.	Discontinue. Call doctor right away.
• Dizziness, blurred vision, swollen feet.	Continue. Call doctor when convenient.
Rare:	
• Blood in urine.	Discontinue. Call doctor right away.
• Increased or painful urination.	Continue. Call doctor when convenient.

WARNINGS & PRECAUTIONS

Don't use if:
You are allergic to any topical anesthetic.

Before you start, consult your doctor:
- If you have skin infection at site of treatment.
- If you have had severe or extensive skin disorders such as eczema or psoriasis.
- If you have bleeding hemorrhoids.

Over age 60:
Adverse reactions and side effects may be more frequent and severe than in younger persons.

Pregnancy:
No proven harm to unborn child. Avoid if possible.

Breast-feeding:
No problems expected.

Infants & children:
Use caution. More likely to be absorbed through skin and cause adverse reactions.

Prolonged use:
Possible excess absorption. Don't use longer than 3 days for any one problem.

Skin & sunlight:
No problems expected.

Driving, piloting or hazardous work:
No problems expected.

Discontinuing:
May be unnecessary to finish medicine. Follow doctor's instructions.

Others:
No problems expected.

POSSIBLE INTERACTION WITH OTHER DRUGS

GENERIC NAME OR DRUG CLASS	COMBINED EFFECT
Sulfa drugs*	Decreased effect of sulfa drugs for infection.

POSSIBLE INTERACTION WITH OTHER SUBSTANCES

INTERACTS WITH	COMBINED EFFECT
Alcohol:	None expected.
Beverages:	None expected.
Cocaine:	Possible nervous-system toxicity. Avoid.
Foods:	None expected.
Marijuana:	None expected.
Tobacco:	None expected.

ANESTHETICS, DENTAL (Topical)

BRAND AND GENERIC NAMES

Americaine
Baby Anbesol
Baby Orajel
BENZOCAINE
BUTACAINE
Butyn
Ethyl aminobenzoate
Hurricane
LIDOCAINE
Orabase with
  Benzocaine

Orajel
Rid-A-Pain
Spec T
T-Caine
Triamcinolone in
  Orabase
Tyrobenz
Xylocaine
Xylocaine Viscous

BASIC INFORMATION

Habit forming? No
Prescription needed? Yes, for some.
Available as generic? Yes for Lidocaine, no
  for others
Drug class: Anesthetic (topical)

 USES

Relieves pain or irritation in mouth caused by
toothache, teething, mouth sores, dentures,
braces, dental appliances. Also relieves pain of
sore throat for short periods of time.

 **DOSAGE & USAGE
INFORMATION**

How to use:
- For mouth problems—Apply to sore places
  with cotton-tipped applicator. Don't swallow.
- For throat—Gargle, but don't swallow.
- For aerosol spray—Don't inhale.

When to use:
As directed by physician or label on package.

If you forget a dose:
Use as soon as you remember.

Continued next column

 OVERDOSE

SYMPTOMS:
Overabsorption by body—Dizziness, blurred
vision, seizures, drowsiness.
WHAT TO DO:
- Dial 0 (operator) or 911 (emergency) for
  an ambulance or medical help. Then give
  first aid immediately.
- Not for internal use. If child accidentally
  swallows, call poison-control center.
- See emergency information on inside covers.

What drug does:
Blocks pain impulses to the brain.

Time lapse before drug works:
Immediately.

Don't use with:
Any other medicine without consulting your
doctor or pharmacist.

 **POSSIBLE
ADVERSE REACTIONS
OR SIDE EFFECTS**

SYMPTOMS	WHAT TO DO
Life-threatening:	
Unusual anxiety, excitement, nervousness, irregular or slow heartbeat.	Discontinue. Seek emergency treatment.
Common:	
Ringing or buzzing in ears.	Discontinue. Call doctor right away.
Infrequent:	
Redness, irritation, sores not present before treatment, rash, itchy skin, hives.	Discontinue. Call doctor right away.
Rare:	
Paleness, sweating.	Discontinue. Call doctor right away.

ANESTHETICS, DENTAL (Topical)

WARNINGS & PRECAUTIONS

Don't use if:
You are allergic to any of the products listed.

Before you start, consult your doctor:
- If you are allergic to anything.
- If you have infection, canker sores or other sores in your mouth.
- If you take medicine for myasthenia gravis, eye drops for glaucoma or any sulfa medicine.

Over age 60:
Adverse reactions and side effects may be more frequent and severe than in younger persons. Ask doctor about smaller doses.

Pregnancy:
No problems expected, but check with doctor.

Breast-feeding:
No problems expected, but check with doctor.

Infants & children:
No problems expected, but check with doctor.

Prolonged use:
Not intended for prolonged use.

Skin & sunlight:
No problems expected.

Driving, piloting or hazardous work:
Wait to see if causes dizziness, sweating, drowsiness or blurred vision. If not, no problems expected.

Discontinuing:
No problems expected.

Others:
- Keep cool, but don't freeze.
- Don't puncture, break or burn aerosol containers.
- Don't eat, drink or chew gum for 1 hour after use.
- Heat and moisture in bathroom medicine cabinet can cause breakdown of medicine. Store someplace else.
- Before anesthesia, tell dentist about any medicines you take or use.

POSSIBLE INTERACTION WITH OTHER DRUGS

GENERIC NAME OR DRUG CLASS	COMBINED EFFECT
So remote, they are not considered clinically significant.	

POSSIBLE INTERACTION WITH OTHER SUBSTANCES

INTERACTS WITH	COMBINED EFFECT
Alcohol:	Adverse reactions more common.
Beverages:	None expected.
Cocaine:	May cause too much nervousness and trembling. Avoid.
Foods:	None expected.
Marijuana:	None expected.
Tobacco:	Avoid. Tobacco makes mouth problems worse.

ANESTHETICS, LOCAL (Ophthalmic)

BRAND AND GENERIC NAMES

Ak-Taine
Alcaine
Kainaire
Ocu-Caine
Ophthaine

Ophthetic
Pontocaine
PROPARACAINE
TETRACAINE

BASIC INFORMATION

Habit forming? No
Prescription needed? Yes
Available as generic? Yes
Drug class: Anesthetic, local (ophthalmic)

 USES

Eliminates pain in eye temporarily to measure pressure in eye to check for glaucoma, remove foreign bodies and stitches and corneal scraping for diagnostic procedures.

 DOSAGE & USAGE INFORMATION

How to use:
Eye drops
- Wash hands.
- Apply pressure to inside corner of eye with middle finger.
- Continue pressure for 1 minute after placing medicine in eye.
- Tilt head backward. Pull lower lid away from eye with index finger of the same hand.
- Drop eye drops into pouch and close eye. Don't blink.
- Keep eyes closed for 1 to 2 minutes.

Eye ointment
- Wash hands.
- Pull lower lid down from eye to form a pouch.
- Squeeze tube to apply thin strip of ointment into pouch.
- Close eye for 1 to 2 minutes.
- Don't touch applicator tip to any surface (including the eye). If you accidentally touch tip, clean with warm soap and water.
- Keep container tightly closed.
- Keep cool, but don't freeze.
- Wash hands immediately after using.

Continued next column

 OVERDOSE

SYMPTOMS:
None expected.
WHAT TO DO:
Not intended for internal use. If child accidentally swallows, call poison-control center.

When to use:
As directed on label.

If you forget a dose:
Use as soon as you remember.

What drug does:
Blocks conduction of pain impulses.

Time lapse before drug works:
13-15 seconds.

Don't use with:
Other drops in eyes such as antiglaucoma eye drops.

 POSSIBLE ADVERSE REACTIONS OR SIDE EFFECTS

SYMPTOMS	WHAT TO DO
Life-threatening: Anaphylaxis (severe itching, hives, wheezing, runny nose, paleness, cold sweats, coma).	See inside covers.
Common: Mild stinging and burning.	Continue. Tell doctor at next visit.
Infrequent: Allergic reaction symptoms—itching, pain, redness, swelling, watery eyes.	Discontinue. Call doctor right away.
Rare (extremely): Symptoms of excess medicine absorbed by body—Weakness, increased sweating, nervousness, difficult breathing, vomiting, nausea, muscle spasms, irregular heartbeat, dizziness, drowsiness.	Discontinue. Call doctor right away.

WARNINGS & PRECAUTIONS

Don't use if:
You are allergic to any eye anesthetic.

Before you start, consult your doctor:
- If you have ever had an allergic reaction to any local anesthetic applied to skin, ears, mucous membranes or injected, such as benzocaine, butacaine, butamben, chloroprocaine, procaine, propoxycaine.
- If you have had an allergic reaction to sunscreens.

Over age 60:
No problems expected.

Pregnancy:
No problems expected, but check with doctor.

Breast-feeding:
No problems expected, but check with doctor.

Infants & children:
Use only under close medical supervision.

Prolonged use:
May retard healing. Avoid if possible.

Skin & sunlight:
No problems expected.

Driving, piloting or hazardous work:
No problems expected.

Discontinuing:
No problems expected.

Others:
- Don't rub or wipe eye until anesthetic has worn off (usually about 20 minutes) or until normal feeling in eye returns.
- Keep cool, but don't freeze.

POSSIBLE INTERACTION WITH OTHER DRUGS

GENERIC NAME OR DRUG CLASS	COMBINED EFFECT
Clinically significant interactions with oral or injected medicines unlikely.	

POSSIBLE INTERACTION WITH OTHER SUBSTANCES

INTERACTS WITH	COMBINED EFFECT
Alcohol:	None expected.
Beverages:	None expected.
Cocaine:	None expected.
Foods:	None expected.
Marijuana:	None expected.
Tobacco:	None expected.

ANGIOTENSIN-CONVERTING ENZYME (ACE) INHIBITORS

BRAND & GENERIC NAMES

See complete list of brand and generic names in the *Brand Name Directory*, page 906.

BASIC INFORMATION

Habit forming? No
Prescription needed? Yes
Available as generic? No
Drug class: Antihypertensive, ACE inhibitor

 ## USES

Treatment for high blood pressure and congestive heart failure.

 ## DOSAGE & USAGE INFORMATION

How to take:
Tablet—Swallow with liquid. Instructions to take on empty stomach mean 1 hour before or 2 hours after eating.

When to take:
At the same times each day, usually 2-3 times daily. Take first dose at bedtime and lie down immediately.

If you forget a dose:
Take as soon as you remember up to 2 hours late. If more than 2 hours, wait for next scheduled dose (don't double this dose).

What drug does:
- Reduces resistance in arteries.
- Strengthens heartbeat.

Time lapse before drug works:
60 to 90 minutes.

Don't take with:
Any other medicine without consulting your doctor or pharmacist.

 ## OVERDOSE

SYMPTOMS:
Low blood pressure, fever, chills, sore throat, fainting, convulstions, coma.
WHAT TO DO:
- Dial 0 (operator) or 911 (emergency) for an ambulance or medical help. Then give first aid immediately.
- See emergency information on inside covers.

 ## POSSIBLE ADVERSE REACTIONS OR SIDE EFFECTS

SYMPTOMS	WHAT TO DO
Life-threatening:	
Hives, rash, intense itching, faintness soon after a dose (anaphylaxis); difficulty breathing.	Seek emergency treatment immediately.
Common:	
Rash, loss of taste.	Discontinue. Call doctor right away.
Infrequent:	
• Swelling of mouth, face, hands or feet.	Discontinue. Seek emergency treatment.
• Dizziness, fainting, chest pain, fast or irregular heartbeat, coughing, confusion, nervousness, numbness and tingling in hands or feet.	Discontinue. Call doctor right away.
• Diarrhea, headache, tiredness.	Continue. Call doctor when convenient.
Rare:	
• Sore throat, cloudy urine, fever, chills.	Discontinue. Call doctor right away.
• Nausea, vomiting, indigestion, abdominal pain.	Continue. Call doctor when convenient.

 ## WARNINGS & PRECAUTIONS

Don't take if:
- You are allergic to captopril, enalapril or lisinopril.
- You have any autoimmune disease, including AIDS or lupus.
- You are receiving blood from a blood bank.
- You take drugs for cancer.
- You will have surgery within 2 months, including dental surgery, requiring general or spinal anesthesia.

Before you start, consult your doctor:
- If you have had a stroke.
- If you have angina or heart or blood-vessel disease.
- If you have high level of potassium in blood.
- If you have kidney or liver disease.
- If you are on severe salt-restricted diet.

Over age 60:
Adverse reactions and side effects may be more frequent and severe than in younger persons.

ANGIOTENSIN-CONVERTING ENZYME (ACE) INHIBITORS

Pregnancy:
Risk to unborn child outweighs drug benefits. Don't use.

Breast-feeding:
Drug passes into milk. Avoid drug or discontinue nursing until you finish medicine. Consult doctor for advice on maintaining milk supply.

Infants & children:
Under close medical supervision only.

Prolonged use:
- May decrease white cells in blood or cause protein loss in urine.
- Request periodic laboratory blood counts and urine tests.

Skin & sunlight:
No problems expected.

Driving, piloting or hazardous work:
Avoid if you become dizzy or faint. Otherwise, no problems expected.

Discontinuing:
Don't discontinue without consulting doctor. Dose may require gradual reduction if you have taken drug for a long time. Doses of other drugs may also require adjustment.

Others:
- Stop taking diuretics or increase salt intake 1 week before starting any ACE inhibitor.
- Avoid exercising in hot weather.
- May affect results in some medical tests.
- Advise any doctor or dentist whom you consult that you take this medicine.

 POSSIBLE INTERACTION WITH OTHER DRUGS

GENERIC NAME OR DRUG CLASS	COMBINED EFFECT
Amiloride	Possible excessive potassium in blood.
Antihypertensives, other*	Increased antihypertensive effect. Dosage of each may require adjustment.
Beta-adrenergic blockers*	Increased antihypertensive effect. Dosage of each may require adjustment.
Carteolol	Increased antihypertensive effects of both drugs. Dosages may require adjustment.
Chloramphenicol	Possible blood disorders.

Diuretics*	Possible severe blood pressure drop with first dose.
Diclofenac	May decrease ACE inhibitor effect.
Guanfacine	Increased effect of both drugs.
Nicardipine	Possible excessive potassium in blood. Dosages may require adjustment.
Nimodipine	Possible excessive potassium in blood. Dangerous blood pressure drop.
Nitrates*	Possible excessive blood pressure drop.
Non-steroidal anti-inflammatory drugs (NSAIDs)*	Decreased ACE inhibitor effect.
Pentamidine	May increase bone marrow depression or make kidney damage more likely.
Pentoxifylline	Increased antihypertensive effect.
Potassium supplements*	Possible increased potassium in blood.
Potassium iodide	May raise potassium levels in blood to toxic levels.

Continued on page 933

 POSSIBLE INTERACTION WITH OTHER SUBSTANCES

INTERACTS WITH	COMBINED EFFECT
Alcohol:	Possible excessive blood pressure drop.
Beverages: Low-salt milk.	Possible excessive potassium in blood.
Cocaine	Increased risk of heart block and high blood pressure.
Foods: Salt substitutes.	Possible excessive potassium.
Marijuana:	Increased dizziness.
Tobacco:	May decrease ACE inhibitor effect.

*See Glossary

53

ANGIOTENSIN-CONVERTING ENZYME (ACE) INHIBITORS & HYDROCHLOROTHIAZIDE

BRAND AND GENERIC NAMES

See complete list of brand and generic names in the *Brand Names Directory*, page 906.

BASIC INFORMATION

Habit forming? No
Prescription needed? Yes
Available as generic? No
Drug class: Antihypertensive, diuretic (thiazide), ACE inhibitor

USES

- Treatment for high blood pressure and congestive heart failure.
- Reduces fluid retention.

DOSAGE & USAGE INFORMATION

How to take:
Tablet—Swallow with liquid. Instructions to take on empty stomach mean 1 hour before or 2 hours after eating.

When to take:
At the same times each day, usually 2 to 3 times daily. Take first dose at bedtime and lie down immediately.

If you forget a dose:
Take as soon as you remember up to 2 hours late. If more than 2 hours, wait for next scheduled dose (don't double this dose).

What drug does:
- Forces sodium and water excretion, reducing body fluid.
- Relaxes muscle cells of small arteries.
- Reduced body fluid and relaxed arteries lower blood pressure.
- Reduces resistance in arteries.
- Strengthens heartbeat.

Continued next column

OVERDOSE

SYMPTOMS:
Cramps, weakness, drowsiness, weak pulse, low blood pressure.
WHAT TO DO:
- **Dial 0 (operator) or 911 (emergency) for an ambulance or medical help. Then give first aid immediately.**
- **See emergency information on inside covers.**

Time lapse before drug works:
4 to 6 hours. May require several weeks to lower blood pressure.

Don't take with:
- Non-prescription drugs without consulting doctor.
- See Interaction column and consult doctor.

POSSIBLE ADVERSE REACTIONS OR SIDE EFFECTS

SYMPTOMS	WHAT TO DO
Life-threatening:	
Irregular heartbeat (fast or uneven); hives, rash, intense itching, faintness soon after a dose (anaphylaxis).	Discontinue. Seek emergency treatment.
Common:	
• Dry mouth, thirst, tiredness, weakness, muscle cramps, vomiting, chest pain, skin rash, coughing, weak pulse.	Discontinue. Call doctor right away.
• Taste loss, dizziness.	Continue. Call doctor when convenient.
Infrequent:	
• Face, mouth, hands swell.	Discontinue. Call doctor right away.
• Nausea, diarrhea.	Continue. Call doctor when convenient.
Rare:	
Jaundice (yellow eyes and skin), bruising, back pain.	Discontinue. Call doctor right away.

WARNINGS & PRECAUTIONS

Don't take if:
- You are allergic to any ACE inhibitor or any thiazide diuretic drug.
- You have any autoimmune disease, including AIDS or lupus.
- You are receiving blood from a blood bank.
- You take drugs for cancer.
- If you will have surgery within 2 months, including dental surgery, requiring general or spinal anesthesia.

Before you start, consult your doctor:
- If you have had a stroke.
- If you have angina, heart or blood-vessel disease, a high level of potassium in blood, lupus, gout, liver, pancreas or kidney disorder.
- If you are on severe salt-restricted diet.
- If you are allergic to any sulfa drug.

ANGIOTENSIN-CONVERTING ENZYME (ACE) INHIBITORS & HYDROCHLOROTHIAZIDE

Over age 60:
Adverse reactions and side effects may be more frequent and severe than in younger persons, especially dizziness and excessive potassium loss.

Pregnancy:
Risk to unborn child outweighs drug benefits. Don't use.

Breast-feeding:
Drug passes into milk. Avoid drug or discontinue nursing until you finish medicine. Consult doctor for advice on maintaining milk supply.

Infants & children:
Not recommended.

Prolonged use:
Talk to your doctor about the need for follow-up medical examinations or laboratory studies to check blood pressure, ECG*, liver function, kidney function.

Skin & sunlight:
May cause rash or intensify sunburn in areas exposed to sun or sunlamp.

Driving, piloting or hazardous work:
Don't drive or pilot aircraft until you learn how medicine affects you. Don't work around dangerous machinery. Don't climb ladders or work in high places. Danger increases if you drink alcohol or take medicine affecting alertness and reflexes, such as antihistamines, tranquilizers, sedatives, pain medicine, narcotics and mind-altering drugs.

Discontinuing:
Don't discontinue without consulting doctor. Dose may require gradual reduction if you have taken drug for a long time. Doses of other drugs may also require adjustment.

Others:
- Hot weather and fever may cause dehydration and drop in blood pressure. Dose may require temporary adjustment. Weigh daily and report any unexpected weight decreases to your doctor.
- May cause rise in uric acid, leading to gout.
- May cause blood-sugar rise in diabetics.

POSSIBLE INTERACTION WITH OTHER DRUGS

GENERIC NAME OR DRUG CLASS	COMBINED EFFECT
Allopurinol	Decreased allopurinol effect.
Amiloride	Possible excessive potassium in blood.

Antidepressants, tricyclic (TCA)*	Dangerous drop in blood pressure. Avoid combination unless under medical supervision.
Antihypertensives, other*	Increased antihypertensive effect. Dosage of each may require adjustment.
Barbiturates*	Increased hydrochlorothiazide effect.
Beta-adrenergic blockers*	Increased antihypertensive effect. Dosage of each may require adjustments.
Carteolol	Increased antihypertensive effects of both drugs. Dosages may require adjustment.
Chloramphenicol	Possible blood disorders.
Cholestyramine	Decreased hydrochlorothiazide effect.
Cortisone drugs*	Excessive potassium loss that causes dangerous heart rhythms.
Digitalis preparations*	Excessive potassium loss that causes dangerous heart rhythms.

Continued page 933

POSSIBLE INTERACTION WITH OTHER SUBSTANCES

INTERACTS WITH	COMBINED EFFECT
Alcohol:	Dangerous blood pressure drop. Avoid.
Beverages: Low-salt milk.	Possible excessive potassium in blood.
Cocaine	Increased risk of heart block and high blood pressure.
Foods: Salt substitutes.	Possible excessive potassium.
Marijuana:	Increased dizziness, may increase blood pressure.
Tobacco:	May decrease blood pressure lowering effect.

*See Glossary

ANTACIDS

BRAND AND GENERIC NAMES

See complete list of brand names in the *Brand Names Directory,* page 906.

BASIC INFORMATION

Habit forming? No
Prescription needed? No
Available as generic? Yes, for some.
Drug class: Antacid

USES

Treatment for hyperacidity in upper gastrointestinal tract, including stomach and esophagus. Symptoms may be heartburn or acid indigestion. Diseases include peptic ulcer, gastritis, esophagitis, hiatal hernia.

DOSAGE & USAGE INFORMATION

How to take:
Follow package instructions.

When to take:
1 to 3 hours after meals unless directed otherwise by your doctor.

If you forget a dose:
Take as soon as you remember, but not simultaneously with any other medicine.

What drug does:
• Neutralizes some of the hydrochloric acid in the stomach.
• Reduces action of pepsin, a digestive enzyme.

Time lapse before drug works:
15 minutes for antacid effect.

Don't take with:
Other medicines at the same time. Decreases absorption of other drugs. Wait 2 hours between doses.

OVERDOSE

SYMPTOMS:
Dry mouth, shallow breathing, diarrhea, weakness, fatigue, stupor, bone pain.
WHAT TO DO:
• **Overdose unlikely to threaten life. Depending on severity of symptoms and amount taken, call doctor, poison-control center or hospital emergency room for instructions.**
• **Dial 0 (operator) or 911 (emergency) for an ambulance or medical help. Then give first aid immediately.**
• **See emergency information on inside covers.**

POSSIBLE ADVERSE REACTIONS OR SIDE EFFECTS

SYMPTOMS	WHAT TO DO
Life-threatening:	
Heartbeat irregularity in patient with heart disease.	Discontinue. Seek emergency treatment.
Common:	
• Constipation, headache, appetite loss, distended stomach.	Discontinue. Call doctor right away.
• Unpleasant taste in mouth, abdominal pain, laxative effect, belching, chalky taste.	Continue. Call doctor when convenient.
Infrequent:	
• Bone pain, frequent urination, dizziness, urgent urination, muscle weakness or pain, nausea, weight gain.	Discontinue. Call doctor right away.
• Tiredness or weakness	Continue. Call Doctor when convenient.
Rare:	
Mood changes, vomiting, nervousness, swollen feet and ankles.	Discontinue. Call doctor right away.

Note: Side effects are rare unless you take too much medicine for a long time.

WARNINGS & PRECAUTIONS

Don't take if:
• You are allergic to any antacid.
• You have a high blood-calcium level.

Before you start, consult your doctor:
If you have kidney disease, chronic constipation, colitis, diarrhea, symptoms of appendicitis, stomach or intestinal bleeding, irregular heartbeat.

Over age 60:
Adverse reactions and side effects may be more frequent and severe than in younger persons. Diarrhea or constipation particularly likely.

Pregnancy:
Risk to unborn child outweighs drug benefits. Don't use.

Breast-feeding:
Drug passes into milk. Avoid drug or discontinue nursing until you finish medicine. Consult doctor for advice on maintaining milk supply.

Infants & children:
Use only under medical supervision.

Prolonged use:
- High blood level of calcium (if your antacid contains calcium) which disturbs electrolyte balance.
- Kidney stones, impaired kidney function.
- Talk to your doctor about the need for follow-up medical examinations or laboratory studies to check kidney function, serum calcium, serum potassium.

Skin & sunlight:
No problems expected.

Driving, piloting or hazardous work:
No problems expected.

Discontinuing:
May be unnecessary to finish medicine. Follow doctor's instructions.

Others:
- Don't take longer than 2 weeks unless under medical supervision.
- May affect results in some medical tests.

 ## POSSIBLE INTERACTION WITH OTHER DRUGS

GENERIC NAME OR DRUG CLASS	COMBINED EFFECT
Chlorpromazine	Decreased chlorpromazine effect.
Ciprofloxacin	May cause kidney dysfunction.
Digitalis preparations*	Decreased digitalis effect.
Iron supplements*	Decreased iron effect.
Isoniazid	Decreased isoniazid effect.
Levodopa	Increased levodopa effect.
Ketoconazole	Reduced ketoconazole effect.
Meperidine	Increased meperidine effect.
Methenamine	Reduced methenamine effect.
Nalidixic acid	Decreased nalidixic acid effect.
Nicardipine	Possible decreased nicardipine effect.
Nizatidine	Decreased nizatidine absorption.
Ofloxacin	Decreased ofloxacin effect.
Oxyphenbutazone	Decreased oxyphenbutazone effect.
Para-aminosalicylic acid (PAS)	Decreased PAS effect.
Penicillins*	Decreased penicillin effect.
Pseudoephedrine	Increased pseudoephedrine effect.
Salicylates*	Increased salicylate effect.
Tetracyclines	Decreased tetracycline effect.
Ticlopidine	Decreased ticlopidine effect.

 ## POSSIBLE INTERACTION WITH OTHER SUBSTANCES

INTERACTS WITH	COMBINED EFFECT
Alcohol:	Decreased antacid effect.
Beverages: Milk	May cause bone discomfort.
Cocaine:	No proven problems.
Foods:	Decreased antacid effect. Wait 1 hour after eating.
Marijuana:	Decreased antacid effect.
Tobacco:	Decreased antacid effect.

*See Glossary

ANTHRALIN (Topical)

BRAND NAMES

Anthra-Derm	Drithocreme HP
Anthraforte	Lasan
Anthranol	Lasan HP
Anthrascalp	Lasan Pomade
Dithranol	Lasan Unguent
Drithocreme	

BASIC INFORMATION

Habit forming? No
Prescription needed? Yes
Available as generic? No
Drug class: Antipsoriasis, hair growth stimulant

 ## USES

- Treats quiescent or chronic psoriasis.
- Stimulates hair growth in some people (not an approved use by the FDA).

 ## DOSAGE & USAGE INFORMATION

How to use:
- Wear plastic gloves for all applications.
- If directed, apply at night.
- Cream, lotion, ointment—Bathe and dry area before use. Apply small amount and rub gently.
- If for short contact, same as above for cream.
- Leave on 20 to 30 minutes. Then remove medicine by bathing or shampooing.
- If for scalp overnight—Shampoo before use to remove scales or medicine. Dry hair. Part hair several times and apply to scalp. Wear plastic cap on head. Clean off next morning with petroleum, then shampoo.

When to use:
As directed.

If you forget a dose:
Use as soon as you remember.

What drug does:
Reduces growth activity within abnormal cells by inhibiting enzymes.

Continued next column

 ## OVERDOSE

SYMPTOMS:
None expected.
WHAT TO DO:
Not for internal use. If child accidentally swallows, call poison-control center.

Time lapse before drug works:
May require several weeks or more.

Don't use with:
Any other medicine without consulting your doctor or pharmacist.

 ## POSSIBLE ADVERSE REACTIONS OR SIDE EFFECTS

SYMPTOMS	WHAT TO DO
Life-threatening: None expected.	
Common: None expected.	
Infrequent: Redness or irritation of skin not present before application, rash.	Discontinue. Call doctor right away.
Rare: None expected.	

WARNINGS & PRECAUTIONS

Don't use if:
• You are allergic to anthralin.
• You have infected skin.

Before you start, consult your doctor:
• If you have chronic kidney disease.
• If you are allergic to anything.

Over age 60:
No problems expected, but check with doctor.

Pregnancy:
No problems expected, but check with doctor.

Breast-feeding:
No problems expected, but check with doctor.

Infants & children:
No problems expected, but check with doctor.

Prolonged use:
No problems expected, but check with doctor.

Skin & sunlight:
May cause rash or intensify sunburn in areas exposed to sun or sunlamp. Avoid undue exposure.

Driving, piloting or hazardous work:
No problems expected.

Discontinuing:
No problems expected.

Others:
• Keep cool, but don't freeze.
• Apply petroleum jelly to normal skin or scalp to protect areas not being treated.
• Will stain hair, clothing, shower, bathtub or sheets. Wash as soon as possible.
• Heat and moisture in bathroom medicine cabinet can cause breakdown of medicine. Store someplace else.

POSSIBLE INTERACTION WITH OTHER DRUGS

GENERIC NAME OR DRUG CLASS	COMBINED EFFECT
Antidiabetic agents*	Increased sensitivity to sun exposure.
Coal tar preparations*	Increased sensitivity to sun exposure.
Diuretics, thiazide*	Increased sensitivity to sun exposure.
Griseofulvin	Increased sensitivity to sun exposure.
Methosalen	Increased sensitivity to sun exposure.
Nalidixic acid	Increased sensitivity to sun exposure.
Phenothiazines*	Increased sensitivity to sun exposure.
Sulfa drugs*	Increased sensitivity to sun exposure.
Tetracyclines*	Increased sensitivity to sun exposure.
Trioxsalen	Increased sensitivity to sun exposure.

POSSIBLE INTERACTION WITH OTHER SUBSTANCES

INTERACTS WITH	COMBINED EFFECT
Alcohol:	None expected.
Beverages:	None expected.
Cocaine:	None expected.
Foods:	None expected.
Marijuana:	None expected.
Tobacco:	None expected.

*See Glossary

ANTI-ACNE (Topical)

BRAND NAMES

See complete list of brand names in the *Brand Name Directory*, page 907.

BASIC INFORMATION

Habit forming? No
Prescription needed? Yes, on some.
Available as generic? Yes
Drug class: Anti-acne (topical)

 ## USES

Treatment for acne, psoriasis, ichthyosis, keratosis, folliculitis, flat warts.

 ## DOSAGE & USAGE INFORMATION

How to use:
- Wash skin with non-medicated soap, pat dry, wait 20 minutes before applying.
- Cream or gel—Apply to affected areas with fingertips and rub in gently.
- Solution—Apply to affected areas with gauze pad or cotton swab. Avoid getting too wet so medicine doesn't drip into eyes, mouth, lips or inside nose.
- Follow manufacturer's directions on container.

When to use:
At the same time each day.

If you forget an application:
Use as soon as you remember.

What drug does:
Increases skin-cell turnover so skin layer peels off more easily.

Time lapse before drug works:
2 to 3 weeks. May require 6 weeks for maximum improvement.

Don't use with:
- Benzoyl peroxide. Apply 12 hours apart.
- Any other medicine without consulting your doctor or pharmacist.

 ## OVERDOSE

SYMPTOMS:
None expected.
WHAT TO DO:
If person swallows drug, call doctor, poison-control center or hospital emergency room for instructions.

 ## POSSIBLE ADVERSE REACTIONS OR SIDE EFFECTS

SYMPTOMS	WHAT TO DO
Life-threatening:	
None expected.	
Common:	
• Pigment change in treated area, warmth or stinging, peeling.	Continue. Tell doctor at next visit.
• Senstivity to wind or cold.	No action necessary.
Infrequent:	
Blistering crusting, severe burning, swelling.	Discontinue. Call doctor right away.
Rare:	
None expected.	

WARNINGS & PRECAUTIONS

Don't take if:
- You are allergic to tretinoin.
- You are sunburned, windburned or have an open skin wound.

Before you start, consult your doctor:
If you have eczema.

Over age 60:
Not recommended.

Pregnancy:
No proven harm to unborn child. Avoid if possible.

Breast-feeding:
No problems expected.

Infants & children:
Not recommended.

Prolonged use:
No problems expected.

Skin & sunlight:
- May cause rash or intensify sunburn in areas exposed to sun or sunlamp.
- In some animal studies, tretinoin caused skin tumors to develop faster when treated area was exposed to ultraviolet light (sunlight or sunlamp). No proven similar effects in humans.

Driving, piloting or hazardous work:
No problems expected.

Discontinuing:
Don't discontinue without doctor's advice until you complete prescribed dose, even though symptoms diminish or disappear.

Others:
Acne may get worse before improvement starts in 2 or 3 weeks. Don't wash face more than 2 or 3 times daily.

POSSIBLE INTERACTION WITH OTHER DRUGS

GENERIC NAME OR DRUG CLASS	COMBINED EFFECT
Anti-acne topical preparations (other)	Severe skin irritation.
Cosmetics (medicated)	Severe skin irritation.
Skin preparations with alcohol	Severe skin irritation.
Soaps or cleansers (abrasive)	Severe skin irritation.

POSSIBLE INTERACTION WITH OTHER SUBSTANCES

INTERACTS WITH	COMBINED EFFECT
Alcohol:	None expected.
Beverages:	None expected.
Cocaine:	None expected.
Foods:	None expected.
Marijuana:	None expected.
Tobacco:	None expected.

ANTI-ACNE, CLEANSING (Topical)

BRAND AND GENERIC NAMES

ALCOHOL
  AND ACETONE
ALCOHOL
  AND SULFUR
Liquimat
Seba-Nil
SULFURATED LIME

Transact
Trans-Plantar
Trans-Ver-Sal
Tyrosum Liquid
Vlem-Dome
Vlemasque
Vlemickx's solution
Xerac

BASIC INFORMATION

Habit forming? No
Prescription needed? Yes
Available as generic? No
Drug class: Anti-acne agent, cleansing
  agent

 ## USES

Treats acne or oily skin.

 ## DOSAGE & USAGE INFORMATION

How to use:
- Lotion, gel or pledget—Start with small amount and wipe over face to remove dirt and surface oil. Don't apply to wounds or burns. Don't rinse with water and avoid contact with eyes. Skin may be more sensitive in dry or cold climates.
- Plaster—Follow package instructions.

When to use:
As directed. May increase frequency up to 3 or more times daily as tolerated. Warm, humid weather may allow more frequent use.

If you forget a dose:
Use as soon as you remember and then go back to regular schedule.

Continued next column

 ## OVERDOSE

SYMPTOMS:
None expected.
WHAT TO DO:
- Not for internal use. If child accidentally swallows, call poison-control center.
- Dial 0 (operator) or 911 (emergency) for an ambulance or medical help. Then give first aid immediately.
- See emergency information on inside covers.

What drug does:
Helps remove oil from skin's surface.

Time lapse before drug works:
Works immediately.

Don't use with:
- Other topical acne treatments unless directed by doctor.
- See Interaction column and consult doctor.

 ## POSSIBLE ADVERSE REACTIONS OR SIDE EFFECTS

SYMPTOMS	WHAT TO DO
Life-threatening: None expected.	
Common: None expected.	
Infrequent: Skin infection, pustules or rash; unusual pain, swelling or redness of treated skin; burning or stinging of skin.	Discontinue. Call doctor right away.
Rare: None expected.	

ANTI-ACNE, CLEANSING (Topical)

WARNINGS & PRECAUTIONS

Don't use if:
You have to apply over a wounded or burned area.

Before you start, consult your doctor:
If you use benzoyl peroxide, resorcinol, salicylic acid, sulfur or tretinoin (vitamin A acid).

Over age 60:
No problems expected.

Pregnancy:
No problems expected, but check with doctor.

Breast-feeding:
No problems expected, but check with doctor.

Infants & children:
No problems expected, but check with doctor. Use only under close medical supervision.

Prolonged use:
Excessive drying of skin.

Skin & sunlight:
No problems expected, but check with doctor.

Driving, piloting or hazardous work:
No problems expected, but check with doctor.

Discontinuing:
No problems expected, but check with doctor.

Others:
Some antiacne agents are flammable. Don't use near fire or while smoking.

POSSIBLE INTERACTION WITH OTHER DRUGS

GENERIC NAME OR DRUG CLASS	COMBINED EFFECT
Abrasive or medicated soaps	Irritation or too much drying.
After-shave lotions	Irritation or too much drying.
Anti-acne topical preparations (other)	Irritation or too much drying.
"Cover-up" cosmetics	Irritation or too much drying.
Drying cosmetic soaps	Irritation or too much drying.
Isoretinoin	Irritation or too much drying.
Mercury compounds	May stain skin black and smell bad.
Perfumed toilet water	Irritation or too much drying.
Preparations containing skin-peeling agents such as benzoyl peroxide, esorcinol, salicylic acid, sulfur, tretinoin	Irritation or too much drying.

POSSIBLE INTERACTION WITH OTHER SUBSTANCES

INTERACTS WITH	COMBINED EFFECT
Alcohol:	None expected.
Beverages:	None expected.
Cocaine:	None expected.
Foods:	None expected.
Marijuana:	None expected.
Tobacco:	None expected.

ANTIBACTERIALS (Ophthalmic)

BRAND AND GENERIC NAMES

See complete list of brand and generic names in the *Brand Name Directory*, page 908.

BASIC INFORMATION

Habit forming? No
Prescription needed? Yes
Available as generic? Yes, for some
Drug class: Antibacterial (ophthalmic)

 ## USES

Helps body overcome eye infections on surface tissues of the eye.

 ## DOSAGE & USAGE INFORMATION

How to use:
Eye drops
- Wash hands.
- Apply pressure to inside corner of eye with middle finger.
- Continue pressure for 1 minute after placing medicine in eye.
- Tilt head backward. Pull lower lid away from eye with index finger of the same hand.
- Drop eye drops into pouch and close eye. Don't blink.
- Keep eyes closed for 1 to 2 minutes.

Eye ointment
- Wash hands.
- Pull lower lid down from eye to form a pouch.
- Squeeze tube to apply thin strip of ointment into pouch.
- Close eye for 1 to 2 minutes.
- Don't touch applicator tip to any surface (including the eye). If you accidentally touch tip, clean with warm soap and water.
- Keep container tightly closed.
- Keep cool, but don't freeze.
- Wash hands immediately after using.

When to use:
As directed. Don't miss doses.

If you forget a dose:
Use as soon as you remember.

Continued next column

 ## OVERDOSE

SYMPTOMS:
None expected.
WHAT TO DO:
Not intended for internal use. If child accidentally swallows, call poison-control center.

What drug does:
Penetrates bacterial cell membrane and prevents cells from multiplying.

Time lapse before drug works:
Begins in 1 hour. May require 7 to 10 days to control infection.

Don't use with:
Any other eye drops or ointment without checking with your ophthalmologist.

 ## POSSIBLE ADVERSE REACTIONS OR SIDE EFFECTS

SYMPTOMS	WHAT TO DO
Life-threatening: None expected.	
Common: Ointments cause blurred vision for a few minutes.	Continue. Tell doctor at next visit.
Infrequent: None expected.	
Rare: None expected.	

ANTIBACTERIALS (Ophthalmic)

WARNINGS & PRECAUTIONS

Don't use if:
You are allergic to any antibiotic used on skin, ears, vagina or rectum.

Before you start, consult your doctor:
If you have had an allergic reaction to any medicine, food or other substances.

Over age 60:
No problems expected.

Pregnancy:
No problems expected, but check with doctor.

Breast-feeding:
No problems expected, but check with doctor.

Infants & children:
No problems expected.

Prolonged use:
Sensitivity reaction may develop.

Skin & sunlight:
No problems expected.

Driving, piloting or hazardous work:
No problems expected.

Discontinuing:
No problems expected.

Others:
- Notify doctor if symptoms fail to improve in 2 to 4 days.
- Keep cool, but don't freeze.

POSSIBLE INTERACTION WITH OTHER DRUGS

GENERIC NAME OR DRUG CLASS	COMBINED EFFECT
Clinically significant interactions with oral or injected medicines unlikely.	

POSSIBLE INTERACTION WITH OTHER SUBSTANCES

INTERACTS WITH	COMBINED EFFECT
Alcohol:	None expected.
Beverages:	None expected.
Cocaine:	None expected.
Foods:	None expected.
Marijuana:	None expected.
Tobacco:	None expected.

ANTIBACTERIALS (Otic)

BRAND AND GENERIC NAMES

CHLORAMPHENICOL
Chloromycetin
Colistin
Neomycin and
  Hydrocortisone
Coly-Mycin S
Cortisporin
DESONIDE AND
  ACETIC ACID
Garamycin
Genoptic
GENTAMICIN (otic)
HYDROCORTISONE
  AND ACETIC ACID
LazerSporin-C

NEOMYCIN,
  POLYMIXIN B AND
  HYDRO-
  CORTISONE
Ortega Otic-M
Oticair
Otic Tridesilon
  Solution
Otobione
Otocort
Otoreid-HC
Pediotic
Pentamycetin
Sopamycetin
Tridesilon Solution
VoSol HC

BASIC INFORMATION

Habit forming? No
Prescription needed? Yes
Available as generic? No
Drug class: Antibacterial (otic)

USES

Ear infections in external ear canal (not middle ear) caused by susceptible germs (bacteria, virus, fungus).

DOSAGE & USAGE INFORMATION

How to use:
Ear drops
- Warm ear drops under running water around the unopened bottle.
- Lie down with affected ear up.
- Adults—Pull ear lobe back and up.
- Children—Pull ear lobe down and back.
- Drop medicine into ear canal until canal is full.
- Stay lying down for 2 minutes.
- Gently insert cotton plug into ear to prevent leaking.

Continued next column

OVERDOSE

SYMPTOMS:
None expected.
WHAT TO DO:
Not intended for internal use. If child accidentally swallows, call poison-control center.

Ear ointment
- Apply small amount to skin just inside the ear canal.
- Use finger or piece of sterile gauze.
- Don't use cotton-tipped applicators.

When to use:
As directed on label.

If you forget a dose:
Use as soon as you remember.

What drug does:
Kills germs that infect the skin of the external ear canal.

Time lapse before drug works:
15 minutes.

Don't use with:
Other ear medications unless directed by your doctor.

POSSIBLE ADVERSE REACTIONS OR SIDE EFFECTS

SYMPTOMS	WHAT TO DO
Life-threatening: None expected.	
Common: None expected.	
Infrequent: Itching, burning, redness, swelling.	Discontinue. Call doctor right away.
Rare: None expected.	

WARNINGS & PRECAUTIONS

Don't use if:
You are allergic to any of the medicines listed.

Before you start, consult your doctor:
If eardrum is punctured.

Over age 60:
No problems expected.

Pregnancy:
No problems expected.

Breast-feeding:
No problems expected.

Infants & children:
No problems expected.

Prolonged use:
Not intended for prolonged use.

Skin & sunlight:
Skin sensitivity more likely.

Driving, piloting or hazardous work:
No problems expected.

Discontinuing:
No problems expected.

Others:
Keep cool, but don't freeze.

 ## POSSIBLE INTERACTION WITH OTHER DRUGS

GENERIC NAME OR DRUG CLASS	COMBINED EFFECT
None expected.	

 ## POSSIBLE INTERACTION WITH OTHER SUBSTANCES

INTERACTS WITH	COMBINED EFFECT
Alcohol:	None expected.
Beverages:	None expected.
Cocaine:	None expected.
Foods:	None expected.
Marijuana:	None expected.
Tobacco:	None expected.

ANTIBACTERIALS (Topical)

BRAND AND GENERIC NAMES

See complete list of brand and generic names in the *Brand Name Directory*, page 909.

BASIC INFORMATION

Habit forming? No
Prescription needed? Yes
Available as generic? Yes
Drug class: Antibacterial (topical)

 USES

Treats skin infections that may accompany burns, superficial boils, insect bites or stings, skin ulcers, minor surgical wounds.

 DOSAGE & USAGE INFORMATION

How to use:
- Cream, lotion, ointment—Bathe and dry area before use. Apply small amount and rub gently.
- May cover with gauze or bandage if desired.

When to use:
3 or 4 times daily, or as directed by doctor.

If you forget a dose:
Use as soon as you remember.

What drug does:
Kills susceptible bacteria by interfering with bacterial DNA and RNA.

Time lapse before drug works:
Begins first day. May require treatment for a week or longer to cure infection.

Don't use with:
Any other medicine without consulting your doctor or pharmacist.

 OVERDOSE

SYMPTOMS:
None expected.
WHAT TO DO:
- Not for internal use. If child accidentally swallows, call poison-control center.
- Dial 0 (operator) or 911 (emergency) for an ambulance or medical help. Then give first aid immediately.
- See emergency information on inside covers.

 POSSIBLE ADVERSE REACTIONS OR SIDE EFFECTS

SYMPTOMS	WHAT TO DO
Life-threatening: None expected.	
Common: None expected.	
Infrequent: Itching, swollen, red skin.	Discontinue. Call doctor right away.
Rare: None expected.	

WARNINGS & PRECAUTIONS

Don't use if:
You are allergic to gentamicin or any topical medication.

Before you start, consult your doctor:
If any of the lesions on the skin are open sores.

Over age 60:
No problems expected.

Pregnancy:
No problems expected, but check with doctor.

Breast-feeding:
No problems expected, but check with doctor.

Infants & children:
No problems expected, but check with doctor.

Prolonged use:
No problems expected, but check with doctor.

Skin & sunlight:
No problems expected, but check with doctor.

Driving, piloting or hazardous work:
No problems expected, but check with doctor.

Discontinuing:
No problems expected, but check with doctor.

Others:
- Heat and moisture in bathroom medicine cabinet can cause breakdown of medicine. Store someplace else.
- Keep cool, but don't freeze.

POSSIBLE INTERACTION WITH OTHER DRUGS

GENERIC NAME OR DRUG CLASS	COMBINED EFFECT
Any other topical medication	Hypersensitivity reactions more likely to occur.

POSSIBLE INTERACTION WITH OTHER SUBSTANCES

INTERACTS WITH	COMBINED EFFECT
Alcohol:	None expected.
Beverages:	None expected.
Cocaine:	None expected.
Foods:	None expected.
Marijuana:	None expected.
Tobacco:	None expected.

*See Glossary

ANTIBACTERIALS, ANTIFUNGALS (Topical)

BRAND AND GENERIC NAMES

See complete list of brand and generic names in the *Brand Name Directory,* page 909.

BASIC INFORMATION

Habit forming? No
Prescription needed? Yes
Available as generic? Yes, some are
Drug class: Antibacterial (topical), antifungal (topical)

 USES

Treats eczema, other inflammatory skin conditions, athlete's foot, skin infections.

 DOSAGE & USAGE INFORMATION

How to use:
- Cream, lotion, ointment—Bathe and dry area before use. Apply small amount and rub gently.
- Keep away from eyes.

When to use:
2 to 4 times a day.

If you forget a dose:
Use as soon as you remember.

What drug does:
Kills some types of fungus and bacteria on contact.

Time lapse before drug works:
2 to 4 weeks, sometimes longer.

Don't use with:
Other ointments, creams or lotions without consulting doctor.

 OVERDOSE

SYMPTOMS:
Severe nausea, vomiting, diarrhea.
WHAT TO DO:
- **Not for internal use. If child accidentally swallows, call poison-control center.**
- **Dial 0 (operator) or 911 (emergency) for an ambulance or medical help. Then give first aid immediately.**
- **See emergency information on inside covers.**

 POSSIBLE ADVERSE REACTIONS OR SIDE EFFECTS

SYMPTOMS	WHAT TO DO
Life-threatening:	
None expected.	
Common:	
May stain skin around nails.	Continue. Tell doctor at next visit.
Infrequent:	
Stomach cramps; hives; itching, burning, peeling, red, stinging, swelling skin.	Discontinue. Call doctor right away.
Rare:	
None expected.	

WARNINGS & PRECAUTIONS

Don't use if:
You are allergic to clioquinol, iodine or any iodine-containing preparation.

Before you start, consult your doctor:
If you are allergic to anything that touches your skin.

Over age 60:
No problems expected.

Pregnancy:
No problems expected, but check with doctor.

Breast-feeding:
No problems expected, but check with doctor.

Infants & children:
No problems expected, but check with doctor.

Prolonged use:
No problems expected, but check with doctor.

Skin & sunlight:
No problems expected, but check with doctor.

Driving, piloting or hazardous work:
No problems expected, but check with doctor.

Discontinuing:
No problems expected, but check with doctor.

Others:
- If not improved in 2 weeks, check with doctor.
- May stain clothing or bed linens.
- May stain hair, skin and nails yellow.
- If accidentally gets into eyes, flush with clear water immediately.
- Tests of thyroid function may yield inaccurate results if you use clioquinol within 1 month before testing.

POSSIBLE INTERACTION WITH OTHER DRUGS

GENERIC NAME OR DRUG CLASS	COMBINED EFFECT
None expected.	

POSSIBLE INTERACTION WITH OTHER SUBSTANCES

INTERACTS WITH	COMBINED EFFECT
Alcohol:	None expected.
Beverages:	None expected.
Cocaine:	None expected.
Foods:	None expected.
Marijuana:	None expected.
Tobacco:	None expected.

ANTIBACTERIALS FOR ACNE (Topical)

BRAND AND GENERIC NAMES

Achromycin
Akne-mycin
A/T/S
Aureomycin
CHLORTETRA-
    CYCLINE (topical)
CLINDAMYCIN
    (topical)
Cleocin T
Dalacin T
EryDerm
Erycette
Erygel

Erymax
Ery-Sol
ERYTHROMYCIN
    (topical)
ETS
Meclan
MECLOCYCLINE
    (topical)
Staticin
T-Stat
TETRACYCLINE
    (topical)
Topicycline

BASIC INFORMATION

Habit forming? No
Prescription needed? Yes
Available as generic? No
Drug class: Antibacterial (topical)

USES

Treats acne by killing skin bacteria that may be part of the cause of acne.

DOSAGE & USAGE INFORMATION

How to use:
- Pledgets and solutions are flammable. Use away from flame or heat.
- Apply medication to entire area, not just to pimples.
- If you use other acne medicines on skin, wait an hour after using erythromycin before applying other medicine.
- Cream, lotion, ointment—Bathe and dry area before use. Apply small amount and rub gently.

When to use:
2 times a day, morning and evening, or as directed by your doctor.

If you forget a dose:
Use as soon as you remember.

What drug does:
Kills bacteria on skin, skin glands or in hair follicles.

Continued next column

OVERDOSE

SYMPTOMS:
None expected.
WHAT TO DO:
Not for internal use. If child accidentally swallows, call poison-control center.

Time lapse before drug works:
3 to 4 weeks to begin improvement.

Don't use with:
- Other skin medicine without telling your doctor.
- See Interaction column and consult doctor.

POSSIBLE ADVERSE REACTIONS OR SIDE EFFECTS

SYMPTOMS	WHAT TO DO
Life-threatening: None expected.	
Common: Stinging or burning of skin for a few minutes after application.	Continue. Tell doctor at next visit.
Infrequent: Red, peeling, itching, irritated skin.	Continue. Call doctor when convenient.
Rare (extremely): Symptoms of excess medicine absorbed by body—Abdominal pain, diarrhea, fever, nausea, vomiting, thirst, weakness, weight loss.	Discontinue. Call doctor right away.

WARNINGS & PRECAUTIONS

Don't use if:
You are allergic to erythromycin.

Before you start, consult your doctor:
- If you are allergic to any substance that touches your skin.
- If you use benzoyl peroxide, resorcinol, salicylic acid, sulfur or tretinoin (vitamin A acid).

Over age 60:
No problems expected.

Pregnancy:
No problems expected, but check with doctor.

Breast-feeding:
No problems expected, but check with doctor.

Infants & children:
No problems expected, but check with doctor.

Prolonged use:
Excess irritation to skin.

Skin & sunlight:
No problems expected, but check with doctor.

Driving, piloting or hazardous work:
No problems expected, but check with doctor.

Discontinuing:
No problems expected, but check with doctor.

Others:
- Use water-base cosmetics.
- Keep medicine away from mouth or eyes.
- If accidentally gets into eyes, flush immediately with clear water.
- Keep away from heat or flame.
- Keep cool, but don't freeze.

POSSIBLE INTERACTION WITH OTHER DRUGS

GENERIC NAME OR DRUG CLASS	COMBINED EFFECT
Abrasive or medicated soaps	Irritation or too much drying.
After-shave lotions	Irritation or too much drying.
Anti-acne topical preparations (other)	Irritation or too much drying.
"Cover-up" cosmetics	Irritation or too much drying.
Drying cosmetic soaps	Irritation or too much drying.
Isoretinoin	Irritation or too much drying.
Mercury compounds	May stain skin black and smell bad.
Perfumed toilet water	Irritation or too much drying.
Preparations containing skin peeling agents such as benzoyl peroxide, esorcinol, salicylic acid, sulfur, tretinoin	Irritation or too much drying.

POSSIBLE INTERACTION WITH OTHER SUBSTANCES

INTERACTS WITH	COMBINED EFFECT
Alcohol:	None expected.
Beverages:	None expected.
Cocaine:	None expected.
Foods:	None expected.
Marijuana:	None expected.
Tobacco:	None expected.

ANTICOAGULANTS (Oral)

BRAND AND GENERIC NAMES

ANISINDIONE	Marevan
Anthrombin-K	Melitoxin
Carfin	Miradon
Coumadin	Panwarfin
Danilone	PHENINDIONE
DICUMAROL	Sofarin
Dufalone	WARFARIN
Hedulin	SODIUM
Liquamar	Warfilone
Marcumar	Warnerin

BASIC INFORMATION

Habit forming? No
Prescription needed? Yes
Available as generic? Yes
Drug class: Anticoagulant

 ## USES

Reduces blood clots. Used for abnormal clotting inside blood vessels.

 ## DOSAGE & USAGE INFORMATION

How to take:
Tablet—Swallow with liquid. If you can't swallow whole, crumble tablet and take with liquid or food.

When to take:
At the same time each day.

If you forget a dose:
Take as soon as you remember up to 12 hours late. If more than 12 hours, wait for next scheduled dose (don't double this dose). Inform your doctor of any missed doses.

What drug does:
Blocks action of vitamin K necessary for blood clotting.

Time lapse before drug works:
36 to 48 hours.

Don't take with:
Any other medicine without consulting your doctor or pharmacist.

 ## OVERDOSE

SYMPTOMS:
Bloody vomit, coughing blood, bloody or black stools, red urine.
WHAT TO DO:
• **Dial 0 (operator) or 911 (emergency) for an ambulance or medical help. Then give first aid immediately.**
• **See emergency information on inside covers.**

 ## POSSIBLE ADVERSE REACTIONS OR SIDE EFFECTS

SYMPTOMS	WHAT TO DO
Life-threatening:	
In case of overdose, see previous column.	
Common:	
Bloating, gas.	Continue. Tell doctor at next visit.
Infrequent:	
• Black stools or bloody vomit, coughing up blood.	Discontinue. Seek emergency treatment.
• Rash, hives, itch, blurred vision, sore throat, easy bruising, bleeding, cloudy or red urine, back pain, jaundice, fever, chills, fatigue, weakness, painful urination, decreased amount of urine, heavy menstruation, bleeding gums.	Discontinue. Call doctor right away.
• Diarrhea, cramps, nausea, vomiting, swollen feet or legs, hair loss.	Continue. Call doctor when convenient.
Rare:	
• Bleeding into and under skin.	Discontinue. Seek emergency treatment
• Dizziness, headache, mouth sores.	Discontinue. Call doctor right away.

 ## WARNINGS & PRECAUTIONS

Don't take if:
• You have been allergic to any oral anticoagulant.
• You have a bleeding disorder.
• You have an active peptic ulcer.
• You have ulcerative colitis.

Before you start, consult your doctor:
• If you take any other drugs, including non-prescription drugs.
• If you have high blood pressure.
• If you have heavy or prolonged menstrual periods.
• If you have diabetes.
• If you have a bladder catheter.
• If you have serious liver or kidney disease.
• If you will have surgery within 2 months, including dental surgery, requiring general or spinal anesthesia.

Over age 60:
Adverse reactions and side effects may be more frequent and severe than in younger persons.

Pregnancy:
Risk to unborn child outweighs drug benefits.
Don't use.

Breast-feeding:
Drug filters into milk. May harm child. Avoid.

Infants & children:
Use only under doctor's supervision.

Prolonged use:
Talk to your doctor about the need for follow-up
medical examinations or laboratory studies to check
prothorombin time, stool and urine for blood.

Skin & sunlight:
No problems expected.

Driving, piloting or hazardous work:
• Avoid hazardous activities that could cause injury.
• Don't drive if you feel dizzy or have blurred vision.

Discontinuing:
Don't discontinue without consulting doctor.
Dose may require gradual reduction if you have
taken drug for a long time. Doses of other
drugs may also require adjustment.

Others:
• Carry identification to state that you take
anticoagulants.
• Advise any doctor or dentist whom you
consult that you take this medicine.

POSSIBLE INTERACTION WITH OTHER DRUGS

GENERIC NAME OR DRUG CLASS	COMBINED EFFECT
Acetaminophen	Increased effect of anticoagulant.
Allopurinol	Increased effect of anticoagulant.
Aminoglutethmide	Decreased effect of anticoagulant.
Amiodarone	Increased effect of anticoagulant.
Androgens*	Increased effect of anticoagulant.
Antacids* (large doses)	Decreased effect of anticoagulant.
Antibiotics*	Increased effect of anticoagulant.
Antidiabetics, oral*	Increased effect of anticoagulant.
Antihistamines*	Unpredictable increased or decreased effect of anticoagulant.
Aspirin	Possible spontaneous bleeding.

Barbiturates*	Decreased effect of anticoagulant.
Benzodiazepines*	Unpredictable increased or decreased effect of anticoagulant.
Bismuth subsalicylate	Increased risk of bleeding.
Calcium supplements*	Decreased effect of anticoagulant.
Carbamazepine	Decreased effect of anticoagulant.
Cefixime	Increased effect of anticoagulant.
Clofibrate	Increased effect of anticoagulant.
Contraceptives*	Decreased effect of anticoagulant.
Dextrothyroxine	Increased effect of anticoagulant.
Diclofenac	Increased risk of bleeding.
Fluconazole	Increased effect of anticoagulant.
Fluoxetine	May cause confusion, agitation, convulsions and high blood pressure. Avoid combining.
Griseofulvin	Decreased effect of anticoagulant.

Continued on page 933

POSSIBLE INTERACTION WITH OTHER SUBSTANCES

INTERACTS WITH	COMBINED EFFECT
Alcohol:	Can increase or decrease effect of anticoagulant. Use with caution.
Beverages:	None expected.
Cocaine:	None expected.
Foods: High in vitamin K such as fish, liver, spinach, cabbage, cauliflower, Brussels sprouts.	May decrease anticoagulant effect.
Marijuana:	None expected.
Tobacco:	None expected.

*See Glossary

ANTICONVULSANTS, DIONE-TYPE

BRAND AND GENERIC NAMES

PARAMETHADIONE
Paradione

TRIMETHADIONE
Tridione

BASIC INFORMATION

Habit forming? No
Prescription needed? Yes
Available as generic? No
Drug class: Anticonvulsant (dione-type)

 ## USES

Controls but does not cure petit mal seizures (absence seizures).

 ## DOSAGE & USAGE INFORMATION

How to take:
Tablets, capsules or liquid: Take with food or milk to lessen stomach irritation.

When to take:
At the same time each day.

If you forget a dose:
Take as soon as you remember up to 2 hours late. If more than 2 hours, wait for next scheduled dose (don't double this dose).

What drug does:
Raises threshold of seizures in cerebral cortex. Does not alter seizure pattern.

Time lapse before drug works:
1 to 3 hours.

Don't take with:
Any other medicine without consulting your doctor or pharmacist.

 ## OVERDOSE

SYMPTOMS:
Bleeding, nausea, drowsiness, ataxia, coma.
WHAT TO DO:
- **Dial 0 (operator) or 911 (emergency) for an ambulance or medical help. Then give first aid immediately.**
- **If patient is unconscious and not breathing, give mouth-to-mouth breathing. If there is no heartbeat, use cardiac massage and mouth-to-mouth breathing (CPR). Don't try to make patient vomit. If you can't get help quickly, take patient to nearest emergency facility.**
- **See emergency information on inside covers.**

 ## POSSIBLE ADVERSE REACTIONS OR SIDE EFFECTS

SYMPTOMS	WHAT TO DO
Life-threatening:	
In case of overdose, see previous column.	
Common:	
Dizziness, drowsiness, headache, rash.	Continue. Call doctor when convenient.
Infrequent:	
Itching, nausea, vomiting, confusion, insomnia, hair loss.	Continue. Call doctor when convenient.
Rare:	
• Changes in vision; sore throat with fever and mouth sores; bleeding gums; easy bleeding or bruising; smoky or bloody urine; jaundice; puffed hands, face, feet or legs; swollen lymph glands; unusual weakness and fatigue.	Discontinue. Call doctor right away.
• Sensitivity to light.	Continue. Call doctor when convenient.

 ## WARNINGS & PRECAUTIONS

Don't take if:
You are allergic to this drug or any anticonvulsant.

Before you start, consult your doctor:
- If you are pregnant or plan pregnancy.
- If you have blood disease.
- If you have liver or kidney disease.
- If you have disease of optic nerve or eye.
- If you will have surgery within 2 months, including dental surgery, requiring general or spinal anesthesia.

Over age 60:
Adverse reactions and side effects may be more frequent and severe than in younger persons.

Pregnancy:
Risk to unborn child outweighs drug benefits. Don't use.

Breast-feeding:
No problems proven. Avoid if possible. Consult doctor.

Infants & children:
Use only under close medical supervision of clinician experienced in convulsive disorders.

Prolonged use:
- Have regular checkups, especially during early months of treatment.
- Talk to your doctor about the need for follow-up medical examinations or laboratory studies to check complete blood counts (white blood cell count, platelet count, red blood cell count, hemoglobin, hematocrit), liver function, kidney function, eyes, urine.

Skin & sunlight:
Increased sensitivity to sunlight or sun lamp. Avoid overexposure.

Driving, piloting or hazardous work:
Don't drive or pilot aircraft until you learn how medicine affects you. Don't work around dangerous machinery. Don't climb ladders or work in high places. Danger increases if you drink alcohol or take medicine affecting alertness and reflexes, such as antihistamines, tranquilizers, sedatives, pain medicine, narcotics and mind-altering drugs. Be especially careful driving at night because medicine can affect vision.

Discontinuing:
Don't discontinue without consulting doctor. Dose may require gradual reduction if you have taken drug for a long time. Doses of other drugs may also require adjustment.

Others:
Arrange for eye exams every 6 months as well as blood counts and kidney-function studies.

POSSIBLE INTERACTION WITH OTHER DRUGS

GENERIC NAME OR DRUG CLASS	COMBINED EFFECT
Any other medicine	Unpredictable effect on seizure prevention.
Amiodarone	Increased or toxic effect of anti-convulsants.
Anticoagulants*	Increased anticonvulsant effect.
Antidepressants, tricyclic (TCA)*	Greater likelihood of seizures.
Antipsychotic medicines*	Greater likelihood of seizures.
Anticonvulsants* (other)	Increased chance of blood toxicity.
Clozapine	Toxic effect on the central nervous system.
Ethinamate	Dangerous increased effects of ethinamate. Avoid combining.

Fluoxetine	Increased depressant effects of both drugs.
Guanfacine	May increase depressant effects of either drug.
Leucovorin	High alcohol content of leucovorin may cause adverse effects.
Methyprylon	Increased sedative effect, perhaps to dangerous level. Avoid.
Sedatives*, sleeping pills, alcohol, pain medicine, antihistamines, tranquilizers, narcotics, mind-altering drugs.	Extreme drowsiness. Avoid.
Sulfadoxine and pyrimethamine	Increased risk of toxicity.

POSSIBLE INTERACTION WITH OTHER SUBSTANCES

INTERACTS WITH	COMBINED EFFECT
Alcohol:	Increased chance of seizures and liver damage. Avoid.
Beverages: Caffeine drinks.	May decrease anticonvulsant effect.
Cocaine:	Increased chance of seizures. Avoid.
Foods:	No problems expected.
Marijuana:	Increased chance of seizures. Avoid.
Tobacco:	Decreased absorption of medicine leading to uneven control of disease.

*See Glossary

ANTIDIABETIC AGENTS

BRAND AND GENERIC NAMES

See complete list of brand and generic names in the *Brand Names Directory*, page 909.

BASIC INFORMATION

Habit forming? No
Prescription needed? Yes
Available as generic? Yes, for some.
Drug class: Antidiabetic (oral), sulfonurea

 ## USES

- Treatment for diabetes in adults who can't control blood sugar by diet, weight loss and exercise.
- Treatment for diabetes insipidus (except CHLORPROPAMIDE).

 ## DOSAGE & USAGE INFORMATION

How to take:
Tablet—Swallow with liquid or food to lessen stomach irritation. If you can't swallow whole, crumble tablet and take with liquid or food.

When to take:
At the same times each day.

If you forget a dose:
Take as soon as you remember up to 2 hours late. If more than 2 hours, wait for next scheduled dose (don't double this dose).

What drug does:
Stimulates pancreas to produce more insulin. Insulin in blood forces cells to use sugar in blood.

Time lapse before drug works:
3 to 4 hours. May require 2 weeks for maximum benefit.

Don't take with:
Any other medicine without consulting your doctor or pharmacist.

 ## OVERDOSE

SYMPTOMS:
Excessive hunger, nausea, anxiety, cool skin, cold sweats, drowsiness, rapid heartbeat, weakness, unconsciousness, coma.
WHAT TO DO:
- **Dial 0 (operator) or 911 (emergency) for an ambulance or medical help. Then give first aid immediately.**
- **See emergency information on inside covers.**

 ## POSSIBLE ADVERSE REACTIONS OR SIDE EFFECTS

SYMPTOMS	WHAT TO DO
Life-threatening:	
In case of overdose, see previous column.	
Common:	
• Dizziness.	Discontinue. Call doctor right away.
• Diarrhea, appetite loss, nausea, stomach pain, heartburn, constipation.	Continue. Call doctor when convenient.
Infrequent:	
• Low blood sugar (hunger, anxiety, cold sweats, rapid pulse), shortness of breath.	Discontinue. Seek emergency treatment.
• Headache.	Discontinue. Call doctor right away.
Rare:	
Fatigue, itchy skin or rash, sore throat, fever, ringing in ears, unusual bleeding or bruising, jaundice, edema, weakness, confusion.	Discontinue. Call doctor right away.

 ## WARNINGS & PRECAUTIONS

Don't take if:
- You are allergic to any sulfonurea.
- You have impaired kidney or liver function.

Before you start, consult your doctor:
- If you have a severe infection.
- If you have thyroid disease.
- If you take insulin.
- If you have heart disease.

Over age 60:
Dose usually smaller than for younger adults. Avoid "low-blood-sugar" episodes because repeated ones can damage brain permanently.

Pregnancy:
No proven harm to unborn child. Avoid if possible.

Breast-feeding:
Drug filters into milk. May lower baby's blood sugar. Avoid.

Infants & children:
Don't give to infants or children.

Prolonged use:
- Adverse effects more likely.
- Talk to your doctor about the need for follow-up medical examinations or laboratory studies to check blood sugar, complete blood counts (white blood cell count, platelet count, red blood cell count, hemoglobin, hematocrit), eyes.

Skin and sunlight:
Increased sensitivity to sunlight.

Driving, piloting or hazardous work:
No problems expected unless you develop hypoglycemia (low blood sugar). If so, avoid driving or hazardous activity.

Discontinuing:
Don't discontinue without consulting doctor. Dose may require gradual reduction if you have taken drug for a long time. Doses of other drugs may also require adjustment.

Others:
- Don't exceed recommended dose. Hypoglycemia (low blood sugar) may occur, even with proper dose schedule. You must balance medicine, diet and exercise.
- May affect results in some medical tests.
- Advise any doctor or dentist whom you consult that you take this medicine.
- Warning: A large study has shown that there is an increase in death rate from heart disease among those who take oral diabetic agents.

POSSIBLE INTERACTION WITH OTHER DRUGS

GENERIC NAME OR DRUG CLASS	COMBINED EFFECT
Androgens*	Increased blood-sugar lowering.
Anticoagulants, oral*	Unpredictable prothrombin times.
Anticonvulsants, hydantoin*	Decreased blood-sugar lowering.
Aspirin	Increased blood-sugar lowering.
Beta-adrenergic blockers*	Increased blood-sugar lowering. Possible increased difficulty in regulating blood-sugar levels.
Bismuth subsalicylate	Increased insulin effect. May require dosage adjustment.
Chloramphenicol	Increased blood-sugar lowering.
Cimetidine	Increased blood-sugar lowering.
Clofibrate	Increased blood-sugar lowering.
Contraceptives, oral*	Decreased blood-sugar lowering.
Cortisone drugs*	Decreased blood-sugar lowering.

Dapsone	Increased risk of adverse effect on blood cells.
Desmopressin	May increase desmopressin effect.
Dextrothyroxine	Antidiabetic may require adjustment.
Digoxin	Possible decreased digoxin effect.
Diuretics* (loop, thiazide)	Decreased blood-sugar lowering.
Epinephrine	Increased blood-sugar lowering.
Estrogens*	Increased blood-sugar lowering.
Fluconazole	Greater than expected drop in blood sugar. If any oral antidiabetic drug is taken with fluconazole, blood sugars must be monitored carefully.
Guanethidine	Unpredictable blood-sugar lowering effect.
Hemolytics*	Increased risk of adverse effect on blood cells.
Insulin	Increased blood-sugar lowering.
Isoniazid	Decreased blood-sugar lowering.
Labetalol	Increased blood-sugar lowering, may mask hypoglycemia.

Continued on page 934

POSSIBLE INTERACTION WITH OTHER SUBSTANCES

INTERACTS WITH	COMBINED EFFECT
Alcohol:	Disulfiram reaction.* Avoid.
Beverages:	None expected.
Cocaine:	No proven problems.
Foods:	None expected.
Marijuana:	Decreased blood-sugar lowering. Avoid.
Tobacco:	None expected.

*See Glossary

ANTIDYSKINETICS

BRAND AND GENERIC NAMES

See complete list of brand and generic names in the *Brand Names Directory*, page 909.

BASIC INFORMATION

Habit forming? No
Prescription needed? Yes
Available as generic? Yes
Drug class: Antidyskinetic, antiparkinsonism

 ## USES

• Treatment of Parkinson's disease.
• Treatment of adverse effects of phenothiazines.

 ## DOSAGE & USAGE INFORMATION

How to take:
• Tablets—Swallow with liquid. If you can't swallow whole, crumble tablet and take with liquid or food. Instructions to take on empty stomach mean 1 hour before or 2 hours after eating.
• Extended-release capsule or elixir—Take with food to lessen stomach irritation.

When to take:
At the same times each day.

If you forget a dose:
Take as soon as you remember up to 2 hours late. If more than 2 hours, wait for next scheduled dose (don't double this dose).

Continued next column

 ## OVERDOSE

SYMPTOMS:
Agitation, dilated pupils, hallucinations, dry mouth, rapid heartbeat, sleepiness.
WHAT TO DO:
• **Dial 0 (operator) or 911 (emergency) for an ambulance or medical help. Then give first aid immediately.**
• **If patient is unconscious and not breathing, give mouth-to-mouth breathing. If there is no heartbeat, use cardiac massage and mouth-to-mouth breathing (CPR). Don't try to make patient vomit. If you can't get help quickly, take patient to nearest emergency facility.**
• **See emergency information on inside covers.**

What drug does:
• Balances chemical reactions necessary to send nerve impulses within base of brain.
• Improves muscle control and reduces stiffness.

Time lapse before drug works:
1 to 2 hours.

Don't take with:
• Non-prescription drugs for colds, cough or allergy.
• See Interaction column and consult doctor.

 ## POSSIBLE ADVERSE REACTIONS OR SIDE EFFECTS

SYMPTOMS	WHAT TO DO
Life-threatening:	
In case of overdose, see previous column.	
Common:	
• Blurred vision, light sensitivity, constipation, nausea, vomiting.	Continue. Call doctor when convenient.
• Painful or difficult urination, dry mouth.	Continue. Tell doctor at next visit.
Infrequent:	
Headache, memory loss, abdominal pain, nervousness, impotence.	Continue. Call Doctor when convenient.
Rare:	
• Rash, eye pain, hives, delusions, hallucinations, amnesia, paranoia, fever, swollen neck glands, weakness and faintness when arising from bed or chair.	Discontinue. Call doctor right away.
• Confusion, dizziness, sore mouth or tongue, muscle cramps, numbness or tingling in hands or feet.	Continue. Call doctor when convenient.

Note: Most symptoms representing side effects either disappear or decrease when dose is reduced.

 ## WARNINGS & PRECAUTIONS

Don't take if:
You are allergic to any antidyskinetic.

Before you start, consult your doctor:
• If you have had glaucoma.
• If you have had high blood pressure or heart disease.
• If you have had impaired liver function.
• If you have had kidney disease or urination difficulty.
• If you have had myasthenia gravis.

Over age 60:
More sensitive to drug. Aggravates symptoms of enlarged prostate. Causes impaired thinking, hallucinations, nightmares. Consult doctor about any of these.

Pregnancy:
Studies inconclusive on harm to unborn child. Animal studies show fetal abnormalities. Decide with your doctor whether drug benefits justify risk to unborn child.

Breast-feeding:
No problems expected.

Infants & children:
Not recommended for children 3 and younger. Use for older children only under doctor's supervision.

Prolonged use:
- Possible glaucoma.
- Talk to your doctor about the need for follow up medical examinations or laboratory studies to check eye pressure.

Skin & sunlight:
No problems expected.

Driving, piloting or hazardous work:
Don't drive or pilot aircraft until you learn how medicine affects you. Don't work around dangerous machinery. Don't climb ladders or work in high places. Danger increases if you drink alcohol or take medicine affecting alertness and reflexes, such as antihistamines, tranquilizers, sedatives, pain medicine, narcotics and mind-altering drugs.

Discontinuing:
Don't discontinue without consulting doctor. Dose may require gradual reduction if you have taken drug for a long time. Doses of other drugs may also require adjustment.

Others:
- Internal eye pressure should be measured regularly.
- Avoid becoming overheated.
- Advise any doctor or dentist whom you consult that you take this medicine.

 POSSIBLE INTERACTION WITH OTHER DRUGS

GENERIC NAME OR DRUG CLASS	COMBINED EFFECT
Amantadine	Increased amantadine effect.
Antacids*	Possible decreased absorption.
Anticholinergics, others*	Increased anticholinergic effect.
Antidepressants, tricyclic (TCA)*	Increased antidyskinetic effect. May cause glaucoma.
Antihistamines*	Increased antidyskinetic effect.
Clozapine	Toxic effect on the central nervous system (except amantadine).
Digoxin	Possible increased toxicity of digoxin.
Disopyramide	Increased anticholinergic effect.
Haloperidol	Possible behavior changes.
Levodopa	Possible increased levodopa effect.
MAO inhibitors*	Increased antidyskinetic effect.
Meperidine	Increased antidyskinetic effect.
Nabilone	Greater depression of central nervous system.
Phenothiazines*	Behavior changes.
Primidone	Excessive sedation.
Quinidine	Increased antidyskinetic effect.
Sertraline	Increased depressive effects of both drugs.
Slow-k (extended-release potassium)	Increased risk of gastric irritation.
Tranquilizers*	Excessive sedation.

 POSSIBLE INTERACTION WITH OTHER SUBSTANCES

INTERACTS WITH	COMBINED EFFECT
Alcohol:	Over sedation. Don't use.
Beverages:	None expected.
Cocaine:	Decreased antidyskinetic effect. Avoid.
Foods:	None expected.
Marijuana:	None expected.
Tobacco:	None expected.

*See Glossary

ANTIFIBRINOLYTIC AGENTS

BRAND AND GENERIC NAMES

Amicar
AMINOCAPROIC
  ACID

Cyclokapron
Epsikapron
TRANEXAMIC ACID

BASIC INFORMATION

Habit forming? No
Prescription needed? Yes
Available as generic? Yes
Drug class: Antifibrinolytic, antihemorrhagic

USES

- Treats serious bleeding, especially occurring after surgery, dental or otherwise.
- Sometimes used before surgery in hopes of preventing excessive bleeding in patients with disorders that increase the chance of serious bleeding.

DOSAGE & USAGE INFORMATION

How to take:
- Tablet—Swallow with liquid or food to lessen stomach irritation. If you can't swallow whole, crumble tablet and take with liquid or food.
- Syrup—Take as directed on label.

When to take:
As directed by your doctor.

If you forget a dose:
Take as soon as you remember. Don't double this dose.

What drug does:
Inhibits activation of plasminogen to cause blood clots to disintegrate.

Time lapse before drug works:
Within 2 hours.

Don't take with:
- Thrombolytic chemicals such as streptokinase, urokinase.
- Any other medicine without consulting your doctor or pharmacist.

OVERDOSE

SYMPTOMS:
None expected for oral forms. Injectable forms may cause drop in blood pressure or slow heartbeat.
WHAT TO DO:
Follow doctor's instructions.

POSSIBLE ADVERSE REACTIONS OR SIDE EFFECTS

SYMPTOMS	WHAT TO DO
Life-threatening: Shortness of breath, slurred speech, leg or arm numbness.	Seek emergency treatment.
Common: Diarrhea, nausea, vomiting, severe menstrual cramps.	Discontinue. Call doctor right away.
Infrequent: Dizziness; headache; muscular pain and weakness; red eyes; ringing in ears; skin rash; abdominal pain; irregular heartbeat; stuffy nose; decreased urine; swelling of feet, face, legs; weight gain; poor coordination.	Discontinue. Call doctor right away.
Rare: • Unusual tiredness, blurred vision. • Clotting of menstrual flow.	Discontinue. Call doctor right away. Continue. Call doctor when convenient.

WARNINGS & PRECAUTIONS

Don't take if:
- You are allergic to aminocaproic acid or tranexamic acid.
- You have a diagnosis of disseminated intravascular coagulation (DIC).

Before you start, consult your doctor:
- If you have heart disease.
- If you have bleeding from the kidney.
- If you have had impaired liver function.
- If you have had kidney disease or urination difficulty.
- If you have blood clots in parts of the body.

Over age 60:
No changes from other age groups expected.

Pregnancy:
Animal studies show fetal abnormalities. Decide with your doctor whether drug benefits justify risk to unborn child.

Breast-feeding:
No problems documented.

Infants & children:
Use for children only under doctor's supervision.

Prolonged use:
Talk to your doctor about the need for follow-up medical examinations or laboratory studies to check eyes.

Skin & sunlight:
No problems expected.

Driving, piloting or hazardous work:
Don't drive or pilot aircraft until you learn how medicine affects you. Don't work around dangerous machinery. Don't climb ladders or work in high places. Danger increases if you drink alcohol or take medicine affecting alertness and reflexes, such as antihistamines, tranquilizers, sedatives, pain medicine, narcotics and mind-altering drugs.

Discontinuing:
Don't discontinue without consulting doctor. Dose may require gradual reduction if you have taken drug for a long time. Doses of other drugs may also require adjustment.

Others:
- Should not be used in patients with disseminated intravascular coagulation.
- Have eyes checked frequently.

 ## POSSIBLE INTERACTION WITH OTHER DRUGS

GENERIC NAME OR DRUG CLASS	COMBINED EFFECT
Contraceptives, oral*	Increased possibility of blood clotting.
Estrogens*	Increased possibility of blood clotting.
Thrombolytic agents* (alteplase, streptokinase, urokinase)	Decreased effects of both drugs.

 ## POSSIBLE INTERACTION WITH OTHER SUBSTANCES

INTERACTS WITH	COMBINED EFFECT
Alcohol:	Decreases effectiveness of thrombolytic agents.
Beverages:	No problems expected.
Cocaine:	Combined effect unknown. Avoid.
Foods:	No problems expected.
Marijuana:	Combined effect unknown. Avoid.
Tobacco:	Combined effect unknown. Avoid.

ANTIFUNGALS (Topical)

BRAND AND GENERIC NAMES

See complete list of brand and generic names in the *Brand Name Directory,* page 909.

BASIC INFORMATION

Habit forming? No
Prescription needed? Yes, for some
Available as generic? No
Drug class: Antifungal (topical)

 USES

Fights fungus infections such as ringworm of the scalp, athlete's foot, jockey itch, "sun fungus," nail fungus and others.

 DOSAGE & USAGE INFORMATION

How to use:
- Cream, lotion, ointment, gel—Bathe and dry area before use. Apply small amount and rub gently.
- Powder—Apply lightly to skin.
- Shampoo—Follow package instructions.
- Don't bandage or cover treated areas with plastic wrap.
- Follow other instructions from manufacturer listed on label.

When to use:
Twice a day, morning and evening, unless otherwise directed by your doctor.

If you forget a dose:
Use as soon as you remember.

What drug does:
Kills fungi by damaging the fungal cell wall.

Time lapse before drug works:
May require 6 to 8 weeks for cure.

Don't use with:
Other skin medicines without telling your doctor.

 OVERDOSE

SYMPTOMS:
None expected.
WHAT TO DO:
- Not for internal use. If child accidentally swallows, call poison-control center.
- Dial 0 (operator) or 911 (emergency) for an ambulance or medical help. Then give first aid immediately.
- See emergency information on inside covers.

 POSSIBLE ADVERSE REACTIONS OR SIDE EFFECTS

SYMPTOMS	WHAT TO DO
Life-threatening: None expected.	
Common: None expected.	
Infrequent: Itching, redness, swelling of treated skin not present before treatment.	Discontinue. Call doctor right away.
Rare: None expected.	

WARNINGS & PRECAUTIONS

Don't use if:
You are allergic to any topical antifungal medicine listed.

Before you start, consult your doctor:
If you are allergic to anything that touches your skin.

Over age 60:
No problems expected.

Pregnancy:
No problems expected, but check with doctor.

Breast-feeding:
No problems expected, but check with doctor.

Infants & children:
No problems expected, but check with doctor.

Prolonged use:
No problems expected, but check with doctor.

Skin & sunlight:
No problems expected, but check with doctor.

Driving, piloting or hazardous work:
No problems expected, but check with doctor.

Discontinuing:
No problems expected, but check with doctor.

Others:
- Avoid contact with eyes.
- Heat and moisture in bathroom medicine cabinet can cause breakdown of medicine. Store someplace else.
- Keep cool, but don't freeze.
- Store away from heat or sunlight.
- Don't use on other members of the family without consulting your doctor.
- If using for jock itch, avoid wearing tight underwear.
- If using for athlete's foot, dry feet carefully after bathing, wear clean cotton socks with sandals or well-ventilated shoes.

 POSSIBLE INTERACTION WITH OTHER DRUGS

GENERIC NAME OR DRUG CLASS	COMBINED EFFECT
None expected.	

 POSSIBLE INTERACTION WITH OTHER SUBSTANCES

INTERACTS WITH	COMBINED EFFECT
Alcohol:	None expected.
Beverages:	None expected.
Cocaine:	None expected.
Foods:	None expected.
Marijuana:	None expected.
Tobacco:	None expected.

ANTIFUNGALS (Vaginal)

BRAND AND GENERIC NAMES

See complete list of brand and generic names in the *Brand Name Directory*, page 909.

BASIC INFORMATION

Habit forming? No
Prescription needed? Yes, for some
Available as generic? Yes, some
Drug class: Antifungal (vaginal)

 USES

Treats fungus infections of the vagina.

 DOSAGE & USAGE INFORMATION

How to use:
- Vaginal creams—Insert into vagina with applicator as illustrated in patient instructions that comes with prescription.
- Vaginal tablets—Insert with applicator as illustrated in instructions.
- Vaginal suppositories—insert as illustrated in instructions.

When to use:
According to instructions. Usually once or twice daily.

If you forget a dose:
Use as soon as you remember.

What drug does:
Destroys fungus cells membrane causing loss of essential elements to sustain fungus cell life.

Time lapse before drug works:
Begins immediately. May require 2 weeks of treatment to cure vaginal fungus infections. Recurrence common.

Don't use with:
Other vaginal preparations or douches unless otherwise instructed by your doctor.

 OVERDOSE

SYMPTOMS:
None expected.
WHAT TO DO:
Overdose unlikely to threaten life.

 POSSIBLE ADVERSE REACTIONS OR SIDE EFFECTS

SYMPTOMS	WHAT TO DO
Life-threatening: None expected.	
Common: None expected.	
Infrequent: Vaginal burning, itching, irriation, swelling of labia, redness, increased discharge (not present before starting medicine).	Discontinue. Call doctor right away.
Rare: Skin rash, hives, irritation of sex partner's penis.	Discontinue. Call doctor right away.

WARNINGS & PRECAUTIONS

Don't use if:
- You are allergic to any of the products listed.
- You have pre-existing liver disease.

Before you start, consult your doctor:
If you are pregnant.

Over age 60:
No problems expected.

Pregnancy:
No problems expected, but check with doctor.

Breast-feeding:
No problems expected.

Infants & children:
Use only under close medical supervision.

Prolonged use:
No problems expected.

Skin & sunlight:
No problems expected.

Driving, piloting or hazardous work:
No problems expected.

Discontinuing:
Recurrence likely if you stop before time suggested.

Others:
- Gentian Violet and some of the other products can stain clothing. Sanitary napkins may protect against staining.
- Keep the genital area clean. Use plain unscented soap.
- Take showers rather than tub baths.
- Wear cotton underpants or pantyhose with a cotton crotch. Avoid underpants made from non-ventilating materials. Wear freshly laundered underpants.
- Don't sit around in wet clothing—especially a wet bathing suit.
- If you will take antibiotics in the future, ask your doctor about eating yogurt, sour cream, buttermilk or taking acidophilus tablets.
- After urination or bowel movements, cleanse by wiping or washing from front to back (vagina to anus).
- Don't douche unless your doctor recommends it.
- If urinating causes burning, urinate through a tubular device, such as a toilet-paper roll or plastic cup with the end cut out.

POSSIBLE INTERACTION WITH OTHER DRUGS

GENERIC NAME OR DRUG CLASS	COMBINED EFFECT

Clinically significant interactions with oral or injected medicines unlikely.

POSSIBLE INTERACTION WITH OTHER SUBSTANCES

INTERACTS WITH	COMBINED EFFECT
Alcohol:	None expected.
Beverages:	None expected.
Cocaine:	None expected.
Foods:	None expected.
Marijuana:	None expected.
Tobacco:	None expected.

ANTIGLAUCOMA, LONG-ACTING (Ophthalmic)

BRAND AND GENERIC NAMES

Apo-Timop
Betoptic
BETAXOLOL
DEMECARIUM
ECHOTHIOPHATE

ISOFLUROPHATE
Floropryl
Humorsol
Phospholine Iodide
TIMOLOL MALEATE

BASIC INFORMATION

Habit forming? No
Prescription needed? Yes
Available as generic? No
Drug class: Antiglaucoma (ophthalmic)

 USES

- Treats glaucoma (open-angle type).
- Treats glaucoma after some forms of eye surgery and a few other eye disorders.

 DOSAGE & USAGE INFORMATION

How to use:
Eye drops
- Wash hands.
- Apply pressure to inside corner of eye with middle finger.
- Continue pressure for 1 minute after placing medicine in eye.
- Tilt head backward. Pull lower lid away from eye with index finger of the same hand.
- Drop eye drops into pouch and close eye. Don't blink.
- Keep eyes closed for 1 to 2 minutes.
- Press finger to tear duct in corner of eye for 2 minutes to prevent possible absorption by body.

Eye ointment
- Wash hands.
- Pull lower lid down from eye to form a pouch.
- Squeeze tube to apply thin strip of ointment into pouch.
- Close eye for 1 to 2 minutes.
- Don't touch applicator tip to any surface (including the eye). If you accidentally touch tip, clean with warm soap and water.
- Keep container tightly closed.

Continued next column

 OVERDOSE

SYMPTOMS:
None expected.
WHAT TO DO:
Not intended for internal use. If child accidentally swallows, call poison-control center.

- Keep cool, but don't freeze.
- Wash hands immediately after using.
- Press finger to tear duct in corner of eye for 2 minutes to prevent possible absorption by body.

When to use:
As directed on label.

If you forget a dose:
Use as soon as you remember.

What drug does:
Inactivates an enzyme to reduce pressure inside the eye.

Time lapse before drug works:
5 to 60 minutes.

Don't use with:
Any other eye medicine without consulting your doctor.

 POSSIBLE ADVERSE REACTIONS OR SIDE EFFECTS

SYMPTOMS	WHAT TO DO
Life-threatening: None expected.	
Common: Pupils become small.	No action necessary.
Infrequent: Blurred vision, change in vision, eye pain, eyelids twitch, headache, watery eyes.	Discontinue. Call doctor right away.
Rare: Decreased vision with veil or curtain appearing, loss of bladder control, slow heartbeat, increased sweating, weakness, difficult breathing, vomiting, nausea, diarrhea.	Discontinue. Call doctor right away.

WARNINGS & PRECAUTIONS

Don't use if:
You are allergic to demecarium, echothiophate, isoflurophate.

Before you start, consult your doctor:
- If you have a history of retinal detachment.
- If you plan surgery under general or local anesthesia.
- If you have asthma, epilepsy, Down's syndrome, eye infection or other eye disease, heart disease, Parkinson's disease, ulcer in stomach or duodenum.

Over age 60:
No problems expected.

Pregnancy:
No problems expected, but check with doctor.

Breast-feeding:
No problems expected, but check with doctor.

Infants & children:
Use under medical supervision only.

Prolonged use:
No problems expected.

Skin & sunlight:
No problems expected.

Driving, piloting or hazardous work:
Don't drive or pilot aircraft until you learn how medicine affects you. Don't work around dangerous machinery. Don't climb ladders or work in high places. Danger increases if you drink alcohol or take medicine affecting alertness and reflexes, such as antihistamines, tranquilizers, sedatives, pain medicine, narcotics and mind-altering drugs.

Discontinuing:
- Discontinue 2 to 3 weeks prior to eye surgery.
- Otherwise, don't discontinue without consulting your doctor. Dose may require gradual reduction if you have used drug for a long time. Doses of other drugs may also require adjustment.

Others:
- Keep appointments for regular eye examinations to measure pressure in the eye.
- Keep cool, but don't freeze.
- Eyeglass prescription may need changing.

POSSIBLE INTERACTION WITH OTHER DRUGS

GENERIC NAME OR DRUG CLASS	COMBINED EFFECT
Atropine (ophthalmic)	May not be safe. Check with doctor.
Cyclopentolate (ophthalmic)	Reduces effect of antiglaucoma eye medicines.
Insecticides or pesticides with organic phosphates	Increased toxic absorption of pesticides.
Medicines to treat myasthenia gravis	Additive toxicity.
Physostigmine (ophthalmic)	Shortens action of antiglaucoma medicines.
Topical anesthetics	Increased risk of toxic effects of antiglaucoma eye medicines.

POSSIBLE INTERACTION WITH OTHER SUBSTANCES

INTERACTS WITH	COMBINED EFFECT
Alcohol:	None expected.
Beverages:	None expected.
Cocaine:	None expected.
Foods:	None expected.
Marijuana:	None expected.
Tobacco:	None expected.

ANTIGLAUCOMA, SHORT-ACTING (Ophthalmic)

BRAND AND GENERIC NAMES

Ayerst Epitrate
Betagan Standard
  Cap
Betagan C Cap B.I.D.
CARBACHOL
DIPIVEFRIN
Epifrin
Epinal
EPINEPHRINE
Epitrate
Eppy/N

Eserine
Glaucon
Isopto Carbachol
Isopto Eserine
LEVOBUNOLOL
METIPRANOLOL
Miostat
Mytrate
Optipranolol
PHYSOSTIGMINE
Propine

BASIC INFORMATION

Habit forming? No
Prescription needed? Yes
Available as generic? Yes, some are
Drug class: Antiglaucoma (ophthalmic)

 ## USES

Treats glaucoma (open-angle, secondary, angle-closure during or after eye surgery).

 ## DOSAGE & USAGE INFORMATION

How to use:
Eye drops
- Wash hands.
- Apply pressure to inside corner of eye with middle finger.
- Continue pressure for 1 minute after placing medicine in eye.
- Tilt head backward. Pull lower lid away from eye with index finger of the same hand.
- Drop eye drops into pouch and close eye. Don't blink.
- Keep eyes closed for 1 to 2 minutes.

Eye ointment
- Wash hands.
- Pull lower lid down from eye to form a pouch.
- Squeeze tube to apply thin strip of ointment into pouch.

Continued next column

 ## OVERDOSE

SYMPTOMS:
None expected.
WHAT TO DO:
Not intended for internal use. If child accidentally swallows, call poison-control center.

- Close eye for 1 to 2 minutes.
- Don't touch applicator tip to any surface (including the eye). If you accidentally touch tip, clean with warm soap and water.
- Keep container tightly closed.
- Keep cool, but don't freeze.
- Wash hands immediately after using.

When to use:
As directed on label.

If you forget a dose:
Use as soon as you remember.

What drug does:
Inactivates enzyme and facilitates movement of fluid (aquemous humor) into and out of the eye.

Time lapse before drug works:
10-30 minutes.

Don't use with:
Any other eye medicine without consulting your doctor.

 ## POSSIBLE ADVERSE REACTIONS OR SIDE EFFECTS

SYMPTOMS	WHAT TO DO
Life-threatening: None expected.	
Common: Headache; stinging, burning, watery eyes.	Continue. Call doctor when convenient.
Infrequent: Eye pain, changes in vision, blurred vision.	Discontinue. Call doctor right away.
Rare: Faintness, increased sweating, irregular or fast heartbeat, paleness.	Discontinue. Call doctor right away.

**WARNINGS &
PRECAUTIONS**

Don't use if:
You are allergic to any eye medicine for glaucoma.

Before you start, consult your doctor:
- If you plan to have eye or dental surgery.
- If you have any eye disease.
- If you have heart problems or high blood pressure.
- If you have diabetes.

Over age 60:
Adverse reactions and side effects may be more frequent and severe than in younger persons. Ask doctor about smaller doses.

Pregnancy:
Safety to unborn child unestablished. Avoid if possible.

Breast-feeding:
Safety unestablished. Avoid if possible.

Infants & children:
Use only under close medical supervision.

Prolonged use:
May be necessary.

Skin & sunlight:
No problems expected.

Driving, piloting or hazardous work:
Don't drive or pilot aircraft until you learn how medicine affects you. Don't work around dangerous machinery. Don't climb ladders or work in high places. Danger increases if you drink alcohol or take medicine affecting alertness and reflexes, such as antihistamines, tranquilizers, sedatives, pain medicine, narcotics and mind-altering drugs.

Discontinuing:
Don't discontinue without consulting your doctor. Dose may require gradual reduction if you have used drug for a long time. Doses of other drugs may also require adjustment.

Others:
- Most normal physical activities, including swimming or other exercise, are okay while you use this medicine.
- Keep cool, but don't freeze.
- Keep appointments for regular eye examinations to measure pressure in the eye.

 **POSSIBLE INTERACTION
WITH OTHER DRUGS**

GENERIC NAME OR DRUG CLASS	COMBINED EFFECT
Clinically significant interactions with oral or injected medicines unlikely.	

 **POSSIBLE INTERACTION
WITH OTHER SUBSTANCES**

INTERACTS WITH	COMBINED EFFECT
Alcohol:	None expected.
Beverages:	None expected.
Cocaine:	None expected.
Foods:	None expected.
Marijuana:	None expected.
Tobacco:	None expected.

ANTIHISTAMINES

BRAND AND GENERIC NAMES

See complete list of brand and generic names in the *Brand Name Directory*, page 910.

BASIC INFORMATION

Habit forming? No
Prescription needed?
  High strength: Yes
  Low strength: No
Available as generic? Yes
Drug class: Antihistamine

 USES

- Reduces allergic symptoms such as hay fever, hives, rash or itching.
- Prevents motion sickness, nausea, vomiting.
- Induces sleep.
- Reduces stiffness and tremors of Parkinson's disease.

 DOSAGE & USAGE INFORMATION

How to take:
Follow label directions.

When to take:
Varies with form. Follow label directions.

If you forget a dose:
Take as soon as you remember up to 2 hours late. If more than 2 hours, wait for next scheduled dose (don't double this dose).

What drug does:
Blocks action of histamine after an allergic response triggers histamine release in sensitive cells.

Time lapse before drug works:
30 minutes.

Don't take with:
Any other medicine without consulting your doctor or pharmacist.

 OVERDOSE

SYMPTOMS:
Convulsions, red face, hallucinations, coma.
WHAT TO DO:
- Dial 0 (operator) or 911 (emergency) for an ambulance or medical help. Then give first aid immediately.
- See emergency information on inside covers.

 POSSIBLE ADVERSE REACTIONS OR SIDE EFFECTS

SYMPTOMS	WHAT TO DO
Life-threatening:	
In case of overdose, see previous column.	
Common:	
Drowsiness (except astemizole); dizziness, dry mouth, nose throat; nausea.	Continue. Tell doctor at next visit.
Infrequent:	
• Change in vision, clumsiness, rash.	Discontinue. Call doctor right away.
• Less tolerance for contact lenses, painful or difficult urination.	Continue. Call doctor when convenient.
• Appetite loss.	Continue. Tell doctor at next visit.
Rare:	
Nightmares, agitation, irritability, sore throat, fever, rapid heartbeat, unusual bleeding or bruising, fatigue, weakness, confusion.	Discontinue. Call doctor right away.

 WARNINGS & PRECAUTIONS

Don't take if:
You are allergic to any antihistamine.

Before you start, consult your doctor:
- If you have glaucoma.
- If you have enlarged prostate.
- If you have asthma.
- If you have kidney disease.
- If you have peptic ulcer.
- If you will have surgery within 2 months, including dental surgery, requiring general or spinal anesthesia.

Over age 60:
Don't exceed recommended dose. Adverse reactions and side effects may be more frequent and severe than in younger persons, especially urination difficulty, diminished alertness and other brain and nervous-system symptoms.

Pregnancy:
No proven harm to unborn child. Avoid if possible.

Breast-feeding:
Drug passes into milk. Avoid drug or discontinue nursing until you finish medicine. Consult doctor for advice on maintaining milk supply.

Infants & children:
Not recommended for premature or newborn infants. Otherwise, no problems expected.

Prolonged use:
Avoid. May damage bone marrow and nerve cells.

Skin & sunlight:
May cause rash or intensify sunburn in areas exposed to sun or sunlamp.

Driving, piloting or hazardous work:
Don't drive or pilot aircraft until you learn how medicine affects you. Don't work around dangerous machinery. Don't climb ladders or work in high places. Danger increases if you drink alcohol or take medicine affecting alertness and reflexes, such as antihistamines, tranquilizers, sedatives, pain medicine, narcotics and mind-altering drugs.

Discontinuing:
No problems expected.

Others:
- May mask symptoms of hearing damage from aspirin, other salicylates, cisplatin, paromomycin, vancomycin or anticonvulsants. Consult doctor if you use these.
- Advise any doctor or dentist whom you consult that you take this medicine.

POSSIBLE INTERACTION WITH OTHER DRUGS

GENERIC NAME OR DRUG CLASS	COMBINED EFFECT
Anticholinergics*	Increased anti-cholinergic effect.
Anticoagulants, oral*	Decreased anti-histamine effect.
Antidepressants*	Excess sedation. Avoid.
Antihistamines, other*	Excess sedation. Avoid.
Carteolol	Decreased anti-histamine effect.
Clozapine	Toxic effect on the central nervous system.
Dronabinol	Increased effects of both drugs. Avoid.
Hypnotics*	Excess sedation. Avoid.
MAO inhibitors*	Increased anti-histamine effect.
Mind-altering drugs*	Excess sedation. Avoid.
Molindone	Increased sedative and antihistamine effect.
Nabilone	Greater depression of central nervous system.
Narcotics*	Excess sedation. Avoid.
Procarbazine	May increase sedation.
Sedatives*	Excess sedation. Avoid.
Sertraline	Increased depressive effects of both drugs.
Sleep inducers*	Excess sedation. Avoid.
Sotalol	Increased antihistamine effect.
Tranquilizers*	Excess sedation. Avoid.

POSSIBLE INTERACTION WITH OTHER SUBSTANCES

INTERACTS WITH	COMBINED EFFECT
Alcohol:	Excess sedation. Avoid.
Beverages: Caffeine drinks.	Less antihistamine sedation.
Cocaine:	Decreased antihistamine effect. Avoid.
Foods:	None expected.
Marijuana:	Excess sedation. Avoid.
Tobacco:	None expected.

ANTI-INFLAMMATORY DRUGS, NON-STEROIDAL (NSAIDs)

BRAND AND GENERIC NAMES

See complete list of brand and generic names in the *Brand Names Directory*, page 912.

BASIC INFORMATION

Habit forming? No
Prescription needed? Yes, for some.
Available as generic? Yes, for some.
Drug class: Anti-inflammatory (non-steroidal)

 ## USES

- Treatment for joint pain, stiffness, inflammation and swelling of arthritis and gout.
- Pain reliever.
- Treatment for dysmenorrhea (painful or difficult menstruation).
- Treats juvenile rheumatoid arthritis.

 ## DOSAGE & USAGE INFORMATION

How to take:
- Tablet or capsule—Swallow with liquid or food to lessen stomach irritation. If you can't swallow whole, crumble tablet and take with liquid or food.
- Liquid—Take as directed on bottle. Don't freeze.
- Rectal Suppositories—Remove wrapper and moisten suppository with water. Gently insert into rectum, large end first. If suppository is too soft, chill in refrigerator or cool water before removing wrapper.

When to take:
At the same times each day.

If you forget a dose:
Take as soon as you remember up to 2 hours late. If more than 2 hours, wait for next scheduled dose (don't double this dose).

Continued next column

 ## OVERDOSE

SYMPTOMS:
Confusion, agitation, severe headache, incoherence, convulsions, possible hemorrhage from stomach or intestine, coma.
WHAT TO DO:
- **Dial 0 (operator) or 911 (emergency) for an ambulance or medical help. Then give first aid immediately.**
- **See emergency information on inside covers.**

What drug does:
Reduces tissue concentration of prostaglandins (hormones which produce inflammation and pain).

Time lapse before drug works:
Begins in 4 to 24 hours. May require 3 weeks regular use for maximum benefit.

Don't take with:
Any other medicine without consulting your doctor or pharmacist.

 ## POSSIBLE ADVERSE REACTIONS OR SIDE EFFECTS

SYMPTOMS	WHAT TO DO
Life-threatening:	
Hives, rash, intense itching, faintness soon after a dose (anaphylaxis in aspirin-sensitive persons).	Seek emergency treatment immediately.
Common:	
• Dizziness, nausea, pain.	Continue. Call doctor when convenient.
• Headache.	Continue. Tell doctor at next visit.
Infrequent:	
• Depression; drowsiness; ringing in ears; swollen feet, face or legs; constipation or diarrhea; vomiting; gaseousness; dry mouth; tremors; insomnia.	Continue. Call doctor when convenient.
• Muscle cramps, numbness or tingling in hands or feet, mouth ulcers, rapid weight gain.	Discontinue. Call doctor right away.
Rare:	
• Convulsions; confusion; rash, hives or itch; blurred vision; black, bloody, tarry stool; difficult breathing; tightness in chest; rapid heartbeat; unusual bleeding or bruising; blood in urine; jaundice; psychosis; frequent, painful urination; fainting; sore throat; fever; chills; diminished hearing; eye pain; nosebleeds; severe abdominal pain.	Discontinue. Call doctor right away.
• Fatigue, weakness, menstrual irregularities.	Continue. Call doctor when convenient.

WARNINGS & PRECAUTIONS

Don't take if:
- You are allergic to aspirin or any non-steroidal, anti-inflammatory drug.
- You have gastritis, peptic ulcer, enteritis, ileitis, ulcerative colitis, asthma, heart failure, high blood pressure or bleeding problems.
- Patient is younger than 15.

Before you start, consult your doctor:
- If you have epilepsy.
- If you have Parkinson's disease.
- If you have been mentally ill.
- If you have impaired kidney or liver function.

Over age 60:
Adverse reactions and side effects may be more frequent and severe than in younger persons.

Pregnancy:
Studies inconclusive on harm to unborn child. Decide with your doctor whether drug benefits justify risk to unborn child.

Breast-feeding:
May harm child. Avoid.

Infants & children:
Not recommended for anyone younger than 15. Use only under medical supervision.

Prolonged use:
- Eye damage.
- Reduced hearing.
- Sore throat, fever.
- Weight gain.
- Talk to your doctor about the need for follow-up medical examinations or laboratory studies to check complete blood counts (white blood cell count, platelet count, red blood cell count, hemoglobin, hematocrit), liver function, stools for blood, eyes.

Skin & sunlight:
Possible increased sensitivity to sunlight.

Driving, piloting or hazardous work:
Don't drive or pilot aircraft until you learn how medicine affects you. Don't work around dangerous machinery. Don't climb ladders or work in high places. Danger increases if you drink alcohol or take medicine affecting alertness and reflexes, such as antihistamines, tranquilizers, sedatives, pain medicine, narcotics and mind-altering drugs.

Discontinuing:
Don't discontinue without consulting doctor. Dose may require gradual reduction if you have taken drug for a long time. Doses of other drugs may also require adjustment.

Others:
Advise any doctor or dentist whom you consult that you take this medicine.

POSSIBLE INTERACTION WITH OTHER DRUGS

GENERIC NAME OR DRUG CLASS	COMBINED EFFECT
ACE inhibitors*: captopril, enalapril, lisinopril	May decrease ACE inhibitor effect.
Antacids*	Decreased pain relief.
Anticoagulants, oral*	Increased risk of bleeding.
Anti-inflammatory pain relievers (any combination of)	Danger of increased side effects, such as stomach bleeding.
Aspirin	Increased risk of stomach ulcer.
Beta-adrenergic blockers*	Decreased antihypertensive effect.
Carteolol	Decreased antihypertensive effect of carteolol.
Cephalosporins*	Increased risk of bleeding.
Cortisone drugs*	Increased risk of stomach ulcer.
Didanosine	Increased risk of pancreatitis (sulindac only).
Diuretics*	May decrease diuretic effect.
Gold compounds*	Increased risk of kidney toxicity.

Continued on page 934

POSSIBLE INTERACTION WITH OTHER SUBSTANCES

INTERACTS WITH	COMBINED EFFECT
Alcohol:	Possible stomach ulcer or bleeding.
Beverages:	None expected.
Cocaine:	None expected.
Foods:	None expected.
Marijuana:	Increased pain relief from NSAIAs.
Tobacco:	None expected.

*See Glossary

ANTI-INFLAMMATORY DRUGS, STEROIDAL (Ophthalmic)

BRAND AND GENERIC NAMES

See complete list of brand and generic names in the *Brand Name Directory,* page 913.

BASIC INFORMATION

Habit forming? No
Prescription needed? Yes
Available as generic? Yes
Drug class: Adrenocorticoid (ophthalmic); anti-inflammatory, steroidal (ophthalmic)

 USES

- Relieves redness and irritation due to allergies or other irritants.
- Prevents damage to eye.

 DOSAGE & USAGE INFORMATION

How to use:
Eye drops
- Wash hands.
- Apply pressure to inside corner of eye with middle finger.
- Continue pressure for 1 minute after placing medicine in eye.
- Tilt head backward. Pull lower lid away from eye with index finger of the same hand.
- Drop eye drops into pouch and close eye. Don't blink.
- Keep eyes closed for 1 to 2 minutes.

Eye ointment
- Wash hands.
- Pull lower lid down from eye to form a pouch.
- Squeeze tube to apply thin strip of ointment into pouch.
- Close eye for 1 to 2 minutes.
- Don't touch applicator tip to any surface (including the eye). If you accidentally touch tip, clean with warm soap and water.
- Keep container tightly closed.
- Keep cool, but don't freeze.
- Wash hands immediately after using.

Continued next column

 OVERDOSE

SYMPTOMS:
None expected.
WHAT TO DO:
Not intended for internal use. If child accidentally swallows, call poison-control center.

When to use:
As directed.

If you forget a dose:
Use as soon as you remember.

What drug does:
Affects cell membranes and decreases response to irritating substances.

Time lapse before drug works:
Immediately.

Don't use with:
Medicines for abdominal cramps or glaucoma without first consulting doctor.

 POSSIBLE ADVERSE REACTIONS OR SIDE EFFECTS

SYMPTOMS	WHAT TO DO
Life-threatening: None expected.	
Common: None expected.	
Infrequent: Watery, stinging, burning eyes.	Continue. Call doctor when convenient.
Rare (extremely): Eye pain, blurred vision, eyelid droops, halos around lights, enlarged pupils.	Discontinue. Call doctor right away.

ANTI-INFLAMMATORY DRUGS, STEROIDAL
(Ophthalmic)

 WARNINGS & PRECAUTIONS

Don't use if:
You are allergic to any cortisone medicine.

Before you start, consult your doctor:
If you have or ever have had any eye infection, glaucoma, virus (herpes) infection of the eye, tuberculosis of the eye. .

Over age 60:
No problems expected.

Pregnancy:
Safety to unborn child unestablished. Avoid if possible.

Breast-feeding:
Safety unestablished. Avoid if possible.

Infants & children:
Use for short periods of time only.

Prolonged use:
Recheck with eye doctor at regular intervals.

Skin & sunlight:
No problems expected.

Driving, piloting or hazardous work:
No problems expected.

Discontinuing:
No problems expected.

Others:
* Cortisone eye medicines should not be used for bacterial, viral, fungal or tubercular infections.
* Keep cool, but don't freeze.
* Notify doctor if condition doesn't improve within 3 days.

 POSSIBLE INTERACTION WITH OTHER DRUGS

GENERIC NAME OR DRUG CLASS	COMBINED EFFECT
Clinically significant interactions with oral or injected medicines unlikely.	

 POSSIBLE INTERACTION WITH OTHER SUBSTANCES

INTERACTS WITH	COMBINED EFFECT
Alcohol:	None expected.
Beverages:	None expected.
Cocaine:	None expected.
Foods:	None expected.
Marijuana:	None expected.
Tobacco:	None expected.

ANTI-INFLAMMATORY DRUGS, STEROIDAL (Otic)

BRAND AND GENERIC NAMES

BETAMETHASONE
  (Otic)
Betnesol
Cortamed
Cortisol
Corti-sporin (Otic)

Decadron
DECAMETHASONE
  (Otic)
HYDROCORTISONE
  (Otic)

BASIC INFORMATION

Habit forming? No
Prescription needed? Yes
Available as generic? No
Drug class: Anti-inflammatory, steroidal
  (otic); adrenocorticoid (otic)

USES

- Treats allergic conditions involving external ear.
- Used together with antibiotics to treat ear infections.
- Treats seborrheic and eczematoid dermatitis involving the ear.

DOSAGE & USAGE INFORMATION

How to use:
Ear drops
- Warm ear drops under running water around the unopened bottle.
- Lie down with affected ear up.
- Adults—Pull ear lobe back and up.
- Children—Pull ear lobe down and back.
- Drop medicine into ear canal until canal is full.
- Stay lying down for 2 minutes.
- Gently insert cotton plug into ear to prevent leaking.

Continued next column

OVERDOSE

SYMPTOMS:
None expected.
WHAT TO DO:
Not intended for internal use. If child accidentally swallows, call poison-control center.

Ear ointment
- Apply small amount to skin just inside the ear canal.
- Use finger or piece of sterile gauze.
- Don't use cotton-tipped applicators.

When to use:
As directed by your doctor.

If you forget a dose:
Use as soon as you remember.

What drug does:
Decreases tissue inflammation, decreases scarring.

Time lapse before drug works:
15 minutes.

Don't use with:
Other ear medications unless directed by your doctor.

POSSIBLE ADVERSE REACTIONS OR SIDE EFFECTS

SYMPTOMS	WHAT TO DO
Life-threatening: None expected.	
Common: None expected.	
Infrequent: Itching, burning, redness, swelling.	Discontinue. Call doctor right away.
Rare: None expected.	

WARNINGS & PRECAUTIONS

Don't use if:
You are allergic to any of the medications listed under Brand and Generic Names.

Before you start, consult your doctor:
If eardrum is punctured.

Over age 60:
No problems expected.

Pregnancy:
No problems expected.

Breast-feeding:
No problems expected.

Infants & children:
Use small amounts only.

Prolonged use:
Not intended for prolonged use.

Skin & sunlight:
No problems expected.

Driving, piloting or hazardous work:
No problems expected.

Discontinuing:
No problems expected.

Others:
Keep cool, but don't freeze.

POSSIBLE INTERACTION WITH OTHER DRUGS

GENERIC NAME OR DRUG CLASS	COMBINED EFFECT
None expected.	

POSSIBLE INTERACTION WITH OTHER SUBSTANCES

INTERACTS WITH	COMBINED EFFECT
Alcohol:	None expected.
Beverages:	None expected.
Cocaine:	None expected.
Foods:	None expected.
Marijuana:	None expected.
Tobacco:	None expected.

*See Glossary

ANTISEBORRHEICS (Topical)

BRAND AND GENERIC NAMES

See complete list of brand and generic names in the *Brand Name Directory*, page 913

BASIC INFORMATION

Habit forming? No
Prescription needed? Yes
Available as generic? No
Drug class: Antiseborrheic

 ## USES

Treats dandruff or seborrheic dermatitis of scalp.

 ## DOSAGE & USAGE INFORMATION

How to use:
* Wet hair and scalp.
* Apply enough medicine to form lather.
* Rub in well. Keep away from eyes.
* Allow to remain on scalp 3 to 5 minutes then rinse.
* Repeat above steps once.

Continued next column

 ## OVERDOSE

SYMPTOMS:
None expected.
WHAT TO DO:
* **Not for internal use. If child accidentally swallows, call poison-control center.**
* **Dial 0 (operator) or 911 (emergency) for an ambulance or medical help. Then give first aid immediately.**
* **See emergency information on inside covers.**

When to use:
As directed by doctor. Twice a week for shampoo is average.

If you forget a dose:
Use as soon as you remember.

What drug does:
Slows cell growth in scales on scalp.

Time lapse before drug works:
Varies a great deal. If no improvement in 2 weeks, notify doctor.

Don't use with:
* Other scalp preparations without notifying doctor.
* Any other medicine without consulting your doctor or pharmacist.

 ## POSSIBLE ADVERSE REACTIONS OR SIDE EFFECTS

SYMPTOMS	WHAT TO DO
Life-threatening: None expected.	
Common: None expected.	
Infrequent:	
• Irritation not present before using, rash.	Discontinue. Call doctor right away.
• Dryness or itching scalp.	Continue. Call doctor when convenient.
Rare: None expected.	

ANTISEBORRHEICS (Topical)

WARNINGS & PRECAUTIONS

Don't use if:
- You have had an allergic reaction to chloroxine, clioquinol (iodochlorhydroxyquin), iodoquinol (diiodohydroxyquin) or edate sodium.
- Scalp is blistered or infected with oozing or raw areas.

Before you start, consult your doctor:
If you are allergic to anything.

Over age 60:
No problems expected.

Pregnancy:
No problems expected, but check with doctor.

Breast-feeding:
No problems expected, but check with doctor.

Infants & children:
No problems expected, but check with doctor.

Prolonged use:
No problems expected, but check with doctor.

Skin & sunlight:
No problems expected, but check with doctor.

Driving, piloting or hazardous work:
No problems expected, but check with doctor.

Discontinuing:
No problems expected, but check with doctor.

Others:
- If medicine accidentally gets into eyes, flush them immediately with cool water.
- Heat and moisture in bathroom medicine cabinet can cause breakdown of medicine. Store someplace else.
- Keep cool, but don't freeze.

POSSIBLE INTERACTION WITH OTHER DRUGS

GENERIC NAME OR DRUG CLASS	COMBINED EFFECT
Other medical shampoos	May accentuate adverse reactions of each medicine.

POSSIBLE INTERACTION WITH OTHER SUBSTANCES

INTERACTS WITH	COMBINED EFFECT
Alcohol:	None expected.
Beverages:	None expected.
Cocaine:	None expected.
Foods:	None expected.
Marijuana:	None expected.
Tobacco:	None expected.

*See Glossary

ANTITHYROID DRUGS

BRAND AND GENERIC NAMES

METHIMAZOLE	Tapazole
PROPYLTHIOURACIL	Thiamazole
Propyl-Thyracil	

BASIC INFORMATION

Habit forming? No
Prescription needed? Yes
Available as generic? Yes
Drug class: Antihyperthyroid

USES

- Treatment of overactive thyroid (hyperthyroidism).
- Treatment of angina in patients who have overactive thyroid.

DOSAGE & USAGE INFORMATION

How to take:
Tablet—Swallow with liquid or food to lessen stomach irritation. If you can't swallow whole, crumble tablet and take with liquid or food.

When to take:
At the same times each day.

If you forget a dose:
Take as soon as you remember up to 2 hours late. If more than 2 hours, wait for next scheduled dose (don't double this dose).

What drug does:
Prevents thyroid gland from producing excess thyroid hormone.

Time lapse before drug works:
10 to 20 days.

Don't take with:
- Anticoagulants
- Any other medicine without consulting your doctor or pharmacist.

OVERDOSE

SYMPTOMS:
Bleeding, spots on skin, jaundice (yellow eyes and skin), loss of consciousness.
WHAT TO DO:
Overdose unlikely to threaten life. If person takes much larger amount than prescribed, call doctor, poison-control center or hospital emergency room for instructions.

POSSIBLE ADVERSE REACTIONS OR SIDE EFFECTS

SYMPTOMS	WHAT TO DO
Life-threatening:	
In case of overdose, see previous column.	
Common:	
Skin rash, itching, dryness.	Discontinue. Call doctor right away.
Infrequent:	
Dizziness, taste loss, sore throat with chills and fever, abdominal pain, constipation, diarrhea.	Discontinue. Call doctor right away.
Rare:	
Headache; enlarged lymph glands; irregular or rapid heartbeat; unusual bruising or bleeding; backache; numbness or tingling in toes, fingers or face; joint pain; muscle aches; menstrual irregularities; jaundice; tired, weak, sleepy, listless; swollen eyes or feet; black stools; excessive cold feeling; puffy skin; irritability.	Discontinue. Call doctor right away.

ANTITHYROID DRUGS

WARNINGS & PRECAUTIONS

Don't take if:
You are allergic to antithyroid medicines.

Before you start, consult your doctor:
- If you have liver disease.
- If you have blood disease.
- If you have an infection.
- If you take anticoagulants.

Over age 60:
Adverse reactions and side effects may be more frequent and severe than in younger persons.

Pregnancy:
Risk to unborn child outweighs drug benefits. Don't use.

Breast-feeding:
Drug filters into milk. May harm child. Don't use.

Infants & children:
Use only under special medical supervision by experienced clinician.

Prolonged use:
- Adverse reactions and side effects more common.
- Talk to your doctor about the need for follow-up medical examinations or laboratory studies to check thyroid function, complete blood counts (white blood cell count, platelet count, red blood cell count, hemoglobin, hematocrit).

Skin & sunlight:
No problems expected.

Driving, piloting or hazardous work:
Don't drive or pilot aircraft until you learn how medicine affects you. Don't work around dangerous machinery. Don't climb ladders or work in high places. Danger increases if you drink alcohol or take medicine affecting alertness and reflexes, such as antihistamines, tranquilizers, sedatives, pain medicine, narcotics and mind-altering drugs.

Discontinuing:
Don't discontinue without consulting doctor. Dose may require gradual reduction if you have taken drug for a long time. Doses of other drugs may also require adjustment.

Others:
No problems expected.

POSSIBLE INTERACTION WITH OTHER DRUGS

GENERIC NAME OR DRUG CLASS	COMBINED EFFECT
Anticoagulants*	Increased effect of anticoagulants.
Antineoplastic drugs*	Increased chance to suppress bone marrow.
Chloramphenicol	Increased chance to suppress bone marrow.
Clozapine	Toxic effect on bone marrow.
Levamisole	Increased risk of bone marrow depression.
Lithium	Decreased thyroid activity.
Thioguanine	More likelihood of toxicity of both drugs.
Tiopronin	Increased risk of toxicity to bone marrow.

POSSIBLE INTERACTION WITH OTHER SUBSTANCES

INTERACTS WITH	COMBINED EFFECT
Alcohol:	Increased possibility of liver toxicity. Avoid.
Beverages:	No problems expected.
Cocaine:	Increased toxicity potential of medicines. Avoid.
Foods:	No problems expected.
Marijuana:	Increased rapid or irregular heartbeat. Avoid.
Tobacco:	Increased chance of rapid heartbeat. Avoid.

ANTIVIRALS (Ophthalmic)

BRAND AND GENERIC NAMES

Herplex Eye Drops
IDOXURIDINE DROPS
  & OINTMENT
Liquifilm

Stoxil Eye Ointment
TRIFLURIDINE
Trifluorothymidine
Viroptic

BASIC INFORMATION

Habit forming? No
Prescription needed? Yes
Available as generic? No
Drug class: Antiviral (ophthalmic)

 USES

Treats virus infections of the eye (usually herpes simplex virus)

 DOSAGE & USAGE INFORMATION

How to use:
Eye drops
- Wash hands.
- Apply pressure to inside corner of eye with middle finger.
- Continue pressure for 1 minute after placing medicine in eye.
- Tilt head backward. Pull lower lid away from eye with index finger of the same hand.
- Drop eye drops into pouch and close eye. Don't blink.
- Keep eyes closed for 1 to 2 minutes.

Eye ointment
- Wash hands.
- Pull lower lid down from eye to form a pouch.
- Squeeze tube to apply thin strip of ointment into pouch.
- Close eye for 1 to 2 minutes.
- Don't touch applicator tip to any surface (including the eye). If you accidentally touch tip, clean with warm soap and water.
- Keep container tightly closed.
- Keep cool, but don't freeze.
- Wash hands immediately after using.

Continued next column

 OVERDOSE

SYMPTOMS:
None expected.
WHAT TO DO:
Not intended for internal use. If child accidentally swallows, call poison-control center.

When to use:
As directed. Usually 1 drop every 2 hours up to maximum of 9 drops daily.

If you forget a dose:
Use as soon as you remember.

What drug does:
Destroys reproductive capacity of virus.

Time lapse before drug works:
Begins work immediately. Usual course of treatment is 7 days.

Don't use with:
Other eye drops, boric acid or ointment without consulting doctor.

 POSSIBLE ADVERSE REACTIONS OR SIDE EFFECTS

SYMPTOMS	WHAT TO DO
Life-threatening	
None expected.	
Common	
Stinging or burning eyes.	Continue. Tell doctor at next visit.
Infrequent	
None expected.	
Rare	
Itchy, red eyes; swollen eyelid or eye; excess flow of tears.	Discontinue. Call doctor right away.

WARNINGS & PRECAUTIONS

Don't use if:
You are allergic to trifluridine or idoxuridine.

Before you start, consult your doctor:
• If you have had any other eye problems.
• If you use eye drops for glaucoma.

Over age 60:
No problems expected.

Pregnancy:
No problems expected, but safety not established.

Breast-feeding:
No problems expected, but safety not established.

Infants & children:
Use only under close medical supervision.

Prolonged use:
Avoid unless directed by your eye doctor.

Skin & sunlight:
No problems expected.

Driving, piloting or hazardous work:
No problems expected.

Discontinuing:
Don't discontinue without consulting doctor.

Others:
• Don't use more often or longer than prescribed.
• Keep cool, but don't freeze.
• If problem doesn't improve within a week, notify your doctor.

 ## POSSIBLE INTERACTION WITH OTHER DRUGS

GENERIC NAME OR DRUG CLASS	COMBINED EFFECT
Clinically significant interactions with oral or injected medicines unlikely.	

 ## POSSIBLE INTERACTION WITH OTHER SUBSTANCES

INTERACTS WITH	COMBINED EFFECT
Alcohol:	None expected.
Beverages:	None expected.
Cocaine:	None expected.
Foods:	None expected.
Marijuana:	None expected.
Tobacco:	None expected.

APPETITE SUPPRESSANTS

BRAND AND GENERIC NAMES

See complete list of brand and generic names in the *Brand Name Directory,* page 913.

BASIC INFORMATION

Habit forming? Yes
Prescription needed? Yes
Available as generic? Yes
Drug class: Appetite suppressant

 ## USES

Suppresses appetite.

 ## DOSAGE & USAGE INFORMATION

How to take:
* Tablet or capsule—Swallow with liquid. You may chew or crush tablet.
* Extended-release tablets or capsules—Swallow each dose whole with liquid; do not crush.
* Elixir—Swallow with liquid.

When to take:
* Long-acting forms—10 to 14 hours before bedtime.
* Short-acting forms—1 hour before meals. Last dose no later than 4 to 6 hours before bedtime.

If you forget a dose:
* Long-acting form—Take as soon as you remember up to 2 hours late. If more than 2 hours, wait for next scheduled dose (don't double this dose).
* Short-acting form—Wait for next scheduled dose. Don't double this dose.

What drug does:
Apparently stimulates brain's appetite-control center.

Continued next column

 ## OVERDOSE

SYMPTOMS:
Irritability, overactivity, trembling, insomnia, mood changes, fever, rapid heartbeat, confusion, disorientation, hallucinations, convulsions, coma.
WHAT TO DO:
* **Dial 0 (operator) or 911 (emergency) for an ambulance or medical help. Then give first aid immediately.**
* **See emergency information on inside covers.**

Time lapse before drug works:
Begins in 1 hour. Short-acting form lasts 4 hours. Long-acting form lasts 14 hours.

Don't take with:
* Non-prescription drugs without consulting doctor.
* See Interaction column and consult doctor.

 ## POSSIBLE ADVERSE REACTIONS OR SIDE EFFECTS

SYMPTOMS	WHAT TO DO
Life-threatening:	
In case of overdose, see previous column.	
Common:	
Irritability, nervousness, insomnia, false sense of well-being.	Continue. Call doctor when convenient.
Infrequent:	
• Irregular or pounding heartbeat, urgent or difficult urination.	Discontinue. Call doctor right away.
• Blurred vision, unpleasant taste or dry mouth, constipation or diarrhea, nausea, vomiting, cramps, changes in sex drive, increased sweating, headache, nightmares, weakness.	Continue. Call doctor when convenient.
Rare:	
• Mood changes, rash or hives, breathing difficulty.	Discontinue. Call doctor right away.
• Hair loss.	Continue. Call doctor when convenient.

106

WARNINGS & PRECAUTIONS

Don't take if:
- You are allergic to any sympathomimetic or phenylpropanolamine.
- You have glaucoma.
- You have taken MAO inhibitors within 2 weeks.
- You plan to become pregnant within medication period.
- You have a history of drug abuse.
- You have irregular or rapid heartbeat.

Before you start, consult your doctor:
- If you have high blood pressure or heart disease.
- If you have an overactive thyroid, nervous tension or "anxiety."
- If you have epilepsy.
- If you will have surgery within 2 months, including dental surgery, requiring general or spinal anesthesia.
- If you take any other over-the-counter medicine.

Over age 60:
Adverse reactions and side effects may be more frequent and severe than in younger persons.

Pregnancy:
Safety not established. Avoid.

Breast-feeding:
Safety not established. Consult doctor.

Infants & children:
Don't give to children younger than 12.

Prolonged use:
- Loses effectiveness. Avoid.
- Talk to your doctor about the need for follow-up medical examinations or laboratory studies.

Skin & sunlight:
No problems expected.

Driving, piloting or hazardous work:
Don't drive or pilot aircraft until you learn how medicine affects you. Don't work around dangerous machinery. Don't climb ladders or work in high places. Danger increases if you drink alcohol or take medicine affecting alertness and reflexes, such as antihistamines, tranquilizers, sedatives, pain medicine, narcotics and mind-altering drugs.

Discontinuing:
Don't discontinue without consulting doctor. Dose may require gradual reduction if you have taken drug for a long time. Doses of other drugs may also require adjustment.

Others:
Don't increase dose.

POSSIBLE INTERACTION WITH OTHER DRUGS

GENERIC NAME OR DRUG CLASS	COMBINED EFFECT
Antihypertensives*	Decreased antihypertensive effect.
Appetite suppressants, other*	Dangerous overstimulation.
Caffeine	Increased stimulant effect.
Furazolidine	Sudden severe increase in blood pressure.
Guanethidine	Decreased guanethidine effect.
Hydralazine	Decreased hydralazine effect.
MAO inhibitors*	Dangerous blood-pressure rise.
Methyldopa	Decreased methyldopa effect.
Molindone	Decreased suppressant effect.
Phenothiazines*	Decreased appetite suppressant effect.
Rauwolfia alkaloids*	Decreased effect of rauwolfia alkaloids.
Sodium bicarbonate	Increased action of appetite suppressants.

POSSIBLE INTERACTION WITH OTHER SUBSTANCES

INTERACTS WITH	COMBINED EFFECT
Alcohol: Beer, Chianti wines, vermouth.	Increased sedation.
Beverages: • Caffeine drinks. • Drinks containing tyramine.*	Excessive stimulation. Blood-pressure rise.
Cocaine	Convulsions or excessive nervousness.
Foods: Foods containing tyramine.*	Blood-pressure rise.
Marijuana:	Frequent use— Irregular heartbeat.
Tobacco:	None expected.

ASPIRIN

BRAND NAMES

See complete list of brand names in the *Brand Name Directory*, page 914.

BASIC INFORMATION

Habit forming? No
Prescription needed? No
Available as generic? Yes
Drug class: Analgesic, anti-inflammatory (non-steroidal)

 ## USES

- Reduces pain, fever, inflammation.
- Relieves swelling, stiffness, joint pain of arthritis or rheumatism.
- Antiplatelet effect to reduce chances of heart attack and/or stroke.

 ## DOSAGE & USAGE INFORMATION

How to take:
- Tablet or capsule—Swallow with liquid or food to lessen stomach irritation.
- Extended-release tablets or capsules—Swallow each dose whole.
- Effervescent tablets—Dissolve in water.
- Chewing gum tablets—Chew completely. Don't swallow whole.
- Suppositories—Remove wrapper and moisten suppository with water. Gently insert into rectum, large end first.

When to take:
Pain, fever, inflammation—As needed, no more often than every 4 hours.

If you forget a dose:
- Pain, fever—Take as soon as you remember. Wait 4 hours for next dose.
- Arthritis—Take as soon as you remember up to 2 hours late. Return to regular schedule.

Continued next column

 ## OVERDOSE

SYMPTOMS:
Ringing in ears; nausea; vomiting; dizziness; fever; deep, rapid breathing; hallucinations; convulsions; coma.
WHAT TO DO:
- **Dial 0 (operator) or 911 (emergency) for an ambulance or medical help. Then give first aid immediately.**
- **See emergency information on inside covers.**

What drug does:
- Affects hypothalamus, the part of the brain which regulates temperature by dilating small blood vessels in skin.
- Prevents clumping of platelets (small blood cells) so blood vessels remain open.
- Decreases prostaglandin effect.
- Suppresses body's pain messages.

Time lapse before drug works:
30 minutes for pain, fever, arthritis.

Don't take with:
- Tetracyclines. Space doses 1 hour apart.
- Any other medicine without consulting your doctor or pharmacist.

 ## POSSIBLE ADVERSE REACTIONS OR SIDE EFFECTS

SYMPTOMS	WHAT TO DO
Life-threatening:	
Black or bloody vomit; blood in urine; difficulty breathing; hives, rash, intense itching, faintness soon after a dose (anaphylaxis).	Seek emergency treatment immediately.
Common:	
• Nausea, vomiting, hearing loss.	Discontinue. Seek emergency treatment.
• Heartburn, indigestion.	Continue. Call doctor when convenient.
• Ringing in ears.	Continue. Tell doctor at next visit.
Infrequent:	
None expected.	
Rare:	
• Black stools, unexplained fever.	Discontinue. Seek emergency treatment.
• Rash, hives, itch, diminished vision, shortness of breath, wheezing, jaundice, mental confusion.	Discontinue. Call doctor right away.
• Drowsiness.	Continue. Call doctor when convenient.

 ## WARNINGS & PRECAUTIONS

Don't take if:
- You need to restrict sodium in your diet. Buffered effervescent tablets and sodium salicylate are high in sodium.
- You are sensitive to aspirin or aspirin has a strong vinegar-like odor, which means it has decomposed.
- You have a peptic ulcer of stomach or duodenum or a bleeding disorder.

Before you start, consult your doctor:
- If you have had stomach or duodenal ulcers.
- If you have had gout.
- If you have asthma or nasal polyps.
- If you have kidney or liver disease.

Over age 60:
More likely to cause hidden bleeding in stomach or intestines. Watch for dark stools.

Pregnancy:
Risk to unborn child outweighs drug benefits. Don't use.

Breast-feeding:
Drug passes into milk. Avoid drug or discontinue nursing until you finish medicine. Consult doctor for advice on maintaining milk supply.

Infants & children:
- Overdose frequent and severe. Keep bottles out of children's reach.
- Consult doctor before giving to persons under age 18 who have fever and discomfort of viral illness, especially chicken pox and influenza. Probably increases risk of Reye's syndrome.

Prolonged use:
Talk to your doctor about the need for follow-up medical examinations or laboratory studies to check liver function, complete blood counts (white blood cell count, platelet count, red blood cell count, hemoglobin, hematocrit).

Skin & sunlight:
Aspirin combined with sunscreen may decrease sunburn.

Driving, piloting or hazardous work:
No restrictions unless you feel drowsy.

Discontinuing:
For chronic illness—Don't discontinue without doctor's advice until you complete prescribed dose, even though symptoms diminish or disappear.

Others:
- Aspirin can complicate surgery, pregnancy, labor and delivery, and illness.
- For arthritis—Don't change dose without consulting doctor.
- Urine tests for blood sugar may be inaccurate.
- Don't take if pills have vinegar-like odor.

 POSSIBLE INTERACTION WITH OTHER DRUGS

GENERIC NAME OR DRUG CLASS	COMBINED EFFECT
Acebutolol	Decreased anti-hypertensive effect of acebutolol.
ACE inhibitors*: captopril, enalapril, lisinopril	Decreased ACE inhibitor effect.
Allopurinol	Decreased allopurinol effect.
Antacids*	Decreased aspirin effect.
Anticoagulants*	Increased anticoagulant effect. Abnormal bleeding.
Antidiabetics, oral*	Low blood sugar.
Bumetanide	Possible aspirin toxicity.
Carteolol	Decreased anti-hypertensive effect of carteolol.
Cortisone drugs*	Increased cortisone effect. Risk of ulcers and stomach bleeding.
Dextrothyroxine (large doses, continuous use)	Increased dextrothyroxine effect.
Diclofenac	Increased risk of stomach ulcer.
Ethacrynic acid	Possible aspirin toxicity.
Furosemide	Possible aspirin toxicity. May decrease furosemide effect.
Gold compounds*	Increased likelihood of kidney damage.
Indomethacin	Risk of stomach bleeding and ulcers.

Continued page 934

 POSSIBLE INTERACTION WITH OTHER SUBSTANCES

INTERACTS WITH	COMBINED EFFECT
Alcohol:	Possible stomach irritation and bleeding. Avoid.
Beverages:	None expected.
Cocaine:	None expected.
Foods:	None expected.
Marijuana:	Possible increased pain relief, but marijuana may slow body's recovery. Avoid.
Tobacco:	None expected.

*See Glossary

ATROPINE

GENERIC NAME

ATROPINE

BASIC INFORMATION

Habit forming? No
Prescription needed?
  Low strength: No
  High strength: Yes
Available as generic? Yes
Drug class: Antispasmodic, anticholinergic

 USES

- Reduces spasms of digestive system, bladder and urethra.
- Treatment of bronchial spasms.

 DOSAGE & USAGE INFORMATION

How to take:
- Tablet—Swallow with liquid or food to lessen stomach irritation.
- Aerosol—Dilute in saline and inhale as nebulizer.

When to take:
30 minutes before meals (unless directed otherwise by doctor).

If you forget a dose:
Take as soon as you remember up to 2 hours late. If more than 2 hours, wait for next scheduled dose (don't double this dose).

What drug does:
Blocks nerve impulses at parasympathetic nerve endings, preventing muscle contractions and gland secretions of organs involved.

Time lapse before drug works:
15 to 30 minutes.

Don't take with:
- Antacids* or antidiarrheals*.
- Any other medicine without consulting your doctor or pharmacist.

 OVERDOSE

SYMPTOMS:
Dilated pupils, rapid pulse and breathing, dizziness, fever, hallucinations, confusion, slurred speech, agitation, flushed face, convulsions, coma.
WHAT TO DO:
- **Dial 0 (operator) or 911 (emergency) for an ambulance or medical help. Then give first aid immediately.**
- **See emergency information on inside covers.**

 POSSIBLE ADVERSE REACTIONS OR SIDE EFFECTS

SYMPTOMS	WHAT TO DO
Life-threatening:	
In case of overdose, see previous column.	
Common:	
• Confusion, delirium, rapid heartbeat.	Discontinue. Call doctor right away.
• Nausea, vomiting, decreased sweating.	Continue. Call doctor when convenient.
• Constipation.	Continue. Tell doctor at next visit.
• Dryness in ears, nose, throat, mouth.	No action necessary.
Infrequent:	
• Headache, difficult or painful urination, nasal congestion, altered taste.	Continue. Call doctor when convenient.
• Lightheadedness.	Discontinue. Call doctor right away.
Rare:	
Rash or hives, eye pain, blurred vision, fever.	Discontinue. Call doctor right away.

 WARNINGS & PRECAUTIONS

Don't take if:
- You are allergic to any anticholinergic.
- You have trouble with stomach bloating.
- You have difficulty emptying your bladder completely.
- You have narrow-angle glaucoma.
- You have severe ulcerative colitis.

Before you start, consult your doctor:
- If you have open-angle glaucoma.
- If you have angina.
- If you have chronic bronchitis or asthma.
- If you have liver, kidney or thyroid disease.
- If you have hiatal hernia.
- If you have enlarged prostate.
- If you have myasthenia gravis.
- If you have peptic ulcer.
- If you will have surgery within 2 months, including dental surgery, requiring general or spinal anesthesia.

Over age 60:
Adverse reactions and side effects may be more frequent and severe than in younger persons.

Pregnancy:
Studies inconclusive on harm to unborn child. Animal studies show fetal abnormalities. Decide with your doctor whether drug benefits justify risk to unborn child.

Breast-feeding:
Drug passes into milk and decreases milk flow. Avoid drug or discontinue nursing until you finish medicine. Consult doctor for advice on maintaining milk supply.

Infants & children:
Use only under medical supervision.

Prolonged use:
Chronic constipation, possible fecal impaction. Consult doctor immediately.

Skin & sunlight:
No problems expected.

Driving, piloting or hazardous work:
Use disqualifies you for piloting aircraft. Otherwise, no problems expected.

Discontinuing:
May be unnecessary to finish medicine. Follow doctor's instructions.

Others:
Advise any doctor or dentist whom you consult that you take this medicine.

 POSSIBLE INTERACTION WITH OTHER DRUGS

GENERIC NAME OR DRUG CLASS	COMBINED EFFECT
Amantadine	Increased atropine effect.
Anticholinergics, other*	Increased atropine effect.
Antidepressants, tricyclic (TCA)*	Increased atropine effect. Increased sedation.
Antihistamines*	Increased atropine effect.
Attapulgite	Decreased atropine effect.
Cortisone drugs*	Increased internal eye pressure.
Disopyramide	Increased atropine effect.
Haloperidol	Increased internal eye pressure.
Ketoconazole	Decreased ketoconazole effect.
MAO inhibitors*	Increased atropine effect.
Meperidine	Increased atropine effect.
Methylphenidate	Increased atropine effect.
Molindone	Increased anticholinergic effect.
Nitrates*	Increased internal eye pressure.
Nizatidine	Increased nizatidine effect.
Orphenadrine	Increased atropine effect.
Phenothiazines*	Increased atropine effect.
Pilocarpine	Loss of pilocarpine effect in glaucoma treatment.
Potassium supplements*	Possible intestinal ulcers with oral potassium tablets.
Quinidine	Increased atropine effect.
Sedatives* or central nervous system (CNS) depressants*	Increased sedative effect of both drugs.
Vitamin C	Decreased atropine effect. Avoid large doses of vitamin C.

 POSSIBLE INTERACTION WITH OTHER SUBSTANCES

INTERACTS WITH	COMBINED EFFECT
Alcohol:	None expected.
Beverages:	None expected.
Cocaine:	Excessively rapid heartbeat. Avoid.
Foods:	None expected.
Marijuana:	Drowsiness and dry mouth.
Tobacco:	None expected.

*See Glossary

ATROPINE, HYOSCYAMINE, METHENAMINE, METHYLENE BLUE, PHENYLSALICYLATE & BENZOIC ACID

BRAND NAMES

Atrosept	Urimed
Dolsed	Urinary
Hexalol	Antiseptic No. 2
Prosed	Urised
Trac Tabs	Urisep
U-Tract	Uritab
UAA	Uritin
Uridon Modified	Uro-Ves

BASIC INFORMATION

Habit forming? No
Prescription needed? Yes
Available as generic? No
Drug class: Analgesic (urinary), antispasmodic, anti-infective (urinary)

 ## USES

A combination medicine to control infection, spasms and pain caused by urinary tract infections.

 ## DOSAGE & USAGE INFORMATION

How to take:
Tablet—Swallow with liquid or food to lessen stomach irritation.

When to take:
30 minutes before meals (unless directed otherwise by doctor).

If you forget a dose:
Take as soon as you remember up to 2 hours late. If more than 2 hours, wait for next scheduled dose (don't double this dose).

Continued next column

 ## OVERDOSE

SYMPTOMS:
Dilated pupils, rapid pulse and breathing, dizziness, fever, hallucinations, confusion, slurred speech, agitation, flushed face, convulsions, coma.
WHAT TO DO:
- **Dial 0 (operator) or 911 (emergency) for an ambulance or medical help. Then give first aid immediately.**
- **See emergency information on inside covers.**

What drug does:
Makes urine acid. Blocks nerve impulses at parasympathetic nerve endings, preventing muscle contractions and gland secretions of organs involved. Methenamine destroys some germs.

Time lapse before drug works:
15 to 30 minutes.

Don't take with:
- Antacids* or antidiarrheals*.
- Any other medicine without consulting your doctor or pharmacist.

 ## POSSIBLE ADVERSE REACTIONS OR SIDE EFFECTS

SYMPTOMS	WHAT TO DO
Life-threatening:	
Heartbeat irregularity, shortness of breath or difficulty breathing.	Seek emergency treatment immediately.
Common:	
Dry mouth, throat, ears, nose.	Continue. Call doctor when convenient.
Infrequent:	
• Flushed, red face; drowsiness; difficult urination; nausea and vomiting; abdominal pain; ringing or buzzing in ears; severe drowsiness; back pain; lightheadedness.	Discontinue. Call doctor right away.
• Headache, nasal congestion, altered taste.	Continue. Call doctor when convenient.
Rare:	
Blurred vision; pain in eyes; skin rash, hives.	Discontinue. Seek emergency treatment.

 ## WARNINGS & PRECAUTIONS

Don't take if:
- You are allergic to any of the ingredients or aspirin.
- Brain damage in child.
- You have glaucoma.

Before you start, consult your doctor:
- If you are on any special diet such as low-sodium.
- If you have had a hiatal hernia, bronchitis, asthma, liver disease, stomach or duodenal ulcers.
- If you have asthma, nasal polyps, bleeding disorder or enlarged prostate.
- If you will have any surgery within 2 months.

ATROPINE, HYOSCYAMINE, METHENAMINE, METHYLENE BLUE, PHENYLSALICYLATE & BENZOIC ACID

Over age 60:
- Adverse reactions and side effects may be more frequent and severe than in younger persons.
- More likely to cause hidden bleeding in stomach or intestines. Watch for dark stools.

Pregnancy:
Risk to unborn child outweighs benefits. Don't use.

Breast-feeding:
Drug passes into milk. Avoid or discontinue nursing until you finish medicine.

Infants & children:
Side effects more likely. Not recommended in children under 12.

Prolonged use:
May lead to constipation or kidney damage. Request lab studies to monitor effects of prolonged use.

Skin & sunlight:
No problems expected.

Driving, piloting or hazardous work:
May disqualify for piloting aircraft during time you take medicine.

Discontinuing:
May be unnecessary to finish medicine. Follow your symptoms and doctor's advice.

Others:
- Salicylates can complicate surgery, pregnancy, labor and delivery, and illness.
- Urine tests for blood sugar may be inaccurate.
- Drink cranberry juice or eat prunes or plums to help make urine more acid.

POSSIBLE INTERACTION WITH OTHER DRUGS

GENERIC NAME OR DRUG CLASS	COMBINED EFFECT
Allopurinol	Decreased allopurinol effect.
Amantadine	Increased atropine and belladonna effect.
Antacids*	Decreased salicylate and methenamine effect.
Anticoagulants*	Increased anti-coagulant effect. Abnormal bleeding.
Anticholinergics, other*	Increased atropine and belladonna effect.
Antidepressants, other*	Increased sedation.
Antidiabetics, oral*	Low blood sugar.
Antihistamines*	Increased atropine and hyoscyamine effect.
Aspirin	Likely salicylate toxicity.
Beta-adrenergic blockers*	Decreased antihypertensive effect.
Carbonic anhydrase inhibitors*	Decreased methenamine effect.
Cortisone drugs*	Increased internal-eye pressure, increased cortisone effect. Risk of ulcers and stomach bleeding.
Diuretics, thiazide*	Decreased urine acidity.
Furosemide	Possible salicylate toxicity.
Gold compounds*	Increased likelihood of kidney damage.
Haloperidol	Increased internal-eye pressure.
Indomethacin	Risk of stomach bleeding and ulcers.
Ketoconazole	Reduced ketoconazole effect.

Continued page 935

POSSIBLE INTERACTION WITH OTHER SUBSTANCES

INTERACTS WITH	COMBINED EFFECT
Alcohol:	Excessive sedation. Possible stomach irritation and bleeding. Avoid.
Beverages:	None expected.
Cocaine:	Excessively rapid heartbeat. Avoid.
Foods:	None expected.
Marijuana:	Drowsiness and dry mouth. May slow body's recovery.
Tobacco:	Dry mouth.

*See Glossary

ATTAPULGITE

BRAND NAMES

Diar-Aid
Diasorb
Kaopectate

Rheaban
St. Joseph
Antidiarrheal

BASIC INFORMATION

Habit forming? No
Prescription needed? No
Available as generic? Yes
Drug class: Antidiarrheal

USES

Treats diarrhea. Used in conjunction with fluids, appropriate diet and rest. Treats symptoms only. Does not cure any disorder that causes diarrhea.

DOSAGE & USAGE INFORMATION

How to take:
Tablets—Swallow with liquid. If you can't swallow whole, crumble tablet and take with liquid or food. Instructions to take on empty stomach mean 1 hour before or 2 hours after eating.

When to take:
2 hours before or 3 hours after taking any other oral medications. Outside of this restriction, take a dose after each loose bowel movement until diarrhea is controlled.

If you forget a dose:
Take as soon as you remember, then resume regular schedule.

What drug does:
Absorbs bacteria and toxins and reduces water loss. Attapulgite does not get absorbed into the body.

Time lapse before drug works:
5 to 8 hours.

Don't take with:
See Interaction column and consult doctor.

OVERDOSE

SYMPTOMS:
None expected.
WHAT TO DO:
Overdose unlikely to threaten life. If person takes much larger amount than prescribed, call doctor, poison-control center or hospital emergency room for instructions.

POSSIBLE ADVERSE REACTIONS OR SIDE EFFECTS

SYMPTOMS	WHAT TO DO
Life-threatening: None expected.	
Common: None expected.	
Infrequent: Constipation (usually mild and of short duration).	Continue. Call doctor when convenient.
Rare: None expected.	

WARNINGS & PRECAUTIONS

Don't take if:
- You are allergic to attapulgite.
- You or your doctor suspects intestinal obstruction.

Before you start, consult your doctor:
If you are dehydrated (signs are a dry mouth, loose skin, sunken eyes and parched lips).

Over age 60:
- Dehydration is more likely in this age group.
- Side effects of constipation are more likely.

Pregnancy:
No proven problems. Consult doctor.

Breast-feeding:
No problems expected, but consult doctor.

Infants & children:
Use only under close medical supervision for children up to 3 years of age. This age group is quite susceptible to fluid and electrolyte loss.

Prolonged use:
Not intended for prolonged use.

Skin & sunlight:
No special problems expected.

Driving, piloting or hazardous work:
No special problems expected.

Discontinuing:
May be unnecessary to finish medicine. Follow doctor's instructions.

Others:
No special problems expected.

POSSIBLE INTERACTION WITH OTHER DRUGS

GENERIC NAME OR DRUG CLASS	COMBINED EFFECT
Digitalis	May decrease effectiveness of digitalis.
Lincomycins*	May decrease effectiveness of lincomycins.
Any other medicine taken by mouth	When taken at the same time, neither drug may be as effective. Take other medicines 2 hours before or 3 hours after attapulgite.

POSSIBLE INTERACTION WITH OTHER SUBSTANCES

INTERACTS WITH	COMBINED EFFECT
Alcohol:	No proven problems.
Beverages:	No proven problems.
Cocaine:	No proven problems.
Foods: Prunes, prune juice and other fruits or foods that may cause diarrhea.	Decreased effect of attapulgite.
Marijuana:	No proven problems.
Tobacco:	No proven problems.

AZATHIOPRINE

BRAND NAMES

Imuran

BASIC INFORMATION

Habit forming? No
Prescription needed? Yes
Available as generic? Yes
Drug class: Immunosuppressant,
antirheumatic

 ## USES

- Protects against rejection of transplanted organs (e.g., kidney, heart).
- Treats severe active rheumatoid arthritis and other immunologic diseases if simpler treatment plans have been ineffective.

 ## DOSAGE & USAGE INFORMATION

How to take:
Tablets—Swallow with liquid. If you can't swallow whole, crumble tablet and take with liquid or food. Instructions to take on empty stomach mean 1 hour before or 2 hours after eating.

When to take:
Follow your doctor's instructions. Usually once a day.

If you forget a dose:
Take as soon as you remember up to 2 hours late. If more than 2 hours, wait for next scheduled dose (don't double this dose).

What drug does:
Unknown; probably inhibits synthesis of DNA and RNA.

Time lapse before drug works:
6 to 8 weeks.

Don't take with:
Any other medicines (including over-the-counter drugs such as cough and cold medicines, laxatives, antacids, diet pills, caffeine, nose drops or vitamins) without consulting your doctor.

 ## OVERDOSE

SYMPTOMS:
None expected.
WHAT TO DO:
Overdose unlikely to threaten life. If person takes much larger amount than prescribed, call doctor, poison-control center or hospital emergency room for instructions.

 ## POSSIBLE ADVERSE REACTIONS OR SIDE EFFECTS

SYMPTOMS	WHAT TO DO
Life-threatening:	
Rapid heart rate, sudden fever, muscle or joint pain, cough, shortness of breath.	Seek emergency treatment immediately.
Common:	
• Infection or low blood count causing fever and chills, back pain, cough, painful urination; anemia (tiredness or weakness); nausea; vomiting.	Discontinue. Call doctor right away.
• Appetite loss.	Continue. Call doctor when convenient.
Infrequent:	
Jaundice (yellow eyes, skin), skin rash.	Discontinue. Call doctor right away.
Rare:	
Low platelet count causing bleeding or bruising, tarry or black stools, bloody urine, red spots under skin; severe abdominal pain; mouth sores.	Discontinue. Call doctor right away.

AZATHIOPRINE

WARNINGS & PRECAUTIONS

Don't take if:
- You have chicken pox.
- You have shingles (herpes zoster).

Before you start, consult your doctor:
- If you have gout.
- If you have liver or kidney disease.
- If you have an infection.

Over age 60:
Adverse reactions and side effects may be more frequent and severe than in younger persons. You may need smaller doses for shorter periods of time.

Pregnancy:
Risk to unborn child outweighs drug benefits. Don't use.

Breast-feeding:
Drug passes into milk. Avoid drug or discontinue nursing until you finish medicine. Consult doctor for advice on maintaining milk supply.

Infants & children:
No special problems expected.

Prolonged use:
- May increase likelihood of problems upon discontinuing.
- Talk to your doctor about the need for follow-up medical examinations or laboratory studies to check thyroid function, liver function, electrolytes (sodium potassium, chloride), blood pressure and complete blood counts (white blood count, platelet count, red blood cell count, hemoglobin, hematocrit) every week during first two months, then once a month.

Skin & sunlight:
No special problems expected.

Driving, piloting or hazardous work:
Avoid if you feel confused, drowsy or dizzy.

Discontinuing:
May still experience symptoms of bone marrow depression, such as: blood in stools, fever or chills, blood spots under the skin, back pain, hoarseness, bloody urine. If any of these occur, call your doctor right away.

Others:
- Advise any doctor or dentist whom you consult that you take this medicine.
- May affect results in some medical tests.

POSSIBLE INTERACTION WITH OTHER DRUGS

GENERIC NAME OR DRUG CLASS	COMBINED EFFECT
Allopurinol	Greatly increased azathioprine activity.
Clozapine	Toxic effect on bone marrow.
Didanosine	Increased risk of pancreatitis.
Tiopronin	Increased risk of toxicity to bone marrow.
Immunosuppressants, other*	Higher risk of developing infection or malignancies.
Levamisole	Increased risk of bone marrow depression.
Vaccines	May decrease effectiveness or cause disease itself.

POSSIBLE INTERACTION WITH OTHER SUBSTANCES

INTERACTS WITH	COMBINED EFFECT
Alcohol:	No special problems expected.
Beverages:	No special problems expected.
Cocaine:	Increased likelihood of adverse reactions. Avoid.
Foods:	No special problems expected.
Marijuana:	Increased likelihood of adverse reactions. Avoid.
Tobacco:	No special problems expected.

BACAMPICILLIN

BRAND NAMES

Penglobe   Spectrobid

BASIC INFORMATION

Habit forming? No
Prescription needed? Yes
Available as generic? No
Drug class: Antibiotic (penicillin)

USES

Treatment of bacterial infections that are
susceptible to bacampicillin.

DOSAGE & USAGE INFORMATION

How to take:

- Capsules—Swallow with liquid on an empty
  stomach 1 hour before meals or 2 hours after
  eating.
- Chewable tablets—Chew well before swallowing.
- Liquid—Take with cold beverage. Liquid form
  is perishable and effective for only 7 days at
  room temperature. Effective for 14 days if
  stored in refrigerator. Don't freeze.

When to take:

Follow instructions on prescription label or side
of package. Doses should be evenly spaced.
For example, 4 times a day means before meals
and at bedtime.

If you forget a dose:

Take as soon as you remember. Continue
regular schedule.

What drug does:

Destroys susceptible bacteria. Does not kill
viruses.

Time lapse before drug works:

May be several days before medicine affects
infection.

Don't take with:

Any other medicine without consulting your
doctor or pharmacist.

OVERDOSE

SYMPTOMS:
Severe diarrhea, nausea or vomiting.
WHAT TO DO:
Overdose unlikely to threaten life. If person
takes much larger amount than prescribed,
call doctor, poison-control center or
hospital emergency room for specific
instructions.

POSSIBLE ADVERSE REACTIONS OR SIDE EFFECTS

SYMPTOMS	WHAT TO DO
Life-threatening:	
Hives, rash, intense itching, faintness soon after a dose (anaphylaxis); difficulty breathing.	Seek emergency treatment immediately.
Common:	
Dark or discolored tongue.	Continue. Tell doctor at next visit.
Infrequent:	
• Mild nausea, vomiting, diarrhea.	Continue. Call doctor when convenient.
• Bloody urine, face and ankle swelling.	Discontinue. Call doctor right away.
Rare:	
Unexplained bleeding or bruising, weakness, sore throat, fever, abdominal cramps, convulsions.	Discontinue. Call doctor right away.

WARNINGS & PRECAUTIONS

Don't take if:
You are allergic to bacampicillin, cephalosporin antibiotics, or other penicillins. Life-threatening reaction may occur.

Before you start, consult your doctor:
- If you are allergic to any substance or drug.
- If you take birth control pills.

Over age 60:
You may have skin reactions, particularly around genitals and anus.

Pregnancy:
Studies inconclusive on harm to unborn child. Animal studies show fetal abnormalities. Decide with your doctor whether drug benefits justify risk to unborn child.

Breast-feeding:
Drug passes into milk. Child may become sensitive to this and all penicillins. Avoid bacampicillin or discontinue nursing until you finish medicine. Consult doctor for advice on maintaining milk supply.

Infants & children:
No problems expected.

Prolonged use:
- You may become more susceptible to infections caused by germs not responsive to bacampicillin. Super-infection also a potential.
- Talk to your doctor about the need for follow-up medical examinations or laboratory studies to check SGPT*, SGOT*.

Skin & sunlight:
No problems expected.

Driving, piloting, or hazardous work:
Usually not dangerous. Most hazardous reactions likely to occur a few minutes after taking bacampicillin.

Discontinuing:
Don't discontinue without doctor's advice until you complete prescribed dose, even though symptoms diminish or disappear.

Others:
- Urine sugar test for diabetes may show false positive result.
- Birth control pills may not be effective. Use additional birth-control methods.

POSSIBLE INTERACTION WITH OTHER DRUGS

GENERIC NAME OR DRUG CLASS	COMBINED EFFECT
Beta-adrenergic blockers*	Increased chance of anaphylaxis (see emergency information on inside front cover).
Birth control pills	Impaired contraceptive efficiency.
Chloramphenicol	Decreased effect of both drugs.
Erythromycins*	Decreased effect of both drugs.
Loperamide	Decreased bacampicillin effect.
Paromomycin	Decreased effect of both drugs.
Probenecid	Increased effect of all penicillins.
Sodium benzoate & sodium phenylacetate	May reduce effect of sodium benzoate & sodium phenylacetate.
Tetracyclines*	Decreased effect of both drugs.
Troleandomycin	Decreased effect of both drugs.

POSSIBLE INTERACTION WITH OTHER SUBSTANCES

INTERACTS WITH	COMBINED EFFECT
Alcohol:	Occasional stomach irritation.
Beverages:	None expected.
Cocaine:	No proven problems.
Foods: Acidic fruits or juices, aged cheese, wines, syrups (if taken with).	Decreased antibiotic effect.
Marijuana:	No proven problems.
Tobacco:	None expected.

BACLOFEN

BRAND NAMES

Lioresal

BASIC INFORMATION

Habit forming? No
Prescription needed? Yes
Available as generic? Yes
Drug class: Muscle relaxant in multiple sclerosis

 ## USES

- Relieves spasms, cramps and spasticity of muscles caused by medical problems, including multiple sclerosis and spine injuries.
- Reduces number and severity of trigeminal neuralgia attacks.

 ## DOSAGE & USAGE INFORMATION

How to take:
Tablet—Swallow with liquid or food to lessen stomach irritation.

When to take:
3 or 4 times daily as directed.

If you forget a dose:
Take as soon as you remember up to 2 hours late. If more than 2 hours, wait for next scheduled dose (don't double this dose).

What drug does:
Blocks body's pain and reflex messages to brain.

Time lapse before drug works:
Variable. Few hours to weeks.

Continued next column

 ## OVERDOSE

SYMPTOMS:
Blurred vision, blindness, difficult breathing, vomiting, drowsiness, muscle weakness, convulsive seizures.
WHAT TO DO:
- **Dial 0 (operator) or 911 (emergency) for an ambulance or medical help. Then give first aid immediately.**
- **If patient is unconscious and not breathing, give mouth-to-mouth breathing. If there is no heartbeat, use cardiac massage and mouth-to-mouth breathing (CPR). Don't try to make patient vomit. If you can't get help quickly, take patient to nearest emergency facility.**
- **See emergency information on inside covers.**

Don't take with:
Any other medicine without consulting your doctor or pharmacist.

 ## POSSIBLE ADVERSE REACTIONS OR SIDE EFFECTS

SYMPTOMS	WHAT TO DO
Life-threatening:	
In case of overdose, see previous column.	
Common:	
Dizziness, lightheadedness, confusion, insomnia, drowsiness, nausea.	Continue. Call doctor when convenient.
Infrequent:	
• Rash with itching, numbness or tingling in hands or feet.	Discontinue. Call doctor right away.
• Headache, abdominal pain, diarrhea or constipation, appetite loss, muscle weakness, difficult or painful urination, male sex problems, nasal congestion, clumsiness, slurred speech, insomnia.	Continue. Call doctor when convenient.
Rare:	
• Fainting, weakness, hallucinations, depression, chest pain, muscle pain, pounding heatbeat.	Discontinue. Call doctor right away.
• Ringing in ears, lowered blood pressure, dry mouth, taste disturbance, euphoria, weight gain.	Continue. Call doctor when convenient.

 ## WARNINGS & PRECAUTIONS

Don't take if:
- You are allergic to any muscle relaxant.
- Muscle spasm due to strain or sprain.

Before you start, consult your doctor:
- If you have Parkinson's disease.
- If you have cerebral palsy.
- If you have had a recent stroke.
- If you have had a recent head injury.
- If you have arthritis.
- If you have diabetes.
- If you have epilepsy.
- If you have psychosis.
- If you have kidney disease.
- If you will have surgery within 2 months, including dental surgery, requiring general or spinal anesthesia.

Over age 60:
Adverse reactions and side effects may be more frequent and severe than in younger persons.

Pregnancy:
Risk to unborn child outweighs drug benefits. Don't use.

Breast-feeding:
Avoid nursing or discontinue until you finish medicine.

Infants & children:
Not recommended.

Prolonged use:
Epileptic patients should be monitored with EEGs. Diabetics should more closely monitor blood sugar levels. Obtain periodic liver function tests.

Skin & sunlight:
No problems expected.

Driving, piloting or hazardous work:
Don't drive or pilot aircraft until you learn how medicine affects you. Don't work around dangerous machinery. Don't climb ladders or work in high places. Danger increases if you drink alcohol or take medicine affecting alertness and reflexes, such as antihistamines, tranquilizers, sedatives, pain medicine, narcotics and mind-altering drugs.

Discontinuing:
Don't discontinue without consulting doctor. Dose may require gradual reduction if you have taken drug for a long time. Doses of other drugs may also require adjustment.

Others:
No problems expected.

POSSIBLE INTERACTION WITH OTHER DRUGS

GENERIC NAME OR DRUG CLASS	COMBINED EFFECT
Anesthetics, general*	Increased sedation. Low blood pressure. Avoid.
Central nervous system (CNS) depressants* (antidepressants,* antihistamines,* narcotics,* other muscle relaxants,* sedatives,* sleeping pills,* tranquilizers*)	Increased sedation. Low blood pressure. Avoid.

Clozapine	Toxic effect on the central nervous system.
Ethinamate	Dangerous increased effects of ethinamate. Avoid combining.
Fluoxetine	Increased depressant effects of both drugs.
Guanfacine	May increase depressant effects of either drug.
Insulin or oral antidiabetic drugs*	Need to adjust diabetes medicine dosage.
Leucovorin	High alcohol content of leucovorin may cause adverse effects.
Methyprylon	Increased sedative effect, perhaps to dangerous level. Avoid.
Nabilone	Greater depression of the central nervous system.
Sertraline	Increased depressive effects of both drug.

POSSIBLE INTERACTION WITH OTHER SUBSTANCES

INTERACTS WITH	COMBINED EFFECT
Alcohol:	Increased sedation. Low blood pressure. Avoid.
Beverages:	No problems expected.
Cocaine:	Increased spasticity. Avoid.
Foods:	No problems expected.
Marijuana:	Increased spasticity. Avoid.
Tobacco:	May interfere with absorption of medicine.

*See Glossary

BARBITURATES

BRAND AND GENERIC NAMES

See complete list of brand and generic names in the *Brand Names Directory,* page 914.

BASIC INFORMATION

Habit forming? Yes
Prescription needed? Yes
Available as generic? No
Drug class: Sedative, hypnotic (barbiturate)

 USES

- Reduces anxiety or nervous tension (low dose).
- Reduces likelihood of seizures in epilepsy.
- Aids sleep at night.

 DOSAGE & USAGE INFORMATION

How to take:
- Capsule—Swallow with liquid. If you can't swallow whole, open capsule and take with liquid or food. Instructions to take on empty stomach mean 1 hour before or 2 hours after eating.
- Elixir—Swallow with liquid.
- Rectal Suppositories—Remove wrapper and moisten suppository with water. Gently insert into rectum, large end first. If suppository is too soft, chill in refrigerator or cool water before removing wrapper.
- Tablet—Swallow with liquid or food to lessen stomach irritation. If you can't swallow whole, crumble tablet and take with liquid or food.

When to take:
At the same times each day.

Continued next column

 OVERDOSE

SYMPTOMS:
Deep sleep, trouble breathing, weak pulse, coma.
WHAT TO DO:
- Dial 0 (operator) or 911 (emergency) for an ambulance or medical help. Then give first aid immediately.
- If patient is unconscious and not breathing, give mouth-to-mouth breathing. If there is no heartbeat use cardiac massage and mouth-to-mouth breathing (CPR). Don't try to make patient vomit. If you can't get help quickly, take patient to nearest emergency facility.
- See emergency information on inside covers.

If you forget a dose:
Take as soon as you remember up to 2 hours late. If more than 2 hours, wait for next scheduled dose (don't double this dose).

What drug does:
May partially block nerve impulses at nerve-cell connections.

Time lapse before drug works:
60 minutes.

Don't take with:
- Non-prescription drugs without consulting doctor.
- See Interaction column and consult doctor.

 POSSIBLE ADVERSE REACTIONS OR SIDE EFFECTS

SYMPTOMS	WHAT TO DO
Life-threatening:	
In case of overdose, see previous column.	
Common:	
Dizziness, drowsiness, "hangover" effect.	Continue. Call doctor when convenient.
Infrequent:	
• Rash or hives; face, lip or eyelid swelling; sore throat; fever.	Discontinue. Call doctor right away.
• Depression, confusion, diarrhea, nausea, vomiting, joint or muscle pain, slurred speech, hallucinations, headache, decreased sex drive.	Continue. Call doctor when convenient.
Rare:	
• Agitation, slow heartbeat, difficult breathing, jaundice, chest pain.	Discontinue. Call doctor right away.
• Unexplained bleeding or bruising.	Continue. Call doctor when convenient.

 WARNINGS & PRECAUTIONS

Don't take if:
- You are allergic to any barbiturate.
- You have porphyria.

Before you start, consult your doctor:
- If you have epilepsy.
- If you have kidney or liver damage.
- If you have asthma.
- If you have anemia.
- If you have chronic pain.
- If you will have surgery within 2 months, including dental surgery, requiring general or spinal anesthesia.

Over age 60:
Adverse reactions and side effects may be more frequent and severe than in younger persons. Use small doses.

Pregnancy:
Risk to unborn child outweighs drug benefits. Don't use.

Breast-feeding:
Drug passes into milk. Avoid drug or discontinue nursing until you finish medicine. Consult doctor for advice on maintaining milk supply.

Infants & children:
Use only under doctor's supervision.

Prolonged use:
- May cause addiction, anemia, chronic intoxication.
- May lower body temperature, making exposure to cold temperatures hazardous.
- Talk to your doctor about the need for follow-up medical examinations or laboratory studies to check blood sugar, kidney function.

Skin & sunlight:
May cause rash or intensify sunburn in areas exposed to sun or sunlamp.

Driving, piloting or hazardous work:
Don't drive or pilot aircraft until you learn how medicine affects you. Don't work around dangerous machinery. Don't climb ladders or work in high places. Danger increases if you drink alcohol or take medicine affecting alertness and reflexes.

Discontinuing:
If you become addicted, don't stop taking barbiturates suddenly. Seek medical help for safe withdrawal.

Others:
- May affect results in some medical tests.
- Barbiturate addiction is common. Withdrawal effects may be fatal.
- Advise any doctor or dentist whom you consult that you take this medicine.

 ## POSSIBLE INTERACTION WITH OTHER DRUGS

GENERIC NAME OR DRUG CLASS	COMBINED EFFECT
Anticoagulants, oral*	Decreased effect of anticoagulant.
Anticonvulsants*	Changed seizure patterns.
Antidepressants, tricyclics (TCA)*	Decreased antidepressant effect. Possible dangerous oversedation.
Antidiabetics, oral*	Increased effect of barbituate.
Antihistamines*	Dangerous sedation. Avoid.
Aspirin	Decreased aspirin effect.

Beta-adrenergic blockers*	Decreased effect of beta-adrenergic blocker.
Carbamazepine	Decreased carbamazepine effect.
Carteolol	Increased barbiturate effect. Dangerous sedation.
Clozapine	Toxic effect on the central nervous system.
Contraceptives, oral*	Decreased contraceptive effect.
Dextrothyroxine	Decreased bariturate effect.
Divalproex	Dangerous sedation. Avoid.
Doxycycline	Decreased doxycycline effect.
Griseofulvin	Decreased griseofulvin effect.
MAO inhibitors*	Increased barbituate effect.
Mind-altering drugs*	Dangerous sedation. Avoid.
Nabilone	Greater depression of central nervous system.
Narcotics*	Dangerous sedation. Avoid.
Pain relievers*	Dangerous sedation. Avoid.
Sedatives*	Dangerous sedation. Avoid.

Continued page 936

 ## POSSIBLE INTERACTION WITH OTHER SUBSTANCES

INTERACTS WITH	COMBINED EFFECT
Alcohol:	Possible fatal oversedation. Avoid.
Beverages:	None expected.
Cocaine:	Decreased barbiturate effect.
Foods:	None expected.
Marijuana:	Excessive sedation. Avoid.
Tobacco:	None expected.

*See Glossary

BECLOMETHASONE

BRAND NAMES

Beclovent
Vanceril
Beclovent Rotacaps

BASIC INFORMATION

Habit forming? No
Prescription needed? Yes
Available as generic? No
Drug class: Cortisone drug (adrenal corticosteroid), antiasthmatic

 USES

Prevents attacks of bronchial asthma and allergic hay fever. Does not stop an active asthma attack.

 DOSAGE & USAGE INFORMATION

How to take:
• Aerosol—Follow package instructions. Don't inhale more than 4 times twice a day. Rinse mouth after use to prevent hoarseness, throat irritation and mouth infection. Wait at least 1 minute between inhalations.
• Use other inhaled asthma drugs before beclomethasone.

When to take:
Regularly at the same times each day.

If you forget a dose:
Take as soon as you remember up to 2 hours late. If more than 2 hours, wait for next scheduled dose (don't double this dose).

What drug does:
Reduces inflammation in bronchial tubes.

Time lapse before drug works:
1 to 4 weeks.

Don't take with:
Any other medicine without consulting your doctor or pharmacist.

 OVERDOSE

SYMPTOMS:
Fluid retention, flushed face, nervousness, stomach irritation.
WHAT TO DO:
Overdose unlikely to threaten life. If person inhales much larger amount than prescribed, call doctor, poison-control center or hospital emergency room for instructions.

 POSSIBLE ADVERSE REACTIONS OR SIDE EFFECTS

SYMPTOMS	WHAT TO DO
Life-threatening:	
In case of overdose, see previous column.	
Common:	
Fungus infection with white patches in mouth, dryness, sore throat, constipation, gaseousness, unpleasant taste, diarrhea, headache, cough, dizziness, hoarseness, appetite loss.	Continue. Call doctor when convenient.
Infrequent:	
• Rash, various infections, nausea or vomiting, swallowing difficulty, hives, increased thirst.	Discontinue. Call doctor right away.
• Spasm of bronchial tubes, facial swelling, dry mouth, euphoria, insomnia, nosebleed.	Continue. Call doctor when convenient.
Rare:	
Unusual weight gain.	Continue. Call doctor when convenient.

WARNINGS & PRECAUTIONS

Don't take if:
- You have bone disease, thyroid disease, colitis, stomach ulcer, diabetes, myasthenia gravis, liver or kidney disease, diverticulitis, glaucoma, heart disease.
- You are allergic to beclomethasone.
- You have had tuberculosis or systemic fungal infection.
- You are having an asthma attack.

Before you start, consult your doctor:
- If you are taking any other prescription or non-prescription medicine.
- If you have an infection.

Over age 60:
More likely to develop lung infections.

Pregnancy:
Risk to unborn child outweighs drug benefits. Don't use.

Breast-feeding:
Drug passes into milk. Avoid drug or discontinue nursing.

Infants & children:
Use only under medical supervision.

Prolonged use:
Talk to your doctor about the need for follow-up medical examinations or laboratory studies to check blood pressure, serum electrolytes, stools for blood.

Skin & sunlight:
No problems expected.

Driving, piloting or hazardous work:
No problems expected.

Discontinuing:
Don't discontinue without doctor's advice until you complete prescribed dose, even though symptoms diminish or disappear.

Others:
- Unrelated illness or injury may require cortisone drugs by mouth or injection. Notify your doctor.
- Consult doctor as soon as possible if your asthma returns while using beclamethasone as a preventive.
- Drug can reactivate tuberculosis or lung fungal infection.
- Consult doctor frequently if changing from oral cortisone drug to beclomethasone inhaler.
- Advise any doctor or dentist whom you consult that you take this medicine.
- Your resistance to infection is less while taking this medicine.

POSSIBLE INTERACTION WITH OTHER DRUGS

GENERIC NAME OR DRUG CLASS	COMBINED EFFECT
Albuterol	Increased beclomethasone effect.
Antiasthmatics, other*	Increased anti-asthmatic effect.
Antidiabetic drugs*	Increased blood glucose level.
Bitolerol	Increased beclomethasone effect.
Digitalis*	Decreased blood potassium.
Diuretics*	Dangerously low potassium in blood.
Ephedrine	Increased beclomethasone effect.
Epinephrine	Increased beclomethasone effect.
Indapamide	Possible excessive potassium loss, causing dangerous heartbeat irregularity.
Isoetharine	Increased beclomethasone effect.
Isoproterenol	Increased beclomethasone effect.
Metaproterenol	Increased beclomethasone effect.
Potassium supplements*	Decreased potassium effect.
Terbutaline	Increased beclomethasone effect.
Theophylline	Increased beclomethasone effect.

POSSIBLE INTERACTION WITH OTHER SUBSTANCES

INTERACTS WITH	COMBINED EFFECT
Alcohol:	None expected.
Beverages:	None expected.
Cocaine:	None expected.
Foods:	None expected.
Marijuana:	Decreased beclomethasone effect.
Tobacco:	Decreased beclomethasone effect.

*See Glossary

BELLADONNA

GENERIC NAME

BELLADONNA

BASIC INFORMATION

Habit forming? No
Prescription needed?
  Low strength: No
  High strength: Yes
Available as generic? Yes
Drug class: Antispasmodic, anticholinergic

 USES

Reduces spasms of digestive system, bladder and urethra.

 DOSAGE & USAGE INFORMATION

How to take:
- Tablet, elixir or capsule—Swallow with liquid or food to lessen stomach irritation.
- Drops—Dilute dose in beverage before swallowing.

When to take:
30 minutes before meals (unless directed otherwise by doctor).

If you forget a dose:
Take as soon as you remember up to 2 hours late. If more than 2 hours, wait for next scheduled dose (don't double this dose).

What drug does:
Blocks nerve impulses at parasympathetic nerve endings, preventing muscle contractions and gland secretions of organs involved.

Time lapse before drug works:
15 to 30 minutes.

Don't take with:
- Antacids* or antidiarrheals*.
- Any other medicine without consulting your doctor or pharmacist.

 OVERDOSE

SYMPTOMS:
Dilated pupils, rapid pulse and breathing, dizziness, fever, hallucinations, confusion, slurred speech, agitation, flushed face, convulsions, coma.
WHAT TO DO:
- **Dial 0 (operator) or 911 (emergency) for an ambulance or medical help. Then give first aid immediately.**
- **See emergency information on inside covers.**

 POSSIBLE ADVERSE REACTIONS OR SIDE EFFECTS

SYMPTOMS	WHAT TO DO
Life-threatening:	
In case of overdose, see previous column.	
Common:	
• Confusion, delirium, rapid heartbeat.	Discontinue. Call doctor right away.
• Nausea, vomiting, decreased sweating,	Continue. Call doctor when convenient.
• Constipation.	Continue. Tell doctor at next visit.
• Dryness in ears, nose, throat, mouth.	No action necessary.
Infrequent:	
• Headache, difficult urination, nasal congestion, altered taste.	Continue. Call doctor when convenient.
• Lightheadedness.	Discontinue. Call doctor right away.
Rare:	
Rash or hives, eye pain, blurred vision.	Discontinue. Call doctor right away.

 WARNINGS & PRECAUTIONS

Don't take if:
- You are allergic to any anticholinergic.
- You have trouble with stomach bloating.
- You have difficulty emptying your bladder completely.
- You have narrow-angle glaucoma.
- You have severe ulcerative colitis.

Before you start, consult your doctor:
- If you have open-angle glaucoma.
- If you have angina or fast heartbeat.
- If you have chronic bronchitis or asthma.
- If you have hiatal hernia; liver, kidney or thyroid disease; enlarged prostate or myasthenia gravis.
- If you will have surgery within 2 months, including dental surgery, requiring general or spinal anesthesia.

Over age 60:
Adverse reactions and side effects may be more frequent and severe than in younger persons.

Pregnancy:
Safety not established. Studies inconclusive on harm to unborn child. Animal studies show fetal abnormalities. Decide with your doctor whether drug benefits justify risk to unborn child. May cause bleeding in neonate.

Breast-feeding:
Drug passes into milk and decreases milk flow. Avoid drug or discontinue nursing until you finish medicine. Consult doctor for advice on maintaining milk supply.

Infants & children:
Use only under medical supervision. Do not use if under 6 months of age.

Prolonged use:
Chronic constipation, possible fecal impaction. Consult doctor immediately.

Skin & sunlight:
No problems expected.

Driving, piloting or hazardous work:
Use disqualifies you for piloting aircraft. Otherwise, no problems expected.

Discontinuing:
May be unnecessary to finish medicine. Follow doctor's instructions.

Others:
Advise any doctor or dentist whom you consult that you take this medicine.

POSSIBLE INTERACTION WITH OTHER DRUGS

GENERIC NAME OR DRUG CLASS	COMBINED EFFECT
Amantadine	Increased belladonna effect.
Anticholinergics, other*	Increased belladonna effect.
Antidepressants, tricyclic (TCA)*	Increased belladonna effect. Increased sedation.
Antihistamines*	Increased belladonna effect.
Attapulgite	Decreased belladonna effect.
Cortisone drugs*	Increased internal eye pressure.
Guanethidine	Decreased belladonna effect.
Haloperidol	Increased internal eye pressure.
Ketoconazole	Decreased ketoconazole effect.
MAO inhibitors*	Increased belladonna effect.
Meperidine	Increased belladonna effect.
Methylphenidate	Increased belladonna effect.
Metoclopramide	May decrease metoclopramide effect.
Molindone	Increased anticholinergic effect.
Nitrates*	Increased internal eye pressure.
Nizatidine	Increased nizatidine effect.
Orphenadrine	Increased belladonna effect.
Phenothiazines*	Increased belladonna effect.
Pilocarpine	Loss of pilocarpine effect in glaucoma treatment.
Potassium supplements*	Possible intestinal ulcers with oral potassium tablets.
Quinidine	Increased belladonna effect.
Reserpine	Decreased belladonna effect.
Sedatives* or central nervous system (CNS) depressants*	Increased sedative effect of both drugs.
Vitamin C	Decreased belladonna effect. Avoid large doses of vitamin C.

POSSIBLE INTERACTION WITH OTHER SUBSTANCES

INTERACTS WITH	COMBINED EFFECT
Alcohol:	None expected.
Beverages:	None expected.
Cocaine:	Excessively rapid heartbeat. Avoid.
Foods:	None expected.
Marijuana:	Drowsiness and dry mouth.
Tobacco:	None expected.

*See Glossary

BELLADONNA ALKALOIDS & BARBITURATES

BRAND AND GENERIC NAMES

See complete list of brand and generic names in the *Brand Name Directory,* page 914.

BASIC INFORMATION

Habit forming? Yes
Prescription needed? Yes
Available as generic? Some yes, some no
Drug class: Antispasmodic, anticholinergic, sedative

 USES

- Reduces spasms of digestive system, bladder and urethra.
- Reduces anxiety or nervous tension (low dose).
- Relieves insomnia (higher bedtime dose).

 DOSAGE & USAGE INFORMATION

How to take:
- Tablet, liquid or capsule—Swallow with liquid or food to lessen stomach irritation. If you can't swallow whole, crumble tablet or open capsule and take with liquid or food.
- Extended-release tablets or capsules— Swallow each dose whole.
- Chewable tablets—Chew well before swallowing.
- Drops—Dilute dose in beverage before swallowing.

When to take:
At the same times each day.

If you forget a dose:
Take as soon as you remember up to 2 hours late. If more than 2 hours, wait for next scheduled dose (don't double this dose).

Continued next column

 OVERDOSE

SYMPTOMS:
Blurred vision, confusion, convulsions, irregular heartbeat, hallucinations, coma.
WHAT TO DO:
- **Dial 0 (operator) or 911 (emergency) for an ambulance or medical help. Then give first aid immediately.**
- **See emergency information on inside covers.**

What drug does:
- May partially block nerve impulses at nerve-cell connections.
- Blocks nerve impulses at parasympathetic nerve endings, preventing muscle contractions and gland secretions of organs involved.

Time lapse before drug works:
15 to 30 minutes.

Don't take with:
- Antacids* or antidiarrheals*.
- Any other medicine without consulting your doctor or pharmacist.

 POSSIBLE ADVERSE REACTIONS OR SIDE EFFECTS

SYMPTOMS	WHAT TO DO
Life-threatening:	
Unusual excitement, restlessness, fast heartbeat, breathing difficulty.	Seek emergency treatment immediately.
Common:	
• Dry mouth, throat, nose; drowsiness; constipation; dizziness; nausea; vomiting; ''hangover'' effect; depression; confusion.	Discontinue. Call doctor right away.
• Reduced sweating, slurred speech, agitation, nasal congestion, altered taste.	Continue. Call doctor when convenient.
Infrequent:	
Difficult urination; difficult swallowing; rash or hives; face, lip or eyelid swelling; joint or muscle pain; lightheadedness.	Discontinue. Call doctor right away.
Rare:	
Jaundice; unusual bruising or bleeding; hives, skin rash; pain in eyes; blurred vision; sore throat, fever, mouth sores; unexplained bleeding or bruising.	Discontinue. Call doctor right away.

WARNINGS & PRECAUTIONS

Don't take if:
- You are allergic to any barbiturate or any anticholinergic.
- You have porphyria, trouble with stomach bloating, difficulty emptying your bladder completely, narrow-angle glaucoma, severe ulcerative colitis.

Before you start, consult your doctor:
- If you have open-angle glaucoma, angina, chronic bronchitis or asthma, hiatal hernia, liver disease, enlarged prostate, myasthenia gravis, peptic ulcer, epilepsy, kidney or liver damage, anemia, chronic pain, thyroid disease.
- If you will have surgery within 2 months, including dental surgery, requiring general or spinal anesthesia.

Over age 60:
Adverse reactions and side effects may be more frequent and severe than in younger persons. Ask your doctor about small doses.

Pregnancy:
Risk to unborn child outweighs drug benefits. Don't use.

Breast-feeding:
Drug passes into milk. Avoid drug or discontinue nursing until you finish medicine.

Infants & children:
Use only under doctor's supervision.

Prolonged use:
- May cause addiction, anemia, chronic intoxication.
- May lower body temperature, making exposure to cold temperatures hazardous.

Skin & sunlight:
May cause rash or intensify sunburn in areas exposed to sun or sunlamp.

Driving, piloting or hazardous work:
Don't drive or pilot aircraft until you learn how medicine affects you. Don't work around dangerous machinery. Don't climb ladders or work in high places. Danger increases if you drink alcohol or take medicine affecting alertness and reflexes.

Discontinuing:
May be unnecessary to finish medicine. Follow doctor's instructions. If you develop withdrawal symptoms of hallucinations, agitation or sleeplessness after discontinuing, call doctor right away.

Others:
- Great potential for abuse.
- Advise any doctor or dentist whom you consult that you take this medicine.

POSSIBLE INTERACTION WITH OTHER DRUGS

GENERIC NAME OR DRUG CLASS	COMBINED EFFECT
Acetaminophen	Possible decreased barbiturate effect.
Amantadine	Increased belladonna effect.
Anticoagulants, oral*	Decreased anti-coagulant effect.
Anticholinergics, other*	Increased belladonna effect.
Anticonvulsants*	Changed seizure patterns.
Antidepressants, tricyclics (TCA)*	Possible dangerous oversedation. Avoid.
Antidiabetics, oral*	Increased barbiturate effect.
Antihistamines*	Dangerous sedation. Avoid.
Aspirin	Decreased aspirin effect.
Attapulgite	Decreased belladonna effect.
Beta-adrenergic blockers*	Decreased effects of beta-adrenergic blocker.
Carteolol	Increased barbiturate effect. Dangerous sedation.

Continued page 936

POSSIBLE INTERACTION WITH OTHER SUBSTANCES

INTERACTS WITH	COMBINED EFFECT
Alcohol:	Possible fatal oversedation. Avoid.
Beverages:	None expected.
Cocaine:	Excessively rapid heartbeat. Avoid.
Foods:	None expected.
Marijuana:	Drowsiness and dry mouth. Avoid.
Tobacco:	Decreased effectiveness of acid reduction in stomach.

*See Glossary

BENZODIAZEPINES

BRAND AND GENERIC NAMES

See complete list of brand and generic names in the *Brand Names Directory*, page 915.

BASIC INFORMATION

Habit forming? Yes
Prescription needed? Yes
Available as generic? Yes, for most.
Drug class: Tranquilizer (benzodiazepine)

 ## USES

- Treatment for nervousness or tension.
- Treatment for muscle spasm.
- Treatment for convulsive disorders.
- Treatment for insomnia.

 ## DOSAGE & USAGE INFORMATION

How to take:
- Tablet, extended-release capsule or liquid— Swallow with liquid.
- Sublingual tablet—Do not chew or swallow. Place under tongue until dissolved.

When to take:
At the same time each day, according to instructions on prescription label.

If you forget a dose:
Take as soon as you remember up to 2 hours late. If more than 2 hours, wait for next scheduled dose (don't double this dose).

What drug does:
Affects limbic system of brain, the part that controls emotions.

Time lapse before drug works:
2 hours. May take 6 weeks for full benefit.

Continued next column

 ## OVERDOSE

SYMPTOMS:
Drowsiness, weakness, tremor, stupor, coma.
WHAT TO DO:
- **Dial 0 (operator) or 911 (emergency) for an ambulance or medical help. Then give first aid immediately.**
- **If patient is unconscious and not breathing, give mouth-to-mouth breathing. If there is no heartbeat, use cardiac massage and mouth-to-mouth breathing (CPR). Don't try to make patient vomit. If you can't get help quickly, take patient to nearest emergency facility.**
- **See emergency information on inside covers.**

Don't take with:
Any other medicine without consulting your doctor or pharmacist.

 ## POSSIBLE ADVERSE REACTIONS OR SIDE EFFECTS

SYMPTOMS	WHAT TO DO
Life-threatening:	
In case of overdose, see previous column.	
Common:	
Clumsiness, drowsiness, dizziness.	Continue. Call doctor when convenient.
Infrequent:	
• Hallucinations, confusion, depression, irritability, rash, itch, vision changes, sore throat, fever, chills, dry mouth.	Discontinue. Call doctor right away.
• Constipation or diarrhea, nausea, vomiting, difficult urination, vivid dreams, behavior changes, abdominal pain, headache.	Continue. Call doctor when convenient.
Rare:	
• Slow heartbeat, breathing difficulty.	Discontinue. Seek emergency treatment.
• Mouth, throat ulcers; jaundice.	Discontinue. Call doctor right away.
• Decreased sex drive.	Continue. Call doctor when convenient.

 ## WARNINGS & PRECAUTIONS

Don't take if:
- You are allergic to any benzodiazepine.
- You have myasthenia gravis.
- You are an active or recovering alcoholic.
- Patient is younger than 6 months.

Before you start, consult your doctor:
- If you have liver, kidney or lung disease.
- If you have diabetes, epilepsy or porphyria.
- If you have glaucoma.

Over age 60:
Adverse reactions and side effects may be more frequent and severe than in younger persons. You may need smaller doses for shorter periods of time. You may develop agitation, rage or "hangover" effect.

Pregnancy:
Risk to unborn child outweighs drug benefits. Don't use.

Breast-feeding:
Drug passes into milk. Avoid drug or discontinue nursing until you finish medicine. Consult doctor for advice on maintaining milk supply.

Infants & children:
Use only under medical supervision for children older than 6 months.

Prolonged use:
May impair liver function.

Skin & sunlight:
No problems expected.

Driving, piloting or hazardous work:
Don't drive or pilot aircraft until you learn how medicine affects you. Don't work around dangerous machinery. Don't climb ladders or work in high places. Danger increases if you drink alcohol or take medicine affecting alertness and reflexes.

Discontinuing:
Don't discontinue without consulting doctor. Dose may require gradual reduction if you have taken drug for a long time. Doses of other drugs may also require adjustment.

Others:
- Hot weather, heavy exercise and profuse sweat may reduce excretion and cause overdose.
- Blood sugar may rise in diabetics, requiring insulin adjustment.
- Don't use for insomnia more than 4-7 days.
- Advise any doctor or dentist whom you consult that you take this medicine.

POSSIBLE INTERACTION WITH OTHER DRUGS

GENERIC NAME OR DRUG CLASS	COMBINED EFFECT
Anticonvulsants*	Change in seizure frequency or severity.
Antidepressants*	Increased sedative effect of both drugs.
Antihistamines*	Increased sedative effect of both drugs.
Antihypertensives*	Excessively low blood pressure.
Clozapine	Toxic effect on the central nervous system.
Contraceptives, oral*	Increased benzodiazepine effect.
Disulfiram	Increased benzodiazepine effect.
Dronabinol	Increased effects of both drugs. Avoid.
Erythromycins*	Increased benzodiazepine effect.
Ketoconazole	Increased benzodiazepine effect.
Levodopa	Possible decreased levodopa effect.
MAO inhibitors*	Convulsions, deep sedation, rage.
Molindone	Increased tranquilizer effect.
Nabilone	Greater depression of central nervous system.
Narcotics*	Increased sedative effect of both drugs.
Nicotine	Increased benzodiazepine effect.
Nizatidine	Increased effect and toxicity of benzodiazepine.
Omeprazole	Delayed excretion of benzodiazepine causing increased amount of benzodiazepine in blood.
Probenecid	Increased benzodiazepine effect.
Sedatives*	Increased sedative effect of both drugs.
Sertraline	Increased depressive effects of both drugs.
Sleep inducers*	Increased sedative effect of both drugs.
Tranquilizers*	Increased sedative effect of both drugs.
Zidovudine	Increased toxicity of zidovudine.

POSSIBLE INTERACTION WITH OTHER SUBSTANCES

INTERACTS WITH	COMBINED EFFECT
Alcohol:	Heavy sedation. Avoid.
Beverages:	None expected.
Cocaine:	Decreased benzodiazepine effect.
Foods:	None expected.
Marijuana:	Heavy sedation. Avoid.
Tobacco:	Decreased benzodiazepine effect.

BENZOYL PEROXIDE

BRAND NAMES

See complete list of brand names in the *Brand Name Directory*, page 915.

BASIC INFORMATION

Habit forming? No
Prescription needed? No
Available as generic? Yes
Drug class: Anti-acne (topical)

 ## USES

- Treatment for acne.
- Treats pressure sores.

 ## DOSAGE & USAGE INFORMATION

How to use:
Cream, gel, pads, sticks, lotion, cleansing bar or facial mask—Wash affected area with plain soap and water. Dry gently with towel. Rub medicine into affected areas. Keep away from eyes, nose, mouth.

When to use:
Apply 1 or more times daily. If you have a fair complexion, start with single application at bedtime.

If you forget an application:
Use as soon as you remember.

What drug does:
Slowly releases oxygen from skin, which controls some skin bacteria. Also causes peeling and drying, helping control blackheads and whiteheads.

Time lapse before drug works:
1 to 2 weeks.

Don't use with:
Any other medicine without consulting your doctor or pharmacist.

 ## OVERDOSE

SYMPTOMS:
None expected.
WHAT TO DO:
- **If person swallows drug, call doctor, poison-control center or hospital emergency room for instructions.**
- **See emergency information on inside covers.**

 ## POSSIBLE ADVERSE REACTIONS OR SIDE EFFECTS

SYMPTOMS	WHAT TO DO
Life-threatening: None expected.	
Common: None expected.	
Infrequent: • Rash, excessive dryness, peeling skin.	Discontinue. Call doctor right away.
• Painful skin irritation.	Continue. Call doctor when convenient.
Rare: None expected.	

132

WARNINGS & PRECAUTIONS

Don't take if:
You are allergic to benzoyl peroxide.

Before you start, consult your doctor:
- If you plan to become pregnant within medication period.
- If you take oral contraceptives.
- If you are using any other prescription or non-prescription medicine for acne.
- If you are using abrasive skin cleansers or medicated cosmetics.

Over age 60:
No problems expected.

Pregnancy:
No proven problems. Consult doctor.

Breast-feeding:
No proven problems. Consult doctor.

Infants & children:
Not recommended.

Prolonged use:
Permanent rash or scarring.

Skin & sunlight:
No problems expected.

Driving, piloting or hazardous work:
No problems expected.

Discontinuing:
- May be unnecessary to finish medicine. Discontinue when acne improves.
- If acne doesn't improve in 2 weeks, call doctor.

Others:
- Keep away from hair and clothing. May bleach.
- Store away from heat in cool, dry place.
- Avoid contact with eyes, lips, nose and sensitive areas of the neck.

POSSIBLE INTERACTION WITH OTHER DRUGS

GENERIC NAME OR DRUG CLASS	COMBINED EFFECT
Antiacne topical preparations, other	Excessive skin irritation.
Skin-peeling agents (salicylic acid, sulfur, resorcinol, tretinoin)	Excessive skin irritation.

POSSIBLE INTERACTION WITH OTHER SUBSTANCES

INTERACTS WITH	COMBINED EFFECT
Alcohol:	None expected.
Beverages:	None expected.
Cocaine:	None expected.
Foods: Cinnamon, foods with benzoic acid.	Skin rash.
Marijuana:	None expected.
Tobacco:	None expected.

BETA-ADRENERGIC BLOCKERS

BRAND AND GENERIC NAMES

See complete list of brand and generic names in the *Brand Names Directory*, page 915.

BASIC INFORMATION

Habit forming? No
Prescription needed? Yes
Available as generic? Yes, for some.
Drug class: Beta-adrenergic blocker

USES

- Reduces angina attacks.
- Stabilizes irregular heartbeat.
- Lowers blood pressure.
- Reduces frequency of vascular headaches. (Does not relieve headache pain.)
- Other uses prescribed by your doctor.

DOSAGE & USAGE INFORMATION

How to take:
Tablet, liquid or extended-release capsule— Swallow with liquid. If you can't swallow whole, crumble tablet or open capsule and take with liquid or food. Don't crush capsule or extended-release tablet.

When to take:
With meals or immediately after.

If you forget a dose:
Take as soon as you remember. Return to regular schedule, but allow 3 hours between doses.

What drug does:
- Blocks certain actions of sympathetic nervous system.
- Lowers heart's oxygen requirements.
- Slows nerve impulses through heart.
- Reduces blood vessel contraction in heart, scalp and other body parts.

Continued next column

OVERDOSE

SYMPTOMS:
Weakness, slow or weak pulse, blood-pressure drop, fainting, difficulty breathing, convulsions, cold and sweaty skin.
WHAT TO DO:
- **Dial 0 (operator) or 911 (emergency) for an ambulance or medical help. Then give first aid immediately.**
- **See emergency information on inside covers.**

Time lapse before drug works:
1 to 4 hours.

Don't take with:
Non-prescription drugs or drugs in Interaction column without consulting doctor.

POSSIBLE ADVERSE REACTIONS OR SIDE EFFECTS

SYMPTOMS	WHAT TO DO
Life-threatening:	
Congestive heart failure (severe shortness of breath, rapid heartbeat).	Discontinue. Seek emergency treatment.
Common:	
• Pulse slower than 50 beats per minute.	Discontinue. Call doctor right away.
• Drowsiness, fatigue, numbness or tingling of fingers or toes, dizziness, diarrhea, nausea, weakness.	Continue. Call doctor when convenient.
• Cold hands or feet; dry mouth, eyes and skin.	Continue. Tell doctor at next visit.
Infrequent:	
• Hallucinations, nightmares, insomnia, headache, difficult breathing, joint pain, anxiety, chest pain.	Discontinue. Call doctor right away.
• Confusion, reduced alertness, depression, impotence, abdominal pain.	Continue. Call doctor when convenient.
• Constipation.	Continue. Tell doctor at next visit.
Rare:	
• Rash, sore throat, fever.	Discontinue. Call doctor right away.
• Unusual bleeding and bruising; dry, burning eyes.	Continue. Call doctor when convenient.

BETA-ADRENERGIC BLOCKERS

WARNINGS & PRECAUTIONS

Don't take if:
- You are allergic to any beta-adrenergic blocker.
- You have asthma.
- You have hay fever symptoms.
- You have taken MAO inhibitors in past 2 weeks.

Before you start, consult your doctor:
- If you have heart disease or poor circulation to the extremities.
- If you have hay fever, asthma, chronic bronchitis, emphysema.
- If you have overactive thyroid function.
- If you have impaired liver or kidney function.
- If you will have surgery within 2 months, including dental surgery, requiring general or spinal anesthesia.
- If you have diabetes or hypoglycemia.

Over age 60:
Adverse reactions and side effects may be more frequent and severe than in younger persons.

Pregnancy:
Risk to unborn child outweighs drug benefits. Don't use.

Breast-feeding:
Drug passes into milk. Avoid drug or discontinue nursing until you finish medicine. Consult doctor for advice on maintaining milk supply.

Infants & children:
Not recommended.

Prolonged use:
- Weakens heart muscle contractions.
- Talk to your doctor about the need for follow-up medical examinations or laboratory studies to check blood pressure, ECG*, kidney function, blood sugar.

Skin & sunlight:
No problems expected.

Driving, piloting or hazardous work:
Don't drive or pilot aircraft until you learn how medicine affects you. Don't work around dangerous machinery. Don't climb ladders or work in high places. Danger increases if you drink alcohol or take medicine affecting alertness and reflexes.

Discontinuing:
Don't discontinue without consulting doctor. Dose may require gradual reduction if you have taken drug for a long time. Doses of other drugs may also require adjustment.

Others:
- May mask hypoglycemia.
- May affect results in some medical tests. Advise any doctor or dentist whom you consult that you take this medicine.

POSSIBLE INTERACTION WITH OTHER DRUGS

GENERIC NAME OR DRUG CLASS	COMBINED EFFECT
ACE inhibitors*: captopril, enalapril, lisinopril	Increased antihypertensive effects of both drugs. Dosages may require adjustment.
Antidiabetics*	Increased antidiabetic effect.
Antihistamines*	Decreased antihistamine effect.
Antihypertensives*	Increased antihypertensive effect.
Barbiturates*	Increased barbiturate effect. Dangerous sedation.
Beta-agonists*	Decreased beta-agonist effect.
Betaxolol eyedrops	Possible increased beta blocker effect.
Calcium channel blockers*	Additional blood pressure drop.
Clonidine	Additional blood pressure drop.
Diazoxide	Additional blood pressure drop.
Dextrothyroxine	Possible decreased beta blocker effect.
Digitalis preparations*	Can either increase or decrease heart rate. Improves irregular heartbeat.

Continued page 937

POSSIBLE INTERACTION WITH OTHER SUBSTANCES

INTERACTS WITH	COMBINED EFFECT
Alcohol:	Excessive blood pressure drop. Avoid.
Beverages:	None expected.
Cocaine:	Irregular heartbeat; decreased beta-adrenergic effect. Avoid.
Foods:	None expected.
Marijuana:	Daily use—Impaired circulation to hands and feet.
Tobacco:	Possible irregular heartbeat.

BETA-ADRENERGIC BLOCKING AGENTS & THIAZIDE DIURETICS

BRAND AND GENERIC NAMES

See complete list of brand and generic names in the *Brand Names Directory*, page 916.

BASIC INFORMATION

Habit forming? No
Prescription needed? Yes
Available as generic? Yes
Drug class: Beta-adrenergic blocker,
diuretic (thiazide)

USES

- Controls, but doesn't cure, high blood pressure.
- Reduces fluid retention (edema).
- Reduces angina attacks.
- Stabilizes irregular heartbeat.
- Lowers blood pressure.
- Reduces frequency of migraine headaches. (Does not relieve headache pain.)
- Other uses prescribed by your doctor.

DOSAGE & USAGE INFORMATION

How to take:
Extended-release capsules—Swallow with liquid. If you can't swallow whole, open capsule and take with liquid or food.

When to take:
At the same time each day.

If you forget a dose:
Take as soon as you remember up to 4 hours late. If more than 4 hours, wait for next scheduled dose (don't double this dose).

What drug does:
- Forces sodium and water excretion, reducing body fluid.
- Relaxes muscle cells of small arteries.
- Reduced body fluid and relaxed arteries lower blood pressure.

Continued next column

OVERDOSE

SYMPTOMS:
Irregular heartbeat (usually too slow), seizures, confusion, fainting, convulsions, coma.
WHAT TO DO:
- **Dial 0 (operator) or 911 (emergency) for an ambulance or medical help. Then give first aid immediately.**
- **See emergency information on inside covers.**

- Blocks some of the actions of sympathetic nervous system.
- Lowers heart's oxygen requirements.
- Slows nerve impulses through heart.
- Reduces blood vessel contraction in heart, scalp and other body parts.

Time lapse before drug works:
- 1 to 4 hours for beta-blocker effect.
- May require several weeks to lower blood pressure.

Don't take with:
Any other medicines, even over-the-counter drugs such as cough/cold medicines, diet pills, nose drops, caffeine, without consulting your doctor.

POSSIBLE ADVERSE REACTIONS OR SIDE EFFECTS

SYMPTOMS	WHAT TO DO
Life-threatening:	
Wheezing, chest pain, seizures, irregular heartbeat.	Seek emergency treatment immediately.
Common:	
• Dry mouth, weak pulse, vomiting, muscle cramps, increased thirst, mood changes, nausea.	Discontinue. Call doctor right away.
• Weakness, tiredness, dizziness, mental depression, diminished sex drive, constipation, nightmares, insomnia.	Continue. Call doctor when convenient.
Infrequent:	
• Cold feet and hands, chest pain, breathing difficulty, anxiety, nervousness, headache, appetite loss, abdominal pain, numbness and tingling in fingers and toes, slow heartbeat.	Discontinue. Call doctor right away.
• Confusion, diarrhea.	Continue. Call doctor when convenient.
Rare:	
• Hives, skin rash; joint pain; jaundice; fever, sore throat, mouth ulcers.	Discontinue. Call doctor right away.
• Impotence, back pain.	Continue. Call doctor when convenient.

BETA-ADRENERGIC BLOCKING AGENTS & THIAZIDE DIURETICS

WARNINGS & PRECAUTIONS

Don't take if:
- You are allergic to any beta-adrenergic blocker or any thiazide diuretic drug.
- You have asthma or hay fever symptoms.
- You have taken MAO inhibitors in past two weeks.

Before you start, consult your doctor:
- If you have heart disease or poor circulation to the extremities.
- If you have hay fever, asthma, chronic bronchitis, emphysema, overactive thyroid function, impaired liver or kidney function, gout, diabetes, hypoglycemia, pancreas disorder, systemic lupus erythematosus.
- If you are allergic to any sulfa drug or tartrazine dye.
- If you will have surgery within 2 months, including dental surgery, requiring general or spinal anesthesia.

Over age 60:
Adverse reactions and side effects may be more frequent and severe than in younger persons, especially dizziness and excessive potassium loss.

Pregnancy:
Risk to unborn child outweighs drug benefits. Don't use.

Breast-feeding:
Drug passes into milk. Avoid drug or discontinue nursing until you finish medicine. Consult doctor for advice on maintaining milk supply.

Infants & children:
Not recommended.

Prolonged use:
- Weakens heart muscle contractions.
- You may need medicine to treat high blood pressure for the rest of your life.
- Talk to your doctor about the need for follow-up medical examinations or laboratory studies.

Skin & sunlight:
May cause rash or intensify sunburn in areas exposed to sun or sunlamp.

Driving, piloting or hazardous work:
Don't drive or pilot aircraft until you learn how medicine affects you. Don't work around dangerous machinery. Don't climb ladders or work in high places. Danger increases if you drink alcohol or take medicine affecting alertness and reflexes, such as antihistamines, tranquilizers, sedatives, pain medicine, narcotics and mind-altering drugs.

Discontinuing:
Don't discontinue without consulting doctor. Dose may require gradual reduction if you have taken drug for a long time. Doses of other drugs may also require adjustment.

Others:
- May mask hypoglycemia symptoms.
- Hot weather and fever may cause dehydration and drop in blood pressure. Dose may require temporary adjustment. Weigh daily and report any unexpected weight decreases to your doctor.
- May cause rise in uric acid, leading to gout.
- May cause blood-sugar rise in diabetics.

POSSIBLE INTERACTION WITH OTHER DRUGS

GENERIC NAME OR DRUG CLASS	COMBINED EFFECT
Allopurinol	Decreased allopurinol effect.
Antidepressants, tricyclic (TCA)*	Dangerous drop in blood pressure. Avoid combination unless under medical supervision.
Antidiabetics*	Increased antidiabetic effect.
Antihistamines*	Decreased antihistamine effect.

Continued page 937

POSSIBLE INTERACTION WITH OTHER SUBSTANCES

INTERACTS WITH	COMBINED EFFECT
Alcohol:	Dangerous blood pressure drop. Avoid.
Beverages:	None expected.
Cocaine:	Irregular heartbeat, decreased beta blocker effect. Avoid.
Foods: Licorice.	Excessive potassium loss that causes dangerous heart rhythms.
Marijuana:	May increase blood pressure.
Tobacco:	May increase blood pressure and make heart work harder. Avoid.

BETA CAROTENE

BRAND NAMES

Solatene
Numerous multiple vitamin and mineral supplements. Check labels.

BASIC INFORMATION

Habit forming? No
Prescription needed? No
Available as generic? No
Drug class: Nutritional supplement

 ## USES

- Used as a nutritional supplement.
- Prevents night blindness.
- Used as an adjunct to the treatment of steatorrhea, chronic fever, obstructive jaundice, pancreatic insufficiency, protein deficiency, total parenteral nutrition and photosensitivity in photo porphyria.

 ## DOSAGE & USAGE INFORMATION

How to take:
Tablet or capsule—Swallow with liquid. If you can't swallow whole, crumble tablet or open capsule and take with liquid or food.

When to take:
At the same time each day, according to directions on package or prescription label.

If you forget a dose:
Take as soon as you remember (don't double this dose).

What drug does:
Enables the body to manufacture vitamin A, which is essential for the normal functioning of the retina, normal growth and development and normal testicular and ovarian function.

Time lapse before drug works:
Total effect may take several weeks.

Don't take with:
No restrictions.

 ## OVERDOSE

SYMPTOMS:
Yellow skin
WHAT TO DO:
Overdose unlikely to threaten life. If person takes much larger amount than prescribed, call doctor, poison-control center or hospital emergency room for instructions.

 ## POSSIBLE ADVERSE REACTIONS OR SIDE EFFECTS

SYMPTOMS	WHAT TO DO
Life-threatening: None expected.	
Common: Yellow palms, hands, soles of feet.	Continue. Call doctor when convenient.
Infrequent: None expected.	
Rare: • Joint pain, unusual bleeding or bruising.	Discontinue. Call doctor right away.
• Diarrhea, dizziness.	Continue. Call doctor when convenient.

WARNINGS & PRECAUTIONS

Don't take if:
You are hypersensitive to beta carotene

Before you start, consult your doctor:
- If you have liver or kidney disease.
- If you have hypervitaminosis*.

Over age 60:
No problems expected.

Pregnancy:
No problems expected.

Breast-feeding:
No problems expected.

Infants & children:
No problems expected.

Prolonged use:
No problems expected.

Skin & sunlight:
Beta carotene is not a sunscreen.

Driving, piloting or hazardous work:
No special problems expected.

Discontinuing:
No special problems expected.

Others:
- Some researchers claim that beta carotene may reduce the occurrence of some cancers. There is insufficient data to substantiate this claim.
- May affect results of some medical tests.

 ## POSSIBLE INTERACTION WITH OTHER DRUGS

GENERIC NAME OR DRUG CLASS	COMBINED EFFECT
Cholestyramine	Decreased absorption of beta carotene.
Colestipol	Decreased absorption of beta carotene.
Mineral oil	Decreased absorption of beta carotene.
Neomycin	Decreased absorption of beta carotene.

 ## POSSIBLE INTERACTION WITH OTHER SUBSTANCES

INTERACTS WITH	COMBINED EFFECT
Alcohol:	None expected.
Beverages:	None expected.
Cocaine:	None expected.
Foods:	None expected.
Marijuana:	None expected.
Tobacco:	None expected.

BETAMETHASONE

BRAND NAMES

See complete list of brand names in the *Brand Name Directory*, page 916.

BASIC INFORMATION

Habit forming? No
Prescription needed? Yes
Available as generic? Yes
Drug class: Cortisone drug (adrenal corticosteroid)

 ## USES

- Reduces inflammation caused by many different medical problems.
- Treatment for some allergic diseases, blood disorders, kidney diseases, asthma and emphysema.
- Replaces corticosteroid deficiencies.

 ## DOSAGE & USAGE INFORMATION

How to take:
- Tablet, extended-release tablet, syrup or liquid—Swallow with liquid or food to lessen stomach irritation. If you can't swallow whole, crumble tablet and take with liquid or food.
- Inhaler—Follow label instructions.

When to take:
At the same times each day. Take once-a-day or once-every-other-day doses in mornings.

If you forget a dose:
- Several-doses-per-day prescription—Take as soon as you remember up to 2 hours late. If more than 2 hours, wait for next scheduled dose (don't double this dose).
- Once-a-day dose or less—Wait for next dose. Double this dose.

What drug does:
Decreases inflammatory responses.

Time lapse before drug works:
2 to 4 days.

Continued in next column

 ## OVERDOSE

SYMPTOMS:
Headache, convulsions, heart failure.
WHAT TO DO:
- **Dial 0 (operator) or 911 (emergency) for an ambulance or medical help. Then give first aid immediately.**
- **See emergency information on inside covers.**

Don't take with:
Any other medicine without consulting your doctor or pharmacist.

 ## POSSIBLE ADVERSE REACTIONS OR SIDE EFFECTS

SYMPTOMS	WHAT TO DO
Life-threatening:	
In case of overdose, see previous column.	
Common:	
Acne, poor wound healing, thirst, indigestion, nausea, vomiting, constipation, gaseousness, unpleasant taste, diarrhea, headache, cough, dizziness, hoarseness, appetite loss.	Continue. Call doctor when convenient.
Infrequent:	
• Bloody or black, tarry stool; various infections; swallowing difficulty; hives.	Discontinue. Seek emergency treatment.
• Blurred vision, halos around lights, sore throat, fever, abdominal pain.	Discontinue. Call doctor right away.
• Mood changes, insomnia, fatigue, restlessness, frequent urination, weight gain, round face, weakness, menstrual irregularities, dry mouth, euphoria, nosebleed.	Continue. Call doctor when convenient.
Rare:	
• Irregular heartbeat.	Discontinue. Seek emergency treatment.
• Rash, TB recurrence.	Discontinue. Call doctor right away.

 ## WARNINGS & PRECAUTIONS

Don't take if:
- You are allergic to any cortisone drug.
- You have tuberculosis or fungus infection.
- You have herpes infection of eyes, lips or genitals.
- You have bone disease, thyroid disease, colitis, stomach ulcer, diabetes, myasthenia gravis, liver or kidney disease, diverticulitis, glaucoma, heart disease.

Before you start, consult your doctor:
- If you are taking any other prescription or non-prescription medicine.
- If you have had tuberculosis.

- If you have an infection, congestive heart failure, diabetes, peptic ulcer, glaucoma, underactive thyroid, high blood pressure, myasthenia gravis, blood clots in legs or lungs.

Over age 60:
Adverse reactions and side effects may be more frequent and severe than in younger persons. Likely to aggravate edema, diabetes or ulcers. Likely to cause cataracts and osteoporosis (softening of the bones).

Pregnancy:
Risk to unborn child outweighs drug benefits. Don't use.

Breast-feeding:
Drug passes into milk. Avoid drug or discontinue nursing until you finish medicine. Consult doctor for advice on maintaining milk supply.

Infants & children:
Use only under medical supervision.

Prolonged use:
- Retards growth in children.
- Possible glaucoma, cataracts, diabetes, fragile bones and thin skin.
- Functional dependence.
- Talk to your doctor about the need for follow-up medical examinations or laboratory studies to check blood pressure, stools for blood, serum electrolytes.

Skin & sunlight:
No problems expected.

Driving, piloting or hazardous work:
No problems expected.

Discontinuing:
- Don't discontinue without doctor's advice until you complete prescribed dose, even though symptoms diminish or disappear.
- Drug affects your response to surgery, illness, injury or stress for up to 2 years after discontinuing. Inform doctor.

Others:
- Avoid immunizations if possible.
- Your resistance to infection is less while taking this medicine.
- Advise any doctor or dentist whom you consult that you take this medicine.

 ## POSSIBLE INTERACTION WITH OTHER DRUGS

GENERIC NAME OR DRUG CLASS	COMBINED EFFECT
Amphotericin B	Potassium depletion.
Anticholinergics*	Possible glaucoma.
Anticoagulants, oral*	Decreased anti-coagulant effect.
Anticonvulsants, hydantoin*	Decreased beta-methasone effect.
Antidiabetics, oral*	Decreased anti-diabetic effect.
Antihistamines*	Decreased beta-methasone effect.
Aspirin	Increased beta-methasone effect.
Barbiturates*	Decreased beta-methasone effect. Oversedation.
Beta-adrenergic blockers*	Decreased beta-methasone effect.
Butmetanide	Potassium depletion.
Chloral hydrate	Decreased beta-methasone effect.
Chlorthalidone	Potassium depletion.
Cholestyramine	Decreased beta-methasone effect.
Cholinergics*	Decreased cholinergic effect.
Colestipol	Decreased beta-methasone effect.
Contraceptives, oral*	Increased beta-methasone effect.
Cyclosporine	May increase cyclosporine effect.
Digitalis preparations*	Dangerous potassium depletion. Possible digitalis toxicity.
Diuretics, thiazide*	Potassium depletion.

Continued page 938

 ## POSSIBLE INTERACTION WITH OTHER SUBSTANCES

INTERACTS WITH	COMBINED EFFECT
Alcohol:	Risk of stomach ulcers.
Beverages:	No proven problems.
Cocaine:	Overstimulation. Avoid.
Foods:	No proven problems.
Marijuana:	Decreased immunity.
Tobacco:	Increased beta-methasone effect. Possible toxicity.

BETHANECHOL

BRAND NAMES

Duvoid   Urecholine
Urabeth

BASIC INFORMATION

Habit forming? No
Prescription needed? Yes
Available as generic? Yes
Drug class: Cholinergic

 USES

- Helps initiate urination following surgery, or for persons with urinary infections or enlarged prostate.
- Treats reflux esophagitis.

 DOSAGE & USAGE INFORMATION

How to take:
Tablet—Swallow with liquid, 1 hour before or 2 hours after eating.

When to take:
At the same times each day.

If you forget a dose:
Take as soon as you remember up to 2 hours late. If more than 2 hours, wait for next scheduled dose (don't double this dose).

What drug does:
Affects chemical reactions in the body that strengthen bladder muscles.

Continued next column

 OVERDOSE

SYMPTOMS:
Shortness of breath, wheezing or chest tightness, unconsciousness, coma.
WHAT TO DO:
- **Dial 0 (operator) or 911 (emergency) for an ambulance or medical help. Then give first aid immediately.**
- **If patient is unconscious and not breathing, give mouth-to-mouth breathing. If there is no heartbeat, use cardiac massage and mouth-to-mouth breathing (CPR). Don't try to make patient vomit. If you can't get help quickly, take patient to nearest emergency facility.**
- **See emergency information on inside covers.**

Time lapse before drug works:
30 to 90 minutes.

Don't take with:
Any other medicine without consulting your doctor or pharmacist.

 POSSIBLE ADVERSE REACTIONS OR SIDE EFFECTS

SYMPTOMS	WHAT TO DO
Life-threatening:	
In case of overdose, see previous column.	
Common:	
None expected.	
Infrequent:	
Dizziness, headache, faintness, blurred or changed vision, diarrhea, nausea, vomiting, stomach discomfort, belching, excessive urge to urinate.	Continue. Call doctor when convenient.
Rare:	
Shortness of breath, wheezing, tightness in chest.	Discontinue. Call doctor right away.

WARNINGS & PRECAUTIONS

Don't take if:
You are allergic to any cholinergic.

Before you start, consult your doctor:
- If you plan to become pregnant within medication period.
- If you have asthma.
- If you have epilepsy.
- If you have heart or blood-vessel disease.
- If you have high or low blood pressure.
- If you have overactive thyroid.
- If you have intestinal blockage.
- If you have Parkinson's disease.
- If you have stomach problems (including ulcer).
- If you have had bladder or intestinal surgery within 1 month.

Over age 60:
Adverse reactions and side effects may be more frequent and severe than in younger persons.

Pregnancy:
Risk to unborn child outweighs drug benefits. Don't use.

Breast-feeding:
Drug filters into milk. May harm child. Avoid.

Infants & children:
Use only under medical supervision.

Prolonged use:
No problems expected.

Skin & sunlight:
No problems expected.

Driving, piloting or hazardous work:
Don't drive or pilot aircraft until you learn how medicine affects you. Don't work around dangerous machinery. Don't climb ladders or work in high places. Danger increases if you drink alcohol or take medicine affecting alertness and reflexes, such as antihistamines, tranquilizers, sedatives, pain medicine, narcotics and mind-altering drugs.

Discontinuing:
May be unnecessary to finish medicine. Follow doctor's instructions.

Others:
- Be cautious about standing up suddenly.
- Interferes with laboratory studies of liver and pancreas function.
- Side effects more likely with injections.

POSSIBLE INTERACTION WITH OTHER DRUGS

GENERIC NAME OR DRUG CLASS	COMBINED EFFECT
Cholinergics, other*	Increased effect of both drugs. Possible toxicity.
Ganglionic blockers*	Decreased blood pressure.
Nitrates*	Decreased bethanechol effect.
Procainamide	Decreased bethanechol effect.
Quinidine	Decreased bethanechol effect.

POSSIBLE INTERACTION WITH OTHER SUBSTANCES

INTERACTS WITH	COMBINED EFFECT
Alcohol:	None expected.
Beverages:	None expected.
Cocaine:	None expected.
Foods:	None expected.
Marijuana:	None expected.
Tobacco:	None expected.

*See Glossary

BISACODYL

BRAND NAMES

Bisac-Evac	Deficol
Bisacolax	Dulcolax
Bisco-Lax	Fleet Bisacodyl
Carter's Little Pills	Fleet Bisacodyl Prep
Clysodrast	Laxit
Dacodyl	Theralax

BASIC INFORMATION

Habit forming? No
Prescription needed? No
Available as generic? Yes
Drug class: Laxative (stimulant)

USES

Constipation relief.

DOSAGE & USAGE INFORMATION

How to take:
- Follow package instructions.
- Tablet—Swallow with liquid, do not crush.
- Suppository—Remove wrapper and moisten suppository with water. Gently insert larger end into rectum. Push well into rectum with finger. Retain in rectum 20-30 minutes.

When to take:
Usually at bedtime with a snack, unless directed otherwise.

If you forget a dose:
Take as soon as you remember.

What drug does:
Acts on smooth muscles of intestine wall to cause vigorous bowel movement.

Time lapse before drug works:
6 to 10 hours.

Don't take with:
- Any other medicine without consulting your doctor or pharmacist.
- Don't take within 2 hours of taking another medicine. Laxative interferes with medicine absorption.

OVERDOSE

SYMPTOMS:
Vomiting, electrolyte depletion.
WHAT TO DO:
Overdose unlikely to threaten life. If person takes much larger amount than prescribed, call doctor, poison-control center or hospital emergency room for instructions.

POSSIBLE ADVERSE REACTIONS OR SIDE EFFECTS

SYMPTOMS	WHAT TO DO
Life-threatening: None expected.	
Common: Rectal irritation.	Continue. Call doctor when convenient.
Infrequent:	
• Dangerous potassium loss (thirst, weakness, heartbeat irregularity, paralysis, nausea and diarrhea).	Discontinue. Call doctor right away.
• Belching, cramps, nausea.	Continue. Call doctor when convenient.
Rare:	
• Irritability, headache, confusion, rash, breathing difficulty, irregular heartbeat, muscle cramps, unusual tiredness or weakness.	Discontinue. Call doctor right away.
• Burning on urination.	Continue. Call doctor when convenient.

WARNINGS & PRECAUTIONS

Don't take if:
- You have symptoms of appendicitis, inflamed bowel or intestinal blockage.
- You are allergic to a stimulant laxative.
- You have missed a bowel movement for only 1 or 2 days.

Before you start, consult your doctor:
- If you have a colostomy or ileostomy.
- If you have congestive heart disease.
- If you have diabetes.
- If you have high blood pressure.
- If you have a laxative habit.
- If you have rectal bleeding.
- If you take other laxatives.

Over age 60:
Adverse reactions and side effects may be more frequent and severe than in younger persons.

Pregnancy:
Risk to mother and unborn child outweighs drug benefits. Don't use.

Breast-feeding:
Drug passes into milk. Avoid drug or discontinue nursing until you finish medicine. Consult doctor for advice on maintaining milk supply.

Infants & children:
Use only under medical supervision.

Prolonged use:
Don't take for more than 1 week unless under doctor's supervision. May cause laxative dependence.

Skin & sunlight:
No problems expected.

Driving, piloting or hazardous work:
No problems expected.

Discontinuing:
May be unnecessary to finish medicine. Follow doctor's instructions.

Others:
Don't take to "flush out" your system or as a "tonic."

POSSIBLE INTERACTION WITH OTHER DRUGS

GENERIC NAME OR DRUG CLASS	COMBINED EFFECT
Antacids*	Tablet coating may dissolve too rapidly, irritating stomach or bowel.
Antihypertensives*	May cause dangerous low potassium level.
Cimetidine	Stomach or bowel irritation.
Diuretics*	May cause dangerous low potassium level.
Famotidine	Stomach or bowel irritation.
Ranitidine	Stomach or bowel irritation.

POSSIBLE INTERACTION WITH OTHER SUBSTANCES

INTERACTS WITH	COMBINED EFFECT
Alcohol:	None expected.
Beverages:	None expected.
Cocaine:	None expected.
Foods:	None expected.
Marijuana:	None expected.
Tobacco:	None expected.

*See Glossary

BISMUTH SUBSALICYLATE

BRAND NAMES

Pepto-Bismol

BASIC INFORMATION

Habit forming? No
Prescription needed? No
Available as generic? No
Drug class: Antidiarrheal, antacid

 USES

- Treats symptoms of diarrhea, heartburn, nausea, acid indigestion.
- Helps prevent traveler's diarrhea.

 DOSAGE & USAGE INFORMATION

How to take:
- Chewable tablets—Chew well before swallowing.
- Liquid—Take as directed on label.

When to take:
As directed on label or by your doctor.

If you forget a dose:
Take as soon as you remember. Don't double this dose.

What drug does:
- Binds toxin of some bacteria.
- Stimulates absorption of fluid and electrolytes across the intestinal wall.
- Decreases inflammation and increased motility of the intestinal muscles and lining.

Time lapse before drug works:
30 minutes to 1 hour.

Don't take with:
Any other medicine without consulting your doctor or pharmacist.

 OVERDOSE

SYMPTOMS:
Anxiety, confusion, speech difficulty, severe headache, muscle spasms, depression, trembling.
WHAT TO DO:
- Dial 0 (operator) or 911 (emergency) for an ambulance or medical help. Then give first aid immediately.
- See emergency information on inside covers.

 POSSIBLE ADVERSE REACTIONS OR SIDE EFFECTS

SYMPTOMS	WHAT TO DO
Life-threatening:	
In case of overdose, see previous column.	
Common:	
Black stools, dark tongue. (These symptoms are normal and medically insignificant.)	No action necessary.
Infrequent:	
• Hearing loss, confusion, dizziness, fast breathing, headache, increased thirst, ringing or buzzing in ears, vision problems.	Discontinue. Call doctor right away.
• Constipation.	Continue. Call doctor when convenient.
Rare:	
Flapping movements of hands, abdominal pain, increased sweating, muscle weakness, drowsiness, anxiety, trembling.	Discontinue. Call doctor right away.

WARNINGS & PRECAUTIONS

Don't take if:
- You are allergic to aspirin, salicylates or other non-steroidal anti-inflammatory drugs.
- You have stomach ulcers that have ever bled.
- The patient is a child with fever.

Before you start, consult your doctor:
- If you are on a low-sodium, low-sugar or other special diet.
- If you have had diarrhea for more than 24 hours. This is especially applicable to infants, children and those over 60.
- If you have had kidney disease.

Over age 60:
- Consult doctor before using.
- May cause severe constipation.

Pregnancy:
- Don't use during last 3 months of pregnancy.
- Studies inconclusive on harm to unborn child. Decide with your doctor whether drug benefits justify risk to unborn child.

Breast-feeding:
- Drug passes into milk. Avoid or discontinue nursing until you finish medicine.
- May harm baby if mother takes large amounts.

Infants & children:
Not recommended for children 3 and younger. May cause constipation.

Prolonged use:
May cause constipation.

Skin & sunlight:
No problems expected.

Driving, piloting or hazardous work:
Don't drive or pilot aircraft if you take high or prolonged dose until you learn how medicine affects you. Don't work around dangerous machinery. Don't climb ladders or work in high places. Danger increases if you drink alcohol or take medicine affecting alertness and reflexes, such as antihistamines, tranquilizers, sedatives, pain medicine, narcotics and mind-altering drugs.

Discontinuing:
No problems expected.

Others:
- Pepto-Bismol contains salicylates. When given to children with flu or chickenpox, salicylates may cause a serious illness called Reye's syndrome. An overdose in children can cause the same problems as aspirin poisoning.
- May cause false urine sugar tests.

POSSIBLE INTERACTION WITH OTHER DRUGS

GENERIC NAME OR DRUG CLASS	COMBINED EFFECT
Anticoagulants*	Increased risk of bleeding.
Insulin or oral antidiabetic drugs*	Increased insulin effect. May require dosage adjustment.
Probenecid	Decreased effect of probenecid.
Salicylates, other*	Increased risk of salicylate toxicity.
Sulfinpyrazone	Decreased effect of sulfinpyrazone.
Tetracylines*	Decreased absorption of tetracycline.
Thrombolytic agents*	Increased risk of bleeding.

POSSIBLE INTERACTION WITH OTHER SUBSTANCES

INTERACTS WITH	COMBINED EFFECT
Alcohol:	None expected.
Beverages:	None expected.
Cocaine:	Decreased Pepto-bismol effect. Avoid.
Foods:	None expected.
Marijuana:	None expected.
Tobacco:	None expected.

*See Glossary

BROMOCRIPTINE

BRAND NAMES

Parlodel

BASIC INFORMATION

Habit forming? No
Prescription needed? Yes
Available as generic? No
Drug class: Antiparkinsonism

 USES

- Controls Parkinson's disease symptoms such as rigidity, tremors and unsteady gait.
- Treats female infertility.
- Treats acromegaly.

 DOSAGE & USAGE INFORMATION

How to take:
Tablet or capsule—Swallow with liquid or food to lessen stomach irritation. If you can't swallow whole, crumble tablet or open capsule and take with liquid or food.

When to take:
At the same times each day.

If you forget a dose:
Take as soon as you remember up to 2 hours late. If more than 2 hours, wait for next scheduled dose (don't double this dose).

Continued next column

 OVERDOSE

SYMPTOMS:
Muscle twitch, spastic eyelid closure, nausea, vomiting, diarrhea, irregular and rapid pulse, weakness, fainting, confusion, agitation, hallucination, coma.
WHAT TO DO:

- **Dial 0 (operator) or 911 (emergency) for an ambulance or medical help. Then give first aid immediately.**
- **If patient is unconscious and not breathing, give mouth-to-mouth breathing. If there is no heartbeat, use cardiac massage and mouth-to-mouth breathing (CPR). Don't try to make patient vomit. If you can't get help quickly, take patient to nearest emergency facility.**
- **See emergency information on inside covers.**

What drug does:
Restores chemical balance necessary for normal nerve impulses.

Time lapse before drug works:
2 to 3 weeks to improve; 6 weeks or longer for maximum benefit.

Don't take with:
Any other medicine without consulting your doctor or pharmacist.

 POSSIBLE ADVERSE REACTIONS OR SIDE EFFECTS

SYMPTOMS	WHAT TO DO
Life-threatening:	
In case of overdose, see previous column.	
Common:	
• Mood changes, uncontrollable body movements, diarrhea, nausea.	Continue. Call doctor when convenient.
• Dry mouth, body odor.	No action necessary.
Infrequent:	
• Fainting, severe dizziness, headache, insomnia, nightmares, rash, itch, vomiting, irregular heartbeat.	Discontinue. Call doctor right away.
• Flushed face, blurred vision, muscle twitching, discolored or dark urine, difficult urination, muscle cramps, appetite loss, abdominal discomfort, nasal congestion, tingling and numbness of hands and feet.	Continue. Call doctor when convenient.
• Constipation, tiredness.	Continue. Tell doctor at next visit.
Rare:	
• High blood pressure, hallucinations, psychosis.	Discontinue. Call doctor right away.
• Anemia, impotence.	Continue. Call doctor when convenient.
• Hair loss.	Continue. Tell doctor at next visit.

WARNINGS & PRECAUTIONS

Don't take if:
- You are allergic to bromocriptine or ergotamine.
- You have taken MAO inhibitors in past 2 weeks.
- You have glaucoma (narrow-angle type).

Before you start, consult your doctor:
- If you have diabetes or epilepsy.
- If you have had high blood pressure, heart or lung disease.
- If you have had liver or kidney disease.
- If you have a peptic ulcer.
- If you will have surgery within 2 months, including dental surgery, requiring general or spinal anesthesia.

Over age 60:
Adverse reactions and side effects may be more frequent and severe than in younger persons.

Pregnancy:
Risk to unborn child outweighs drug benefits. Don't use.

Breast-feeding:
Drug filters into milk. May harm child. Avoid.

Infants & children:
Not recommended if under 15 years old.

Prolonged use:
- May lead to uncontrolled movements of head, face, mouth, tongue, arms or legs.
- Talk to your doctor about the need for follow-up medical examinations or laboratory studies to check blood pressure, x-rays, growth hormone levels.

Skin & sunlight:
No problems expected.

Driving, piloting or hazardous work:
Don't drive or pilot aircraft until you learn how medicine affects you. Don't work around dangerous machinery. Don't climb ladders or work in high places. Danger increases if you drink alcohol or take medicine affecting alertness and reflexes, such as antihistamines, tranquilizers, sedatives, pain medicine, narcotics and mind-altering drugs.

Discontinuing:
Don't discontinue without doctor's advice until you complete prescribed dose, even though symptoms diminish or disappear.

Others:
Expect to start with small doses and increase gradually to lessen frequency and severity of adverse reactions.

POSSIBLE INTERACTION WITH OTHER DRUGS

GENERIC NAME OR DRUG CLASS	COMBINED EFFECT
Antihypertensives*	May decrease blood pressure.
Antiparkinsonism drugs, other*	Increased bromo-criptine effect.
Contraceptives, oral*	Decreased bromo-criptine effect.
Guanfacine	Increased effect of both drugs.
Haloperidol	Decreased bromo-criptine effect.
Levodopa	Decreased anti-parkinson effect.
MAO inhibitors*	Dangerous rise in blood pressure.
Methyldopa	Decreased bromo-criptine effect.
Papaverine	Decreased bromo-criptine effect.
Phenothiazines*	Decreased bromo-criptine effect.
Pyridoxine (Vitamin B-6)	Decreased bromo-criptine effect.
Rauwolfia alkaloids*	Decreased bromo-criptine effect.

POSSIBLE INTERACTION WITH OTHER SUBSTANCES

INTERACTS WITH	COMBINED EFFECT
Alcohol:	Decreased alcohol tolerance.
Beverages:	None expected.
Cocaine:	Decreased bromo-criptine effect. Avoid.
Foods:	None expected.
Marijuana:	Increased fatigue, lethargy, fainting. Avoid.
Tobacco:	Interferes with absorption. Avoid.

BRONCHODILATORS, ADRENERGIC

BRAND AND GENERIC NAMES

See complete list of brand and generic names in the *Brand Name Directory*, page 916.

BASIC INFORMATION

Habit forming? No
Prescription needed? Yes, for most.
Available as generic? Yes, for some.
Drug class: Sympathomimetic

 ## USES

- Relieves bronchial asthma.
- Decreases congestion of breathing passages.
- Suppresses allergic reactions.

 ## DOSAGE & USAGE INFORMATION

How to take:
- Tablet or capsule—Swallow with liquid. You may chew or crush tablet.
- Extended-release tablets or capsules—Swallow each dose whole.
- Syrup—Take as directed on bottle.
- Drops—Dilute dose in beverage.
- Aerosol inhalor—Follow directions in package.

When to take:
As needed, no more often than every 4 hours.

If you forget a dose:
Take up to 2 hours late. If more than 2 hours, wait for next dose (don't double this dose).

What drug does:
- Prevents cells from releasing allergy-causing chemicals (histamines).
- Relaxes muscles of bronchial tubes.
- Decreases blood-vessel size and blood flow, thus causing decongestion.

Time lapse before drug works:
30 to 60 minutes.

Continued next column

 ## OVERDOSE

SYMPTOMS:
Severe anxiety, confusion, delirium, muscle tremors, rapid and irregular pulse.
WHAT TO DO:
- **Dial 0 (operator) or 911 (emergency) for an ambulance or medical help. Then give first aid immediately.**
- **See emergency information on inside covers.**

Don't take with:
- Non-prescription drugs with ephedrine, pseudoephedrine or epinephrine.
- Non-prescription drugs for cough, cold, allergy or asthma without consulting doctor.
- Any other medicine without consulting your doctor or pharmacist.

 ## POSSIBLE ADVERSE REACTIONS OR SIDE EFFECTS

SYMPTOMS	WHAT TO DO
Life-threatening:	
In case of overdose, see previous column.	
Common:	
Nervousness, headache, paleness, rapid heartbeat, trembling, dry mouth.	Continue. Call doctor when convenient.
Insomnia, large pupils, increased blood pressure.	Continue. Tell doctor at next visit.
Infrequent:	
Irregular heartbeat, chest pain, hallucinations.	Discontinue. Call doctor right away.
Dizziness, appetite loss, nausea, vomiting, painful or difficult urination, coughing.	Continue. Call doctor when convenient.
Rare:	
Muscle cramps.	Discontinue. Call doctor right away.

 ## WARNINGS & PRECAUTIONS

Don't take if:
You are allergic to ephedrine or any bronchodilator* drug.

Before you start, consult your doctor:
- If you have high blood pressure.
- If you have diabetes.
- If you have overactive thyroid gland.
- If you have difficulty urinating.
- If you have taken any MAO inhibitor in past 2 weeks.
- If you have taken digitalis preparations in the last 7 days.
- If you will have surgery within 2 months, including dental surgery, requiring general or spinal anesthesia.

Over age 60:
More likely to develop high blood pressure, heart-rhythm disturbances, angina and to feel drug's stimulant effects.

Pregnancy:
No proven harm to unborn child. Avoid if possible.

Breast-feeding:
Drug passes into milk. Avoid drug or discontinue nursing until you finish medicine. Consult doctor for advice on maintaining milk supply.

Infants & children:
No problems expected.

Prolonged use:
- Excessive doses—Rare toxic psychosis.
- Men with enlarged prostate gland may have more urination difficulty.
- Talk to your doctor about the need for follow-up medical examinations or laboratory studies to check ECG*, blood pressure.

Skin & sunlight:
No problems expected.

Driving, piloting or hazardous work:
Avoid if you feel dizzy. Otherwise, no problems expected.

Discontinuing:
May be unnecessary to finish medicine. Follow doctor's instructions.

Others:
May affect results in some medical tests.

 POSSIBLE INTERACTION WITH OTHER DRUGS

GENERIC NAME OR DRUG CLASS	COMBINED EFFECT
Antidepressants, tricyclic (TCA)*	Increased effect of bronchodilator. Excessive stimulation of heart and blood pressure.
Antihypertensives*	Decreased antihypertensive effect.
Beta-adrenergic blockers*	Decreased effects of both drugs.
Digitalis preparations*	Serious heart-rhythm disturbances.
Epinephrine	Increased bronchodilator effect.
Ergot preparations*	Serious blood-pressure rise.
Furazolidine	Sudden severe increase in blood pressure.
Guanadrel	Decreased effect of both drugs.
Guanethidine	Decreased effect of both drugs.
MAO inhibitors*	Increased bronchodilator effect. Dangerous blood-pressure rise.
Methyldopa	Possible increased blood pressure.
Nitrates*	Possible decreased effects of both drugs.
Phenothiazines*	Possible increased bronchodilator toxicity. Possible decreased bronchodilator effect.
Pseudoephedrine	Increased bronchodilator effect.
Rauwolfia	Decreased rauwolfia effect.
Sympathomimetics*	Increased bronchodilator effect.
Terazosin	Decreases effectiveness of terazosin.
Theophylline	Increased gastrointestinal intolerance.
Thyroid Drugs	Increased bronchodilator effect.

 POSSIBLE INTERACTION WITH OTHER SUBSTANCES

INTERACTS WITH	COMBINED EFFECT
Alcohol:	None expected.
Beverages: Caffeine drinks.	Nervousness or insomnia.
Cocaine:	High risk of heartbeat irregularities and high blood pressure.
Foods:	None expected.
Marijuana:	Rapid heartbeat, possible heart-rhythm disturbance.
Tobacco:	None expected.

BRONCHODILATORS, XANTHINE

BRAND AND GENERIC NAMES

See complete list of brand and generic names in the *Brand Name Directory*, page 916.

BASIC INFORMATION

Habit forming? No
Prescription needed?
U.S.: High strength—Yes
Low strength—No
Canada: No
Available as generic? Yes
Drug class: Bronchodilator (xanthine)

 USES

Treatment for bronchial asthma symptoms.

 DOSAGE & USAGE
INFORMATION

How to take:
- Tablet or capsule—Swallow with liquid.
- Extended-release tablets or capsules—Swallow each dose whole. If you take regular tablets, you may chew or crush them.
- Suppositories—Remove wrapper and moisten suppository with water. Gently insert larger end into rectum. Push well into rectum with finger.
- Syrup—Take as directed on bottle.
- Enema—Use as directed on label.

When to take:
Most effective taken on empty stomach 1 hour before or 2 hours after eating. However, may take with food to lessen stomach upset.

If you forget a dose:
Take as soon as you remember up to 2 hours late. If more than 2 hours, wait for next scheduled dose (don't double this dose).

Continued next column

 OVERDOSE

SYMPTOMS:
Restlessness, irritability, confusion, black or tarry stool, breathing difficulty, pounding and irregular heartbeat, vomiting blood, delirium, convulsions, rapid pulse, coma.
WHAT TO DO:
- **Dial 0 (operator) or 911 (emergency) for an ambulance or medical help. Then give first aid immediately.**
- **See emergency information on inside covers.**

What drug does:
Relaxes and expands bronchial tubes.

Time lapse before drug works:
15 to 30 minutes.

Don't take with:
Any other medicine without consulting your doctor or pharmacist.

 POSSIBLE
ADVERSE REACTIONS
OR SIDE EFFECTS

SYMPTOMS	WHAT TO DO
Life-threatening:	
In case of overdose, see previous column.	
Common:	
Headache, irritability, nervousness, nausea, restlessness, insomnia, vomiting, stomach pain.	Continue. Call doctor when convenient.
Infrequent:	
• Rash or hives, flushed face, diarrhea, appetite loss, rapid breathing, irregular heartbeat.	Discontinue. Call doctor right away.
• Dizziness or lightheadedness.	Continue. Call doctor when convenient.
Rare:	
Frequent urination.	Continue. Call doctor when convenient.

 WARNINGS &
PRECAUTIONS

Don't take if:
- You are allergic to any bronchodilator.
- You have an active peptic ulcer.

Before you start, consult your doctor:
- If you have had impaired kidney or liver function.
- If you have gastritis.
- If you have a peptic ulcer.
- If you have high blood pressure or heart disease.
- If you take medication for gout.

Over age 60:
Adverse reactions and side effects may be more frequent and severe than in younger persons.

Pregnancy:
Risk to unborn child outweighs drug benefits. Don't use.

Breast-feeding:
Drug passes into milk. Avoid drug or discontinue nursing until you finish medicine. Consult doctor for advice on maintaining milk supply.

BRONCHODILATORS, XANTHINE

Infants & children:
Use only under medical supervision.

Prolonged use:
Stomach irritation.

Skin & sunlight:
No problems expected.

Driving, piloting or hazardous work:
Avoid if lightheaded or dizzy. Otherwise, no problems expected.

Discontinuing:
May be unnecessary to finish medicine. Follow doctor's instructions.

Others:
No problems expected.

 POSSIBLE INTERACTION WITH OTHER DRUGS

GENERIC NAME OR DRUG CLASS	COMBINED EFFECT
Allopurinol	Increased allopurinol effect.
Aminoglutethimide	Possible decreased bronchodilator effect.
Beta-agonists*	Increased effect of both drugs.
Beta-adrenergic blockers*	Decreased broncho-dilator effect.
Cimetidine	Increased broncho-dilator effect.
Ciprofloxin	Increased xanthine bronchodilator in blood. Dosage adjustments necessary.
Clarithromycin	Increased concentration of theophylline.
Clindamycin	May increase bronchodilator effect.
Corticosteroids*	Possible increased bronchodilator effect.
Erythromicin	Increased broncho-dilator effect.
Finasteride	Decreased theophylline effect.
Furosemide	Increased furosemide effect.
Lincomycins*	May increase bronchodilator effect.
Lithiuim	Decreased lithiuim effect.
Moricizine	Decreased bronchodilator effect.
Norfloxacin	Increased xanthine bronchodilator in blood. Dosage adjustments necessary.
Phenobarbital	Decreased broncho-dilator effect.
Phenytoin	Decreased broncho-dilator effect.
Probenecid	Increased effect of dyphylline.
Ranitidine	Possible increased bronchodilator effect and toxicity.
Rauwolfia alkaloids*	Rapid heartbeat.
Rifampin	Decreased broncho-dilator effect.
Sulfinpyrazone	Increased effect of dyphylline.
Sympathomimetics*	Possible increased bronchodilator effect.
Ticlopidine	Increased theophylline effect.
Troleandomycin	Increased broncho-dilator effect.

 POSSIBLE INTERACTION WITH OTHER SUBSTANCES

INTERACTS WITH	COMBINED EFFECT
Alcohol:	None expected.
Beverages: Caffeine drinks.	Nervousness and insomnia.
Cocaine:	Excess stimulation. Avoid.
Foods:	None expected.
Marijuana:	Slightly increased antiasthmatic effect of bronchodilator. Decreased effect with chronic use.
Tobacco:	Decreased broncho-dilator effect.

*See Glossary

BUCLIZINE

BRAND NAMES

Bucladin-S

BASIC INFORMATION

Habit forming? No
Prescription needed?
 U.S.: No
 Canada: Yes
Available as generic? No
Drug class: Antihistamine, antiemetic, anti-motion sickness

 USES

Prevents motion sickness.

 DOSAGE & USAGE INFORMATION

How to take:
Tablet—Swallow with liquid or food to lessen stomach irritation. If you can't swallow whole, crumble tablet and chew or take with liquid or food.

When to take:
30 minutes to 1 hour before traveling.

If you forget a dose:
Take as soon as you remember. Wait 4 hours for next dose.

What drug does:
Reduces sensitivity of nerve endings in inner ear, blocking messages to brain's vomiting center.

Time lapse before drug works:
30 to 60 minutes.

Don't take with:
Any other medicine without consulting your doctor or pharmacist.

 OVERDOSE

SYMPTOMS:
Drowsiness, confusion, incoordination, stupor, coma, weak pulse, shallow breathing, hallucinations.
WHAT TO DO:
• **Dial 0 (operator) or 911 (emergency) for an ambulance or medical help. Then give first aid immediately.**
• **See emergency information on inside covers.**

 POSSIBLE ADVERSE REACTIONS OR SIDE EFFECTS

SYMPTOMS	WHAT TO DO
Life-threatening:	
In case of overdose, see previous column.	
Common:	
Drowsiness.	Continue. Tell doctor at next visit.
Infrequent:	
• Headache, diarrhea or constipation, fast heartbeat.	Continue. Call doctor when convenient.
• Dry mouth, nose, throat.	Continue. Tell doctor at next visit.
Rare:	
• Rash or hives.	Discontinue. Call doctor right away.
• Restlessness, excitement, insomnia, blurred vision, frequent urination, difficult urination, hallucinations.	Continue. Call doctor when convenient.
• Appetite loss, nausea.	Continue. Tell doctor at next visit.

 WARNINGS & PRECAUTIONS

Don't take if:
• You are allergic to meclizine, buclizine or cyclizine.
• You have taken MAO inhibitors in the past 2 weeks.

Before you start, consult your doctor:
• If you have glaucoma.
• If you have prostate enlargement.
• If you have reacted badly to any antihistamine.

Over age 60:
Adverse reactions and side effects may be more frequent and severe than in younger persons, especially impaired urination from enlarged prostate gland.

Pregnancy:
Studies inconclusive on harm to unborn child. Animal studies show fetal abnormalities. Decide with your doctor whether drug benefits justify risk to unborn child.

Breast-feeding:
Drug passes into milk. Avoid drug or discontinue nursing until you finish medicine. Consult doctor for advice on maintaining milk supply.

Infants & children:
Safety not established. Avoid if less than 12 years old.

Prolonged use:
No problems expected.

Skin & sunlight:
No problems expected.

Driving, piloting or hazardous work:
Don't fly aircraft. Don't drive until you learn how medicine affects you. Don't work around dangerous machinery. Don't climb ladders or work in high places. Danger increases if you drink alcohol or take medicine affecting alertness and reflexes, such as antihistamines, tranquilizers, sedatives, pain medicine, narcotics and mind-altering drugs.

Discontinuing:
No problems expected.

Others:
Buclizine contains tartrazine dye. Avoid if allergic (especially aspirin hypersensitivity).

POSSIBLE INTERACTION WITH OTHER DRUGS

GENERIC NAME OR DRUG CLASS	COMBINED EFFECT
Amphetamines*	May decrease drowsiness caused by buclizine.
Anticholinergics*	Increased effect of both drugs.
Antidepressants, tricyclic (TCA)*	Increased effect of both drugs.
Carteolol	Decreased anti-histamine effect.
Clozapine	Toxic effect on the central nervous system.
Dronabinol	Increases effect of buclizine.
Ethinamate	Dangerous increased effects of ethinamate. Avoid combining.
Fluoxetine	Increased depressant effects of both drugs.
Guanfacine	May increase depressant effects of either drug.
MAO inhibitors*	Increased buclizine effect.

Methyprylon	Increased sedative effect, perhaps to dangerous level. Avoid.
Nabilone	Greater depression of central nervous system.
Narcotics*	Increased effect of both drugs.
Pain relievers*	Increased effect of both drugs.
Sedatives*	Increased effect of both drugs.
Sertraline	Increased depressive effects of both drugs.
Sleep inducers*	Increased effect of both drugs.
Sotalol	Increased antihistamine effect.
Tranquilizers*	Increased effect of both drugs.

POSSIBLE INTERACTION WITH OTHER SUBSTANCES

INTERACTS WITH	COMBINED EFFECT
Alcohol:	Increased sedation. Avoid.
Beverages: Caffeine drinks.	May decrease drowsiness.
Cocaine:	None expected.
Foods:	None expected.
Marijuana:	Increased drowsiness, dry mouth.
Tobacco:	None expected.

*See Glossary

BUPROPION

BRAND AND GENERIC NAMES

AMFEBUTAMONE   **Wellbutrin**

BASIC INFORMATION

Habit forming? No
Prescription needed? Yes
Available as generic? No
Drug class: Antidepressant

 USES

Relieves severe mental depression.

 DOSAGE & USAGE INFORMATION

How to take:
Tablets—Swallow with liquid. If you can't
swallow whole, crumble tablet and take with
liquid or food. Instructions to take on empty
stomach mean 1 hour before or 2 hours after
eating.

When to take:
At the same time each day, according to
instructions on prescription label.

If you forget a dose:
Take as soon as you remember up to 2 hours
late. If more than 2 hours, wait for next
scheduled dose (don't double this dose).

What drug does:
Blocks dopamine uptake.

Time lapse before drug works:
4 to 6 weeks.

Don't take with:
Any other medicine without consulting your
doctor or pharmacist.

 OVERDOSE

SYMPTOMS:
Confusion, agitation, seizures, coma.
WHAT TO DO:
- **Dial 0 (operator) or 911 (emergency) for
  an ambulance or medical help. Then give
  first aid immediately.**
- **See emergency information on inside
  covers.**

 POSSIBLE ADVERSE REACTIONS OR SIDE EFFECTS

SYMPTOMS	WHAT TO DO
Life-threatening:	
Seizures.	Seek emergency treatment immediately.
Common:	
Excitement, anxiety, insomnia, restlessness, confusion, heartbeat irregularity, headaches.	Continue. Call doctor when convenient.
Infrequent:	
Rash, blurred vision, drowsiness, chills, fever, hallucinations, fatigue, nightmares.	Discontinue. Call doctor right away.
Rare:	
Fainting, hostility.	Discontinue. Call doctor right away.

WARNINGS & PRECAUTIONS

Don't take if:
- You have anorexia nervosa or bulimia.
- You have had recent head injury.
- You have convulsions (seizures).
- You have a brain or spinal cord tumor.

Before you start, consult your doctor:
- If you have manic phases to your illness.
- If you abuse drugs.
- If you have liver, kidney or heart disease.

Over age 60:
See Interaction column and consult doctor.

Pregnancy:
No proven harm to unborn child, but avoid if possible.

Breast-feeding:
Effect not documented. Consult your doctor.

Infants & children:
Effect not documented. Consult your doctor.

Prolonged use:
Talk to your doctor about the need for follow-up medical examinations or laboratory studies to check kidney function, liver function and serum bupropion levels in blood.

Skin & sunlight:
No problems expected.

Driving, piloting or hazardous work:
Don't drive or pilot aircraft until you learn how medicine affects you. Don't work around dangerous machinery. Don't climb ladders or work in high places. Danger increases if you drink alcohol or take medicine affecting alertness and reflexes.

Discontinuing:
No special problems expected.

Others:
- May affect results in some medical tests.
- Advise any doctor or dentist whom you consult that you take this medicine.

POSSIBLE INTERACTION WITH OTHER DRUGS

GENERIC NAME OR DRUG CLASS	COMBINED EFFECT
Antidepressants, tricyclic (TCA)*	Increased risk of major seizures.
Cimetidine	Increased bupropion effect.
Haloperidol	Increased risk of major seizures.
Lithium	Increased risk of major seizures.
Loxapine	Increased risk of major seizures.
MAO inhibitors*	Increased risk of bupropion toxicity.
Molindone	Increased risk of major seizures.
Phenothiazines*	Increased risk of major seizures.
Thioxanthenes*	Increased risk of major seizures.

POSSIBLE INTERACTION WITH OTHER SUBSTANCES

INTERACTS WITH	COMBINED EFFECT
Alcohol:	Increased risk of seizures. Avoid.
Beverages: Coffee, tea, cocoa.	Increased side effects such as restlessness, insomnia.
Cocaine:	Increased risk of seizures. Avoid.
Foods:	No special problems expected.
Marijuana:	Increased risk of seizures. Avoid.
Tobacco:	No special problems expected.

*See Glossary

BUSPIRONE

BRAND NAMES

BuSpar

BASIC INFORMATION

Habit forming? Unknown
Prescription needed? Yes
Available as generic? No
Drug class: Tranquilizer

 USES

Treats anxiety disorders with nervousness or tension. Not intended for treatment of ordinary stress of daily living. Causes less sedation than some anti-anxiety drugs.

 DOSAGE & USAGE INFORMATION

How to take:
Tablets—Take with a glass of liquid.

When to take:
As directed. Usually 3 times daily. Food does not interfere with absorption.

If you forget a dose:
Take as soon as you remember, but skip this dose and don't double the next dose if it is almost time for the next dose.

What drug does:
Chemical family azaspirodecanedione; *not* a benzodiazepine. Probably has an effect on neurotransmitter systems.

Time lapse before drug works:
1 or 2 weeks before beneficial effects may be observed.

Don't take with:
Alcohol, other tranquilizers, antihistamines, muscle relaxants, sedatives or narcotics.

 OVERDOSE

SYMPTOMS:
Severe drowsiness or nausea, vomiting, small pupils, unconsciousness.
WHAT TO DO:
- Dial 0 (operator) or 911 (emergency) for an ambulance or medical help. Then give first aid immediately.
- See emergency information on inside covers.

 POSSIBLE ADVERSE REACTIONS OR SIDE EFFECTS

SYMPTOMS	WHAT TO DO
Life-threatening:	
Chest pain; pounding, fast heartbeat (rare).	Discontinue. Seek emergency treatment.
Common:	
Lightheadedness, headache, nausea, restlessness, dizziness.	Discontinue. Call doctor right away.
Infrequent:	
Drowsiness, dry mouth, ringing in ears, nightmares or vivid dreams, unusual fatigue.	Continue. Call doctor when convenient.
Rare:	
Numbness or tingling in feet or hands; sore throat; fever; depression or confusion; uncontrollable movements of tongue, lips, arms and legs; slurred speech; psychosis; blurred vision.	Discontinue. Call doctor right away.

BUSPIRONE

WARNINGS & PRECAUTIONS

Don't take if:
If you are allergic to buspirone.

Before you start, consult your doctor:
- If you have ever been addicted to any substance.
- If you have chronic kidney or liver disease.
- If you are already taking *any* medicine.

Over age 60:
Adverse reactions and side effects may be more frequent and severe than in younger persons.

Pregnancy:
No problems expected, but better to avoid if possible.

Breast-feeding:
Buspirone passes into milk of lactating experimental animals. Avoid if possible.

Infants & children:
Safety and efficacy not established for under 18 years old.

Prolonged use:
- Not recommended for prolonged use. Adverse side effects more likely.
- Request follow-up studies to check kidney function, blood counts, and platelet counts.

Skin & sunlight:
No problems expected.

Driving, piloting or hazardous work:
Don't drive or pilot aircraft until you learn how medicine affects you. Don't work around dangerous machinery. Don't climb ladders or work in high places. Danger increases if you drink alcohol or take medicine affecting alertness and reflexes, such as antihistamines, tranquilizers, sedatives, pain medicine, narcotics and mind-altering drugs.

Discontinuing:
No problems expected.

Others:
Before elective surgery requiring local or general anesthesia, tell your dentist, surgeon or anesthesiologist that you take buspirone.

POSSIBLE INTERACTION WITH OTHER DRUGS

GENERIC NAME OR DRUG CLASS	COMBINED EFFECT
Antihistamines*	Excessive sedation. Sedative effect of both drugs may be increased.
Barbiturates*	Excessive sedation. Sedative effect of both drugs may be increased.
MAO inhibitors*	May increase blood pressure.
Muscle relaxants*	Excessive sedation. Sedative effect of both drugs may be increased.
Narcotics*	Excessive sedation. Sedative effect of both drugs may be increased.
Sedatives*	Excessive sedation. Sedative effect of both drugs may be increased.
Tranquilizers, other*	Excessive sedation. Sedative effect of both drugs may be increased.

POSSIBLE INTERACTION WITH OTHER SUBSTANCES

INTERACTS WITH	COMBINED EFFECT
Alcohol:	Excess sedation. Avoid.
Beverages: Caffeine-containing drinks.	Avoid. Decreased anti-anxiety effect of busiprone.
Cocaine:	Avoid. Decreased anti-anxiety effect of busiprone.
Foods:	None expected.
Marijuana:	Avoid. Decreased anti-anxiety effect of busiprone.
Tobacco:	Avoid. Decreased antianxiety effect of busiprone.

BUSULFAN

BRAND NAMES

Myleran

BASIC INFORMATION

Habit forming? No
Prescription needed? Yes
Available as generic? No
Drug class: Antineoplastic,
immunosuppressant

 USES

- Treatment for some kinds of cancer.
- Suppresses immune response after transplant and in immune disorders.

 DOSAGE & USAGE INFORMATION

How to take:
Tablet—Swallow with liquid after light meal.
Don't drink fluids with meals. Drink extra fluids between meals. Avoid sweet or fatty foods.

When to take:
At the same time each day.

If you forget a dose:
Take as soon as you remember. Don't ever double dose.

What drug does:
Inhibits abnormal cell reproduction. May suppress immune system.

Time lapse before drug works:
Up to 6 weeks for full effect.

Don't take with:
Any other medicine without consulting your doctor or pharmacist.

 OVERDOSE

SYMPTOMS:
Bleeding, chills, fever, collapse, stupor, seizure.
WHAT TO DO:
- Dial 0 (operator) or 911 (emergency) for an ambulance or medical help. Then give first aid immediately.
- If patient is unconscious and not breathing, give mouth-to-mouth breathing. If there is no heartbeat, use cardiac massage and mouth-to-mouth breathing (CPR). Don't try to make patient vomit. If you can't get help quickly, take patient to nearest emergency facility.
- See emergency information on inside covers.

 POSSIBLE ADVERSE REACTIONS OR SIDE EFFECTS

SYMPTOMS	WHAT TO DO
Life-threatening:	
In case of overdose, see previous column.	
Common:	
• Unusual bleeding or bruising, mouth sores with sore throat, chills and fever, black stools, lip sores, menstrual irregularities.	Discontinue. Call doctor right away.
• Hair loss.	Continue. Call doctor when convenient.
• Nausea, vomiting, diarrhea (almost always occurs), tiredness, weakness.	Continue. Tell doctor at next visit.
Infrequent:	
• Mental confusion, shortness of breath.	Continue. Call doctor when convenient.
• Cough, joint pain, dizziness, appetite loss.	Continue. Tell doctor at next visit.
Rare:	
• Jaundice, cataracts, symptoms of myasthenia gravis.*	Discontinue. Call doctor right away.
• Swollen breasts.	Continue. Call doctor when convenient.

WARNINGS & PRECAUTIONS

Don't take if:
- You have had hypersensitivity to alkylating antineoplastic drugs.
- Your physician has not explained the serious nature of your medical problem and risks of taking this medicine.

Before you start, consult your doctor:
- If you have gout.
- If you have had kidney stones.
- If you have active infection.
- If you have impaired kidney or liver function.
- If you have taken other antineoplastic drugs or had radiation treatment in last 3 weeks.

Over age 60:
Adverse reactions and side effects may be more frequent and severe than in younger persons.

Pregnancy:
Consult doctor. Risk to child is significant.

Breast-feeding:
Drug passes into milk. Don't nurse.

Infants & children:
Use only under care of medical supervisors who are experienced in anticancer drugs.

Prolonged use:
- Adverse reactions more likely the longer drug is required.
- Talk to your doctor about the need for follow-up medical examinations or laboratory studies to check complete blood counts (white blood cell count, platelet count, red blood cell count, hemoglobin, hematocrit), serum uric acid.

Skin & sunlight:
No problems expected.

Driving, piloting or hazardous work:
No problems expected.

Discontinuing:
Don't discontinue without doctor's advice until you complete prescribed dose, even though symptoms diminish or disappear. Some side effects may follow discontinuing. Report to doctor blurred vision, convulsions, confusion, persistent headache.

Others:
- May cause sterility.
- May increase chance of developing leukemia.

POSSIBLE INTERACTION WITH OTHER DRUGS

GENERIC NAME OR DRUG CLASS	COMBINED EFFECT
Antigout drugs*	Decreased antigout effect.
Antineoplastic drugs, other*	Increased effect of all drugs (may be beneficial).
Chloramphenicol	Increased likelihood of toxic effects of both drugs.
Clozapine	Toxic effect on bone marrow.
Lovastatin	Increased heart and kidney damage.
Tiopronin	Increased risk of toxicity to bone marrow.

POSSIBLE INTERACTION WITH OTHER SUBSTANCES

INTERACTS WITH	COMBINED EFFECT
Alcohol:	May increase chance of intestinal bleeding.
Beverages:	No problems expected.
Cocaine:	Increases chance of toxicity.
Foods:	Reduces irritation in stomach.
Marijuana:	No problems expected.
Tobacco:	Increases lung toxicity.

BUTALBITAL & ASPIRIN
(Also contains caffeine)

BRAND AND GENERIC NAMES

See complete list of brand and generic names in the *Brand Names Directory*, page 917.

BASIC INFORMATION

Habit forming? Yes
Prescription needed? Yes
Available as generic? Yes
Drug class: Analgesic, anti-inflammatory (non-steroidal), sedative

USES

- Reduces anxiety or nervous tension (low dose).
- Reduces pain, fever, inflammation.

DOSAGE & USAGE INFORMATION

How to take:
Tablet or capsule—Swallow with liquid or food to lessen stomach irritation. If you can't swallow whole, crumble tablet or open capsule and take with liquid or food.

When to take:
At the same times each day. No more often than every 4 hours.

If you forget a dose:
Take as soon as you remember up to 2 hours late. If more than 2 hours, wait for next scheduled dose (don't double this dose).

What drug does:
- May partially block nerve impulses at nerve-cell connections.
- Affects hypothalamus, the part of the brain which regulates temperature by dilating small blood vessels in skin.
- Prevents clumping of platelets (small blood cells) so blood vessels remain open.

Continued next column

OVERDOSE

SYMPTOMS:
Deep sleep, weak pulse, ringing in ears, nausea, vomiting, dizziness, fever, deep and rapid breathing, hallucinations, convulsions, coma.
WHAT TO DO:
- **Dial 0 (operator) or 911 (emergency) for an ambulance or medical help. Then give first aid immediately.**
- **See emergency information on inside covers.**

- Decreases prostaglandin effect.
- Suppresses body's pain messages.

Time lapse before drug works:
30 minutes.

Don't take with:
- Non-prescription drugs without consulting doctor.
- See Interaction column and consult doctor.

POSSIBLE ADVERSE REACTIONS OR SIDE EFFECTS

SYMPTOMS	WHAT TO DO
Life-threatening:	
Hives, rash, intense itching, faintness soon after a dose (anaphylaxis); wheezing; tightness in chest; black or bloody vomit; black stools; shortness of breath.	Seek emergency treatment immediately.
Common:	
Dizziness, drowsiness, heartburn.	Continue. Call doctor when convenient.
Infrequent:	
Jaundice; vomiting blood; easy bruising; skin rash, hives; confusion; depression; sore throat, fever, mouth sores; hearing loss; slurred speech; decreased vision.	Discontinue. Call doctor right away.
Rare:	
• Diminished vision, blood in urine, unexplained fever.	Discontinue. Call doctor right away.
• Insomnia, nightmares, constipation, headache, jaundice, nervousness.	Continue. Call doctor when convenient.

WARNINGS & PRECAUTIONS

Don't take if:
- You are allergic to any barbiturate or aspirin.
- You have a peptic ulcer of stomach or duodenum, bleeding disorder, porphyria.

Before you start, consult your doctor:
- If you have had stomach or duodenal ulcers.
- If you have asthma, nasal polyps, epilepsy, kidney or liver damage, anemia, chronic pain.
- If you will have surgery within 2 months, including dental surgery, requiring general or spinal anesthesia.

Over age 60:
- Adverse reactions and side effects may be more frequent and severe than in younger persons.
- More likely to cause hidden bleeding in stomach or intestines. Watch for dark stools.

Pregnancy:
Risk to unborn child outweighs drug benefits. Don't use.

Breast-feeding:
Drug passes into milk. Avoid drug or discontinue nursing until you finish medicine. Consult doctor for advice on maintaining milk supply.

Infants & children:
- Overdose frequent and severe. Keep bottles out of children's reach.
- Use only under doctor's supervision.
- Consult doctor before giving to persons under age 18 who have fever and discomfort of viral illness, especially chicken pox and influenza. Probably increases risk of Reye's syndrome.

Prolonged use:
- Kidney damage. Periodic kidney-function test recommended.
- May cause addiction, anemia, chronic intoxication.
- May lower body temperature, making exposure to cold temperatures hazardous.

Skin & sunlight:
May cause rash or intensify sunburn in areas exposed to sun or sunlamp.

Driving, piloting or hazardous work:
Don't drive or pilot aircraft until you learn how medicine affects you. Don't work around dangerous machinery. Don't climb ladders or work in high places. Danger increases if you drink alcohol or take medicine affecting alertness and reflexes, such as antihistamines, tranquilizers, sedatives, pain medicine, narcotics and mind-altering drugs.

Discontinuing:
May be unnecessary to finish medicine. Follow doctor's instructions. If you develop withdrawal symptoms of hallucinations, agitation or sleeplessness after discontinuing, call doctor right away.

Others:
- Aspirin can complicate surgery; illness; pregnancy, labor and delivery.
- For arthritis—Don't change dose without consulting doctor.
- Urine tests for blood sugar may be inaccurate.
- Great potential for abuse.

POSSIBLE INTERACTION WITH OTHER DRUGS

GENERIC NAME OR DRUG CLASS	COMBINED EFFECT
Allopurinol	Decreased allopurinol effect.
Antacids*	Decreased aspirin effect.
Anticoagulants, oral*	Increased anticoagulant effect. Abnormal bleeding.
Anticonvulsants*	Changed seizure patterns.
Antidepressants*	Decreased antidepressant effect. Possible dangerous oversedation.
Antidiabetics, oral*	Increased butalbital effect. Low blood sugar.
Antihistamines*	Dangerous sedation. Avoid.
Aspirin, other	Likely aspirin toxicity.
Beta-adrenergic blockers*	Decreased effect of beta-adrenergic blocker.
Contraceptives, oral*	Decreased contraceptive effect.

Continued page 938

POSSIBLE INTERACTION WITH OTHER SUBSTANCES

INTERACTS WITH	COMBINED EFFECT
Alcohol:	Possible stomach irritation and bleeding, possible fatal oversedation. Avoid.
Beverages:	None expected.
Cocaine:	Decreased butalbital effect.
Foods:	None expected.
Marijuana:	Possible increased pain relief, but marijuana may slow body's recovery. Avoid.
Tobacco:	None expected.

BUTALBITAL, ASPIRIN & CODEINE
(Also contains caffeine)

BRAND NAMES

ABC Compound
with Codeine

Ascomp with
Codeine No. 3

B-A-C with Codeine

Butinal with
Codeine No. 3

Fiomor with Codeine

Fiorgen with Codeine

Fiorinal with Codeine

Isollyl with Codeine

BASIC INFORMATION

Habit forming? Yes
Prescription needed? Yes
Available as generic? No
Drug class: Narcotic, analgesic

 ## USES

- Reduces anxiety or nervous tension (low dose).
- Reduces pain, fever, inflammation.

 ## DOSAGE & USAGE INFORMATION

How to take:
- Tablet or capsule—Swallow with liquid or food to lessen stomach irritation. If you can't swallow whole, crumble tablet or open capsule and take with liquid or food.
- Extended-release tablets or capsules— Swallow each dose whole.

When to take:
When needed. No more often than every 4 hours.

Continued next column

 ## OVERDOSE

SYMPTOMS:
Deep sleep, slow and weak pulse, ringing in ears, nausea, vomiting, dizziness, fever, deep and rapid breathing, hallucinations, convulsions, coma.
WHAT TO DO:
- **Dial 0 (operator) or 911 (emergency) for an ambulance or medical help. Then give first aid immediately.**
- **If patient is unconscious and not breathing, give mouth-to-mouth breathing. if there is no heartbeat, use cardiac massage and mouth-to-mouth breathing (CPR). Don't try to make patient vomit. If you can't get help quickly, take patient to nearest emergency facility.**
- **See emergency information on inside covers.**

If you forget a dose:
Take as soon as you remember. Wait 4 hours for next dose.

What drug does:
- May partially block nerve impulses at nerve-cell connections.
- Affects hypothalamus, the part of the brain which regulates temperature by dilating small blood vessels in skin.
- Prevents clumping of platelets (small blood cells) so blood vessels remain open.
- Decreases prostaglandin effect.
- Blocks pain messages to brain and spinal cord.
- Reduces sensitivity of brain's cough-control center.

Time lapse before drug works:
30 minutes.

Don't take with:
- Non-prescription drugs without consulting doctor.
- See Interaction column and consult doctor.

 ## POSSIBLE ADVERSE REACTIONS OR SIDE EFFECTS

SYMPTOMS	WHAT TO DO
Life-threatening: Wheezing, tightness in chest, pinpoint pupils.	Seek emergency treatment immediately.
Common: Dizziness, drowsiness, heartburn, flushed face, depression, false sense of well-being, increased urination.	Continue. Call doctor when convenient.
Infrequent: Jaundice; vomiting blood; easy bruising; skin rash, hives; confusion; depression; sore throat, fever, mouth sores; difficult urination; hearing loss; slurred speech; blood in urine; decreased vision.	Discontinue. Call doctor right away.
Rare: Insomnia, nightmares, constipation, headache, nervousness, flushed face, increased sweating, unusual tiredness.	Continue. Call doctor when convenient.

BUTALBITAL, ASPIRIN & CODEINE
(Also contains caffeine)

WARNINGS & PRECAUTIONS

Don't take if:
- You are allergic to any barbiturate or narcotic.
- You have a peptic ulcer of stomach or duodenum, bleeding disorder, porphyria.

Before you start, consult your doctor:
- If you have had stomach or duodenal ulcers.
- If you have asthma, epilepsy, kidney or liver damage, anemia, chronic pain, gout.
- If you will have surgery within 2 months, including dental surgery, requiring general or spinal anesthesia.

Over age 60:
- Adverse reactions and side effects may be more frequent and severe than in younger persons.
- More likely to cause hidden bleeding in stomach or intestines. Watch for dark stools.
- More likely to be drowsy, dizzy, unsteady or constipated. Use only if absolutely necessary.

Pregnancy:
Risk to unborn child outweighs drug benefits. Don't use.

Breast-feeding:
Drug passes into milk. Avoid drug or discontinue nursing until you finish medicine. Consult doctor for advice on maintaining milk supply.

Infants & children:
- Overdose frequent and severe. Keep bottles out of children's reach.
- Use only under doctor's supervision.
- Consult doctor before giving to persons under age 18 who have fever and discomfort of viral illness, especially chicken pox and influenza. Probably increases risk of Reye's syndrome.

Prolonged use:
- Kidney damage. Periodic kidney-function test recommended.
- May cause addiction, anemia, chronic intoxication.
- May lower body temperature, making exposure to cold temperatures hazardous.

Skin & sunlight:
May cause rash or intensify sunburn in areas exposed to sun or sunlamp.

Driving, piloting or hazardous work:
Don't drive or pilot aircraft until you learn how medicine affects you. Don't work around dangerous machinery. Don't climb ladders or work in high places. Danger increases if you drink alcohol or take medicine affecting alertness and reflexes, such as antihistamines, tranquilizers, sedatives, pain medicine, narcotics and mind-altering drugs.

Discontinuing:
May be unnecessary to finish medicine. Follow doctor's instructions. If you develop withdrawal symptoms of hallucinations, agitation or sleeplessness after discontinuing, call doctor right away.

Others:
- Aspirin can complicate surgery; illness; pregnancy, labor and delivery.
- For arthritis—Don't change dose without consulting doctor.
- Urine tests for blood sugar may be inaccurate.
- Great potential for abuse.

POSSIBLE INTERACTION WITH OTHER DRUGS

GENERIC NAME OR DRUG CLASS	COMBINED EFFECT
Allopurinol	Decreased allopurinol effect.
Analgesics, other*	Increased analgesic effect.
Antacids*	Decreased aspirin effect.
Anticoagulants, oral*	Increased anticoagulant effect. Abnormal bleeding.
Anticonvulsants*	Changed seizure patterns.

Continued page 939

POSSIBLE INTERACTION WITH OTHER SUBSTANCES

INTERACTS WITH	COMBINED EFFECT
Alcohol:	Possible stomach irritation and bleeding, possible fatal oversedation. Avoid.
Beverages:	None expected.
Cocaine:	Increased cocaine toxic effects. Avoid.
Foods:	None expected.
Marijuana:	Possible increased pain relief, but marijuana may slow body's recovery. Impairs physical and mental performance. Avoid.
Tobacco:	None expected.

*See Glossary

CAFFEINE

See complete list of brand names in the *Brand Name Directory*, page 917.

BRAND NAMES

See complete list of brand names in the
Brand Name Directory, page 917.

BASIC INFORMATION

Habit forming? Yes
Prescription needed? No
Available as generic? Yes
Drug class: Stimulant (xanthine),
vasoconstrictor

 USES

- Treatment for drowsiness and fatigue.
- Treatment for migraine and other vascular headaches in combination with ergot.

 DOSAGE & USAGE INFORMATION

How to take:
- Tablet or liquid—Swallow with liquid or food to lessen stomach irritation. If you can't swallow whole, crumble tablet and take with liquid or food.
- Extended-release capsules—Swallow whole with liquid.

When to take:
At the same times each day.

If you forget a dose:
Take as soon as you remember up to 2 hours late. If more than 2 hours, wait for next scheduled dose (don't double this dose).

What drug does:
- Constricts blood-vessel walls.
- Stimulates central nervous system.

Time lapse before drug works:
30 minutes.

Continued next column

 OVERDOSE

SYMPTOMS:
Excitement, insomnia, rapid heartbeat
(infants can have slow heartbeat),
confusion, fever, hallucinations,
convulsions, coma.
WHAT TO DO:
- Dial 0 (operator) or 911 (emergency) for an ambulance or medical help. Then give first aid immediately.
- See emergency information on inside covers.

Don't take with:
- Non-prescription drugs without consulting doctor.
- See Interaction column and consult doctor.

 POSSIBLE ADVERSE REACTIONS OR SIDE EFFECTS

SYMPTOMS	WHAT TO DO
Life-threatening:	
In case of overdose, see previous column.	
Common:	
• Rapid heartbeat, low blood sugar (hunger, anxiety, cold sweats, rapid pulse) with tremor, irritability (mild).	Discontinue. Call doctor right away.
• Nervousness, insomnia.	Continue. Tell doctor at next visit.
• Increased urination.	No action necessary.
Infrequent:	
• Confusion, irritability (severe).	Discontinue. Call doctor right away.
• Nausea, indigestion, burning feeling in stomach.	Continue. Call doctor when convenient.
Rare:	
None expected.	

WARNINGS & PRECAUTIONS

Don't take if:
- You are allergic to any stimulant.
- You have heart disease.
- You have active peptic ulcer of stomach or duodenum.

Before you start, consult your doctor:
- If you have irregular heartbeat.
- If you have hypoglycemia (low blood sugar).
- If you have epilepsy.
- If you have high blood pressure.
- If you have insomnia.

Over age 60:
Adverse reactions and side effects may be more frequent and severe than in younger persons.

Pregnancy:
Risk to unborn child outweighs drug benefits. Don't use.

Breast-feeding:
Drug passes into milk. Avoid drug or discontinue nursing until you finish medicine. Consult doctor for advice on maintaining milk supply.

Infants & children:
Not recommended.

Prolonged use:
Stomach ulcers.

Skin & sunlight:
No problems expected.

Driving, piloting or hazardous work:
No problems expected.

Discontinuing:
Will cause withdrawal symptoms of headache, irritability, drowsiness. Discontinue gradually if you use caffeine for a month or more.

Others:
May produce or aggravate fibrocystic disease of the breast in women.

POSSIBLE INTERACTION WITH OTHER DRUGS

GENERIC NAME OR DRUG CLASS	COMBINED EFFECT
Cimetidine	Increased caffeine effect.
Contraceptives, oral*	Increased caffeine effect.
Isoniazid	Increased caffeine effect.
MAO inhibitors*	Dangerous blood-pressure rise.
Sedatives*	Decreased sedative effect.
Sleep inducers*	Decreased sedative effect.
Sympathomimetics*	Overstimulation.
Thyroid hormones*	Increased thyroid effect.
Tranquilizers*	Decreased tranquilizer effect.

POSSIBLE INTERACTION WITH OTHER SUBSTANCES

INTERACTS WITH	COMBINED EFFECT
Alcohol:	Decreased alcohol effect.
Beverages: Caffeine drinks (coffee, tea, or soft drinks).	Increased caffeine effect.
Cocaine	Convulsions or excessive nervousness.
Foods:	No proven problems.
Marijuana:	Increased effect of both drugs. May lead to dangerous, rapid heartbeat. Avoid.
Tobacco:	Increased heartbeat. Avoid. Decreased caffeine effect.

*See Glossary

CALCIUM CHANNEL BLOCKERS

BRAND AND GENERIC NAMES

See complete list of brand and generic names in *Brand Name Directory*, page 917.

BASIC INFORMATION

Habit forming? No
Prescription needed? Yes
Available as generic? Yes
Drug class: Calcium channel blocker, antiarrhythmic, antianginal

USES

- Prevents angina attacks.
- Stabilizes irregular heartbeat.
- Treats high blood pressure.

DOSAGE & USAGE INFORMATION

How to take:
- Tablet or capsule—Swallow with liquid. You may chew or crush tablet.
- Extended-release tablets or capsules—Swallow each dose whole with liquid; do not crush.

When to take:
At the same times each day. Take verapamil with food.

If you forget a dose:
Take as soon as you remember up to 2 hours late. If more than 2 hours, wait for next scheduled dose (don't double this dose).

What drug does:
- Reduces work that heart must perform.
- Reduces normal artery pressure.
- Increases oxygen to heart muscle.

Continued in next column

OVERDOSE

SYMPTOMS:
Unusually fast or unusually slow heartbeat, loss of consciousness, cardiac arrest.
WHAT TO DO:
- **Dial 0 (operator) or 911 (emergency) for an ambulance or medical help. Then give first aid immediately.**
- **If patient is unconscious and not breathing, give mouth-to-mouth breathing. If there is no heartbeat, use cardiac massage and mouth-to-mouth breathing (CPR). Don't try to make patient vomit. If you can't get help quickly, take patient to nearest emergency facility.**
- **See emergency information on inside covers.**

Time lapse before drug works:
1 to 2 hours.

Don't take with:
Any other medicine without consulting your doctor or pharmacist.

POSSIBLE ADVERSE REACTIONS OR SIDE EFFECTS

SYMPTOMS	WHAT TO DO
Life-threatening:	
In case of overdose. see previous column.	
Common:	
Tiredness.	Continue. Tell doctor at next visit.
Infrequent:	
• Unusually fast or unusually slow heartbeat, wheezing, cough, shortness of breath.	Discontinue. Call doctor right away.
• Dizziness; numbness or tingling in hands and feet; swollen feet, ankles or legs; difficult urination.	Continue. Call doctor when convenient.
• Nausea, constipation.	Continue. Tell doctor at next visit.
Rare:	
• Fainting, depression, psychosis, rash, jaundice.	Discontinue. Call doctor right away.
• Headache, insomnia, vivid dreams, hair loss.	Continue. Tell doctor at next visit.

WARNINGS & PRECAUTIONS

Don't take if:
- You are allergic to calcium channel blockers.
- You have very low blood pressure.

Before you start, consult your doctor:
- If you have kidney or liver disease.
- If you have high blood pressure.
- If you have heart disease other than coronary artery disease.

Over age 60:
Adverse reactions and side effects may be more frequent and severe than in younger persons.

Pregnancy:
Risks to unborn child outweigh benefits. Don't use.

Breast-feeding:
Safety not established. Avoid if possible.

Infants & children:
Not recommended.

all activities
function of cells.
for bone, nerve

ollow-up
to check
, ECG*.

ks:

oblems

ours have passed

consulting your

e until
ugh

CTIONS
CTS
AT TO DO

drops
ke drug

continue. Seek
ergency treatment.

ON

EFFECT

continue. Call
or right away.

ssive
olood.
require

continue. Call
or right away.

ased
icity of

ased
effect.

ect.

e drop.
require

ular
con-
failure.

um level.

eased
um
er.

ur doctor:
ease, kidney
sis, malabsorption.

e effect

ased
um
er.

k your doctor.

oxicity.

italis
ed to

supervision.

Disopyramide	May cause dangerously slow, fast or irregular heartbeat.
Diuretics*	Dangerous blood pressure drop. Dosages may require adjustment.
Encainide	Increased effect of toxicity on heart muscle.
Lithium	Possible decreased lithium effect.
Nicardipine	Possible increased effect and toxicity of each drug.
Nimodipine	Dangerous blood pressure drop.
Nitrates*	Reduced angina attacks.
Propafenone	Increased effect of both drugs and increased risk of toxicity.
Quinidine	Increased quinidine effect.
Rifampin	Decreased effect of calcium channel blocker.
Theophylline	May increase effect and toxicity of theophylline.
Phenytoin	Possible decreased calcium channel blocker effect.
Vitamin D	Decreased effect of calcium channel blockers.

 POSSIBLE INTERACTION WITH OTHER SUBSTANCES

INTERACTS WITH	COMBINED EFFECT
Alcohol:	Dangerously low blood pressure. Avoid.
Beverages:	None expected.
Cocaine:	Possible irregular heartbeat. Avoid.
Foods:	None expected.
Marijuana:	Possible irregular heartbeat. Avoid.
Tobacco:	Possible rapid heartbeat. Avoid.

BRAND AND GENERIC NAMES

See complete list of brand and generic names in the *Brand Name Directory*, page 917.

BASIC INFORMATION

Habit forming? No
Prescription needed? For some
Available as generic? Yes
Drug class: Antihypocalcemic, dietary replacement

USES

- Treats or prevents osteoporosis (thin, porous, easily fractured bones). Frequently prescribed with estrogen beginning at menopause.
- Helps heart, muscle and nervous system to work properly.
- Dietary supplement when calcium ingestion is insufficient or there is a deficiency such as osteomalacia or rickets.

DOSAGE & USAGE INFORMATION

How to take:
- Take in addition to foods high in calcium (milk, yogurt, sardines, cheese, canned salmon, turnip greens, broccoli, shrimp, tofu).
- Tablet—Swallow with liquid or food to lessen stomach irritation. If you can't swallow whole, crumble tablet and take with food or liquid.
- Syrup—Take before meals.
- Suspension—Swallow with liquid or food to lessen stomach irritation.

When to take:
As directed. Don't take within 2 hours of any other medicine you take by mouth.

If you forget a dose:
Use as soon as you remember.

Continued next column

OVERDOSE

SYMPTOMS:
Confusion, irregular heartbeat, depression, bone pain, coma.
WHAT TO DO:
- **Dial 0 (operator) or 911 (emergency) for an ambulance or medical help. Then give first aid immediately.**
- **See emergency information on inside covers.**

What drug does:
- Participates in metabolism essential for normal life and
- Provides calcium necessary function.

Time lapse before drug wo
15 to 30 minutes.

Don't take with:
- Any other medicine until 2 since taking calcium.
- Any other medicine without doctor or pharmacist.

POSSIBLE ADVERSE REA OR SIDE EFFE

SYMPTOMS	W
Life-threatening:	
Irregular or very slow heart rate.	Dis em
Common:	
None expected.	
Infrequent:	
Constipation, diarrhea, drowsiness, headache, appetite loss, dry mouth, weakness.	Dis do
Rare:	
Frequent, painful or difficult urination; increased thirst; nausea, vomiting; rash; urine frequency increased and volume larger; confusion; high blood pressure; eyes sensitive to light.	Dis do

WARNINGS & PRECAUTIONS

Don't take if:
- You are allergic to calcium
- You have a high blood-calc

Before you start, consult y
If you have diarrhea, heart di stones, kidney disease, sarcoid

Over age 60:
No problems expected.

Pregnancy:
No problems expected, but a

Breast-feeding:
No problems expected.

Infants & children:
Use only under close medica

Prolonged use:
- Side effects more likely.
- Talk to your doctor about the need for follow-up medical examinations or laboratory studies to check serum calcium determinations, blood pressure, urine.

Skin & sunlight:
No problems expected.

Driving, piloting or hazardous work:
No problems expected.

Discontinuing:
No problems expected.

Others:
- Exercise, along with vitamin D from sunshine and calcium, helps prevent osteoporosis.
- Don't use bone meal or dolomite as a source for calcium supplement (they may contain lead).

 POSSIBLE INTERACTION WITH OTHER DRUGS

GENERIC NAME OR DRUG CLASS	COMBINED EFFECT
Anticoagulants, oral*	Decreased anti-coagulant effect.
Calcitonin	Decreased calcitonin effect.
Chlorpromazine	Decreased chlor-promazine effect.
Corticosteroids*	Decreased calcium absorption and effect.
Digitalis preparations*	Decreased digitalis effect.
Diuretics, thiazide*	Increased calcium in blood.
Estrogens and birth control pills*	May increase absorption of calcium—frequently a desirable combined effect.
Iron supplements*	Decreased iron effect.
Meperidine	Increased meperidine effect.
Mexiletine	May slow elimination of mexiletine and cause need to adjust dosage.
Nalidixic acid	Decreased effect of nalidixic acid.
Nicardipine	Possible decreased nicardipine effect.
Nimodipine	Possible decreased nimodipine effect.
Oxyphenbutazone	Decreased oxyphen-butazone effect.
Para-aminosalicylic acid (PAS)	Decreased PAS effect.
Penicillins*	Decreased penicillin effect.
Pentobarbital	Decreased pento-barbital effect.
Phenylbutazone	Decreased phenyl-butazone effect.
Phenytoin	Decreased phenytoin absorption.
Pseudoephedrine	Increased pseudo-ephedrine effect.
Quinidine	Increased quinidine effect.
Salicylates*	Increased salicylate effect.
Sulfa drugs*	Decreased sulfa effect.
Tetracyclines*	Decreased tetracycline effect.
Vitamin A	Decreased vitamin effect.
Vitamin D	Increased vitamin absorption, some-times excessively.

 POSSIBLE INTERACTION WITH OTHER SUBSTANCES

INTERACTS WITH	COMBINED EFFECT
Alcohol:	Decreased absorption of calcium.
Beverages:	No problems expected.
Cocaine:	No proven problems.
Foods: Don't take within 1 or 2 hours of eating.	Decreased absorption of calcium.
Marijuana:	Decreased absorption of calcium.
Tobacco:	Decreased absorption of calcium.

CAPSAICIN

BRAND NAMES

Axsain   Zotrix-HP
Zotrix

BASIC INFORMATION

Habit forming? No
Prescription needed? No
Available as generic? No
Drug class: Analgesic (topical)

 ## USES

- Treats neuralgias, such as pain that occurs following shingles (herpes zoster) or neuropathy of the feet, ankles and fingers (common in diabetes).
- Treats discomfort caused by arthritis.

 ## DOSAGE & USAGE INFORMATION

How to use:
Cream—Apply a small amount and rub carefully on the affected areas. Use every day. Wash hands after applying. Don't apply to irritated skin. Don't bandage over treated areas.

When to use:
Apply 3 or 4 times a day.

If you forget a dose:
Use as soon as you remember.

What drug does:
Blocks transmission of pain impulses.

Time lapse before drug works:
Begins to work immediately. Frequently takes 2 to 3 weeks for full benefit, but may take up to 6 or 8 weeks.

Don't use with:
No problems expected.

 ## OVERDOSE

SYMPTOMS:
None expected.
WHAT TO DO:
Not intended for internal use. If child accidentally swallows, call poison-control center.

 ## POSSIBLE ADVERSE REACTIONS OR SIDE EFFECTS

SYMPTOMS	WHAT TO DO
Life-threatening: None expected.	
Common: Stinging or burning sensation at application site.	Nothing. It usually improves in 2 to 3 days or becomes less severe the longer you use the drug.
Infrequent: None expected.	
Rare: None expected.	

WARNINGS & PRECAUTIONS

Don't use if:
You are allergic to capsaicin or to the fruit of capsaicin plants (for example, hot peppers).

Before you start, consult your doctor:
If you have any allergies.

Over age 60:
No problems expected.

Pregnancy:
No problems expected.

Breast-feeding:
No problems expected.

Infants & children:
Not recommended for children under age 2.

Prolonged use:
No problems expected.

Skin & sunlight:
No problems expected.

Driving, piloting or hazardous work:
No problems expected.

Discontinuing:
Discontinue if there are no signs of improvement within a month.

Others:
- Capsaicin is not a local anesthetic*.
- Although capsaicin may help relieve the pain of neuropathy, it does not cure any disorder.
- If you accidently get some capsaicin in your eye, flush with water.

POSSIBLE INTERACTION WITH OTHER DRUGS

GENERIC NAME OR DRUG CLASS	COMBINED EFFECT
None expected	

POSSIBLE INTERACTION WITH OTHER SUBSTANCES

INTERACTS WITH	COMBINED EFFECT
Alcohol:	No proven problems.
Beverages:	No proven problems.
Cocaine:	No proven problems.
Foods:	No proven problems.
Marijuana:	No proven problems.
Tobacco:	No proven problems.

*See Glossary

CARBAMAZEPINE

BRAND NAMES

Apo-Carbamazepine   Mazepine
Epitol   Tegretol
Novocarbamaz

BASIC INFORMATION

Habit forming? No
Prescription needed? Yes
Available as generic? Yes
Drug class: Analgesic, anticonvulsant

USES

- Decreased frequency, severity and duration of attacks of tic douloureaux.*
- Prevents seizures.

DOSAGE & USAGE INFORMATION

How to take:
Regular or chewable tablet—Swallow with liquid or food to lessen stomach irritation.

When to take:
At the same times each day.

If you forget a dose:
Take as soon as you remember up to 2 hours late. If more than 2 hours, wait for next scheduled dose (don't double this dose).

What drug does:
- Reduces transmission of pain messages at certain nerve terminals.
- Reduces excitability of nerve fibers in brain, thus inhibiting repetitive spread of nerve impulses.

Continued next column

OVERDOSE

SYMPTOMS:
Involuntary movements, irregular bleeding, decreased urination, decreased blood pressure, dilated pupils, flushed skin, stupor, coma.
WHAT TO DO:
- **Dial 0 (operator) or 911 (emergency) for an ambulance or medical help. Then give first aid immediately.**
- **If patient is unconscious and not breathing, give mouth-to-mouth breathing. If there is no heartbeat, use cardiac massage and mouth-to-mouth breathing (CPR). Don't try to make patient vomit. If you can't get help quickly, take patient to nearest emergency facility.**
- **See emergency information on inside covers.**

Time lapse before drug works:
- Tic douloureaux—24 to 72 hours.
- Seizures—1 to 2 weeks.

Don't take with:
Any other medicine without consulting your doctor or pharmacist.

POSSIBLE ADVERSE REACTIONS OR SIDE EFFECTS

SYMPTOMS	WHAT TO DO
Life-threatening:	
In case of overdose, see previous column.	
Common:	
Blurred vision.	Continue. Call doctor when convenient.
Back-and-forth eye movements.	Discontinue. Call doctor right away.
Infrequent:	
Confusion, slurred speech, fainting, depression, headache, hallucinations, hives, rash, mouth sores, sore throat, fever, unusual bleeding or bruising, unusual fatigue, jaundice.	Discontinue. Call doctor right away.
Diarrhea, nausea, vomiting, constipation, dry mouth, impotence.	Continue. Call doctor when convenient.
Rare:	
Breathing difficulty; irregular, pounding or slow heartbeat; chest pain; uncontrollable body jerks; numbness, weakness or tingling in hands and feet; tender, bluish legs or feet; less urine; swollen lymph glands.	Discontinue. Call doctor right away.
Frequent urination, muscle pains, joint aches.	Continue. Call doctor when convenient.

WARNINGS & PRECAUTIONS

Don't take if:
- You are allergic to carbamazepine.
- You have had liver or bone-marrow disease.
- You have taken MAO inhibitors in the past 2 weeks.

Before you start, consult your doctor:
- If you have high blood pressure, thrombophlebitis or heart disease.
- If you have glaucoma.
- If you have emotional or mental problems.

- If you have liver or kidney disease.
- If you drink more than 2 alcoholic drinks per day.

Over age 60:
Adverse reactions and side effects may be more frequent and severe than in younger persons.

Pregnancy:
Studies inconclusive on harm to unborn child. Animal studies show fetal abnormalities. Decide with your doctor whether drug benefits justify risk to unborn child.

Breast-feeding:
Drug passes into milk. Avoid drug or discontinue nursing until you finish medicine. Consult doctor for advice on maintaining milk supply.

Infants & children:
Not recommended.

Prolonged use:
- Jaundice and liver damage.
- Hair loss.
- Ringing in ears.
- Lower sex drive.
- Talk to your doctor about the need for follow-up medical examinations or laboratory studies to check complete blood counts (white blood cell count, platelet count, red blood cell count, hemoglobin, hematocrit), serum iron.

Skin & sunlight:
May cause rash or intensify sunburn in areas exposed to sun or sunlamp.

Driving, piloting or hazardous work:
Don't drive or pilot aircraft until you learn how medicine affects you. Don't work around dangerous machinery. Don't climb ladders or work in high places. Danger increases if you drink alcohol or take medicine affecting alertness and reflexes.

Discontinuing:
Don't discontinue without doctor's advice until you complete prescribed dose, even though symptoms diminish or disappear.

Others:
- Use only if less-hazardous drugs are not effective. Stay under medical supervision.
- Periodic blood tests are needed.

 POSSIBLE INTERACTION WITH OTHER DRUGS

GENERIC NAME OR DRUG CLASS	COMBINED EFFECT
Anticoagulants, oral*	Decreased anticoagulant effect.
Anticonvulsants, hydantoin*	Decreased effect of both drugs.
Antidepressants, tricyclic (TCA)*	Confusion. Possible psychosis.

Cimetidine	Increased carbamazepine effect.
Clozapine	Toxic effect on bone marrow and central nervous system.
Contraceptives, oral*	Reduced contraceptive protection. Use another birth-control method.
Cortisone*	Decreased cortisone effect.
Desmopressin	May increase desmopressin effect.
Digitalis preparations*	Excess slowing of heart.
Doxycycline	Decreased doxycycline effect.
Erythromycins*	Increased carbamazepine effect.
Ethinamate	Dangerous increased effects of ethinamate. Avoid combining.
Fluoxetine	Increased depressant effects of both drugs.
Guanfacine	May increase depressant effects of either drug.
Isoniazid	Increased risk of liver damage.
Leucovorin	High alcohol content of leucovorin may cause adverse effects.

Continued page 940

 POSSIBLE INTERACTION WITH OTHER SUBSTANCES

INTERACTS WITH	COMBINED EFFECT
Alcohol:	Increased sedative effect of alcohol. Avoid.
Beverages:	None expected.
Cocaine:	Increased adverse effects of carbamazepine. Avoid.
Foods:	None expected.
Marijuana:	Increased adverse effects of carbamazepine. Avoid.
Tobacco:	None expected.

*See Glossary

CARBENICILLIN

BRAND NAMES

Geocillin   Geopen Oral
Geopen   Pyopen

BASIC INFORMATION

Habit forming? No
Prescription needed? Yes
Available as generic? No
Drug class: Antibiotic (penicillin)

 ## USES

Treatment of bacterial urinary tract infections that are susceptible to carbenicillin.

 ## DOSAGE & USAGE INFORMATION

How to take:
Tablet—Swallow with liquid on an empty stomach 1 hour before or 2 hours after eating.

When to take:
Follow instructions on prescription label or side of package. Doses should be evenly spaced. For example, 4 times a day means every 6 hours.

If you forget a dose:
Take as soon as you remember. Continue regular schedule.

What drug does:
Destroys susceptible bacteria. Does not kill viruses.

Time lapse before drug works:
May be several days before medicine affects infection.

Don't take with:
Any other medicine without consulting your doctor or pharmacist.

 ## OVERDOSE

SYMPTOMS:
Severe diarrhea, nausea or vomiting.
WHAT TO DO:
Overdose unlikely to threaten life. If person takes much larger amount than prescribed, call doctor, poison-control center or hospital emergency room for instructions.

 ## POSSIBLE ADVERSE REACTIONS OR SIDE EFFECTS

SYMPTOMS	WHAT TO DO
Life-threatening:	
Hives, rash, intense itching, faintness soon after a dose (anaphylaxis).	Seek emergency treatment immediately.
Common:	
Dark or discolored tongue.	Continue. Tell doctor at next visit.
Infrequent:	
• Mild nausea, vomiting, diarrhea.	Continue. Call doctor when convenient.
• Bloody urine, face and ankle swelling.	Discontinue. Call doctor right away.
Rare:	
Unexplained bleeding or bruising, weakness, sore throat, fever, abdominal cramps, convulsions.	Discontinue. Call doctor right away.

WARNINGS & PRECAUTIONS

Don't take if:
You are allergic to carbenicillin, cephalosporin antibiotics, or other penicillins. Life-threatening reaction may occur.

Before you start, consult your doctor:
- If you are allergic to any substance or drug.
- If you take birth control pills.

Over age 60:
You may have skin reactions, particularly around genitals and anus.

Pregnancy:
Studies inconclusive on harm to unborn child. Animal studies show fetal abnormalities. Decide with your doctor whether drug benefits justify risk to unborn child.

Breast-feeding:
Drug passes into milk. Child may become sensitive to penicillins and have allergic reactions to penicillin drugs. Avoid carbenicillin or discontinue nursing until you finish medicine. Consult doctor for advice on maintaining milk supply.

Infants & children:
No problems expected.

Prolonged use:
- You may become more susceptible to infections caused by germs not responsive to carbenicillin.
- Talk to your doctor about the need for follow-up medical examinations or laboratory studies to check SGPT*, SGOT*.

Skin & sunlight:
No problems expected.

Driving, piloting or hazardous work:
Usually not dangerous. Most hazardous reactions likely to occur a few minutes after taking carbenicillin.

Discontinuing:
Don't discontinue without doctor's advice until you complete prescribed dose, even though symptoms diminish or disappear.

Others:
- Injection forms may cause fluid retention (edema) with weakness and low potassium in the blood.
- May interfere with the accuracy of some medical tests.
- Birth control pills may not be effective. Use additional birth-control methods.

POSSIBLE INTERACTION WITH OTHER DRUGS

GENERIC NAME OR DRUG CLASS	COMBINED EFFECT
Beta-adrenergic blockers*	Increased chance of anaphylaxis (see emergency information on inside front cover).
Birth control pills.	Impaired contraceptive efficiency.
Chloramphenicol	Decreased effect of both drugs.
Cholestyramine	May decrease carbenicillin effect.
Colestipol	May decrease carbenicillin effect.
Erythromycins*	Decreased effect of both drugs.
Paromomycin	Decreased effect of both drugs.
Probenecid	Increased effect of all penicillins.
Sodium benzoate & sodium phenylacetate	May reduce effect of sodium benzoate & sodium phenylacetate.
Tetracyclines*	Decreased effect of both drugs.
Troleandomycin	Decreased effect of both drugs.

POSSIBLE INTERACTION WITH OTHER SUBSTANCES

INTERACTS WITH	COMBINED EFFECT
Alcohol:	Occasional stomach irritation.
Beverages:	None expected.
Cocaine:	No proven problems.
Foods: Acidic fruits or juices, aged cheese, wines, syrups (if taken with).	Decreased antibiotic effect.
Marijuana:	No proven problems.
Tobacco:	None expected.

*See Glossary

CARBIDOPA & LEVODOPA

BRAND NAMES

Sinemet   **Sinemet CR**

BASIC INFORMATION

Habit forming? No
Prescription needed? Yes
Available as generic? No
Drug class: Antiparkinsonism

USES

Controls Parkinson's disease symptoms such as rigidity, tremor and unsteady gait.

DOSAGE & USAGE INFORMATION

How to take:
Tablet—Swallow with liquid or food to lessen stomach irritation. If you can't swallow whole, crumble tablet and take with liquid or food.

When to take:
At the same times each day.

If you forget a dose:
Take as soon as you remember up to 2 hours late. If more than 2 hours, wait for next scheduled dose (don't double this dose).

What drug does:
Restores chemical balance necessary for normal nerve impulses.

Continued next column

OVERDOSE

SYMPTOMS:
Muscle twitch, spastic eyelid closure, nausea, vomiting, diarrhea, irregular and rapid pulse, weakness, fainting, confusion, agitation, hallucination, coma.
WHAT TO DO:
- **Dial 0 (operator) or 911 (emergency) for an ambulance or medical help. Then give first aid immediately.**
- **If patient is unconscious and not breathing, give mouth-to-mouth breathing. If there is no heartbeat, use cardiac massage and mouth-to-mouth breathing (CPR). Don't try to make patient vomit. If you can't get help quickly, take patient to nearest emergency facility.**
- **See emergency information on inside covers.**

Time lapse before drug works:
2 to 3 weeks to improve; 6 weeks or longer for maximum benefit.

Don't take with:
Any other medicine without consulting your doctor or pharmacist.

POSSIBLE ADVERSE REACTIONS OR SIDE EFFECTS

SYMPTOMS	WHAT TO DO
Life-threatening:	
In case of overdose, see previous column.	
Common:	
• Mood changes, uncontrollable body movements, diarrhea.	Continue. Call doctor when convenient.
• Dry mouth, body odor.	No action necessary.
Infrequent:	
• Fainting, severe dizziness, headache, insomnia, nightmares, rash, itch, nausea, vomiting, irregular heartbeat.	Discontinue. Call doctor right away.
• Flushed face, blurred vision, muscle twitching, discolored or dark urine, difficult urination.	Continue. Call doctor when convenient.
• Constipation, tiredness.	Continue. Tell doctor at next visit.
Rare:	
• High blood pressure.	Discontinue. Call doctor right away.
• Upper abdominal pain, anemia.	Continue. Call doctor when convenient.

WARNINGS & PRECAUTIONS

Don't take if:
- You are allergic to levodopa or carbidopa.
- You have taken MAO inhibitors in past 2 weeks.
- You have glaucoma (narrow-angle type).

Before you start, consult your doctor:
- You have diabetes or epilepsy.
- If you have had high blood pressure, heart or lung disease.
- If you have had liver or kidney disease.
- If you have a peptic ulcer.
- If you have malignant melanoma.
- If you will have surgery within 2 months, including dental surgery, requiring general or spinal anesthesia.

Over age 60:
Adverse reactions and side effects may be more frequent and severe than in younger persons.

Pregnancy:
Risk to unborn child outweighs drug benefits. Don't use.

Breast-feeding:
Drug filters into milk. May harm child. Avoid.

Infants & children:
Not recommended.

Prolonged use:
- May lead to uncontrolled movements of head, face, mouth, tongue, arms or legs.
- Talk to your doctor about the need for follow-up medical examinations or laboratory studies to check complete blood counts (white blood cell count, platelet count, red blood cell count, hemoglobin, hematocrit), liver function, eyes, kidney function.

Skin & sunlight:
No problems expected.

Driving, piloting or hazardous work:
Don't drive or pilot aircraft until you learn how medicine affects you. Don't work around dangerous machinery. Don't climb ladders or work in high places. Danger increases if you drink alcohol or take medicine affecting alertness and reflexes, such as antihistamines, tranquilizers, sedatives, pain medicine, narcotics and mind-altering drugs.

Discontinuing:
Don't discontinue without doctor's advice until you complete prescribed dose, even though symptoms diminish or disappear.

Others:
Expect to start with small dose and increase gradually to lessen frequency and severity of adverse reactions.

 POSSIBLE INTERACTION WITH OTHER DRUGS

GENERIC NAME OR DRUG CLASS	COMBINED EFFECT
Antidepressants*	Weakness or faintness when arising from bed or chair.
Antihypertensives*	Decreased blood pressure and effect of carbidopa and levodopa.
Antiparkinsonism drugs, other*	Increased effect of carbidopa and levodopa.

Haloperidol	Decreased effect of carbidopa and levodopa.
MAO inhibitors*	Dangerous rise in blood pressure.
Methyldopa	Decreased effect of carbidopa and levodopa.
Papaverine	Decreased effect of carbidopa and levodopa.
Phenothiazines*	Decreased effect of carbidopa and levodopa.
Phenytoin	Decreased effect of carbidopa and levodopa.
Pyridoxine (Vitamin B-6)	Decreased effect of carbidopa and levodopa.
Rauwolfia alkaloids*	Decreased effect of carbidopa and levodopa.

 POSSIBLE INTERACTION WITH OTHER SUBSTANCES

INTERACTS WITH	COMBINED EFFECT
Alcohol:	None expected.
Beverages:	None expected.
Cocaine:	Decreased carbidopa and levodopa effect. High rise of heartbeat irregularities. Avoid.
Foods:	None expected.
Marijuana:	Increased fatigue, lethargy, fainting.
Tobacco:	None expected.

*See Glossary

CARBOL-FUCHSIN (Topical)

BRAND NAMES

Castellani Paint   Castel Plus

BASIC INFORMATION

Habit forming? No
Prescription needed? No
Available as generic? Yes
Drug class: Antifungal (topical), drying
  agent (topical)

 ## USES

Treats fungus infections of skin and nails.

 ## DOSAGE & USAGE INFORMATION

How to use:
Topical solution—Wash and dry affected areas.
Use an applicator or swab to apply to affected
areas only. Don't bandage. You may need to
apply for several months to cure.

When to use:
As directed, usually 1 to 3 times a day.

If you forget a dose:
Apply as soon as remember.

What drug does:
• Kills spores of fungus and some bacteria.
• Stimulates growth of new skin.

Time lapse before drug works:
2 to 3 weeks or more.

Don't use with:
Any other topical medicine without telling your
doctor.

 ## OVERDOSE

SYMPTOMS:
None expected unless accidentally
swallowed.
WHAT TO DO:
If accidentally swallowed, call nearest
poison-control center or your doctor.

 ## POSSIBLE ADVERSE REACTIONS OR SIDE EFFECTS

SYMPTOMS	WHAT TO DO
Life-threatening: None expected.	
Common: Skin irritation.	Discontinue. Call doctor right away.
Infrequent: Mild stinging where applied.	No action necessary.
Rare: None expected.	

CARBOL-FUCHSIN (Topical)

WARNINGS & PRECAUTIONS

Don't use if:
No special problems expected.

Before you start, consult your doctor:
If you are taking any other prescription or non-prescription medicine.

Over age 60:
No special problems expected.

Pregnancy:
No special problems expected.

Breast-feeding:
No special problems expected.

Infants & children:
Don't use more than once daily.

Prolonged use:
No special problems expected.

Skin & sunlight:
No special problems expected.

Driving, piloting or hazardous work:
No special problems expected.

Discontinuing:
No special problems expected.

Others:
Advise any doctor or dentist whom you consult that you take this medicine.

POSSIBLE INTERACTION WITH OTHER DRUGS

GENERIC NAME OR DRUG CLASS	COMBINED EFFECT
None expected.	

POSSIBLE INTERACTION WITH OTHER SUBSTANCES

INTERACTS WITH	COMBINED EFFECT
Alcohol:	None expected.
Beverages:	None expected.
Cocaine:	None expected.
Foods:	None expected.
Marijuana:	None expected.
Tobacco:	None expected.

CARBONIC ANHYDRASE INHIBITORS

BRAND AND GENERIC NAMES

Acetazolam
ACETAZOLAMIDE
Ak-Zol
Apo-Acetazolamide
Daranide
Dazamide

Diamox
DICHLOR-
 PHENAMIDE
METHAZOLAMIDE
Neptazane

BASIC INFORMATION

Habit forming? No
Prescription needed? Yes
Available as generic? Yes
Drug class: Carbonic anhydrase inhibitor

USES

- Treatment of glaucoma.
- Treatment of epileptic seizures.
- Treatment of body-fluid retention.
- Treatment for shortness of breath, insomnia and fatigue in high altitudes.

DOSAGE & USAGE INFORMATION

How to take:
- Sustained-release tablets—Swallow whole with liquid or food to lessen stomach irritation.
- Extended-release capsules—Swallow whole with liquid.

When to take:
- 1 dose per day—At the same time each morning.
- More than 1 dose per day—Take last dose several hours before bedtime.

If you forget a dose:
Take as soon as you remember. Continue regular schedule.

Continued next column

OVERDOSE

SYMPTOMS:
Drowsiness, confusion, excitement, nausea, vomiting, numbness in hands and feet, coma.
WHAT TO DO:
- **Call your doctor or poison-control center for advice if you suspect overdose, even if not sure. Symptoms may not appear until damage has occurred.**
- **See emergency information on inside covers.**

What drug does:
- Inhibits action of carbonic anhydrase, an enzyme. This lowers the internal eye pressure by decreasing fluid formation in the eye.
- Forces sodium and water excretion, reducing body fluid.

Time lapse before drug works:
2 hours.

Don't take with:
- Non-prescription drugs without consulting doctor.
- See Interaction column and consult doctor.

POSSIBLE ADVERSE REACTIONS OR SIDE EFFECTS

SYMPTOMS	WHAT TO DO
Life-threatening: Convulsions.	Seek emergency treatment immediately.
Common: None expected.	
Infrequent:	
• Back pain, sedation.	Discontinue. Call doctor right away.
• Fatigue, weakness, tingling or burning in feet or hands.	Continue. Call doctor when convenient.
Rare:	
• Headache; mood changes; nervousness; clumsiness; trembling; confusion; hives, itch, rash; sores; ringing in ears; hoarseness; dry mouth; thirst; sore throat; fever; appetite change; nausea; vomiting; black, tarry stool; breathing difficulty; irregular or weak heartbeat; easy bleeding or bruising; muscle cramps; painful or frequent urination; blood in urine.	Discontinue. Call doctor right away.
• Depression, loss of libido.	Continue. Call doctor when convenient.

CARBONIC ANHYDRASE INHIBITORS

WARNINGS & PRECAUTIONS

Don't take if:
- You are allergic to any carbonic anhydrase inhibitor.
- You have liver or kidney disease.
- You have Addison's disease (adrenal gland failure).
- You have diabetes.

Before you start, consult your doctor:
- If you have gout or lupus.
- If you are allergic to any sulfa drug.
- If you will have surgery within 2 months, including dental surgery, requiring general or spinal anesthesia.

Over age 60:
- Don't exceed recommended dose.
- If you take a digitalis preparation, eat foods high in potassium content or take a potassium supplement.

Pregnancy:
No proven harm to unborn child. Avoid if possible, especially first 3 months.

Breast-feeding:
Avoid drug or don't nurse your infant.

Infants & children:
Not recommended for children younger than 12.

Prolonged use:
May cause kidney stones, vision change, loss of taste and smell, jaundice or weight loss.

Skin & sunlight:
No problems expected.

Driving, piloting or hazardous work:
Avoid if you feel drowsy or dizzy. Otherwise, no problems expected.

Discontinuing:
Don't discontinue without medical advice.

Others:
Medicine may increase sugar levels in blood and urine. Diabetics may need insulin adjustment.

POSSIBLE INTERACTION WITH OTHER DRUGS

GENERIC NAME OR DRUG CLASS	COMBINED EFFECT
Amphetamines*	Increased amphetamine effect.
Anticonvulsants*	Increased loss of bone minerals.
Antidepressants, tricyclic (TCA)*	Increased anti-depressant effect.
Antidiabetics, oral*	Increased potassium loss.
Aspirin	Decreased aspirin effect.
Ciprofloxacin	May cause kidney dysfunction.
Cortisone drugs*	Increased potassium loss.
Digitalis preparations*	Possible digitalis toxicity.
Diuretics*	Increased potassium loss.
Lithium	Decreased lithium effect.
Methenamine	Decreased methenamine effect.
Mexiletene	May slow elimination of mexilitene and cause need to adjust dosage.
Quinidine	Increased quinidine effect.
Salicylates*	Salicylate toxicity.
Sympathomimetics*	Increased sympatho-mimetic effect.

POSSIBLE INTERACTION WITH OTHER SUBSTANCES

INTERACTS WITH	COMBINED EFFECT
Alcohol:	None expected.
Beverages:	None expected.
Cocaine:	Avoid. Decreased carbonic anhydrase inhibitor effect.
Foods: Potassium-rich foods.*	Eat these to decrease potassium loss.
Marijuana:	Avoid. Increased carbonic anhydrase inhibitor effect.
Tobacco:	May decrease absorption of carbonic anhydrase inhibitors.

CASCARA

BRAND NAMES

Aromatic Cascara
  Fluidextract
Cascara Sagrada

Caroid Laxative
Nature's Remedy

BASIC INFORMATION

Habit forming? No
Prescription needed? No
Available as generic? Yes
Drug class: Laxative (stimulant)

 USES

Constipation relief.

 DOSAGE & USAGE INFORMATION

How to take:
* Follow package instructions.
* Tablet—Swallow with liquid. If you can't swallow whole, chew or crumble tablet and take with liquid or food.
* Liquid—Drink 6 to 8 glasses of water each day, in addition to one taken with each dose.

When to take:
Usually at bedtime with a snack, unless directed otherwise.

If you forget a dose:
Take as soon as you remember.

What drug does:
Acts on smooth muscles of intestine wall to cause vigorous bowel movement.

Time lapse before drug works:
6 to 10 hours.

Don't take with:
* Any other medicine without consulting your doctor or pharmacist.
* Don't take within 2 hours of taking another medicine. Laxative interferes with medicine absorption.

 OVERDOSE

SYMPTOMS:
Vomiting, electrolyte depletion.
WHAT TO DO:
Overdose unlikely to threaten life. If person takes much larger amount than prescribed, call doctor, poison-control center or hospital emergency room for instructions.

 POSSIBLE ADVERSE REACTIONS OR SIDE EFFECTS

SYMPTOMS	WHAT TO DO
Life-threatening: None expected.	
Common: Rectal irritation.	Continue. Call doctor when convenient.
Infrequent:	
• Dangerous potassium loss (thirst, weakness, heartbeat irregularity, paralysis, nausea and diarrhea).	Discontinue. Call doctor right away.
• Belching, cramps, nausea.	Continue. Call doctor when convenient.
Rare:	
• Irritability, confusion, headache, rash, breathing difficulty, irregular heartbeat, muscle cramps, unusual tiredness or weakness.	Discontinue. Call doctor right away.
• Burning on urination.	Continue. Call doctor when convenient.
• Discoloration of urine.	No action necessary.

WARNINGS & PRECAUTIONS

Don't take if:
- You have symptoms of appendicitis, inflamed bowel or intestinal blockage.
- You are allergic to a stimulant laxative.
- You have missed a bowel movement for only 1 or 2 days.

Before you start, consult your doctor:
- If you have a colostomy or ileostomy.
- If you have congestive heart disease.
- If you have diabetes.
- If you have high blood pressure.
- If you have a laxative habit.
- If you have rectal bleeding.
- If you take other laxatives.

Over age 60:
Adverse reactions and side effects may be more frequent and severe than in younger persons.

Pregnancy:
Risk to mother and unborn child outweighs drug benefits. Don't use.

Breast-feeding:
Drug passes into milk. Avoid drug or discontinue nursing until you finish medicine. Consult doctor for advice on maintaining milk supply.

Infants & children:
Use only under medical supervision.

Prolonged use:
Don't take for more than 1 week unless under a doctor's supervision. May cause laxative dependence.

Skin & sunlight:
No problems expected.

Driving, piloting or hazardous work:
No problems expected.

Discontinuing:
May be unnecessary to finish medicine. Follow doctor's instructions.

Others:
Don't take to "flush out" your system or as a "tonic."

POSSIBLE INTERACTION WITH OTHER DRUGS

GENERIC NAME OR DRUG CLASS	COMBINED EFFECT
Antacids*	Irritation of stomach or small intestine.
Digoxin	Increased toxicity due to decreased potassium level.
Diuretics*	May cause dangerous low potassium level.
Ranitidine	Irritation of stomach or small intestine.

POSSIBLE INTERACTION WITH OTHER SUBSTANCES

INTERACTS WITH	COMBINED EFFECT
Alcohol:	None expected.
Beverages:	None expected.
Cocaine:	None expected.
Foods:	None expected.
Marijuana:	None expected.
Tobacco:	None expected.

*See Glossary

CASTOR OIL

BRAND NAMES

Alphamul
Emulsoil
Fleet Flavored
  Castor Oil
Kellogg's Castor Oil
Neoloid
Purge

BASIC INFORMATION

Habit forming? No
Prescription needed? No
Available as generic? Yes
Drug class: Laxative (stimulant)

 USES

Constipation relief.

 DOSAGE & USAGE INFORMATION

How to take:
- Follow package instructions.
- Liquid or capsules—Drink 6 to 8 glasses of water each day, in addition to one taken with each dose.

When to take:
Usually at bedtime with a snack, unless directed otherwise.

If you forget a dose:
Take as soon as you remember.

What drug does:
Acts on smooth muscles of intestine wall to cause vigorous bowel movement.

Time lapse before drug works:
2 to 6 hours.

Don't take with:
- Any other medicine without consulting your doctor or pharmacist.
- Don't take within 2 hours of taking another medicine. Laxative interferes with medicine absorption.

 OVERDOSE

SYMPTOMS:
Vomiting, electrolyte depletion.
WHAT TO DO:
Overdose unlikely to threaten life. If person takes much larger amount than prescribed, call doctor, poison-control center or hospital emergency room for instructions.

 POSSIBLE ADVERSE REACTIONS OR SIDE EFFECTS

SYMPTOMS	WHAT TO DO
Life-threatening:	
None expected.	
Common:	
Rectal irritation.	Continue. Call doctor when convenient.
Infrequent:	
• Dangerous potassium loss (thirst, weakness, heartbeat irregularities, paralysis, nausea and diarrhea).	Discontinue. Call doctor right away.
• Belching, cramps, nausea.	Continue. Call doctor when convenient.
Rare:	
• Irritability, headache, confusion, rash, breathing difficulty, irregular heartbeat, muscle cramps, unusual tiredness or weakness.	Discontinue. Call doctor right away.
• Burning on urination.	Continue. Call doctor when convenient.

WARNINGS & PRECAUTIONS

Don't take if:
- You have symptoms of appendicitis, inflamed bowel or intestinal blockage.
- You are allergic to a stimulant laxative.
- You have missed a bowel movement for only 1 or 2 days.

Before you start, consult your doctor:
- If you have a colostomy or ileostomy.
- If you have congestive heart disease.
- If you have diabetes.
- If you have high blood pressure.
- If you have a laxative habit.
- If you have rectal bleeding.
- If you take other laxatives.

Over age 60:
Adverse reactions and side effects may be more frequent and severe than in younger persons.

Pregnancy:
Risk to mother and unborn child outweighs drug benefits. Don't use.

Breast-feeding:
Drug passes into milk. Avoid drug or discontinue nursing until you finish medicine. Consult doctor for advice on maintaining milk supply.

Infants & children:
Use only under medical supervision.

Prolonged use:
Don't take for more than 1 week unless under doctor's supervision. May cause laxative dependence.

Skin & sunlight:
No problems expected.

Driving, piloting or hazardous work:
No problems expected.

Discontinuing:
May be unnecessary to finish medicine. Follow doctor's instructions.

Others:
Don't take to "flush out" your system or as a "tonic."

 POSSIBLE INTERACTION WITH OTHER DRUGS

GENERIC NAME OR DRUG CLASS	COMBINED EFFECT
Antihypertensives*	May cause dangerous low potassium level.
Diuretics*	May cause dangerous low potassium level.

 POSSIBLE INTERACTION WITH OTHER SUBSTANCES

INTERACTS WITH	COMBINED EFFECT
Alcohol:	None expected.
Beverages:	None expected.
Cocaine:	None expected.
Foods:	None expected.
Marijuana:	None expected.
Tobacco:	None expected.

*See Glossary

CELLULOSE SODIUM PHOSPHATE

BRAND NAMES

Calcibind

BASIC INFORMATION

Habit forming? No
Prescription needed? Yes
Available as generic? No
Drug class: Antiurolithic

 ## USES

Prevents formation of calcium kidney stones.

 ## DOSAGE & USAGE INFORMATION

How to take:
Oral suspension—Dissolve in full glass of liquid and swallow. *Note:* Drink 8 ounces of water or other liquid every hour while you are awake.

When to take:
- According to instructions on prescription label. Usually 3 times a day *with* meals.
- Don't take within 1-1/2 hours of taking any laxative or antacid containing magnesium.

If you forget a dose:
Take as soon as you remember up to 2 hours late. If more than 2 hours, wait for next scheduled dose (don't double this dose).

What drug does:
Combines with calcium in food to prevent absorption into the bloodstream.

Time lapse before drug works:
None. Works right away.

Don't take with:
Any other medicines (including over-the-counter drugs such as cough and cold medicines, laxatives, antacids, diet pills, caffeine, nose drops or vitamins) without consulting your doctor.

 ## OVERDOSE

SYMPTOMS:
Drowsiness, mental changes, muscle spasms, seizures.
WHAT TO DO:
- **Dial 0 (operator) or 911 (emergency) for an ambulance or medical help. Then give first aid immediately.**
- **See emergency information on inside covers.**

 ## POSSIBLE ADVERSE REACTIONS OR SIDE EFFECTS

SYMPTOMS	WHAT TO DO
Life-threatening:	
In case of overdose, see previous column.	
Common:	
Loose bowel movements.	Continue. Call doctor when convenient.
Infrequent:	
Abdominal pain.	Discontinue. Call doctor right away.
Rare:	
None expected.	

CELLULOSE SODIUM PHOSPHATE

WARNINGS & PRECAUTIONS

Don't take if:
- You have bone disease.
- You have hyperparathyroidism.
- You have too little calcium in your blood.

Before you start, consult your doctor:
- If you have heart disease.
- If you have kidney disease.

Over age 60:
No special problems expected.

Pregnancy:
Risk to unborn child outweighs drug benefits. Don't use.

Breast-feeding:
No special problems expected.

Infants & children:
Not recommended up to age 16.

Prolonged use:
Talk to your doctor about the need for follow-up medical examinations or laboratory studies to check serum calcium and magnesium concentrations (every 6 months), serum parathyroid hormone, urinary calcium and urinary oxalate levels (occasionally).

Skin & sunlight:
No problems expected.

Driving, piloting or hazardous work:
Avoid if you feel confused, drowsy or dizzy

Discontinuing:
No special problems expected.

Others:
Advise any doctor or dentist whom you consult that you take this medicine.

POSSIBLE INTERACTION WITH OTHER DRUGS

GENERIC NAME OR DRUG CLASS	COMBINED EFFECT
Magnesium-containing medicines (includes many laxatives* and antacids*)	Decreased magnesium effect.
Vitamin C (ascorbic acid)	Decreased vitamin C effect.

POSSIBLE INTERACTION WITH OTHER SUBSTANCES

INTERACTS WITH	COMBINED EFFECT
Alcohol:	No special problems expected.
Beverages: Milk or other dairy products or tea.	Decreases effectiveness of cellulose sodium phosphate.
Cocaine:	No special problems expected.
Foods: Spinach, broccoli, rhubarb.	Decreases effectiveness of cellulose sodium phosphate.
Marijuana:	No special problems expected.
Tobacco:	No special problems expected.

CEPHALOSPORINS

BRAND NAMES

Anspor	C-Lexin
Apo-Cephalex	Ceporex
Ceclor	Duricef
CEFACLOR	Entacef
CEFADROXIL	Keflet
Cefanex	Keflex
CEFIXIME	Keftab
CEFPODOXIME	Novolexin
CEFPROZIL	Nu-Cephalex
Ceftin	Ro-ceph
CEFUROXIME	Suprax
Cefzil	Ultracef
CEPHALEXIN	Vantin
CEPHRADINE	Velosef

BASIC INFORMATION

Habit forming? No
Prescription needed? Yes
Available as generic? Yes
Drug class: Antibiotic (cephalosporin)

USES

Treatment of bacterial infections. Will not cure viral infections such as cold and flu.

DOSAGE & USAGE INFORMATION

How to take:
- Capsule—Swallow with liquid. If you can't swallow whole, open capsule and take with liquid or food.
- Liquid—Use measuring spoon.

When to take:
- At same times each day, 1 hour before or 2 hours after eating.
- Take until gone or as directed.

If you forget a dose:
Take as soon as you remember or double next dose. Return to regular schedule.

Continued next column

OVERDOSE

SYMPTOMS:
Abdominal cramps, nausea, vomiting, severe diarrhea with mucus or blood in stool, convulsions.
WHAT TO DO:
Overdose unlikely to threaten life. If person takes much larger amount than prescribed, call doctor, poison-control center or hospital emergency room for instructions.

What drug does:
Kills susceptible bacteria.

Time lapse before drug works:
May require several days to affect infection.

Don't take with:
Any other medicine without consulting your doctor or pharmacist.

POSSIBLE ADVERSE REACTIONS OR SIDE EFFECTS

SYMPTOMS	WHAT TO DO
Life-threatening:	
Hives, rash, intense itching, faintness soon after a dose (anaphylaxis); difficulty breathing.	Seek emergency treatment immediately.
Common:	
• Rash, redness, itching.	Discontinue. Call doctor right away.
• Diarrhea (mild).	Continue. Call doctor when convenient.
Infrequent:	
Rectal itching, oral or vaginal white spots.	Continue. Call doctor when convenient.
Rare:	
Mild nausea, vomiting, cramps, severe diarrhea with mucus or blood in stool, unusual weakness, tiredness, weight loss, fever, bleeding or bruising, abdominal cramping pain, increased thirst, joint pain, appetite loss.	Discontinue. Call doctor right away.

WARNINGS & PRECAUTIONS

Don't take if:
You are allergic to any cephalosporin antibiotic.

Before you start, consult your doctor:
- If you are allergic to any penicillin antibiotic.
- If you have a kidney disorder.
- If you have colitis or enteritis.

Over age 60:
Adverse reactions and side effects may be more frequent and severe than in younger persons. More likely to itch around rectum and genitals.

Pregnancy:
No proven harm to unborn child. Avoid if possible.

Breast-feeding:
Drug passes into milk. Avoid drug or discontinue nursing until you finish medicine. Consult doctor for advice on maintaining milk supply.

Infants & children:
No special warnings.

Prolonged use:
- Kills beneficial bacteria that protect body against other germs. Unchecked germs may cause secondary infections.
- Talk to your doctor about the need for follow-up medical examinations or laboratory studies to check prothrombin time.

Skin & sunlight:
No problems expected.

Driving, piloting or hazardous work:
No problems expected.

Discontinuing:
Don't discontinue without doctor's advice until you complete prescribed dose, even though symptoms diminish or disappear.

Others:
No problems expected.

POSSIBLE INTERACTION WITH OTHER DRUGS

GENERIC NAME OR DRUG CLASS	COMBINED EFFECT
Anticoagulants*	Increased anticoagulant effect.
Erythromycins*	Decreased antibiotic effect of cephalosporin.
Chloramphenicol	Decreased antibiotic effect of cephalosporin.
Clindamycin	Decreased antibiotic effect of cephalosporin.
Non-steroidal anti-inlammatory drugs (NSAIDs)*	Increased risk of peptic ulcer.
Probenecid	Increased cephalosporin effect.
Tetracyclines*	Decreased antibiotic effect of cephalosporin.

POSSIBLE INTERACTION WITH OTHER SUBSTANCES

INTERACTS WITH	COMBINED EFFECT
Alcohol:	Increased kidney toxicity, likelihood of disulfiram-like* effect.
Beverages:	None expected.
Cocaine:	None expected, but cocaine may slow body's recovery. Avoid.
Foods:	Slow absorption. Take with liquid 1 hour before or 2 hours after eating.
Marijuana:	None expected, but marijuana may slow body's recovery. Avoid.
Tobacco:	None expected.

*See Glossary

CHARCOAL, ACTIVATED

BRAND NAMES

Acta-Char
Acta-Char Liquid
Actidose-Aqua
Aqueous Charcodote
Charcoaid

Charcocaps
Charcodote
Insta-Char
Liqui-Char
SuperChar

BASIC INFORMATION

Habit forming? No
Prescription needed? No
Available as generic? Yes
Drug class: Antidote (adsorbent)

 ## USES

- Treatment of poisonings from medication.
- Treatment (infrequent) for diarrhea or excessive gaseousness.

 ## DOSAGE & USAGE INFORMATION

How to take:
- Tablet or capsule—Swallow with liquid. If you can't swallow whole, crumble tablet or open capsule and take with liquid or food.
- Liquid—Take as directed on label. Don't mix with chocolate syrup, ice cream or sherbet.

When to take:
- For poisoning—Take immediately after poisoning. If your doctor or emergency poison control center has also recommended syrup of ipecac, don't take charcoal for 30 minutes or until vomiting from ipecac stops.
- For diarrhea or gas—Take at same times each day.
- Take one or more hours after taking other medicines.

If you forget a dose:
- For poisonings—Not applicable.
- For diarrhea or gas—Take as soon as you remember up to 2 hours late. If more than 2 hours, wait for next scheduled dose (don't double this dose).

Continued next column

 ## OVERDOSE

SYMPTOMS:
None expected.
WHAT TO DO:
Overdose unlikely to threaten life. If person takes much larger amount than prescribed, call doctor, poison-control center or hospital emergency room for instructions.

What drug does:
- Helps prevent poison from being absorbed from stomach and intestines.
- Helps absorb gas in intestinal tract.

Time lapse before drug works:
Begins immediately.

Don't take with:
Ice cream or sherbet.

 ## POSSIBLE ADVERSE REACTIONS OR SIDE EFFECTS

SYMPTOMS	WHAT TO DO
Life-threatening: None expected.	
Always: Black bowel movements.	No action necessary.
Infrequent: None expected.	
Rare: Unless taken with cathartic, can cause constipation when taken for overdose of other medicine.	Take a laxative after crisis is over.

WARNINGS & PRECAUTIONS

Don't take if:
The poison was lye or other strong alkali, strong acids (such as sulfuric acid), cyanide, iron, ethyl alcohol or methyl alcohol. Charcoal will not prevent these poisons from causing ill effects.

Before you start, consult your doctor:
If you are taking it as an antidote for poison.

Over age 60:
No problems expected.

Pregnancy:
No problems expected.

Breast-feeding:
No problems expected.

Infants & children:
Don't give to children for more than 3 or 4 days for diarrhea. Continuing for longer periods can interfere with normal nutrition.

Prolonged use:
No problems expected.

Skin & sunlight:
No problems expected.

Driving, piloting or hazardous work:
No problems expected.

Discontinuing:
No problems expected.

Others:
No problems expected.

POSSIBLE INTERACTION WITH OTHER DRUGS

GENERIC NAME OR DRUG CLASS	COMBINED EFFECT
Any medicine taken at the same time	May decrease absorption of medicine.

POSSIBLE INTERACTION WITH OTHER SUBSTANCES

INTERACTS WITH	COMBINED EFFECT
Alcohol:	None expected.
Beverages:	None expected.
Cocaine:	None expected.
Foods: Chocolate syrup, ice cream or sherbet.	Decreased charcoal effect.
Marijuana:	None expected.
Tobacco:	None expected.

*See Glossary

CHENODIOL

BRAND NAMES

Chenix

BASIC INFORMATION

Habit forming? No
Prescription needed? Yes
Available as generic? No
Drug class: Anticholelithic

 USES

Treats cholesterol gallstone disease in patients who, for any reason, can't have surgery.

 DOSAGE & USAGE INFORMATION

How to take:
Tablets—Swallow with liquid. If you can't swallow whole, crumble tablet and take with liquid or food. Instructions to take on empty stomach mean 1 hour before or 2 hours after eating.

When to take:
Usually twice a day (morning and night) with food or milk.

If you forget a dose:
Take as soon as you remember up to 2 hours late. If more than 2 hours, wait for next scheduled dose (don't double this dose).

What drug does:
Reduces cholesterol saturation in blood and dissolves gallstones.

Time lapse before drug works:
1 to 2 hours.

Don't take with:
Any other medicines (including over-the-counter drugs such as cough and cold medicines, laxatives, antacids, diet pills, caffeine, nose drops or vitamins) without consulting your doctor or pharmacist.

 OVERDOSE

SYMPTOMS:
None expected.
WHAT TO DO:
Overdose unlikely to threaten life. If person takes much larger amount than prescribed, call doctor, poison-control center or hospital emergency room for instructions.

 POSSIBLE ADVERSE REACTIONS OR SIDE EFFECTS

SYMPTOMS	WHAT TO DO
Life-threatening: None expected.	
Common: Mild diarrhea.	Continue. Call doctor when convenient.
Infrequent: Constipation, indigestion, appetite loss, abdominal pain, gaseousness.	Continue. Call doctor when convenient.
Rare: Severe diarrhea.	Discontinue. Call doctor right away.

WARNINGS & PRECAUTIONS

Don't take if:
- You have hardening of the arteries (atherosclerosis).
- You are jaundiced.

Before you start, consult your doctor:
- If you have pancreatitis.
- If you have bile duct disease.
- If you have liver disease.
- If you have spastic colitis.

Over age 60:
No special problems expected.

Pregnancy:
Not recommended.

Breast-feeding:
No problems expected.

Infants & children:
Effect not documented. Consult your pediatrician.

Prolonged use:
Talk to your doctor about the need for follow-up medical examinations or laboratory studies to check continued presence of gallstones (sonograms or cholecystograms), liver function and serum cholesterol levels (every 6 months).

Skin & sunlight:
No problems expected.

Driving, piloting or hazardous work:
No problems expected.

Discontinuing:
No special problems expected.

Others:
- Advise any doctor or dentist whom you consult that you take this medicine.
- May affect results in some medical tests.

POSSIBLE INTERACTION WITH OTHER DRUGS

GENERIC NAME OR DRUG CLASS	COMBINED EFFECT
Antacids with magnesium*	Severe diarrhea.
Laxatives*	Decreased chenodiol effect.

POSSIBLE INTERACTION WITH OTHER SUBSTANCES

INTERACTS WITH	COMBINED EFFECT
Alcohol:	Decreased chenodiol effect.
Beverages:	No special problems expected.
Cocaine:	No special problems expected.
Foods:	No special problems expected.
Marijuana:	No special problems expected.
Tobacco:	No special problems expected.

CHLOPHEDIANOL

BRAND NAMES

Ulone

BASIC INFORMATION

Habit forming? No
Prescription needed? Yes
Available as generic? No
Drug class: Cough suppressant

 ## USES

Reduces non-productive cough due to bronchial irritation.

 ## DOSAGE & USAGE INFORMATION

How to take:
Take syrup without diluting. Don't drink fluids immediately after medicine.

When to take:
3 or 4 times a day when needed. No more often than every 3 hours.

If you forget a dose:
Take as soon as you remember up to 2 hours late. If more than 2 hours, wait for next scheduled dose (don't double this dose).

What drug does:
Reduces cough reflex by direct effect on cough center in brain, and by local anesthetic action.

Time lapse before drug works:
30 minutes to 1 hour.

Don't take with:
• Alcohol or brain depressant or stimulant drugs.
• Any other medicine without consulting your doctor or pharmacist.

 ## OVERDOSE

SYMPTOMS:
Blurred vision, hallucinations, coma.
WHAT TO DO:
• **Dial 0 (operator) or 911 (emergency) for an ambulance or medical help. Then give first aid immediately.**
• **If patient is unconscious and not breathing, give mouth-to-mouth breathing. If there is no heartbeat, use cardiac massage and mouth-to-mouth breathing (CPR). Don't try to make patient vomit. If you can't get help quickly, take patient to nearest emergency facility.**
• **See emergency information on inside covers.**

 ## POSSIBLE ADVERSE REACTIONS OR SIDE EFFECTS

SYMPTOMS	WHAT TO DO
Life-threatening:	
In case of overdose, see previous column.	
Common:	
Difficult urination in older men with enlarged prostate.	Continue. Call doctor when convenient.
Infrequent:	
None expected.	
Rare:	
• Hallucinations, drowsiness, rash or hives, nausea, vomiting, irregular heartbeat.	Discontinue. Call doctor right away.
• Nightmares, excitement or irritability, blurred vision, dry mouth.	Continue. Call doctor when convenient.

CHLOPHEDIANOL

WARNINGS & PRECAUTIONS

Don't take if:
You are allergic to chlophedianol.

Before you start, consult your doctor:
- If medicine is for hyperactive child who takes medicine for treatment.
- If your cough brings up sputum (phlegm).
- If you have heart disease.
- If you will have surgery within 2 months, including dental surgery, requiring general or spinal anesthesia.

Over age 60:
Adverse reactions and side effects may be more frequent and severe than in younger persons.

Pregnancy:
Risk to unborn child outweighs drug benefits. Don't use.

Breast-feeding:
Unknown whether medicine filters into milk. Consult doctor.

Infants & children:
Not recommended for children under age 2.

Prolonged use:
Not recommended. If cough persists despite medicine, consult doctor.

Skin & sunlight:
No problems expected.

Driving, piloting or hazardous work:
Don't drive or pilot aircraft until you learn how medicine affects you. Don't work around dangerous machinery. Don't climb ladders or work in high places. Danger increases if you drink alcohol or take medicine affecting alertness and reflexes, such as antihistamines, tranquilizers, sedatives, pain medicine, narcotics and mind-altering drugs.

Discontinuing:
May be unnecessary to finish medicine. Follow doctor's instructions.

Others:
Consult doctor if cough persists despite medication for 7 days or if fever, skin rash or headache accompany cough.

POSSIBLE INTERACTION WITH OTHER DRUGS

GENERIC NAME OR DRUG CLASS	COMBINED EFFECT
Anticonvulsants*	Interferes with actions of both.
Antidepressants, tricyclic (TCA)*	Excess sedation.
Appetite suppressants*	Excess stimulation.
Central nervous system depressants* (antidepressants,* antihistamines,* muscle relaxants,* narcotics,* pain pills, sedatives,* sleeping pills, tranquilizers*)	Excess sedation.
MAO inhibitors*	Excess sedation.
Sympathomimetics*	Excess stimulation.

POSSIBLE INTERACTION WITH OTHER SUBSTANCES

INTERACTS WITH	COMBINED EFFECT
Alcohol:	Excess sedation. Avoid.
Beverages: Coffee, tea, cocoa, cola.	Excess stimulation. Avoid.
Cocaine:	Increased chance of toxic stimulation. Avoid.
Foods:	None expected.
Marijuana:	Increased chance of toxic stimulation. Avoid.
Tobacco:	Decreased effect of chlophedianol.

CHLORAL HYDRATE

BRAND NAMES

Aquachloral   Novochlorhydrate
Noctec

BASIC INFORMATION

Habit forming? Yes
Prescription needed? Yes
Available as generic? Yes
Drug class: Hypnotic

 USES

- Reduces anxiety.
- Relieves insomnia.

 DOSAGE & USAGE INFORMATION

How to take:
- Syrup or capsule—Swallow with milk or food to lessen stomach irritation.
- Suppositories—Remove wrapper and moisten suppository with water. Gently insert larger end into rectum. Push well into rectum with finger.

When to take:
At the same time each day.

If you forget a dose:
Take as soon as you remember up to 2 hours late. If more than 2 hours, wait for next scheduled dose (don't double this dose).

Continued next column

 OVERDOSE

SYMPTOMS:
Confusion, weakness, breathing difficulty, throat irritation, jaundice, stagger, slow or irregular heartbeat, unconsciousness, convulsions, coma.
WHAT TO DO:
- **Dial 0 (operator) or 911 (emergency) for an ambulance or medical help. Then give first aid immediately.**
- **If patient is unconscious and not breathing, give mouth-to-mouth breathing. If there is no heartbeat, use cardiac massage and mouth-to-mouth breathing (CPR). Don't try to make patient vomit. If you can't get help quickly, take patient to nearest emergency facility.**
- **See emergency information on inside covers.**

What drug does:
Affects brain centers that control wakefulness and alertness.

Time lapse before drug works:
30 to 60 minutes.

Don't take with:
Any other medicine without consulting your doctor or pharmacist.

 POSSIBLE ADVERSE REACTIONS OR SIDE EFFECTS

SYMPTOMS	WHAT TO DO
Life-threatening: In case of overdose, see previous column.	
Common: Nausea, stomach pain, vomiting.	Discontinue. Call doctor right away.
Infrequent: "Hangover" effect, clumsiness or unsteadiness, drowsiness, dizziness, lightheadedness, diarrhea.	Continue. Call doctor when convenient.
Rare: • Hallucinations, agitation, confusion. leukopenia (white blood cells causing sore throat and fever).	Discontinue. Call doctor right away.
• Hives, rash.	Continue. Call doctor when convenient.

 WARNINGS & PRECAUTIONS

Don't take if:
You are allergic to chloral hydrate.

Before you start, consult your doctor:
- If you have had liver, kidney or heart trouble.
- If you are prone to stomach upsets (if medicine is in oral form).
- If you are allergic to tartrazine dye.
- If you have colitis or a rectal inflammation (if medicine is in suppository form).

Over age 60:
Adverse reactions and side effects may be more frequent and severe than in younger persons. More likely to have "hangover" effect.

Pregnancy:
Risk to unborn child outweighs drug benefits. Unborn child may become addicted to drug. Don't use.

Breast-feeding:
Drug filters into milk. May harm child. Avoid.

Infants & children:
Use only under medical supervision.

Prolonged use:
Addiction and possible kidney damage.

Skin & sunlight:
No problems expected.

Driving, piloting or hazardous work:
Don't drive or pilot aircraft until you learn how medicine affects you. Don't work around dangerous machinery. Don't climb ladders or work in high places. Danger increases if you drink alcohol or take medicine affecting alertness and reflexes, such as antihistamines, tranquilizers, sedatives, pain medicine, narcotics and mind-altering drugs.

Discontinuing:
Don't discontinue without consulting doctor. Dose may require gradual reduction if you have taken drug for a long time. Doses of other drugs may also require adjustment.

Others:
Frequent kidney-function tests recommended when drug is used for long time.

 POSSIBLE INTERACTION WITH OTHER DRUGS

GENERIC NAME OR DRUG CLASS	COMBINED EFFECT
Anticoagulants, oral*	Possible hemorrhaging.
Antidepressants*	Increased chloral hydrate effect.
Antihistamines*	Increased chloral hydrate effect.
Clozapine	Toxic effect on the central nervous system.
Ethinamate	Dangerous increased effects of ethinamate. Avoid combining.
Fluoxetine	Increased depressant effects of both drugs.
Guanfacine	May increase depressant effects of either drug.
Leucovorin	High alcohol content of leucovorin may cause adverse effects.

MAO inhibitors*	Increased chloral hydrate effect.
Methyprylon	Increased sedative effect, perhaps to dangerous level. Avoid.
Mind-altering drugs*	Increased chloral hydrate effect.
Molindone	Increased tranquilizer effect.
Nabilone	Greater depression of central nervous system.
Narcotics*	Increased chloral hydrate effect.
Pain relievers*	Increased chloral hydrate effect.
Phenothiazines*	Increased chloral hydrate effect.
Sedatives*	Increased chloral hydrate effect.
Sertraline	Increased depressive effects of both drugs.
Sleep inducers*	Increased chloral hydrate effect.
Tranquilizers*	Increased chloral hydrate effect.

 POSSIBLE INTERACTION WITH OTHER SUBSTANCES

INTERACTS WITH	COMBINED EFFECT
Alcohol:	Increased sedative effect of both. Avoid.
Beverages:	None expected.
Cocaine:	Decreased chloral hydrate effect. Avoid.
Foods:	None expected.
Marijuana:	May severely impair mental and physical functioning. Avoid.
Tobacco:	None expected.

CHLORAMBUCIL

BRAND NAMES

Leukeran

BASIC INFORMATION

Habit forming? No
Prescription needed? Yes
Available as generic? No
Drug class: Antineoplastic,
immunosuppressant

 ## USES

- Treatment for some kinds of cancer.
- Suppresses immune response after transplant and in immune disorders.

 ## DOSAGE & USAGE INFORMATION

How to take:
Tablet—Swallow with liquid after light meal. Don't drink fluids with meals. Drink extra fluids between meals. Avoid sweet or fatty foods.

When to take:
At the same time each day.

If you forget a dose:
Take as soon as you remember. Don't ever double dose.

What drug does:
Inhibits abnormal cell reproduction. May suppress immune system.

Time lapse before drug works:
Up to 6 weeks for full effect.

Don't take with:
Any other medicine without consulting your doctor or pharmacist.

 ## OVERDOSE

SYMPTOMS:
Bleeding, chills, fever, vomiting, abdominal pain, ataxia, collapse, stupor, seizure.
WHAT TO DO:
- Dial 0 (operator) or 911 (emergency) for an ambulance or medical help. Then give first aid immediately.
- If patient is unconscious and not breathing, give mouth-to-mouth breathing. If there is no heartbeat, use cardiac massage and mouth-to-mouth breathing (CPR). Don't try to make patient vomit. If you can't get help quickly, take patient to nearest emergency facility.
- See emergency information on inside covers.

 ## POSSIBLE ADVERSE REACTIONS OR SIDE EFFECTS

SYMPTOMS	WHAT TO DO
Life-threatening:	
In case of overdose, see previous column.	
Common:	
• Unusual bleeding or bruising, mouth sores with sore throat, chills and fever, black stools, mouth and lip sores, menstrual irregularities, back pain.	Discontinue. Call doctor right away.
• Hair loss, joint pain.	Continue. Call doctor when convenient.
• Nausea, vomiting, diarrhea, tiredness, weakness.	Continue. Tell doctor at next visit.
Infrequent:	
• Mental confusion, shortness of breath.	Continue. Call doctor when convenient.
• Cough, rash, foot swelling.	Continue. Tell doctor at next visit.
Rare:	
Jaundice, convulsions, hallucinations, muscle twitching.	Discontinue. Call doctor right away.

WARNINGS & PRECAUTIONS

Don't take if:
- You have had hypersensitivity to alkylating antineoplastic drugs.
- Your physician has not explained serious nature of your medical problem and risks of taking this medicine.

Before you start, consult your doctor:
- If you have gout.
- If you have had kidney stones.
- If you have active infection.
- If you have impaired kidney or liver function.
- If you have taken other antineoplastic drugs or had radiation treatment in last 3 weeks.

Over age 60:
Adverse reactions and side effects may be more frequent and severe than in younger persons.

Pregnancy:
Consult doctor. Risk to child is significant.

Breast-feeding:
Drug passes into milk. Don't nurse.

Infants & children:
Use only under care of medical supervisors who are experienced in anticancer drugs.

Prolonged use:
- Adverse reactions more likely the longer drug is required.
- Talk to your doctor about the need for follow-up medical examinations or laboratory studies to check complete blood counts (white blood cell count, platelet count, red blood cell count, hemoglobin, hematocrit).

Skin & sunlight:
No problems expected.

Driving, piloting or hazardous work:
No problems expected.

Discontinuing:
Don't discontinue without doctor's advice until you complete prescribed dose, even though symptoms diminish or disappear. Some side effects may follow discontinuing. Report to doctor blurred vision, convulsions, confusion, persistent headache.

Others:
- May cause sterility.
- May increase chance of developing leukemia.

POSSIBLE INTERACTION WITH OTHER DRUGS

GENERIC NAME OR DRUG CLASS	COMBINED EFFECT
Antigout drugs*	Decreased antigout effect.
Antineoplastic drugs, other*	Increased effect of all drugs (may be beneficial).
Chloramphenicol	Increased likelihood of toxic effects of both drugs.
Clozapine	Toxic effect on bone marrow.
Cyclosporine	May increase risk of infection.
Immuno-suppressants*	Increased chance of infection.
Lovastatin	Increased heart and kidney damage.
Tiopronin	Increased risk of toxicity to bone marrow.

POSSIBLE INTERACTION WITH OTHER SUBSTANCES

INTERACTS WITH	COMBINED EFFECT
Alcohol:	May increase chance of intestinal bleeding.
Beverages:	No problems expected.
Cocaine:	Increases chance of toxicity.
Foods:	Reduces irritation in stomach.
Marijuana:	No problems expected.
Tobacco:	Increases lung toxicity.

*See Glossary

CHLORAMPHENICOL

BRAND NAMES

Chloromycetin   Novochlorocap

BASIC INFORMATION

Habit forming? No
Prescription needed? Yes
Available as generic? Yes
Drug class: Antibiotic

 ## USES

Treatment of infections susceptible to chloramphenicol.

 ## DOSAGE & USAGE INFORMATION

How to take:
• Suspension or capsule—Swallow with liquid.
• Eye or ear solution or cream—Follow label instructions.

When to take:
Capsule or suspension—1 hour before or 2 hours after eating.

If you forget a dose:
Take as soon as you remember up to 2 hours late. If more than 2 hours, wait for next scheduled dose (don't double this dose).

What drug does:
Prevents bacteria from growing and reproducing. Will not kill viruses.

Time lapse before drug works:
2 to 5 days, depending on type and severity of infection.

Don't take with:
Any other medicine without consulting your doctor or pharmacist.

 ## OVERDOSE

SYMPTOMS:
Nausea, vomiting, diarrhea.
WHAT TO DO:
Overdose unlikely to threaten life. If person takes much larger amount than prescribed, call doctor, poison-control center or hospital emergency room for instructions.

 ## POSSIBLE ADVERSE REACTIONS OR SIDE EFFECTS

SYMPTOMS	WHAT TO DO
Life-threatening: Hives, rash, intense itching, faintness soon after a dose (anaphylaxis).	Seek emergency treatment immediately.
Common: None expected.	
Infrequent: • Swollen face or extremities; diarrhea; nausea; vomiting; numbness, tingling, burning pain or weakness in hands and feet, pale skin, unusual bleeding or bruising.	Discontinue. Call doctor right away.
• Headache, confusion.	Continue. Call doctor when convenient.
Rare: • Pain, blurred vision, possible vision loss, delirium, rash, sore throat, fever, jaundice, anemia.	Discontinue. Call doctor right away.
• In babies: Bloated stomach, uneven breathing, drowsiness, low temperature, gray skin.	Discontinue. Call doctor right away.

 ## WARNINGS & PRECAUTIONS

Don't take if:
• You are allergic to chloramphenicol.
• It is prescribed for a minor disorder such as flu, cold or mild sore throat.

Before you start, consult your doctor:
• If you have had a blood disorder or bone-marrow disease.
• If you have had kidney or liver disease.
• If you have diabetes.

Over age 60:
Adverse reactions and side effects may be more frequent and severe than in younger persons, particularly skin irritation around rectum.

Pregnancy:
Risk to unborn child outweighs drug benefits.
Don't use.

Breast-feeding:
Drug passes into milk. Avoid drug or
discontinue nursing until you finish medicine.
Consult doctor for advice on maintaining milk
supply.

Infants & children:
Don't give to infants younger than 2.

Prolonged use:
- You may become more susceptible to
  infections caused by germs not responsive to
  chloramphenicol.
- Talk to your doctor about the need for follow-
  up medical examinations or laboratory studies
  to check complete blood counts (white blood
  cell count, platelet count, red blood cell
  count, hemoglobin, hematocrit), chloramphenicol
  serum levels.

Skin & sunlight:
No problems expected.

Driving, piloting or hazardous work:
Don't drive or pilot aircraft until you learn how
medicine affects you. Don't work around
dangerous machinery. Don't climb ladders or
work in high places. Danger increases if you
drink alcohol or take medicine affecting
alertness and reflexes.

Discontinuing:
Don't discontinue without doctor's advice until
you complete prescribed dose, even though
symptoms diminish or disappear.

Others:
- Chloramphenicol can cause serious anemia.
  Frequent laboratory blood studies, liver and
  kidney tests recommended.
- Second medical opinion recommended
  before starting.

POSSIBLE INTERACTION WITH OTHER DRUGS

GENERIC NAME OR DRUG CLASS	COMBINED EFFECT
Anticoagulants*	Increased anticoagulant effect.
Antidiabetics, oral*	Increased antidiabetic effect.
Anticonvulsants*	Increased chance of toxicity to bone marrow.
Cefiximine	Decreased antibiotic effect of cefiximine.

Cephalosporins*	Decreased chloramphenicol effect.
Clozapine	Toxic effect on bone marrow.
Cyclophosphamide	Increased cyclophos-phamide effect.
Didanosine	Increased risk of peripheral neuropathy.
Flecainide	Possible decreased blood cell production in bone marrow.
Levamisole	Increased risk of bone marrow depression.
Lisinopril	Possible blood disorders.
Penicillins*	Decreased penicillin effect.
Phenobarbital	Increased phenobarbital effect.
Phenytoin	Increased phenytoin effect.
Rifampin	Decreased chloram-phenicol effect.
Thioguanine	More likelihood of toxicity of both drugs.
Tiopronin	Increased risk of toxicity to bone marrow.
Tocainide	Possible decreased blood-cell production in bone marrow.

POSSIBLE INTERACTION WITH OTHER SUBSTANCES

INTERACTS WITH	COMBINED EFFECT
Alcohol:	Possible liver problems. May cause disulfiram reaction.*
Beverages:	None expected.
Cocaine:	No proven problems.
Foods:	None expected.
Marijuana:	None expected.
Tobacco:	None expected.

CHLORDIAZEPOXIDE & AMITRIPTYLINE

BRAND NAMES

Limbitrol　　　　**Limbitrol DS**

BASIC INFORMATION

Habit forming? Yes
Prescription needed? Yes
Available as generic? No
Drug class: Antidepressant, tranquilizer (benzodiazepine)

 USES

- Treatment for nervousness or tension.
- Gradually relieves, but doesn't cure, symptoms of depression.

 DOSAGE & USAGE INFORMATION

How to take:
Tablet—Swallow with liquid. If you can't swallow whole, crumble tablet and take with liquid or food.

When to take:
At the same time each day, according to instructions on prescription label.

If you forget a dose:
Bedtime dose—If you forget your once-a-day bedtime dose, don't take it more than 3 hours late. If more than 3 hours, wait for next scheduled dose (don't double this dose).

What drug does:
Affects limbic system of brain—part that controls emotions.

Continued next column

 OVERDOSE

SYMPTOMS:
Drowsiness, weakness, tremor, enlarged pupils, fast heartbeat, fever, hallucinations, severe vomiting, convulsions, stupor, coma.
WHAT TO DO:
- **Dial 0 (operator) or 911 (emergency) for an ambulance or medical help. Then give first aid immediately.**
- **If patient is unconscious and not breathing, give mouth-to-mouth breathing. If there is no heartbeat, use cardiac massage and mouth-to-mouth breathing (CPR). Don't try to make patient vomit. If you can't get help quickly, take patient to nearest emergency facility.**
- **See emergency information on inside covers.**

Time lapse before drug works:
Begins in 1 to 2 weeks. May require 4 to 6 weeks for maximum benefit.

Don't take with:
- Non-prescription drugs without consulting doctor.
- See Interaction column and consult doctor.

 POSSIBLE ADVERSE REACTIONS OR SIDE EFFECTS

SYMPTOMS	WHAT TO DO
Life-threatening: In case of overdose, see previous column.	
Common: ● Clumsiness, drowsiness, dizziness, headache, insomnia, dry mouth or unpleasant taste, constipation, fatigue, weakness.	Continue. Call doctor when convenient.
● "Sweet tooth," weight gain.	Continue. Tell doctor at next visit.
Infrequent: ● Hallucinations, confusion, irritability, depression, rash, itch, vision changes, blurred vision, eye pain, jaundice, fainting, irregular heartbeat, tremors.	Discontinue. Call doctor right away.
● Constipation, difficult urination, diarrhea, nausea, vomiting, vivid dreams, indigestion, bloating.	Continue. Call doctor when convenient.
Rare: ● Mouth or throat ulcers, fever.	Discontinue. Call doctor right away.
● Decreased libido, sensitivity to sunlight.	Continue. Call doctor when convenient.

 WARNINGS & PRECAUTIONS

Don't take if:
- You are allergic to any benzodiazepine or tricyclic antidepressant.
- You have myasthenia gravis, glaucoma, taken MAO inhibitors within 2 weeks, had a heart attack within 6 weeks.
- You are active or recovering alcoholic.
- Patient is younger than 12.

CHLORDIAZEPOXIDE & AMITRIPTYLINE

Before you start, consult your doctor:
- If you have liver, kidney or lung disease, diabetes, epilepsy, porphyria, enlarged prostate, heart disease, high blood pressure, stomach or intestinal problems, overactive thyroid, asthma.
- If you will have surgery within 2 months, including dental surgery, requiring general or spinal anesthesia.

Over age 60:
More likely to develop urination difficulty and more side effects.

Pregnancy:
Risk to unborn child outweighs drug benefits. Don't use.

Breast-feeding:
Drug passes into milk. Avoid drug or discontinue nursing until you finish medicine. Consult doctor for advice on maintaining milk supply.

Infants & children:
Use only under medical supervision for children older than 6 months.

Prolonged use:
- May impair liver function.
- Talk to your doctor about the need for follow-up medical examinations or laboratory studies to check complete blood counts (white blood cell count, platelet count, red blood cell count, hemoglobin, hematocrit), liver function, blood pressure.

Skin & sunlight:
May cause rash or intensify sunburn in areas exposed to sun or sunlamp.

Driving, piloting or hazardous work:
Don't drive or pilot aircraft until you learn how medicine affects you. Don't work around dangerous machinery. Don't climb ladders or work in high places. Danger increases if you drink alcohol or take medicine affecting alertness and reflexes, such as antihistamines, tranquilizers, sedatives, pain medicine, narcotics and mind-altering drugs.

Discontinuing:
Don't discontinue without consulting doctor. Dose may require gradual reduction if you have taken drug for a long time. Doses of other drugs may also require adjustment.

Others:
- Hot weather, heavy exercise and profuse sweat may reduce excretion and cause overdose.
- Blood sugar may rise in diabetics, requiring insulin adjustment.
- Advise any doctor or dentist whom you consult that you take this medicine.
- For relief of dry mouth, use sugarless candy or gum or melt ice chips in your mouth.

POSSIBLE INTERACTION WITH OTHER DRUGS

GENERIC NAME OR DRUG CLASS	COMBINED EFFECT
Addictive drugs*	Increased risk of addiction.
Anticoagulants, oral*	Increased anti-coagulant effect.
Anticonvulsants*	Change in seizure frequency or severity.
Anticholinergics*	Increased anti-cholinergic effect.
Antidepressants*	Increased sedative effect of both drugs.
Antihistamines*	Increased sedative effect of both drugs.
Antihypertensives*	Excessively low blood pressure.
Antithyroid drugs*	Increased risk of bone-marrow damage.
Barbiturates*	Decreased anti-depressant effect.
Cimetidine	Excess sedation.
Clonidine	Decreased clonidine effect.
Contraceptives, oral*	Increased chlor-diazepoxide effect.
Disulfiram	Increased chlor-diazepoxide effect.
Diuretics*	Increased anti-depressant effect.

Continued page 941

POSSIBLE INTERACTION WITH OTHER SUBSTANCES

INTERACTS WITH	COMBINED EFFECT
Alcohol: Beverages or medicines with alcohol.	Excessive intoxication. Avoid.
Beverages:	None expected.
Cocaine:	Excessive intoxication. Avoid.
Foods:	None expected.
Marijuana:	Excessive drowsiness. Avoid.
Tobacco:	Decreased chlor-diazepoxide effect.

*See Glossary

205

CHLORDIAZEPOXIDE & CLIDINIUM

BRAND NAMES

Apo-Chlorax
Clindex
Clinoxide
Clipoxide

Corium
Librax
Lidox

BASIC INFORMATION

Habit forming? Yes
Prescription needed? Yes
Available as generic? Yes
Drug class: Tranquilizer (benzodiazepine), antispasmodic, anticholinergic

 USES

- Reduces spasms of digestive system, bladder and urethra.
- Treatment for nervousness or tension.
- Treatment for muscle spasm.

 DOSAGE & USAGE INFORMATION

How to take:
Capsule—Swallow with liquid. If you can't swallow whole, open capsule and take with liquid or food.

When to take:
At the same time each day, according to instructions on prescription label.

If you forget a dose:
Take as soon as you remember up to 2 hours late. If more than 2 hours, wait for next scheduled dose (don't double this dose).

Continued next column

 OVERDOSE

SYMPTOMS:
Dilated pupils, rapid pulse and breathing, dizziness, drowsiness, weakness, tremor, stupor, fever, hallucinations, confusion, slurred speech, agitation, flushed face, convulsions, coma.
WHAT TO DO:
- **Dial 0 (operator) or 911 (emergency) for an ambulance or medical help. Then give first aid immediately.**
- **If patient is unconscious and not breathing, give mouth-to-mouth breathing. If there is no heartbeat, use cardiac massage and mouth-to-mouth breathing (CPR). Don't try to make patient vomit. If you can't get help quickly, take patient to nearest emergency facility.**
- **See emergency information on inside covers.**

What drug does:
- Blocks nerve impulses at parasympathetic nerve endings, preventing muscle contractions and gland secretions of organs involved.
- Affects limbic system of brain—part that controls emotions.

Time lapse before drug works:
15 to 30 minutes.

Don't take with:
Any other medicine without consulting your doctor or pharmacist.

 POSSIBLE ADVERSE REACTIONS OR SIDE EFFECTS

SYMPTOMS	WHAT TO DO
Life-threatening:	
In case of overdose, see previous column.	
Common:	
• Clumsiness, drowsiness, dizziness, delirium.	Discontinue. Call doctor right away.
• Dry mouth, throat, nose; bloating; headache.	Continue. Tell doctor at next visit.
Infrequent:	
• Hallucinations, confusion, irritability, depression, rash, itch, vision changes, vomiting, shortness of breath, sore throat, fever, insomnia, memory loss, weakness.	Discontinue. Call doctor right away.
• Constipation, diarrhea, nausea, urination difficulty, vivid dreams, impotence.	Continue. Call doctor when convenient.
Rare:	
• Jaundice, rash or hives, eye pain, blurred vision.	Discontinue. Call doctor right away.
• Decreased libido.	Continue. Call doctor when convenient.

 WARNINGS & PRECAUTIONS

Don't take if:
- You are allergic to any anticholinergic or any benzodiazepine.
- You have trouble with stomach bloating, difficulty emptying your bladder completely, narrow-angle glaucoma, severe ulcerative colitis, myasthenia gravis.
- You are active or recovering alcoholic.
- Patient is younger than 6 months.

CHLORDIAZEPOXIDE & CLIDINIUM

Before you start, consult your doctor:
- If you have open-angle glaucoma, angina, chronic bronchitis or asthma, hiatal hernia, enlarged prostate, myasthenia gravis, peptic ulcer, liver, kidney or lung disease, diabetes, epilepsy or porphyria.
- If you will have surgery within 2 months, including dental surgery, requiring general or spinal anesthesia.

Over age 60:
Adverse reactions and side effects may be more frequent and severe than in younger persons.

Pregnancy:
Risk to unborn child outweighs drug benefits. Don't use.

Breast-feeding:
Drug passes into milk. Avoid drug or discontinue nursing until you finish medicine. Consult doctor for advice on maintaining milk supply.

Infants & children:
Use only under medical supervision.

Prolonged use:
- Chronic constipation, possible fecal impaction.
- May impair liver function.
- Talk to your doctor about the need for follow-up medical examinations or laboratory studies to check complete blood counts (white blood cell count, platelet count, red blood cell count, hemoglobin, hematocrit), liver function, eyes.

Skin & sunlight:
No problems expected.

Driving, piloting or hazardous work:
Don't drive or pilot aircraft until you learn how medicine affects you. Don't work around dangerous machinery. Don't climb ladders or work in high places. Danger increases if you drink alcohol or take medicine affecting alertness and reflexes, such as antihistamines, tranquilizers, sedatives, pain medicine, narcotics and mind-altering drugs.

Discontinuing:
Don't discontinue without consulting doctor. Dose may require gradual reduction if you have taken drug for a long time. Doses of other drugs may also require adjustment.

Others:
- Hot weather, heavy exercise and profuse sweat may reduce excretion and cause overdose.
- Blood sugar may rise in diabetics, requiring insulin adjustment.

 POSSIBLE INTERACTION WITH OTHER DRUGS

GENERIC NAME OR DRUG CLASS	COMBINED EFFECT
Amantadine	Increased clidinium effect.
Antacids*	Decreased clidinium effect.
Anticholinergics, other*	Increased clidinium effect.
Antidepressants*	Increased sedative effect of both drugs.
Antihistamines*	Increased sedative effect of both drugs.
Antihypertensives*	Excessively low blood pressure.
Attapulgite	Increased clidinium effect.
Contraceptives, oral*	Increased chlordiazepoxide effect.
Disulfiram	Increased chlordiazepoxide effect.
Dronabinol	Increased effects of both drugs. Avoid.
Erythromycins*	Increased chlordiazepoxide effect.
Haloperidol	Increased internal-eye pressure.
Ketoconazole	Increased chlordiazepoxide effect.
Levodopa	Possible decreased levodopa effect.

Continued page 941

 POSSIBLE INTERACTION WITH OTHER SUBSTANCES

INTERACTS WITH	COMBINED EFFECT
Alcohol:	Heavy sedation. Avoid.
Beverages:	None expected.
Cocaine:	Excessively rapid heartbeat. Avoid.
Foods:	None expected.
Marijuana:	Drowsiness and dry mouth, heavy sedation. Avoid.
Tobacco:	Decreased chlordiazepoxide effect.

CHLOROQUINE

BRAND NAMES

Aralen

BASIC INFORMATION

Habit forming? No
Prescription needed? Yes
Available as generic? Yes
Drug class: Antiprotozoal, antirheumatic

 ## USES

- Treatment for protozoal infections, such as malaria and amebiasis.
- Treatment for some forms of arthritis and lupus.

 ## DOSAGE & USAGE INFORMATION

How to take:
Tablet—Swallow with food or milk to lessen stomach irritation.

When to take:
- Depends on condition. Is adjusted during treatment.
- Malaria prevention—Begin taking medicine 2 weeks before entering areas with malaria.

If you forget a dose:
- 1 or more doses a day—Take as soon as you remember up to 2 hours late. If more than 2 hours, wait for next scheduled dose (don't double this dose).
- 1 dose weekly—Take as soon as possible, then return to regular dosing schedule.

What drug does:
- Inhibits parasite multiplication.
- Decreases inflammatory response in diseased joint.

Time lapse before drug works:
1 to 2 hours.

Don't take with:
Any other medicine without consulting your doctor or pharmacist.

 ## OVERDOSE

SYMPTOMS:
Severe breathing difficulty, drowsiness, faintness, headache, seizures.
WHAT TO DO:
- Dial 0 (operator) or 911 (emergency) for an ambulance or medical help. Then give first aid immediately.
- See emergency information on inside covers.

 ## POSSIBLE ADVERSE REACTIONS OR SIDE EFFECTS

SYMPTOMS	WHAT TO DO
Life-threatening:	
In case of overdose, see previous column.	
Common:	
Headache, appetite loss, abdominal pain.	Continue. Tell doctor at next visit.
Infrequent:	
• Blurred or changed vision.	Discontinue. Call doctor right away.
• Rash or itch, diarrhea, nausea, vomiting, decreased blood pressure, hair loss, blue-black skin or mouth, dizziness, nervousness.	Continue. Call doctor when convenient.
Rare:	
• Mood or mental changes, seizures, sore throat, fever, unusual bleeding or bruising, muscle weakness, convulsions.	Discontinue. Call doctor right away.
• Ringing or buzzing in ears, hearing loss.	Continue. Call doctor when convenient.

208

WARNINGS & PRECAUTIONS

Don't take if:
You are allergic to chloroquine or hydroxychloroquine.

Before you start, consult your doctor:
- If you plan to become pregnant within the medication period.
- If you have blood disease.
- If you have eye or vision problems.
- If you have a G6PD deficiency.
- If you have liver disease.
- If you have nerve or brain disease (including seizure disorders).
- If you have porphyria.
- If you have psoriasis.
- If you have stomach or intestinal disease.
- If you drink more than 3 oz. of alcohol daily.

Over age 60:
Adverse reactions and side effects may be more frequent and severe than in younger persons.

Pregnancy:
Risk to unborn child outweighs drug benefits. Don't use.

Breast-feeding:
Drug passes into milk. Avoid drug or discontinue nursing.

Infants & children:
Not recommended. Dangerous.

Prolonged use:
- Permanent damage to the retina (back part of the eye) or nerve deafness.
- Talk to your doctor about the need for follow-up medical examinations or laboratory studies to check complete blood counts (white blood cell count, platelet count, red blood cell count, hemoglobin, hematocrit), eyes.

Skin & sunlight:
May cause rash or intensify sunburn in areas exposed to sun or sunlamp.

Driving, piloting or hazardous work:
Don't drive or pilot aircraft until you learn how medicine affects you. Don't work around dangerous machinery. Don't climb ladders or work in high places. Danger increases if you drink alcohol or take medicine affecting alertness and reflexes.

Discontinuing:
Don't discontinue without doctor's advice until you complete prescribed dose, even though symptoms diminish or disappear.

Others:
- Periodic physical and blood examinations recommended.
- If you are in a malaria area for a long time, you may need to change to another preventive drug every 2 years.

POSSIBLE INTERACTION WITH OTHER DRUGS

GENERIC NAME OR DRUG CLASS	COMBINED EFFECT
Penicillamine	Possible blood or kidney toxicity.

POSSIBLE INTERACTION WITH OTHER SUBSTANCES

INTERACTS WITH	COMBINED EFFECT
Alcohol:	Possible liver toxicity. Avoid.
Beverages:	None expected.
Cocaine:	None expected.
Foods:	None expected.
Marijuana:	None expected.
Tobacco:	None expected.

*See Glossary

CHLORPROTHIXENE

BRAND NAMES

Taractan   Tarasan

BASIC INFORMATION

Habit forming? No
Prescription needed? Yes
Available as generic? No
Drug class: Tranquilizer (thioxanthene),
antiemetic

USES

- Reduces anxiety, agitation, psychosis.
- Stops vomiting, hiccups.

DOSAGE & USAGE INFORMATION

How to take:
- Tablet or sustained-release capsule—Swallow with liquid. If you can't swallow whole, crumble tablet and take with liquid or food.
- Syrup—Dilute dose in beverage before swallowing.

When to take:
At the same time each day.

If you forget a dose:
Take as soon as you remember up to 2 hours late. If more than 2 hours, wait for next scheduled dose (don't double this dose).

What drug does:
Corrects imbalance of nerve impulses.

Time lapse before drug works:
3 weeks.

Continued next column

OVERDOSE

SYMPTOMS:
Drowsiness, dizziness, weakness, muscle rigidity, twitching, tremors, confusion, dry mouth, blurred vision, rapid pulse, shallow breathing, low blood pressure, convulsions, coma.
WHAT TO DO:
- **Dial 0 (operator) or 911 (emergency) for an ambulance or medical help. Then give first aid immediately.**
- **If patient is unconscious and not breathing, give mouth-to-mouth breathing. If there is no heartbeat, use cardiac massage and mouth-to-mouth breathing (CPR). Don't try to make patient vomit. If you can't get help quickly, take patient to nearest emergency facility.**
- **See emergency information on inside covers.**

Don't take with:
Any other medicine without consulting your doctor or pharmacist.

POSSIBLE ADVERSE REACTIONS OR SIDE EFFECTS

SYMPTOMS	WHAT TO DO
Life-threatening:	
Uncontrollable movements of head, neck, arms, legs (rarely).	Discontinue. Seek emergency treatment.
Common:	
Fainting; jerky, involuntary movements; restlessness; blurred vision; rapid heartbeat.	Discontinue. Call doctor right away.
Dizziness, drowsiness, constipation, muscle spasms, shuffling walk, decreased sweating, increased appetite, weight gain, sensitivity to light.	Continue. Call doctor when convenient.
Dry mouth, stuffy nose.	Continue. Tell doctor at next visit.
Infrequent:	
Rash.	Discontinue. Call doctor right away.
Less sexual ability, difficult urination.	Continue. Call doctor when convenient.
Menstrual irregularities, swollen breasts, breast milk secretion.	Continue. Tell doctor at next visit.
Rare:	
Sore throat, fever, jaundice, abdominal pain, lip smacking, cheek puffing, chewing movements of mouth, heatstroke, unusual bleeding or bruising.	Discontinue. Call doctor right away.

WARNINGS & PRECAUTIONS

Don't take if:
- You are allergic to any thioxanthine or phenothiazine tranquilizer.
- You have serious blood disorder.
- You have Parkinson's disease.
- Patient is younger than 12.

Before you start, consult your doctor:
- If you have had liver or kidney disease.
- If you have epilepsy, glaucoma or prostate trouble.
- If you have high blood pressure or heart disease (especially angina).
- If you use alcohol daily.
- If you will have surgery within 2 months, including dental surgery, requiring general or spinal anesthesia.

Over age 60:
Adverse reactions and side effects may be more frequent and severe than in younger persons.

Pregnancy:
No proven harm to unborn child. Avoid if possible.

Breast-feeding:
Studies inconclusive. Consult your doctor.

Infants & children:
Not recommended.

Prolonged use:
- Pigment deposits in lens and retina of eye.
- Involuntary movements of jaws, lips, tongue (tardive dyskinesia).
- Talk to your doctor about the need for follow-up medical examinations or laboratory studies to check complete blood counts (white blood cell count, platelet count, red blood cell count, hemoglobin, hematocrit), liver function, eyes.

Skin & sunlight:
May cause rash or intensify sunburn in areas exposed to sun or sunlamp.

Driving, piloting or hazardous work:
Don't drive or pilot aircraft until you learn how medicine affects you. Don't work around dangerous machinery. Don't climb ladders or work in high places. Danger increases if you drink alcohol or take medicine affecting alertness and reflexes.

Discontinuing:
Don't discontinue without consulting doctor. Dose may require gradual reduction if you have taken drug for a long time. Doses of other drugs may also require adjustment.

Others:
Hot temperatures increase chance of heat stroke.

POSSIBLE INTERACTION WITH OTHER DRUGS

GENERIC NAME OR DRUG CLASS	COMBINED EFFECT
Anticholinergics*	Increased anticholinergic effect.
Anticonvulsants*	Change in seizure pattern.
Antidepressants, tricyclic (TCA)*	Increased chlorprothixene effect. Excessive sedation.
Antihistamines*	Increased chlorprothixene effect. Excessive sedation.
Antihypertensives*	Excessively low blood pressure.
Barbiturates*	Increased chlorprothixene effect. Excessive sedation.
Bethanechol	Decreased bethanechol effect.
Bupropion	Increased risk of major seizures.
Dronabinol	Increased effects of both drugs. Avoid.
Epinephrine	Low blood pressure and rapid heartbeat.
Guanethidine	Decreased guanethidine effect.
Levodopa	Decreased levodopa effect.
MAO inhibitors*	Excessive sedation.
Mind-altering drugs*	Increased chlorprothixene effect. Excessive sedation.
Narcotics*	Increased chlorprothixene effect. Excessive sedation.
Pergolide	Decreased pergolide effect.
Procarbazine	Increased sedation.
Sedatives*	Increased chlorprothixene effect. Excessive sedation.
Sleep inducers*	Increased chlorprothixene effect. Excessive sedation.
Tranquilizers*	Increased chlorprothixene effect. Excessive sedation.

POSSIBLE INTERACTION WITH OTHER SUBSTANCES

INTERACTS WITH	COMBINED EFFECT
Alcohol:	Excessive brain depression. Avoid.
Beverages:	None expected.
Cocaine:	Decreased chlorprothixene effect. Avoid.
Foods:	None expected.
Marijuana:	Daily use—Fainting likely, possible psychosis.
Tobacco:	None expected.

*See Glossary

CHLORZOXAZONE & ACETAMINOPHEN

BRAND NAMES

See complete list of brand names in the *Brand Names Directory*, page 917.

BASIC INFORMATION

Habit forming? Possibly
Prescription needed? Yes
Available as generic? Yes
Drug class: Muscle relaxant, analgesic, fever-reducer

 USES

- Adjunctive treatment to rest, analgesics and physical therapy for muscle spasms.
- Treatment of mild to moderate pain and fever.

 DOSAGE & USAGE INFORMATION

How to take:
Tablet—Swallow with liquid.

When to take:
As needed, no more often than every 3 hours.

If you forget a dose:
Take as soon as you remember. Wait 3 hours for next dose.

What drug does:
- Blocks body's pain messages to brain. Also causes sedation.
- May affect hypothalamus, the part of the brain that helps regulate body heat and receives body's pain messages.

Continued next column

 OVERDOSE

SYMPTOMS:
Nausea, vomiting, diarrhea, anorexia, headache, severe weakness, unusual increase in sweating, fainting, breathing difficulty, irritability, convulsions, sensation of paralysis, coma.
WHAT TO DO:
- **Overdose unlikely to threaten life. Depending on severity of symptoms and amount taken, call doctor, poison-control center or hospital emergency room for instructions.**
- **Dial 0 (operator) or 911 (emergency) for an ambulance or medical help. Then give first aid immediately.**
- **See emergency information on inside covers.**

Time lapse before drug works:
15 to 30 minutes. May last 4 hours.

Don't take with:
- Other drugs with acetaminophen. Too much acetaminophen can damage liver and kidneys.
- Any other medicine without consulting your doctor or pharmacist.

 POSSIBLE ADVERSE REACTIONS OR SIDE EFFECTS

SYMPTOMS	WHAT TO DO
Life-threatening:	
Hives, rash, intense itching, faintness soon after a dose (anaphylaxis); extreme weakness, transient paralysis, temporary loss of vision.	Seek emergency treatment immediately.
Common:	
Dizziness, lightheadedness, drowsiness.	Discontinue. Call doctor right away.
Infrequent:	
• Difficult or frequent urination, severe back pain, cloudy urine.	Discontinue. Call doctor right away.
• Nervousness, restlessnes, irritability, headache, indigestion, depression, agitation, constipation, tiredness, weakness.	Continue. Call doctor when convenient.
Rare:	
• Sudden decrease in urine output; swelling of lips, face or tongue.	Discontinue. Seek emergency treatment.
• Bloody or black stools, jaundice, unusual bleeding or bruising, sore mouth or throat, fever, hiccups, skin rash, hives.	Discontinue. Call doctor right away.

 WARNINGS & PRECAUTIONS

Don't take if:
- You are allergic to any skeletal-muscle relaxant or acetaminophen.
- Your symptoms don't improve after 2 days use. Call your doctor.

Before you start, consult your doctor:
- If you have had liver disease.
- If you have kidney disease or liver damage.
- If you plan pregnancy within medication period.
- If you are allergic to tartrazine dye.

CHLORZOXAZONE & ACETAMINOPHEN

Over age 60:
- Adverse reactions and side effects may be more frequent and severe than in younger persons.
- Don't exceed recommended dose. You can't eliminate drug as efficiently as younger persons.

Pregnancy:
Safety not proven. Avoid if possible.

Breast-feeding:
Drug passes into milk. Avoid drug or discontinue nursing until you finish medicine. Consult doctor for advice on maintaining milk supply.

Infants & children:
Not recommended.

Prolonged use:
- May affect blood system and cause anemia. Limit use to 5 days for children 12 and under, and 10 days for adults.
- Talk to your doctor about the need for follow-up medical examinations or laboratory studies to check complete blood counts (white blood cell count, platelet count, red blood cell count, hemoglobin, hematocrit), liver function.

Skin & sunlight:
No problems expected.

Driving, piloting or hazardous work:
Don't drive or pilot aircraft until you learn how medicine affects you. Don't work around dangerous machinery. Don't climb ladders or work in high places. Danger increases if you drink alcohol or take medicine affecting alertness and reflexes, such as antihistamines, tranquilizers, sedatives, pain medicine, narcotics and mind-altering drugs.

Discontinuing:
Don't discontinue without consulting your doctor. Dose may require gradual reduction if you have taken drug for a long time. Doses of other drugs may also require adjustment.

Others:
Periodic liver-function tests recommended if you use this drug for a long time.

POSSIBLE INTERACTION WITH OTHER DRUGS

GENERIC NAME OR DRUG CLASS	COMBINED EFFECT
Anticoagulants, oral*	May increase anti-coagulant effect. If combined frequently, prothrombin time should be monitored.
Antidepressants*	Increased sedation.
Antihistamines*	Increased sedation.
Clozapine	Toxic effect on the central nervous system.
Dronabinol	Increased effect of dronabinol on central nervous system. Avoid combination.
MAO inhibitors*	Increased effect (but safety not established) of both drugs.
Mind-altering drugs*	Increased sedation.
Muscle relaxants, others*	Increased sedation.
Narcotics*	Increased sedation.
Phenobarbital	Quicker elimination and decreased effects of acetaminophen.
Sedatives*	Increased sedation.
Sertraline	Increased depressive effects of both drugs.
Sleep inducers*	Increased sedation.
Tetracyclines* (effervescent granules or tablets)	May slow tetracycline absorption. Space doses 2 hours apart.
Tranquilizers*	Increased sedation.
Zidovudine	Increased toxicity of zidovudine.

POSSIBLE INTERACTION WITH OTHER SUBSTANCES

INTERACTS WITH	COMBINED EFFECT
Alcohol:	Drowsiness, increased sedation. Long-term use may cause toxic effect in liver.
Beverages:	No problems expected.
Cocaine:	Lack of coordination. May slow body's recovery. Avoid.
Foods:	No problems expected.
Marijuana:	Increased pain relief, lack of coordination, drowsiness, fainting. May slow body's recovery. Avoid.
Tobacco:	No problems expected.

*See Glossary

CHOLESTYRAMINE

BRAND NAMES

Cholybar
Questran

Questran Light

BASIC INFORMATION

Habit forming? No
Prescription needed? Yes
Available as generic? No
Drug class: Antihyperlipidemic, antipruritic

 USES

- Removes excess bile acids that occur with some liver problems. Reduces persistent itch caused by bile acids.
- Lowers cholesterol level.
- Treatment of one form of colitis (rare).

 DOSAGE & USAGE INFORMATION

How to take:
Powder, granules—Sprinkle into 8 oz. liquid. Let stand for 2 minutes, then mix with liquid before swallowing. Or mix with cereal, soup or pulpy fruit. Don't swallow dry.

When to take:
- 3 or 4 times a day on an empty stomach, 1 hour before or 2 hours after eating.
- If taking other medicines, take 1 hour before or 4 to 6 hours after taking cholestyramine.

If you forget a dose:
Take as soon as you remember up to 2 hours late. If more than 2 hours, wait for next scheduled dose (don't double this dose).

What drug does:
Binds with bile acids to prevent their absorption.

Time lapse before drug works:
- Cholesterol reduction—1 day.
- Bile-acid reduction—3 to 4 weeks.

Continued in next column

 OVERDOSE

SYMPTOMS:
Increased side effects and adverse reactions.
WHAT TO DO:
Overdose unlikely to threaten life. Depending on severity of symptoms and amount taken, call doctor, poison-control center or hospital emergency room for instructions.

Don't take with:
- Any drug or vitamin simultaneously. Space doses 2 hours apart.
- Any other medicine without consulting your doctor or pharmacist.

 POSSIBLE ADVERSE REACTIONS OR SIDE EFFECTS

SYMPTOMS	WHAT TO DO
Life-threatening:	
In case of overdose, see previous column.	
Common:	
Constipation.	Continue. Call doctor when convenient.
Infrequent:	
• Belching, bloating, diarrhea, mild nausea, vomiting, stomach pain, rapid weight gain.	Discontinue. Call doctor right away.
• Heartburn (mild).	Continue. Call doctor when convenient.
Rare:	
• Severe stomach pain; black, tarry stool.	Discontinue. Seek emergency treatment.
• Rash, hives, hiccups.	Discontinue. Call doctor right away.
• Sore tongue.	Continue. Call doctor when convenient.

WARNINGS & PRECAUTIONS

Don't take if:
You are allergic to cholestyramine.

Before you start, consult your doctor:
- If you plan to become pregnant within medication period.
- If you have angina, heart or blood-vessel disease.
- If you have stomach problems (including ulcer).
- If you have tartrazine sensitivity.
- If you have constipation or hemorrhoids.
- If you have kidney disease.

Over age 60:
Adverse reactions and side effects may be more frequent and severe than in younger persons.

Pregnancy:
No proven harm to unborn child. Avoid if possible.

Breast-feeding:
No problems expected, but consult doctor.

Infants & children:
Not recommended.

Prolonged use:
- May decrease absorption of folic acid.
- Talk to your doctor about the need for follow-up medical examinations or laboratory studies to check serum cholesterol and triglycerides.

Skin & sunlight:
No problems expected.

Driving, piloting or hazardous work:
No problems expected.

Discontinuing:
Don't discontinue without doctor's advice until you complete prescribed dose, even though symptoms diminish or disappear.

Others:
No problems expected.

POSSIBLE INTERACTION WITH OTHER DRUGS

GENERIC NAME OR DRUG CLASS	COMBINED EFFECT
Anticoagulants, oral*	Increased anticoagulant effect.
Beta carotene	Decreased absorption of beta carotene.
Dextrothyroxine	Decreased dextrothyroxine effect.
Digitalis preparations*	Decreased digitalis effect.
Indapamide	Decreased indapamide effect.
Thiazides*	Decreased absorption of cholestyramine.
Thyroid hormones*	Decreased thyroid effect.
Trimethoprim	Decreased absorption of cholestyramine.
Ursodiol	Decreased absorption of ursodiol.
Vancomycin	Increased chance of hearing loss or kidney damage. Decreased therapeutic effect of vancomycin.
Vitamins	Decreased absorption of fat-soluble vitamins (A,D,E,K).
All other medicines	Decreased absorption, so dosages or dosage intervals may require adjustment.

POSSIBLE INTERACTION WITH OTHER SUBSTANCES

INTERACTS WITH	COMBINED EFFECT
Alcohol:	None expected.
Beverages:	None expected.
Cocaine:	None expected.
Foods:	Absorption of vitamins in foods decreased. Take vitamin supplements, particularly A, D, E & K.
Marijuana:	None expected.
Tobacco:	None expected.

CINOXACIN

BRAND NAMES

Cinobac

BASIC INFORMATION

Habit forming? No
Prescription needed? Yes
Available as generic? No
Drug class: Anti-infective (urinary)

 USES

Treatment for urinary-tract infections.

 DOSAGE & USAGE INFORMATION

How to take:
Capsules—Swallow with food or milk to lessen stomach irritation. If you can't swallow whole, open capsule and take with liquid or food.

When to take:
At the same times each day.

If you forget a dose:
Take as soon as you remember up to 2 hours late. If more than 2 hours, wait for next scheduled dose (don't double this dose).

What drug does:
Destroys bacteria susceptible to cinoxacin.

Time lapse before drug works:
1 to 2 weeks.

Don't take with:
Any other medicine without consulting your doctor or pharmacist.

 OVERDOSE

SYMPTOMS:
Lethargy, stomach upset, behavioral changes, convulsions and stupor.
WHAT TO DO:
- Dial 0 (operator) or 911 (emergency) for an ambulance or medical help. Then give first aid immediately.
- If patient is unconscious and not breathing, give mouth-to-mouth breathing. If there is no heartbeat, use cardiac massage and mouth-to-mouth breathing (CPR). Don't try to make patient vomit. If you can't get help quickly, take patient to nearest emergency facility.
- See emergency information on inside covers.

 POSSIBLE ADVERSE REACTIONS OR SIDE EFFECTS

SYMPTOMS	WHAT TO DO
Life-threatening:	
Hives, rash, intense itching, faintness soon after a dose (anaphylaxis).	Seek emergency treatment immediately.
Common:	
Rash, itch; decreased, blurred or double vision; halos around lights or excess brightness; changes in color vision; nausea, vomiting, diarrhea.	Discontinue. Call doctor right away.
Infrequent:	
Dizziness, drowsiness, headache, ringing in ears, insomnia, appetite loss.	Continue. Call doctor when convenient.
Rare:	
Severe stomach pain, seizures, psychosis, joint pain, numbness or tingling in hands or feet (infants and children).	Discontinue. Call doctor right away.

WARNINGS & PRECAUTIONS

Don't take if:
- You are allergic to cinoxacin or nalidixic acid.
- You have a seizure disorder (epilepsy, convulsions).

Before you start, consult your doctor:
- If you plan to become pregnant during medication period.
- If you have or have had kidney or liver disease.
- If you have impaired circulation to the brain (hardened arteries).

Over age 60:
Adverse reactions and side effects may be more frequent and severe than in younger persons.

Pregnancy:
Risk to unborn child outweighs drug benefits. Don't use, especially during first 3 months.

Breast-feeding:
No problems expected, unless you have impaired kidney function. Consult doctor.

Infants & children:
Don't give to infants younger than 3 months.

Prolonged use:
Talk to your doctor about the need for follow-up medical examinations or laboratory studies to check kidney function, liver function.

Skin & sunlight:
- May cause sunlight to hurt eyes.
- May cause rash or intensify sunburn in areas exposed to sun or sunlamp.

Driving, piloting or hazardous work:
Avoid if you feel drowsy, dizzy or have vision problems. Otherwise, no problems expected.

Discontinuing:
Don't discontinue without consulting doctor. Dose may require gradual reduction if you have taken drug for a long time. Doses of other drugs may also require adjustment.

Others:
May interfere with the accuracy of some medical tests.

POSSIBLE INTERACTION WITH OTHER DRUGS

GENERIC NAME OR DRUG CLASS	COMBINED EFFECT
Probenecid	Decreased elimination.

POSSIBLE INTERACTION WITH OTHER SUBSTANCES

INTERACTS WITH	COMBINED EFFECT
Alcohol:	Impaired alertness, judgment and coordination.
Beverages:	None expected.
Cocaine:	Impaired judgment and coordination.
Foods:	None expected.
Marijuana:	Impaired alertness, judgment and coordination.
Tobacco:	None expected.

CIPROFLOXACIN

BRAND NAMES

Cipro

BASIC INFORMATION

Habit forming? No
Prescription needed? Yes
Available as generic? No
Drug class: Antibacterial (antibiotic), fluoroquinolone

USES

Treats a wide range of germs that may cause diarrhea, pneumonia, skin and soft tissue infections, urinary tract infections, bone infections.

DOSAGE & USAGE INFORMATION

How to take:
Tablets—Take with full glass of water on empty stomach.

When to take:
As directed by your doctor.

If you forget a dose:
Take as soon as you remember up to 2 hours late. If more than 2 hours, wait for next scheduled dose (don't double this dose).

What drug does:
Destroys bacteria in the body, probably by promoting DNA breakage in germs.

Time lapse before drug works:
1 to 2 hours.

Don't take with:
• Food or antacids.
• Any other medicine without consulting your doctor or pharmacist.

OVERDOSE

SYMPTOMS:
Convulsions.
WHAT TO DO:
• Dial 0 (operator) or 911 (emergency) for an ambulance or medical help. Then give first aid immediately.
• If patient is unconscious and not breathing, give mouth-to-mouth breathing. If there is no heartbeat, use cardiac massage and mouth-to-mouth breathing (CPR). Don't try to make patient vomit. If you can't get help quickly, take patient to nearest emergency facility.
• See emergency information on inside covers.

POSSIBLE ADVERSE REACTIONS OR SIDE EFFECTS

SYMPTOMS	WHAT TO DO
Life-threatening:	
Hives, rash, intense itching, faintness soon after a dose (anaphylaxis).	Seek emergency treatment immediately.
Common:	
Abdominal discomfort, diarrhea, vomiting	Discontinue. Call doctor right away.
Infrequent:	
• Blood in urine, back pain, pain while urinating.	Discontinue. Call doctor right away.
• Drowsiness, joint pain, skin rash, insomnia.	Continue. Call doctor when convenient.
Rare:	
Sun sensitivity, visual disturbances.	Discontinue. Call doctor right away.

WARNINGS & PRECAUTIONS

Don't take if:
You are allergic to ciprofloxacin, nalidixic acid or norfloxacin.

Before you start, consult your doctor:
If you have any disorder of the central nervous system such as epilepsy or stroke.

Over age 60:
Adverse reactions and side effects may be more frequent and severe than in younger persons. You may need smaller doses for shorter periods of time.

Pregnancy:
Studies inconclusive on harm to unborn child. Not recommended for use during pregnancy.

Breast-feeding:
Not recommended.

Infants & children:
Not recommended.

Prolonged use:
No documented problems.

Skin & sunlight:
Rare adverse reaction to sunlight or sun lamp. Avoid over-exposure.

Driving, piloting or hazardous work:
Don't drive or pilot aircraft until you learn how medicine affects you. Don't work around dangerous machinery. Don't climb ladders or work in high places. Danger increases if you drink alcohol or take medicine affecting alertness and reflexes, such as antihistamines, tranquilizers, sedatives, pain medicine, narcotics and mind-altering drugs.

Discontinuing:
Don't discontinue without consulting doctor. Dose may require gradual reduction if you have taken drug for a long time. Doses of other drugs may also require adjustment.

Others:
May affect accuracy of laboratory test values for SGOT, serum bilirubin, serum creatinine and LDH.

POSSIBLE INTERACTION WITH OTHER DRUGS

GENERIC NAME OR DRUG CLASS	COMBINED EFFECT
Antacids*	May cause kidney dysfunction.
Carbonic anyhdrase inhibitors*	May cause kidney dysfunction.
Probenecid	May cause kidney dysfunction.
Theophylline	May increase possibility of central nervous system poisoning, such as nausea, vomiting, restlessness, palpitations.

POSSIBLE INTERACTION WITH OTHER SUBSTANCES

INTERACTS WITH	COMBINED EFFECT
Alcohol:	Increased possibility of central nervous system poisoning.
Beverages:	None expected.
Cocaine:	Increased possibility of central nervous system poisoning.
Foods:	None expected.
Marijuana:	Increased possibility of central nervous system poisoning.
Tobacco:	Increased possibility of central nervous system poisoning.

*See Glossary

CITRATES

BRAND AND GENERIC NAMES

Albright's Solution
Bicitra
Citra Forte
Citrolith
Efricon Expectorant
  Liquid
Lanatuss
  Expectorant
Modified Shohl's
  Solution
Oracit
Phanadex
Phanatuss
Polycitra
Polycitra-K
Polycitra-LC-
  Sugar-free

POTASSIUM
  CITRATE
POTASSIUM
  CITRATE &
  CITRIC ACID
POTASSIUM
  CITRATE &
  SODIUM CITRATE
SODIUM CITRATE
  & CITRIC ACID
TRICITRATES
Tricodene NN Cough
  & Cold Medication
Tussirex with
  Codeine liquid
Urocit-K

BASIC INFORMATION

Habit forming? No
Prescription needed? Yes
Available as generic? No
Drug class: Urinary alkalizer, antiurolithic

 ## USES

- To make urine more alkaline (less acid).
- To treat or prevent recurrence of some types of kidney stones.

 ## DOSAGE & USAGE INFORMATION

How to take:
Tablets or liquid—Take right after a meal or with a bedtime snack.

When to take:
On full stomach, usually after meals or with food.

If you forget a dose:
Take as soon as you remember up to 2 hours late. If more than 2 hours, wait for next scheduled dose (don't double this dose).

Continued next column

 ## OVERDOSE

SYMPTOMS:
Convulsions, coma.
WHAT TO DO:
- **Dial 0 (operator) or 911 (emergency) for an ambulance or medical help. Then give first aid immediately.**
- **See emergency information on inside covers.**

What drug does:
Increases urinary alkalinity by excretion of bicarbonate ions.

Time lapse before drug works:
1 hour.

Don't take with:
- Any medicine that will decrease mental alertness or reflexes, such as alcohol, other mind-altering drugs, cough/cold medicines, antihistamines, allergy medicine, sedatives, tranquilizers (sleeping pills or "downers"), barbiturates, seizure medicine, narcotics, other prescription medicine for pain, muscle relaxants, anesthetics.
- See Interaction column and consult doctor.

 ## POSSIBLE ADVERSE REACTIONS OR SIDE EFFECTS

SYMPTOMS	WHAT TO DO
Life-threatening:	
Black, tarry stools; vomiting blood; severe abdominal cramps; irregular heartbeat; shortness of breath.	Discontinue. Seek emergency treatment.
Common:	
Nausea or vomiting.	Continue. Call doctor when convenient.
Infrequent:	
Confusion, dizziness, swollen feet and ankles, irritability, depression, muscle pain, nervousness, numbness or tingling in hands or feet, unpleasant taste, weakness.	Discontinue. Call doctor right away.
Rare:	
Slow breathing, tiredness.	Discontinue. Call doctor right away.

WARNINGS & PRECAUTIONS

Don't take if:
You are allergic to any citrate.

Before you start, consult your doctor:
- If you have any disease involving the adrenal glands, diabetes, chronic diarrhea, heart problems, hypertension, kidney disease, stomach ulcer or gastritis, urinary tract infection, toxemia of pregnancy.
- If you plan strenuous exercise.

Over age 60:
Adverse reactions and side effects may be more frequent and severe than in younger persons. Ask doctor about smaller doses.

Pregnancy:
Safety to unborn child unestablished. Avoid if possible.

Breast-feeding:
Safety during lactation not established. Consult doctor.

Infants & children:
Use only under close medical supervision.

Prolonged use:
- Adverse reactions more likely.
- Talk to your doctor about the need for follow-up medical examinations or laboratory studies to check complete blood counts (white blood cell count, platelet count, red blood cell count, hemoglobin, hematocrit), serum electrolytes, urine.

Skin & sunlight:
No problems expected.

Driving, piloting or hazardous work:
Don't drive or pilot aircraft until you learn how medicine affects you. Don't work around dangerous machinery. Don't climb ladders or work in high places. Danger increases if you drink alcohol or take medicine affecting alertness and reflexes, such as antihistamines, tranquilizers, sedatives, pain medicine, narcotics and mind-altering drugs.

Discontinuing:
Don't discontinue without consulting doctor. Dose may require gradual reduction if you have taken drug for a long time. Doses of other drugs may also require adjustment.

Others:
- Drink at least 8 ounces of water or other liquid (except milk) every hour while awake.
- Liquid may be chilled (don't freeze) to improve taste.
- Monitor potassium in blood with frequent laboratory studies.

POSSIBLE INTERACTION WITH OTHER DRUGS

GENERIC NAME OR DRUG CLASS	COMBINED EFFECT
Amphetamines*	Increased amphetamine effect.
Antacids*	Toxic effect of citrates (alkalosis).
Calcium supplements*	Increases risk of kidney stones.
Digitalis*	Increased risk of too much potassium in blood.
Methenamine	Decreases effects of methenamine.
Mexiletine	May slow elimination of mexiletine and cause need to adjust dosage.
Quinidine	Prolongs quinidine effect.

POSSIBLE INTERACTION WITH OTHER SUBSTANCES

INTERACTS WITH	COMBINED EFFECT
Alcohol:	Will decrease mental alertness.
Beverages: Salt-free milk.	May cause potassium toxicity.
Cocaine:	No proven problems.
Foods: Milk, cheese, ice cream, yogurt, buttermilk, salty foods, salt, salt substitutes.	May increase likelihood of kidney stones.
Marijuana:	No proven problems.
Tobacco:	Increases likelihood of stomach irritation.

*See Glossary

CLARITHROMYCIN

BRAND NAMES

Biaxin

BASIC INFORMATION

Habit forming? No
Prescription needed? Yes
Available as generic? No
Drug class: Antibacterial (macrolide)

 USES

Treats infections including bronchitis, pharyngitis, pneumonia, sinusitis, skin infections and Legionnaire's disease.

 DOSAGE & USAGE INFORMATION

How to take:
Tablets—Swallow with liquid. If you can't swallow whole, crumble tablet and take with liquid or food.

When to take:
At the same time each day.

If you forget a dose:
- If you take 3 or more doses daily—Take as soon as you remember, then resume regular schedule.
- If you take 2 doses daily—Take as soon as you remember. Wait 5 to 6 hours for next dose. Return to regular schedule.

What drug does:
Prevents growth and reproduction of susceptible bacteria.

Time lapse before drug works:
Usually within 2 hours. Will take 2 to 5 days for noticeable effect.

Don't take with:
Any other medicine without consulting your doctor.

 OVERDOSE

SYMPTOMS:
Nausea, vomiting, abdominal discomfort, diarrhea.
WHAT TO DO:
Overdose unlikely to threaten life. If person takes much larger amount than prescribed, call doctor, poison-control center or hospital emergency room for instructions.

 POSSIBLE ADVERSE REACTIONS OR SIDE EFFECTS

SYMPTOMS	WHAT TO DO
Life-threatening: None expected.	
Common: Headache.	Continue. Call doctor when convenient.
Infrequent: Abdominal discomfort, diarrhea, nausea.	Discontinue. Call doctor right away.
Rare: None expected.	

CLARITHROMYCIN

WARNINGS & PRECAUTIONS

Don't take if:
You are allergic to clarithromycin or erythromycins*.

Before you start, consult your doctor:
If you have significant kidney disease

Over age 60:
Adverse reactions and side effects may be more frequent and severe than in younger persons.

Pregnancy:
No proven harm to unborn child. Avoid if possible.

Breast-feeding:
Drug passes into milk. Avoid drug or discontinue nursing until you finish medicine. Consult doctor for advice on maintaining milk supply.

Infants & children:
Use only under medical supervision.

Prolonged use:
- You may become more susceptible to infections caused by germs that are not responsive to clarithromycin.
- Talk to your doctor about the need for follow-up medical examinations or laboratory studies to check liver function.

Skin & sunlight:
No special problems expected.

Driving, piloting or hazardous work:
No special problems expected.

Discontinuing:
Take drug for the full amount of time prescribed by doctor.

Others:
No problems expected.

POSSIBLE INTERACTION WITH OTHER DRUGS

GENERIC NAME OR DRUG CLASS	COMBINED EFFECT
Theophylline	Increased concentration of theophylline.
Zidovudine	Decreased effect of zidovudine.

POSSIBLE INTERACTION WITH OTHER SUBSTANCES

INTERACTS WITH	COMBINED EFFECT
Alcohol:	Possible liver damage.
Beverages: Caffeine drinks	Increased caffeine toxicity. Avoid.
Cocaine:	No proven problems.
Foods:	No proven problems.
Marijuana:	No proven problems.
Tobacco:	No proven problems.

CLIDINIUM

BRAND NAMES

Clipoxide   Quarzan
Librax

BASIC INFORMATION

Habit forming? No
Prescription needed?
  Low strength: No
  High strength: Yes
Available as generic? No
Drug class: Antispasmodic, anticholinergic

USES

Reduces spasms of digestive system, bladder and urethra.

DOSAGE & USAGE INFORMATION

How to take:
Capsule—Swallow with liquid or food to lessen stomach irritation.

When to take:
30 minutes before meals (unless directed otherwise by doctor).

If you forget a dose:
Take as soon as you remember up to 2 hours late. If more than 2 hours, wait for next scheduled dose (don't double this dose).

What drug does:
Blocks nerve impulses at parasympathetic nerve endings, preventing muscle contractions and gland secretions of organs involved.

Time lapse before drug works:
15 to 30 minutes.

Don't take with:
Any other medicine without consulting your doctor or pharmacist.

OVERDOSE

SYMPTOMS:
Dilated pupils, rapid pulse and breathing, dizziness, fever, hallucinations, confusion, slurred speech, agitation, flushed face, convulsions, coma.
WHAT TO DO:
- Dial 0 (operator) or 911 (emergency) for an ambulance or medical help. Then give first aid immediately.
- See emergency information on inside covers.

POSSIBLE ADVERSE REACTIONS OR SIDE EFFECTS

SYMPTOMS	WHAT TO DO
Life-threatening:	
In case of overdose, see previous column.	
Common:	
• Confusion, delirium, rapid heartbeat.	Discontinue. Call doctor right away.
• Nausea, vomiting, decreased sweating.	Continue. Call doctor when convenient.
• Constipation.	Continue. Tell doctor at next visit.
• Dryness in ears, nose, throat, mouth.	No action necessary.
Infrequent:	
• Nasal congestion, altered taste, difficult urination, headache, impotence.	Continue. Call doctor when convenient.
• Lightheadedness.	Discontinue. Call doctor right away.
Rare:	
Rash or hives, eye pain, blurred vision.	Discontinue. Call doctor right away.

WARNINGS & PRECAUTIONS

Don't take if:
- You are allergic to any anticholinergic.
- You have trouble with stomach bloating.
- You have difficulty emptying your bladder completely (enlarged prostate).
- You have narrow-angle glaucoma.
- You have severe ulcerative colitis.

Before you start, consult your doctor:
- If you have open-angle glaucoma.
- If you have angina, chronic bronchitis or asthma, kidney or thyroid disease, hiatal hernia, liver disease, enlarged prostate, myasthenia gravis, peptic ulcer.
- If you will have surgery within 2 months, including dental surgery, requiring general or spinal anesthesia.

Over age 60:
Adverse reactions and side effects may be more frequent and severe than in younger persons.

Pregnancy:
Studies inconclusive on harm to unborn child. Animal studies show fetal abnormalities. Decide with your doctor whether drug benefits justify risk to unborn child.

Breast-feeding:
Drug passes into milk and decreases milk flow. Avoid drug or discontinue nursing until you finish medicine. Consult doctor for advice on maintaining milk supply.

Infants & children:
Use only under medical supervision.

Prolonged use:
Chronic constipation, possible fecal impaction. Consult doctor immediately.

Skin & sunlight:
No problems expected.

Driving, piloting or hazardous work:
Don't drive or pilot aircraft until you learn how medicine affects you. Don't work around dangerous machinery. Don't climb ladders or work in high places. Danger increases if you drink alcohol or take medicine affecting alertness and reflexes, such as antihistamines, tranquilizers, sedatives, pain medicine, narcotics, or mind-altering drugs.

Discontinuing:
May be unnecessary to finish medicine. Follow doctor's instructions.

Others:
Advise any doctor or dentist whom you consult that you take this medicine.

POSSIBLE INTERACTION WITH OTHER DRUGS

GENERIC NAME OR DRUG CLASS	COMBINED EFFECT
Amantadine	Increased clidinium effect.
Antacids*	Decreased clidinium effect.
Anticholinergics, other*	Increased clidinium effect.
Antidepressants, tricyclic (TCA)*	Increased clidinium effect. Increased sedation.
Antidiarrheals*	Increased clidinium effect.
Antihistamines*	Increased clidinium effect.
Attapulgite	Decreased clidinium effect.
Haloperidol	Increased internal eye pressure.
Ketoconazole	Decreased ketoconazole effect.
MAO inhibitors*	Increased clidinium effect.
Meperidine	Increased clidinium effect.
Methylphenidate	Increased clidinium effect.
Molindone	Increased anti-cholinergic effect.
Nitrates*	Increased internal eye pressure.
Nizatidine	Increased nizatidine effect.

Continued page 941

POSSIBLE INTERACTION WITH OTHER SUBSTANCES

INTERACTS WITH	COMBINED EFFECT
Alcohol:	None expected.
Beverages:	None expected.
Cocaine:	Excessively rapid heartbeat. Avoid.
Foods:	None expected.
Marijuana:	Drowsiness and dry mouth.
Tobacco:	None expected.

*See Glossary

CLINDAMYCIN

BRAND NAMES

Cleocin

BASIC INFORMATION

Habit forming? No
Prescription needed? Yes
Available as generic? No
Drug class: Antibiotic (lincomycin)

 USES

- Treatment of bacterial infections that are susceptible to clindamycin.
- Topical treatment for acne. Follow instructions on package.

 DOSAGE & USAGE INFORMATION

How to take:
Capsule or liquid—Swallow with liquid 1 hour before or 2 hours after eating.

When to take:
At the same times each day.

If you forget a dose:
Take as soon as you remember up to 2 hours late. If more than 2 hours, wait for next scheduled dose (don't double this dose).

What drug does:
Destroys susceptible bacteria. Does not kill viruses.

Time lapse before drug works:
3 to 5 days.

Don't take with:
Any other medicine without consulting your doctor or pharmacist.

 OVERDOSE

SYMPTOMS:
Severe nausea, vomiting, diarrhea.
WHAT TO DO:
Overdose unlikely to threaten life. If person takes much larger amount than prescribed, call doctor, poison-control center or hospital emergency room for instructions.

 POSSIBLE ADVERSE REACTIONS OR SIDE EFFECTS

SYMPTOMS	WHAT TO DO
Life-threatening:	
Hives, wheezing, faintness, itching, coma.	Seek emergency treatment immediately.
Common:	
Bloating.	Discontinue. Call doctor right away.
Infrequent:	
• Unusual thirst; vomiting; stomach cramps; severe and watery diarrhea with blood or mucus; weight loss, painful, swollen joints; fever; jaundice; tiredness; weakness.	Discontinue. Call doctor right away.
• White patches in mouth; rash, itch around groin, rectum or armpits; vaginal discharge, itching.	Continue. Call doctor when convenient.
Rare:	
None expected.	

226

WARNINGS & PRECAUTIONS

Don't take if:
- You are allergic to lincomycins.
- You have had ulcerative colitis.
- Prescribed for infant under 1 month old.

Before you start, consult your doctor:
- If you have had yeast infections of mouth, skin or vagina.
- If you will have surgery within 2 months, including dental surgery, requiring general or spinal anesthesia.
- If you have kidney or liver disease.
- If you have allergies of any kind.

Over age 60:
Adverse reactions and side effects may be more frequent and severe than in younger persons.

Pregnancy:
Risk to unborn child outweighs drug benefits. Don't use.

Breast-feeding:
Drug passes into milk. Avoid drug or discontinue nursing until you finish medicine. Consult doctor for advice on maintaining milk supply.

Infants & children:
Don't give to infants younger than 1 month. Use for children only under medical supervision.

Prolonged use:
- Severe colitis with diarrhea and bleeding.
- You may become more susceptible to infections caused by germs not responsive to clindamycin.
- Talk to your doctor about the need for follow-up medical examinations or laboratory studies to check stool exams and perform proctosigmoidoscopy.

Skin & sunlight:
No problems expected.

Driving, piloting or hazardous work:
No problems expected.

Discontinuing:
Don't discontinue without doctor's advice until you complete prescribed dose, even though symptoms diminish or disappear.

Others:
May interfere with the accuracy of some medical tests.

POSSIBLE INTERACTION WITH OTHER DRUGS

GENERIC NAME OR DRUG CLASS	COMBINED EFFECT
Antidiarrheal preparations*	Decreased clindamycin effect.
Cefixime	Decreased antibiotic effect of cefixime.
Chloramphenicol	Decreased clindamycin effect.
Diphenoxylate	May delay removal of toxins from colon in cases of diarrhea caused by side effects of clindamycin.
Erythromycins*	Decreased clindamycin effect.
Loperamide	May delay removal of toxins from colon in cases of diarrhea caused by side effects of clindamycin.
Muscle-blocking drugs*	Increased actions of muscle blockers to unsafe degree. Avoid.

POSSIBLE INTERACTION WITH OTHER SUBSTANCES

INTERACTS WITH	COMBINED EFFECT
Alcohol:	None expected.
Beverages:	None expected.
Cocaine:	None expected.
Foods:	None expected.
Marijuana:	None expected.
Tobacco:	None expected.

*See Glossary

CLOFIBRATE

BRAND NAMES

Atromid-S   Novofibrate
Claripex

BASIC INFORMATION

Habit forming? No
Prescription needed? Yes
Available as generic? Yes
Drug class: Antihyperlipidemic

 ## USES

Reduces fatty substances in the blood
(triglycerides).

 ## DOSAGE & USAGE INFORMATION

How to take:
Capsule—Swallow with liquid or food to lessen
stomach irritation.

When to take:
At the same times each day.

If you forget a dose:
Take as soon as you remember up to 2 hours
late. If more than 2 hours, wait for next
scheduled dose (don't double this dose).

What drug does:
Inhibits formation of fatty substances.

Time lapse before drug works:
3 months or more.

Don't take with:
Any other medicine without consulting your
doctor or pharmacist.

 ## OVERDOSE

SYMPTOMS:
Diarrhea, headache, muscle pain.
WHAT TO DO:
Overdose unlikely to threaten life. If person
takes much larger amount than prescribed,
call doctor, poison-control center or
hospital emergency room for instructions.

 ## POSSIBLE ADVERSE REACTIONS OR SIDE EFFECTS

SYMPTOMS	WHAT TO DO
Life-threatening:	
None expected.	
Common:	
None expected.	
Infrequent:	
• Chest pain, shortness of breath, irregular heartbeat, gallstones, nausea, flu-like illness, vomiting.	Discontinue. Call doctor right away.
• Diarrhea, abdominal pain.	Continue. Call doctor when convenient.
Rare:	
• Cardiac arrythmias, angina.	Discontinue. Seek emergency treatment.
• Rash, itch; mouth or lip sores; sore throat; swollen feet, legs; blood in urine; painful urination; fever; chills, anemia.	Discontinue. Call doctor right away.
• Dizziness, weakness, drowsiness, muscle cramps, headache, diminished sex drive, hair loss, dry mouth.	Continue. Call doctor when convenient.

CLOFIBRATE

WARNINGS & PRECAUTIONS

Don't take if:
- You are allergic to any clofibrate.
- You have had serious liver disease.

Before you start, consult your doctor:
- If you have had liver or kidney disease.
- If you have had peptic-ulcer disease.
- If you have diabetes.

Over age 60:
Adverse reactions and side effects may be more frequent and severe than in younger persons. May develop flu-like symptoms.

Pregnancy:
Risk to unborn child outweighs drug benefits. Don't use.

Breast-feeding:
May harm child. Avoid.

Infants & children:
Not recommended.

Prolonged use:
- May cause gall bladder infection.
- Possible cause of stomach cancer.
- Talk to your doctor about the need for follow-up medical examinations or laboratory studies to check complete blood counts (white blood cell count, platelet count, red blood cell count, hemoglobin, hematocrit), serum low-density lipoprotein.

Skin & sunlight:
No problems expected.

Driving, piloting or hazardous work:
Avoid if you feel drowsy or dizzy. Otherwise, no problems expected.

Discontinuing:
Don't discontinue without doctor's advice until you complete prescribed dose, even though symptoms diminish or disappear.

Others:
- Periodic blood-cell counts and liver-function studies recommended if you take clofibrate for a long time.
- Some studies question effectiveness. Many studies warn against toxicity.

POSSIBLE INTERACTION WITH OTHER DRUGS

GENERIC NAME OR DRUG CLASS	COMBINED EFFECT
Anticoagulants, oral*	Increased anti-coagulant effect. Dose reduction of anticoagulant necessary.
Antidiabetics, oral*	Increased antidiabetic effect.
Contraceptives, oral*	Decreased clofibrate effect.
Desmopressin	May decrease desmopressin effect.
Estrogens*	Decreased clofibrate effect.
Furosemide	Possible toxicity of both drugs.
Insulin	Increased insulin effect.
Probenecid	Increased effect and toxicity of clofibrate.
Thyroid hormones*	Increased clofibrate effect.
Ursodiol	Decreased effect of ursodiol.

POSSIBLE INTERACTION WITH OTHER SUBSTANCES

INTERACTS WITH	COMBINED EFFECT
Alcohol:	None expected.
Beverages:	None expected.
Cocaine:	None expected.
Foods: Fatty foods.	Decreased clofibrate effect.
Marijuana:	None expected.
Tobacco:	None expected.

CLOMIPHENE

BRAND NAMES

Clomid   Serophene
Milophene

BASIC INFORMATION

Habit forming? No
Prescription needed? Yes
Available as generic? No
Drug class: Gonad stimulant

 USES

- Treatment for men with low sperm counts.
- Treatment for ovulatory failure in women who wish to become pregnant.

 DOSAGE & USAGE INFORMATION

How to take:
Tablet—Swallow with liquid.

When to take:
- Men—Take at the same time each day.
- Women—Follow physician's instructions carefully.

If you forget a dose:
Take as soon as you remember. If you forget a day, double next dose. If you miss 2 or more doses, consult doctor.

What drug does:
Antiestrogen effect stimulates ovulation and sperm production.

Time lapse before drug works:
Usually 3 to 6 months. Ovulation may occur 6 to 10 days after last day of treatment in any cycle.

Don't take with:
No restrictions.

 OVERDOSE

SYMPTOMS:
Increased severity of adverse reactions and side effects.
WHAT TO DO:
Overdose unlikely to threaten life. If person takes much larger amount than prescribed, call doctor, poison-control center or hospital emergency room for instructions.

 POSSIBLE ADVERSE REACTIONS OR SIDE EFFECTS

SYMPTOMS	WHAT TO DO
Life-threatening:	
Sudden shortness of breath.	Seek emergency treatment.
Common:	
• Bloating, abdominal pain, pelvic pain.	Discontinue. Call doctor right away.
• Hot flashes.	Continue. Tell doctor at next visit.
Infrequent:	
• Rash, itch, vomiting, jaundice.	Discontinue. Call doctor right away.
• Constipation, diarrhea, increased appetite, heavy menstrual flow, frequent urination, breast discomfort, weight change, hair loss, nausea.	Continue. Call doctor when convenient.
Rare:	
• Vision changes.	Discontinue. Call doctor right away.
• Dizziness, headache, tiredness, depression, nervousness.	Continue. Call doctor when convenient.

WARNINGS & PRECAUTIONS

Don't take if:
You are allergic to clomiphene.

Before you start, consult your doctor:
- If you have an ovarian cyst, fibroid uterine tumors or unusual vaginal bleeding.
- If you have inflamed veins caused by blood clots.
- If you have liver disease.
- If you are depressed.

Over age 60:
Not recommended.

Pregnancy:
Stop taking at first sign of pregnancy.

Breast-feeding:
Not used.

Infants & children:
Not used.

Prolonged use:
- Not recommended.
- Talk to your doctor about the need for follow-up medical examinations or laboratory studies to check basal body temperature, endometrial biopsy, kidney function, eyes.

Skin & sunlight:
Eyes more sensitive to light.

Driving, piloting or hazardous work:
- Avoid if you feel dizzy.
- May cause blurred vision.

Discontinuing:
May be unnecessary to finish medicine. Follow doctor's instructions.

Others:
- Have a complete pelvic examination before treatment.
- If you become pregnant, twins or triplets are possible.

 ## POSSIBLE INTERACTION WITH OTHER DRUGS

GENERIC NAME OR DRUG CLASS	COMBINED EFFECT
Thyroglobulin	May increase serum thyroglobulin.
Thyroxine (T-4)	May increase serum thyroxine.

 ## POSSIBLE INTERACTION WITH OTHER SUBSTANCES

INTERACTS WITH	COMBINED EFFECT
Alcohol:	None expected.
Beverages:	None expected.
Cocaine:	None expected.
Foods:	None expected.
Marijuana:	None expected.
Tobacco:	None expected.

CLONIDINE

BRAND NAMES

Catapres   Dixarit
Catapres-TTS

BASIC INFORMATION

Habit forming? No
Prescription needed? Yes
Available as generic? Yes
Drug class: Antihypertensive

 USES

- Treatment of high blood pressure and congestive heart failure.
- Treatment of dysmenorrhea and menopausal "hot flashes."
- Treatment of narcotic withdrawal syndrome.
- Prevention of vascular headaches.

 DOSAGE & USAGE INFORMATION

How to take:
- Tablet—Swallow with liquid.
- Patches that attach to skin—Apply to clean, dry, hairless skin on arm or trunk.

When to take:
Daily dose at bedtime.

If you forget a dose:
Bedtime dose—If you forget your once-a-day dose, take it as soon as you remember. *Don't* double dose.

What drug does:
Relaxes and allows expansion of blood vessel walls.

Continued next column

 OVERDOSE

SYMPTOMS:
Vomiting, fainting, slow heartbeat, coma, diminished reflexes, shortness of breath, dizziness, extreme tiredness.
WHAT TO DO:
- **Dial 0 (operator) or 911 (emergency) for an ambulance or medical help. Then give first aid immediately.**
- **If patient is unconscious and not breathing, give mouth-to-mouth breathing. If there is no heartbeat, use cardiac massage and mouth-to-mouth breathing (CPR). Don't try to make patient vomit. If you can't get help quickly, take patient to nearest emergency facility.**
- **See emergency information on inside covers.**

Time lapse before drug works:
1 to 3 hours.

Don't take with:
- Non-prescription medicines containing alcohol.
- Any other medicine without consulting your doctor or pharmacist.

 POSSIBLE ADVERSE REACTIONS OR SIDE EFFECTS

SYMPTOMS	WHAT TO DO
Life-threatening:	
In case of overdose, see previous column.	
Common:	
• Dizziness, weight gain, drowsiness, lightheadedness upon rising from sitting or lying, swollen breasts.	Continue. Call doctor when convenient.
• Dry mouth, tiredness.	Continue. Tell doctor at next visit.
Infrequent:	
• Abnormal heart rhythm.	Discontinue. Call doctor right away.
• Headache; painful glands in neck; nightmares; nausea; vomiting; cold fingers and toes; dry, burning eyes; depression.	Continue. Call doctor when convenient.
• Insomnia, constipation, appetite loss, diminished sex drive, nervousness.	Continue. Tell doctor at next visit.
Rare:	
Rash, itch.	Discontinue. Call doctor right away.

 WARNINGS & PRECAUTIONS

Don't take if:
- You are allergic to any alpha-adrenergic blocker.
- You are under age 12.

Before you start, consult your doctor:
- If you will have surgery within 2 months, including dental surgery, requiring general or spinal anesthesia.
- If you have heart disease or chronic kidney disease.
- If you have a peripheral circulation disorder (intermittent claudication, Buerger's disease).
- If you have history of depression.

Over age 60:
Adverse reactions and side effects may be more frequent and severe than in younger persons.

Pregnancy:
Studies inconclusive on harm to unborn child. Animal studies show fetal abnormalities. Decide with your doctor whether drug benefits justify risk to unborn child.

Breast-feeding:
Unknown whether safe or not. Consult doctor.

Infants & children:
Use only under careful medical supervision after age 12. Avoid before age 12.

Prolonged use:
- Don't discontinue without consulting doctor. Dose may require gradual reduction if you have taken drug for a long time. Doses of other drugs may also require adjustment.
- Continued use may cause fluid retention, requiring addition of diuretic to treatment program.
- Request yearly eye examinations.
- Talk to your doctor about the need for follow-up medical examinations or laboratory studies.

Skin & sunlight:
No problems expected.

Driving, piloting or hazardous work:
Don't drive or pilot aircraft until you learn how medicine affects you. Don't work around dangerous machinery. Don't climb ladders or work in high places. Danger increases if you drink alcohol or take medicine affecting alertness and reflexes.

Discontinuing:
Don't discontinue abruptly. May cause rebound high blood pressure, anxiety, chest pain, insomnia, headache, nausea, irregular heartbeat, flushed face, sweating.

Others:
No problems expected.

 POSSIBLE INTERACTION
WITH OTHER DRUGS

GENERIC NAME OR DRUG CLASS	COMBINED EFFECT
ACE inhibitors*: captopril, enalapril, lisinopril	Possible excessive potassium in blood.
Antidepressants, tricyclic (TCA)*	Decreased clonidine effect.
Antihypertensives, other*	Excessive blood pressure drop.
Appetite suppressants*	Decreased clonidine effect.
Beta-adrenergic blockers*	Possible precipitous change in blood pressure.

Carteolol	Increased antihypertensive effect.
Clozapine	Toxic effect on the central nervous system.
Diuretics*	Excessive blood pressure drop.
Ethinamate	Dangerous increased effects of ethinamate. Avoid combining.
Fenfluramine	Possible increased clonidine effect.
Fluoxetine	Increased depressant effects of both drugs.
Guanfacine	Blood pressure control impaired.
Leucovorin	High alcohol content of leucovorin may cause adverse effects.
Methyprylon	Increased sedative effect, perhaps to dangerous level. Avoid.
Nabilone	Greater depression of central nervous system.
Nicardipine	Blood pressure drop. Dosages may require adjustment.

Continued on page 942

 POSSIBLE INTERACTION
WITH OTHER SUBSTANCES

INTERACTS WITH	COMBINED EFFECT
Alcohol:	Increased sensitivity to sedative effect of alcohol and very low blood pressure. Avoid.
Beverages: Caffeine-containing drinks.	Decreased clonidine effect.
Cocaine	Increased risk of heart block and high blood pressure.
Foods:	No problems expected.
Marijuana:	Weakness on standing.
Tobacco:	No problems expected.

*See Glossary

CLONIDINE & CHLORTHALIDONE

BRAND NAMES

Combipres

BASIC INFORMATION

Habit forming? No
Prescription needed? Yes
Available as generic? No
Drug class: Antihypertensive

 USES

- Treatment of high blood pressure.
- Reduces fluid retention (edema) caused by conditions such as heart disorders and liver disease.

 DOSAGE & USAGE INFORMATION

How to take:
Tablet—Swallow with liquid. If you can't swallow whole, crumble tablet and take with liquid or food. Don't exceed dose.

When to take:
At the same time each day.

If you forget a dose:
Take as soon as you remember up to 2 hours late. If more than 2 hours, wait for next scheduled dose (don't double this dose).

What drug does:
- Relaxes and allows expansion of blood vessel walls.

Continued next column

 OVERDOSE

SYMPTOMS:
Vomiting; fainting; rapid, irregular, slow heartbeat; diminished reflexes; cramps; shortness of breath; weakness; drowsiness; weak pulse; coma.
WHAT TO DO:
- **Dial 0 (operator) or 911 (emergency) for an ambulance or medical help. Then give first aid immediately.**
- **If patient is unconscious and not breathing, give mouth-to-mouth breathing. If there is no heartbeat, use cardiac massage and mouth-to-mouth breathing (CPR). Don't try to make patient vomit. If you can't get help quickly, take patient to nearest emergency facility.**
- **See emergency information on inside covers.**

- Forces sodium and water excretion, reducing body fluid.
- Reduced body fluid and relaxed arteries lower blood pressure.

Time lapse before drug works:
4 to 6 hours. May require several weeks to lower blood pressure.

Don't take with:
Any medicine that will decrease mental alertness such as alcohol, antihistamines, cold/cough medicines, sedatives, tranquilizers, narcotics, prescription pain medicine, barbiturates, seizure medicine, anesthetics.

 POSSIBLE ADVERSE REACTIONS OR SIDE EFFECTS

SYMPTOMS	WHAT TO DO
Life-threatening: Irregular heartbeat, weak pulse.	Discontinue. Seek emergency treatment.
Common: Dry mouth, increased thirst, muscle cramps, nausea or vomiting, mood changes, drowsiness.	Discontinue. Call doctor right away.
Infrequent: Vomiting, diminished sex desire and performance, insomnia, dizziness, diarrhea, constipation, appetite loss.	Continue. Call doctor when convenient.
Rare: • Jaundice; easy bruising or bleeding; sore throat, fever, mouth ulcers; rash or hives; joint pain; flank pain; abdominal pain.	Discontinue. Call doctor right away.
• Cold fingers and toes, nightmares.	Continue. Call doctor when convenient.

 WARNINGS & PRECAUTIONS

Don't take if:
- You are allergic to any thiazide diuretic drug or alpha-adrenergic blocker.
- You are under age 12.

Before you start, consult your doctor:
- If you are allergic to any sulfa drug.
- If you have gout, liver, pancreas or kidney disorder, a peripheral circulation disorder (intermittent claudication, Buerger's disease), history of depression, heart disease.

- If you will have surgery within 2 months, including dental surgery, requiring general or spinal anesthesia.

Over age 60:
Adverse reactions and side effects may be more frequent and severe than in younger persons, especially dizziness and excessive potassium loss.

Pregnancy:
Risk to unborn child outweighs drug benefits. Don't use.

Breast-feeding:
Drug passes into milk. Avoid drug or discontinue nursing until you finish medicine. Consult doctor for advice on maintaining milk supply.

Infants & children:
Use only after careful medical supervision after age 12. Avoid before age 12.

Prolonged use:
- Don't discontinue without consulting doctor. Dose may require gradual reduction if you have taken drug for a long time. Doses of other drugs may also require adjustment.
- Continued use may cause fluid retention, requiring addition of diuretic to treatment program.
- Request yearly eye examinations.
- Talk to your doctor about the need for follow-up medical examinations or laboratory studies.

Skin & sunlight:
May cause rash or intensify sunburn in areas exposed to sun or sunlamp.

Driving, piloting or hazardous work:
Don't drive or pilot aircraft until you learn how medicine affects you. Don't work around dangerous machinery. Don't climb ladders or work in high places. Danger increases if you drink alcohol or take medicine affecting alertness and reflexes, such as antihistamines, tranquilizers, sedatives, pain medicine, narcotics and mind-altering drugs.

Discontinuing:
Don't discontinue abruptly. May cause rebound high blood pressure, anxiety, chest pain, insomnia, headache, nausea, irregular heartbeat, flushed face, sweating.

Others:
- Hot weather and fever may cause dehydration and drop in blood pressure. Dose may require temporary adjustment. Weigh daily and report any unexpected weight decreases to your doctor.
- May cause rise in uric acid, leading to gout.
- May cause blood-sugar rise in diabetics.

POSSIBLE INTERACTION WITH OTHER DRUGS

GENERIC NAME OR DRUG CLASS	COMBINED EFFECT
ACE inhibitors*: captopril, enalapril, lisinopril	Possible excessive potassium in blood.
Allopurinol	Decreased allopurinol effect.
Antidepressants, tricyclic (TCA)*	Dangerous drop in blood pressure. Avoid combination unless under medical supervision.
Antihypertensives, other*	Excessive blood pressure drop.
Appetite suppressants*	Decreased clonidine effect.
Barbiturates*	Increased chlorthalidone effect.
Beta-adrenergic blockers*	Possible precipitous change in blood pressure.
Carteolol	Increased antihypertensive effect.

Continued page 942

POSSIBLE INTERACTION WITH OTHER SUBSTANCES

INTERACTS WITH	COMBINED EFFECT
Alcohol:	Increased sensitivity to sedative effect of alcohol and very low blood pressure. Avoid.
Beverages: Caffeine-containing drinks.	Decreased clonidine effect.
Cocaine	Increased risk of heart block and high blood pressure.
Foods: Licorice.	Excessive potassium loss that causes dangerous heart rhythm.
Marijuana:	Weakness on standing. May increase blood pressure.
Tobacco:	None expected.

*See Glossary

CLOTRIMAZOLE (Oral-Local)

BRAND NAMES

Mycelex

BASIC INFORMATION

Habit forming? No
Prescription needed? Yes
Available as generic? No
Drug class: Antifungal

USES

- Treats thrush, white mouth (candidiasis).
- Used primarily in immunosuppressed patients to treat and prevent mouth infection.

DOSAGE & USAGE INFORMATION

How to take:
Lozenges—Dissolve slowly and completely in the mouth, 5 times a day. Swallow saliva during this time. Don't swallow lozenge whole and don't chew.

When to take:
14 days or longer.

If you forget a dose:
Take as soon as you remember up to 2 hours late. If more than 2 hours, wait for next scheduled dose (don't double this dose).

What drug does:
Kills fungus by interfering with cell wall membrane and its permeability.

Time lapse before drug works:
1 to 3 hours.

Don't take with:
Any other medicine without consulting your doctor or pharmacist.

OVERDOSE

SYMPTOMS:
None expected, but if large dose has been taken, follow instructions below.
WHAT TO DO:
- Dial 0 (operator) or 911 (emergency) for an ambulance or medical help. Then give first aid immediately.
- See emergency information on inside covers.

POSSIBLE ADVERSE REACTIONS OR SIDE EFFECTS

SYMPTOMS	WHAT TO DO
Life-threatening: None expected.	
Common: None expected.	
Infrequent: Abdominal pain, diarrhea, nausea, vomiting.	Discontinue. Call doctor right away.
Rare: None expected.	

CLOTRIMAZOLE (Oral-Local)

WARNINGS & PRECAUTIONS

Don't take if:
You have severe liver disease.

Before you start, consult your doctor:
If you have had a recent organ transplant.

Over age 60:
Adverse reactions and side effects may be more frequent and severe than in younger persons. You may need smaller doses for shorter periods of time.

Pregnancy:
Risk to unborn child outweighs drug benefits. Don't use.

Breast-feeding:
Drug passes into milk. Avoid drug or discontinue nursing until you finish medicine. Consult doctor for advice on maintaining milk supply.

Infants & children:
Use only under medical supervision for children younger than 4 or 5 years.

Prolonged use:
No problems expected.

Skin & sunlight:
No problems expected.

Driving, piloting or hazardous work:
Don't drive or pilot aircraft until you learn how medicine affects you. Don't work around dangerous machinery. Don't climb ladders or work in high places. Danger increases if you drink alcohol or take medicine affecting alertness and reflexes.

Discontinuing:
Don't discontinue without consulting doctor. Dose may require gradual reduction if you have taken drug for a long time. Doses of other drugs may also require adjustment.

Others:
• Continue for full term of treatment. May require several months.
• Check with physician if not improved in 1 week.

POSSIBLE INTERACTION WITH OTHER DRUGS

GENERIC NAME OR DRUG CLASS	COMBINED EFFECT
None expected.	

POSSIBLE INTERACTION WITH OTHER SUBSTANCES

INTERACTS WITH	COMBINED EFFECT
Alcohol:	Decreased effects of clotrimazole.
Beverages:	None expected.
Cocaine:	Decreased effects of clotrimazole.
Foods:	None expected.
Marijuana:	Decreased effects of clotrimazole.
Tobacco:	Decreased effects of clotrimazole.

CLOXACILLIN

BRAND NAMES

Apo-Cloxi	Orbenin
Cloxapen	Tegopen
Novocloxin	

BASIC INFORMATION

Habit forming? No
Prescription needed? Yes
Available as generic? Yes
Drug class: Antibiotic (penicillin)

USES

Treatment of bacterial infections that are susceptible to cloxacillin.

DOSAGE & USAGE INFORMATION

How to take:
- Capsules—Swallow with liquid on an empty stomach 1 hour before or 2 hours after eating.
- Liquid—Take with cold beverage. Liquid form is perishable and effective for only 7 days at room temperature. Effective for 14 days if stored in refrigerator. Don't freeze.

When to take:
Follow instructions on prescription label or side of package. Doses should be evenly spaced. For example, 4 times a day means every 6 hours.

If you forget a dose:
Take as soon as you remember. Continue regular schedule.

What drug does:
Destroys susceptible bacteria. Does not kill viruses.

Time lapse before drug works:
May be several days before medicine affects infection.

Don't take with:
Any other medicine without consulting your doctor or pharmacist.

OVERDOSE

SYMPTOMS:
Severe diarrhea, nausea or vomiting.
WHAT TO DO:
Overdose unlikely to threaten life. If person takes much larger amount than prescribed, call doctor, poison-control center or hospital emergency room for instructions.

POSSIBLE ADVERSE REACTIONS OR SIDE EFFECTS

SYMPTOMS	WHAT TO DO
Life-threatening:	
Hives, rash, intense itching, faintness soon after a dose (anaphylaxis).	Seek emergency treatment immediately.
Common:	
Dark or discolored tongue.	Continue. Tell doctor at next visit.
Infrequent:	
• Mild nausea, vomiting, diarrhea.	Continue. Call doctor when convenient.
• Bloody urine, face and ankle swelling.	Discontinue. Call doctor right away.
Rare:	
Unexplained bleeding or bruising, weakness, sore throat, fever, abdominal cramps, convulsions.	Discontinue. Call doctor right away.

WARNINGS & PRECAUTIONS

Don't take if:
You are allergic to cloxacillin, cephalosporin antibiotics, other penicillins or penicillamine. Life-threatening reaction may occur.

Before you start, consult your doctor:
- If you are allergic to any substance or drug.
- If you take birth control pills.

Over age 60:
You may have skin reactions, particularly around genitals and anus.

Pregnancy:
Studies inconclusive on harm to unborn child. Animal studies show fetal abnormalities. Decide with your doctor whether drug benefits justify risk to unborn child.

Breast-feeding:
Drug passes into milk. Child may become sensitive to penicillins and have allergic reactions to penicillin drugs. Avoid cloxacillin or discontinue nursing until you finish medicine. Consult doctor for advice on maintaining milk supply.

Infants & children:
No problems expected.

Prolonged use:
- You may become more susceptible to infections caused by germs not responsive to cloxacillin.
- Talk to your doctor about the need for follow-up medical examinations or laboratory studies to check SGPT*, SGOT*.

Skin & sunlight:
No problems expected.

Driving, piloting or hazardous work:
Usually not dangerous. Most hazardous reactions likely to occur a few minutes after taking cloxacillin.

Discontinuing:
Don't discontinue without doctor's advice until you complete prescribed dose, even though symptoms diminish or disappear.

Others:
- May interfere with the accuracy of some medical tests.
- Birth control pills may not be effective. Use additional birth-control methods.

POSSIBLE INTERACTION WITH OTHER DRUGS

GENERIC NAME OR DRUG CLASS	COMBINED EFFECT
Beta-adrenergic blockers*	Increased chance of anaphylaxis (see emergency information on inside front cover).
Birth control pills	Impaired contraceptive efficiency.
Chloramphenicol	Decreased effect of both drugs.
Erythromycins*	Decreased effect of both drugs.
Loperamide	Decreased cloxacillin effect.
Paromomycin	Decreased effect of both drugs.
Probenecid	Increased effect of all penicillins.
Sodium benzoate & sodium phenylacetate	May reduce effect of sodium benzoate & sodium phenylacetate.
Tetracyclines*	Decreased effect of both drugs.
Troleandomycin	Decreased effect of both drugs.

POSSIBLE INTERACTION WITH OTHER SUBSTANCES

INTERACTS WITH	COMBINED EFFECT
Alcohol:	Occasional stomach irritation.
Beverages:	None expected.
Cocaine:	No proven problems.
Foods: Acidic fruits or juices, aged cheese, wines, syrups (if taken with).	Decreased antibiotic effect.
Marijuana:	No proven problems.
Tobacco:	None expected.

CLOZAPINE

BRAND NAMES

Clozaril   Leponex

BASIC INFORMATION

Habit forming? No
Prescription needed? Yes. Prescribed only
through a special program.
Available as generic? No
Drug class: Antipsychotic

 ## USES

Treats severe schizophrenia in patients not
helped by other medicines.

 ## DOSAGE & USAGE
INFORMATION

How to take:
Tablet—Swallow with liquid. If you can't swallow
whole, crumble tablet and take with liquid or
food.

When to take:
Once or twice daily as directed.

If you forget a dose:
Take as soon as you remember up to 2 hours
late. If more than 2 hours, wait for next
scheduled dose (don't double this dose).

What drug does:
Interferes with binding of dopamine. May
produce significant improvement, but may at
times also make schizophrenia worse.

Time lapse before drug works:
1 to 6 hours.

Don't take with:
Any other prescription drug, non-prescription
drug or alcohol without first checking with your
doctor.

 ## OVERDOSE

SYMPTOMS:
Heartbeat fast, slow, irregular;
hallucinations; restlessness;
excitement; drowsiness; breathing difficulty.
WHAT TO DO:
- **Dial 0 (operator) or 911 (emergency) for**
  an ambulance or medical help. Then give
  first aid immediately.
- **See emergency information on inside**
  covers.

 ## POSSIBLE
ADVERSE REACTIONS
OR SIDE EFFECTS

SYMPTOMS	WHAT TO DO
Life-threatening:	
Seizures (rare).	Seek emergency treatment immediately.
Common:	
• Fast or irregular heartbeat, dizziness or fainting, fever.	Continue, but call doctor right away.
• Constipation, lightheadedness, increased salivation, heartburn, nausea, weight gain.	Continue. Call doctor when convenient.
Infrequent:	
Abdominal discomfort, increased sweating, anxiety, confusion, mild restlessness, blurred vision, unusual bleeding.	Discontinue. Call doctor right away.
Rare:	
Chills, fever, sore throat, mouth ulcers; difficult urination; rigid muscles; muscle tremors; mental depression; insomnia; lip-smacking, cheek puffing, uncontrolled tongue movements.	Discontinue. Call doctor right away.

WARNINGS & PRECAUTIONS

Don't take if:
- You are significantly mentally depressed.
- You have bone marrow depression from other drugs.
- You have glaucoma.

Before you start, consult your doctor:
- If you have an enlarged prostate gland.
- If you have ever had seizures from any cause.
- If you have liver, heart or gastrointestinal disease.

Over age 60:
Possible greater risk of weakness or dizziness upon standing after sitting or lying down. Greater risk of excitement, confusion. Great risk of difficulty in urination.

Pregnancy:
Safety not established. Consult doctor.

Breast-feeding:
May cause sedation, restlessness or irritability in the nursing infant. Avoid.

Infants & children:
Safety not established. Consult doctor.

Prolonged use:
Effects unknown.

Skin & sunlight:
No problems expected.

Driving, piloting or hazardous work:
Don't drive or pilot aircraft until you learn how medicine affects you. Don't work around dangerous machinery. Don't climb ladders or work in high places. Danger increases if you drink alcohol or take medicine affecting alertness and reflexes.

Discontinuing:
Don't discontinue without consulting doctor. Dose may require gradual reduction if you have taken drug for a long time. Doses of other drugs may also require adjustment.

Others:
- In 1991 this medicine is available only through a special management program for monitoring and distributing this drug.
- You will need laboratory studies each week for white blood cell and differential counts.

POSSIBLE INTERACTION WITH OTHER DRUGS

GENERIC NAME OR DRUG CLASS	COMBINED EFFECT
Bone marrow depressants*	Toxic bone marrow depression.
Central nervous system (CNS) depressants*	Toxic effects on the central nervous system.
Lithium	Increased risk of seizures.

POSSIBLE INTERACTION WITH OTHER SUBSTANCES

INTERACTS WITH	COMBINED EFFECT
Alcohol:	Avoid. Increases toxic effect on the central nervous system.
Beverages: Caffeine drinks.	Excess (more than 3 cups of coffee or equivalent) increases risk of heartbeat irregularities.
Cocaine:	Increased risk of heartbeat irregularities.
Foods:	No special problems expected.
Marijuana:	Increased risk of heartbeat irregularities.
Tobacco:	Decreased serum concentration of clozapine. Avoid.

---

*See Glossary

COAL TAR (Topical)

BRAND AND GENERIC NAMES

See complete list of brand and generic names in the *Brand Name Directory*, page 917.

BASIC INFORMATION

Habit forming? No
Prescription needed? No (for most)
Available as generic? Yes
Drug class: Antiseborrheic, antipsoriatic, keratolytic

 ## USES

Applied to the skin to treat dandruff, seborrhea, dermatitis, eczema and other skin diseases.

 ## DOSAGE & USAGE INFORMATION

How to use:
- Follow package instructions.
- Don't apply to blistered, oozing, infected or raw skin.
- Keep away from eyes.
- Protect treated area from sunshine for 72 hours.

When to use:
According to package instructions.

If you forget a dose:
Use as soon as you remember.

What drug does:
- Kills bacteria and fungus organisms on contact.
- Suppresses overproduction of skin cells.

Time lapse before drug works:
None. Works immediately. May take several days before maximum effect.

Don't take with:
Any other medicine without consulting your doctor or pharmacist.

 ## OVERDOSE

SYMPTOMS:
None expected.
WHAT TO DO:
Overdose unlikely to threaten life. If person takes much larger amount than prescribed, call doctor, poison-control center or hospital emergency room for instructions.

 ## POSSIBLE ADVERSE REACTIONS OR SIDE EFFECTS

SYMPTOMS	WHAT TO DO
Life-threatening: None expected.	
Common: Skin stinging.	Continue. Call doctor when convenient.
Infrequent: Skin more irritated.	Continue. Call doctor when convenient.
Rare: Pus forms in lesions on skin.	Continue. Call doctor when convenient.

WARNINGS & PRECAUTIONS

Don't use if:
You have intolerance to coal tar.

Before you start, consult your doctor:
If you have infected skin or open wounds.

Over age 60:
No special problems expected.

Pregnancy:
No special problems expected.

Breast-feeding:
No special problems expected.

Infants & children:
Don't use on infants.

Prolonged use:
No special problems expected.

Skin & sunlight:
Protect treated area from direct sunlight for 72 hours.

Driving, piloting or hazardous work:
No problems expected.

Discontinuing:
No special problems expected.

Others:
May affect results in some medical tests.

POSSIBLE INTERACTION WITH OTHER DRUGS

GENERIC NAME OR DRUG CLASS	COMBINED EFFECT
Psoralens (methoxsalen, trioxsalen)	Excess sensitivity to sun.

POSSIBLE INTERACTION WITH OTHER SUBSTANCES

INTERACTS WITH	COMBINED EFFECT
Alcohol:	No special problems expected.
Beverages:	No special problems expected.
Cocaine:	No special problems expected.
Foods:	No special problems expected.
Marijuana:	No special problems expected.
Tobacco:	No special problems expected.

COCAINE

GENERIC NAMES

COCAINE

BASIC INFORMATION

Habit forming? Yes
Prescription needed? Yes
Available as generic? Yes
Drug class: Anesthetic (local)

 ## USES

Provides local anesthesia to the nose, mouth or throat to allow some types of surgery or examinations without pain.

 ## DOSAGE & USAGE INFORMATION

How to use:
Used only under doctor's supervision, it's applied by spray or cotton swab directly to the area being anesthetized.

When to use:
Immediately before special examinations or surgery.

If you forget a dose:
Not applicable.

What drug does:
- Blocks conduction of nerve impulses to brain.
- Reduces swelling, bleeding and congestion at operation site.

Time lapse before drug works:
Immediate.

Don't use with:
Any other medicine without consulting your doctor or pharmacist.

 ## OVERDOSE

SYMPTOMS:
Abdominal pain, chills, confusion, light-headedness, dizziness, severe nervousness or restlessness, fast or irregular heartbeat, severe headache, sweating, twitching, dilated pupils, bulging eyes.
WHAT TO DO:
- **Tell your doctor immediately if any of the above occurs after cocaine has been applied.**
- **Dial 0 (operator) or 911 (emergency) for an ambulance or medical help. Then give first aid immediately.**
- **See emergency information on inside covers.**

 ## POSSIBLE ADVERSE REACTIONS OR SIDE EFFECTS

SYMPTOMS	WHAT TO DO
Life-threatening: Blue discoloration of skin, lips, nails; irregular, weak heartbeat; chest pain; seizure; loss of bowel and bladder control.	Seek emergency treatment immediately.
Common: Abdominal pain, dizziness, confusion, agitation, irritability, hallucinations, fast or irregular heartbeat, headache, euphoria, psychotic behavior, trembling, large pupils, chills and fever, twitching, stuffy nose.	Discontinue. Seek medical help if symptoms don't quickly subside.
Infrequent: Loss of taste or smell after application to nose or mouth.	Nothing. This is a normal effect.
Rare: Death.	

WARNINGS & PRECAUTIONS

Don't take if:
You are allergic to cocaine.

Before you start, consult your doctor:
- If you are allergic to anything.
- If you are taking *any* other medicine.
- If you have any acute illness or history of cancer, convulsions, irregular heartbeat, heart disease, blood vessel disease, high blood pressure, liver disease, heart attack history, hyperthyroidism (overactive thyroid gland).
- If you have recently used an insecticide.
- If you have had glaucoma or are using eye drops for glaucoma (such as Betoptic, Betagan, Timoptic).
- If you have a throat infection.

Over age 60:
More sensitive to drug. May cause impaired thinking, hallucinations, nightmares. Consult doctor about any of these.

Pregnancy:
Risk to unborn child outweighs any possible drug benefits. Don't use.

Breast-feeding:
Risk outweighs any possible drug benefits. Don't use.

Infants & children:
Not recommended for children 6 and younger. Use for older children only under doctor's supervision.

Prolonged use:
Addiction.

Skin & sunlight:
No problems expected.

Driving, piloting or hazardous work:
Don't drive or pilot aircraft for 24 hours after cocaine has been used for local anesthesia. Don't work around dangerous machinery. Don't climb ladders or work in high places. Danger increases if you drink alcohol or take medicine affecting alertness and reflexes, such as antihistamines, tranquilizers, sedatives, pain medicine, narcotics and mind-altering drugs.

Discontinuing:
No problems expected.

Others:
- In some people, even small amounts of cocaine can cause serious adverse reactions.
- Cocaine is used only under the direct supervision of your doctor.
- May interfere with the accuracy of some medical tests, such as blood sugar, blood pressure, heart rate.

POSSIBLE INTERACTION WITH OTHER DRUGS

GENERIC NAME OR DRUG CLASS	COMBINED EFFECT
Anesthetics*	Increased risk of heartbeat irregularity.
Antidepressants, tricyclic (TCA)*	Increased risk of heartbeat irregularity.
Antihypertensives*	Increased risk of heart block and high blood pressure.
Beta-blockers*	Decreased beta-blocker effect.
Central nervous system stimulants*	Convulsions or excessive nervousness.
Digitalis preparations*	Increased risk of heartbeat irregularity.
Insecticides	Increased risk of toxicity.
Levodopa	Increased risk of heartbeat irregularity.
MAO inhibitors*	Increased risk of toxicity.
Methyldopa	Increased risk of heartbeat irregularity.
Nitrates*	Reduced effectiveness of nitrates.
Sympathomimetics*	High risk of heartbeat irregularities and high blood pressure.

POSSIBLE INTERACTION WITH OTHER SUBSTANCES

INTERACTS WITH	COMBINED EFFECT
Alcohol:	Dangerous interaction. Don't use.
Beverages: Caffeine drinks.	Dangerous interaction. Don't use.
Cocaine: Orally.	Increased chance of adverse reactions or death.
Foods:	No proven problems.
Marijuana:	Dangerous interaction. Don't use.
Tobacco:	Increased likelihood of irregular or rapid heartbeat.

*See Glossary

COLCHICINE

BRAND NAMES

ColBenemid   Col-Probenecid

BASIC INFORMATION

Habit forming? No
Prescription needed? Yes
Available as generic? Yes
Drug class: Antigout

 USES

- Relieves joint pain, inflammation, swelling of gout.
- Also used for familial Mediterranean fever, dermatitis herpetiformis.

 DOSAGE & USAGE INFORMATION

How to take:
Tablet—Swallow with liquid or food to lessen stomach irritation.

When to take:
- As prescribed. Stop taking when pain stops or at first sign of digestive upset. Wait at least 3 days between treatments.
- Don't take more than 8 doses.

If you forget a dose:
Don't double next dose. Consult doctor.

What drug does:
Decreases acidity of joint tissues and prevents deposits of uric-acid crystals.

Time lapse before drug works:
12 to 48 hours.

Don't take with:
Any other medicine without consulting your doctor or pharmacist.

 OVERDOSE

SYMPTOMS:
Bloody urine, diarrhea, burning feeling in stomach, muscle weakness, fever, shortness of breath, stupor, convulsions, coma.
WHAT TO DO:
- **Dial 0 (operator) or 911 (emergency) for an ambulance or medical help. Then give first aid immediately.**
- **See emergency information on inside covers.**

 POSSIBLE ADVERSE REACTIONS OR SIDE EFFECTS

SYMPTOMS	WHAT TO DO
Life-threatening:	
In case of overdose, see previous column.	
Common:	
Diarrhea, nausea, vomiting, abdominal pain.	Discontinue. Call doctor right away.
Infrequent:	
• Rash, itch, unusual bruising, blood in urine.	Discontinue. Call doctor right away.
• Numbness, tingling, pain or weakness in hands or feet; unusual tiredness or weakness; fever; hair loss; appetite loss.	Continue. Call doctor when convenient.
Rare:	
Jaundice, aplastic anemia (low red blood cells), agranulocytosis (low white blood cells).	Discontinue. Call doctor right away.

246

WARNINGS & PRECAUTIONS

Don't take if:
You are allergic to colchicine.

Before you start, consult your doctor:
- If you have had peptic ulcers or ulcerative colitis.
- If you have heart, liver or kidney disease.
- If you will have surgery within 2 months, including dental surgery, requiring general or spinal anesthesia.

Over age 60:
Adverse reactions and side effects may be more frequent and severe than in younger persons. Colchicine has a narrow margin of safety for people in this age group.

Pregnancy:
Risk to unborn child outweighs drug benefits. Don't use.

Breast-feeding:
No problems expected, but consult doctor.

Infants & children:
Not recommended.

Prolonged use:
- Hair loss.
- Numbness or tingling in hands and feet.
- Talk to your doctor about the need for follow-up medical examinations or laboratory studies to check complete blood counts (white blood cell count, platelet count, red blood cell count, hemoglobin, hematocrit).

Skin & sunlight:
No problems expected.

Driving, piloting or hazardous work:
Don't drive or pilot aircraft until you learn how medicine affects you. Don't work around dangerous machinery. Don't climb ladders or work in high places. Danger increases if you drink alcohol or take medicine affecting alertness and reflexes, such as antihistamines, tranquilizers, sedatives, pain medicine, narcotics and mind-altering drugs.

Discontinuing:
- May be unnecessary to finish medicine. Follow doctor's instructions.
- Stop taking if digestive upsets occur before symptoms are relieved.

Others:
- Limit each course of treatment to 8 mg. Don't exceed 3 mg. per 24 hours.
- May cause decreased sperm production in males.
- May interfere with the accuracy of some medical tests.

POSSIBLE INTERACTION WITH OTHER DRUGS

GENERIC NAME OR DRUG CLASS	COMBINED EFFECT
Anticoagulants*	Increased anticoagulant effect.
Clozapine	Toxic effect on bone marrow.
Diuretics*	Decreased antigout effect of colchicine.
Levamisole	Increased risk of bone marrow depression.
Phenylbutazone	Increased chance of ulcers in gastro-intestinal tract.
Thioguanine	May need increased dosage of colchicine.
Tiopronin	Increased risk of toxicity to bone marrow.
Vitamin B-12	Decreased absorption of vitamin B-12.

POSSIBLE INTERACTION WITH OTHER SUBSTANCES

INTERACTS WITH	COMBINED EFFECT
Alcohol:	Increased risk of gastrointestinal toxicity.
Beverages: Herbal teas.	Increased colchicine effect. Avoid.
Cocaine:	Overstimulation. Avoid.
Foods:	No proven problems.
Marijuana:	Decreased colchicine effect.
Tobacco:	No proven problems.

*See Glossary

COLESTIPOL

BRAND NAMES

Colestid

BASIC INFORMATION

Habit forming? No
Prescription needed? Yes
Available as generic? No
Drug class: Antihyperlipidemic

 USES

- Reduces cholesterol level in blood in patients with type IIa hyperlipidemia.
- Treats overdose of digitalis.
- Reduces skin itching associated with some forms of liver disease.
- Treats diarrhea after some surgical operations.
- Treatment of one form of colitis (rare).

 DOSAGE & USAGE INFORMATION

How to take:

Mix well with 6 ounces or more or water or liquid, or in soups, pulpy fruits, with milk or in cereals. Will not dissolve.

When to take:

- Before meals.
- If taking other medicine, take it 1 hour before or 4 to 6 hours after taking colestipol.

If you forget a dose:

Take as soon as you remember up to 2 hours late. If more than 2 hours, wait for next scheduled dose (don't double this dose).

What drug does:

Binds with bile acids in intestines, preventing reabsorption.

Time lapse before drug works:

3 to 12 months.

Don't take with:

Any other medicine without consulting your doctor or pharmacist.

 OVERDOSE

SYMPTOMS:
Fecal impaction.
WHAT TO DO:
Overdose unlikely to threaten life. If person takes much larger amount than prescribed, call doctor, poison-control center or hospital emergency room for instructions.

 POSSIBLE ADVERSE REACTIONS OR SIDE EFFECTS

SYMPTOMS	WHAT TO DO
Life-threatening:	
None expected.	
Common:	
None expected.	
Infrequent:	
• Black, tarry stools from gastrointestinal bleeding.	Discontinue. Seek emergency treatment.
• Severe abdominal pain.	Discontinue. Call doctor right away.
• Constipation, belching, diarrhea, nausea, unexpected weight loss.	Continue. Call doctor when convenient.
Rare:	
Hives, skin rash, hiccups.	Discontinue. Call doctor right away.

WARNINGS & PRECAUTIONS

Don't take if:
You are allergic to colestipol.

Before you start, consult your doctor:
- If you have liver disease such as cirrhosis.
- If you are jaundiced.
- If you will have surgery within 2 months, including dental surgery, requiring general or spinal anesthesia.
- If you are constipated.
- If you have peptic ulcer.
- If you have coronary artery disease.

Over age 60:
Constipation more likely. Other adverse effects more likely.

Pregnancy:
No proven harm to unborn child. Avoid if possible.

Breast-feeding:
No proven harm to child. Consult doctor.

Infants & children:
Only under expert medical supervision.

Prolonged use:
- Request lab studies to determine serum cholesterol and serum triglycerides.
- May decrease absorption of folic acid.

Skin & sunlight:
No problems expected.

Driving, piloting or hazardous work:
No problems expected.

Discontinuing:
Don't discontinue without consulting doctor. Dose may require gradual reduction if you have taken drug for a long time. Doses of other drugs may also require adjustment, particularly digitalis.

Others:
- This medicine does not cure disorders, but helps to control them.
- May interfere with the accuracy of some medical tests.

POSSIBLE INTERACTION WITH OTHER DRUGS

GENERIC NAME OR DRUG CLASS	COMBINED EFFECT
Anticoagulants, oral*	Decreased anti-coagulant effect.
Beta carotene	Decreased absorption of beta carotene.
Dextrothyroxine	Decreased dextro-thyroxine effect.
Digitalis preparations*	Decreased absorption of digitalis preparations.
Diuretics, thiazide*	Decreased absorption of thiazide diuretics.
Penicillins*	Decreased absorption of penicillins.
Tetracyclines*	Decreased absorption of tetracyclines.
Thiazides*	Decreased absorption of colestipol.
Trimethoprim	Decreased absorption of colestipol.
Ursodiol	Decreased absorption of ursodiol.
Vancomycin	Increased chance of hearing loss or kidney damage. Decreased therapeutic effect of vancomycin.
Vitamins	Decreased absorption of fat-soluble vitamins (A,D,E,K)
Other medicines	May delay or reduce absorption.

POSSIBLE INTERACTION WITH OTHER SUBSTANCES

INTERACTS WITH	COMBINED EFFECT
Alcohol:	None expected.
Beverages:	None expected.
Cocaine:	None expected.
Foods:	Interferes with absorption of vitamins. Take supplements.
Marijuana:	None expected.
Tobacco:	None expected.

*See Glossary

CONTRACEPTIVES, ORAL

BRAND AND GENERIC NAMES

See complete list of brand and generic names in the *Brand Name Directory*, page 918.

BASIC INFORMATION

Habit forming? No
Prescription needed? Yes
Available as generic? No
Drug class: Female sex hormone,
contraceptive (oral)

 ## USES

- Prevents pregnancy.
- Regulates menstrual periods.

 ## DOSAGE & USAGE INFORMATION

How to take:
Tablet—Swallow with liquid or food to lessen stomach irritation.

When to take:
At same time each day according to prescribed instructions, usually for 21 days of 28-day cycle.

If you forget a dose:
Call doctor's office for advice about additional protection against pregnancy.

What drug does:
- Alters mucus at cervix entrance to prevent sperm entry.
- Alters uterus lining to resist implantation of fertilized egg.
- Creates same chemical atmosphere in blood that exists during pregnancy, suppressing pituitary hormones which stimulate ovulation.

Time lapse before drug works:
10 days or more to provide contraception.

Don't take with:
- Tobacco
- Any other medicine without consulting your doctor or pharmacist.

 ## OVERDOSE

SYMPTOMS:
Drowsiness, nausea, vomiting, vaginal bleeding.
WHAT TO DO:
Overdose unlikely to threaten life. If person takes much larger amount than prescribed, call doctor, poison-control center or hospital emergency room for instructions.

 ## POSSIBLE ADVERSE REACTIONS OR SIDE EFFECTS

SYMPTOMS	WHAT TO DO
Life-threatening:	
Stroke, chest pain, coughing blood, sudden severe headache, severe leg pain, shortness of breath.	Seek emergency treatment immediately.
Common:	
Brown blotches on skin; vaginal discharge, itch; fluid retention; breakthrough bleeding; acne.	Continue. Call doctor when convenient.
Infrequent:	
• Headache; pain, swelling in leg (possible blood clots in leg vein); muscle, joint pain; depression; severe abdominal pain; bulging eyes; fainting; frequent urination; breast lumps.	Discontinue. Call doctor right away.
• Blue tinge to objects, lights; appetite change; nausea; bloating; vomiting; pain; changed sex drive.	Continue. Call doctor when convenient.
Rare:	
• Jaundice, rash, hives, itch, fever, hypercalcemia in breast cancer, intolerance of contact lenses, excess hair growth, voice change, enlarged clitoris in women.	Discontinue. Call doctor right away.
• Amenorrhea, insomnia, hair loss.	Continue. Call doctor when convenient.

 ## WARNINGS & PRECAUTIONS

Don't take if:
- You are allergic to any female hormone.
- You have had heart disease, blood clots or stroke.
- You have liver disease.
- You have cancer of breast, uterus or ovaries.
- You have unexplained vaginal bleeding.
- You smoke cigarettes.

Before you start, consult your doctor:
- If you have fibrocystic disease of breast.
- If you have migraine headaches.
- If you have fibroid tumors of uterus.
- If you have epilepsy.

- If you have asthma.
- If you have high blood pressure.
- If you will have surgery within 2 months, including dental surgery, requiring general or spinal anesthesia.
- If you have endometriosis.
- If you have diabetes.
- If you have sickle-cell anemia.
- If you are over age 35.

Over age 60:
Not used.

Pregnancy:
May harm child. Discontinue at first sign of pregnancy.

Breast-feeding:
Drug passes into milk. Avoid drug or discontinue nursing.

Infants & children:
Not recommended.

Prolonged use:
- Gallstones.
- Gradual blood-pressure rise.
- Possible difficulty becoming pregnant after discontinuing.
- Talk to your doctor about the need for follow-up medical examinations or laboratory studies to check blood pressure, liver function, pap smear.

Skin & sunlight:
May cause rash or intensify sunburn in areas exposed to sun or sunlamp.

Driving, piloting or hazardous work:
No problems expected.

Discontinuing:
Don't become pregnant for 6 months after discontinuing.

Others:
- Failure to take oral contraceptives for 1 day may cancel pregnancy protection. If you forget a dose, use other contraceptive measures and call doctor for instructions on re-starting oral contraceptive.
- May interfere with the accuracy of some medical tests.
- May cause some vitamin deficiencies.

 POSSIBLE INTERACTION WITH OTHER DRUGS

GENERIC NAME OR DRUG CLASS	COMBINED EFFECT
Ampicillin	Decreased contraceptive effect.
Anticoagulants*	Decreased anticoagulant effect.
Anticonvulsants, hydantoin*	Decreased contraceptive effect.
Antidepressants, tricyclic (TCA)*	Increased toxicity of antidepressants.
Antidiabetics*	Decreased antidiabetic effect.
Antifibronolytic agents*	Increased possibility of blood clotting.
Antihistamines*	Decreased contraceptive effect.
Barbiturates*	Decreased contraceptive effect.
Chloramphenicol	Decreased contraceptive effect.
Clofibrate	Decreased clofibrate effect.
Dextrothyroxine	Decreased dextrothyroxine effect.
Guanethidine	Decreased guanethidine effect.
Hypoglycemics, oral*	Decreased effect of hypoglycemics.
Insulin	Possibly decreased insulin effect.
Meperidine	Increased meperidine effect.
Meprobamate	Decreased contraceptive effect.
Mineral oil	Decreased contraceptive effect.

Continued on page 942

 POSSIBLE INTERACTION WITH OTHER SUBSTANCES

INTERACTS WITH	COMBINED EFFECT
Alcohol:	No proven problems.
Beverages:	No proven problems.
Cocaine:	No proven problems.
Foods: Salt.	Increased edema (fluid retention).
Marijuana:	Increased bleeding between periods. Avoid.
Tobacco:	Possible heart attack, blood clots and stroke. If you take "the pill," *don't* smoke.

BRAND AND GENERIC NAMES

See complete list of brand and generic names in the *Brand Name Directory*, page 918.

BASIC INFORMATION

Habit forming? No
Prescription needed? Not for most
Available as generic? Most aren't
Drug class: Contraceptive (vaginal)

USES

- Provides a degree of protection against pregnancy.
- Protects against some sexually transmitted diseases, such as those caused by chlamydia, gardnerella, mycoplasma, neisseria, trichomonas, ureaplasma and possibly herpes virus.

DOSAGE & USAGE INFORMATION

How to take:
Read package insert carefully. Some cautions to remember:
- Do not douche for 6 to 8 hours after intercourse.
- Do not remove sponge, cervical cap or diaphragm for 6 to 8 hours after intercourse.
- Follow product label instructions for storage.

When to take:
Consistently with every sexual exposure.

If you forget to use:
Contact your doctor to consider using another form of pregnancy protection, such as the "morning-after" pill.

What drug does:
Forms a chemical barrier between sperm in semen and the mucous membranes in the vagina. The chemical acts to inactivate viable sperm and also kills some bacteria, viruses, yeast and fungus.

Time lapse before vaginal contraceptive works:
- Immediate for foam, gels, jellies and sponges.
- 5 to 15 minutes for film and suppositories.

Don't use with:
Not applicable.

OVERDOSE

SYMPTOMS:
None expected.

POSSIBLE ADVERSE REACTIONS OR SIDE EFFECTS

SYMPTOMS	WHAT TO DO
Life-threatening:	
Toxic shock syndrome (chills; fever; skin rash; muscle aches; extreme weakness; confusion; redness of vagina, inside of mouth, nose, throat or eyes). (Very rare.)	Seek emergency treatment immediately.
Common:	
None expected.	
Infrequent:	
None expected.	
Rare:	
Vaginal discharge, irritation or rash; painful urination; cloudy or bloody urine.	Discontinue. Call doctor right away.

CONTRACEPTIVES, VAGINAL (Spermicides)

WARNINGS & PRECAUTIONS

Don't take if:
You are allergic to any form of octoxynol, nonoxynol or benzalkonium chloride.

Before you start, consult your doctor:
If you desire complete protection against pregnancy, a combination of methods gives better protection than vaginal contraceptives alone.

Over age 60:
Adverse reactions and side effects may be more frequent and severe than in younger persons.

Pregnancy:
No special problems expected.

Breast-feeding:
Safety not established. Consult doctor.

Infants & children:
Not recommended.

Prolonged use:
Allergic reactions and irritation more likely.

Skin & sunlight:
No problems expected.

Driving, piloting or hazardous work:
No special problems expected.

Discontinuing:
No special problems expected.

Others:
- Failure rate when used alone is relatively high. Therefore a vaginal cream, sponge, suppository, foam, gel, jelly or other product should be used with a mechanical barrier, such as a condom, cervical cap, vaginal diaphragm or other form of pregnancy protection.
- Don't use a cervical cap, sponge or diaphragm during menstruation. Consider using a condom instead if additional protection is desired.
- Vaginal contraceptives usually also have spermicidal effects and may partially protect against sexually transmitted diseases.

POSSIBLE INTERACTION WITH OTHER DRUGS

GENERIC NAME OR DRUG CLASS	COMBINED EFFECT
Topical vaginal medications that include any of the following: sulfa drugs, soaps or disinfectants, nitrates*, permanganates, lanolin, hydrogen peroxide, iodides, cotton dressings, aluminum citrates, salicylates*	Spermicidal activity may be reduced or negated. Avoid combinations.
Vaginal douche products	May prevent spermicidal effect. Avoid until 8 hours following intercourse.

POSSIBLE INTERACTION WITH OTHER SUBSTANCES

INTERACTS WITH	COMBINED EFFECT
Alcohol:	None expected.
Beverages:	None expected.
Cocaine:	None expected.
Foods:	None expected.
Marijuana:	None expected.
Tobacco:	None expected.

*See Glossary

CORTISONE

BRAND NAMES

Cortone   Cortone Acetate

BASIC INFORMATION

Habit forming? No
Prescription needed? Yes
Available as generic? Yes
Drug class: Cortisone drug (adrenal corticosteroid)

 USES

- Reduces inflammation caused by many different medical problems.
- Treatment for some allergic diseases, blood disorders, kidney diseases, asthma and emphysema.
- Replaces corticosteroid deficiencies.

 DOSAGE & USAGE INFORMATION

How to take:
Tablet—Swallow with liquid or food to lessen stomach irritation. If you can't swallow whole, crumble tablet and take with liquid or food.

When to take:
At the same times each day. Take once-a-day or once-every-other-day doses in mornings.

If you forget a dose:
- Several-doses-per-day prescription—Take as soon as you remember up to 2 hours late. If more than 2 hours, wait for next scheduled dose (don't double this dose).
- Once-a-day dose or less—Wait for next dose. Double this dose.

What drug does:
- Decreases inflammatory responses.
- Replaces cortisone in patients with adrenal insufficiency.

Time lapse before drug works:
2 to 4 days.

Don't take with:
Any other medicine without consulting your doctor or pharmacist.

 OVERDOSE

SYMPTOMS:
Headache, convulsions, fluid retention, heart failure.
WHAT TO DO:
- **Dial 0 (operator) or 911 (emergency) for an ambulance or medical help. Then give first aid immediately.**
- **See emergency information on inside covers.**

 POSSIBLE ADVERSE REACTIONS OR SIDE EFFECTS

SYMPTOMS	WHAT TO DO
Life-threatening:	
Hives, rash, intense itching, faintness soon after a dose (anaphylaxis).	Seek emergency treatment immediately.
Common:	
Acne, thirst, nausea, indigestion, vomiting, poor wound healing.	Continue. Call doctor when convenient.
Infrequent:	
• Bloody or black, tarry stool.	Discontinue. Seek emergency treatment.
• Blurred vision; halos around lights; sore throat, fever; muscle cramps; swollen legs, feet.	Discontinue. Call doctor right away.
• Mood changes, insomnia, fatigue, restlessness, frequent urination, weight gain, round face, weakness, irregular menstrual periods.	Continue. Call doctor when convenient.
Rare:	
• Irregular heartbeat.	Discontinue. Seek emergency treatment.
• Rash, hallucinations, thrombophlebitis, pancreatitis, numbness or tingling in hands or feet, convulsions.	Discontinue. Call doctor right away.

 WARNINGS & PRECAUTIONS

Don't take if:
- You are allergic to any cortisone drug.
- You have tuberculosis or fungus infection.
- You have herpes infection of eyes, lips or genitals.

Before you start, consult your doctor:
- If you have had tuberculosis.
- If you have congestive heart failure.
- If you have diabetes, peptic ulcer, glaucoma, underactive thyroid, high blood pressure, myasthenia gravis, blood clots in legs or lungs.

Over age 60:
- Adverse reactions and side effects may be more frequent and severe than in younger persons.
- Likely to aggravate edema, diabetes or ulcers.
- Likely to cause cataracts and osteoporosis (softening of the bones).

CORTISONE

Pregnancy:
Risk to unborn child outweighs drug benefits. Don't use.

Breast-feeding:
Drug passes into milk. Avoid drug or discontinue nursing until you finish medicine. Consult doctor for advice on maintaining milk supply.

Infants & children:
Use only under medical supervision.

Prolonged use:
- Retards growth in children.
- Possible glaucoma, cataracts, diabetes, fragile bones and thin skin.
- Functional dependence.
- Talk to your doctor about the need for follow-up medical examinations or laboratory studies to check blood sugar, eyes, serum electrolytes, stools for blood.

Skin & sunlight:
No problems expected.

Driving, piloting or hazardous work:
No problems expected.

Discontinuing:
- Don't discontinue without doctor's advice until you complete prescribed dose, even though symptoms diminish or disappear.
- Drug affects your response to surgery, illness, injury or stress for 2 years after discontinuing. Tell anyone who takes medical care of you within 2 years about drug.

Others:
- Avoid immunizations if possible.
- Your resistance to infection is less while taking this medicine.
- Advise any doctor or dentist whom you consult that you take this medicine.
- Those who have inactive or "cured" tuberculosis may be subjected to a possible recurrence of active tuberculosis.
- Children who must take cortisone drugs may grow less well.

 POSSIBLE INTERACTION WITH OTHER DRUGS

GENERIC NAME OR DRUG CLASS	COMBINED EFFECT
Amphotericin B	Potassium depletion.
Anticholinergics*	Possible glaucoma.
Anticoagulants, oral*	Decreased anti-coagulant effect.
Anticonvulsants, hydantoin*	Decreased cortisone effect.
Antidiabetics, oral*	Decreased anti-diabetic effect.
Antihistamines*	Decreased cortisone effect.
Aspirin	Increased cortisone effect.
Attenuated virus vaccines*	Possible viral infection.
Barbiturates*	Decreased cortisone effect. Oversedation.
Chloral hydrate	Decreased cortisone effect.
Chlorthalidone	Potassium depletion.
Cholinergics*	Decreased cholinergic effect.
Cholestyramine	Decreased cortisone absorption effect.
Colestipol	Decreased cortisone abosrption effect.
Contraceptives, oral*	Increased cortisone effect.
Cyclosporine	Increased risk of infection.
Diclofenac	Increased risk of stomach ulcer.
Digitalis preparations*	Dangerous potassium depletion. Possible digitalis toxicity.
Diuretics, thiazide*	Potassium depletion.
Ephedrine	Decreased cortisone effect.
Estrogens*	Increased cortisone effect.
Ethacrynic acid	Potassium depletion.
Furosemide	Potassium depletion.
Glutethimide	Decreased cortisone effect.

Continued page 942

 POSSIBLE INTERACTION WITH OTHER SUBSTANCES

INTERACTS WITH	COMBINED EFFECT
Alcohol:	Risk of stomach ulcers.
Beverages:	No proven problems.
Cocaine:	Overstimulation. Avoid.
Foods:	No proven problems.
Marijuana:	Decreased immunity.
Tobacco:	Increased cortisone effect. Possible toxicity.

*See Glossary

255

CROMOLYN

BRAND NAMES

Fivent
Gastrocrom
Intal
Nalcrom
Nasalcrom

Opticrom
Rynacrom
Sodium
   Cromoglycate

BASIC INFORMATION

Habit forming? No
Prescription needed? Yes
Available as generic? No
Drug class: Antiasthmatic, anti-inflammatory
(non-steroidal)

USES

- Powdered form and nebulizer solution prevent asthma attacks. Will not stop an active asthma attack.
- Eye drops treat inflammation of covering to eye and cornea.
- Nasal spray reduces nasal allergic symptoms.
- Capsules prevent allergic symptoms.

DOSAGE & USAGE INFORMATION

How to take:
Inhaler
Follow instructions enclosed with inhaler. Don't swallow cartridges for inhaler. Gargle and rinse mouth after inhalations.

Eye drops
- Wash hands.
- Apply pressure to inside corner of eye with middle finger.
- Continue pressure for 1 minute after placing medicine in eye.
- Tilt head backward. Pull lower lid away from eye with index finger of the same hand.
- Drop eye drops into pouch and close eye.
- Don't blink. Keep eyes closed for 1 to 2 minutes.
- Don't touch applicator tip to any surface (including the eye). If you accidentally touch tip, clean with warm soap and water.

Continued in next column

OVERDOSE

SYMPTOMS:
Increased side effects and adverse reactions listed.
WHAT TO DO:
Overdose unlikely to threaten life. If person inhales much larger amount than prescribed, call doctor, poison-control center or hospital emergency room for instructions.

- Keep container tightly closed.
- Keep cool, but don't freeze.
- Wash hands immediately after using.

Nasal solution
Follow prescription instructions.

Capsules
Swallow with liquid. If you can't swallow whole, open capsule and take with liquid or food.

When to take:
At the same times each day. If you also use a bronchodilator inhaler, use the bronchodilator before the cromolyn.

If you forget a dose:
Take as soon as you remember up to 2 hours late. If more than 2 hours, wait for next scheduled dose (don't double this dose).

What drug does:
Blocks histamine release from mast cells.

Time lapse before drug works:
- For inhaler forms: 4 weeks for prevention of asthma attacks. However, if taken 10-15 minutes after exercise or exposure to known allergens, may prevent wheezing.
- 1 to 2 weeks for nasal symptoms; only a few days for eye symptoms.

Don't take with:
Any other medicine without consulting your doctor or pharmacist.

POSSIBLE ADVERSE REACTIONS OR SIDE EFFECTS

SYMPTOMS	WHAT TO DO
Life-threatening:	
Hives, rash, intense itching, faintness soon after a dose (anaphylaxis).	Seek emergency treatment immediately.
Common:	
Cough, dry mouth.	Continue. Call doctor when convenient.
Infrequent:	
• Rash, hives, swallowing difficulty, nausea, vomiting, increased wheezing, joint pain or swelling, sneezing, nasal burning, weakness, muscle pain, difficult or painful urination.	Discontinue. Call doctor right away.
• Drowsiness, dizziness, headache, watery eyes, stuffy nose, throat irritation, insomnia.	Continue. Call doctor when convenient.

Rare:

Nosebleed, numbness or tingling in feet or hands, hoarseness.

Continue. Call doctor when convenient.

WARNINGS & PRECAUTIONS

Don't take if:
You use the dry powder form of cromolyn and if you are allergic to cromolyn, lactose, milk or milk products.

Before you start, consult your doctor:
- If you plan to become pregnant within medication period.
- If you have kidney or liver disease.

Over age 60:
Adverse reactions and side effects may be more frequent and severe than in younger persons.

Pregnancy:
No proven harm to unborn child, but avoid if possible.

Breast-feeding:
Effects unknown. Confer with your doctor.

Infants & children:
Use only under medical supervision.

Prolonged use:
No problems expected.

Skin & sunlight:
No problems expected.

Driving, piloting or hazardous work:
No problems expected.

Discontinuing:
No problems expected.

Others:
- Inhaler must be cleaned and work well for drug to be effective.
- Treatment with inhalation cromolyn does not stop an acute asthma attack. It may aggravate it.

POSSIBLE INTERACTION WITH OTHER DRUGS

GENERIC NAME OR DRUG CLASS	COMBINED EFFECT
Cortisone drugs*	Increased cortisone effect in treating asthma. Cortisone dose may be decreased.
Ipratroprium	Increased cromolyn effect.

POSSIBLE INTERACTION WITH OTHER SUBSTANCES

INTERACTS WITH	COMBINED EFFECT
Alcohol:	None expected.
Beverages:	None expected.
Cocaine:	None expected.
Foods:	None expected.
Marijuana:	None expected.
Tobacco:	None expected, but tobacco smoke aggravates asthma and eye irritation. Avoid.

---

*See Glossary

CYCLACILLIN

BRAND NAMES

Cyclapen-W

BASIC INFORMATION

Habit forming? No
Prescription needed? Yes
Available as generic? No
Drug class: Antibiotic (penicillin)

USES

Treatment of bacterial infections that are susceptible to cyclacillin.

DOSAGE & USAGE INFORMATION

How to take:
- Tablet—Swallow with liquid on an empty stomach 1 hour before or 2 hours after eating.
- Liquid—Take with cold beverage. Liquid form is perishable and effective for only 7 days at room temperature. Effective for 14 days if stored in refrigerator. Don't freeze.

When to take:
Follow instructions on prescription label or side of package. Doses should be evenly spaced. For example, 4 times a day means every 6 hours.

If you forget a dose:
Take as soon as you remember. Continue regular schedule.

What drug does:
Destroys susceptible bacteria. Does not kill viruses.

Time lapse before drug works:
May be several days before medicine affects infection.

Don't take with:
Any other medicine without consulting your doctor or pharmacist.

OVERDOSE

SYMPTOMS:
Severe diarrhea, nausea or vomiting.
WHAT TO DO:
Overdose unlikely to threaten life. If person takes much larger amount than prescribed, call doctor, poison-control center or hospital emergency room for instructions.

POSSIBLE ADVERSE REACTIONS OR SIDE EFFECTS

SYMPTOMS	WHAT TO DO
Life-threatening:	
Hives, rash, intense itching, faintness soon after a dose (anaphylaxis).	Seek emergency treatment immediately.
Common:	
Dark or discolored tongue.	Continue. Tell doctor at next visit.
Infrequent:	
• Mild nausea, vomiting, diarrhea.	Continue. Call doctor when convenient.
• Bloody urine, face and ankle swelling.	Discontinue. Call doctor right away.
Rare:	
Unexplained bleeding or bruising, weakness, sore throat, fever, abdominal cramps, convulsions.	Discontinue. Call doctor right away.

WARNINGS & PRECAUTIONS

Don't take if:
Your are allergic to cyclacillin, cephalosporin antibiotics, other penicillins or penicillamine. Life-threatening reaction may occur.

Before you start, consult your doctor:
- If you are allergic to any substance or drug.
- If you take birth control pills.

Over age 60:
You may have skin reactions, particularly around genitals and anus.

Pregnancy:
Studies inconclusive on harm to unborn child. Animal studies show fetal abnormalities. Decide with your doctor whether drug benefits justify risk to unborn child.

Breast-feeding:
Drug passes into milk. Child may become sensitive to penicillins and have allergic reactions to penicillin drugs. Avoid cyclacillin or discontinue nursing until you finish medicine. Consult doctor for advice on maintaining milk supply.

Infants & children:
No problems expected.

Prolonged use:
- You may become more susceptible to infections caused by germs not responsive to cyclacillin.
- Talk to your doctor about the need for follow-up medical examinations or laboratory studies to check SGPT*, SGOT*.

Skin & sunlight:
No problems expected.

Driving, piloting or hazardous work:
Usually not dangerous. Most hazardous reactions likely to occur a few minutes after taking cyclacillin.

Discontinuing:
Don't discontinue without doctor's advice until you complete prescribed dose, even though symptoms diminish or disappear.

Others:
- Birth control pills may not be effective. Use additional birth-control methods.
- May interfere with the accuracy of some medical tests.

POSSIBLE INTERACTION WITH OTHER DRUGS

GENERIC NAME OR DRUG CLASS	COMBINED EFFECT
Beta-adrenergic blockers*	Increased chance of anaphylaxis (see emergency information on inside front cover).
Birth control pills	Impaired contraceptive efficiency.
Chloramphenicol	Decreased effect of both drugs.
Erythromycins*	Decreased effect of both drugs.
Loperamide	Decreased cyclacillin effect.
Paromomycin	Decreased effect of both drugs.
Probenecid	Increased effect of all penicillins.
Tetracyclines*	Decreased effect of both drugs.
Troleandomycin	Decreased effect of both drugs.

POSSIBLE INTERACTION WITH OTHER SUBSTANCES

INTERACTS WITH	COMBINED EFFECT
Alcohol:	Occasional stomach irritation.
Beverages:	None expected.
Cocaine:	No proven problems.
Foods: Acidic fruits or juices, aged cheese, wines, syrups (if taken with).	Decreased antibiotic effect.
Marijuana:	No proven problems.
Tobacco:	None expected.

---

*See Glossary

CYCLANDELATE

BRAND NAMES

Cyclospasmol   Cyraso-400

BASIC INFORMATION

Habit forming? No
Prescription needed?
  U.S.: Yes
  Canada: No
Available as generic? Yes
Drug class: Vasodilator

USES

Improves poor blood flow to extremities.

DOSAGE & USAGE INFORMATION

How to take:
Tablet or capsule—Swallow with liquid. If you can't swallow whole, crumble tablet or open capsule and take with liquid or food.

When to take:
At the same time each day.

If you forget a dose:
Take as soon as you remember up to 2 hours late. If more than 2 hours, wait for next scheduled dose (don't double this dose).

What drug does:
Increases blood flow by relaxing and expanding blood-vessel walls.

Time lapse before drug works:
3 weeks.

Don't take with:
Any other medicine without consulting your doctor or pharmacist.

OVERDOSE

SYMPTOMS:
Severe headache, dizziness; nausea, vomiting; flushed, hot face.
WHAT TO DO:
Overdose unlikely to threaten life. If person takes much larger amount than prescribed, call doctor, poison-control center or hospital emergency room for instructions.

POSSIBLE ADVERSE REACTIONS OR SIDE EFFECTS

SYMPTOMS	WHAT TO DO
Life-threatening:	
In case of overdose, see previous column.	
Common:	
None expected.	
Infrequent:	
• Rapid heartbeat.	Discontinue. Call doctor right away.
• Dizziness; headache; weakness; flushed face; tingling in face, fingers or toes; unusual sweating.	Continue. Call doctor when convenient.
• Belching, heartburn, nausea or stomach pain.	Continue. Tell doctor at next visit.
Rare:	
None expected.	

WARNINGS & PRECAUTIONS

Don't take if:
You have had allergic reaction to cyclandelate.

Before you start, consult your doctor:
- If you have glaucoma.
- If you have had heart attack or stroke.

Over age 60:
Adverse reactions and side effects may be more frequent and severe than in younger persons.

Pregnancy:
No proven harm to unborn child. Avoid if possible.

Breast-feeding:
No proven problems. Consult doctor.

Infants & children:
Not recommended.

Prolonged use:
No problems expected.

Skin & sunlight:
No problems expected.

Driving, piloting or hazardous work:
Avoid if you feel dizzy or weak. Otherwise, no problems expected.

Discontinuing:
Don't discontinue without doctor's advice until you complete prescribed dose, even though symptoms diminish or disappear.

Others:
Response to drug varies. If your symptoms don't improve after 3 weeks of use, consult doctor.

POSSIBLE INTERACTION WITH OTHER DRUGS

GENERIC NAME OR DRUG CLASS	COMBINED EFFECT
None expected.	

POSSIBLE INTERACTION WITH OTHER SUBSTANCES

INTERACTS WITH	COMBINED EFFECT
Alcohol:	None expected.
Beverages:	None expected.
Cocaine:	Decreased cyclandelate effect. Avoid.
Foods:	None expected.
Marijuana:	None expected.
Tobacco:	May decrease cyclandelate effect.

CYCLIZINE

BRAND NAMES

Marezine   **Marzine**

BASIC INFORMATION

Habit forming? No
Prescription needed?
 U.S.: No
 Canada: Yes
Available as generic? No
Drug class: Antiemetic, anti-motion
 sickness

 ## USES

Prevents motion sickness.

 ## DOSAGE & USAGE
INFORMATION

How to take:
Tablet—Swallow with liquid or food to lessen
stomach irritation. If you can't swallow whole,
crumble tablet and chew or take with liquid or
food.

When to take:
30 minutes to 1 hour before traveling.

If you forget a dose:
Take as soon as you remember. Wait 4 hours
for next dose.

What drug does:
Reduces sensitivity of nerve endings in inner
ear, blocking messages to brain's vomiting
center.

Time lapse before drug works:
30 to 60 minutes.

Don't take with:
Any other medicine without consulting your
doctor or pharmacist.

 ## OVERDOSE

SYMPTOMS:
**Drowsiness, confusion, incoordination,
stupor, coma, weak pulse, shallow
breathing hallucinations.**
WHAT TO DO:
• **Dial 0 (operator) or 911 (emergency) for
an ambulance or medical help. Then give
first aid immediately.**
• **See emergency information on inside
covers.**

 ## POSSIBLE
ADVERSE REACTIONS
OR SIDE EFFECTS

SYMPTOMS	WHAT TO DO
Life-threatening:	
In case of overdose, see previous column.	
Common:	
Drowsiness.	Continue. Tell doctor at next visit.
Infrequent:	
• Headache, diarrhea or constipation, nausea, fast heartbeat.	Continue. Call doctor when convenient.
• Dry mouth, nose, throat; dizziness.	Continue. Tell doctor at next visit.
Rare:	
• Rash or hives, jaundice.	Discontinue. Call doctor right away.
• Restlessness, excitement, insomnia, blurred vision, frequent or difficult urination, hallucinations.	Continue. Call doctor when convenient.
• Appetite loss, nausea.	Continue. Tell doctor at next visit.

 ## WARNINGS &
PRECAUTIONS

Don't take if:
• You are allergic to meclizine, buclizine or
cyclizine.
• You have taken MAO inhibitors in the past 2
weeks.

Before you start, consult your doctor:
• If you have glaucoma.
• If you have prostate enlargement.
• If you have reacted badly to any antihistamine.

Over age 60:
Adverse reactions and side effects may be more
frequent and severe than in younger persons,
especially impaired urination from enlarged
prostate gland.

Pregnancy:
Studies inconclusive on harm to unborn child.
Animal studies show fetal abnormalities. Decide
with your doctor whether drug benefits justify
risk to unborn child.

Breast-feeding:
Drug passes into milk. Avoid drug or discontinue
nursing until you finish medicine. Consult doctor
for advice on maintaining milk supply.

Infants & children:
Safety not established. Avoid if under age 12.

Prolonged use:
No problems expected.

Skin & sunlight:
No problems expected.

Driving, piloting or hazardous work:
Don't fly aircraft. Don't drive until you learn how medicine affects you. Don't work around dangerous machinery. Don't climb ladders or work in high places. Danger increases if you drink alcohol or take medicine affecting alertness and reflexes, such as antihistamines, tranquilizers, sedatives, pain medicine, narcotics and mind-altering drugs.

Discontinuing:
No problems expected.

Others:
- Some products contain tartrazine dye. Avoid if allergic (especially aspirin hypersensitivity).
- May interfere with the accuracy of some medical tests.

POSSIBLE INTERACTION WITH OTHER DRUGS

GENERIC NAME OR DRUG CLASS	COMBINED EFFECT
Amphetamines*	May decrease drowsiness caused by cyclizine.
Anticholinergics*	Increased effect of both drugs.
Antidepressants, tricyclic (TCA)*	Increased effect of both drugs.
Carteolol	Decreased antihistamine effect.
Clozapine	Toxic effect on the central nervous system.
Dronabinol	Increased cyclizine effect.
Ethinamate	Dangerous increased effects of ethinamate. Avoid combining.
Fluoxetine	Increased depressant effects of both drugs.
Guanfacine	May increase depressant effects of either drug.
Leucovorin	High alcohol content of leucovorin may cause adverse effects.

MAO inhibitors*	Increased cyclizine effect.
Methyprylon	Increased sedative effect, perhaps to dangerous level. Avoid.
Nabilone	Greater depression of central nervous system.
Narcotics*	Increased effect of both drugs.
Pain relievers*	Increased effect of both drugs.
Sedatives*	Increased effect of both drugs.
Sertraline	Increased depressive effect of both drugs.
Sleep inducers*	Increased effect of both drugs.
Sotalol	Increased antihistamine effect.
Tranquilizers*	Increased effect of both drugs.

POSSIBLE INTERACTION WITH OTHER SUBSTANCES

INTERACTS WITH	COMBINED EFFECT
Alcohol:	Increased sedation. Avoid.
Beverages: Caffeine drinks.	May decrease drowsiness.
Cocaine:	None expected.
Foods:	None expected.
Marijuana:	Increased drowsiness, dry mouth.
Tobacco:	None expected.

CYCLOBENZAPRINE

BRAND NAMES

Flexeril

BASIC INFORMATION

Habit forming? No
Prescription needed? Yes
Available as generic? No
Drug class: Muscle relaxant

 USES

Treatment for pain and limited motion caused by spasms in voluntary muscles.

 DOSAGE & USAGE INFORMATION

How to take:
Tablet—Swallow with liquid.

When to take:
At the same time each day or according to label instructions.

If you forget a dose:
Take as soon as you remember. Wait 4 hours for next dose.

What drug does:
Blocks body's pain messages to brain. May also sedate.

Time lapse before drug works:
30 to 60 minutes.

Continued next column

 OVERDOSE

SYMPTOMS:
Drowsiness, confusion, difficulty concentrating, visual problems, vomiting, blood-pressure drop, low body temperature, weak and rapid pulse, convulsions, coma.
WHAT TO DO:
● **Dial 0 (operator) or 911 (emergency) for an ambulance or medical help. Then give first aid immediately.**
● **If patient is unconscious and not breathing, give mouth-to-mouth breathing. If there is no heartbeat, use cardiac massage and mouth-to-mouth breathing (CPR). Don't try to make patient vomit. If you can't get help quickly, take patient to nearest emergency facility.**
● **See emergency information on inside covers.**

Don't take with:
● Non-prescription drugs without consulting doctor.
● See Interaction column and consult doctor.

 POSSIBLE ADVERSE REACTIONS OR SIDE EFFECTS

SYMPTOMS	WHAT TO DO
Life-threatening:	
In case of overdose, see previous column.	
Common:	
Drowsiness, dizziness, dry mouth.	Continue. Call doctor when convenient.
Infrequent:	
● Blurred vision, fast heartbeat.	Discontinue. Call doctor right away.
● Insomnia, numbness in extremities, bad taste in mouth, fatigue, nausea, sweating.	Continue. Call doctor when convenient.
Rare:	
● Unsteadiness, confusion, depression, hallucinations, rash, itch, swelling, breathing difficulty.	Discontinue. Call doctor right away.
● Difficult urination, rash.	Continue. Call doctor when convenient.

 WARNINGS & PRECAUTIONS

Don't take if:
● You are allergic to any skeletal-muscle relaxant.
● You have taken MAO inhibitors* in last 2 weeks.
● You have had a heart attack within 6 weeks, or suffer from congestive heart failure.
● You have overactive thyroid.

Before you start, consult your doctor:
● If you have a heart problem.
● If you have reacted to tricyclic antidepressants.
● If you have glaucoma.
● If you have a prostate condition and urination difficulty.
● If you intend to pilot aircraft.

Over age 60:
Adverse reactions and side effects may be more frequent and severe than in younger persons. Avoid extremes of heat and cold.

Pregnancy:
Risk to unborn child outweighs drug benefits. Don't use.

Breast-feeding:
Drug passes into milk. Avoid drug or discontinue nursing until you finish medicine. Consult doctor for advice on maintaining milk supply.

Infants & children:
Don't use for children younger than 15.

Prolonged use:
Do not take for longer than 2 to 3 weeks.

Skin & sunlight:
May cause rash or intensify sunburn in areas exposed to sun or sunlamp.

Driving, piloting or hazardous work:
Don't drive or pilot aircraft until you learn how medicine affects you. Don't work around dangerous machinery. Don't climb ladders or work in high places. Danger increases if you drink alcohol or take medicine affecting alertness and reflexes.

Discontinuing:
May be unnecessary to finish medicine. Follow doctor's instructions.

Others:
No problems expected.

 POSSIBLE INTERACTION WITH OTHER DRUGS

GENERIC NAME OR DRUG CLASS	COMBINED EFFECT
Anticholinergics*	Increased anti-cholinergic effect.
Antidepressants*	Increased sedation.
Antihistamines*	Increased anti-histamine effect.
Barbiturates*	Increased sedation.
Cimetidine	Possible increased cyclobenzaprine effect.
Clonidine	Decreased clonidine effect.
Dronabinol	Increased effect of dronabinol on central nervous system. Avoid combination.
Guanethidine	Decreased guanethidine effect.
MAO inhibitors*	High fever, convulsions, possible death.
Methyldopa	Decreased methyldopa effect.
Mind-altering drugs*	Increased mind-altering effect.
Narcotics*	Increased sedation.
Pain relievers*	Increased pain reliever effect.
Procainamide	Possible increased conduction disturbance.
Quinidine	Possible increased conduction disturbance.
Rauwolfia alkaloids*	Decreased effect of rauwolfia alkaloids.
Sedatives*	Increased sedative effect.
Sleep inducers*	Increased sedation.
Tranquilizers*	Increased tranquilizer effect.

 POSSIBLE INTERACTION WITH OTHER SUBSTANCES

INTERACTS WITH	COMBINED EFFECT
Alcohol:	Depressed brain function. Avoid.
Beverages:	None expected.
Cocaine:	Decreased cyclobenzaprine effect.
Foods:	None expected.
Marijuana:	Occasional use—Drowsiness. Frequent use—Severe mental and physical impairment.
Tobacco:	None expected.

*See Glossary

CYCLOPEGIC, MYDRIATIC (Ophthalmic)

BRAND AND GENERIC NAMES

AK Homatropine
Atropair
ATROPINE
Atropine Care Eye
  Drops & Ointment
Atropine Sul
Atropisol
Dispersa
Homatrine
HOMATROPINE
I-Homatropine

Isopto
Isopto Atropine
Isopto Homatropine
Isopto Hyoscine
I-Tropine
Minims
Minims Atropine
Ocu-Tropine
S.M.P. Atropine
SCOPOLAMINE
Spectro-
  Homatropine

BASIC INFORMATION

Habit forming? No
Prescription needed? Yes
Available as generic? Yes, some
Drug class: Cyclopegic, mydriatic

 USES

- Dilates pupil of the eye.
- Used before some eye examinations, before and after some eye surgical procedures and, rarely, to treat some eye problems such as glaucoma.

 DOSAGE & USAGE INFORMATION

How to use:
Eye drops
- Wash hands.
- Apply pressure to inside corner of eye with middle finger.
- Continue pressure for 1 minute after placing medicine in eye.
- Tilt head backward. Pull lower lid away from eye with index finger of the same hand.
- Drop eye drops into pouch and close eye. Don't blink.
- Keep eyes closed for 1 to 2 minutes.

Continued next column

 OVERDOSE

SYMPTOMS:
None expected.
WHAT TO DO:
Not intended for internal use. If child accidentally swallows, call poison-control center.

Eye ointment
- Wash hands.
- Pull lower lid down from eye to form a pouch.
- Squeeze tube to apply thin strip of ointment into pouch.
- Close eye for 1 to 2 minutes.
- Don't touch applicator tip to any surface (including the eye). If you accidentally touch tip, clean with warm soap and water.
- Keep container tightly closed.
- Keep cool, but don't freeze.
- Wash hands immediately after using.

When to use:
As directed on label.

If you forget a dose:
Use as soon as you remember.

What drug does:
Blocks normal response to sphincter muscle of the iris of the eye and the accommodative muscle of the ciliary body.

Time lapse before drug works:
Begins within 1 minute. Residual effects may last up to 14 days.

Don't use with:
Other eye medicines such as carbachol, demecarium, echothiopate, isoflurophate, physostigmine, pilocarpine.

 POSSIBLE ADVERSE REACTIONS OR SIDE EFFECTS

SYMPTOMS	WHAT TO DO
Life-threatening: None expected.	
Common: • Increased sensitivity to light.	Continue. Call doctor when convenient.
• Burning eyes.	Continue. Tell doctor at next visit.
Infrequent: None expected.	
Rare (extremely): Symptoms of excess medicine absorbed by the body—Clumsiness, confusion, fever, flushed face, hallucinations, rash, slurred speech, swollen stomach (children), drowsiness, fast heartbeat.	Discontinue. Seek emergency treatment.

CYCLOPEGIC, MYDRIATIC (Ophthalmic)

WARNINGS & PRECAUTIONS

Don't use if:
You are allergic to cyclopentolate.

Before you start, consult your doctor:
- If medicine is for a brain-damaged child or child with Down's syndrome.
- If prescribed for a child with spastic paralysis.

Over age 60:
No problems expected.

Pregnancy:
Safety to unborn child unestablished. Avoid if possible.

Breast-feeding:
Safety unestablished. Avoid if possible.

Infants & children:
Use only under close medical supervision.

Prolonged use:
Avoid. May increase absorption into body.

Skin & sunlight:
Wear sunglasses to protect from sunlight and bright light.

Driving, piloting or hazardous work:
Don't drive or pilot aircraft until you learn how medicine affects you. Don't work around dangerous machinery. Don't climb ladders or work in high places. Danger increases if you drink alcohol or take medicine affecting alertness and reflexes, such as antihistamines, tranquilizers, sedatives, pain medicine, narcotics and mind-altering drugs.

Discontinuing:
Effects may last up to 14 days later.

Others:
Keep cool, but don't freeze.

POSSIBLE INTERACTION WITH OTHER DRUGS

GENERIC NAME OR DRUG CLASS	COMBINED EFFECT
Clinically significant interactions with oral or injected medicines unlikely.	

POSSIBLE INTERACTION WITH OTHER SUBSTANCES

INTERACTS WITH	COMBINED EFFECT
Alcohol:	None expected.
Beverages:	None expected.
Cocaine:	None expected.
Foods:	None expected.
Marijuana:	None expected.
Tobacco:	None expected.

CYCLOPENTOLATE (Ophthalmic)

BRAND NAMES

Ak-Pentolate
Cyclogyl
I-Pentolate
Minims
  Cyclopentolate

Ocu-Pentolate
Pentolair
Spectro-Pentolate

BASIC INFORMATION

Habit forming? No
Prescription needed? Yes
Available as generic? Yes
Drug class: Cyclopegic, mydriatic

 ## USES

- Enlarges (dilates) pupil.
- Temporarily paralyzes the normal pupil accommodation to light before eye examinations and to treat some eye conditions.

 ## DOSAGE & USAGE INFORMATION

How to use:
Eye drops
- Wash hands.
- Apply pressure to inside corner of eye with middle finger.
- Continue pressure for 1 minute after placing medicine in eye.
- Tilt head backward. Pull lower lid away from eye with index finger of the same hand.
- Drop eye drops into pouch and close eye. Don't blink.
- Keep eyes closed for 1 to 2 minutes.
- Don't touch applicator tip to any surface (including the eye). If you accidentally touch tip, clean with warm soap and water.
- Keep container tightly closed.
- Keep cool, but don't freeze.
- Wash hands immediately after using.

When to use:
As directed on bottle.

Continued next column

 ## OVERDOSE

SYMPTOMS:
None expected.
WHAT TO DO:
Not intended for internal use. If child accidentally swallows, call poison-control center.

If you forget a dose:
Use as soon as you remember.

What drug does:
Blocks sphincter muscle of the iris and ciliary body.

Time lapse before drug works:
Within 30 to 60 minutes. Effects usually disapper in 24 hours.

Don't use with:
Other eye medicines such as carbachol, demecarium, echothiopate, isoflurophate, physostigmine, pilocarpine.

 ## POSSIBLE ADVERSE REACTIONS OR SIDE EFFECTS

SYMPTOMS	WHAT TO DO
Life-threatening:	
None expected.	
Common:	
• Increased sensitivity to light.	Continue. Call doctor when convenient.
• Burning eyes.	Continue. Tell doctor at next visit.
Infrequent:	
None expected.	
Rare (extremely):	
Symptoms of excess medicine absorbed by the body—Clumsiness, confusion, fever, flushed face, hallucinations, rash, slurred speech, swollen stomach (children), drowsiness, fast heartbeat.	Discontinue. Seek emergency treatment.

CYCLOPENTOLATE (Ophthalmic)

WARNINGS & PRECAUTIONS

Don't use if:
You are allergic to cyclopentolate.

Before you start, consult your doctor:
- If medicine is for a brain-damaged child or child with Down's syndrome.
- If prescribed for a child with spastic paralysis.

Over age 60:
No problems expected.

Pregnancy:
Safety to unborn child unestablished. Avoid if possible.

Breast-feeding:
Safety unestablished. Avoid if possible.

Infants & children:
Use only under close medical supervision.

Prolonged use:
Avoid. May increase absorption into body.

Skin & sunlight:
Wear sunglasses to protect from sunlight and bright light.

Driving, piloting or hazardous work:
Don't drive or pilot aircraft until you learn how medicine affects you. Don't work around dangerous machinery. Don't climb ladders or work in high places. Danger increases if you drink alcohol or take medicine affecting alertness and reflexes, such as antihistamines, tranquilizers, sedatives, pain medicine, narcotics and mind-altering drugs.

Discontinuing:
If effects last longer than 36 hours after last drops, consult doctor.

Others:
Keep cool, but don't freeze.

POSSIBLE INTERACTION WITH OTHER DRUGS

GENERIC NAME OR DRUG CLASS	COMBINED EFFECT
Clinically significant interactions with oral or injected medicines unlikely.	

POSSIBLE INTERACTION WITH OTHER SUBSTANCES

INTERACTS WITH	COMBINED EFFECT
Alcohol:	None expected.
Beverages:	None expected.
Cocaine:	None expected.
Foods:	None expected.
Marijuana:	None expected.
Tobacco:	None expected.

*See Glossary

CYCLOPHOSPHAMIDE

BRAND NAMES

Cytoxan   Procytox
Neosar

BASIC INFORMATION

Habit forming? No
Prescription needed? Yes
Available as generic? No
Drug class: Immunosuppressant

 ## USES

- Treatment for cancer.
- Treatment for severe rheumatoid arthritis.
- Treatment for blood-vessel disease.
- Treatment for skin disease.

 ## DOSAGE & USAGE INFORMATION

How to take:
Tablet or liquid—Swallow with liquid. If you can't swallow whole, crumble tablet and take with liquid or food.

When to take:
Works best if taken first thing in morning. However, may take with food to lessen stomach irritation. Don't take at bedtime.

If you forget a dose:
Take as soon as you remember up to 12 hours late. If more than 12 hours, wait for next scheduled dose (don't double this dose).

What drug does:
- Kills cancer cells.
- Suppresses spread of cancer cells.
- Suppresses immune system.

Time lapse before drug works:
7 to 10 days continual use.

Don't take with:
Any other medicine without consulting your doctor or pharmacist.

 ## OVERDOSE

SYMPTOMS:
Bloody urine, water retention, weight gain, severe infection.
WHAT TO DO:
Overdose unlikely to threaten life. If person takes much larger amount than prescribed, call doctor, poison-control center or hospital emergency room for instructions.

 ## POSSIBLE ADVERSE REACTIONS OR SIDE EFFECTS

SYMPTOMS	WHAT TO DO
Life-threatening:	
Hives, rash, intense itching, faintness soon after a dose (anaphylaxis).	Seek emergency treatment immediately.
Common:	
• Sore throat, fever.	Discontinue. Call doctor right away.
• Dark skin, nails; nausea; appetite loss; vomiting; missed menstrual period.	Continue. Call doctor when convenient.
Infrequent:	
• Rash, hives, itch; shortness of breath; rapid heartbeat; cough; blood in urine, painful urination; pain in side; bleeding; bruising; increased sweating; hoarseness; foot or ankle swelling.	Discontinue. Call doctor right away.
• Confusion, agitation, headache, dizziness, flushed face, stomach pain, joint pain, fatigue, weakness, diarrhea.	Continue. Call doctor when convenient.
Rare:	
• Mouth, lip sores; black stool; unusual thirst; jaundice.	Discontinue. Call doctor right away.
• Blurred vision, increased urination, hair loss.	Continue. Call doctor when convenient.

CYCLOPHOSPHAMIDE

WARNINGS & PRECAUTIONS

Don't take if:
- You are allergic to any alkylating agent.
- You have an infection.
- You have bloody urine.
- You will have surgery within 2 months, including dental surgery, requiring general or spinal anesthesia.

Before you start, consult your doctor:
- If you have impaired liver or kidney function.
- If you have impaired bone-marrow or blood-cell production.
- If you have had chemotherapy or X-ray therapy.
- If you have taken cortisone drugs in the past year.

Over age 60:
Adverse reactions and side effects may be more frequent and severe than in younger persons. To reduce risk of chemical bladder inflammation, drink 8 to 10 glasses of water daily.

Pregnancy:
Risk to unborn child outweighs drug benefits. Don't use.

Breast-feeding:
Drug passes into milk. Avoid drug or discontinue nursing until you finish medicine. Consult doctor for advice on maintaining milk supply.

Infants & children:
Use only under medical supervision.

Prolonged use:
- Development of fibrous lung tissue.
- Possible jaundice.
- Swelling of feet, lower legs.
- Cancer.
- Infertility in men.
- Talk to your doctor about the need for follow-up medical examinations or laboratory studies to check complete blood counts (white blood cell count, platelet count, red blood cell count, hemoglobin, hematocrit), urine, liver function.

Skin & sunlight:
No problems expected.

Driving, piloting or hazardous work:
Avoid if you feel dizzy or have blurred vision. Otherwise, no problems expected.

Discontinuing:
Don't discontinue without consulting doctor. Dose may require gradual reduction if you have taken drug for a long time. Doses of other drugs may also require adjustment.

Others:
- Frequently causes hair loss. After treatment ends, hair should grow back.
- Avoid vaccinations.

POSSIBLE INTERACTION WITH OTHER DRUGS

GENERIC NAME OR DRUG CLASS	COMBINED EFFECT
Allopurinol or other medicines to treat gout	Possible anemia; decreased anti-gout effect.
Antidiabetics, oral*	Increased antidiabetic effect.
Clozapine	Toxic effect on bone marrow.
Cyclosporine	May increase risk of infection.
Digoxin	Possible decreased digoxin absorption.
Immuno-suppressants,* other	Increased risk of infection.
Insulin	Increased insulin effect.
Levamisole	Increased risk of bone marrow depression.
Lovastatin	Increased heart and kidney damage.
Phenobarbital	Increased cyclophosphamide effect.
Tiopronin	Increased risk of toxicity to bone marrow.

POSSIBLE INTERACTION WITH OTHER SUBSTANCES

INTERACTS WITH	COMBINED EFFECT
Alcohol:	No problems expected.
Beverages:	No problems expected. Drink at least 2 quarts fluid every day.
Cocaine:	Increased danger of brain damage.
Foods:	None expected.
Marijuana:	Increased impairment of immunity.
Tobacco:	None expected.

*See Glossary

CYCLOSERINE

BRAND NAMES

Seromycin

BASIC INFORMATION

Habit forming? No
Prescription needed? Yes
Available as generic? No
Drug class: Antibacterial (antibiotic)

 USES

- Treats urinary tract infections.
- Treats tuberculosis.

 DOSAGE & USAGE INFORMATION

How to take:

Capsules—Swallow with liquid or food to lesson stomach irritation. If you can't swallow whole, open capsule and take with liquid or food.

When to take:

- Once or twice daily.
- At the same time each day after meals to prevent stomach irritation.

If you forget a dose:

Take as soon as you remember up to 2 hours late. If more than 2 hours, wait for next scheduled dose (don't double this dose).

What drug does:

Interferes with bacterial wall synthesis and keeps germs from multiplying.

Time lapse before drug works:

3 to 4 hours.

Don't take with:

Any other medicine without consulting your doctor or pharmacist.

 OVERDOSE

SYMPTOMS:
Seizures.
WHAT TO DO:

- Dial 0 (operator) or 911 (emergency) for an ambulance or medical help. Then give first aid immediately.
- See emergency information on inside covers.

 POSSIBLE ADVERSE REACTIONS OR SIDE EFFECTS

SYMPTOMS	WHAT TO DO
Life-threatening:	
Seizures, muscle twitching or trembling.	Seek emergency treatment immediately.
Common:	
Gum inflammation, pale skin, depression, confusion, dizziness, restlessness, anxiety, nightmares, severe headache, drowsiness.	Discontinue. Call doctor right away.
Infrequent:	
Visual changes; sun sensitivity; skin rash; numbness, tingling or burning in hands and feet; jaundice; eye pain.	Continue. Call doctor when convenient.
Rare:	
Seizures, thoughts of suicide.	Discontinue. Seek emergency treatment.

CYCLOSERINE

WARNINGS & PRECAUTIONS

Don't take if:
- You are an alcoholic.
- You have a convulsive disorder.

Before you start, consult your doctor:
- If you are depressed.
- If you have kidney disease.
- If you have severe anxiety.

Over age 60:
Adverse reactions and side effects may be more frequent and severe than in younger persons. You may need smaller doses for shorter periods of time.

Pregnancy:
Safety not established. Consult your doctor.

Breast-feeding:
Drug passes into milk. Avoid drug or discontinue nursing until you finish medicine. Consult doctor for advice on maintaining milk supply.

Infants & children:
No information available.

Prolonged use:
- May cause liver or kidney damage.
- May cause anemia.

Skin & sunlight:
May cause hypersensitivity to sun exposure.

Driving, piloting or hazardous work:
Don't drive or pilot aircraft until you learn how medicine affects you. Don't work around dangerous machinery. Don't climb ladders or work in high places. Danger increases if you drink alcohol or take medicine affecting alertness and reflexes.

Discontinuing:
Don't discontinue without consulting doctor. Dose may require gradual reduction if you have taken drug for a long time. Doses of other drugs may also require adjustment.

Others:
- May have to take anticonvulsants, sedatives and/or pyridoxine to prevent or minimize toxic effects on the brain.
- If you must take more than 500 mg per day, toxicity is much more likely to occur.
- Talk to your doctor about taking pyridoxine as a supplement.

POSSIBLE INTERACTION WITH OTHER DRUGS

GENERIC NAME OR DRUG CLASS	COMBINED EFFECT
Ethionamide	Increased risk of seizures.
Isoniazid	Increased risk of central nervous system effects.
Pyridoxine	Reduces effects of pyridoxine. Since pyridoxine is a vital vitamin, patients on cycloserine require pyridoxine supplements to prevent anemia or peripheral neuritis.

POSSIBLE INTERACTION WITH OTHER SUBSTANCES

INTERACTS WITH	COMBINED EFFECT
Alcohol:	Toxic. May increase risk of seizures. Avoid.
Beverages:	None expected. All beverages except those with alcohol.
Cocaine:	Toxic. Avoid.
Foods:	None expected.
Marijuana:	May increase risk of seizures.
Tobacco:	May decrease effect of cycloserine.

CYCLOSPORINE

BRAND NAMES

Sandimmune

BASIC INFORMATION

Habit forming? No
Prescription needed? Yes
Available as generic? No
Drug class: Immunosuppressant

 ## USES

Suppresses the immune response in patients who have transplants of the heart, lung, kidney, liver, pancreas. Cyclosporine treats rejection as well as helps prevent it.

 ## DOSAGE & USAGE INFORMATION

How to take:
- Oral solution—Take after meals with liquid to decrease stomach irritation. May mix with milk, chocolate milk or orange juice. Don't mix in styrofoam cups. Use special dropper for exact dosage.
- Capsules—Take with water or other fluid. Don't break capsule open.

When to take:
At the same time each day, according to instructions on prescription label.

If you forget a dose:
Take as soon as you remember up to 2 hours late. If more than 2 hours, wait for next scheduled dose (don't double this dose).

What drug does:
Exact mechanism is unknown, but believed to inhibit interluken II to affect T-lymphocytes.

Time lapse before drug works:
3 to 3-1/2 hours.

Don't take with:
Any other medicine without consulting your doctor or pharmacist.

 ## OVERDOSE

SYMPTOMS:
Irregular heartbeat, seizures, coma.
WHAT TO DO:
- **Dial 0 (operator) or 911 (emergency) for an ambulance or medical help. Then give first aid immediately.**
- **See emergency information on inside covers.**

 ## POSSIBLE ADVERSE REACTIONS OR SIDE EFFECTS

SYMPTOMS	WHAT TO DO
Life-threatening: Seizures, wheezing with shortness of breath, convulsions.	Discontinue. Seek emergency treatment.
Common: • Gum inflammation, blood in urine, jaundice, tremors.	Continue. Call doctor when convenient.
• Increased hair growth.	Continue. Tell doctor at next visit.
Infrequent: • Fever, chills, sore throat, shortness of breath.	Call doctor right away.
• Frequent urination, headache, leg cramps.	Continue. Call doctor when convenient.
Rare: • Confusion, irregular heartbeat, numbness of hands and feet, nervousness, face flushing, severe abdominal pain, weakness.	Call doctor right away.
• Acne, headache.	Continue. Call doctor when convenient.

 ## WARNINGS & PRECAUTIONS

Don't take if:
- You have chicken pox.
- You have shingles (herpes zoster).

Before you start, consult your doctor:
- If you have liver problems.
- If you have an infection.
- If you have kidney disease.

Over age 60:
No special problems expected.

Pregnancy:
Safety not established. Consult your doctor.

Breast-feeding:
Drug passes into milk. Avoid drug or discontinue nursing until you finish medicine. Consult doctor for advice on maintaining milk supply.

Infants & children:
No problems expected.

Prolonged use:
- Can cause reduced function of kidney.
- Talk to your doctor about the need for follow-up medical examinations or laboratory studies to check blood pressure, kidney function, liver function.

Skin & sunlight:
No problems expected.

Driving, piloting or hazardous work:
Don't drive or pilot aircraft until you learn how medicine affects you. Don't work around dangerous machinery. Don't climb ladders or work in high places. Danger increases if you drink alcohol or take medicine affecting alertness and reflexes.

Discontinuing:
Don't discontinue without consulting doctor. You probably will require this medicine for the remainder of your life.

Others:

- Request regular laboratory studies to measure levels of potassium, cyclosporine in blood, and to evaluate liver and kidney function.
- Check blood pressure. Cyclosporine sometimes causes hypertension.
- Don't store solution in the refrigerator.
- Avoid any immunizations except those specifically recommended by your doctor.
- Maintain good dental hygiene. Cyclosporine can cause gum problems.
- Kidney toxicity occurs commonly after 12 months of taking cyclosporine.
- Don't mix in styrofoam cups.

POSSIBLE INTERACTION WITH OTHER DRUGS

GENERIC NAME OR DRUG CLASS	COMBINED EFFECT
Androgens	Increased effect of cyclosporine.
Anticonvulsants*	Decreased effect of cyclosporine.
Cimetidine	Increased effect of cyclosporine.
Danazol	Increased effect of cyclosporine.
Diltiazem	Increased effect of cyclosporine.
Diuretics, potassium-sparing	Increased effect of cyclosporine.
Erythromycin	Increased effect of cyclosporine.
Estrogens	Increased effect of cyclosporine.
Fluconazole	Increased effect of cyclosporine. Cyclosporine dosage must be adjusted.

GENERIC NAME OR DRUG CLASS	COMBINED EFFECT
Immuno-suppressants* (adrenocorticoids, azathioprine, chlorambucil, cyclophosphamide, mercaptopurine, muromonab-CD3)	May increase risk of infection.
Ketoconazole	Increased risk of toxicity to kidney.
Lovastatin	Increased heart and kidney damage.
Medicines that may be toxic to kidneys (gold*, NSAIDs* sulfonamides*)	Increased risk of toxicity to kidneys.
Nimodipine	Increased cyclosporine toxicity.
Rifampin	Decreased effect of cyclosporine.
Tiopronin	Increased risk of toxicity to kidneys.
Vancomycin	Increased chance of hearing loss or kidney damage.
Virus vaccines	Increased adverse reactions to vaccine.

POSSIBLE INTERACTION WITH OTHER SUBSTANCES

INTERACTS WITH	COMBINED EFFECT
Alcohol:	May increase possibility of toxic effects. Avoid.
Beverages:	None expected.
Cocaine:	May increase possibility of toxic effects. Avoid.
Foods:	None expected.
Marijuana:	May increase possibility of toxic effects. Avoid.
Tobacco:	May increase possibility of toxic effects. Avoid.

*See Glossary

DANAZOL

BRAND NAMES

Cyclomen   Danocrine

BASIC INFORMATION

Habit forming? No
Prescription needed? Yes
Available as generic? No
Drug class: Gonadotropin inhibitor

 USES

Treatment of endometriosis, fibrocystic breast
disease, angioneurotic edema except in
pregnant women, gynecomastia, infertility,
excessive menstruation, precocious puberty.

 **DOSAGE & USAGE
INFORMATION**

How to take:
Capsule—Swallow with liquid or food to lessen
stomach irritation. If you can't swallow whole,
open capsule and take with liquid or food.

When to take:
At the same times each day.

If you forget a dose:
Take as soon as you remember (don't double
dose).

What drug does:
Partially prevents output of pituitary follicle-
stimulating hormone and lutenizing hormone
reducing estrogen production.

Time lapse before drug works:
- 2 to 3 months to treat endometriosis.
- 1 to 2 months to treat other disorders.

Don't take with:
- Birth control pills.
- Any other medicine without consulting your
  doctor or pharmacist.

 OVERDOSE

SYMPTOMS:
None expected.
WHAT TO DO:
Overdose unlikely to threaten life. If person
takes much larger amount than prescribed,
call doctor, poison-control center or
hospital emergency room for instructions.

 **POSSIBLE
ADVERSE REACTIONS
OR SIDE EFFECTS**

SYMPTOMS	WHAT TO DO
Life-threatening:	
None expected.	
Common:	
Menstrual irregularities.	Continue. Call doctor when convenient.
Infrequent:	
• Unnatural hair growth in women, nosebleeds, bleeding gums, sore throat and chills.	Discontinue. Call doctor right away.
• Dizziness; deepened voice; hoarseness; flushed or red skin; muscle cramps; enlarged clitoris; decreased testicle size; vaginal burning, itching; swollen feet; decreased breast size; increased or decreased sex drive.	Continue. Call doctor when convenient.
• Headache, acne, weight gain, vision changes.	Continue. Tell doctor at next visit.
Rare:	
Jaundice, flushing, sweating, vaginitis, rash, nausea, vomiting, constipation, abdominal pain.	Discontinue. Call doctor right away.

DANAZOL

WARNINGS & PRECAUTIONS

Don't take if:
- You become pregnant.
- You have breast cancer.

Before you start, consult your doctor:
- If you take birth control pills.
- If you have diabetes.
- If you have heart disease.
- If you have epilepsy.
- If you have kidney disease.
- If you have liver disease.
- If you have migraine headaches.

Over age 60:
Adverse reactions and side effects may be more frequent and severe than in younger persons.

Pregnancy:
Risk to unborn child outweighs drug benefits. Don't use. Stop if you get pregnant.

Breast-feeding:
Unknown whether medicine filters into milk. Consult doctor.

Infants & children:
Not recommended.

Prolonged use:
- Required for full effect. Don't discontinue without consulting doctor.
- Talk to your doctor about the need for follow-up medical examinations or laboratory studies to check liver function, mammogram.

Skin & sunlight:
No problems expected.

Driving, piloting or hazardous work:
No problems expected.

Discontinuing:
Don't discontinue without consulting doctor. Menstrual periods may be absent for 2 to 3 months after discontinuation.

Others:
- May alter blood-sugar levels in diabetic persons.
- May interfere with the accuracy of some medical tests.

POSSIBLE INTERACTION WITH OTHER DRUGS

GENERIC NAME OR DRUG CLASS	COMBINED EFFECT
Anticoagulants, oral*	Increased anticoagulant effect.
Antidiabetic agents, oral*	Decreased antidiabetic effect.
Cyclosporine	Increased risk of kidney damage.
Insulin	Decreased insulin effect.

POSSIBLE INTERACTION WITH OTHER SUBSTANCES

INTERACTS WITH	COMBINED EFFECT
Alcohol:	Excessive nervous system depression. Avoid.
Beverages: Caffeine.	Rapid, irregular heartbeat. Avoid.
Cocaine:	May interfere with expected action of danazol. Avoid.
Foods:	No problems expected.
Marijuana:	May interfere with expected action of danazol. Avoid.
Tobacco:	Rapid, irregular heartbeat. Avoid. Increased leg cramps.

DANTHRON AND DOCUSATE

BRAND NAMES

Regulex-D Doss

BASIC INFORMATION

Habit forming? No
Prescription needed? No
Available as generic? No
Drug class: Laxative (stimulant)

 USES

Constipation relief.

 DOSAGE & USAGE INFORMATION

How to take:
- Tablet—Swallow with liquid or food.
- Liquid—Drink 6 to 8 glasses of water each day, in addition to one taken with each dose.

When to take:
Usually at bedtime with a snack, unless directed otherwise.

If you forget a dose:
Take as soon as you remember.

What drug does:
Acts on smooth muscles of intestine wall to cause vigorous bowel movement.

Time lapse before drug works:
6 to 10 hours.

Don't take with:
- Don't take within 2 hours of taking another medicine. Laxative interferes with medicine absorption.
- Any other medicine without consulting your doctor or pharmacist.

 OVERDOSE

SYMPTOMS:
Vomiting, electrolyte depletion.
WHAT TO DO:
Overdose unlikely to threaten life. If person takes much larger amount than prescribed, call doctor, poison-control center or hospital emergency room for instructions.

 POSSIBLE ADVERSE REACTIONS OR SIDE EFFECTS

SYMPTOMS	WHAT TO DO
Life-threatening: None expected.	
Common: Rectal irritation.	Continue. Call doctor when convenient.
Infrequent:	
• Dangerous potassium loss (thirst, weakness, heartbeat irregularity, paralysis and diarrhea).	Discontinue. Call doctor right away.
• Belching, cramps, nausea.	Continue. Call doctor when convenient.
Rare:	
• Irritability, confusion, headache, rash breathing difficulty, irregular heartbeat, muscle cramps, unusual tiredness, weakness.	Discontinue. Call doctor right away.
• Burning on urination.	Continue. Call doctor when convenient.

WARNINGS & PRECAUTIONS

Don't take if:
- You have symptoms of appendicitis, inflamed bowel or intestinal blockage.
- You are allergic to a stimulant laxative.
- You have missed a bowel movement for only 1 or 2 days.

Before you start, consult your doctor:
- If you have a colostomy or ileostomy.
- If you have congestive heart disease.
- If you have diabetes.
- If you have high blood pressure.
- If you have a laxative habit.
- If you have rectal bleeding.
- If you take other laxatives.

Over age 60:
Adverse reactions and side effects may be more frequent and severe than in younger persons.

Pregnancy:
Risk to mother and unborn child outweighs drug benefits. Don't use.

Breast-feeding:
Drug passes into milk. Avoid drug or discontinue nursing until you finish medicine. Consult doctor for advice on maintaining milk supply.

Infants & children:
Use only under medical supervision.

Prolonged use:
Don't take for more than 1 week unless under a doctor's supervision. May cause laxative dependence.

Skin & sunlight:
No problems expected.

Driving, piloting or hazardous work:
No problems expected.

Discontinuing:
May be unnecessary to finish medicine. Follow doctor's instructions.

Others:
Don't take to "flush out" your system or as a "tonic."

POSSIBLE INTERACTION WITH OTHER DRUGS

GENERIC NAME OR DRUG CLASS	COMBINED EFFECT
Antihypertensives*	May cause dangerous low potassium level.
Digoxin	Increased possibility of digitalis toxicity.
Diuretics*	May cause dangerous low potassium level.
Docusate calcium	Liver toxicity.
Docusate sodium	Liver toxicity.

POSSIBLE INTERACTION WITH OTHER SUBSTANCES

INTERACTS WITH	COMBINED EFFECT
Alcohol:	None expected.
Beverages:	None expected.
Cocaine:	None expected.
Foods:	None expected.
Marijuana:	None expected.
Tobacco:	None expected.

*See Glossary

DANTROLENE

BRAND NAMES

Dantrium

BASIC INFORMATION

Habit forming? No
Prescription needed? Yes
Available as generic? No
Drug class: Muscle relaxant, antispastic

 USES

- Relieves muscle spasticity caused by diseases such as multiple sclerosis, cerebral palsy, stroke.
- Relieves muscle spasticity caused by injury to spinal cord.
- Relieves or prevents excess body temperature brought on by some surgical procedures.

 DOSAGE & USAGE INFORMATION

How to take:
Capsules—Swallow with liquid.

When to take:
Once a day for muscle spasticity during first 6 days. Later, every 6 hours. For excess body temperature, follow label instructions.

If you forget a dose:
Take as soon as you remember up to 2 hours late. If more than 2 hours, wait for next scheduled dose (don't double this dose).

Continued next column

 OVERDOSE

SYMPTOMS:
Shortness of breath, bloody urine, chest pain, convulsions.
WHAT TO DO:
- Dial 0 (operator) or 911 (emergency) for an ambulance or medical help. Then give first aid immediately.
- If patient is unconscious and not breathing, give mouth-to-mouth breathing. If there is no heartbeat, use cardiac massage and mouth-to-mouth breathing (CPR). Don't try to make patient vomit. If you can't get help quickly, take patient to nearest emergency facility.
- See emergency information on inside covers.

What drug does:
Acts directly on muscles to prevent excess contractions.

Time lapse before drug works:
1 or more weeks.

Don't take with:
Any other medicine without consulting your doctor or pharmacist.

 POSSIBLE ADVERSE REACTIONS OR SIDE EFFECTS

SYMPTOMS	WHAT TO DO
Life-threatening:	
Seizure.	Seek emergency treatment immediately.
Common:	
Drowsiness, dizziness, weakness.	Discontinue. Call doctor right away.
Infrequent:	
• Rash, hives; black or bloody stools; chest pain; fast heartbeat; backache; blood in urine; painful, swollen feet; chills; fever; shortness of breath.	Discontinue. Call doctor right away.
• Depression, confusion, headache, slurred speech, insomnia, nervousness, diarrhea, blurred vision, difficult swallowing, appetite loss, difficult urination, decreased sexual function in males.	Continue. Call doctor when convenient.
Rare:	
• Jaundice, abdominal cramps, double vision.	Discontinue. Call doctor right away.
• Constipation.	Continue. Call doctor when convenient.

DANTROLENE

WARNINGS & PRECAUTIONS

Don't take if:
You are allergic to dantrolene or any muscle relaxant or antispastic medication.

Before you start, consult your doctor:
- If you have liver disease.
- If you have heart disease.
- If you have lung disease (especially emphysema).
- If you are over age 35.
- If you will have surgery within 2 months, including dental surgery, requiring general or spinal anesthesia.

Over age 60:
Adverse reactions and side effects may be more frequent and severe than in younger persons.

Pregnancy:
No proven harm to unborn child. Avoid if possible.

Breast-feeding:
Avoid nursing or discontinue until you finish drug.

Infants & children:
Only under close medical supervision.

Prolonged use:
Recommended periodically during prolonged use—Blood counts, G6PD tests before treatment begins in Negroes and Caucasians of Mediterranean heritage, liver function studies.

Skin & sunlight:
May cause rash or intensify sunburn in areas exposed to sun or sunlamp.

Driving, piloting or hazardous work:
Don't drive or pilot aircraft until you learn how medicine affects you. Don't work around dangerous machinery. Don't climb ladders or work in high places. Danger increases if you drink alcohol or take medicine affecting alertness and reflexes, such as antihistamines, tranquilizers, sedatives, pain medicine, narcotics and mind-altering drugs.

Discontinuing:
Don't discontinue without consulting doctor. Dose may require gradual reduction if you have taken drug for a long time. Doses of other drugs may also require adjustment.

Others:
No problems expected.

POSSIBLE INTERACTION WITH OTHER DRUGS

GENERIC NAME OR DRUG CLASS	COMBINED EFFECT
Central nervous system (CNS) depressants * (antidepressants,* antihistamines,* narcotics,* other muscle relaxants,* sedatives,* sleeping pills,* tranquilizers*)	Increased sedation, low blood pressure. Avoid.
Dronabinol	Increased effect of dronabinol on central nervous system. Avoid.

POSSIBLE INTERACTION WITH OTHER SUBSTANCES

INTERACTS WITH	COMBINED EFFECT
Alcohol:	Increased sedation, low blood pressure. Avoid.
Beverages:	No problems expected.
Cocaine:	Increased spasticity. Avoid.
Foods:	No problems expected.
Marijuana:	Increased spasticity. Avoid.
Tobacco:	May interfere with absorption of medicine.

*See Glossary

DAPSONE

BRAND NAMES

Avlosulfon　　　　**DDS**

BASIC INFORMATION

Habit forming? No
Prescription needed? Yes
Available as generic? Yes
Drug class: Antibacterial (antileprosy),
　　sulfone

USES

- Treatment of dermatitis herpetiformis.
- Treatment of leprosy.
- Prevention and treatment of pneumocystis carnii pneumonia.
- Other uses include granuloma annulare, pemphigoid, pyoderma gangrenosum, polychondritis, eye ulcerations, systemic lupus erythematosus.

DOSAGE & USAGE INFORMATION

How to take:
Tablet—Swallow with liquid or food to lessen stomach irritation.

When to take:
Once a day at same time.

If you forget a dose:
Take as soon as you remember up to 2 hours late. If more than 2 hours, wait for next scheduled dose (don't double this dose).

Continued next column

OVERDOSE

SYMPTOMS:
Bleeding, vomiting, seizures, cyanosis, coma.
WHAT TO DO:
- **Dial 0 (operator) or 911 (emergency) for an ambulance or medical help. Then give first aid immediately.**
- **If patient is unconscious and not breathing, give mouth-to-mouth breathing. If there is no heartbeat, use cardiac massage and mouth-to-mouth breathing (CPR). Don't try to make patient vomit. If you can't get help quickly, take patient to nearest emergency facility.**
- **See emergency information on inside covers.**

What drug does:
Inhibits enzymes. Kills leprosy germs.

Time lapse before drug works:
- 3 years for leprosy.
- 1 to 2 weeks for dermatitis herpetiformis.

Don't take with:
Any other medicine without consulting your doctor or pharmacist.

POSSIBLE ADVERSE REACTIONS OR SIDE EFFECTS

SYMPTOMS	WHAT TO DO
Life-threatening:	
In case of overdose, see previous column.	
Common:	
• Rash, abdominal pain.	Discontinue. Call doctor right away.
• Appetite loss.	Continue. Call doctor when convenient.
Infrequent:	
Pale.	Discontinue. Call doctor right away.
Rare:	
• Dizziness; mental changes; sore throat; fever; difficult breathing; bleeding; jaundice; numbness, tingling, pain or burning in hands or feet; swelling of feet, hands, eyelids; blurred vision; anemia; peeling skin.	Discontinue. Call doctor right away.
• Headache; itching; nausea; vomiting; blue fingernails, lips.	Continue. Call doctor when convenient.

WARNINGS & PRECAUTIONS

Don't take if:
- You have G6PD deficiency.
- You are allergic to furosemide, thiazide diuretics, sulfonureas, carbonic anhydrase inhibitors, sulfonamides.

Before you start, consult your doctor:
- If you take any other medicine.
- If you are anemic.
- If you have liver or kidney disease.
- If you are Negro or Caucasian with Mediterranean heritage.
- If you will have surgery within 2 months, including dental surgery, requiring general or spinal anesthesia.

Over age 60:
Adverse reactions and side effects may be more frequent and severe than in younger persons.

Pregnancy:
No problems expected, although there haven't been adequate human studies reported.

Breast-feeding:
Consult doctor.

Infants & children:
Under close medical supervision only.

Prolonged use:
- Request liver function studies.
- Talk to your doctor about the need for follow-up medical examinations or laboratory studies to check complete blood counts (white blood cell count, platelet count, red blood cell count, hemoglobin, hematocrit).

Skin & sunlight:
Exposure may cause illness with swelling, spots on skin, fever.

Driving, piloting or hazardous work:
Don't drive or pilot aircraft until you learn how medicine affects you. Don't work around dangerous machinery. Don't climb ladders or work in high places. Danger increases if you drink alcohol or take medicine affecting alertness and reflexes, such as antihistamines, tranquilizers, sedatives, pain medicine, narcotics and mind-altering drugs.

Discontinuing:
Don't discontinue without consulting doctor. Dose may require gradual reduction if you have taken drug for a long time. Doses of other drugs may also require adjustment.

Others:
- Dapsone may rarely cause liver damage.
- For full effect you may need to take dapsone for many months or years.

POSSIBLE INTERACTION WITH OTHER DRUGS

GENERIC NAME OR DRUG CLASS	COMBINED EFFECT
Aminobenzoic acid (PABA)	Decreased dapsone effect. Avoid.
Didanosine	Increased risk of peripheral neuropathy. Reduced absorption of both drugs.
Dideoxyinosine (ddl)	Decreased dapsone effect.
Hemolytics*	May increase adverse effects on blood cells.
Methotrexate	May increase blood toxicity.
Probenecid	Increased toxicity of dapsone.
Pyrimethamine	May increase blood toxicity.
Rifampin	Decreased effect of dapsone.
Trimethoprim	May increase blood toxicity.

POSSIBLE INTERACTION WITH OTHER SUBSTANCES

INTERACTS WITH	COMBINED EFFECT
Alcohol:	Increased chance of toxicity to liver.
Beverages:	No problems expected.
Cocaine:	Increased chance of toxicity. Avoid.
Foods:	No problems expected.
Marijuana:	Increased chance of toxicity. Avoid.
Tobacco:	May interfere with absorption of medicine.

*See Glossary

DECONGESTANTS (Ophthalmic)

BRAND AND GENERIC NAMES

Ak-Con
Albalon
Allerest
Clear Eyes
Comfort
Degest 2
Estivin II
I-Naphline
Murine
Muro's Opcon
Nafazair

NAPHAZOLINE
Naphcon
Naphcon Forte
Napholine
Ocu-Zoline
Opcon
TETRAHYDROZILINE
VasoClear
Vasocon
Visine

BASIC INFORMATION

Habit forming? No
Prescription needed? Yes, for some
Available as generic? Yes
Drug class: Decongestant (ophthalmic)

USES

Treats eye redness, itching, burning or other irritation due to dust, colds, allergies, rubbing eyes, wearing contact lenses, swimming or eye strain from close work, watching TV, reading.

DOSAGE & USAGE INFORMATION

How to use:
Eye drops
- Wash hands.
- Apply pressure to inside corner of eye with middle finger.
- Tilt head backward. Pull lower lid away from eye with index finger of the same hand.
- Drop eye drops into pouch and close eye. Don't blink.
- Keep eyes closed for 1 to 2 minutes.
- Continue pressure for 1 minute after placing medicine in eye.
- Don't touch applicator tip to any surface (including the eye). If you accidentally touch tip, clean with warm soap and water.
- Keep container tightly closed.
- Keep cool, but don't freeze.
- Wash hands immediately after using.

Continued next column

OVERDOSE

SYMPTOMS:
None expected.
WHAT TO DO:
Not intended for internal use. If child accidentally swallows, call poison-control center.

When to use:
As directed. Usually every 3 or 4 hours.

If you forget a dose:
Use as soon as you remember.

What drug does:
Acts on small blood vessels to make them constrict or become smaller.

Time lapse before drug works:
2 to 10 minutes.

Don't use with:
Other eye drops without consulting your doctor.

POSSIBLE ADVERSE REACTIONS OR SIDE EFFECTS

SYMPTOMS	WHAT TO DO
Life-threatening: None expected.	
Common: Increased eye irritation.	Discontinue. Call doctor right away.
Infrequent: None expected.	
Rare: Blurred vision, large pupils, weakness, drowsiness, decreased body temperature, slow heartbeat, dizziness, headache, nervousness, nausea.	Discontinue. Call doctor right away.

DECONGESTANTS (Ophthalmic)

WARNINGS & PRECAUTIONS

Don't use if:
You are allergic to any decongestant eye drops.

Before you start, consult your doctor:
- If you take antidepressants or maprolitine.
- If you have eye disease, infection or injury.
- If you have heart disease, high blood pressure, thyroid disease.

Over age 60:
No problems expected.

Pregnancy:
No problems expected, but check with doctor.

Breast-feeding:
No problems expected, but check with doctor.

Infants & children:
Don't use.

Prolonged use:
Don't use for more than 3 or 4 days.

Skin & sunlight:
No problems expected.

Driving, piloting or hazardous work:
No problems expected.

Discontinuing:
May not need all the medicine in container. If symptoms disappear, stop using.

Others:
- Keep cool, but don't freeze.
- Check with your doctor if eye irritation continues or becomes worse.

POSSIBLE INTERACTION WITH OTHER DRUGS

GENERIC NAME OR DRUG CLASS	COMBINED EFFECT
Clinically significant interactions with oral or injected medicines unlikely.	

POSSIBLE INTERACTION WITH OTHER SUBSTANCES

INTERACTS WITH	COMBINED EFFECT
Alcohol:	None expected.
Beverages:	None expected.
Cocaine:	None expected.
Foods:	None expected.
Marijuana:	None expected.
Tobacco:	Smoke may increase eye irritation. Avoid.

DEHYDROCHOLIC ACID

BRAND NAMES

Bilax	Hepahydrin
Cholan-HMB	Neolax
Decholin	Trilax

BASIC INFORMATION

Habit forming? No
Prescription needed? No
Available as generic? Yes
Drug class: Laxative (stimulant)

 USES

Constipation relief.

 DOSAGE & USAGE INFORMATION

How to take:
Tablet or capsule—Swallow with liquid.

When to take:
Usually at bedtime with a snack, unless directed otherwise.

If you forget a dose:
Take as soon as you remember.

What drug does:
Acts on smooth muscles of intestine wall to cause vigorous bowel movement.

Time lapse before drug works:
6 to 10 hours.

Don't take with:
- Any other medicine without consulting your doctor or pharmacist.
- Don't take within 2 hours of taking another medicine. Laxative interferes with medicine absorption.

 OVERDOSE

SYMPTOMS:
Vomiting, electrolyte depletion.
WHAT TO DO:
Overdose unlikely to threaten life. If person takes much larger amount than prescribed, call doctor, poison-control center or hospital emergency room for instructions.

 POSSIBLE ADVERSE REACTIONS OR SIDE EFFECTS

SYMPTOMS	WHAT TO DO
Life-threatening: None expected.	
Common: Rectal irritation.	Continue. Call doctor when convenient.
Infrequent:	
• Dangerous potassium loss (thirst, weakness, heartbeat irregularity, paralysis and diarrhea).	Discontinue. Call doctor right away.
• Belching, cramps, nausea.	Continue. Call doctor when convenient.
Rare:	
• Irritability, confusion, headache, rash, breathing difficulty, irregular heartbeat, muscle cramps, unusual tiredness or weakness.	Discontinue. Call doctor right away.
• Burning on urination.	Continue. Call doctor when convenient.

WARNINGS & PRECAUTIONS

Don't take if:
- You have symptoms of appendicitis, inflamed bowel or intestinal blockage.
- You are allergic to a stimulant laxative.
- You have missed a bowel movement for only 1 or 2 days.
- You have liver disease.

Before you start, consult your doctor:
- If you have a colostomy or ileostomy.
- If you have congestive heart disease.
- If you have diabetes.
- If you have an enlarged prostate.
- If you have a laxative habit.
- If you have rectal bleeding.
- If you take other laxatives.

Over age 60:
Adverse reactions and side effects may be more frequent and severe than in younger persons.

Pregnancy:
Risk to mother and unborn child outweighs drug benefits. Don't use.

Breast-feeding:
Drug passes into milk. Avoid drug or discontinue nursing until you finish medicine. Consult doctor for advice on maintaining milk supply.

Infants & children:
Use only under medical supervision.

Prolonged use:
Don't take for more than 1 week unless under a doctor's supervision. May cause laxative dependence.

Skin & sunlight:
No problems expected.

Driving, piloting or hazardous work:
No problems expected.

Discontinuing:
May be unnecessary to finish medicine. Follow doctor's instructions.

Others:
Don't take to "flush out" your system or as a "tonic."

POSSIBLE INTERACTION WITH OTHER DRUGS

GENERIC NAME OR DRUG CLASS	COMBINED EFFECT
Antihypertensives*	May cause dangerous low potassium level.
Diuretics*	May cause dangerous low potassium level.

POSSIBLE INTERACTION WITH OTHER SUBSTANCES

INTERACTS WITH	COMBINED EFFECT
Alcohol:	None expected.
Beverages:	None expected.
Cocaine:	None expected.
Foods:	None expected.
Marijuana:	None expected.
Tobacco:	None expected.

*See Glossary

DESMOPRESSIN

BRAND NAMES

DDAVP   **Stimate**

BASIC INFORMATION

Habit forming? No
Prescription needed? Yes
Available as generic? No
Drug class: Antidiuretic, antihemorrhagic

 ## USES

- Prevents and controls symptoms associated with central diabetes insipidus.
- Treats primary nocturnal enuresis (bedwetting during sleep).

 ## DOSAGE & USAGE INFORMATION

How to take:
Nasal spray—Fill the rhinyle (a flexible, calibrated catheter) with a measured dose of the nasal spray. Blow on the other end of the catheter to deposit the solution deep in the nasal cavity. For infants and children, an air-filled syringe may be used.

When to take:
At the same time each day, according to instructions on prescription label.

If you forget a dose:
Take as soon as you remember up to 2 hours late. If more than 2 hours, wait for next scheduled dose. Don't double this dose.

What drug does:
Increases water reabsorption in the kidney and decreases urine output.

Time lapse before drug works:
Within 1 hour. Effect may last from 6 to 24 hours.

Don't take with:
Any other medicine without consulting your doctor or pharmacist.

 ## OVERDOSE

SYMPTOMS:
Confusion, coma, seizures.
WHAT TO DO:
Overdose unlikely to threaten life. If person takes much larger amount than prescribed, call doctor, poison-control center or hospital emergency room for instructions.

 ## POSSIBLE ADVERSE REACTIONS OR SIDE EFFECTS

SYMPTOMS	WHAT TO DO
Life-threatening: None expected.	
Common: Headache.	Continue. Call doctor when convenient.
Infrequent: • Flushed or red skin, nausea.	Discontinue. Call doctor right away.
• Abdominal cramps.	Continue. Call doctor when convenient.
Rare: • Water intoxication (confusion, drowsiness, headache, seizures, rapid weight gain).	Discontinue. Seek emergency treatment.
• Increased blood pressure.	Discontinue. Call doctor right away.

WARNINGS & PRECAUTIONS

Don't take if:
You know that you are sensitive to desmopressin.

Before you start, consult your doctor:
- If you have allergic rhinitis.
- If you have nasal congestion.
- If you have a cold or other upper respiratory infection.
- If you have heart disease or high blood pressure.

Over age 60:
Increased risk of water intoxication.

Pregnancy:
No proven harm to unborn child, but avoid if possible.

Breast-feeding:
Drug passes into milk. Avoid drug or discontinue nursing until you finish medicine. Consult doctor for advice on maintaining milk supply.

Infants & children:
More sensitive to effect.

Prolonged use:
May require increasing dosage for same effect.

Skin & sunlight:
No special problems expected.

Driving, piloting or hazardous work:
Don't drive or pilot aircraft until you learn how medicine affects you. Don't work around dangerous machinery. Don't climb ladders or work in high places. Danger increases if you drink alcohol or take medicine affecting alertness and reflexes.

Discontinuing:
No special problems expected.

Others:
- Advise any doctor or dentist whom you consult that you take this medicine.
- Fluid intake may need to be adjusted.

POSSIBLE INTERACTION WITH OTHER DRUGS

GENERIC NAME OR DRUG CLASS	COMBINED EFFECT
Carbamazepine	May increase desmopressin effect.
Chlorpropamide	May increase desmopressin effect.
Clofibrate	May increase desmopressin effect.
Demeclocycline	May decrease desmopressin effect.
Lithium	May decrease desmopressin effect.
Norepinephrine	May decrease desmopressin effect.

POSSIBLE INTERACTION WITH OTHER SUBSTANCES

INTERACTS WITH	COMBINED EFFECT
Alcohol:	May decrease desmopressin effect.
Beverages: Caffeine drinks.	May decrease desmopressin effect.
Cocaine:	May decrease desmopressin effect.
Foods:	None expected.
Marijuana:	May decrease desmopressin effect.
Tobacco:	May decrease desmopressin effect.

DEXAMETHASONE

BRAND NAMES

See complete list of brand names in the *Brand Name Directory*, page 918.

BASIC INFORMATION

Habit forming? No
Prescription needed? Yes
Available as generic? Yes
Drug class: Cortisone drug (adrenal corticosteroid)

USES

- Reduces inflammation caused by many different medical problems.
- Treatment for some allergic diseases, blood disorders, kidney diseases, asthma and emphysema.
- Replaces corticosteroid deficiencies.

DOSAGE & USAGE INFORMATION

How to take:
- Tablet or liquid—Swallow with liquid or food to lessen stomach irritation. If you can't swallow whole, crumble tablet and take with liquid or food.
- Inhaler—Follow label instructions.

When to take:
At the same times each day. Take once-a-day or once-every-other-day doses in mornings.

If you forget a dose:
- Several-doses-per-day prescription—Take as soon as you remember up to 2 hours late. If more than 2 hours, wait for next scheduled dose (don't double this dose).
- Once-a-day dose or less—Wait for next dose. Double this dose.

What drug does:
Decreases inflammatory responses.

Time lapse before drug works:
2 to 4 days.

Continued next column

OVERDOSE

SYMPTOMS:
Headache, convulsions, fluid retention, heart failure.
WHAT TO DO:
- **Dial 0 (operator) or 911 (emergency) for an ambulance or medical help. Then give first aid immediately.**
- **See emergency information on inside covers.**

Don't take with:
Any other medicine without consulting your doctor or pharmacist.

POSSIBLE ADVERSE REACTIONS OR SIDE EFFECTS

SYMPTOMS	WHAT TO DO
Life-threatening:	
Hives, rash, intense itching, faintness soon after a dose (anaphylaxis).	Seek emergency treatment immediately.
Common:	
Poor wound healing, acne, thirst, nausea, indigestion, vomiting.	Continue. Call doctor when convenient.
Infrequent:	
• Bloody or black, tarry stool.	Discontinue. Seek emergency treatment.
• Blurred vision; halos around lights; sore throat, fever; muscle cramps; swollen legs, feet.	Discontinue. Call doctor right away.
• Mood changes, insomnia, fatigue, restlessness, frequent urination, weight gain, round face, weakness, irregular menstrual periods.	Continue. Call doctor when convenient.
Rare:	
• Irregular heartbeat.	Discontinue. Seek emergency treatment.
• Rash, pancreatitis, numbness or tingling in hands or feet, thrombophlebitis, hallucinations, hiccups, convulsions.	Discontinue. Call doctor right away.

WARNINGS & PRECAUTIONS

Don't take if:
- You are allergic to any cortisone drug.
- You have tuberculosis or fungus infection.
- You have herpes infection of eyes, lips or genitals.

Before you start, consult your doctor:
- If you have had tuberculosis.
- If you have congestive heart failure, diabetes, peptic ulcer, glaucoma, underactive thyroid, high blood pressure, myasthenia gravis.
- If you have blood clots in legs or lungs.

Over age 60:
Adverse reactions and side effects may be more frequent and severe than in younger persons. Likely to aggravate edema, diabetes or ulcers. Likely to cause cataracts and osteoporosis (softening of the bones).

Pregnancy:
Risk to unborn child outweighs drug benefits. Don't use.

Breast-feeding:
Drug passes into milk. Avoid drug or discontinue nursing until you finish medicine. Consult doctor for advice on maintaining milk supply.

Infants & children:
Use only under medical supervision.

Prolonged use:
- Retards growth in children.
- Possible glaucoma, cataracts, diabetes, fragile bones and thin skin.
- Functional dependence.
- Talk to your doctor about the need for follow-up medical examinations or laboratory studies to check blood sugar, eyes, serum electrolytes, stools for blood.

Skin & sunlight:
No problems expected.

Driving, piloting or hazardous work:
No problems expected.

Discontinuing:
- Don't discontinue without doctor's advice until you complete prescribed dose, even though symptoms diminish or disappear.
- Drug affects your response to surgery, illness, injury or stress for 2 years after discontinuing. Tell anyone who takes medical care of you within 2 years about drug.

Others:
- Avoid immunizations if possible.
- Your resistance to infection is less while taking this medicine.
- Advise any doctor or dentist whom you consult that you take this medicine.
- Those who have inactive or ''cured'' tuberculosis* may be subjected to a possible recurrence of active tuberculosis.
- Children who must take cortisone drugs may grow less well.

POSSIBLE INTERACTION WITH OTHER DRUGS

GENERIC NAME OR DRUG CLASS	COMBINED EFFECT
Aminoglutethimide	Dexamethasone effect decreased by half.
Amphotericin B	Potassium depletion.
Anticholinergics*	Possible glaucoma.
Anticoagulants, oral*	Decreased anti-coagulant effect.
Anticonvulsants, hydantoin*	Decreased dexa-methasone effect.
Antidiabetics, oral*	Decreased anti-diabetic effect.
Antihistamines*	Decreased dexa-methasone effect.
Aspirin	Increased dexa-methasone effect.
Attenuated virus vaccines*	Possible viral infection.
Barbiturates*	Decreased dexa-methasone effect. Oversedation.
Chloral hydrate	Decreased dexa-methasone effect.
Chlorthalidone	Potassium depletion.
Cholestyramine	Decreased dexa-methasone effect.
Cholinergics*	Decreased cholinergic effect.
Colestipol	Decreased dexa-methasone absorption.
Contraceptives, oral*	Increased dexa-methasone effect.
Digitalis preparations*	Dangerous potassium depletion. Possible digitalis toxicity.
Diuretics, thiazide*	Potassium depletion.
Ephedrine	Decreased dexa-methasone effect.

Continued page 943

POSSIBLE INTERACTION WITH OTHER SUBSTANCES

INTERACTS WITH	COMBINED EFFECT
Alcohol:	Risk of stomach ulcers.
Beverages:	No proven problems.
Cocaine:	Overstimulation. Avoid.
Foods:	No proven problems.
Marijuana:	Decreased immunity.
Tobacco:	Increased dexa-methasone effect. Possible toxicity.

*See Glossary

DEXTROMETHORPHAN

BRAND NAMES

See complete list of brand names in the *Brand Name Directory,* page 918.

BASIC INFORMATION

Habit forming? No
Prescription needed? No
Available as generic? No
Drug class: Cough suppressant

 ## USES

Suppresses cough associated with allergies or infections such as colds, bronchitis, flu and lung disorders.

 ## DOSAGE & USAGE INFORMATION

How to take:
- Chewable tablet—Chew well before swallowing.
- Lozenges or syrups—Take as directed on label.

When to take:
As needed, no more often than every 3 hours.

If you forget a dose:
Take as soon as you remember. Wait 3 hours for next dose.

What drug does:
Reduces sensitivity of brain's cough-control center, suppressing urge to cough.

Time lapse before drug works:
15 to 30 minutes.

Don't take with:
Any other medicine without consulting your doctor or pharmacist.

 ## OVERDOSE

SYMPTOMS:
Euphoria, overactivity, sense of intoxication, visual and auditory hallucinations, lack of coordination, stagger, stupor, shallow breathing.
WHAT TO DO:
- **Dial 0 (operator) or 911 (emergency) for an ambulance or medical help. Then give first aid immediately.**
- **See emergency information on inside covers.**

 ## POSSIBLE ADVERSE REACTIONS OR SIDE EFFECTS

SYMPTOMS	WHAT TO DO
Life-threatening:	
In case of overdose, see previous column.	
Common:	
None expected.	
Infrequent:	
Confusion, excitement or nervousness.	Discontinue. Call doctor right away.
Rare:	
Dizziness, drowsiness, rash, diarrhea, nausea or vomiting, abdominal pain.	Discontinue. Call doctor right away.

WARNINGS & PRECAUTIONS

Don't take if:
You are allergic to any cough syrup containing dextromethorphan.

Before you start, consult your doctor:
- If you have asthma attacks.
- If you have impaired liver function.

Over age 60:
Adverse reactions and side effects may be more frequent and severe than in younger persons. You may require smaller doses for shorter periods of time.

Pregnancy:
No proven harm to unborn child. Avoid if possible.

Breast-feeding:
No proven problems. Consult doctor.

Infants & children:
Use only as label directs.

Prolonged use:
No problems expected.

Skin & sunlight:
No problems expected.

Driving, piloting or hazardous work:
Don't drive or pilot aircraft until you learn how medicine affects you. Don't work around dangerous machinery. Don't climb ladders or work in high places. Danger increases if you drink alcohol or take medicine affecting alertness and reflexes, such as antihistamines, tranquilizers, sedatives, pain medicine, narcotics and mind-altering drugs.

Discontinuing:
May be unnecessary to finish medicine. Follow doctor's instructions.

Others:
- If cough persists or if you cough blood or brown-yellow, thick mucus, call your doctor.
- Excessive use may lead to functional dependence.

 ## POSSIBLE INTERACTION WITH OTHER DRUGS

GENERIC NAME OR DRUG CLASS	COMBINED EFFECT
MAO inhibitors*	Disorientation, high fever, drop in blood pressure and loss of consciousness.
Sedatives* and other central nervous system (CNS) depressants*	Increased sedative effect of both drugs.

 ## POSSIBLE INTERACTION WITH OTHER SUBSTANCES

INTERACTS WITH	COMBINED EFFECT
Alcohol:	None expected.
Beverages:	None expected.
Cocaine:	Decreased dextromethorphan effect. Avoid.
Foods:	None expected.
Marijuana:	None expected.
Tobacco:	None expected.

DEXTROSE & ELECTROLYTES

BRAND NAMES

Gastrolyte
Lytren
Pedialyte

Rapolyte
Rehyrdralyte
Resol

BASIC INFORMATION

Habit forming? No
Prescription needed? Not for all
Available as generic? Yes
Drug class: Electrolyte replenisher

 ## USES

Replenishes fluids and electrolytes (salts) in dehydrated children and adults.

 ## DOSAGE & USAGE INFORMATION

How to take:
Follow package instructions.

When to take:
According to doctor's instructions. Frequency of need varies greatly.

If you forget a dose:
Take as soon as you remember up to 2 hours late. If more than 2 hours, wait for next scheduled dose (don't double this dose).

What drug does:
Prevents and treats electrolyte imbalance due to severe diarrhea.

Time lapse before drug works:
8 to 12 hours.

Don't take with:
Any other medicines (including over-the-counter drugs such as cough and cold medicines, laxatives, antacids, diet pills, caffeine, nose drops or vitamins) without consulting your doctor.

 ## OVERDOSE

SYMPTOMS:
Seizures.
WHAT TO DO:
- Dial 0 (operator) or 911 (emergency) for an ambulance or medical help. Then give first aid immediately.
- See emergency information on inside covers.

 ## POSSIBLE ADVERSE REACTIONS OR SIDE EFFECTS

SYMPTOMS	WHAT TO DO
Life-threatening:	
In case of overdose, see previous column.	
Common:	
Vomiting.	Continue treatment.
Infrequent:	
Failure to improve.	Continue.
Rare:	
• Too-high blood sodium causing convulsions.	Discontinue. Seek emergency treatment.
• Overhydration (puffy eyes).	Discontinue. Call doctor right away.

WARNINGS & PRECAUTIONS

Don't take if:
- Kidneys are not functioning.
- Patient is unable to drink.
- There is severe and sustained vomiting.

Before you start, consult your doctor:
If patient is younger than 6 months.

Over age 60:
No problems expected; well-tolerated by older patients.

Pregnancy:
No problems expected.

Breast-feeding:
No problems expected.

Infants & children:
Safe and effective in young; not yet evaluated in premature infants.

Prolonged use:
Talk to your doctor about the need for follow-up medical examinations or laboratory studies to check body weight, blood pressure, serum electrolytes and serum pH.

Skin & sunlight:
No problems expected.

Driving, piloting or hazardous work:
No problems expected.

Discontinuing:
No special problems expected.

Others:
- Advise any doctor or dentist whom you consult that you take this medicine.
- May affect results in some medical tests.

POSSIBLE INTERACTION WITH OTHER DRUGS

GENERIC NAME OR DRUG CLASS	COMBINED EFFECT
None expected.	

POSSIBLE INTERACTION WITH OTHER SUBSTANCES

INTERACTS WITH	COMBINED EFFECT
Alcohol:	Dangerous. Avoid.
Beverages:	Continuing milk all right. Others as tolerated.
Cocaine:	Dangerous. Avoid.
Foods: Rice, cereal, bananas, cooked potatoes or other carbohydrate-rich foods as tolerated.	Helps maintain nutrition.
Marijuana:	Dangerous. Avoid.
Tobacco:	May increase diarrhea. Avoid.

*See Glossary

DEXTROTHYROXINE

BRAND NAMES·

Choloxin

BASIC INFORMATION

Habit forming? No
Prescription needed? Yes
Available as generic? No
Drug class: Antihyperlipidemic

USES

Lowers blood cholesterol and low-density lipoprotein in patients who don't respond to low-fat diet and weight loss alone.

DOSAGE & USAGE INFORMATION

How to take:
Tablets—Swallow with liquid. If you can't swallow whole, crumble tablet and take with liquid or food. Instructions to take on empty stomach mean 1 hour before or 2 hours after eating.

When to take:
According to your doctor's instructions.

If you forget a dose:
Take as soon as you remember up to 2 hours late. If more than 2 hours, wait for next scheduled dose (don't double this dose).

What drug does:
Increases breakdown of LDL (low-density lipoprotein).

Time lapse before drug works:
1 to 2 months.

Don't take with:
Any other medicines (including over-the-counter drugs such as cough and cold medicines, laxatives, antacids, diet pills, caffeine, nose drops or vitamins) without consulting your doctor.

OVERDOSE

SYMPTOMS:
None expected.
WHAT TO DO:
Overdose unlikely to threaten life. If person takes much larger amount than prescribed, call doctor, poison-control center or hospital emergency room for instructions.

POSSIBLE ADVERSE REACTIONS OR SIDE EFFECTS

SYMPTOMS	WHAT TO DO
Life-threatening: None expected.	
Common: • Tremor, headache, irritability, insomnia.	Discontinue. Call doctor right away.
• Appetite change, diarrhea, leg cramps, menstrual irregularities, fever, heat sensitivity, unusual sweating, weight loss.	Continue. Call doctor when convenient.
Infrequent: Hives, rash, vomiting, chest pain, rapid and irregular heartbeat, shortness of breath.	Discontinue. Call doctor right away.
Rare: None expected.	

WARNINGS & PRECAUTIONS

Don't take if:
• You have had a heart attack within 6 weeks.
• You have no thyroid deficiency, but want to use this to lose weight.

Before you start, consult your doctor:
• If you have heart disease or high blood pressure.
• If you have diabetes.
• If you have Addison's disease, have had adrenal gland deficiency or use epinephrine, ephedrine or isoproterenol for asthma.

Over age 60:
More sensitive to thyroid hormone. May need smaller doses.

Pregnancy:
Considered safe if for thyroid deficiency only.

Breast-feeding:
Present in milk. Considered safe if dose is correct.

Infants & children:
Use only under medical supervision.

Prolonged use:
• No problems expected, if dose is correct.
• Talk to your doctor about the need for follow-up medical examinations or laboratory studies to check serum cholesterol and triglycerides.

Skin & sunlight:
No problems expected.

Driving, piloting or hazardous work:
No problems expected.

Discontinuing:
Don't discontinue without consulting doctor. Dose may require gradual reduction if you have taken drug for a long time. Doses of other drugs may also require adjustment.

Others:
- Digestive upsets, tremors, cramps, nervousness, insomnia or diarrhea may indicate need for dose adjustment.
- Advise any doctor or dentist whom you consult that you take this medicine.
- May affect results in some medical tests.
- Stay on a low-fat diet.

POSSIBLE INTERACTION WITH OTHER DRUGS

GENERIC NAME OR DRUG CLASS	COMBINED EFFECT
Amphetamines*	Increased amphetamine effect.
Anticoagulants, oral*	Increased anticoagulant effect.
Antidepressants, tricyclic (TCA)*	Increased anti-depressant effect. Irregular heartbeat.
Antidiabetics*	Antidiabetic may require adjustment.
Aspirin (large doses, continuous use)	Increased dextrothyroxine effect.
Barbiturates*	Decreased barbiturate effect.
Beta-adrenergic blockers*	Possible decreased beta blockers effect.
Cholestyramine	Decreased dextrothyroxine effect.
Colestipol	Decreased dextrothyroxine effect.
Contraceptives, oral*	Decreased dextrothyroxine effect.
Cortisone drugs*	Requires dose adjustment to prevent cortisone deficiency.
Digitalis preparations*	Decreased digitalis effect.
Ephedrine	Increased ephedrine effect.
Epinephrine	Increased epinephrine effect.
Estrogens*	Decreased dextrothyroxine effect.
Methylphenidate	Increased methylphenidate effect.
Phenytoin	Possible decreased dextrothyroxine effect.

POSSIBLE INTERACTION WITH OTHER SUBSTANCES

INTERACTS WITH	COMBINED EFFECT
Alcohol:	None expected.
Beverages:	None expected.
Cocaine:	Excess stimulation. Avoid.
Foods: Soybeans.	Heavy consumption interferes with thyroid function.
Marijuana:	None expected.
Tobacco:	None expected.

*See Glossary

DICLOXACILLIN

BRAND NAMES

Dycill   Pathocil
Dynapen

BASIC INFORMATION

Habit forming? No
Prescription needed? Yes
Available as generic? Yes
Drug class: Antibiotic (penicillin)

 USES

Treatment of bacterial infections that are
susceptible to dicloxacillin.

 DOSAGE & USAGE INFORMATION

How to take:
- Capsules—Swallow with liquid on an empty
  stomach 1 hour before or 2 hours after
  eating.
- Liquid—Take with cold beverage. Liquid form
  is perishable and effective for only 7 days at
  room temperature. Effective for 14 days if
  stored in refrigerator. Don't freeze.

When to take:
Follow instructions on prescription label or side
of package. Doses should be evenly spaced.
For example, 4 times a day means every 6
hours.

If you forget a dose:
Take as soon as you remember. Continue
regular schedule.

What drug does:
Destroys susceptible bacteria. Does not kill
viruses.

Time lapse before drug works:
May be several days before medicine affects
infection.

Don't take with:
Any other medicine without consulting your
doctor or pharmacist.

 OVERDOSE

SYMPTOMS:
Severe diarrhea, nausea or vomiting.
WHAT TO DO:
**Overdose unlikely to threaten life. If person
takes much larger amount than prescribed,
call doctor, poison-control center or
hospital emergency room for instructions.**

 POSSIBLE ADVERSE REACTIONS OR SIDE EFFECTS

SYMPTOMS	WHAT TO DO
Life-threatening:	
Hives, rash, intense itching, faintness soon after a dose (anaphylaxis).	Seek emergency treatment immediately.
Common:	
Dark or discolored tongue.	Continue. Tell doctor at next visit.
Infrequent:	
• Mild nausea, vomiting, diarrhea.	Continue. Call doctor when convenient.
• Bloody urine, face and ankle swelling.	Discontinue. Call doctor right away.
Rare:	
Unexplained bleeding or bruising, weakness, sore throat, fever, abdominal cramps, convulsions.	Discontinue. Call doctor right away.

WARNINGS & PRECAUTIONS

Don't take if:
You are allergic to dicloxacillin, cephalosporin antibiotics, other penicillins or penicillamine. Life-threatening reaction may occur.

Before you start, consult your doctor:
- If you are allergic to any substance or drug.
- If you take birth control pills.

Over age 60:
You may have skin reactions, particularly around genitals and anus.

Pregnancy:
Studies inconclusive on harm to unborn child. Animal studies show fetal abnormalities. Decide with your doctor whether drug benefits justify risk to unborn child.

Breast-feeding:
Drug passes into milk. Child may become sensitive to penicillins and have allergic reactions to penicillin drugs. Avoid dicloxacillin or discontinue nursing until you finish medicine. Consult doctor for advice on maintaining milk supply.

Infants & children:
No problems expected.

Prolonged use:
- You may become more susceptible to infections caused by germs not responsive to dicloxacillin.
- Talk to your doctor about the need for follow-up medical examinations or laboratory studies to check SGPT*, SGOT*.

Skin & sunlight:
No problems expected.

Driving, piloting or hazardous work:
Usually not dangerous. Most hazardous reactions likely to occur a few minutes after taking dicloxacillin.

Discontinuing:
Don't discontinue without doctor's advice until you complete prescribed dose, even though symptoms diminish or disappear.

Others:
- May interfere with the accuracy of some medical tests.
- Birth control pills may not be effective. Use additional birth-control methods.

POSSIBLE INTERACTION WITH OTHER DRUGS

GENERIC NAME OR DRUG CLASS	COMBINED EFFECT
Beta-adrenergic blockers*	Increased chance of anaphylaxis (see emergency information on inside front cover).
Birth control pills	Impaired contraceptive efficiency.
Chloramphenicol	Decreased effect of both drugs.
Erythromycins*	Decreased effect of both drugs.
Loperamlde	Decreased dicloxacillin effect.
Paromomycin	Decreased effect of both drugs.
Probenecid	Increased effect of all penicillins.
Tetracyclines*	Decreased effect of both drugs.
Sodium benzoate & sodium phenylacetate	May reduce effect of sodium benzoate & sodium phenylacetate.
Troleandomycin	Decreased effect of both drugs.

POSSIBLE INTERACTION WITH OTHER SUBSTANCES

INTERACTS WITH	COMBINED EFFECT
Alcohol:	Occasional stomach irritation.
Beverages:	None expected.
Cocaine:	No proven problems.
Foods: Acidic fruits or juices, aged cheese, wines, syrups (if taken with).	Decreased antibiotic effect.
Marijuana:	No proven problems.
Tobacco:	None expected.

DICYCLOMINE

BRAND NAMES

See complete list of brand names in the *Brand Name Directory*, page 919.

BASIC INFORMATION

Habit forming? No
Prescription needed?
 Low strength: No
 High strength: Yes
Available as generic? Yes
Drug class: Antispasmodic, anticholinergic

 ## USES

Reduces spasms of digestive system, bladder and urethra.

 ## DOSAGE & USAGE INFORMATION

How to take:
Tablet, syrup or capsule—Swallow with liquid or food to lessen stomach irritation.

When to take:
30 minutes before meals (unless directed otherwise by doctor).

If you forget a dose:
Take as soon as you remember up to 2 hours late. If more than 2 hours, wait for next scheduled dose (don't double this dose).

What drug does:
Blocks nerve impulses at parasympathetic nerve endings, preventing muscle contractions and gland secretions of organs involved.

Time lapse before drug works:
15 to 30 minutes.

Don't take with:
Any other medicine without consulting your doctor or pharmacist.

 ## OVERDOSE

SYMPTOMS:
Dilated pupils, blurred vision, rapid pulse and breathing, dizziness, fever, hallucinations, confusion, slurred speech, agitation, flushed face, convulsions, coma.
WHAT TO DO:
- **Dial 0 (operator) or 911 (emergency) for an ambulance or medical help. Then give first aid immediately.**
- **See emergency information on inside covers.**

 ## POSSIBLE ADVERSE REACTIONS OR SIDE EFFECTS

SYMPTOMS	WHAT TO DO
Life-threatening:	
Hives, rash, intense itching, faintness soon after a dose (anaphylaxis).	Seek emergency treatment immediately.
Common:	
• Confusion, delirium, rapid heartbeat.	Discontinue. Call doctor right away.
• Nausea, vomiting, decreased sweating.	Continue. Call doctor when convenient.
• Constipation, loss of taste.	Continue. Tell doctor at next visit.
• Dry ears, nose, throat, mouth.	No action necessary.
Infrequent:	
• Headache, difficult urination, nasal congestion, altered taste.	Continue. Call doctor when convenient.
• Lightheadedness.	Discontinue. Call doctor right away.
Rare:	
Rash or hives, eye pain, blurred vision.	Discontinue. Call doctor right away.

 ## WARNINGS & PRECAUTIONS

Don't take if:
- You are allergic to any anticholinergic.
- You have trouble with stomach bloating.
- You have difficulty emptying your bladder completely.
- You have narrow-angle glaucoma.
- You have severe ulcerative colitis.

Before you start, consult your doctor:
- If you have open-angle glaucoma.
- If you have angina, chronic bronchitis or asthma.
- If you have hiatal hernia, liver disease, kidney or thyroid disease, enlarged prostate, myasthenia gravis, peptic ulcer.
- If you will have surgery within 2 months, including dental surgery, requiring general or spinal anesthesia.

Over age 60:
Adverse reactions and side effects may be more frequent and severe than in younger persons.

Pregnancy:
Studies inconclusive on harm to unborn child. Animal studies show fetal abnormalities. Decide with your doctor whether drug benefits justify risk to unborn child.

Breast-feeding:
Drug passes into milk and decreases milk flow. Avoid drug or discontinue nursing until you finish medicine. Consult doctor for advice on maintaining milk supply.

Infants & children:
Use only under medical supervision.

Prolonged use:
Chronic constipation, possible fecal impaction. Consult doctor immediately.

Skin & sunlight:
No problems expected.

Driving, piloting or hazardous work:
Use disqualifies you for piloting aircraft. Otherwise, no problems expected.

Discontinuing:
May be unnecessary to finish medicine. Follow doctor's instructions.

Others:
Advise any doctor or dentist whom you consult that you take this medicine.

 POSSIBLE INTERACTION WITH OTHER DRUGS

GENERIC NAME OR DRUG CLASS	COMBINED EFFECT
Amantadine	Increased dicyclomine effect.
Antacids*	Decreased dicyclomine effect.
Anticholinergics, other*	Increased dicyclomine effect.
Antidepressants, tricyclic (TCA)*	Increased dicyclomine effect. Increased sedation.
Antidiarrheals*	Decreased dicyclomine effect.
Antihistamines*	Increased dicyclomine effect.
Attapulgite	Decreased dicyclomine effect.
Buclizine	Increased dicyclomine effect.
Cortisone drugs*	Increased internal-eye pressure.
Digitalis	Possible decreased absorption of digitalis.
Haloperidol	Increased internal-eye pressure.
Ketoconazole	Decreased ketoconazole effect.

MAO inhibitors*	Increased dicyclomine effect.
Meperidine	Increased dicyclomine effect.
Methylphenidate	Increased dicyclomine effect.
Nitrates*	Increased internal-eye pressure.
Nizatidine	Increased nizatidine effect.
Orphenadrine	Increased dicyclomine effect.
Phenothiazines*	Increased dicyclomine effect.
Pilocarpine	Loss of pilocarpine effect in glaucoma treatment.
Potassium supplements*	Possible intestinal ulcers with oral potassium tablets.
Quinidine	Increased dicyclomine effect.
Sedatives* or central nervous system (CNS) depressants*	Increased sedative effect of both drugs.
Vitamin C	Decreased dicyclomine effect. Avoid large doses of vitamin C.

 POSSIBLE INTERACTION WITH OTHER SUBSTANCES

INTERACTS WITH	COMBINED EFFECT
Alcohol:	None expected.
Beverages:	None expected.
Cocaine:	Excessively rapid heartbeat. Avoid.
Foods:	None expected.
Marijuana:	Drowsiness and dry mouth.
Tobacco:	None expected.

*See Glossary

DIDANOSINE

BRAND NAMES

Videx

BASIC INFORMATION

Habit forming? No
Prescription needed? Yes
Available as generic? No
Drug class: Antiviral

 ## USES

- Treats human immunodeficiency virus (HIV).
- Treats acquired immunodeficiency syndrome (AIDS).

 ## DOSAGE & USAGE INFORMATION

How to take:
Tablets—Swallow with liquid. If you can't swallow whole, crumble tablet, mix with at least 1 ounce of water and swallow immediately.

When to take:
At the same times each day, according to instructions on prescription label.

If you forget a dose:
Take as soon as you remember up to 2 hours late. If more than 2 hours, wait for next scheduled dose (don't double this dose).

What drug does:
Suppresses replication of human immunodeficiency virus.

Time lapse before drug works:
90 minutes.

Don't take with:
See Interaction column and consult doctor.

 ## OVERDOSE

SYMPTOMS:
Seizures.
WHAT TO DO:
- Dial 0 (operator) or 911 (emergency) for an ambulance or medical help. Then give first aid immediately.
- See emergency information on inside covers.

 ## POSSIBLE ADVERSE REACTIONS OR SIDE EFFECTS

SYMPTOMS	WHAT TO DO
Life-threatening:	
Seizures.	Seek emergency treatment immediately.
Common:	
• Tingling, numbness and burning in the feet and ankles.	Discontinue. Call doctor right away.
• Headache, restlessness, digestive disturbances, diarrhea.	Continue. Call doctor when convenient.
Infrequent:	
Unusual tiredness and weakness, fever, chills, sore throat, unusual bleeding or bruising, yellow skin and eyes, skin rash.	Discontinue. Call doctor right away.
Rare:	
None expected.	

 ## WARNINGS & PRECAUTIONS

Don't take if:
You are allergic to didanosine.

Before you start, consult your doctor:
- If you are an alcoholic.
- If you have hypertriglyceridemia or pancreatitis.
- If you have any condition requiring sodium restriction.
- If you have liver disease, impaired liver function or peripheral neuropathy.

Over age 60:
No special problems expected.

Pregnancy:
Unknown effect.

Breast-feeding:
Unknown effect.

Infants & children:
May cause depigmentation of the retina.

Prolonged use:
No special problems expected.

Skin & sunlight:
No special problems expected.

Driving, piloting or hazardous work:
Don't drive or pilot aircraft until you learn how medicine affects you. Don't work around dangerous machinery. Don't climb ladders or work in high places. Danger increases if you drink alcohol or take medicine affecting alertness and reflexes, such as antihistamines, tranquilizers, sedatives, pain medicines, narcotics and mind-altering drugs.

Discontinuing:
Don't discontinue without consulting doctor. Dose may require gradual reduction if you have taken drug for a long time. Doses of other drugs may require adjustment.

Others:
- Advise any doctor or dentist whom you consult that you take this medicine.
- Avoid sexual intercourse or use condoms to help prevent the transmission of HIV.
- Don't share needles or injectable equipment with other persons.
- The drug zidovudine should be used as the initial treatment for HIV infection since there are no controlled studies as yet on the effectiveness of didanosine in prolonging survival or decreasing the incidence of opportunistic infections.

POSSIBLE INTERACTION WITH OTHER DRUGS

GENERIC NAME OR DRUG CLASS	COMBINED EFFECT
Asparaginase	Increased risk of pancreatitis.
Azathioprine	Increased risk of pancreatitis.
Chloramphenicol	Increased risk of peripheral neuropathy.
Dapsone	Increased risk of peripheral neuropathy. Reduced absorption of both drugs.
Diuretics, thiazide*	Increased risk of pancreatitis.
Estrogens*	Increased risk of pancreatitis.
Ethambutol	Increased risk of peripheral neuropathy.
Ethionamide	Increased risk of peripheral neuropathy.
Fluoroquinolone antibacterials (antibiotics)*	Reduced antibiotic effect.

Furosemide	Increased risk of pancreatitis.
Hydralazine	Increased risk of peripheral neuropathy.
Isoniazid	Increased risk of peripheral neuropathy.
Ketoconazole	Reduced absorption of both drugs. Increased risk of pancreatitis.
Lithium	Increased risk of peripheral neuropathy.
Methyldopa	Increased risk of pancreatitis.
Metronidazole	Increased risk of peripheral neuropathy.
Nitrofurantoin	Increased risk of pancreatitis and peripheral neuropathy.
Phenytoin	Increased risk of peripheral neuropathy.
Sulfonamides*	Increased risk of pancreatitis.
Sulindac	Increased risk of pancreatitis.
Valproic acid	Increased risk of pancreatitis.
Vincristine	Increased risk of peripheral neuropathy.

POSSIBLE INTERACTION WITH OTHER SUBSTANCES

INTERACTS WITH	COMBINED EFFECT
Alcohol:	Increased chance of pancreatitis or peripheral neuropathy.
Beverages:	No proven problems.
Cocaine:	No proven problems.
Foods:	No proven problems.
Marijuana:	No proven problems.
Tobacco:	No proven problems.

*See Glossary

DIFENOXIN & ATROPINE

BRAND NAMES

Motofen

BASIC INFORMATION

Habit forming? Yes
Prescription needed? Yes
Available as generic? No
Drug class: Antidiarrheal

USES

- Reduces spasms of digestive system.
- Treats severe diarrhea.

DOSAGE & USAGE INFORMATION

How to take:
Tablet—Swallow with liquid or food to lessen stomach irritation.

When to take:
After each loose stool or every 3 to 4 hours. No more than 5 tablets in 12 hours.

If you forget a dose:
Take as soon as you remember. Don't double this dose.

What drug does:
- Blocks nerve impulses at parasympathetic nerve endings, preventing muscle contractions and gland secretions of organs involved.
- Acts on brain to decrease spasm of smooth muscle.

Time lapse before drug works:
40 to 60 minutes.

Don't take with:
- Any medicine that will decrease mental alertness or reflexes, such as alcohol, other mind-altering drugs, cough/cold medicines, antihistamines, allergy medicine, sedatives, tranquilizers (sleeping pills or "downers")

Continued next column

OVERDOSE

SYMPTOMS:
Dilated pupils, rapid pulse and breathing, dizziness, fever, hallucinations, confusion, slurred speech, agitation, flushed face, convulsions, coma.
WHAT TO DO:
- **Dial 0 (operator) or 911 (emergency) for an ambulance or medical help. Then give first aid immediately.**
- **See emergency information on inside covers.**

barbiturates, seizure medicine, narcotics, other prescription medicine for pain, muscle relaxants, anesthetics.
- See Interaction column and consult doctor.

POSSIBLE ADVERSE REACTIONS OR SIDE EFFECTS

SYMPTOMS	WHAT TO DO
Life-threatening:	
Shortness of breath, agitation, nervousness.	Discontinue. Seek emergency treatment.
Common:	
Dizziness, drowsiness.	Continue. Call doctor when convenient.
Infrequent:	
• Bloating; constipation; appetite loss; abdominal pain; blurred vision; warm, flushed skin; fast heartbeat; dry mouth.	Discontinue. Call doctor right away.
• Frequent urination, light-headedness, dry skin, headache, insomnia.	Continue. Call doctor when convenient.
Rare:	
Weakness, confusion, fever.	Continue. Call doctor when convenient.

WARNINGS & PRECAUTIONS

Don't take if:
- You are allergic to any anticholinergic.
- You have trouble with stomach bloating, difficulty emptying your bladder completely, narrow-angle glaucoma, severe ulcerative colitis.
- You are dehydrated.

Before you start, consult your doctor:
- If you have open-angle glaucoma, angina, chronic bronchitis, asthma, liver disease, hiatal hernia, enlarged prostate, myasthenia gravis, peptic ulcer.
- If you will have surgery within 2 months, including dental surgery, requiring general or spinal anesthesia.

Over age 60:
Adverse reactions and side effects may be more frequent and severe than in younger persons.

Pregnancy:
Studies inconclusive on harm to unborn child. Animal studies show fetal abnormalities. Decide with your doctor whether drug benefits justify risk to unborn child.

Breast-feeding:
Drug passes into milk. Avoid drug or discontinue nursing until you finish medicine. Consult doctor for advice on maintaining milk supply.

Infants & children:
Use only under medical supervision.

Prolonged use:
- Chronic constipation, possible fecal impaction. Consult doctor immediately.
- Talk to your doctor about the need for follow-up medical examinations or laboratory studies to check liver function.

Skin & sunlight:
No problems expected.

Driving, piloting or hazardous work:
Use disqualifies you for piloting aircraft. Otherwise, no problems expected.

Discontinuing:
May be unnecessary to finish medicine. Follow doctor's instructions.

Others:
Atropine included at doses below therapeutic level to prevent abuse.

 ## POSSIBLE INTERACTION WITH OTHER DRUGS

GENERIC NAME OR DRUG CLASS	COMBINED EFFECT
Addictive substances (narcotics,* others)	Increased chance of abuse.
Amantadine	Increased atropine effect.
Anticholinergics, other*	Increased atropine effect.
Antidepressants, tricyclic (TCA)*	Increased atropine effect. Increased sedation.
Antihistamines*	Increased atropine effect.
Antihypertensives*	Increased sedation.
Clozapine	Toxic effect on the central nervous system.
Cortisone drugs*	Increased internal-eye pressure.
Ethinamate	Dangerous increased effects of ethinamate. Avoid combining.
Fluoxetine	Increased depressant effects of both drugs.
Guanfacine	May increase depressant effects of either drug.
Haloperidol	Increased internal-eye pressure.
Leucovorin	High alcohol content of leucovorin may cause adverse effects.
MAO inhibitors*	Increased atropine effect.
Meperidine	Increased atropine effect.
Methylphenidate	Increased atropine effect.
Methyprylon	Increased sedative effect, perhaps to dangerous level. Avoid.
Nabilone	Greater depression of central nervous system.
Naltrexone	Triggers withdrawal symptoms.
Narcotics*	Increased sedation. Avoid.
Nitrates*	Increased internal-eye pressure.
Orphenadrine	Increased atropine effect.
Phenothiazines*	Increased atropine effect.
Pilocarpine	Loss of pilocarpine effect in glaucoma treatment.
Potassium supplements*	Possible intestinal ulcers with oral potassium tablets.
Procainamide	Increased atropine effect.
Sertraline	Increased depressive effects of both drugs.
Vitamin C	Decreased atropine effect. Avoid large doses of vitamin C.

 ## POSSIBLE INTERACTION WITH OTHER SUBSTANCES

INTERACTS WITH	COMBINED EFFECT
Alcohol:	Increased sedation. Avoid.
Beverages:	None expected.
Cocaine:	Excessively rapid heartbeat. Avoid.
Foods:	None expected.
Marijuana:	Drowsiness and dry mouth.
Tobacco:	May increase diarrhea. Avoid.

*See Glossary

DIGITALIS PREPARATIONS
(Digitalis Glycosides)

BRAND AND GENERIC NAMES

Crystodigin
DIGITALIS
DIGITOXIN
DIGOXIN

Lanoxicaps
Lanoxin
Novodigoxin

BASIC INFORMATION

Habit forming? No
Prescription needed? Yes
Available as generic? Yes
Drug class: Digitalis preparation

 USES

- Strengthens weak heart-muscle contractions to prevent congestive heart failure.
- Corrects irregular heartbeat.

 DOSAGE & USAGE INFORMATION

How to take:
- Tablet or capsule—Swallow with liquid. If you can't swallow whole, crumble tablet or open capsule and take with liquid or food.
- Liquid—Dilute dose in beverage before swallowing.

When to take:
At the same time each day.

If you forget a dose:
Take as soon as you remember up to 12 hours late. If more than 12 hours, wait for next scheduled dose (don't double this dose).

What drug does:
- Strengthens heart-muscle contraction.
- Delays nerve impulses to heart.

Time lapse before drug works:
May require regular use for a week or more.

Continued next column

 OVERDOSE

SYMPTOMS:
Nausea, vomiting, diarrhea, vision disturbances, halos around lights, fatigue, irregular heartbeat, confusion, hallucinations, convulsions.
WHAT TO DO:
- Dial 0 (operator) or 911 (emergency) for an ambulance or medical help. Then give first aid immediately.
- See emergency information on inside covers.

Don't take with:
- Non-prescription drugs without consulting doctor.
- See Interaction column and consult doctor.

 POSSIBLE ADVERSE REACTIONS OR SIDE EFFECTS

SYMPTOMS	WHAT TO DO
Life-threatening:	
In case of overdose, see previous column.	
Common:	
Appetite loss, diarrhea.	Continue. Call doctor when convenient.
Infrequent:	
Extreme drowsiness, lethargy, disorientation, headache, fainting.	Discontinue. Call doctor right away.
Rare:	
• Rash, hives, cardiac arrhythmias, hallucinations, psychosis.	Discontinue. Call doctor right away.
• Double or yellow-green vision; enlarged, sensitive male breasts; tiredness; weakness; depression; decreased sex drive.	Continue. Call doctor when convenient.

 WARNINGS & PRECAUTIONS

Don't take if:
- You are allergic to any digitalis preparation.
- Your heartbeat is slower than 50 beats per minute.

Before you start, consult your doctor:
- If you have taken another digitalis preparation in past 2 weeks.
- If you have taken a diuretic within 2 weeks.
- If you have liver or kidney disease.
- If you have a thyroid disorder.
- If you will have surgery within 2 months, including dental surgery, requiring general or spinal anesthesia.

Over age 60:
Adverse reactions and side effects may be more frequent and severe than in younger persons.

Pregnancy:
Studies inconclusive on harm to unborn child. Consult your doctor.

Breast-feeding:
Drug filters into milk. May harm child. Avoid.

Infants & children:
Use only under medical supervision.

DIGITALIS PREPARATIONS
(Digitalis Glycosides)

Prolonged use:
Talk to your doctor about the need for follow-up medical examinations or laboratory studies to check ECG*, liver function, kidney function, serum electrolytes.

Skin & sunlight:
No problems expected.

Driving, piloting or hazardous work:
Possible vision disturbances. Otherwise, no problems expected.

Discontinuing:
Don't stop without doctor's advice.

Others:
Some digitalis products contain tartrazine dye. Avoid, especially if you are allergic to aspirin.

 POSSIBLE INTERACTION WITH OTHER DRUGS

GENERIC NAME OR DRUG CLASS	COMBINED EFFECT
Amiodarone	Increased digitalis effect.
Amphotericin B	Decreased potassium. Increased toxicity of amphotericin B.
Antacids*	Decreased digitalis effect.
Anticonvulsants, hydantoin*	Increased digitalis effect at first, then decreased.
Anticholinergics*	Possible increased digitalis effect.
Attapulgite	May decrease effectiveness of digitalis.
Beta-adrenergic blockers*	Increased digitalis effect.
Beta-agonists*	Increased risk of heartbeat irregularity.
Calcium supplements*	Decreased digitalis effects.
Carteolol	Can either increase or decrease heart rate. Improves irregular heartbeat.
Cholestyramine	Decreased digitalis effect.
Colestipol	Decreased digitalis effect.
Cortisone drugs*	Digitalis toxicity.
Dextrothyroxine	Decreased digitalis effect.
Disopyramide	Possible decreased digitalis effect.
Diuretics*	Possible digitalis toxicity. Excessive potassium loss that may cause irregular heartbeat.
Ephedrine	Disturbed heart rhythm. Avoid.
Epinephrine	Disturbed heart rhythm. Avoid.
Erythromycins*	May increase digitalis absorption.
Flecainide	May increase digitalis blood level.
Fluoxetine	May cause confusion, agitation, convulsions and high blood pressure. Avoid combining.
Hydroxychloroquine	Possible increased digitalis toxicity.
Laxatives*	Decreased digitalis effect.
Metoclopramide	Decreased digitalis absorption.

Continued page 943

 POSSIBLE INTERACTION WITH OTHER SUBSTANCES

INTERACTS WITH	COMBINED EFFECT
Alcohol:	None expected.
Beverages: Caffeine drinks.	Irregular heartbeat. Avoid.
Cocaine:	Irregular heartbeat. Avoid.
Foods: Prune juice, bran cereals, foods high in fiber.	Decreased digitalis effect.
Marijuana:	Decreased digitalis effect.
Tobacco:	Irregular heartbeat. Avoid.

*See Glossary

DIMETHYL SULFOXIDE (DMSO)

BRAND NAMES

Rimso-50

BASIC INFORMATION

Habit forming? No
Prescription needed? Yes
Available as generic? Yes
Drug class: Anti-inflammatory (local)

 USES

When applied directly to the bladder's membrane lining, DMSO relieves symptoms of bladder inflammation.

 DOSAGE & USAGE INFORMATION

How to use:
Under doctor's guidance, directly instill into urinary bladder using a catheter or aseptic syringe. Allow to remain in bladder about 15 minutes, then void. *Note:* Follow doctor's instructions.

When to use:
Follow doctor's instructions.

If you forget a dose:
Take as soon as you remember up to 2 hours late. If more than 2 hours, wait for next scheduled dose (don't double this dose).

What drug does:
Reduces inflammation by unknown mechanism.

Time lapse before drug works:
Works quickly (within minutes).

Don't take with:
Any other medicines (including over-the-counter drugs such as cough and cold medicines, laxatives, antacids, diet pills, caffeine, nose drops or vitamins) without consulting your doctor.

 OVERDOSE

SYMPTOMS:
None expected.
WHAT TO DO:
Overdose unlikely to threaten life. If person takes much larger amount than prescribed, call doctor, poison-control center or hospital emergency room for instructions.

 POSSIBLE ADVERSE REACTIONS OR SIDE EFFECTS

SYMPTOMS	WHAT TO DO
Life-threatening:	
Breathing difficulty.	Seek emergency treatment immediately.
Common:	
Garlic-like taste for up to 72 hours.	No action necessary.
Infrequent:	
Vision problems (not documented in humans, but well-documented in animals).	Continue. Call doctor when convenient.
Rare:	
Nasal congestion, itching, hives, facial swelling.	Discontinue. Seek emergency treatment.

WARNINGS & PRECAUTIONS

Don't use if:
- You have a bladder malignancy.
- You are allergic to DMSO.

Before you start, consult your doctor:
If you have visual problems.

Over age 60:
No special problems expected.

Pregnancy:
Risk to unborn child outweighs drug benefits. Don't use.

Breast-feeding:
Effect not documented. Consult your doctor.

Infants & children:
Not recommended.

Prolonged use:
Talk to your doctor about the need for follow-up medical examinations or laboratory studies to check liver and kidney function, complete blood counts (white blood cell count, platelet count, red blood cell count, hemoglobin, hematocrit) and vision.

Skin & sunlight:
No special problems expected.

Driving, piloting or hazardous work:
No special problems expected.

Discontinuing:
No special problems expected.

Others:
Although readily available in impure forms, DMSO has *not* proven effective or safe for sprains, strains, arthritis, scleroderma, gout, skin infections, burns or other uses. Many studies are underway for safety and efficacy for conditions other than bladder inflammation.

POSSIBLE INTERACTION WITH OTHER DRUGS

GENERIC NAME OR DRUG CLASS	COMBINED EFFECT
Any other drug used inside the bladder	Increased effect of both medicines.

POSSIBLE INTERACTION WITH OTHER SUBSTANCES

INTERACTS WITH	COMBINED EFFECT
Alcohol:	No special problems expected.
Beverages:	No special problems expected.
Cocaine:	No special problems expected.
Foods:	No special problems expected.
Marijuana:	No special problems expected.
Tobacco:	No special problems expected.

DINOPROSTONE (Vaginal)

BRAND NAMES

Prostin E2

BASIC INFORMATION

Habit forming? No
Prescription needed? Yes
Available as generic? No
Drug class: Abortifacient (a prostoglandin), uterine stimulant

 USES

- To induce abortion from 12th through 20th week of pregnancy. Sometimes used with other substances such as urea, hypertonic saline, oxytocin.
- To empty uterus of a dead fetus, resulting from a missed abortion.
- Reduces blood loss after delivery (sometimes).

 DOSAGE & USAGE INFORMATION

How to use:
- Allow suppository to warm to room temperature prior to use.
- Insert suppository into vagina and remain lying down for 10 minutes.
- Take prescribed medicines for vomiting and diarrhea prior to taking dinoprostone.
- Frequently used during hospitalization to allow close monitoring of pulse, blood pressure and temperature.

When to use:
As directed by your doctor.

What drug does:
Stimulates contractions of the uterus and softens the cervix.

Time lapse before drug works:
Varies from patient to patient.

Don't use with:
Oxytocin or other medications to induce abortions.

 OVERDOSE

SYMPTOMS:
Drop in blood pressure, wheezing, tightness in chest.
WHAT TO DO:
This medication is used only under medical supervision, so the necessary steps to treat overdose or hypersensitivity will be recognized and used by your doctor.

 POSSIBLE ADVERSE REACTIONS OR SIDE EFFECTS

SYMPTOMS	WHAT TO DO
Life-threatening:	
Excessive bleeding.	Discontinue. Seek emergency treatment.
Common:	
• Fever that doesn't return to normal by 6 hours after using (about 50%).	Discontinue. Call doctor right away.
• Diarrhea (about 40%).	Continue. Call doctor when convenient.
• Nausea and vomiting (about 67%).	Continue. Call doctor when convenient.
Infrequent:	
Chills, headache.	Continue. Call doctor when convenient.
Rare:	
None expected.	

DINOPROSTONE (Vaginal)

WARNINGS & PRECAUTIONS

Don't use if:
- You have had allergic or unusual reaction previously to dinoprostone.
- Membranes have ruptured.
- You have heart, liver or kidney disease.

Before you start, consult your doctor:
If you have anemia, asthma, lung disease, active heart disease, high blood pressure, low blood pressure, cervical stenosis, past surgery on the uterus, infected cervix, diabetes, epilepsy, glaucoma, liver disease, history of jaundice, acute pelvic inflammatory disease, kidney disease.

Over age 60:
Not used.

Infants & children:
Not used.

Prolonged use:
Not used.

Skin & sunlight:
No problems expected.

Driving, piloting or hazardous work:
Don't drive or pilot aircraft until you learn how medicine affects you. Don't work around dangerous machinery. Don't climb ladders or work in high places. Danger increases if you drink alcohol or take medicine affecting alertness and reflexes, such as antihistamines, tranquilizers, sedatives, pain medicine, narcotics and mind-altering drugs.

Discontinuing:
Some symptoms may be experienced such as unusual bleeding, fever, chills, foul-smelling vaginal discharge, abdominal pain. If any occur, notify your doctor immediately.

Others:
Make sure in your own mind that you are using this medication of your own free will, not the will of others imposed on you.

POSSIBLE INTERACTION WITH OTHER DRUGS

GENERIC NAME OR DRUG CLASS	COMBINED EFFECT
Clinically significant interactions with oral or injected medicines unlikely.	

POSSIBLE INTERACTION WITH OTHER SUBSTANCES

INTERACTS WITH	COMBINED EFFECT
Alcohol:	None expected.
Beverages:	None expected.
Cocaine:	None expected.
Foods:	None expected.
Marijuana:	None expected.
Tobacco:	None expected.

DIPHENIDOL

BRAND NAMES

Vontrol

BASIC INFORMATION

Habit forming? No
Prcription needed? Yes
Available as generic? No
Drug class: Antiemetic, antivertigo

 ## USES

- Prevents motion sickness.
- Controls nausea and vomiting (do not use during pregnancy).

 ## DOSAGE & USAGE INFORMATION

How to take:
Tablet—Swallow with liquid or food to lessen stomach irritation. If you can't swallow whole, crumble tablet and chew or take with liquid or food.

When to take:
30 to 60 minutes before traveling.

If you forget a dose:
Take as soon as you remember. Wait 4 hours for next dose.

What drug does:
Reduces sensitivity of nerve endings in inner ear, blocking messages to brain's vomiting center.

Time lapse before drug works:
30 to 60 minutes.

Don't take with:
Any other medicine without consulting your doctor or pharmacist.

 ## OVERDOSE

SYMPTOMS:
Drowsiness, confusion, incoordination, weak pulse, shallow breathing, stupor, coma.
WHAT TO DO:
- Dial 0 (operator) or 911 (emergency) for an ambulance or medical help. Then give first aid immediately.
- See emergency information on inside covers.

 ## POSSIBLE ADVERSE REACTIONS OR SIDE EFFECTS

SYMPTOMS	WHAT TO DO
Life-threatening:	
In case of overdose, see previous column.	
Common:	
Drowsiness.	Continue. Tell doctor at next visit.
Infrequent:	
• Headache, diarrhea or constipation, fast heartbeat, heartburn.	Continue. Call doctor when convenient.
• Dry mouth, nose, throat, dizziness.	Continue. Tell doctor at next visit.
Rare:	
• Hallucinations, confusion.	Discontinue. Seek emergency treatment.
• Rash or hives, depression, jaundice.	Discontinue. Call doctor right away.
• Restlessness; excitement; insomnia; blurred vision; urgent, painful or difficult urination.	Continue. Call doctor when convenient.
• Appetite loss, nausea, weakness.	Continue. Tell doctor at next visit.

WARNINGS & PRECAUTIONS

Don't take if:
- You have severe kidney disease.
- You are allergic to diphenidol or meclizine.

Before you start, consult your doctor:
- If you have prostate enlargement.
- If you have glaucoma.
- If you have heart disease.
- If you have intestinal obstruction or ulcers in the gastrointestinal tract.
- If you have kidney disease.
- If you have low blood pressure.
- If you will have surgery within 2 months, including dental surgery, requiring general or spinal anesthesia.

Over age 60:
Adverse reactions and side effects may be more frequent and severe than in younger persons.

Pregnancy:
Animal studies show fetal abnormalities. Decide with your doctor whether drug benefits justify risk to unborn child.

Breast-feeding:
Drug passes into milk. Avoid drug or discontinue nursing until you finish medicine. Consult doctor for advice on maintaining milk supply.

Infants & children:
No problems expected.

Prolonged use:
No problems expected.

Skin & sunlight:
No problems expected.

Driving, piloting or hazardous work:
Don't fly aircraft. Don't drive until you learn how medicine affects you. Don't work around dangerous machinery. Don't climb ladders or work in high places. Danger increases if you drink alcohol or take medicine affecting alertness and reflexes, such as antihistamines, tranquilizers, sedatives, pain medicine, narcotics and mind-altering drugs.

Discontinuing:
No problems expected.

Others:
No problems expected.

POSSIBLE INTERACTION WITH OTHER DRUGS

GENERIC NAME OR DRUG CLASS	COMBINED EFFECT
Anticonvulsants*	Increased effect of both drugs.
Antidepressants, tricyclic (TCA)*	Increased sedative effect of both drugs.
Antihistamines*	Increased sedative effect of both drugs.
Atropine	Increased chance of toxic effect of atropine and atropine-like medicines.
Narcotics*	Increased sedative effect of both drugs.
Sedatives*	Increased sedative effect of both drugs.
Tranquilizers*	Increased sedative effect of both drugs.

POSSIBLE INTERACTION WITH OTHER SUBSTANCES

INTERACTS WITH	COMBINED EFFECT
Alcohol:	Increased sedation. Avoid.
Beverages: Caffeine.	May decrease drowsiness.
Cocaine:	Increased chance of toxic effects of cocaine. Avoid.
Foods:	None expected.
Marijuana:	Increased drowsiness, dry mouth.
Tobacco:	None expected.

*See Glossary

DIPHENOXYLATE & ATROPINE

BRAND NAMES

Diphenatol	Lonox
Lofene	Lo-Trol
Logen	Low-Quel
Lomanate	Nor-Mil
Lomotil	

BASIC INFORMATION

Habit forming? Yes
Prescription needed? Yes
Available as generic? Yes
Drug class: Antidiarrheal

USES

Relieves diarrhea and intestinal cramps.

DOSAGE & USAGE INFORMATION

How to take:
- Tablet—Swallow with liquid or food to lessen stomach irritation.
- Drops or liquid—Follow label instructions and use marked dropper.

When to take:
No more often than directed on label.

If you forget a dose:
Take as soon as you remember up to 2 hours late. If more than 2 hours, wait for next scheduled dose (don't double this dose).

What drug does:
Blocks digestive tract's nerve supply, which reduces propelling movements.

Continued next column

OVERDOSE

SYMPTOMS:
Excitement, constricted pupils, shallow breathing, coma.
WHAT TO DO:
- Dial 0 (operator) or 911 (emergency) for an ambulance or medical help. Then give first aid immediately.
- If patient is unconscious and not breathing, give mouth-to-mouth breathing. If there is no heartbeat, use cardiac massage and mouth-to-mouth breathing (CPR). Don't try to make patient vomit. If you can't get help quickly, take patient to nearest emergency facility.
- See emergency information on inside covers.

Time lapse before drug works:
May require 12 to 24 hours of regular doses to control diarrhea.

Don't take with:
Any other medicine without consulting your doctor or pharmacist.

POSSIBLE ADVERSE REACTIONS OR SIDE EFFECTS

SYMPTOMS	WHAT TO DO
Life-threatening:	
Hives, rash, intense itching, faintness soon after a dose (anaphylaxis).	Seek emergency treatment immediately.
Common:	
None expected.	
Infrequent:	
• Dry mouth, swollen gums, rapid heartbeat.	Discontinue. Call doctor right away.
• Dizziness, depression, drowsiness, rash or itch, blurred vision, decreased urination.	Continue. Call doctor when convenient.
Rare:	
Restlessness, flush, fever, headache, stomach pain, nausea, vomiting, bloating, constipation, numbness of hands or feet.	Discontinue. Call doctor right away.

WARNINGS & PRECAUTIONS

Don't take if:
- You are allergic to diphenoxylate and atropine or any narcotic or anticholinergic.
- You have jaundice.
- You have infectious diarrhea or antibiotic-associated diarrhea.
- Patient is younger than 2.

Before you start, consult your doctor:
- If you have had liver problems.
- If you have ulcerative colitis.
- If you plan to become pregnant within medication period.
- If you have any medical disorder.
- If you take any medication, including non-prescription drugs.

Over age 60:
Adverse reactions and side effects may be more frequent and severe than in younger persons.

Pregnancy:
No proven harm to unborn child. Avoid because of many side effects.

Breast-feeding:
Drug passes into milk. Avoid drug or discontinue nursing until you finish medicine. Consult doctor for advice on maintaining milk supply.

Infants & children:
Don't give to infants or toddlers. Use only under doctor's supervision for children older than 2.

Prolonged use:
- Habit forming.
- Talk to your doctor about the need for follow-up medical examinations or laboratory studies to check liver function.

Skin & sunlight:
No problems expected.

Driving, piloting or hazardous work:
Don't drive or pilot aircraft until you learn how medicine affects you. Don't work around dangerous machinery. Don't climb ladders or work in high places. Danger increases if you drink alcohol or take medicine affecting alertness and reflexes.

Discontinuing:
- May be unnecessary to finish medicine. Follow doctor's instructions.
- After discontinuing, consult doctor if you experience muscle cramps, nausea, vomiting, trembling, stomach cramps or unusual sweating.

Others:
If diarrhea lasts longer than 4 days, discontinue and call doctor.

POSSIBLE INTERACTION WITH OTHER DRUGS

GENERIC NAME OR DRUG CLASS	COMBINED EFFECT
Barbiturates*	Increased effect of both drugs.
Clozapine	Toxic effect on the central nervous system.
Ethinamate	Dangerous increased effects of ethinamate. Avoid combining.

Fluoxetine	Increased depressant effects of both drugs.
Guanfacine	May increase depressant effects of either drug.
Leucovorin	High alcohol content of leucovorin may cause adverse effects.
MAO inhibitors*	May increase blood pressure excessively.
Methyprylon	Increased sedative effect, perhaps to dangerous level. Avoid.
Naltrexone	Triggers withdrawal symptoms.
Narcotics*	Increased sedation. Avoid.
Sedatives*	Increased effect of both drugs.
Sertraline	Increased depressive effects of both drugs.
Tranquilizers*	Increased effect of both drugs.

POSSIBLE INTERACTION WITH OTHER SUBSTANCES

INTERACTS WITH	COMBINED EFFECT
Alcohol:	Depressed brain function. Avoid.
Beverages:	None expected.
Cocaine:	Decreased effect of diphenoxylate and atropine.
Foods:	None expected.
Marijuana:	None expected.
Tobacco:	None expected.

DIPYRIDAMOLE

BRAND NAMES

Apo-Dipyridamole
Dipimol
Dipridacot
Novodipiradol

Persantin
Persantine
Pyridamole

BASIC INFORMATION

Habit forming? No
Prescription needed?
 U.S.: Yes
 Canada: No
Available as generic? Yes
Drug class: Platelet aggregation inhibitor

 USES

- May reduce frequency and intensity of angina attacks.
- Prevents blood clots after heart surgery.

 DOSAGE & USAGE INFORMATION

How to take:
Tablet—Swallow with liquid. If you can't swallow whole, crumble tablet and take with liquid.

When to take:
1 hour before meals.

If you forget a dose:
Take as soon as you remember up to 2 hours late. If more than 2 hours, wait for next scheduled dose (don't double this dose).

Continued next column

 OVERDOSE

SYMPTOMS:
Decreased blood pressure; weak, rapid pulse; cold, clammy skin; collapse.
WHAT TO DO:
- Dial 0 (operator) or 911 (emergency) for an ambulance or medical help. Then give first aid immediately.
- If patient is unconscious and not breathing, give mouth-to-mouth breathing. If there is no heartbeat, use cardiac massage and mouth-to-mouth breathing (CPR). Don't try to make patient vomit. If you can't get help quickly, take patient to nearest emergency facility.
- See emergency information on inside covers.

What drug does:
- Probably dilates blood vessels to increase oxygen to heart.
- Prevents platelet clumping, which causes blood clots.

Time lapse before drug works:
3 months of continual use.

Don't take with:
Any other medicine without consulting your doctor or pharmacist.

 POSSIBLE ADVERSE REACTIONS OR SIDE EFFECTS

SYMPTOMS	WHAT TO DO
Life-threatening:	
In case of overdose, see previous column.	
Common:	
Dizziness.	Continue. Call doctor when convenient.
Infrequent:	
• Fainting, headache.	Discontinue. Call doctor right away.
• Red flush, rash, nausea, vomiting, cramps, weakness.	Continue. Call doctor when convenient.
Rare:	
Chest pain.	Discontinue. Call doctor right away.

WARNINGS & PRECAUTIONS

Don't take if:
• You are allergic to dipyridamole.
• You are recovering from a heart attack.

Before you start, consult your doctor:
• If you have low blood pressure.
• If you have liver disease.

Over age 60:
Begin treatment with small doses.

Pregnancy:
No proven harm to unborn child. Avoid if possible.

Breast-feeding:
No proven problems. Consult doctor.

Infants & children:
Not recommended.

Prolonged use:
Talk to your doctor about the need for follow-up medical examinations or laboratory studies.

Skin & sunlight:
No problems expected.

Driving, piloting or hazardous work:
Avoid if you feel dizzy. Otherwise, no problems expected.

Discontinuing:
Don't discontinue without doctor's advice until you complete prescribed dose, even though symptoms diminish or disappear.

Others:
Drug increases your ability to be active without angina pain. Avoid excessive physical exertion that might injure heart.

POSSIBLE INTERACTION WITH OTHER DRUGS

GENERIC NAME OR DRUG CLASS	COMBINED EFFECT
Anticoagulants, oral*	Increased anticoagulant effect. Bleeding tendency.
Aspirin and combination drugs containing aspirin	Increased dipyridamole effect. Dose may need adjustment.

POSSIBLE INTERACTION WITH OTHER SUBSTANCES

INTERACTS WITH	COMBINED EFFECT
Alcohol:	May lower blood pressure excessively.
Beverages:	None expected.
Cocaine:	No proven problems.
Foods:	Decreased dipyridamole absorption unless taken 1 hour before eating.
Marijuana:	Daily use— Decreased dipyridamole effect.
Tobacco: Nicotine.	May decrease dipyridamole effect.

*See Glossary

DISOPYRAMIDE

BRAND NAMES

Norpace	Rythmodan
Norpace CR	Rythmodan-LA

BASIC INFORMATION

Habit forming? No
Prescription needed? Yes
Available as generic? Yes
Drug class: Antiarrhythmic

USES

Corrects heart rhythm disorders.

DOSAGE & USAGE INFORMATION

How to take:
Extended-release tablet or capsule—Swallow with liquid. If you can't swallow whole, crumble tablet or open capsule and take with liquid or food.

When to take:
At the same times each day.

If you forget a dose:
Take as soon as you remember up to 2 hours late. If more than 2 hours, wait for next scheduled dose (don't double this dose).

What drug does:
Delays nerve impulses to heart to regulate heartbeat.

Time lapse before drug works:
Begins in 30 to 60 minutes. Must use for 5 to 7 days to determine effectiveness.

Don't take with:
Any other medicine without consulting your doctor or pharmacist.

OVERDOSE

SYMPTOMS:
Blood-pressure drop, irregular heartbeat, apnea, loss of consciousness.
WHAT TO DO:
- **Dial 0 (operator) or 911 (emergency) for an ambulance or medical help. Then give first aid immediately.**
- **If patient is unconscious and not breathing, give mouth-to-mouth breathing. If there is no heartbeat, use cardiac massage and mouth-to-mouth breathing (CPR). Don't try to make patient vomit. If you can't get help quickly, take patient to nearest emergency facility.**
- **See emergency information on inside covers.**

POSSIBLE ADVERSE REACTIONS OR SIDE EFFECTS

SYMPTOMS	WHAT TO DO
Life-threatening:	
Hives, rash, intense itching, faintness soon after a dose (anaphylaxis).	Seek emergency treatment immediately.
Common:	
• Hypoglycemia (cold sweats, fast heartbeat, extreme hunger, shakiness and nervousness, anxiety, cool and pale skin, drowsiness, headache).	Discontinue. Call doctor right away.
• Dry mouth, constipation, painful or difficult urination, rapid weight gain, blurred vision.	Continue. Call doctor when convenient.
Infrequent:	
• Dizziness, fainting, confusion, chest pain, nervousness, depression, slow or fast heartbeat.	Discontinue. Call doctor right away.
• Swollen feet.	Continue. Call doctor when convenient.
Rare:	
• Shortness of breath, psychosis.	Discontinue. Seek emergency treatment.
• Rash, sore throat, fever, headache, jaundice, muscle weakness.	Discontinue. Call doctor right away.
• Eye pain, diminished sex drive, numbness or tingling of hands and feet, bleeding tendency.	Continue. Call doctor when convenient.

WARNINGS & PRECAUTIONS

Don't take if:
- You are allergic to disopyramide or any antiarrhythmic.
- You have second- or third-degree heart block.
- You have heart failure.

Before you start, consult your doctor:
- If you react unfavorably to other antiarrhythmic drugs.
- If you have had heart disease.
- If you have low blood pressure.
- If you have liver disease.
- If you have glaucoma.

- If you have enlarged prostate.
- If you have myasthenia gravis.
- If you take digitalis preparations or diuretics.

Over age 60:
- May require reduced dose.
- More likely to have difficulty urinating or be constipated.
- More likely to have blood-pressure drop.

Pregnancy:
No proven harm to unborn child. Avoid if possible.

Breast-feeding:
Drug passes into milk. Avoid drug or discontinue nursing until you finish medicine. Consult doctor for advice on maintaining milk supply.

Infants & children:
Safety not established. Don't use.

Prolonged use:
Talk to your doctor about the need for follow-up medical examinations or laboratory studies to check liver function, kidney function, ECG*, blood pressure, serum potassium.

Skin & sunlight:
No problems expected.

Driving, piloting or hazardous work:
Don't drive or pilot aircraft until you learn how medicine affects you. Don't work around dangerous machinery. Don't climb ladders or work in high places. Danger increases if you drink alcohol or take medicine affecting alertness and reflexes, such as antihistamines, tranquilizers, sedatives, pain medicine, narcotics, or mind-altering drugs.

Discontinuing:
Don't discontinue without doctor's advice until you complete prescribed dose, even though symptoms diminish or disappear.

Others:
If new illness, injury or surgery occurs, tell doctors of disopyramide use.

POSSIBLE INTERACTION WITH OTHER DRUGS

GENERIC NAME OR DRUG CLASS	COMBINED EFFECT
Antiarrhythmics*	May increase effect and toxicity of each drug.
Anticholinergics*	Increased anticholinergic effect.
Anticoagulants, oral*	Possible increased anticoagulant effect.
Antihypertensives*	Increased antihypertensive effect.
Encainide	Increased effect of toxicity on the heart muscle.
Flecainide	Possible irregular heartbeat.
Nicardipine	May cause dangerously slow, fast or irregular heartbeat.
Nimodipine	May cause dangerous irregular, slow or fast heartbeat.
Phenobarbital	Increased metabolism, decreased disopyramide effect.
Phenytoin	Increased metabolism, decreased disopyramide effect.
Propafenone	Increased effect of both drugs and increased risk of toxicity.
Rifampin	Increased metabolism, decreased disopyramide effect.
Tocainide	Increased likelihood of adverse reactions with either drug.

POSSIBLE INTERACTION WITH OTHER SUBSTANCES

INTERACTS WITH	COMBINED EFFECT
Alcohol:	Decreased blood pressure and blood sugar. Use caution.
Beverages:	None expected.
Cocaine:	Irregular heartbeat.
Foods:	None expected.
Marijuana:	Unpredictable. May decrease disopyramide effect.
Tobacco:	May decrease disopyramide effect.

*See Glossary

DISULFIRAM

BRAND NAMES

Antabuse

BASIC INFORMATION

Habit forming? No
Prescription needed? Yes
Available as generic? Yes
Drug class: None

 USES

Treatment for alcoholism. Will not cure alcoholism, but is a powerful deterrent to drinking.

 DOSAGE & USAGE INFORMATION

How to take:
Tablet—Swallow with liquid.

When to take:
Morning or bedtime. Avoid if you have used *any* alcohol, tonics, cough syrups, fermented vinegar, after-shave lotion or backrub solutions within 12 hours.

If you forget a dose:
Take as soon as you remember up to 12 hours late. If more than 12 hours, wait for next scheduled dose (don't double this dose).

What drug does:
In combination with alcohol, produces a metabolic change that causes severe, temporary toxicity.

Time lapse before drug works:
3 to 12 hours.

Don't take with:
• See Interaction column and consult doctor.
• Non-prescription drugs that contain *any* alcohol.
• Any other central nervous system (CNS) depressant drugs*.

 OVERDOSE

SYMPTOMS:
Memory loss, behavior disturbances, lethargy, confusion and headaches; nausea, vomiting, stomach pain and diarrhea; weakness and unsteady walk; temporary paralysis.
WHAT TO DO:
• **Dial 0 (operator) or 911 (emergency) for an ambulance or medical help. Then give first aid immediately.**
• **See emergency information on inside covers.**

 POSSIBLE ADVERSE REACTIONS OR SIDE EFFECTS

SYMPTOMS	WHAT TO DO
Life-threatening:	
In case of overdose, see previous column.	
Common:	
Drowsiness.	Continue. Tell doctor at next visit.
Infrequent:	
• Eye pain, vision changes, abdominal discomfort, throbbing headache, numbness in hands and feet.	Continue. Call doctor when convenient.
• Mood change, decreased sexual ability in men, tiredness.	Continue. Tell doctor at next visit.
• Bad taste in mouth (metal or garlic).	No action necessary.
Rare:	
Rash, jaundice.	Discontinue. Call doctor right away.

 WARNINGS & PRECAUTIONS

Don't take if:
• You are allergic to disulfiram (alcohol-disulfiram combination is not an allergic reaction).
• You have used alcohol in any form or amount within 12 hours.
• You have taken paraldehyde within 1 week.
• You have heart disease.

Before you start, consult your doctor:
• If you have allergies.
• If you plan to become pregnant within medication period.
• If no one has explained to you how disulfiram reacts.
• If you think you cannot avoid drinking.
• If you have diabetes, epilepsy, liver or kidney disease.
• If you take other drugs.

DISULFIRAM

Over age 60:
Adverse reactions and side effects may be more frequent and severe than in younger persons.

Pregnancy:
Risk to unborn child outweighs drug benefits. Don't use.

Breast-feeding:
Studies inconclusive. Consult your doctor.

Infants & children:
Not recommended.

Prolonged use:
Periodic blood-cell counts and liver-function tests recommended if you take this drug a long time.

Skin & sunlight:
No problems expected.

Driving, piloting or hazardous work:
Avoid if you feel drowsy or have vision side effects. Otherwise, no restrictions.

Discontinuing:
Don't discontinue without consulting doctor. Dose may require gradual reduction if you have taken drug for a long time. Doses of other drugs may also require adjustment. Avoid alcohol at least 14 days following last dose.

Others:
Check all liquids that you take or rub on for presence of alcohol.

POSSIBLE INTERACTION WITH OTHER DRUGS

GENERIC NAME OR DRUG CLASS	COMBINED EFFECT
Anticoagulants*	Possible unexplained bleeding.
Anticonvulsants*	Excessive sedation.
Barbiturates*	Excessive sedation.
Cephalosporins*	Disulfiram reaction.*
Clozapine	Toxic effect on the central nervous system.
Ethinamate	Dangerous increased effects of ethinamate. Avoid combining.
Fluoxetine	Increased depressant effects of both drugs.
Guanfacine	May increase depressant effects of either drug.
Isoniazid	Unsteady walk and disturbed behavior.
Leucovorin	High alcohol content of leucovorin may cause adverse effects.
Methyprylon	Increased sedative effect, perhaps to dangerous level. Avoid.
Metronidazole	Disulfiram reaction.*
Nabilone	Greater depression of central nervous system.
Paraldehyde	Increased paraldehyde effect. Avoid simultaneous use.
Sedatives*	Excessive sedation.
Sertraline	Increased depressive effects of both drugs.

POSSIBLE INTERACTION WITH OTHER SUBSTANCES

INTERACTS WITH	COMBINED EFFECT
Alcohol: *Any* form or amount.	Possible life-threatening toxicity. See disulfiram reaction.*
Beverages: Punch or fruit drink that may contain alcohol.	Disulfiram reaction.*
Cocaine:	Increased disulfiram effect.
Foods: Sauces, fermented vinegar, marinades, desserts or other foods prepared with *any* alcohol.	Disulfiram reaction.*
Marijuana:	None expected.
Tobacco:	None expected.

*See Glossary

DIURETICS, LOOP

BRAND AND GENERIC NAMES

Apo-Furosemide	Furoside
Bumex	Lasix
BUMETANIDE	Lasix Special
Edecrin	Myrosemide
ETHACRYNIC ACID	Novosemide
FUROSEMIDE	Uritol

BASIC INFORMATION

Habit forming? No
Prescription needed? Yes
Available as generic? Yes
Drug class: Diuretic (loop), antihypertensive

 USES

- Lowers high blood pressure.
- Decreases fluid retention.

 DOSAGE & USAGE INFORMATION

How to take:
Tablet or liquid—Swallow with liquid. If you can't swallow whole, crumble tablet and take with liquid or food.

When to take:
- 1 dose a day—Take after breakfast.
- More than 1 dose a day—Take last dose no later than 6 p.m. unless otherwise directed.

If you forget a dose:
- 1 dose a day—Take as soon as you remember up to 12 hours late. If more than 12 hours, wait for next scheduled dose (don't double this dose).
- More than 1 dose a day—Take as soon as you remember up to 2 hours late. If more than 2 hours, wait for next scheduled dose (don't double this dose).

What drug does:
Increases elimination of sodium and water from body. Decreased body fluid reduces blood pressure.

Continued next column

 OVERDOSE

SYMPTOMS:
Weakness, lethargy, dizziness, confusion, nausea, vomiting, leg muscle cramps, thirst, stupor, deep sleep, weak and rapid pulse, cardiac arrest.
WHAT TO DO:
- **Dial 0 (operator) or 911 (emergency) for an ambulance or medical help. Then give first aid immediately.**
- **See emergency information on inside covers.**

Time lapse before drug works:
1 hour to increase water loss. Requires 2 to 3 weeks to lower blood pressure.

Don't take with:
- Non-prescription drugs with aspirin.
- Any other medicine without consulting your doctor.

 POSSIBLE ADVERSE REACTIONS OR SIDE EFFECTS

SYMPTOMS	WHAT TO DO
Life-threatening:	
In case of overdose, see previous column.	
Common:	
Dizziness.	Continue. Call doctor when convenient.
Infrequent:	
Mood change, fatigue, appetite loss, diarrhea, irregular heartbeat, muscle cramps, low blood pressure, abdominal pain, weakness.	Discontinue. Call doctor right away.
Rare:	
Rash or hives, yellow vision, ringing in ears, hearing loss, sore throat, fever, dry mouth, thirst, side or stomach pain, nausea, vomiting, unusual bleeding or bruising, joint pain, jaundice, numbness or tingling in hands or feet.	Discontinue. Call doctor right away.

 WARNINGS & PRECAUTIONS

Don't take if:
You are allergic to loop diuretics.

Before you start, consult your doctor:
- If you are taking any other prescription or non-prescription medicine.
- If you are allergic to any sulfa drug.
- If you have liver or kidney disease.
- If you have gout, diabetes or impaired hearing.
- If you will have surgery within 2 months, including dental surgery, requiring general or spinal anesthesia.

Over age 60:
Adverse reactions and side effects may be more frequent and severe than in younger persons.

Pregnancy:
Risk to unborn child outweighs drug benefits. Don't use.

Breast-feeding:
Drug filters into milk. May harm child. Avoid.

Infants & children:
Use only under medical supervision.

Prolonged use:
- Impaired balance of water, salt and potassium in blood and body tissues.
- Possible diabetes.

Skin & sunlight:
May cause rash or intensify sunburn in areas exposed to sun or sunlamp.

Driving, piloting or hazardous work:
No problems expected.

Discontinuing:
Don't discontinue without doctor's advice until you complete prescribed dose, even though symptoms diminish or disappear.

Others:
Frequent laboratory studies to monitor potassium level in blood recommended. Eat foods rich in potassium or take potassium supplements. Consult doctor.

POSSIBLE INTERACTION WITH OTHER DRUGS

GENERIC NAME OR DRUG CLASS	COMBINED EFFECT
ACE inhibitors*: captopril, enalapril, llsinopril	Possible excessive potassium in blood.
Allopurinol	Decreased allopurinol effect.
Amiodarone	Increased risk of heartbeat irregularity due to low potassium.
Anticoagulants*	Abnormal clotting.
Antidepressants, tricyclic (TCA)*	Excessive blood-pressure drop.
Antidiabetics, oral*	Decreased anti-diabetic effect.
Antihypertensives*	Increased antihypertensive effect. Dosages may require adjustment.
Barbiturates*	Low blood pressure.
Beta-adrenergic blockers*	Increased antihypertensive effect. Dosages may require adjustment.

Corticosteroids*	Decreased potassium.
Cortisone drugs*	Excessive potassium loss.
Digitalis preparations*	Excessive potassium loss could lead to serious heart rhythm disorders.
Diuretics, other*	Increased diuretic effect.
Hypokalemia-causing medicines*	Increased risk of excessive potassium loss.
Insulin	Decreased insulin effect.
Lithium	Increased lithium toxicity.
Narcotics*	Dangerous low blood pressure. Avoid.
Nephrotoxics*	Incresed risk of toxicity.
Nimodipine	Dangerous blood pressure drop.
Nitrates*	Excessive blood pressure drop.
Non-steroidal anti-inflammatory drugs (NSAIDs)*	Decreased diuretic effect.
Phenytoin	Decreased diuretic effect.
Potassium supplements*	Decreased potassium effect.
Probenecid	Decreased probenecid effect.
Salicylates* (including aspirin)	Dangerous salicylate retention.
Sedatives*	Increased diuretic effect.

POSSIBLE INTERACTION WITH OTHER SUBSTANCES

INTERACTS WITH	COMBINED EFFECT
Alcohol:	Blood pressure drop. Avoid.
Beverages:	None expected.
Cocaine:	Dangerous blood pressure drop. Avoid.
Foods:	None expected.
Marijuana:	Increased thirst and urinary frequency, fainting.
Tobacco:	Decreased furosemide effect.

*See Glossary

DIURETICS, THIAZIDE

BRAND AND GENERIC NAMES

See complete list of brand and generic names in the *Brand Names Directory,* page 919.

BASIC INFORMATION

Habit forming? No
Prescription needed? Yes
Available as generic? Yes, for some.
Drug class: Antihypertensive, diuretic (thiazide)

 USES

- Controls, but doesn't cure, high blood pressure.
- Reduces fluid retention (edema) caused by conditions such as heart disorders and liver disease.

 DOSAGE & USAGE INFORMATION

How to take:
Tablet or liquid—Swallow with liquid. If you can't swallow whole, crumble tablet and take with liquid or food. Don't exceed dose.

When to take:
At the same time each day.

If you forget a dose:
Take as soon as you remember up to 2 hours late. If more than 2 hours, wait for next scheduled dose (don't double this dose).

What drug does:
- Forces sodium and water excretion, reducing body fluid.
- Relaxes muscle cells of small arteries.
- Reduced body fluid and relaxed arteries lower blood pressure.

Time lapse before drug works:
4 to 6 hours. May require several weeks to lower blood pressure.

Don't take with:
- Non-prescription drugs without consulting doctor.
- See Interaction column and consult doctor.

 OVERDOSE

SYMPTOMS:
Cramps, weakness, drowsiness, weak pulse, coma.
WHAT TO DO:
- **Dial 0 (operator) or 911 (emergency) for an ambulance or medical help. Then give first aid immediately.**
- **See emergency information on inside covers.**

 POSSIBLE ADVERSE REACTIONS OR SIDE EFFECTS

SYMPTOMS	WHAT TO DO
Life-threatening:	
In case of overdose, see previous column.	
Common:	
Muscle cramps.	Discontinue. Call doctor right away.
Infrequent:	
• Blurred vision, severe abdominal pain, nausea, vomiting, irregular heartbeat, weak pulse.	Discontinue. Call doctor right away.
• Dizziness, mood changes, headaches, weakness, tiredness, weight changes, decreased sex drive, diarrhea.	Continue. Call doctor when convenient.
• Dry mouth, thirst.	Continue. Tell doctor at next visit.
Rare:	
• Rash or hives.	Discontinue. Seek emergency treatment.
• Jaundice, joint pain, black stools.	Discontinue. Call doctor right away.
• Sore throat, fever.	Continue. Tell doctor at next visit.

 WARNINGS & PRECAUTIONS

Don't take if:
You are allergic to any thiazide diuretic drug.

Before you start, consult your doctor:
- If you are allergic to any sulfa drug or tartrazine dye.
- If you have gout, systemic lupus erythematosis.
- If you have liver, pancreas, diabetes or kidney disorder.

Over age 60:
Adverse reactions and side effects may be more frequent and severe than in younger persons, especially dizziness and excessive potassium loss.

Pregnancy:
Risk to unborn child outweighs drug benefits. Don't use.

Breast-feeding:
Drug passes into milk. Avoid drug or discontinue nursing.

Infants & children:
No problems expected.

Prolonged use:
- You may need medicine to treat high blood pressure for the rest of your life.
- Talk to your doctor about the need for follow-up medical examinations or laboratory studies to check blood sugar, kidney function, blood pressure, serum electrolytes.

Skin & sunlight:
May cause rash or intensify sunburn in areas exposed to sun or sunlamp.

Driving, piloting or hazardous work:
Don't drive or pilot aircraft until you learn how medicine affects you. Don't work around dangerous machinery. Don't climb ladders or work in high places. Danger increases if you drink alcohol or take medicine affecting alertness and reflexes, such as antihistamines, tranquilizers, sedatives, pain medicine, narcotics and mind-altering drugs.

Discontinuing:
Don't discontinue without medical advice.

Others:
- Hot weather and fever may cause dehydration and drop in blood pressure. Dose may require temporary adjustment. Weigh daily and report any unexpected weight decreases to your doctor.
- May cause rise in uric acid, leading to gout.
- May cause blood-sugar rise in diabetics.
- May affect results in some medical tests.
- Advise any doctor or dentist whom you consult that you take this medicine.

POSSIBLE INTERACTION WITH OTHER DRUGS

GENERIC NAME OR DRUG CLASS	COMBINED EFFECT
ACE inhibitors*: captopril, enalapril, lisinopril	Decreased blood pressure.
Allopurinol	Decreased allopurinol effect.
Amiodarone	Increased risk of heartbeat irregularity due to low potassium.
Amphotericin B	Increased potassium.
Antidepressants, tricyclic (TCA)*	Dangerous drop in blood pressure. Avoid combination unless under medical supervision.
Antidiabetic agents, oral*	Increased blood sugar.
Antihypertensives*	Increased hypertensive effect.

Barbiturates*	Increased anti-hypertensive effect.
Beta-adrenergic blockers*	Increased antihypertensive effect. Dosages of both drugs may require adjustments.
Calcium supplements*	Increased calcium in blood.
Carteolol	Increased antihypertensive effect.
Cholestyramine	Decreased antihypertensive effect.
Colestipol	Decreased antihypertensive effect.
Cortisone drugs*	Excessive potassium loss that causes dangerous heart rhythms.
Didanosine	Increased risk of pancreatitis.
Digitalis preparations*	Excessive potassium loss that causes dangerous heart rhythms.
Diuretics, thiazide*	Increased effect of other thiazide diuretics.
Indapamide	Increased diuretic effect.
Indomethacin	Decreased antihypertensive effect
Lithium	Increased effect of lithium.

Continued page 944

POSSIBLE INTERACTION WITH OTHER SUBSTANCES

INTERACTS WITH	COMBINED EFFECT
Alcohol:	Dangerous blood pressure drop.
Beverages:	None expected.
Cocaine	Increased risk of heart block and high blood pressure.
Foods: Licorice.	Excessive potassium loss that causes dangerous heart rhythms.
Marijuana:	May increase blood pressure.
Tobacco:	None expected.

DIVALPROEX

BRAND NAMES

Depakote   Epival

BASIC INFORMATION

Habit forming? No
Prescription needed? Yes
Available as generic? No
Drug class: Anticonvulsant

 ## USES

Controls petit mal (absence) seizures in treatment of epilepsy.

 ## DOSAGE & USAGE INFORMATION

How to take:
Tablet—Swallow with liquid or food to lessen stomach irritation.

When to take:
Once a day.

If you forget a dose:
Take as soon as you remember. Don't ever double dose.

What drug does:
Increases concentration of gamma aminobutyric acid, which inhibits nerve transmission in parts of brain.

Time lapse before drug works:
1 to 4 hours.

Don't take with:
Any other medicine without consulting your doctor or pharmacist.

 ## OVERDOSE

SYMPTOMS:
Coma.
WHAT TO DO:
- Dial 0 (operator) or 911 (emergency) for an ambulance or medical help. Then give first aid immediately.
- If patient is unconscious and not breathing, give mouth-to-mouth breathing. If there is no heartbeat, use cardiac massage and mouth-to-mouth breathing (CPR). Don't try to make patient vomit. If you can't get help quickly, take patient to nearest emergency facility.
- See emergency information on inside covers.

 ## POSSIBLE ADVERSE REACTIONS OR SIDE EFFECTS

SYMPTOMS	WHAT TO DO
Life-threatening:	
In case of overdose, see previous column.	
Common:	
Menstrual irregularities, nausea, vomiting, abdominal cramps, diarrhea, tremor, weight gain.	Continue. Call doctor when convenient.
Infrequent:	
• Rash, bloody spots under skin, hair loss, bleeding, easy bruising.	Discontinue. Call doctor right away.
• Drowsiness, weakness, easily upset emotionally, depression, psychic changes, headache, incoordination, appetite change, constipation.	Continue. Call doctor when convenient.
Rare:	
• Double vision, unusual movements of eyes (nystagmus), jaundice, increased bleeding tendency, edema (swelling of feet and legs).	Discontinue. Call doctor right away.
• Anemia (paleness, fatigue).	Continue. Call doctor when convenient.

WARNINGS & PRECAUTIONS

Don't take if:
You are allergic to divalproex.

Before you start, consult your doctor:
- If you have blood, kidney or liver disease.
- If you will have surgery within 2 months, including dental surgery, requiring general or spinal anesthesia.

Over age 60:
Adverse reactions and side effects may be more frequent and severe than in younger persons.

Pregnancy:
No proven harm to unborn child. Avoid if possible.

Breast-feeding:
Unknown effect.

Infants & children:
Under close medical supervision only.

Prolonged use:
Request periodic blood tests, liver and kidney function tests.

Skin & sunlight:
No problems expected.

Driving, piloting or hazardous work:
Don't drive or pilot aircraft until you learn how medicine affects you. Don't work around dangerous machinery. Don't climb ladders or work in high places. Danger increases if you drink alcohol or take medicine affecting alertness and reflexes, such as antihistamines, tranquilizers, sedatives, pain medicine, narcotics and mind-altering drugs.

Discontinuing:
Don't discontinue without consulting doctor. Dose may require gradual reduction if you have taken drug for a long time. Doses of other drugs may also require adjustment.

Others:
No problems expected.

POSSIBLE INTERACTION WITH OTHER DRUGS

GENERIC NAME OR DRUG CLASS	COMBINED EFFECT
Anticoagulants*	Increases chance of bleeding.
Aspirin	Increases chance of bleeding.
Central nervous system (CNS) depressants* (antidepressants,* antihistamines,* muscle relaxants,* narcotics,* sedatives,* sleeping pills,* tranquilizers*)	Increases sedative effect.
Clonazepam	May prolong seizure.
Dipyridamole	Increases chance of bleeding.
MAO inhibitors*	Increases sedative effect.
Nabilone	Greater depression of central nervous system.
Phenobarbital	Increases chance of toxicity.
Phenytoin	Unpredictable. May require increased or decreased dosage.
Primidone	Increases chance of toxicity.
Sertraline	Increased depressive effect of both drugs.
Sulfinpyrazone	Increases chance of bleeding.

POSSIBLE INTERACTION WITH OTHER SUBSTANCES

INTERACTS WITH	COMBINED EFFECT
Alcohol:	Deep sedation. Avoid.
Beverages:	No problems expected.
Cocaine:	Increased brain sensitivity. Avoid.
Foods:	No problems expected.
Marijuana:	Increased brain sensitivity. Avoid.
Tobacco:	Increased brain sensitivity. Avoid.

*See Glossary

DOCUSATE CALCIUM

BRAND NAMES

Docucal-P
Doxidan

Pro-Cal-Sof
Surfak

BASIC INFORMATION

Habit forming? No
Prescription needed? No
Available as generic? Yes
Drug class: Laxative (stool softener)

 USES

Constipation relief.

 DOSAGE & USAGE INFORMATION

How to take:
Capsule—Swallow with liquid. Don't open capsules.

When to take:
At the same time each day, preferably bedtime.

If you forget a dose:
Take as soon as you remember. Wait 12 hours for next dose. Return to regular schedule.

What drug does:
Makes stool hold fluid so it is easier to pass.

Time lapse before drug works:
2 to 3 days of continual use.

Don't take with:
Any other medicine without consulting your doctor or pharmacist.

 OVERDOSE

SYMPTOMS:
Appetite loss, nausea, vomiting, diarrhea.
WHAT TO DO:
Overdose unlikely to threaten life. If person takes much larger amount than prescribed, call doctor, poison-control center or hospital emergency room for instructions.

 POSSIBLE ADVERSE REACTIONS OR SIDE EFFECTS

SYMPTOMS	WHAT TO DO
Life-threatening:	
None expected.	
Common:	
None expected.	
Infrequent:	
Abdominal cramps.	Continue. Call doctor when convenient.
Rare:	
Rash.	Discontinue. Call doctor right away.

DOCUSATE CALCIUM

 ## WARNINGS & PRECAUTIONS

Don't take if:
- You are allergic to any emollient laxative.
- You have abdominal pain and fever that might be appendicitis.

Before you start, consult your doctor:
- If you are taking other laxatives.
- To be sure constipation isn't a sign of a serious disorder.

Over age 60:
You must drink 6 to 8 glasses of fluid every 24 hours for drug to work.

Pregnancy:
No problems expected. Consult doctor.

Breast-feeding:
No problems expected.

Infants & children:
Not recommended.

Prolonged use:
Avoid. Overuse of laxatives may damage intestine lining.

Skin & sunlight:
No problems expected.

Driving, piloting or hazardous work:
No problems expected.

Discontinuing:
May be unnecessary to finish medicine. Follow doctor's instructions.

Others:
No problems expected.

 ## POSSIBLE INTERACTION WITH OTHER DRUGS

GENERIC NAME OR DRUG CLASS	COMBINED EFFECT
Danthron	Possible liver damage.
Digitalis preparations*	Toxic absorption of digitalis.
Mineral oil	Increased mineral oil absorption into bloodstream. Avoid. May cause tumor-like deposits in tissues.
Phenolphthalein	Increased phenolphthalein absorption. Possible toxicity.

 ## POSSIBLE INTERACTION WITH OTHER SUBSTANCES

INTERACTS WITH	COMBINED EFFECT
Alcohol:	None expected.
Beverages:	None expected.
Cocaine:	None expected.
Foods:	None expected.
Marijuana:	None expected.
Tobacco:	None expected.

*See Glossary

DOCUSATE POTASSIUM

BRAND NAMES

Dialose   Kasof
Diocto-K

BASIC INFORMATION

Habit forming? No
Prescription needed? No
Available as generic? Yes
Drug class: Laxative (stool softener)

USES

Constipation relief.

DOSAGE & USAGE INFORMATION

How to take:
Capsule—Swallow with liquid. Don't open capsules.

When to take:
At the same time each day, preferably bedtime.

If you forget a dose:
Take as soon as you remember. Wait 12 hours for next dose. Return to regular schedule.

What drug does:
Makes stool hold fluid so it is easier to pass.

Time lapse before drug works:
2 to 3 days of continual use.

Don't take with:
- Other medicines at same time. Wait 2 hours.
- Any other medicine without consulting your doctor or pharmacist.

OVERDOSE

SYMPTOMS:
Appetite loss, nausea, vomiting, diarrhea.
WHAT TO DO:
Overdose unlikely to threaten life. If person takes much larger amount than prescribed, call doctor, poison-control center or hospital emergency room for instructions.

POSSIBLE ADVERSE REACTIONS OR SIDE EFFECTS

SYMPTOMS	WHAT TO DO
Life-threatening: None expected.	
Common: None expected.	
Infrequent: Abdominal cramps.	Continue. Call doctor when convenient.
Rare: Rash.	Discontinue. Call doctor right away.

DOCUSATE POTASSIUM

WARNINGS & PRECAUTIONS

Don't take if:
- You are allergic to any emollient laxative.
- You have abdominal pain and fever that might be appendicitis.

Before you start, consult your doctor:
- If you are taking other laxatives.
- To be sure constipation isn't a sign of a serious disorder.

Over age 60:
You must drink 6 to 8 glasses of fluid every 24 hours for drug to work.

Pregnancy:
No problems expected. Consult doctor.

Breast-feeding:
No problems expected.

Infants & children:
No problems expected.

Prolonged use:
Avoid. Overuse of laxatives may damage intestine lining.

Skin & sunlight:
No problems expected.

Driving, piloting or hazardous work:
No problems expected.

Discontinuing:
May be unnecessary to finish medicine. Follow doctor's instructions.

Others:
No problems expected.

POSSIBLE INTERACTION WITH OTHER DRUGS

GENERIC NAME OR DRUG CLASS	COMBINED EFFECT
Danthron	Possible liver damage.
Digitalis preparations*	Toxic absorption of digitalis.
Mineral oil	Increased mineral oil absorption into bloodstream. Avoid. May cause tumor-like deposits in tissues.
Phenolphthalein	Increased phenolphthalein absorption. Possible toxicity.

POSSIBLE INTERACTION WITH OTHER SUBSTANCES

INTERACTS WITH	COMBINED EFFECT
Alcohol:	None expected.
Beverages:	None expected.
Cocaine:	None expected.
Foods:	None expected.
Marijuana:	None expected.
Tobacco:	None expected.

*See Glossary

DOCUSATE SODIUM

BRAND NAMES

See complete list of brand names in the *Brand Name Directory*, page 920.

BASIC INFORMATION

Habit forming? No
Prescription needed? No
Available as generic? Yes
Drug class: Laxative (stool softener)

 ## USES

Constipation relief.

 ## DOSAGE & USAGE INFORMATION

How to take:
- Tablet or capsule—Swallow with liquid. Don't open capsules.
- Syrup—Take as directed on bottle.
- Effervescent granules—Dissolve granules in 4 oz. cool water. Drink all the water.

When to take:
At the same time each day, preferably bedtime.

If you forget a dose:
Take as soon as you remember. Wait 12 hours for next dose. Return to regular schedule.

What drug does:
Makes stool hold fluid so it is easier to pass.

Time lapse before drug works:
2 to 3 days of continual use.

Don't take with:
- Other medicines at same time. Wait 2 hours.
- Any other medicine without consulting your doctor or pharmacist.

 ## OVERDOSE

SYMPTOMS:
Appetite loss, nausea, vomiting, diarrhea.
WHAT TO DO:
Overdose unlikely to threaten life. If person takes much larger amount than prescribed, call doctor, poison-control center or hospital emergency room for instructions.

 ## POSSIBLE ADVERSE REACTIONS OR SIDE EFFECTS

SYMPTOMS	WHAT TO DO
Life-threatening: None expected.	
Common: None expected.	
Infrequent: Throat irritation (liquid only), intestinal and stomach cramps.	Continue. Call doctor when convenient.
Rare: Rash.	Discontinue. Call doctor right away.

WARNINGS & PRECAUTIONS

Don't take if:
- You are allergic to any emollient laxative.
- You have abdominal pain and fever that might be appendicitis.

Before you start, consult your doctor:
- If you are taking other laxatives.
- To be sure constipation isn't a sign of a serious disorder.

Over age 60:
You must drink 6 to 8 glasses of fluid every 24 hours for drug to work.

Pregnancy:
No problems expected. Consult doctor.

Breast-feeding:
No problems expected.

Infants & children:
No problems expected.

Prolonged use:
Avoid. Overuse of laxatives may damage intestine lining.

Skin & sunlight:
No problems expected.

Driving, piloting or hazardous work:
No problems expected.

Discontinuing:
May be unnecessary to finish medicine. Follow doctor's instructions.

Others:
No problems expected.

POSSIBLE INTERACTION WITH OTHER DRUGS

GENERIC NAME OR DRUG CLASS	COMBINED EFFECT
Danthron	Possible liver damage.
Digitalis preparations*	Toxic absorption of digitalis.
Mineral oil	Increased mineral oil absorption into bloodstream. Avoid. May cause tumor-like deposits in tissues.
Phenolphthalein	Increased phenolphthalein absorption. Possible toxicity.

POSSIBLE INTERACTION WITH OTHER SUBSTANCES

INTERACTS WITH	COMBINED EFFECT
Alcohol:	None expected.
Beverages:	None expected.
Cocaine:	None expected.
Foods:	None expected.
Marijuana:	None expected.
Tobacco:	None expected.

*See Glossary

DOXAZOSIN

BRAND NAMES

Cardura

BASIC INFORMATION

Habit forming? No
Prescription needed? Yes
Available as generic? Yes
Drug class: Antihypertensive

 USES

- Treatment for high blood pressure.
- May improve congestive heart failure.
- Treatment for Raynaud's disease.

 DOSAGE & USAGE INFORMATION

How to take:
Tablet or capsule—Swallow with liquid. If you can't swallow whole, crumble tablet or open capsule and take with liquid or food.

When to take:
At the same times each day.

If you forget a dose:
Take as soon as you remember up to 2 hours late. If more than 2 hours, wait for next scheduled dose (don't double this dose).

What drug does:
Expands and relaxes blood vessel walls to lower blood pressure.

Time lapse before drug works:
30 minutes.

Don't take with:
Any other medicine without consulting your doctor or pharmacist.

 OVERDOSE

SYMPTOMS:
Extreme weakness; loss of consciousness; cold, sweaty skin; weak, rapid pulse; coma.
WHAT TO DO:
- **Dial 0 (operator) or 911 (emergency) for an ambulance or medical help. Then give first aid immediately.**
- **If patient is unconscious and not breathing, give mouth-to-mouth breathing. If there is no heartbeat, use cardiac massage and mouth-to-mouth breathing (CPR). Don't try to make patient vomit. If you can't get help quickly, take patient to nearest emergency facility.**
- **See emergency information on inside covers.**

 POSSIBLE ADVERSE REACTIONS OR SIDE EFFECTS

SYMPTOMS	WHAT TO DO
Life-threatening:	
In case of overdose, see previous column.	
Common:	
• Rapid heartbeat.	Discontinue. Call doctor right away.
• Vivid dreams, drowsiness, dizziness.	Continue. Call doctor when convenient.
Infrequent:	
• Rash or itchy skin, blurred vision, shortness of breath, difficult breathing, chest pain.	Discontinue. Call doctor right away.
• Appetite loss, constipation or diarrhea, abdominal pain, nausea, vomiting, fluid retention, joint or muscle aches, weakness and faintness when arising from bed or chair.	Continue. Call doctor when convenient.
• Headache, irritability, depression, dry mouth, stuffy nose, increased urination.	Continue. Tell doctor at next visit.
Rare:	
Decreased sexual function, numbness or tingling in hands or feet.	Continue. Call doctor when convenient.

DOXAZOSIN

 ## WARNINGS & PRECAUTIONS

Don't take if:
- You are allergic to prazosin.
- You are depressed.
- You will have surgery within 2 months, including dental surgery, requiring general or spinal anesthesia.

Before you start, consult your doctor:
- If you experience lightheadedness or fainting with other antihypertensive drugs.
- If you are easily depressed.
- If you have impaired brain circulation or have had a stroke.
- If you have coronary heart disease (with or without angina).
- If you have kidney disease or impaired liver function.

Over age 60:
Begin with no more than 1 mg. per day for first 3 days. Increases should be gradual and supervised by your doctor. Don't stand while taking. Sudden changes in position may cause falls. Sit or lie down promptly if you feel dizzy. If you have impaired brain circulation or coronary heart disease, excessive lowering of blood pressure should be avoided. Report problems to your doctor immediately.

Pregnancy:
Studies inconclusive on harm to unborn child. Consult doctor.

Breast-feeding:
No proven problems. Consult doctor.

Infants & children:
Not recommended.

Prolonged use:
Talk to your doctor about the need for follow-up medical examinations or laboratory studies.

Skin & sunlight:
No problems expected.

Driving, piloting or hazardous work:
Don't drive or pilot aircraft until you learn how medicine affects you. Don't work around dangerous machinery. Don't climb ladders or work in high places.

Discontinuing:
Don't discontinue without doctor's advice until you complete prescribed dose, even though symptoms diminish or disappear.

Others:
First dose likely to cause fainting. Take it at night and get out of bed slowly next morning.

 ## POSSIBLE INTERACTION WITH OTHER DRUGS

GENERIC NAME OR DRUG CLASS	COMBINED EFFECT
Amphetamines*	Decreased doxazosin effect.
Antihypertensives, other*	Increased antihypertensive effect. Dosages may require adjustments.
Estrogen	Decreased effect of doxazosin.
Non-steroidal anti-inflammatory drugs (NSAIDs)*	Decreased effect of doxazosin.
Sympathomimetics*	Decreased effect of doxazosin.

 ## POSSIBLE INTERACTION WITH OTHER SUBSTANCES

INTERACTS WITH	COMBINED EFFECT
Alcohol:	Excessive blood pressure drop.
Beverages:	None expected.
Cocaine:	Increased risk of heart block and high blood pressure.
Foods:	None expected.
Marijuana:	Possible fainting. Avoid.
Tobacco:	Possible spasm of coronary arteries. Avoid.

*See Glossary

DRONABINOL (THC, Marijuana)

BRAND NAMES

Marinol

BASIC INFORMATION

Habit forming? Yes
Prescription needed? Yes
Available as generic? No
Drug class: Antiemetic

USES

Prevents nausea and vomiting that may accompany taking anticancer medication (cancer chemotherapy). Should not be used unless other antinausea medicines fail.

DOSAGE & USAGE INFORMATION

How to take:
Capsule—Swallow with liquid.

When to take:
Under supervision, a total of no more than 4 to 6 doses per day, every 2 to 4 hours after cancer chemotherapy for prescribed number of days.

If you forget a dose:
Take as soon as you remember up to 2 hours late. If more than 2 hours, wait for next scheduled dose (don't double this dose).

What drug does:
Affects nausea and vomiting center in brain to make it less irritable following cancer chemotherapy. Exact mechanism is unknown.

Time lapse before drug works:
2 to 4 hours.

Don't take with:
• Non-prescription drugs without consulting doctor.
• Drugs in interaction column without consulting doctor.

OVERDOSE

SYMPTOMS:
Pounding, rapid heart rate; high or low blood pressure; confusion; hallucinations; drastic mood changes; nervousness or anxiety.
WHAT TO DO:
Overdose unlikely to threaten life. If person takes much larger amount than prescribed, call doctor, poison-control center or hospital emergency room for instructions.

POSSIBLE ADVERSE REACTIONS OR SIDE EFFECTS

SYMPTOMS	WHAT TO DO
Life-threatening:	
In case of overdose, see previous column.	
Common:	
• Rapid, pounding heartbeat.	Discontinue. Call doctor right away.
• Dizziness, irritability, drowsiness, euphoria, decreased coordination.	Continue. Call doctor when convenient.
• Red eyes, dry mouth.	No action necessary.
Infrequent:	
• Depression, anxiety, nervousness, headache, hallucinations, dramatic mood changes.	Discontinue. Call doctor right away.
• Blurred or changed vision.	Continue. Call doctor when convenient.
Rare:	
• Rapid heartbeat, fainting, frequent or difficult urination, convulsions, shortness of breath.	Discontinue. Call doctor right away.
• Paranoia, nausea, loss of appetite, dizziness when standing after sitting or lying down, diarrhea.	Continue. Call doctor when convenient.

WARNINGS & PRECAUTIONS

Don't take if:
• Your nausea and vomiting is caused by anything other than cancer chemotherapy.
• You are sensitive or allergic to any form of marijuana or sesame oil.
• Your cycle of chemotherapy is longer than 7 consecutive days. Harmful side effects may occur.

Before you start, consult your doctor:
• If you have heart disease or high blood pressure.
• If you are an alcoholic or drug addict.
• If you are pregnant or intend to become pregnant.
• If you are nursing an infant.
• If you have schizophrenia or a manic-depressive disorder.

DRONABINOL (THC, Marijuana)

Over age 60:
Adverse reactions and side effects may be more frequent and severe than in younger persons.

Pregnancy:
No studies in humans. Avoid if possible.

Breast-feeding:
No studies in humans. Avoid if possible.

Infants & children:
Not recommended.

Prolonged use:
- Avoid. Habit forming.
- Talk to your doctor about the need for follow-up medical examinations or laboratory studies to check heart function.

Skin & sunlight:
No problems expected.

Driving, piloting or hazardous work:
Don't drive or pilot aircraft until you learn how medicine affects you. Don't work around dangerous machinery. Don't climb ladders or work in high places. Danger increases if you drink alcohol or take medicine affecting alertness and reflexes, such as antihistamines, tranquilizers, sedatives, pain medicine, narcotics and mind-altering drugs.

Discontinuing:
Withdrawal effects such as irritability, insomnia, restlessness, sweating, diarrhea, hiccups, loss of appetite and hot flashes may follow abrupt withdrawal within 12 hours. Should they occur, these symptoms will probably subside within 96 hours.

Others:
Store in refrigerator.

POSSIBLE INTERACTION WITH OTHER DRUGS

GENERIC NAME OR DRUG CLASS	COMBINED EFFECT
Anesthetics*	Oversedation.
Anticonvulsants*	Oversedation.
Antidepressants, tricyclics (TCA)*	Oversedation.
Antihistamines*	Oversedation.
Barbiturates*	Oversedation.
Clozapine	Toxic effect on the central nervous system.
Ethinamate	Dangerous increased effects of ethinamate. Avoid combining.
Fluoxetine	Increased depressant effects of both drugs.
Guanfacine	May increase depressant effects of either drug.
Leucovorin	High alcohol content of leucovorin may cause adverse effects.
Methyprylon	Increased sedative effect, perhaps to dangerous level. Avoid.
Molindone	Increased effects of both drugs. Avoid.
Muscle relaxants*	Oversedation.
Nabilone	Greater depression of central nervous system.
Narcotics*	Oversedation.
Sedatives*	Oversedation.
Sertraline	Increased depressive effects of both drugs.
Tranquilizers*	Oversedation.

POSSIBLE INTERACTION WITH OTHER SUBSTANCES

INTERACTS WITH	COMBINED EFFECT
Alcohol:	Oversedation.
Beverages:	No problems expected.
Cocaine:	No problems expected.
Foods:	No problems expected.
Marijuana:	Oversedation.
Tobacco:	No problems expected.

*See Glossary

ENCAINIDE

BRAND NAMES

Enkaid

BASIC INFORMATION

Habit forming? No
Prescription needed? Yes
Available as generic? No
Drug class: Antiarrhythmic

 USES

Stabilizes irregular heartbeat.

 DOSAGE & USAGE INFORMATION

How to take:
Capsules—Swallow with liquid or food to lessen stomach irritation. If you can't swallow whole, open capsule and take with liquid or food.

When to take:
At the same time each day, according to instructions on prescription label.

If you forget a dose:
Take as soon as you remember up to 2 hours late. If more than 2 hours, wait for next scheduled dose (don't double this dose).

What drug does:
- Increases refractory between muscle fiber contractions in the heart.
- Decreases excitability throughout the conducting system of the heart.

Time lapse before drug works:
1 to 3 hours. Peak effect in 30 to 90 minutes.

Don't take with:
Any other medicine without consulting your doctor or pharmacist.

 OVERDOSE

SYMPTOMS:
Very slow heartbeat, extreme weakness, seizures, loss of consciousness, cardiac arrest.
WHAT TO DO:
- Dial 0 (operator) or 911 (emergency) for an ambulance or medical help. Then give first aid immediately.
- See emergency information on inside covers.

 POSSIBLE ADVERSE REACTIONS OR SIDE EFFECTS

SYMPTOMS	WHAT TO DO
Life-threatening:	
Very fast or irregular heartbeat.	Seek emergency treatment immediately.
Common:	
None expected.	
Infrequent:	
• Chest pain, blurred or double vision, skin rash.	Discontinue. Call doctor right away.
• Dizziness, headache, tiredness or weakness, nausea, arm or leg pain.	Continue. Call doctor when convenient.
Rare:	
• Shortness of breath.	Discontinue. Call doctor right away.
• Swelling of lower legs and feet, trembling or shaking.	Continue. Call doctor when convenient.

338

WARNINGS & PRECAUTIONS

Don't take if:
- You have atrioventricular block and you do not have a pacemaker.
- You have right bundle branch block (by ECG*).

Before you start, consult your doctor:
- If you have cardiomyopathy or congestive heart failure.
- If you have had a recent heart attack.
- If you have liver or kidney disease.
- If you have sick sinus syndrome.*
- If you have an alteration in potassium levels.

Over age 60:
No special problems expected.

Pregnancy:
No proven harm to unborn child, but avoid if possible.

Breast-feeding:
Drug passes into milk. Avoid drug or discontinue nursing until you finish medicine. Consult doctor for advice on maintaining milk supply.

Infants & children:
Effect not documented. Consult your doctor.

Prolonged use:
Talk to your doctor about the need for follow-up medical examinations or laboratory studies to check heart rhythms (by Holter monitor or ECG*).

Skin & sunlight:
No problems expected.

Driving, piloting or hazardous work:
Don't drive or pilot aircraft until you learn how medicine affects you. Don't work around dangerous machinery. Don't climb ladders or work in high places. Danger increases if you drink alcohol or take medicine affecting alertness and reflexes.

Discontinuing:
Don't discontinue without consulting doctor. Dose may require gradual reduction if you have taken drug for a long time. Doses of other drugs may also require adjustment.

Others:
Adverse effects may be dose related.

POSSIBLE INTERACTION WITH OTHER DRUGS

GENERIC NAME OR DRUG CLASS	COMBINED EFFECT
Antiarrhythmics*	Increased effect or toxicity on heart muscle.
Carteolol	Increased effect of toxicity on heart muscle.
Cimetidine	Increased effect of cimetidine.
Guanfacine	Increased effect of both drugs.
Nicardipine	Increased effect of toxicity on heart muscle.
Nizatidine	Increased effect of nizatidine.
Propafenone	Increased effect of both drugs and increased risk of toxicity.
Sotalol	Increased effect of toxicity on heart muscle.

POSSIBLE INTERACTION WITH OTHER SUBSTANCES

INTERACTS WITH	COMBINED EFFECT
Alcohol:	Heartbeat irregularities may increase.
Beverages:	None expected.
Cocaine:	Heartbeat irregularities may increase.
Foods:	No special problems expected.
Marijuana:	Heartbeat irregularities may increase.
Tobacco:	Heartbeat irregularities may increase.

*See Glossary

EPHEDRINE

BRAND NAMES

See complete list of brand names in the *Brand Name Directory*, page 920.

BASIC INFORMATION

Habit forming? No
Prescription needed?
  Low Strength: No
  High Strength: Yes
Available as generic? Yes, for some.
Drug class: Sympathomimetic

 USES

- Relieves bronchial asthma.
- Decreases congestion of breathing passages.
- Suppresses allergic reactions.

 DOSAGE & USAGE INFORMATION

How to take:
- Tablet or capsule—Swallow with liquid. You may chew or crush tablet.
- Extended-release tablets or capsules— Swallow each dose whole.
- Syrup—Take as directed on bottle.
- Drops—Dilute dose in beverage.

When to take:
As needed, no more often than every 4 hours.

If you forget a dose:
Take up to 2 hours late. If more than 2 hours, wait for next dose (don't double this dose).

What drug does:
- Prevents cells from releasing allergy-causing chemicals (histamines).
- Relaxes muscles of bronchial tubes.
- Decreases blood-vessel size and blood flow, thus causing decongestion.

Time lapse before drug works:
30 to 60 minutes.

Continued next column

 OVERDOSE

SYMPTOMS:
Severe anxiety, confusion, delirium, muscle tremors, rapid and irregular pulse.
WHAT TO DO:
- **Dial 0 (operator) or 911 (emergency) for an ambulance or medical help. Then give first aid immediately.**
- **See emergency information on inside covers.**

Don't take with:
- Non-prescription drugs with ephedrine, pseudoephedrine or epinephrine.
- Non-prescription drugs for cough, cold, allergy or asthma without consulting doctor.
- See Interaction column and consult doctor.

 POSSIBLE ADVERSE REACTIONS OR SIDE EFFECTS

SYMPTOMS	WHAT TO DO
Life-threatening:	
In case of overdose, see previous column.	
Common:	
Nervousness, headache, paleness, rapid heartbeat.	Continue. Call doctor when convenient.
Insomnia.	Continue. Tell doctor at next visit.
Infrequent:	
Irregular heartbeat.	Discontinue. Call doctor right away.
Dizziness, appetite loss, nausea, vomiting, painful or difficult urination.	Continue. Call doctor when convenient.
Rare:	
None expected.	

 WARNINGS & PRECAUTIONS

Don't take if:
You are allergic to ephedrine or any sympathomimetic* drug.

Before you start, consult your doctor:
- If you have high blood pressure.
- If you have diabetes.
- If you have overactive thyroid gland.
- If you have difficulty urinating.
- If you have taken any MAO inhibitor in past 2 weeks.
- If you have taken digitalis preparations in the last 7 days.
- If you will have surgery within 2 months, including dental surgery, requiring general or spinal anesthesia.

Over age 60:
More likely to develop high blood pressure, heart-rhythm disturbances, angina and to feel drug's stimulant effects.

Pregnancy:
No proven harm to unborn child. Avoid if possible.

Breast-feeding:
Drug passes into milk. Avoid drug or discontinue nursing until you finish medicine. Consult doctor for advice on maintaining milk supply.

Infants & children:
No problems expected.

Prolonged use:
- Excessive doses—Rare toxic psychosis.
- Men with enlarged prostate gland may have more urination difficulty.

Skin & sunlight:
o problems expected.

Driving, piloting or hazardous work:
Avoid if you feel dizzy. Otherwise, no problems expected.

Discontinuing:
May be unnecessary to finish medicine. Follow doctor's instructions.

Others:
No problems expected.

 POSSIBLE INTERACTION WITH OTHER DRUGS

GENERIC NAME OR DRUG CLASS	COMBINED EFFECT
Antidepressants, tricyclic (TCA)*	Increased effect of ephedrine. Excessive stimulation of heart and blood pressure.
Antihypertensives*	Decreased antihypertensive effect.
Beta-adrenergic blockers*	Decreased effects of both drugs.
Dextrothyroxine	Increased ephedrine effect.
Digitalis preparations*	Serious heart-rhythm disturbances.
Epinephrine	Increased epinephrine effect.
Ergot preparations*	Serious blood-pressure rise.
Furazolidine	Sudden, severe increase in blood pressure.
Guanadrel	Decreased effect of both drugs.
Guanethidine	Decreased effect of both drugs.

MAO inhibitors*	Increased ephedrine effect. Dangerous blood-pressure rise.
Methyldopa	Possible increased blood pressure.
Nitrates*	Possible decreased effects of both drugs.
Phenothiazines*	Possible increased ephedrine toxicity. Possible decreased ephedrine effect.
Pseudoephedrine	Increased pseudoephedrine effect.
Rauwolfia	Decreased rauwolfia effect.
Sympathomimetics*	Increased ephedrine effect.
Terazosin	Decreases effectiveness of terazosin.
Theophylline	Increased gastrointestinal intolerance.

 POSSIBLE INTERACTION WITH OTHER SUBSTANCES

INTERACTS WITH	COMBINED EFFECT
Alcohol:	None expected.
Beverages: Caffeine drinks.	Nervousness or insomnia.
Cocaine:	High risk of heartbeat irregularities and high blood pressure.
Foods:	None expected.
Marijuana:	Rapid heartbeat, possible heart-rhythm disturbance.
Tobacco:	None expected.

ERGOLOID MESYLATES

BRAND NAMES

Hydergine
Hydergine LC
Niloric

BASIC INFORMATION

Habit forming? No
Prescription needed? Yes
Available as generic? Yes
Drug class: Ergot preparation

 USES

Treatment for reduced alertness, poor memory, confusion, depression or lack of motivation in the elderly.

 DOSAGE & USAGE INFORMATION

How to take:
- Tablet—Swallow with liquid. If you can't swallow whole, crumble tablet and take with liquid or food.
- Liquid—Take as directed on label.
- Sublingual tablets—Dissolve tablet under tongue.

When to take:
At the same times each day.

If you forget a dose:
Take as soon as you remember up to 2 hours late. If more than 2 hours, wait for next scheduled dose (don't double this dose).

What drug does:
Stimulates brain-cell metabolism to increase use of oxygen and nutrients.

Time lapse before drug works:
Gradual improvements over 3 to 4 months.

Continued next column

 OVERDOSE

SYMPTOMS:
Headache, flushed face, nasal congestion, nausea, vomiting, blood-pressure drop, blurred vision, weakness, collapse, coma.
WHAT TO DO:
- Dial 0 (operator) or 911 (emergency) for an ambulance or medical help. Then give first aid immediately.
- See emergency information on inside covers.

Don't take with:
- Non-prescription drugs containing alcohol without consulting doctor.
- Any other medication without consulting your doctor or pharmacist.

 POSSIBLE ADVERSE REACTIONS OR SIDE EFFECTS

SYMPTOMS	WHAT TO DO
Life-threatening:	
In case of overdose, see previous column.	
Common:	
Runny nose, skin flushing, headache.	Continue. Tell doctor at next visit.
Infrequent:	
• Slow heartbeat, tingling fingers.	Discontinue. Call doctor right away.
• Nervousness, hostility, confusion, depression, blurred vision.	Continue. Call doctor when convenient.
Rare:	
• Fainting.	Discontinue. Seek emergency treatment.
• Rash, nausea, vomiting, stomach cramps.	Discontinue. Call doctor right away.
• Dizziness when getting up, fever, drowsiness, soreness under tongue, appetite loss.	Continue. Call doctor when convenient.

WARNINGS & PRECAUTIONS

Don't use if:
- If you are allergic to any ergot preparation.
- Your heartbeat is less than 60 beats per minute.
- Your systolic blood pressure is consistently below 100.

Before you start, consult your doctor:
If you have had low blood pressure.

Over age 60:
Primarily used in persons older than 60. Results unpredictable, but many patients show improved brain function.

Pregnancy:
Not recommended.

Breast-feeding:
Risk to nursing child outweighs drug benefits. Don't use.

Infants & children:
Not recommended.

Prolonged use:
Talk to your doctor about the need for follow-up medical examinations or laboratory studies.

Skin & sunlight:
No problems expected.

Driving, piloting or hazardous work:
Avoid if you feel dizzy, faint or have blurred vision. Otherwise, no problems expected.

Discontinuing:
No problems expected.

Others:
No problems expected.

POSSIBLE INTERACTION WITH OTHER DRUGS

GENERIC NAME OR DRUG CLASS	COMBINED EFFECT
Ergot preparations, other	May cause decreased circulation to arms, legs, feet and hands. Avoid.
Sympathomimetics*	May cause decreased circulation to arms, legs, feet and hands. Avoid.

POSSIBLE INTERACTION WITH OTHER SUBSTANCES

INTERACTS WITH	COMBINED EFFECT
Alcohol:	Use caution. May drop blood pressure excessively.
Beverages:	None expected.
Cocaine:	Overstimulation. Avoid.
Foods:	None expected.
Marijuana:	Decreased effect of ergot alkaloids.
Tobacco:	Decreased ergoloid effect. Don't smoke.

*See Glossary

ERGONOVINE

BRAND NAMES

Ergometrine
Ergotrate

Ergotrate Maleate

BASIC INFORMATION

Habit forming? No
Prescription needed? Yes
Available as generic? Yes
Drug class: Ergot preparation (uterine stimulant)

USES

Retards excessive post-delivery bleeding.

DOSAGE & USAGE INFORMATION

How to take:
Tablet—Swallow with liquid or food to lessen stomach irritation.

When to take:
At the same times each day.

If you forget a dose:
Don't take missed dose and don't double next one. Wait for next scheduled dose.

What drug does:
Causes smooth-muscle cells of uterine wall to contract and surround bleeding blood vessels of relaxed uterus.

Time lapse before drug works:
Tablets—20 to 30 minutes.

Don't take with:
Any other medicine without consulting your doctor or pharmacist.

OVERDOSE

SYMPTOMS:
Vomiting, diarrhea, weak pulse, low blood pressure, difficult breathing, angina, convulsions.
WHAT TO DO:
* **Dial 0 (operator) or 911 (emergency) for an ambulance or medical help. Then give first aid immediately.**
* **If patient is unconscious and not breathing, give mouth-to-mouth breathing. If there is no heartbeat, use cardiac massage and mouth-to-mouth breathing (CPR). Don't try to make patient vomit. If you can't get help quickly, take patient to nearest emergency facility.**
* **See emergency information on inside covers.**

POSSIBLE ADVERSE REACTIONS OR SIDE EFFECTS

SYMPTOMS	WHAT TO DO
Life-threatening:	
In case of overdose, see previous column.	
Common:	
Nausea, vomiting, severe lower abdominal menstrual-like cramps.	Discontinue. Call doctor right away.
Infrequent:	
• Confusion, ringing in ears, diarrhea, muscle cramps.	Discontinue. Call doctor right away.
• Unusual sweating.	Continue. Call doctor when convenient.
Rare:	
Sudden, severe headache; shortness of breath; chest pain; numb, cold hands and feet.	Discontinue. Seek emergency treatment.

WARNINGS & PRECAUTIONS

Don't take if:
You are allergic to any ergot preparation.

Before you start, consult your doctor:
- If you have coronary-artery or blood-vessel disease.
- If you have liver or kidney disease.
- If you have high blood pressure.
- If you have postpartum infection.

Over age 60:
Not recommended.

Pregnancy:
Risk to unborn child outweighs drug benefits. Don't use.

Breast-feeding:
Drug passes into milk. Avoid drug or discontinue nursing until you finish medicine. Consult doctor for advice on maintaining milk supply.

Infants & children:
Not recommended.

Prolonged use:
Talk to your doctor about the need for follow-up medical examinations or laboratory studies to check blood pressure, ECG*.

Skin & sunlight:
No problems expected.

Driving, piloting or hazardous work:
No problems expected.

Discontinuing:
May be unnecessary to finish medicine. Follow doctor's instructions.

Others:
Drug should be used for short time only following childbirth or miscarriage.

POSSIBLE INTERACTION WITH OTHER DRUGS

GENERIC NAME OR DRUG CLASS	COMBINED EFFECT
Beta-adrenergic blockers*	Possible vasospasm (peripheral and cardiac).
Ergot preparations, other	May cause decreased circulation to arms, legs, feet and hands. Avoid.
Sympathomimetics*	May cause decreased circulation to arms, legs, feet and hands. Avoid.

POSSIBLE INTERACTION WITH OTHER SUBSTANCES

INTERACTS WITH	COMBINED EFFECT
Alcohol:	None expected.
Beverages:	None expected.
Cocaine:	None expected.
Foods:	None expected.
Marijuana:	None expected.
Tobacco:	Decreased ergonovine effect. Don't smoke.

*See Glossary

ERGOTAMINE

BRAND NAMES

Ergomar
Ergostat

Gynergen
Lingraine

BASIC INFORMATION

Habit forming? No
Prescription needed? Yes
Available as generic? No
Drug class: Vasoconstrictor, ergot
   preparation

 USES

Relieves pain of migraines and other headaches
caused by dilated blood vessels. Will not
prevent headaches.

 DOSAGE & USAGE INFORMATION

How to take:
- Tablet or sublingual tablet—Swallow with
  liquid, or let dissolve under tongue. If you
  can't swallow whole, crumble tablet and take
  with liquid or food.
- Suppositories—Remove wrapper and moisten
  suppository with water. Gently insert larger
  end into rectum. Push well into rectum with
  finger.
- Aerosol inhaler—Use only as directed on
  prescription label.
- Lie down in quiet, dark room after taking.

When to take:
At first sign of vascular or migraine headache.

If you forget a dose:
Take as soon as you remember. Wait 4 hours
for next dose.

Continued next column

 OVERDOSE

SYMPTOMS:
**Tingling, cold extremities and muscle pain.
Progresses to nausea, vomiting, diarrhea,
cold skin, rapid and weak pulse, severe
numbness of extremities, confusion,
convulsions, coma.**
WHAT TO DO:
- **Dial 0 (operator) or 911 (emergency) for
  an ambulance or medical help. Then give
  first aid immediately.**
- **See emergency information on inside
  covers.**

What drug does:
Constricts blood vessels in the head.

Time lapse before drug works:
30 to 60 minutes.

Don't take with:
Any other medicine without consulting your
doctor or pharmacist.

 POSSIBLE ADVERSE REACTIONS OR SIDE EFFECTS

SYMPTOMS	WHAT TO DO
Life-threatening:	
In case of overdose, see previous column.	
Common:	
• Dizziness, nausea, diarrhea, vomiting, increased frequency or severity of headaches.	Continue. Call doctor when convenient.
• Feet and ankle swelling.	Discontinue. Call doctor right away.
Infrequent:	
Itchy or swollen skin; cold, pale hands or feet; pain or weakness in arms, legs, back.	Discontinue. Call doctor right away.
Rare:	
Anxiety or confusion; red or purple blisters, especially on hands, feet; change in vision; extreme thirst; stomach pain or bloating; unusually fast or slow heartbeat; chest pain; numbness or tingling in face, fingers, toes.	Discontinue. Call doctor right away.

WARNINGS & PRECAUTIONS

Don't take if:
You are allergic to any ergot preparation.

Before you start, consult your doctor:
- If you plan to become pregnant within medication period.
- If you have an infection.
- If you have angina, heart problems, high blood pressure, hardening of the arteries or vein problems.
- If you have kidney or liver disease.
- If you are allergic to other spray inhalants.

Over age 60:
Adverse reactions and side effects may be more frequent and severe than in younger persons.

Pregnancy:
Risk to unborn child outweighs drug benefits. Don't use.

Breast-feeding:
Drug filters into milk. May harm child. Avoid.

Infants & children:
Studies inconclusive on harm to children. Consult your doctor.

Prolonged use:
Cold skin, muscle pain, gangrene of hands and feet. This medicine not intended for uninterrupted use.

Skin & sunlight:
No problems expected.

Driving, piloting or hazardous work:
Don't drive or pilot aircraft until you learn how medicine affects you. Don't work around dangerous machinery. Don't climb ladders or work in high places. Danger increases if you drink alcohol or take medicine affecting alertness and reflexes, such as antihistamines, tranquilizers, sedatives, pain medicine, narcotics and mind-altering drugs.

Discontinuing:
May be unnecessary to finish medicine. Follow doctor's instructions.

Others:
Impaired blood circulation can lead to gangrene in intestines or extremities. Never exceed recommended dose.

POSSIBLE INTERACTION WITH OTHER DRUGS

GENERIC NAME OR DRUG CLASS	COMBINED EFFECT
Amphetamines*	Dangerous blood pressure rise.
Beta-adrenergic blockers*	Narrowed arteries in heart if ergotamine is taken in high doses.
Ephedrine	Dangerous blood pressure rise.
Epinephrine	Dangerous blood pressure rise.
Ergot preparations, other	May cause decreased circulation to arms, legs, feet and hands. Avoid.
Pseudoephedrine	Dangerous blood pressure rise.
Sympathomimetics*	May cause decreased circulation to arms, legs, feet and hands. Avoid.
Troleandomycin	Increased adverse reactions of ergotamine.

POSSIBLE INTERACTION WITH OTHER SUBSTANCES

INTERACTS WITH	COMBINED EFFECT
Alcohol:	Dilates blood vessels. Makes headache worse.
Beverages: Caffeine drinks.	May help relieve headache.
Cocaine:	Decreased ergotamine effect.
Foods: Any to which you are allergic.	May make headache worse. Avoid.
Marijuana:	Occasional use—Cool extremities. Regular use—Persistent chill.
Tobacco:	Decreased effect of ergotamine. Makes headache worse.

*See Glossary

ERGOTAMINE, BELLADONNA & PHENOBARBITAL

BRAND NAMES

Bellergal   Bellergal Spacetabs
Bellergal-S

BASIC INFORMATION

Habit forming? Yes
Prescription needed? Yes
Available as generic? No
Drug class: Analgesic, antispasmodic, vasoconstrictor

 USES

Reduces anxiety or nervous tension (low dose).

 DOSAGE & USAGE INFORMATION

How to take:
- Tablet or extended-release tablet—Swallow with liquid, or let dissolve under tongue. If you can't swallow whole, crumble tablet or open capsule and take with liquid or food.
- Lie down in quiet, dark room after taking.

When to take:
At first sign of vascular or migraine headache.

If you forget a dose:
Take as soon as you remember. Wait 4 hours for next dose.

What drug does:
- Constricts blood vessels in the head.
- Blocks nerve impulses at parasympathetic nerve endings, preventing muscle contractions and gland secretions of organs involved.

Continued next column

 OVERDOSE

SYMPTOMS:
Tingling, cold extremities; muscle pain; nausea; vomiting; diarrhea; cold skin; rapid and weak pulse; severe numbness of extremities; confusion; dilated pupils; rapid pulse and breathing; dizziness; fever; hallucinations; slurred speech; agitation; flushed face; convulsions; coma.
WHAT TO DO:
- **Dial 0 (operator) or 911 (emergency) for an ambulance or medical help. Then give first aid immediately.**
- **See emergency information on inside covers.**

Time lapse before drug works:
15 to 30 minutes.

Don't take with:
Non-prescription drugs without consulting doctor.

 POSSIBLE ADVERSE REACTIONS OR SIDE EFFECTS

SYMPTOMS	WHAT TO DO
Life-threatening:	
In case of overdose, see previous column.	
Common:	
• Flushed skin, fever, drowsiness, bloating, depression, frequent urination.	Discontinue. Call doctor right away.
• Constipation, dizziness, drowsiness, "hangover" effect, increased frequency or severity of headaches.	Continue. Call doctor when convenient.
Infrequent:	
• Swollen feet and ankles, numbness or tingling in hands or feet, cold hands and feet, rash.	Discontinue. Call doctor right away.
• Nasal congestion, altered taste.	Continue. Call doctor when convenient.
Rare:	
Jaundice, weak legs, swallowing difficulty, dry mouth, increased sensitivity to sunlight, nausea, vomiting, decreased sweating.	Discontinue. Call doctor right away.

 WARNINGS & PRECAUTIONS

Don't take if:
- You are allergic to any barbiturate, tartrazine dye, anticholinergic or ergot preparation.
- You have porphyria, trouble with stomach bloating, difficulty emptying your bladder completely, narrow-angle glaucoma, severe ulcerative colitis, enlarged prostate.

Before you start, consult your doctor:
- If you have epilepsy; kidney, thyroid or liver damage; anemia; chronic pain; open-angle glaucoma; angina; fast heartbeat; heart problems; high blood pressure; hardening of the arteries; vein problems; chronic bronchitis; asthma; hiatal hernia; enlarged prostate; myasthenia gravis; peptic ulcer; an infection.

ERGOTAMINE, BELLADONNA & PHENOBARBITAL

- If you plan to become pregnant within medication period.
- If you will have surgery within 2 months, including dental surgery, requiring general or spinal anesthesia.

Over age 60:
Adverse reactions and side effects may be more frequent and severe than in younger persons.

Pregnancy:
Risk to unborn child outweighs drug benefits. Don't use.

Breast-feeding:
Drug passes into milk. Avoid drug or discontinue nursing until you finish medicine. Consult doctor for advice on maintaining milk supply.

Infants & children:
Not recommended.

Prolonged use:
- May cause addiction, anemia, chronic intoxication.
- May lower body temperature, making exposure to cold temperatures hazardous.
- Chronic constipation, possible fecal impaction.
- Cold skin, muscle pain, gangrene of hands and feet. This medicine not intended for uninterrupted use.

Skin & sunlight:
May cause rash or intensify sunburn in areas exposed to sun or sunlamp.

Driving, piloting or hazardous work:
Don't drive or pilot aircraft until you learn how medicine affects you. Don't work around dangerous machinery. Don't climb ladders or work in high places. Danger increases if you drink alcohol or take medicine affecting alertness and reflexes, such as antihistamines, tranquilizers, sedatives, pain medicine, narcotics and mind-altering drugs.

Discontinuing:
May be unnecessary to finish medicine. Follow doctor's instructions. If you develop withdrawal symptoms of hallucinations, agitation or sleeplessness after discontinuing, call doctor right away.

Others:
Impaired blood circulation can lead to gangrene in intestines or extremities. Never exceed recommended dose.

POSSIBLE INTERACTION WITH OTHER DRUGS

GENERIC NAME OR DRUG CLASS	COMBINED EFFECT
Amantadine	Increased belladonna effect.
Amphetamines*	Dangerous blood pressure rise.
Anticholinergics, other*	Increased belladonna effect.
Anticoagulants, oral*	Decreased anticoagulant effect.
Anticonvulsants*	Changed seizure patterns.
Antidepressants, tricyclics (TCA)*	Decreased antidepressant effect. Possible dangerous oversedation.
Antidiabetics, oral*	Increased phenobarbital effect.
Antihistamines*	Dangerous sedation. Avoid.
Aspirin	Decreased aspirin effect.
Beta-adrenergic blockers*	Narrowed arteries in heart if taken in large doses.
Contraceptives, oral*	Decreased contraceptive effect.
Cortisone drugs*	Decreased cortisone effect. Increased internal eye pressure.

Continued page 944

POSSIBLE INTERACTION WITH OTHER SUBSTANCES

INTERACTS WITH	COMBINED EFFECT
Alcohol:	Possible fatal oversedation. Avoid.
Beverages:	None expected.
Cocaine:	Excessively rapid heartbeat. Avoid.
Foods:	None expected.
Marijuana:	Drowsiness and dry mouth, excessive sedation. Avoid.
Tobacco:	None expected.

ERGOTAMINE & CAFFEINE

BRAND NAMES

Cafatine	Ergo-Caff
Cafergot	Gotamine
Cafermine	Migergot
Ercaf	Wigraine
Ercatabs	

BASIC INFORMATION

Habit forming? No
Prescription needed? Yes
Available as generic? No
Drug class: Analgesic, stimulant (xanthine), vasoconstrictor

 USES

Relieves pain of migraines and other headaches caused by dilated blood vessels. Will not prevent headaches.

 DOSAGE & USAGE INFORMATION

How to take:
- Tablet—Swallow with liquid, or let dissolve under tongue. If you can't swallow whole, crumble tablet and take with liquid or food.
- Suppositories—Remove wrapper and moisten suppository with water. Gently insert larger end into rectum. Push well into rectum with finger.
- Lie down in quiet, dark room after taking.

When to take:
At first sign of vascular or migraine headache.

If you forget a dose:
Take as soon as you remember up to 2 hours late. If more than 2 hours, wait for next scheduled dose (don't double this dose).

What drug does:
- Constricts blood vessels in the head.
- Constricts blood-vessel walls.
- Stimulates central nervous system.

Continued next column

 OVERDOSE

SYMPTOMS:
Tingling, cold extremities; muscle pain; nausea; vomiting; diarrhea; cold skin; severe numbness of extremities; confusion; excitement; rapid heartbeat; insomnia; hallucinations; convulsions; coma.
WHAT TO DO:
- Dial 0 (operator) or 911 (emergency) for an ambulance or medical help. Then give first aid immediately.
- See emergency information on inside covers.

Time lapse before drug works:
30 to 60 minutes.

Don't take with:
- Non-prescription drugs containing alcohol without consulting doctor.
- Any other medicine without consulting your doctor or pharmacist.

 POSSIBLE ADVERSE REACTIONS OR SIDE EFFECTS

SYMPTOMS	WHAT TO DO
Life-threatening:	
In case of overdose, see previous column.	
Common:	
• Fast heartbeat, feet or ankle swelling.	Discontinue. Call doctor right away.
• Dizziness, nausea, diarrhea, vomiting, nervousness, increased frequency or severity of headaches.	Continue. Call doctor when convenient.
Infrequent:	
Itchy skin; abdominal pain; cold hands and feet; weakness in arms, legs, back; confusion; irritability; indigestion; low blood sugar with weakness and trembling.	Discontinue. Call doctor right away.
Rare:	
Anxiety; red or purple blisters, especially on on hands and feet; change in vision; extreme thirst; numbness or tingling in hands or feet.	Discontinue. Call doctor right away.

 WARNINGS & PRECAUTIONS

Don't take if:
- You are allergic to any stimulant or any ergot preparation.
- You have heart disease.
- You have active peptic ulcer of stomach or duodenum.

Before you start, consult your doctor:
- If you have irregular heartbeat, angina, heart problems, high blood pressure, hardening of the arteries or vein problems.
- If you have hypoglycemia (low blood sugar), epilepsy, an infection, kidney or liver disease.
- If you are allergic to spray inhalants.
- If you plan to become pregnant within medication period.

Over age 60:
Adverse reactions and side effects may be more frequent and severe than in younger persons, especially dizziness and excessive potassium loss.

Pregnancy:
Risk to unborn child outweighs drug benefits. Don't use.

Breast-feeding:
Drug passes into milk. Avoid drug or discontinue nursing until you finish medicine. Consult doctor for advice on maintaining milk supply.

Infants & children:
Not recommended.

Prolonged use:
Cold skin, muscle pain, stomach ulcers, gangrene of hands and feet. This medicine not intended for uninterrupted use.

Skin & sunlight:
No problems expected.

Driving, piloting or hazardous work:
Don't drive or pilot aircraft until you learn how medicine affects you. Don't work around dangerous machinery. Don't climb ladders or work in high places. Danger increases if you drink alcohol or take medicine affecting alertness and reflexes, such as antihistamines, tranquilizers, sedatives, pain medicine, narcotics and mind-altering drugs.

Discontinuing:
Will cause withdrawal symptoms of headache, irritability, drowsiness. Discontinue gradually if you use caffeine for a month or more.

Others:
- May produce or aggravate fibrocystic breast disease in women.
- Impaired blood circulation can lead to gangrene in intestines or extremities. Never exceed recommended dose.

 ## POSSIBLE INTERACTION WITH OTHER DRUGS

GENERIC NAME OR DRUG CLASS	COMBINED EFFECT
Amphetamines*	Dangerous blood pressure rise.
Beta-adrenergic blockers*	Narrowed arteries in heart if taken in large doses.
Cimetidine	Increased caffeine effect.
Contraceptives, oral*	Increased caffeine effect.
Ephedrine	Dangerous blood pressure rise.
Epinephrine	Dangerous blood pressure rise.
Isoniazid	Increased caffeine effect.
MAO inhibitors*	Dangerous blood pressure rise.
Pseudoephedrine	Dangerous blood pressure rise.
Sedatives*	Decreased sedative effect.
Sleep inducers*	Decreased sedative effect.
Sympathomimetics*	Overstimulation.
Thyroid hormones*	Increased thyroid effect.
Tranquilizers*	Decreased tranquilizer effect.
Troleandomycin	Increased adverse reactions of ergotamine.

 ## POSSIBLE INTERACTION WITH OTHER SUBSTANCES

INTERACTS WITH	COMBINED EFFECT
Alcohol:	Dilates blood vessels. Makes headache worse.
Beverages: Caffeine drinks.	May help relieve headache.
Cocaine:	Overstimulation. Avoid.
Foods: Any to which you are allergic.	May make headache worse. Avoid.
Marijuana:	Occasional use—Cool extremities. Regular use—Persistent chill. Increased effect of both drugs. May lead to dangerous, rapid heartbeat. Avoid.
Tobacco:	Decreased effect of ergotamine and caffeine. Makes headache worse. Avoid.

*See Glossary

ERGOTAMINE, CAFFEINE, BELLADONNA & PENTOBARBITAL

BRAND NAMES

Cafatine PB
Cafergot-PB

Cafetrate PB
Migergot-PB

BASIC INFORMATION

Habit forming? Yes
Prescription needed? Yes
Available as generic? No
Drug class: Vasoconstrictor, stimulant (xanthine), sedative, antispasmodic

 ## USES

- Relieves pain of migraines and other headaches caused by dilated blood vessels. Will not prevent headaches.
- Reduces anxiety or nervous tension (low dose).

 ## DOSAGE & USAGE INFORMATION

How to take:
- Tablet—Swallow with liquid, or let dissolve under tongue. If you can't swallow whole, crumble tablet and take with liquid or food.
- Suppositories—Remove wrapper and moisten suppository with water. Gently insert larger end into rectum. Push well into rectum with finger.
- Lie down in quiet, dark room after taking.

When to take:
At first sign of vascular or migraine headache.

Continued next column

 ## OVERDOSE

SYMPTOMS:
Tingling, cold extremities and muscle pain. Progresses to nausea, vomiting, diarrhea, insomnia, cold skin, rapid and weak pulse, severe numbness of extremities, confusion, convulsions, coma.
WHAT TO DO:
- **Dial 0 (operator) or 911 (emergency) for an ambulance or medical help. Then give first aid immediately.**
- **See emergency information on inside covers.**

If you forget a dose:
Take as soon as you remember up to 2 hours late. If more than 2 hours, wait for next scheduled dose (don't double this dose).

What drug does:
- Blocks nerve impulses at parasympathetic nerve endings, preventing muscle contractions and gland secretions of organs involved.
- May partially block nerve impulses at nerve-cell connections.
- Constricts blood-vessel walls.
- Stimulates central nervous system.

Time lapse before drug works:
15 to 30 minutes.

Don't take with:
- Non-prescription drugs without consulting doctor.
- Any other medicine without consulting your doctor or pharmacist.

 ## POSSIBLE ADVERSE REACTIONS OR SIDE EFFECTS

SYMPTOMS	WHAT TO DO
Life-threatening:	
In case of overdose, see previous column.	
Common:	
• Moderately fast heartbeat.	Discontinue. Call doctor right away.
• Dizziness, nausea, diarrhea, vomiting, nervousness, "hang-over" effect, increased frequency or severity of headaches.	Continue. Call doctor when convenient.
Infrequent:	
• Itchy skin; rash; abdominal pain; cold hands and feet; weakness in arms, back legs; confusion; irritability; indigestion; low blood sugar with weakness and trembling.	Discontinue. Call doctor right away.
• Nasal congestion, altered taste.	Continue. Call doctor when convenient.
Rare:	
Anxiety; red or purple blisters, especially in hands and feet; change in vision; extreme thirst; numbness or tingling in hands or feet; jaundice.	Discontinue. Call doctor right away.

ERGOTAMINE, CAFFEINE, BELLADONNA & PENTOBARBITAL

WARNINGS & PRECAUTIONS

Don't take if:
- You are allergic to any stimulant, ergot preparation, barbiturate or anticholinergic.
- You have heart disease, peptic ulcer of stomach or duodenum, porphyria, trouble with stomach bloating, difficulty emptying your bladder completely, narrow-angle glaucoma, severe ulcerative colitis.

Before you start, consult your doctor:
- If you have hypoglycemia (low blood sugar), an infection, angina, heart problems, high blood pressure, hardening of the arteries, vein problems, kidney or liver disease, epilepsy, asthma, anemia, chronic pain, open-angle glaucoma, chronic bronchitis, hiatal hernia, enlarged prostate, myasthenia gravis, peptic ulcer.
- If you plan to become pregnant within medication period.
- If you will have surgery within 2 months, including dental surgery, requiring general or spinal anesthesia.

Over age 60:
Adverse reactions and side effects may be more frequent and severe than in younger persons, especially dizziness and excessive potassium loss.

Pregnancy:
Risk to unborn child outweighs drug benefits. Don't use.

Breast-feeding:
Drug filters into milk. May harm child. Avoid.

Infants & children:
Not recommended.

Prolonged use:
- Stomach ulcers.
- Cold skin, muscle pain, gangrene of hands and feet. This medicine not intended for uninterrupted use.
- May cause addiction, anemia, chronic intoxication.
- May lower body temperature, making exposure to cold temperatures hazardous.
- Chronic constipation, possible fecal impaction.

Skin & sunlight:
May cause rash or intensify sunburn in areas exposed to sun or sunlamp.

Driving, piloting or hazardous work:
Don't drive or pilot aircraft until you learn how medicine affects you. Don't work around dangerous machinery. Don't climb ladders or work in high places. Danger increases if you drink alcohol or take medicine affecting alertness and reflexes, such as antihistamines, tranquilizers, sedatives, pain medicine, narcotics and mind-altering drugs.

Discontinuing:
May be unnecessary to finish medicine. Follow doctor's instructions. If you develop withdrawal symptoms of hallucinations, headache, agitation or sleeplessness after discontinuing, call doctor right away.

Others:
- Great potential for abuse.
- May produce or aggravate fibrocystic breast disease in women.
- Impaired blood circulation can lead to gangrene in intestines or extremities. Never exceed recommended dose.

POSSIBLE INTERACTION WITH OTHER DRUGS

GENERIC NAME OR DRUG CLASS	COMBINED EFFECT
Amantadine	Increased belladonna effect.
Amphetamines*	Dangerous blood pressure rise.
Anticoagulants, oral*	Decreased anti-coagulant effect.

Continued page 945

POSSIBLE INTERACTION WITH OTHER SUBSTANCES

INTERACTS WITH	COMBINED EFFECT
Alcohol:	Dilates blood vessels. Makes headache worse. Possible fatal oversedation. Avoid.
Beverages: Caffeine drinks.	May help relieve headache.
Cocaine:	Excessively rapid heartbeat. Avoid.
Foods: Any to which you are allergic.	May make headache worse. Avoid.
Marijuana:	Drowsiness and dry mouth, excessive sedation. Avoid. Occasional use—Cool extremities. Regular use—Persistent chill.
Tobacco:	Decreased effect of ergotamine. Makes headache worse.

*See Glossary

ERYTHROMYCINS

BRAND AND GENERIC NAMES

See complete list of brand and generic names in the *Brand Name Directory*, page 920.

BASIC INFORMATION

Habit forming? No
Prescription needed? Yes
Available as generic? Yes
Drug class: Antibiotic (erythromycin)

 ## USES

Treatment of infections responsive to erythromycin.

 ## DOSAGE & USAGE INFORMATION

How to take:
- Tablet or capsule—Swallow with liquid.
- Extended-release tablets or capsules— Swallow each dose whole. If you take regular tablets, you may chew or crush them.
- Liquid, drops, granules, skin ointment, eye ointment, skin solution—Follow prescription label directions.

When to take:
At the same times each day, 1 hour before or 2 hours after eating.

If you forget a dose:
- If you take 3 or more doses daily—Take as soon as you remember. Return to regular schedule.
- If you take 2 doses daily—Take as soon as you remember. Wait 5 to 6 hours for next dose. Return to regular schedule.

What drug does:
Prevents growth and reproduction of susceptible bacteria.

Time lapse before drug works:
2 to 5 days.

Don't take with:
Any other medicine without consulting your doctor or pharmacist.

 ## OVERDOSE

SYMPTOMS:
Nausea, vomiting, abdominal discomfort, diarrhea.
WHAT TO DO:
Overdose unlikely to threaten life. If person takes much larger amount than prescribed, call doctor, poison-control center or hospital emergency room for instructions.

 ## POSSIBLE ADVERSE REACTIONS OR SIDE EFFECTS

SYMPTOMS	WHAT TO DO
Life-threatening:	
None expected.	
Common:	
Mild nausea.	Continue. Call doctor when convenient.
Infrequent:	
• Diarrhea, abdominal cramps, discomfort, vomiting, rash.	Discontinue. Call doctor right away.
• Skin dryness, irritation, itch, stinging with use of skin solution, sore mouth or tongue.	Continue. Call doctor when convenient.
Rare:	
• Jaundice in adults, hearing loss.	Discontinue. Call doctor right away.
• Unusual tiredness or weakness.	Continue. Call doctor when convenient.

WARNINGS & PRECAUTIONS

Don't take if:
- You are allergic to any erythromycin.
- You have had liver disease or impaired liver function.

Before you start, consult your doctor:
If you have taken erythromycin estolate in the past.

Over age 60:
Adverse reactions and side effects may be more frequent and severe than in younger persons, especially skin reactions around genitals and anus.

Pregnancy:
No proven harm to unborn child. Avoid if possible.

Breast-feeding:
Drug passes into milk. Avoid drug or discontinue nursing until you finish medicine. Consult doctor for advice on maintaining milk supply.

Infants & children:
Use only under medical supervision.

Prolonged use:
- You may become more susceptible to infections caused by germs not responsive to erythromycin.
- Talk to your doctor about the need for follow-up medical examinations or laboratory studies to check liver function.

Skin & sunlight:
No problems expected.

Driving, piloting or hazardous work:
No problems expected.

Discontinuing:
You must take full dose at least 10 consecutive days for streptococcal or staphylococcal infections.

Others:
No problems expected.

POSSIBLE INTERACTION WITH OTHER DRUGS

GENERIC NAME OR DRUG CLASS	COMBINED EFFECT
Aminophylline	Increased effect of aminophylline in blood.
Caffeine	Increased effect of caffeine.
Cefixime	Decreased antibiotic effect of cefixime.
Cyclosporins	May increase cyclosporin toxicity.
Ketoconazole	Possible heartbeat irregularity
Lincomycins*	Decreased lincomycin effect.
Oxtriphylline	Increased level of oxtriphylline in blood.
Penicillins*	Decreased penicillin effect.
Theophylline	Increased level of theophylline in blood.
Warfarin	Increased risk of bleeding.

POSSIBLE INTERACTION WITH OTHER SUBSTANCES

INTERACTS WITH	COMBINED EFFECT
Alcohol:	Possible liver damage.
Beverages: Caffeine containing.	Increased caffeine toxicity. Avoid.
Cocaine:	None expected.
Foods: Wines, syrup, acidic fruits or juices (if taken with).	Decreased antibiotic effect.
Marijuana:	None expected.
Tobacco:	None expected.

*See Glossary

ERYTHROMYCIN & SULFISOXAZOLE

BRAND NAMES

Pediazole

BASIC INFORMATION

Habit forming? No
Prescription needed? Yes
Available as generic? No
Drug class: Antibiotic (erythromycin), sulfa (sulfonamide)

USES

Treatment of infections responsive to erythromycin and sulfa.

DOSAGE & USAGE INFORMATION

How to take:
Suspension—Swallow with liquid. Instructions to take on empty stomach mean 1 hour before or 2 hours after eating. Shake carefully before measuring.

When to take:
At the same times each day, 1 hour before or 2 hours after eating.

If you forget a dose:
Take as soon as you remember up to 2 hours late. If more than 2 hours, wait for next scheduled dose (don't double this dose).

What drug does:
Prevents growth and reproduction of susceptible bacteria.

Time lapse before drug works:
2 to 5 days to affect infection.

Don't take with:
Any other medicine without consulting your doctor or pharmacist.

OVERDOSE

SYMPTOMS:
Less urine, bloody urine, nausea, skin rash, vomiting, abdominal discomfort, diarrhea, coma.
WHAT TO DO:
- **Dial 0 (operator) or 911 (emergency) for an ambulance or medical help. Then give first aid immediately.**
- **See emergency information on inside covers.**

POSSIBLE ADVERSE REACTIONS OR SIDE EFFECTS

SYMPTOMS	WHAT TO DO
Life-threatening:	
In case of overdose, see previous column.	
Common:	
• Headache, dizziness, itchy skin, rash, appetite loss, vomiting.	Discontinue. Call doctor right away.
• Mild nausea.	Continue. Call doctor when convenient.
Infrequent:	
• Dryness, irritation, stinging with use of skin solution, mouth or tongue sore.	Continue. Call doctor when convenient.
• Diarrhea, nausea, abdominal cramps, swallowing difficulty.	Discontinue. Call doctor right away.
Rare:	
• Jaundice, painful or difficult urination, muscle or joint pain, unusual tiredness, blood in urine, swelling of neck.	Discontinue. Call doctor right away.
• Weakness.	Continue. Call doctor when convenient.

WARNINGS & PRECAUTIONS

Don't take if:
- You are allergic to any sulfa drug or any erythromycin.
- You have had liver disease or impaired liver function.

Before you start, consult your doctor:
- If you are allergic to carbonic anhydrase inhibitors, oral antidiabetics or thiazide diuretics.
- If you are allergic by nature.
- If you have liver or kidney disease, porphyria, developed anemia from use of any drug, taken erythromycin estolate in the past.

Over age 60:
Adverse reactions and side effects may be more frequent and severe than in younger persons, especially skin reactions around genitals and anus.

Pregnancy:
Risk to unborn child outweighs drug benefits. Don't use.

ERYTHROMYCIN & SULFISOXAZOLE

Breast-feeding:
Drug passes into milk. Avoid drug or discontinue nursing until you finish medicine. Consult doctor for advice on maintaining milk supply.

Infants & children:
Don't give to infants younger than 1 month.

Prolonged use:
- May enlarge thyroid gland.
- Request frequent blood counts, liver- and kidney-function studies.
- You may become more susceptible to infections caused by germs not responsive to erythromycin or sulfa.

Skin & sunlight:
May cause rash or intensify sunburn in areas exposed to sun or sunlamp.

Driving, piloting or hazardous work:
Avoid if you feel dizzy. Otherwise, no problems expected.

Discontinuing:
Don't discontinue without doctor's advice until you complete prescribed dose, even though symptoms diminish or disappear.

Others:
- Drink extra liquid each day to prevent adverse reactions, such as kidney damage.
- If you require surgery, tell anesthetist you take sulfa.

POSSIBLE INTERACTION WITH OTHER DRUGS

GENERIC NAME OR DRUG CLASS	COMBINED EFFECT
Aminobenzoate potassium	Possible decreased sulfisoxazole effect.
Aminophylline	Increased effect of aminophylline in blood.
Anticoagulants, oral*	Increased anticoagulant effect.
Anticonvulsants, hydantoin*	Toxic effect on brain.
Aspirin	Increased sulfa effect.
Flecainide	Possible decreased blood-cell production in bone marrow.
Isoniazid	Possible anemia.
Lincomycins*	Decreased lincomycin effect.
Methenamine	Possible kidney blockage.

Methotrexate	Increased possibility of toxic side effects from methotrexate.
Oxtriphylline	Increased level of oxtriphylline in blood.
Oxyphenbutazone	Increased sulfa effect.
Para-aminosalicylic acid (PAS)	Decreased sulfa effect.
Penicillins*	Decreased penicillin effect.
Phenylbutazone	Increased sulfa effect.
Probenecid	Increased sulfa effect.
Sulfinpyrazone	Increased sulfa effect.
Theophylline	Increased level of theophylline in blood.
Tocainide	Possible decreased blood-cell production in bone marrow.
Trimethoprim	Increased sulfa effect.

POSSIBLE INTERACTION WITH OTHER SUBSTANCES

INTERACTS WITH	COMBINED EFFECT
Alcohol:	Increased alcohol effect. Possible liver damage.
Beverages:	None expected.
Cocaine:	None expected.
Foods: Wines, syrups, acidic fruits or juices (if taken with).	Decreased antibiotic effect.
Marijuana:	None expected.
Tobacco:	None expected.

*See Glossary

ESTRAMUSTINE

BRAND NAMES

Emcyt

BASIC INFORMATION

Habit forming? No
Prescription needed? Yes
Available as generic? No
Drug class: Antineoplastic

 USES

Treats prostate cancer.

 DOSAGE & USAGE INFORMATION

How to take:
Capsule—Swallow with liquid. If you can't swallow whole, open capsule and take with liquid or food. Instructions to take on empty stomach mean 1 hour before or 2 hours after eating.

When to take:
According to doctor's instructions. Try to take 1 hour before or 2 hours after eating or drinking any milk products.

If you forget a dose:
Skip dose. Never double dose.

What drug does:
Suppresses growth of cancer cells.

Time lapse before drug works:
Within 20 hours.

Don't take with:
Any other medicines (including over-the-counter drugs such as cough and cold medicines, laxatives, antacids, diet pills, caffeine, nose drops or vitamins) without consulting your doctor.

 OVERDOSE

SYMPTOMS:
None expected.
WHAT TO DO:
Overdose unlikely to threaten life. If person takes much larger amount than prescribed, call doctor, poison-control center or hospital emergency room for instructions.

 POSSIBLE ADVERSE REACTIONS OR SIDE EFFECTS

SYMPTOMS	WHAT TO DO
Life-threatening:	
Sudden headaches, chest pain, shortness of breath, leg pain, vision changes, slurred speech.	Seek emergency treatment immediately.
Common:	
• Skin rash, itching	Discontinue. Call doctor right away.
• Increased sun sensitivity.	Decrease sun exposure. Call doctor when convenient.
• Diarrhea, dizziness, nausea, vomiting, headache.	Continue. Call doctor when convenient.
Infrequent:	
• Joint or muscle pain, difficulty swallowing, sore throat and fever, peeling skin, jaundice.	Discontinue. Call doctor right away.
• Mouth or tongue irritation.	Continue. Call doctor when convenient.
Rare:	
Bloody urine, hearing loss, back pain, abdominal pain.	Discontinue. Call doctor right away.

WARNINGS & PRECAUTIONS

Don't take if:
- You have chicken pox.
- You have shingles (herpes zoster).
- You have had a recent heart attack.
- You have active thrombophlebitis.

Before you start, consult your doctor:
- If you have jaundice.
- If you have history of thrombophlebitis.
- If you have peptic ulcer.
- If you have mental depression.
- If you have migraine headaches.

Over age 60:
Adverse reactions and side effects may be more frequent and severe than in younger persons. You may need smaller doses for shorter periods of time.

Pregnancy:
Used in men only.

Breast-feeding:
Used in men only.

Infants & children:
Not used.

Prolonged use:
Talk to your doctor about the need for follow-up medical examinations or laboratory studies to check complete blood counts (white blood cell count, platelet count, red blood cell count, hemoglobin, hematocrit), blood pressure, liver function, serum acid, serum calcium and alkaline phosphatase.

Skin & sunlight:
No problems expected.

Driving, piloting or hazardous work:
No special problems expected.

Discontinuing:
No special problems expected.

Others:
- Advise any doctor or dentist whom you consult that you take this medicine.
- May affect results in some medical tests.
- May decrease sperm count in males.

POSSIBLE INTERACTION WITH OTHER DRUGS

GENERIC NAME OR DRUG CLASS	COMBINED EFFECT
Calcium supplements*	Decreased absorption of estramustine.
Hepatotoxic medications*	Increased risk of liver toxicity.

POSSIBLE INTERACTION WITH OTHER SUBSTANCES

INTERACTS WITH	COMBINED EFFECT
Alcohol:	Increased "hangover effect" and other gastrointestinal symptoms.
Beverages: Milk and milk products.	Decreased absorption of estramustine.
Cocaine:	No special problems expected.
Foods: Foods high in calcium.	Decreased absorption of estramustine.
Marijuana:	No special problems expected.
Tobacco:	Increased risk of heart attack and blood clots.

*See Glossary

ESTROGENS

BRAND AND GENERIC NAMES

See complete list of brand and generic names in *Brand Name Directory*, page 920.

BASIC INFORMATION

Habit forming? No
Prescription needed? Yes
Available as generic? Yes
Drug class: Female sex hormone (estrogen)

USES

- Treatment for estrogen deficiency.
- Treatment for symptoms of menopause and menstrual cycle irregularity.
- Treatment for estrogen-deficiency osteoporosis (bone softening from calcium loss).
- Treatment for vulvar squamous hyperplasia.
- Treatment for atrophic vaginitis.
- Treatment for prostate cancer.

DOSAGE & USAGE INFORMATION

How to take:
- Tablet or capsule—Take with or after food to reduce nausea. Swallow with liquid. If you can't swallow whole, crumble tablet or open capsule and take with liquid or food.
- Vaginal cream or suppositories—Use as directed on label.
- By injection under medical supervision.
- Transdermal patches—Follow package instructions.

When to take:
At the same time each day.

If you forget a dose:
Take as soon as you remember up to 12 hours late. If more than 12 hours, wait for next scheduled dose (don't double this dose).

What drug does:
- Restores normal estrogen level in tissues.
- Combined with progestins for contraception.

Continued in next column

OVERDOSE

SYMPTOMS:
Nausea, vomiting, fluid retention, breast enlargement and discomfort, abnormal vaginal bleeding.
WHAT TO DO:
Overdose unlikely to threaten life. If person takes much larger amount than prescribed, call doctor, poison-control center or hospital emergency room for instructions.

Time lapse before drug works:
10 to 20 days.

Don't take with:
Any other medicine without consulting your doctor or pharmacist.

POSSIBLE ADVERSE REACTIONS OR SIDE EFFECTS

SYMPTOMS	WHAT TO DO
Life-threatening:	
Profuse bleeding.	Seek emergency treatment.
Common:	
• Stomach cramps.	Discontinue. Call doctor right away.
• Appetite loss.	Continue. Call doctor when convenient.
• Nausea; diarrhea; swollen feet and ankles; tender, swollen breasts; acne; intolerance of contact lenses; change in menstruation.	Continue. Tell doctor at next visit.
Infrequent:	
• Rash, stomach or side pain, joint or muscle pain, bloody skin blisters, breast lumps.	Discontinue. Call doctor right away.
• Depression, dizziness, migraine headache, irritability, vomiting.	Continue. Call doctor when convenient.
• Brown blotches, hair loss, vaginal discharge or bleeding, changes in sex drive.	Continue. Tell doctor at next visit.
Rare:	
• Jaundice, hypercalcemia in breast cancer.	Discontinue. Call doctor right away.
• Involuntary movements.	

WARNINGS & PRECAUTIONS

Don't take if:
- You are allergic to any estrogen-containing drugs.
- You have impaired liver function.
- You have had blood clots, stroke or heart attack.
- You have unexplained vaginal bleeding.

Before you start, consult your doctor:
- If you have had cancer of the breast or reproductive organs, fibrocystic breast disease, fibroid tumors of the uterus or endometriosis.
- If you have had migraine headaches, epilepsy or porphyria.

- If you have diabetes, high blood pressure, asthma, congestive heart failure, kidney disease or gallstones.
- If you plan to become pregnant within 3 months.

Over age 60:
Controversial. You and your doctor must decide if risks of drug outweigh benefits.

Pregnancy:
Risk to unborn child outweighs benefits of drug. Don't use.

Breast-feeding:
Drug filters into milk. May harm child. Avoid.

Infants & children:
Not recommended.

Prolonged use:
- Increased growth of fibroid tumors of uterus. Possible association with cancer of uterus.
- Talk to your doctor about the need for follow-up medical examinations or laboratory studies to check pap smear, liver function, mammogram.

Skin & sunlight:
May cause rash or intensify sunburn in areas exposed to sun or sunlamp.

Driving, piloting or hazardous work:
No problems expected.

Discontinuing:
You may need to discontinue estrogens periodically. Consult your doctor.

Others:
- In rare instances, may cause blood clot in lung, brain or leg. Symptoms are *sudden* severe headache, coordination loss, vision change, chest pain, breathing difficulty, slurred speech, pain in legs or groin. Seek emergency treatment immediately.
- Carefully read the paper called "Information for the Patient" that was given to you with your prescription. If you lose it, ask your pharmacist for a copy.

 POSSIBLE INTERACTION WITH OTHER DRUGS

GENERIC NAME OR DRUG CLASS	COMBINED EFFECT
Anticoagulants, oral*	Decreased anti-coagulant effect.
Anticonvulsants, hydantoin*	Decreased estrogen effect.
Antidepressants, tricyclic (TCA)*	Increased toxicity of antidepressants.
Antidiabetics, oral*	Unpredictable increase or decrease in blood sugar.

Antifibrinolytic agents*	Increased possibility of blood clotting.
Carbamazepine	Decreased estrogen effect.
Clofibrate	Decreased clofibrate effect.
Dextrothyroxine	Decreased dextrothyroxine effect.
Didanosine	Increased risk of pancreatitis.
Guanfacine	May decrease antihypertensive effects of guanfacine.
Insulin	Possible decreased insulin effect. May require dosage adjustment.
Meprobamate	Increased estrogen effect.
Phenobarbital	Decreased estrogen effect.
Primidone	Decreased estrogen effect.
Rifampin	Decreased estrogen effect.
Tamoxifen	Decreased tamoxifen effect.
Terazosin	Decreased effectiveness of terazosin.
Thyroid hormones*	Decreased thyroid effect.
Ursodiol	Decreased effect of ursodiol.
Vitamin C	Possible increased estrogen effect.

 POSSIBLE INTERACTION WITH OTHER SUBSTANCES

INTERACTS WITH	COMBINED EFFECT
Alcohol:	None expected.
Beverages:	None expected.
Cocaine:	No proven problems.
Foods:	None expected.
Marijuana:	Possible menstrual irregularities and bleeding between periods.
Tobacco:	Increased risk of blood clots leading to stroke or heart attack.

*See Glossary

ETHCHLORVYNOL

BRAND NAMES

Placidyl

BASIC INFORMATION

Habit forming? Yes
Prescription needed? Yes
Available as generic? No
Drug class: Sleep inducer (hypnotic)

 USES

Treatment of insomnia for short periods.
Prolonged use is not recommended.

 DOSAGE & USAGE INFORMATION

How to take:
Capsules—Take with food or milk to lessen side effects.

When to take:
At or near bedtime.

If you forget a dose:
Bedtime dose—If you forget your once-a-day bedtime dose, don't take it more than 3 hours late.

What drug does:
Affects brain centers that control waking and sleeping.

Time lapse before drug works:
30 to 60 minutes.

Don't take with:
Any other medicine without consulting your doctor or pharmacist.

 OVERDOSE

SYMPTOMS:
Excitement, delirium, incoordination, shortness of breath, slow heartbeat, excessive drowsiness, deep coma.
WHAT TO DO:
● **Dial 0 (operator) or 911 (emergency) for an ambulance or medical help. Then give first aid immediately.**
● **If patient is unconscious and not breathing, give mouth-to-mouth breathing. If there is no heartbeat, use cardiac massage and mouth-to-mouth breathing (CPR). Don't try to make patient vomit. If you can't get help quickly, take patient to nearest emergency facility.**
● **See emergency information on inside covers.**

 POSSIBLE ADVERSE REACTIONS OR SIDE EFFECTS

SYMPTOMS	WHAT TO DO
Life-threatening:	
In case of overdose, see previous column.	
Common:	
● Indigestion, nausea, vomiting, stomach pain.	Discontinue. Call doctor right away.
● Blurred vision, dizziness.	Continue. Call doctor when convenient.
● Unpleasant taste in mouth, fatigue, weakness.	Continue. Tell doctor at next visit.
Infrequent:	
Jitters, clumsiness, unsteadiness, drowsiness, confusion, rash, hives, unusual bleeding or bruising, facial numbness.	Discontinue. Call doctor right away.
Rare:	
Slow heartbeat, difficult breathing, fainting, jaundice, slurred speech, trembling, uncontrolled eye movements.	Discontinue. Call doctor right away.

 WARNINGS & PRECAUTIONS

Don't take if:
● You are allergic to any hypnotic.
● You have porphyria.
● Patient is younger than 12.

Before you start, consult your doctor:
● If you plan to become pregnant within medication period.
● If you have kidney or liver disease.

Over age 60:
Adverse reactions and side effects, especially a "hangover" effect, may be more frequent and severe than in younger persons.

Pregnancy:
Risk to unborn child outweighs drug benefits. Don't use.

Breast-feeding:
No problems expected, but observe child and ask doctor for guidance.

Infants & children:
Not recommended.

Prolonged use:
Impaired vision.

Skin & sunlight:
No problems expected.

Driving, piloting or hazardous work:
Don't drive or pilot aircraft until you learn how medicine affects you. Don't work around dangerous machinery. Don't climb ladders or work in high places. Danger increases if you drink alcohol or take medicine affecting alertness and reflexes.

Discontinuing:
- Don't discontinue without consulting doctor. Dose may require gradual reduction if you have taken drug for a long time. Doses of other drugs may also require adjustment.
- Many side effects may occur when you stop taking this drug, including irritability, muscle twitching, hallucinations or seizures. Consult your doctor.

Others:
No problems expected.

POSSIBLE INTERACTION WITH OTHER DRUGS

GENERIC NAME OR DRUG CLASS	COMBINED EFFECT
Anticoagulants, oral*	Decreased anti-coagulant effect.
Antidepressants, tricyclic (TCA)*	Delirium and deep sedation.
Antihistamines*	Increased antihistamine effect.
Clozapine	Toxic effect on the central nervous system.
Ethinamate	Dangerous increased effects of ethinamate. Avoid combining.
Fluoxetine	Increased depressant effects of both drugs.
Guanfacine	May increase depressant effects of either drug.

Leucovorin	High alcohol content of leucovorin may cause adverse effects.
MAO inhibitors*	Increased sedation.
Methyprylon	Increased sedative effect, perhaps to dangerous level. Avoid.
Molindone	Increased sedative effect.
Nabilone	Greater depression of central nervous system.
Narcotics*	Increased narcotic effect.
Pain relievers*	Increased effect of pain reliever.
Sedatives*	Increased sedative effect.
Sertraline	Increased depressive effects of both drugs.
Tranquilizers*	Increased tranquilizer effect.

POSSIBLE INTERACTION WITH OTHER SUBSTANCES

INTERACTS WITH	COMBINED EFFECT
Alcohol:	Excessive depressant and sedative effect. Avoid.
Beverages:	None expected.
Cocaine:	Decreased ethchlorvynol effect.
Foods:	None expected.
Marijuana:	Occasional use— Drowsiness, unsteadiness, depressed function. Frequent use—Severe drowsiness, impaired physical and mental function.
Tobacco:	None expected.

ETHINAMATE

BRAND NAMES

Valmid

BASIC INFORMATION

Habit forming? Yes
Prescription needed? Yes
Available as generic? No
Drug class: Sedative (hypnotic)

 ## USES

Treats insomnia for short periods. Prolonged use is not recommended.

 ## DOSAGE & USAGE INFORMATION

How to take:
Capsules—Swallow with liquid or food to lessen stomach irritation. If you can't swallow whole, open capsule and take with liquid or food.

When to take:
At bedtime.

If you forget a dose:
Skip dose. Never double-dose.

What drug does:
Helps sleeplessness by an unknown mechanism of action.

Time lapse before drug works:
30 to 40 minutes.

Don't take with:
Any other medicine without consulting your doctor or pharmacist.

 ## OVERDOSE

SYMPTOMS:
Oversedation, slow heartbeat, difficult breathing, coma.
WHAT TO DO:
- **Dial 0 (operator) or 911 (emergency) for an ambulance or medical help. Then give first aid immediately.**
- **See emergency information on inside covers.**

 ## POSSIBLE ADVERSE REACTIONS OR SIDE EFFECTS

SYMPTOMS	WHAT TO DO
Life-threatening:	
Coma, shortness of breath, slow heartbeat.	Seek emergency treatment immediately.
Common:	
Confusion, staggering.	Discontinue. Call doctor right away.
Infrequent:	
• Unusual excitement (especially in children).	Discontinue. Seek emergency treatment.
• Skin rash, upper abdominal discomfort, vomiting.	Discontinue. Call doctor right away.
Rare:	
• Excessive bleeding.	Discontinue. Call doctor right away.
• Daytime drowsiness.	Continue. Call doctor when convenient.

ETHINAMATE

WARNINGS & PRECAUTIONS

Don't take if:
- You are an alcoholic.
- You have a history of drug abuse of any sort.

Before you start, consult your doctor:
- If you have ever had significant depression.
- If you have uncontrolled pain.

Over age 60:
Adverse reactions and side effects may be more frequent and severe than in younger persons. You may need smaller doses for shorter periods of time.

Pregnancy:
Risk to unborn child outweighs drug benefits. Don't use.

Breast-feeding:
Unknown effects. Avoid.

Infants & children:
Not recommended.

Prolonged use:
May lead to habituation.

Skin & sunlight:
No problems expected.

Driving, piloting or hazardous work:
Don't drive or pilot aircraft until you learn how medicine affects you. Don't work around dangerous machinery. Don't climb ladders or work in high places. Danger increases if you drink alcohol or take medicine affecting alertness and reflexes.

Discontinuing:
Discontinue after maximum of 7 days. Don't resume without your doctor's recommendation.

Others:
Has not been shown to be effective after 1 week. If treatment must be repeated, allow 1 or more weeks between treatment periods.

POSSIBLE INTERACTION WITH OTHER DRUGS

GENERIC NAME OR DRUG CLASS	COMBINED EFFECT
Central nervous system (CNS) depressants*	Will dangerously increase the effects of ethinamate and any of the CNS drugs. Avoid combining.
Clozapine	Toxic effect on the central nervous system.
Fluoxetine	Increased depressant effects of both drugs.
Guanfacine	May increase depressant effects of either drug.
Leucovorin	High alcohol content of leucovorin may cause adverse effects.
Methyprylon	Increased sedative effect, perhaps to dangerous level. Avoid.
Nabilone	Greater depression of central nervous system.
Sertraline	Increased depressive effects of both drugs.

POSSIBLE INTERACTION WITH OTHER SUBSTANCES

INTERACTS WITH	COMBINED EFFECT
Alcohol:	Dangerous oversedation. Avoid.
Beverages: Any containing caffeine, such as coffee, tea or cocoa.	Decreases effects of ethinamate.
Cocaine:	Decreases effects of ethinamate and increases chance of toxicity. Avoid.
Foods:	No special problems expected.
Marijuana:	Decreases effects of ethinamate.
Tobacco:	No special problems expected.

*See Glossary

ETHIONAMIDE

BRAND NAMES

Trecator-SC

BASIC INFORMATION

Habit forming? No
Prescription needed? Yes
Available as generic? No
Drug class: Antimycobacterial
(antituberculosis)

 ## USES

Treats tuberculosis. Used in combination with
other antituberculosis drugs such as isoniazid,
streptomycin, nifampin, ethambutol.

 ## DOSAGE & USAGE
INFORMATION

How to take:
Tablets—Swallow with liquid or food to lessen
stomach irritation. If you can't swallow whole,
crumble tablet and take with liquid or food.

When to take:
Usually every 8 to 12 hours, with or after meals.

If you forget a dose:
Take as soon as you remember up to 2 hours
late. If more than 2 hours, wait for next
scheduled dose. Don't double this dose.

What drug does:
Kills germs that cause tuberculosis.

Time lapse before drug works:
Within 3 hours.

Don't take with:
Any other medicine without consulting your
doctor or pharmacist.

 ## OVERDOSE

SYMPTOMS:
None expected.
WHAT TO DO:
**Overdose unlikely to threaten life. If person
takes much larger amount than prescribed,
call doctor, poison-control center or
hospital emergency room for instructions.**

 ## POSSIBLE
ADVERSE REACTIONS
OR SIDE EFFECTS

SYMPTOMS	WHAT TO DO
Life-threatening:	
None expected.	
Common:	
• Vomiting.	Discontinue. Call doctor right away.
• Dizziness, sore mouth, nausea, metallic taste.	Continue. Call doctor when convenient.
Infrequent:	
Jaundice (yellow eyes and skin); numbness, tingling, pain in hands or feet; depression; confusion.	Discontinue. Call doctor right away.
Rare:	
• Hunger, shakiness, rapid heartbeat; blurred vision; vision changes; skin rash.	Discontinue. Call doctor right away.
• Gradual swelling in the neck (thyroid gland).	Continue. Call doctor when convenient.
• Enlargement of breasts (male).	No action necessary.

WARNINGS & PRECAUTIONS

Don't take if:
You know you are hypersensitive to ethionamide.

Before you start, consult your doctor:
- If you have diabetes mellitus.
- If you have liver disease.

Over age 60:
No information available.

Pregnancy:
Risk to unborn child outweighs possible benefits. Don't use.

Breast-feeding:
Effect not documented. Consult your family doctor or pediatrician.

Infants & children:
Effect not documented. Consult your family doctor or pediatrician.

Prolonged use:
No special problems expected.

Skin & sunlight:
No special problems expected.

Driving, piloting or hazardous work:
Don't drive or pilot aircraft until you learn how medicine affects you. Don't work around dangerous machinery. Don't climb ladders or work in high places. Danger increases if you drink alcohol or take medicine affecting alertness and reflexes.

Discontinuing:
Don't discontinue without consulting doctor.

Others:
- Advise any doctor or dentist whom you consult that you take this medicine.
- Request occasional laboratory studies for liver function.
- Request occasional eye examinations.
- Treatment may take months or years.
- You should take pyridoxine (vitamin B-6) supplements while taking ethionamide.

POSSIBLE INTERACTION WITH OTHER DRUGS

GENERIC NAME OR DRUG CLASS	COMBINED EFFECT
Cycloserine	Increased risk of seizures.
Pyridoxine	Increased excretion by kidney. (Should take pyridoxine supplements while on ethionamide to prevent development of neuritis in feet and hands).

POSSIBLE INTERACTION WITH OTHER SUBSTANCES

INTERACTS WITH	COMBINED EFFECT
Alcohol:	Increased incidence of liver diseases.
Beverages: Any alcoholic beverage.	Increased incidence of liver diseases.
Cocaine:	None expected.
Foods:	None expected.
Marijuana:	No interaction expected, but may slow body's recovery.
Tobacco:	No interaction expected, but may slow body's recovery.

ETHOSUXIMIDE

BRAND NAMES

Zarontin

BASIC INFORMATION

Habit forming? No
Prescription needed? Yes
Available as generic? No
Drug class: Anticonvulsant (succinimide)

 USES

Controls seizures in treatment of some forms of epilepsy.

 DOSAGE & USAGE INFORMATION

How to take:
Capsule or syrup—Swallow with liquid or food to lessen stomach irritation.

When to take:
Every day in regularly-spaced doses, according to prescription.

If you forget a dose:
Take as soon as you remember up to 2 hours late. If more than 2 hours, wait for next scheduled dose (don't double this dose).

What drug does:
Depresses nerve transmissions in part of brain that controls muscles.

Time lapse before drug works:
3 hours.

Don't take with:
Any other medicine without consulting your doctor or pharmacist.

 OVERDOSE

SYMPTOMS:
Coma
WHAT TO DO:
- Dial 0 (operator) or 911 (emergency) for an ambulance or medical help. Then give first aid immediately.
- If patient is unconscious and not breathing, give mouth-to-mouth breathing. If there is no heartbeat, use cardiac massage and mouth-to-mouth breathing (CPR). Don't try to make patient vomit. If you can't get help quickly, take patient to nearest emergency facility.
- See emergency information on inside covers.

 POSSIBLE ADVERSE REACTIONS OR SIDE EFFECTS

SYMPTOMS	WHAT TO DO
Life-threatening:	
In case of overdose, see previous column.	
Common:	
Nausea, vomiting, appetite loss, dizziness, drowsiness, hiccups, abdominal pain.	Continue. Call doctor when convenient.
Infrequent:	
Headache, irritability, mood change, tiredness, increased sex drive.	Continue. Call doctor when convenient.
Rare:	
• Sore throat, fever, rash, unusual bleeding or bruising, eye or gum swelling, blood in urine, vaginal bleeding, depression, confusion.	Discontinue. Call doctor right away.
• Swollen lymph glands.	Continue. Call doctor when convenient.

WARNINGS & PRECAUTIONS

Don't take if:
You are allergic to any succinimide anticonvulsant.

Before you start, consult your doctor:
- If you plan to become pregnant within medication period.
- If you take other anticonvulsants.
- If you have blood disease.
- If you have kidney or liver disease.

Over age 60:
Adverse reactions and side effects may be more frequent and severe than in younger persons.

Pregnancy:
Risk to unborn child outweighs drug benefits. Don't use.

Breast-feeding:
Drug passes into milk. Avoid drug or discontinue nursing.

Infants & children:
Use only under medical supervision.

Prolonged use:
Talk to your doctor about the need for follow-up medical examinations or laboratory studies to check complete blood counts (white blood cell count, platelet count, red blood cell count, hemoglobin, hematocrit), liver function, kidney function, urine.

Skin & sunlight:
No problems expected.

Driving, piloting or hazardous work:
Don't drive or pilot aircraft until you learn how medicine affects you. Don't work around dangerous machinery. Don't climb ladders or work in high places. Danger increases if you drink alcohol or take medicine affecting alertness and reflexes, such as antihistamines, tranquilizers, sedatives, pain medicine, narcotics and mind-altering drugs.

Discontinuing:
Don't discontinue without doctor's advice until you complete prescribed dose, even though symptoms diminish or disappear.

Others:
- Your response to medicine should be checked regularly by your doctor. Dose and schedule may have to be altered frequently to fit individual needs.
- Periodic blood-cell counts, kidney- and liver-function studies recommended.
- May discolor urine pink to red-brown. No action necessary.

 POSSIBLE INTERACTION WITH OTHER DRUGS

GENERIC NAME OR DRUG CLASS	COMBINED EFFECT
Anticonvulsants, other*	Increased effect of both drugs.
Antidepressants, tricyclic (TCA)*	May provoke seizures.
Antipsychotics*	May provoke seizures.
Haloperidol	Decreased haloperidol effect; changed seizure pattern.

 POSSIBLE INTERACTION WITH OTHER SUBSTANCES

INTERACTS WITH	COMBINED EFFECT
Alcohol:	May provoke seizures.
Beverages:	None expected.
Cocaine:	May provoke seizures.
Foods:	None expected.
Marijuana:	May provoke seizures.
Tobacco:	None expected.

*See Glossary

ETHOTOIN

BRAND NAMES

Peganone

BASIC INFORMATION

Habit forming? No
Prescription needed? Yes
Available as generic? No
Drug class: Anticonvulsant (hydantoin)

 USES

- Prevents some forms of epileptic seizures.
- Stabilizes irregular heartbeat.

 DOSAGE & USAGE INFORMATION

How to take:
- Tablet—Swallow with liquid.
- Chewable tablets—Chew well before swallowing.
- Suspension—Shake well before taking with liquid.

When to take:
At the same time each day.

If you forget a dose:
- If drug taken 1 time per day—Take as soon as you remember up to 12 hours late. If more than 12 hours, wait for next scheduled dose (don't double this dose).
- If taken several times per day—Take as soon as possible, then return to regular schedule.

What drug does:
Promotes sodium loss from nerve fibers. This lessens excitability and inhibits spread of nerve impulses.

Time lapse before drug works:
7 to 10 days continual use.

Don't take with:
Any other medicine without consulting your doctor or pharmacist.

 OVERDOSE

SYMPTOMS:
Jerky eye movements; stagger; slurred speech; imbalance; drowsiness; blood-pressure drop; slow, shallow breathing; coma.
WHAT TO DO:
- **Dial 0 (operator) or 911 (emergency) for an ambulance or medical help. Then give first aid immediately.**
- **See emergency information on inside covers.**

 POSSIBLE ADVERSE REACTIONS OR SIDE EFFECTS

SYMPTOMS	WHAT TO DO
Life-threatening:	
In case of overdose, see previous column.	
Common:	
Mild dizziness; drowsiness; nausea; vomiting; constipation; bleeding, swollen or tender gums.	Continue. Call doctor when convenient.
Infrequent:	
• Hallucinations, confusion, slurred speech, stagger, rash, change in vision, agitation.	Discontinue. Call doctor right away.
• Headache, diarrhea, muscle twitching.	Continue. Call doctor when convenient.
• Increased body and facial hair, breast swelling, insomnia.	Continue. Tell doctor at next visit.
Rare:	
Sore throat, fever, unusual bleeding or bruising, abdominal pain, jaundice, swollen lymph glands.	Discontinue. Call doctor right away.

 WARNINGS & PRECAUTIONS

Don't take if:
You are allergic to any hydantoin anticonvulsant.

Before you start, consult your doctor:
- If you have had impaired liver function or disease.
- If you will have surgery within 2 months, including dental surgery, requiring general or spinal anesthesia.

Over age 60:
Adverse reactions and side effects may be more frequent and severe than in younger persons.

Pregnancy:
Risk to unborn child outweighs drug benefits. Don't use.

Breast-feeding:
Drug passes into milk. Avoid drug or discontinue nursing until you finish medicine. Consult doctor for advice on maintaining milk supply.

Infants & children:
Use only under medical supervision.

Prolonged use:
- Weakened bones.
- Lymph gland enlargement.
- Possible liver damage.

- Numbness and tingling of hands and feet.
- Continual back-and-forth eye movements.
- Talk to your doctor about the need for follow-up medical examinations or laboratory studies to check complete blood counts (white blood cell count, platelet count, red blood cell count, hemoglobin, hematocrit), liver function, EEG*.

Skin & sunlight:
May cause rash or intensify sunburn in areas exposed to sun or sunlamp.

Driving, piloting or hazardous work:
Don't drive or pilot aircraft until you learn how medicine affects you. Don't work around dangerous machinery. Don't climb ladders or work in high places. Danger increases if you drink alcohol or take medicine affecting alertness and reflexes.

Discontinuing:
Don't discontinue without consulting doctor. Dose may require gradual reduction if you have taken drug for a long time. Doses of other drugs may also require adjustment.

Others:
May cause learning disability.

POSSIBLE INTERACTION WITH OTHER DRUGS

GENERIC NAME OR DRUG CLASS	COMBINED EFFECT
Anticoagulants*	Increased effect of both drugs.
Antidepressants, tricyclic (TCA)*	Need to adjust ethotoin dose.
Barbiturates*	Changed seizure pattern.
Carbamazepine	Possible increased ethotoin metabolism.
Carbonic anhydrase inhibitors*	Increased chance of bone disease.
Central nervous system (CNS) depressants*	Oversedation.
Chloramphenicol	Increased ethotoin effect.
Cimetidine	Increased ethotoin toxicity.
Contraceptives, oral*	Increased seizures.
Cortisone drugs*	Decreased cortisone effect.
Cyclosporine	May decrease cyclosporine effect.
Digitalis preparations*	Decreased digitalis effect.
Disopyramide	Decreased disopyramide effect.
Disulfiram	Increased ethotoin effect.
Estrogens*	Increased estrogen effect.
Furosemide	Decreased furosemide effect.
Glutethimide	Decreased ethotoin effect.
Griseofulvin	Increased griseofulvin effect.
Hypoglycemics, other*	Possible decreased hypoglycemic effect.
Isoniazid	Increased ethotoin effect.
Methadone	Decreased methadone effect.
Methotrexate	Increased methotrexate effect.
Methylphenidate	Increased ethotoin effect.
Nicardipine	Increased anticonvulsant effect.
Nimodipine	Increased anticonvulsant effect.
Oxyphenbutazone	Increased ethotoin effect.
Para-aminosalicylic acid (PAS)	Increased ethotoin effect.
Phenothiazines*	Increased ethotoin effect.

Continued on page 946

POSSIBLE INTERACTION WITH OTHER SUBSTANCES

INTERACTS WITH	COMBINED EFFECT
Alcohol:	Possible decreased anticonvulsant effect. Use with caution.
Beverages:	None expected.
Cocaine:	Possible seizures.
Foods:	None expected.
Marijuana:	Drowsiness, unsteadiness, decreased anticonvulsant effect.
Tobacco:	None expected.

*See Glossary

ETIDRONATE

BRAND NAMES

Didronel   **EHDP**

BASIC INFORMATION

Habit forming? No
Prescription needed? Yes
Available as generic? No
Drug class: Antihypercalcemic

 ## USES

- Treats Paget's disease of the bone.
- Aids healing following hip replacement or spinal cord injury.
- Treats postmenopausal osteoporosis.

 ## DOSAGE & USAGE INFORMATION

How to take:
Tablet—Swallow with water. Do not take with milk.

When to take:
According to doctor's instructions. Take 1 hour before or 2 hours after eating.

If you forget a dose:
Take as soon as you remember up to 6 hours late. If more than 6 hours, wait for next dose (don't double this dose).

What drug does:
Unknown. Appears to retard bone loss and stimulates bone formation.

Time lapse before drug works:
- Paget's disease—1 month.
- Other uses—1 day to several months.

Don't take with:
Any other medicine without consulting your doctor or pharmacist.

 ## OVERDOSE

SYMPTOMS:
None expected.
WHAT TO DO:
Overdose unlikely to threaten life. If person takes much larger amount than prescribed, call doctor, poison control center or hospital emergency room for instructions.

 ## POSSIBLE ADVERSE REACTIONS OR SIDE EFFECTS

SYMPTOMS	WHAT TO DO
Life-threatening:	
None expected.	
Common:	
Tenderness or pain in bones, diarrhea, nausea.	Continue. Call doctor when convenient.
Infrequent:	
None expected.	
Rare:	
Rash; hives; swelling of hands, feet, lips, throat.	Discontinue. Call doctor right away.

WARNINGS & PRECAUTIONS

Don't take if:
You are allergic to etidronate.

Before you start, consult your doctor:
If you have kidney disease, heart failure, bone fractures or colitis.

Over age 60:
No special problems expected.

Pregnancy:
Safety not established. Consult doctor.

Breast-feeding:
Safety not established. Consult doctor.

Infants & children:
Use only under supervision of a medical professional.

Prolonged use:
No special problems expected.

Skin & sunlight:
No special problems expected.

Driving, piloting or hazardous work:
No special problems expected.

Discontinuing:
Don't discontinue without doctor's advice, even though symptoms diminish or disappear.

Others:
- Medicine may be prescribed for 2 weeks, stopped for 2 to 3 months, then started again.
- Have regular check-ups with your doctor even if you currently are not undergoing treatment.

POSSIBLE INTERACTION WITH OTHER DRUGS

GENERIC NAME OR DRUG CLASS	COMBINED EFFECT
Antacids*	Decreased effect of etidronate.
Mineral supplements*	Decreased effect of etidronate.

POSSIBLE INTERACTION WITH OTHER SUBSTANCES

INTERACTS WITH	COMBINED EFFECT
Alcohol:	None expected.
Beverages: Milk.	Decreased effect of etidronate.
Cocaine:	None expected.
Foods: Dairy products or foods containing high levels of calcium.	Decreased effect of etidronate.
Marijuana:	None expected.
Tobacco:	None expected.

ETOPOSIDE

BRAND NAMES

VePesid

BASIC INFORMATION

Habit forming? No
Prescription needed? Yes
Available as generic? No
Drug class: Antineoplastic

 USES

- Treats testicle, lung and bladder cancer.
- Treats Hodgkin's disease and some other forms of cancer.

 DOSAGE & USAGE INFORMATION

How to take:
- Capsules—Swallow with liquid. If you can't swallow whole, open capsule and take with liquid or food. Instructions to take on empty stomach mean 1 hour before or 2 hours after eating.
- Injection—Given under doctor's supervision.

When to take:
According to your doctor's instructions.

If you forget a dose:
Skip this dose. Never double dose. Resume regular schedule.

What drug does:
Inhibits DNA in cancer cells.

Time lapse before drug works:
Unpredictable.

Don't take with:
Any other medicines (including over-the-counter drugs such as cough and cold medicines, laxatives, antacids, diet pills, caffeine, nose drops or vitamins) without consulting your doctor.

 OVERDOSE

SYMPTOMS:
Rapid pulse, shortness of breath, wheezing, fainting, coma.
WHAT TO DO:
- **Dial 0 (operator) or 911 (emergency) for an ambulance or medical help. Then give first aid immediately.**
- **See emergency information on inside covers.**

 POSSIBLE ADVERSE REACTIONS OR SIDE EFFECTS

SYMPTOMS	WHAT TO DO
Life-threatening: In case of overdose, see previous column.	
Common: Appetite loss, nausea, vomiting.	Continue. Call doctor when convenient.
Infrequent: Symptoms of low white blood cell count and low platelet count: black, tarry stools; bloody urine; cough; chills or fever; low back pain; bruising.	Discontinue. Call doctor right away.
Rare: Mouth sores.	Continue. Call doctor when convenient.

WARNINGS & PRECAUTIONS

Don't take if:
- You have chicken pox.
- You have shingles (herpes zoster).

Before you start, consult your doctor:
If you have liver or kidney disease.

Over age 60:
No special problems expected.

Pregnancy:
Risk to unborn child outweighs drug benefits. Don't use.

Breast-feeding:
Drug passes into milk. Avoid drug or discontinue nursing until you finish medicine. Consult doctor for advice on maintaining milk supply.

Infants & children:
Effect not documented. Consult your doctor.

Prolonged use:
- Talk to your doctor about the need for follow-up medical examinations or laboratory studies to check complete blood counts (white blood cell count, platelet count, red blood cell count, hemoglobin, hematocrit).
- Check mouth frequently for ulcers.

Skin & sunlight:
No problems expected.

Driving, piloting or hazardous work:
Avoid if you feel confused, drowsy or dizzy.

Discontinuing:
May still experience symptoms of bone marrow depression, such as: blood in stools, fever or chills, blood spots under the skin, back pain, hoarseness, bloody urine. If any of these occur, call your doctor right away.

Others:
- Advise any doctor or dentist whom you consult that you take this medicine.
- May affect results in some medical tests.
- Etoposide may be used in combinations with other antineoplastic treatment plans. The incidence and severity of side effects may be different when used in combinations such as doxorubicin, procarbazine and etoposide (APE); etoposide, cyclophosphamide, doxorubicin and vincristine (CAVE, ECHO, CAPO, EVAC or VOCA); cyclophosphamide, doxorubicin and etoposide (CAE or ACE); cisplatin, bleomycin, doxorubicin and etoposide; cisplatin, bleomycin and etoposide; cisplatin and etoposide. For further information regarding these combinations, consult your doctor.

POSSIBLE INTERACTION WITH OTHER DRUGS

GENERIC NAME OR DRUG CLASS	COMBINED EFFECT
ACE inhibitors*	May increase bone marrow depression or make kidney damage more likely.
Antineoplastic (cancer-treating) drugs*	May increase bone marrow depression or make kidney damage more likely.
Clozapine	Toxic effect on bone marrow.
Tiopronin	Increased risk of toxicity to bone marrow.

POSSIBLE INTERACTION WITH OTHER SUBSTANCES

INTERACTS WITH	COMBINED EFFECT
Alcohol:	Increased likelihood of adverse reactions. Avoid.
Beverages:	No special problems expected.
Cocaine:	Increased likelihood of adverse reactions. Avoid.
Foods:	No special problems expected.
Marijuana:	Increased likelihood of adverse reactions. Avoid.
Tobacco:	No special problems expected.

*See Glossary

ETRETINATE

BRAND NAMES

Tegison

BASIC INFORMATION

Habit forming? No
Prescription needed? Yes
Available as generic? No
Drug class: Antipsoriatic

 USES

- Treats psoriasis in patients who don't respond well to standard or usual treatment.
- Treats arthritic symptoms sometimes associated with psoriasis.
- Treats ichthyosis.

 DOSAGE & USAGE INFORMATION

How to take:
Capsules—Swallow with liquid or food to lessen stomach irritation. If you can't swallow whole, open capsule and take with liquid or food.

When to take:
At the same time each day, according to instructions on prescription label.

If you forget a dose:
Take as soon as you remember up to 2 hours late. If more than 2 hours, wait for next scheduled dose (don't double this dose).

What drug does:
- Mechanism of action on skin is unknown, but positive effects on the disease have been documented. It probably reduces the production of protein in the outer layers of skin. It is chemically related to Retin-A.
- Also functions as an anti-inflammatory agent.

Continued next column

 OVERDOSE

SYMPTOMS:
None documented. If overdose is suspected, follow instructions below.
WHAT TO DO:
- **Dial 0 (operator) or 911 (emergency) for an ambulance or medical help. Then give first aid immediately.**
- **See emergency information on inside covers.**

Time lapse before drug works:
- 2 to 6 hours for effects to begin.
- Prolonged treatment, up to 2 to 4 weeks (sometimes with psoralens, ultraviolet light may be necessary to develop maximum benefit).

Don't take with:
Any other medicine without consulting your doctor or pharmacist.

 POSSIBLE ADVERSE REACTIONS OR SIDE EFFECTS

SYMPTOMS	WHAT TO DO
Life-threatening:	
None expected.	
Common:	
• Bone and joint pain, eye irritation on exposure to sunlight.	Discontinue. Call doctor right away.
• Dry skin and eyes, nosebleeds, hair loss.	Continue. Call doctor when convenient.
Infrequent:	
Muscle cramps, blurred vision, hearing loss, dark-colored urine, jaundice, unusual bleeding or bruising.	Discontinue. Call doctor right away.
Rare:	
• Itching, peeling skin; inflamed nails; nausea; vomiting; headache.	Discontinue. Call doctor right away.
• Confusion, depression, anxiety, erection difficulties in males.	Continue. Call doctor when convenient.

 WARNINGS & PRECAUTIONS

Don't take if:
If you are pregnant or expect to get pregnant soon.

Before you start, consult your doctor:
- If you have heart or blood vessel disease.
- If you have immediate family members with heart or blood vessel disease.
- If you have high plasma triglycerides.
- If you are an alcoholic.
- If you have diabetes mellitus.
- If you have liver disease.

Over age 60:
Adverse reactions and side effects may be more frequent and severe than in younger persons. You may need smaller doses for shorter periods of time.

Pregnancy:
Risk to unborn child outweighs drug benefits. Don't use.

Breast-feeding:
Drug passes into milk. Avoid drug or discontinue nursing until you finish medicine. Consult doctor for advice on maintaining milk supply.

Infants & children:
Don't use.

Prolonged use:
- No problems expected, if used for no more than 4 months per treatment session.
- Talk to your doctor about the need for follow-up medical examinations or laboratory studies to check blood lipids, liver function.

Skin & sunlight:
May cause increased sensitivity to sunlight. Avoid when possible.

Driving, piloting or hazardous work:
Don't drive or pilot aircraft until you learn how medicine affects you. Don't work around dangerous machinery. Don't climb ladders or work in high places. Danger increases if you drink alcohol or take medicine affecting alertness and reflexes.

Discontinuing:
Don't discontinue without consulting doctor. Dose may require gradual reduction if you have taken drug for a long time. Doses of other drugs may also require adjustment.

Others:
- Courses of treatment are usually limited to 4 months, and repeating, if necessary, after a 4-month rest period.
- Don't donate blood during treatment or for several years thereafter.
- Likelihood of producing cancer is very low.
- During early treatment, psoriasis may appear to worsen.
- May cause changes in cholesterol levels in blood.
- May cause calcium deposits in tendons and ligaments.

POSSIBLE INTERACTION WITH OTHER DRUGS

GENERIC NAME OR DRUG CLASS	COMBINED EFFECT
Abrasive soaps or cleaners	Excessive drying effect on skin.
Acne preparations*	Excessive drying effect on skin.
Any topical preparation containing alcohol, such as after-shave lotions	Excessive drying effect on skin.
Isoniazid	Increased risk of liver damage.
Isoretinoin	Increased toxicity.
Medicated cosmetics	Excessive drying effect on skin.
Methotrexate	Increased toxicity to liver.
Tetracyclines*	Increased adverse reactions of etretinate.
Tretinoin	Increased toxicity.
Vitamin A	Increased toxicity.

POSSIBLE INTERACTION WITH OTHER SUBSTANCES

INTERACTS WITH	COMBINED EFFECT
Alcohol:	May cause hypertriglyceridemia.
Beverages: Milk	Aids absorption of etretinate.
Cocaine:	None expected.
Foods: High-fat diet or milk products.	Aids absorption of etretinate.
Marijuana:	None expected.
Tobacco:	None expected.

FINASTERIDE

BRAND NAMES

Proscar

BASIC INFORMATION

Habit forming? No
Prescription needed? Yes
Available as generic? No
Drug class: Dihydrotestosterone inhibitor

USES

- Treats non-cancerous enlargement of the prostate gland in men (benign prostatic hypertrophy or BPH).
- Theoretically, may prevent the development of prostate cancer.

DOSAGE & USAGE INFORMATION

How to take:
Tablets—Swallow with liquid. If you can't swallow whole, crumble tablet and take with liquid or food.

When to take:
Once a day or as directed, with or without meals.

If you forget a dose:
Take as soon as you remember up to 2 hours late. If more than 2 hours, wait for next scheduled dose (don't double this dose).

What drug does:
Inhibits the enzyme needed for the conversion of testosterone to dihydrotestosterone. Dihydrotestosterone is required for the development of benign prostatic hypertrophy.

Time lapse before drug works:
May require up to 6 months for full therapeutic effect.

Don't take with:
Any other medicine without consulting your doctor or pharmacist.

OVERDOSE

SYMPTOMS:
None expected.
WHAT TO DO:
Overdose unlikely to threaten life.

POSSIBLE ADVERSE REACTIONS OR SIDE EFFECTS

SYMPTOMS	WHAT TO DO
Life-threatening: None expected.	
Common: None expected.	
Infrequent: Decreased volume of ejaculation.	Continue. Tell doctor at next visit.
Rare: Impotence, decreased libido.	Continue. Call doctor when convenient.

WARNINGS & PRECAUTIONS

Don't take if:
You are allergic to finasteride.

Before you start, consult your doctor:
- If you have not had a blood test to check for prostate cancer.
- If your wife is pregnant or may become pregnant.
- If you have a liver disorder.

Over age 60:
No special problems expected.

Pregnancy:
- Not recommended for women.
- Pregnant women should not handle the crushed tablets.
- Avoid exposure to mate's semen if he takes finasteride.

Breast-feeding:
Not recommended for women.

Infants & children:
Not recommended.

Prolonged use:
Talk to your doctor about the need for follow-up medical examinations or laboratory studies to check the effectiveness of the treatment.

Skin & sunlight:
No special problems expected.

Driving, piloting or hazardous work:
No special problems expected.

Discontinuing:
Don't discontinue without medical advice.

Others:
- Advise any doctor or dentist whom you consult that you take this medicine.
- May affect results of some medical tests.
- For those who respond well, the drug must be continued indefinitely.

POSSIBLE INTERACTION WITH OTHER DRUGS

GENERIC NAME OR DRUG CLASS	COMBINED EFFECT
Theophylline	Decreased theophylline effect.

POSSIBLE INTERACTION WITH OTHER SUBSTANCES

INTERACTS WITH	COMBINED EFFECT
Alcohol:	No proven problems.
Beverages:	No proven problems.
Cocaine:	No proven problems.
Foods:	No proven problems.
Marijuana:	No proven problems.
Tobacco:	No proven problems.

FLAVOXATE

BRAND NAMES

Urispas

BASIC INFORMATION

Habit forming? No
Prescription needed? Yes
Available as generic? No
Drug class: Antispasmodic (urinary tract)

 USES

Relieves urinary pain, urgency, nighttime urination, unusual frequency of urination associated with urinary system disorders.

 DOSAGE & USAGE INFORMATION

How to take:
Tablet—Swallow with liquid or food to lessen stomach irritation.

When to take:
30 minutes before meals (unless directed otherwise by doctor).

If you forget a dose:
Take as soon as you remember up to 2 hours late. If more than 2 hours, wait for next scheduled dose (don't double this dose).

What drug does:
Blocks nerve impulses at smooth muscle nerve endings, preventing muscle contractions and gland secretions of organs involved.

Time lapse before drug works:
15 to 30 minutes.

Don't take with:
Any other medicine without consulting your doctor or pharmacist.

 OVERDOSE

SYMPTOMS:
Dilated pupils, rapid pulse and breathing, dizziness, fever, hallucinations, confusion, slurred speech, agitation, flushed face, convulsions, coma.
WHAT TO DO:
- **Dial 0 (operator) or 911 (emergency) for an ambulance or medical help. Then give first aid immediately.**
- **See emergency information on inside covers.**

 POSSIBLE ADVERSE REACTIONS OR SIDE EFFECTS

SYMPTOMS	WHAT TO DO
Life-threatening:	
In case of overdose, see previous column.	
Common:	
• Confusion, delirium, rapid heartbeat.	Discontinue. Call doctor right away.
• Nausea, vomiting, less perspiration, drowsiness.	Continue. Call doctor when convenient.
• Constipation.	Continue. Tell doctor at next visit.
• Dry ears, nose, throat.	No action necessary.
Infrequent:	
• Unusual excitement, irritability, restlessness, clumsiness, hallucinations.	Discontinue. Call doctor right away.
• Headache, increased sensitivity to light, painful or difficult urination.	Continue. Call doctor when convenient.
Rare:	
• Shortness of breath.	Discontinue. Seek emergency treatment.
• Rash or hives; eye pain; blurred vision; sore throat, fever, mouth sores; abdominal pain.	Discontinue. Call doctor right away.
• Dizziness.	Continue. Call doctor when convenient.

WARNINGS & PRECAUTIONS

Don't take if:
- You are allergic to any anticholinergic.
- You have trouble with stomach bloating.
- You have difficulty emptying your bladder completely.
- You have narrow-angle glaucoma.
- You have severe ulcerative colitis.

Before you start, consult your doctor:
- If you have open-angle glaucoma.
- If you have angina.
- If you have chronic bronchitis or asthma.
- If you have liver disease.
- If you have hiatal hernia.
- If you have enlarged prostate.
- If you have myasthenia gravis.
- If you have peptic ulcer.
- If you will have surgery within 2 months, including dental surgery, requiring general or spinal anesthesia.

Over age 60:
Adverse reactions and side effects, particularly mental confusion, may be more frequent and severe than in younger persons.

Pregnancy:
Studies inconclusive on harm to unborn child. Animal studies show fetal abnormalities. Decide with your doctor whether drug benefits justify risk to unborn child.

Breast-feeding:
Drug passes into milk. Avoid drug or discontinue nursing until you finish medicine. Consult doctor for advice on maintaining milk supply.

Infants & children:
Use only under medical supervision.

Prolonged use:
Chronic constipation, possible fecal impaction. Consult doctor immediately.

Skin & sunlight:
No problems expected.

Driving, piloting or hazardous work:
Use disqualifies you for piloting aircraft. Otherwise, no problems expected.

Discontinuing:
May be unnecessary to finish medicine. Follow doctor's instructions.

Others:
No problems expected.

POSSIBLE INTERACTION WITH OTHER DRUGS

GENERIC NAME OR DRUG CLASS	COMBINED EFFECT
Antimuscarinics*	Increased effect of flavoxate.
Central nervous system (CNS) depressants, other*	Increased effect of both drugs.
Clozapine	Toxic effect on the central nervous system.
Ethinamate	Dangerous increased effects of ethinamate. Avoid combining.
Fluoxetine	Increased depressant effects of both drugs.
Guanfacine	May increase depressant effects of either drug.
Leucovorin	High alcohol content of leucovorin may cause adverse effects.
Methyprylon	Increased sedative effect, perhaps to dangerous level. Avoid.
Nabilone	Greater depression of central nervous system.
Nizatidine	Increased nizatidine effect.
Sertraline	Increased depressive effects of both drugs.

POSSIBLE INTERACTION WITH OTHER SUBSTANCES

INTERACTS WITH	COMBINED EFFECT
Alcohol:	None expected.
Beverages:	None expected.
Cocaine:	Excessively rapid heartbeat. Avoid.
Foods:	None expected.
Marijuana:	Drowsiness, dry mouth.
Tobacco:	None expected.

*See Glossary

FLECAINIDE ACETATE

BRAND NAMES

Tambocor

BASIC INFORMATION

Habit forming? No
Prescription needed? Yes
Available as generic? No
Drug class: Antiarrhythmic

USES

Stabilizes irregular heartbeat.

DOSAGE & USAGE INFORMATION

How to take:
Tablet—Swallow with liquid. If you can't swallow whole, crumble tablet and take with liquid or food.

When to take:
At the same time each day, according to instructions on prescription label. Take tablets approximately 12 hours apart.

If you forget a dose:
Take as soon as you remember up to 4 hours late. If more than 4 hours, wait for next scheduled dose (don't double this dose).

What drug does:
Decreases conduction of abnormal electrical activity in the heart muscle or its regulating systems.

Time lapse before drug works:
1 to 6 hours. May need doses daily for 2 to 3 days for maximum effect.

Continued next column

OVERDOSE

SYMPTOMS:
Low blood pressure or unconsciousness, irregular or rapid heartbeat, sleepiness, tremor, sweating.
WHAT TO DO:
- **Dial 0 (operator) or 911 (emergency) for an ambulance or medical help. Then give first aid immediately.**
- **If patient is unconscious and not breathing, give mouth-to-mouth breathing. If there is no heartbeat, use cardiac massage and mouth-to-mouth breathing (CPR). Don't try to make patient vomit. If you can't get help quickly, take patient to nearest emergency facility.**
- **See emergency information on inside covers.**

Don't take with:
Any other medicine without consulting your doctor or pharmacist.

POSSIBLE ADVERSE REACTIONS OR SIDE EFFECTS

SYMPTOMS	WHAT TO DO
Life-threatening:	
In case of overdose, see previous column.	
Common:	
Blurred vision, dizziness.	Continue. Call doctor when convenient.
Infrequent:	
• Chest pain, irregular heartbeat.	Discontinue. Seek emergency treatment.
• Shakiness, rash, nausea, vomiting.	Discontinue. Call doctor right away.
• Anxiety; depression; weakness; headache; appetite loss; weakness in muscles, bones, joints; swollen feet, ankles or legs; loss of taste; numbness or tingling in hands or feet, abdominal pain.	Continue. Call doctor when convenient.
• Constipation.	Continue. Tell doctor at next visit.
Rare:	
• Shortness of breath.	Discontinue. Seek emergency treatment.
• Sore throat, jaundice, fever.	Discontinue. Call doctor right away.

WARNINGS & PRECAUTIONS

Don't take if:
You are allergic to flecainide or a local anesthetic such as novocaine, xylocaine or other drug whose generic name ends with "caine."

Before you start, consult your doctor:
- If you have kidney disease.
- If you have liver disease.
- If you have had a heart attack in past 3 weeks.
- If you have a pacemaker.

Over age 60:
Adverse reactions and side effects may be more frequent and severe than in younger persons.

Pregnancy:
Studies inconclusive on harm to unborn child. Animal studies show fetal abnormalities. Decide with your doctor whether drug benefits justify risk to unborn child.

Breast-feeding:
No proven problems.

Infants & children:
Not recommended. Safety and dosage have not been established.

Prolonged use:
Talk to your doctor about the need for follow-up medical examinations or laboratory studies to check complete blood counts (white blood cell count, platelet count, red blood cell count, hemoglobin, hematocrit), ECG*.

Skin & sunlight:
No problems expected.

Driving, piloting or hazardous work:
Don't drive or pilot aircraft until you learn how medicine affects you. Don't work around dangerous machinery. Don't climb ladders or work in high places. Danger increases if you drink alcohol or take medicine affecting alertness and reflexes, such as antihistamines, tranquilizers, sedatives, pain medicine, narcotics and mind-altering drugs.

Discontinuing:
Don't discontinue without consulting doctor. Dose may require gradual reduction if you have taken drug for a long time. Doses of other drugs may also require adjustment.

Others:
Wear identification bracelet or carry an identification card with inscription of medicine you take.

POSSIBLE INTERACTION WITH OTHER DRUGS

GENERIC NAME OR DRUG CLASS	COMBINED EFFECT
Antacids* (high dose)	Possible increased flecainide acetate effect.
Antiarrhythmics, other*	Possible irregular heartbeat.
Beta-adrenergic blockers*	Possible decreased efficiency of heart-muscle contraction, leading to congestive heart failure.
Bone marrow depressants*	Possible decreased production of blood cells in bone marrow.
Carbonic anhydrase inhibitors*	Possible increased flecainide acetate effect.
Cimetidine	Increased effect of cimetidine.
Digitalis preparations*	Possible increased digitalis effect. Possible irregular heartbeat.
Disopyramide	Possible decreased efficiency of heart-muscle contraction, leading to congestive heart failure.
Encainide	Increased effect of toxicity on the heart muscle.
Nicardipine	Possible increased effect and toxicity of each drug.

Continued page 946

POSSIBLE INTERACTION WITH OTHER SUBSTANCES

INTERACTS WITH	COMBINED EFFECT
Alcohol:	May further depress normal heart function.
Beverages: Caffeine-containing beverages.	Possible decreased flecainide effect.
Cocaine:	Possible decreased flecainide effect.
Foods:	None expected.
Marijuana:	Possible decreased flecainide effect.
Tobacco:	Possible decreased flecainide effect.

*See Glossary

FLUCONAZOLE

BRAND NAMES

Difulcan

BASIC INFORMATION

Habit forming? No
Prescription needed? Yes
Available as generic? No
Drug class: Antifungal

 USES

- Treats meningitis.
- Treats candidiasis (thrush) whether in the mouth or esophagus or widely disseminated throughout the body.

 DOSAGE & USAGE INFORMATION

How to take:
Tablets—Swallow with liquid. If you can't swallow whole, crumble tablet and take with liquid or food. Instructions to take on empty stomach mean 1 hour before or 2 hours after eating.

When to take:
Once a day, probably for 10 to 12 weeks, depending on the disease being treated and your kidney function status.

If you forget a dose:
Take as soon as you remember up to 2 hours late. If more than 2 hours, wait for next scheduled dose (don't double this dose).

What drug does:
Changes the cell membranes of susceptible fungus germs.

Time lapse before drug works:
1 to 2 hours. Several weeks of treatment are necessary for full benefit.

Don't take with:
Other antifungal drugs in the azole family (ketoconazole, miconazole or itraconazole).

 OVERDOSE

SYMPTOMS:
Overdose not expected to threaten life, but if accidental or purposeful overdose occurs, follow the directions below.
WHAT TO DO:
- **Dial 0 (operator) or 911 (emergency) for an ambulance or medical help. Then give first aid immediately.**
- **See emergency information on inside covers.**

 POSSIBLE ADVERSE REACTIONS OR SIDE EFFECTS

SYMPTOMS	WHAT TO DO
Life-threatening:	
In case of overdose, see previous column.	
Common:	
None expected.	
Infrequent:	
Diarrhea, nausea, vomiting.	Continue. Call doctor when convenient.
Rare:	
Skin rash, blistering, peeling skin.	Discontinue. Call doctor right away.

WARNINGS & PRECAUTIONS

Don't take if:
You are allergic to similar drugs, such as ketoconazole, miconazole or itraconazole.

Before you start, consult your doctor:
- If you have kidney disease.
- If you have liver disease.

Over age 60:
No studies available, but dosage may need adjustment if there is any age-related kidney impairment

Pregnancy:
Safety not established. Consult doctor.

Breast-feeding:
Safety not established. Consult doctor.

Infants & children:
Safety not established. Consult doctor.

Prolonged use:
No special problems expected.

Skin & sunlight:
No special problems expected.

Driving, piloting or hazardous work:
No special problems expected

Discontinuing:
Don't discontinue without consulting doctor. Dose may require gradual reduction if you have taken drug for a long time. Doses of other drugs may also require adjustment.

Others:
- Advise any doctor or dentist whom you consult that you take this medicine.
- May affect results of some medical tests.
- Does not alter male hormone activity. (A similar drug, ketoconazole, does alter male hormone activity.)

POSSIBLE INTERACTION WITH OTHER DRUGS

GENERIC NAME OR DRUG CLASS	COMBINED EFFECT
Antidiabetics*	Greater than expected drop in blood sugar. If any antidiabetic agent is taken with fluconazole, blood sugars must be monitored carefully.
Cyclosporine	Increased cyclosporine effect.
Phenytoin	Increased phenytoin effect.
Warfarin	Increased warfarin effect.

POSSIBLE INTERACTION WITH OTHER SUBSTANCES

INTERACTS WITH	COMBINED EFFECT
Alcohol:	None expected.
Beverages:	None expected.
Cocaine:	None expected.
Foods:	None expected.
Marijuana:	None expected.
Tobacco:	None expected.

*See Glossary

FLUOROURACIL (Topical)

BRAND NAMES

Efudex   Fluoroplex

BASIC INFORMATION

Habit forming? No
Prescription needed? Yes
Available as generic? No
Drug class: Antineoplastic (topical)

 ## USES

- Treats precancerous actinic keratoses on skin.
- Treats superficial basal cell carcinomas (skin cancers that don't spread to distant organs and, therefore, do not threaten life).

 ## DOSAGE & USAGE INFORMATION

How to use:
- Apply with cotton-tipped applicator.
- Cream, lotion, ointment—Bathe and dry area before use. Apply small amount and rub gently.
- Wash hands (if fingertips are used to apply) after applying medicine to other parts of body.

When to use:
Once or twice a day or as directed by doctor.

If you forget a dose:
Apply as soon as you remember. Resume basic schedule.

What drug does:
Selectively destroys actively proliferating cells.

Time lapse before drug works:
2 to 3 days.

Don't use with:
Other topical medications unless prescribed by your doctor.

 ## OVERDOSE

SYMPTOMS:
None expected.
WHAT TO DO:
Not for internal use. If child accidentally swallows, call poison-control center.

 ## POSSIBLE ADVERSE REACTIONS OR SIDE EFFECTS

SYMPTOMS	WHAT TO DO
Life-threatening	
None expected.	
Common	
• Skin redness or swelling.	Discontinue. Call doctor right away.
• After 1 or 2 weeks of use—Skin itching or oozing; rash, tenderness, soreness.	Continue. Call doctor when convenient.
Infrequent	
Skin darkening or scaling.	Continue. Call doctor when convenient.
Rare	
Watery eyes.	Discontinue. Call doctor right away.

FLUOROURACIL (Topical)

WARNINGS & PRECAUTIONS

Don't use if:
You are allergic to fluorouracil.

Before you start, consult your doctor:
- If you have cloasma or acne rosacea.
- If you have any other skin problems.

Over age 60:
No problems expected.

Pregnancy:
No problems expected, but check with doctor.

Breast-feeding:
No problems expected, but check with doctor.

Infants & children:
No problems expected, but check with doctor.

Prolonged use:
No problems expected, but check with doctor.

Skin & sunlight:
Increased sensitivity to sunlight during treatment and for 1 to 2 months following. Avoid exposure if possible.

Driving, piloting or hazardous work:
No problems expected, but check with doctor.

Discontinuing:
Pink, smooth area remains after treatment (usually fades in 1 to 2 months).

Others:
- Skin lesions may need biopsy before treatment.
- Keep medicine out of eyes or mouth.
- Heat and moisture in bathroom medicine cabinet can cause breakdown of medicine. Store someplace else.

POSSIBLE INTERACTION WITH OTHER DRUGS

GENERIC NAME OR DRUG CLASS	COMBINED EFFECT
None expected.	

POSSIBLE INTERACTION WITH OTHER SUBSTANCES

INTERACTS WITH	COMBINED EFFECT
Alcohol:	None expected.
Beverages:	None expected.
Cocaine:	None expected.
Foods:	None expected.
Marijuana:	None expected.
Tobacco:	None expected.

FLUOXETINE

BRAND NAMES

Prozac

BASIC INFORMATION

Habit forming? No
Prescription needed? Yes
Available as generic? No
Drug class: Antidepressant

 ## USES

Treats mental depression, particularly in people who do not tolerate tricyclic antidepressants.

 ## DOSAGE & USAGE INFORMATION

How to take:
- Capsules—Swallow with liquid or food to lessen stomach irritation. If you can't swallow whole, open capsule and take with liquid or food.
- Oral solution—Follow Instructions on prescription.

When to take:
In the morning at the same time each day.

If you forget a dose:
Take as soon as you remember up to 2 hours late. If more than 2 hours, wait for next scheduled dose (don't double this dose).

What drug does:
- Inhibits serotonin uptake in the central nervous system, preventing depression.
- Causes loss of appetite.

Time lapse before drug works:
1 to 3 weeks.

Don't take with:
- Any medicine that will change your level of consciousness or reflexes.
- Any other medicine without consulting your doctor or pharmacist.

 ## OVERDOSE

SYMPTOMS:
Seizures, agitation, violent vomiting.
WHAT TO DO:
- Dial 0 (operator) or 911 (emergency) for an ambulance or medical help. Then give first aid immediately.
- See emergency information on inside covers.

 ## POSSIBLE ADVERSE REACTIONS OR SIDE EFFECTS

SYMPTOMS	WHAT TO DO
Life-threatening:	
Rash, itchy skin, breathing difficulty (allergic reaction), chest pain.	Seek emergency treatment immediately.
Common:	
Diarrhea, nervousness, drowsiness, headache, increased sweating, insomnia.	Continue. Call doctor when convenient.
Infrequent:	
• Chills, fever, joint or muscle pain, enlarged lymph glands, unusual excitability, blurred vision, chest pain.	Discontinue. Call doctor right away.
• Nightmares, taste changes, vision changes, decreased sex drive, dry mouth, skin flushing, urinating frequently, dysmenorrhea, stuffy nose, tremors.	Continue. Call doctor when convenient.
Rare:	
• Convulsions.	Discontinue. Seek emergency treatment.
• Fast heartbeat, abdominal pain.	Discontinue. Call doctor right away.
• Nausea, vomiting, constipation, cough, increased appetite.	Continue. Call doctor when convenient.

WARNINGS & PRECAUTIONS

Don't take if:
You have severe liver or kidney disease.

Before you start, consult your doctor:
If you have history of seizure disorders.

Over age 60:
Adverse reactions and side effects may be more frequent and severe than in younger persons. You may need smaller doses for shorter periods of time.

Pregnancy:
No proven effects. Don't take unless essential.

Breast-feeding:
Unknown effects.

Infants & children:
Not recommended.

Prolonged use:
No problems expected.

Skin & sunlight:
No problems expected.

Driving, piloting or hazardous work:
Don't drive or pilot aircraft until you learn how medicine affects you. Don't work around dangerous machinery. Don't climb ladders or work in high places. Danger increases if you drink alcohol or take medicine affecting alertness and reflexes.

Discontinuing:
Don't discontinue without consulting doctor. Dose may require gradual reduction if you have taken drug for a long time. Doses of other drugs may also require adjustment.

Others:
No problems expected.

POSSIBLE INTERACTION WITH OTHER DRUGS

GENERIC NAME OR DRUG CLASS	COMBINED EFFECT
Anticoagulants*	May cause confusion, agitation, convulsions, high blood pressure.
Central nervous system (CNS) depressants*	Increases depressant effect of both drugs.
Digitalis preparations*	May cause confusion, agitation, convulsions, high blood pressure.
MAO inhibitors*	May cause confusion, agitation, convulsions, high blood pressure.
Tryptophan	Increased chance of agitation, restlessness, stomach upsets.

POSSIBLE INTERACTION WITH OTHER SUBSTANCES

INTERACTS WITH	COMBINED EFFECT
Alcohol:	Possible toxicity of both drugs.
Beverages:	Decreases effect of fluoxetine.
Cocaine:	Decreases effect of fluoxetine.
Foods:	None expected.
Marijuana:	Decreases effect of fluoxetine.
Tobacco:	Decreases effect of fluoxetine.

FLUTAMIDE

BRAND NAMES

Eulexin   Euflex

BASIC INFORMATION

Habit forming? No
Prescription needed? Yes
Available as generic? No
Drug class: Antineoplastic

 ## USES

Treats prostate cancer when used with
leuteinizing hormone-releasing hormone (LHRH).

 ## DOSAGE & USAGE INFORMATION

How to take:
Tablet or capsule—Swallow with liquid.

When to take:
According to doctor's instructions.

If you forget a dose:
Take as soon as you remember up to 2 hours
late. If more than 2 hours, wait for next
scheduled dose (don't double this dose).

What drug does:
Interferes with utilization of androgen
(testosterone) by body cells.

Time lapse before drug works:
2 hours.

Don't take with:
Any other medicines (including over-the-counter
drugs such as cough and cold medicines,
laxatives, antacids, diet pills, caffeine, nose
drops or vitamins) without consulting your
doctor.

 ## OVERDOSE

SYMPTOMS:
None expected.
WHAT TO DO:
Overdose unlikely to threaten life. If person
takes much larger amount than prescribed,
call doctor, poison-control center or
hospital emergency room for instructions.

 ## POSSIBLE ADVERSE REACTIONS OR SIDE EFFECTS

SYMPTOMS	WHAT TO DO
Life-threatening: None expected.	
Common: Decreased sex drive, diarrhea, appetite loss, sweating and hot flashes.	Continue. Call doctor when convenient.
Infrequent: Hands and feet tingling or numb, swollen breasts, swollen feet and legs.	Continue. Call doctor when convenient.
Rare: Jaundice (yellow eyes and skin).	Continue. Call doctor right away.

WARNINGS & PRECAUTIONS

Don't take if:
You can't tolerate flutamide.

Before you start, consult your doctor:
If you have liver disease.

Over age 60:
Adverse reactions and side effects may be more frequent and severe than in younger persons. You may need smaller doses for shorter periods of time.

Pregnancy:
Not intended for use in women.

Breast-feeding:
Not intended for use in women.

Infants & children:
Not intended for use in infants and children.

Prolonged use:
Talk to your doctor about the need for follow-up medical examinations or laboratory studies to check liver function.

Skin & sunlight:
No problems expected.

Driving, piloting or hazardous work:
No problems expected.

Discontinuing:
No special problems expected.

Others:
- Advise any doctor or dentist whom you consult that you take this medicine.
- May affect results in some medical tests.
- May decrease sperm count.

 ## POSSIBLE INTERACTION WITH OTHER DRUGS

GENERIC NAME OR DRUG CLASS	COMBINED EFFECT
None expected.	

 ## POSSIBLE INTERACTION WITH OTHER SUBSTANCES

INTERACTS WITH	COMBINED EFFECT
Alcohol:	Jaundice more likely.
Beverages:	No special problems expected.
Cocaine:	No special problems expected.
Foods:	No special problems expected.
Marijuana:	No special problems expected.
Tobacco:	No special problems expected.

FOLIC ACID (Vitamin B-9)

BRAND NAMES

Apo-Folic   **Novofolacid**
Folvite
Numerous other multiple vitamin-mineral supplements. Check labels.

BASIC INFORMATION

Habit forming? No
Prescription needed?
  High strength: Yes
  Vitamin mixtures: No
Available as generic? Yes
Drug class: Vitamin supplement

 ## USES

- Dietary supplement to promote normal growth, development and good health.
- Treatment for anemias due to folic-acid deficiency occurring from alcoholism, liver disease, hemolytic anemia, sprue, infants on artificial formula, pregnancy, breast-feeding and oral-contraceptive use.

 ## DOSAGE & USAGE INFORMATION

How to take:
Tablet—Swallow with liquid or food to lessen stomach irritation. If you can't swallow whole, crumble tablet and take with liquid or food.

When to take:
At the same time each day.

If you forget a dose:
Take when you remember. Don't double next dose. Resume regular schedule.

What drug does:
Essential to normal red-blood-cell formation.

Time lapse before drug works:
Not determined.

Don't take with:
Any other medicine without consulting your doctor or pharmacist.

 ## OVERDOSE

SYMPTOMS:
None expected.
WHAT TO DO:
Overdose unlikely to threaten life.

 ## POSSIBLE ADVERSE REACTIONS OR SIDE EFFECTS

SYMPTOMS	WHAT TO DO
Life-threatening:	
None expected.	
Common:	
Large dose may produce yellow urine.	Continue. Tell doctor at next visit.
Infrequent:	
None expected.	
Rare:	
Rash, itching, bronchospasm.	Discontinue. Call doctor right away.

WARNINGS & PRECAUTIONS

Don't take if:
You are allergic to any B vitamin.

Before you start, consult your doctor:
- If you have liver disease.
- If you have pernicious anemia. (Folic acid corrects anemia, but nerve damage of pernicious anemia continues.)

Over age 60:
No problems expected.

Pregnancy:
No problems expected.

Breast-feeding:
No problems expected.

Infants & children:
No problems expected.

Prolonged use:
No problems expected.

Skin & sunlight:
No problems expected.

Driving, piloting or hazardous work:
No problems expected.

Discontinuing:
Don't discontinue without doctor's advice until you complete prescribed dose, even though symptoms diminish or disappear.

Others:
- Folic acid removed by kidney dialysis. Dialysis patients should increase intake to 300% of RDA.
- A balanced diet should provide all the folic acid a healthy person needs and make supplements unnecessary. Best sources are green, leafy vegetables; fruits; liver and kidney.

POSSIBLE INTERACTION WITH OTHER DRUGS

GENERIC NAME OR DRUG CLASS	COMBINED EFFECT
Analgesics*	Decreased effect of folic acid.
Anticonvulsants*	Decreased effect of folic acid. Possible increased seizure frequency.
Chloramphenicol	Possible decreased folic acid effect.
Contraceptives, oral*	Decreased effect of folic acid.
Cortisone drugs*	Decreased effect of folic acid.
Methotrexate	Decreased effect of folic acid.
Para-aminosalicylic acid (PAS)	Decreased effect of folic acid.
Pyrimethamine	Decreased effect of folic acid.
Sulfasalazine	Decreased dietary absorption of folic acid.
Triamterene	Decreased effect of folic acid.
Trimethoprim	Decreased effect of folic acid.
Zinc supplements	Increased need for zinc.

POSSIBLE INTERACTION WITH OTHER SUBSTANCES

INTERACTS WITH	COMBINED EFFECT
Alcohol:	None expected.
Beverages:	None expected.
Cocaine:	None expected.
Foods:	None expected.
Marijuana:	None expected.
Tobacco:	None expected.

FURAZOLIDONE

BRAND NAMES

Furoxone   Furoxone Liquid

BASIC INFORMATION

Habit forming? No
Prescription needed? Yes
Available as generic? No
Drug class: Antiprotozoal, antibacterial

USES

- As an adjunct in treating most germs that infect the gastrointestinal tract such as cholera, salmonellosis, E. coli, proteus infections, and other bacterial causes of diarrhea.
- Treats giardiasis.

DOSAGE & USAGE INFORMATION

How to take:
- Liquid—Use a measuring spoon to ensure correct dose.
- Tablet—Swallow with liquid or food to lessen stomach irritation. If you can't swallow whole, crumble tablet and take with liquid or food.

When to take:
At the same time each day, according to instructions on prescription label.

If you forget a dose:
Take as soon as you remember up to 2 hours late. If more than 2 hours, wait for next scheduled dose. Don't double this dose.

What drug does:
Kills microscopic germs.

Time lapse before drug works:
Immediate.

Don't take with:
Any other medicine without consulting your doctor or pharmacist.

OVERDOSE

SYMPTOMS:
None expected.
WHAT TO DO:
Overdose unlikely to threaten life. If person takes much larger amount than prescribed, call doctor, poison-control center or hospital emergency room for instructions.

POSSIBLE ADVERSE REACTIONS OR SIDE EFFECTS

SYMPTOMS	WHAT TO DO
Life-threatening:	
None expected except when taken with forbidden foods (see Possible Interaction with Other Substances).	
Common:	
• Nausea, vomiting.	Continue. Call doctor when convenient.
• Dark yellow or brown urine.	No action necessary.
Infrequent:	
• Abdominal pain.	Discontinue. Call doctor right away.
• Headache.	Continue. Call doctor when convenient.
Rare:	
Sore throat, fever, skin rash, itching, joint pain.	Discontinue. Call doctor right away.

WARNINGS & PRECAUTIONS

Don't take if:
- You have G6PD deficiency.
- You have hypersensitivity to furazolidone, nitrofurantoin (Furadantin), or nitrofurazone (Furacin).

Before you start, consult your doctor:
If you are taking any other prescription or non-prescription medicine.

Over age 60:
No special problems expected.

Pregnancy:
No proven harm to unborn child, but avoid if possible.

Breast-feeding:
Drug passes into milk. Avoid drug or discontinue nursing until you finish medicine. Consult doctor for advice on maintaining milk supply.

Infants & children:
Don't use for infants without specific instructions from your doctor.

Prolonged use:
No special problems expected.

Skin & sunlight:
No special problems expected.

Driving, piloting or hazardous work:
No special problems expected.

Discontinuing:
Food restrictions outlined in Possible Interaction with Other Substances must be continued for at least 2 weeks after furazolidone is discontinued.

Others:
- Should not be taken with foods or drinks high in tyramine (see Possible Interaction with Other Substances).
- Advise any doctor or dentist whom you consult that you take this medicine.

POSSIBLE INTERACTION WITH OTHER DRUGS

GENERIC NAME OR DRUG CLASS	COMBINED EFFECT
Antidepressants (tricyclic)*	Sudden, severe increase in blood pressure.
MAO inhibitors*	Sudden, severe increase in blood pressure.
Sympathomimetics*	Sudden, severe increase in blood pressure.

POSSIBLE INTERACTION WITH OTHER SUBSTANCES

INTERACTS WITH	COMBINED EFFECT
Alcohol:	Flushed face, shortness of breath, fever, tightness in chest. Avoid.
Beverages: Any alcoholic beverage.	Flushed face, shortness of breath, fever, tightness in chest. Avoid.
Cocaine:	High blood pressure. Avoid.
Foods: Aged cheese; dark beer; red wine (especially Chianti); sherry; liqueurs; caviar; yeast or protein extracts; fava beans; smoked or pickled meat, poultry, fish; pepperoni, salami, summer sausage; over-ripe fruit.	Sudden, severe high blood pressure that may be life-threatening. Avoid.
Marijuana:	High blood pressure. Avoid.
Tobacco:	No special problems expected.

GALLBLADDER X-RAY TEST DRUGS
(Cholecystographic Agents)

BRAND AND GENERIC NAMES

Bilivist
Bilopaque
Cholebrine
IOCETAMIC ACID
IOPANOIC ACID

IPODATE
Oragrafin Calcium
Oragrafin Sodium
Telepaque
TYROPANOATE

BASIC INFORMATION

Habit forming? No
Prescription needed? Yes
Available as generic? No
Drug class: Diagnostic aid, radiopaque

 USES

To check for problems with the gallbladder or the bile ducts.

 DOSAGE & USAGE INFORMATION

How to take:
- Take tablets or liquid as directed after the evening meal on the evening before special x-rays will be taken.
- Don't eat or drink anything (except water) after taking.

When to take:
As directed.

If you forget a dose:
Take as soon as you remember.

What drug does:
These are organic iodine compounds which get absorbed into the blood stream, get concentrated in a healthy gallbladder and make the gallbladder and gallstones (if present) visible on special x-rays.

Time lapse before drug works:
10 to 15 hours.

Continued next column

 OVERDOSE

SYMPTOMS:
Severe diarrhea, nausea or vomiting; difficult urination.
WHAT TO DO:
Not life-threatening. Discontinue and call doctor right away.

Don't take with:
- Other medicines unless directed by your doctor or x-ray specialist.
- If you take cholestyramine, discontinue it for 48 hours before taking the radiopaque drug.

 POSSIBLE ADVERSE REACTIONS OR SIDE EFFECTS

SYMPTOMS	WHAT TO DO
Life-threatening:	
Faintness; swelling of lips, hands, face; difficult breathing.	Discontinue. Seek emergency treatment.
Common:	
Difficult or painful urination, increased urinary frequency.	No action necessary.
Infrequent:	
Abdominal cramps, diarrhea, dizziness, headache, indigestion, vomiting, nausea.	Discontinue. Call doctor right away.
Rare:	
Itching, unusual bleeding or bruising, hives or rash.	Discontinue. Call doctor right away.

GALLBLADDER X-RAY TEST DRUGS
(Cholecystographic Agents)

 WARNINGS & PRECAUTIONS

Don't take if:
You are allergic to any iodine compound or other radiopaque chemicals.

Before you start, consult your doctor:
If you are allergic to anything, including shellfish, cabbage, kale, turnips, iodized salt.

Over age 60:
Adverse reactions and side effects may be more frequent and severe than in younger persons. Ask doctor about smaller doses.

Pregnancy:
X-rays should not be taken unless absolutely necessary during pregnancy.

Breast-feeding:
No problems expected, but ask doctor.

Infants & children:
No problems expected, but ask doctor.

Prolonged use:
Not intended for prolonged use.

Skin & sunlight:
No problems expected.

Driving, piloting or hazardous work:
Don't drive or pilot aircraft until you learn how medicine affects you. Don't work around dangerous machinery. Don't climb ladders or work in high places. Danger increases if you drink alcohol or take medicine affecting alertness and reflexes, such as antihistamines, tranquilizers, sedatives, pain medicine, narcotics and mind-altering drugs.

Discontinuing:
No problems expected.

Others:
- Special diets and laxatives or enemas before x-rays may be ordered. Follow instructions.
- Tests on your thyroid gland may be made inaccurate for 8 weeks because of the iodine contained in radiopaque substances. Keep this in mind if your doctor orders thyroid tests.
- Results of other lab studies may be inaccurate.

 POSSIBLE INTERACTION WITH OTHER DRUGS

GENERIC NAME OR DRUG CLASS	COMBINED EFFECT
Cholestyramine	Unsuccessful gallbladder test.

 POSSIBLE INTERACTION WITH OTHER SUBSTANCES

INTERACTS WITH	COMBINED EFFECT
Alcohol:	None expected.
Beverages:	None expected.
Cocaine:	None expected.
Foods:	None expected.
Marijuana:	None expected.
Tobacco:	None expected.

GEMFIBROZIL

BRAND NAMES

Lopid

BASIC INFORMATION

Habit forming? No
Prescription needed? Yes
Available as generic? No
Drug class: Antihyperlipidemic

 ## USES

Reduces fatty substances in the blood
(triglycerides).

 ## DOSAGE & USAGE
INFORMATION

How to take:
Capsule—Swallow with liquid or food to lessen
stomach irritation.

When to take:
At the same times each day.

If you forget a dose:
Take as soon as you remember up to 2 hours
late. If more than 2 hours, wait for next
scheduled dose (don't double this dose).

What drug does:
Inhibits formation of fatty substances.

Time lapse before drug works:
3 months or more.

Don't take with:
Any other medicine without consulting your
doctor or pharmacist.

 ## OVERDOSE

SYMPTOMS:
Diarrhea, headache, muscle pain.
WHAT TO DO:
**Overdose unlikely to threaten life. If person
takes much larger amount than prescribed,
call doctor, poison-control center or
hospital emergency room for instructions.**

 ## POSSIBLE
ADVERSE REACTIONS
OR SIDE EFFECTS

SYMPTOMS	WHAT TO DO
Life-threatening: None expected.	
Common: Indigestion.	Continue. Call doctor when convenient.
Infrequent: Chest pain, shortness of breath, irregular heartbeat, nausea, vomiting, diarrhea, stomach pain.	Discontinue. Call doctor right away.
Rare: • Rash, itch; sores in mouth, on lips; sore throat; swollen feet, legs; blood in urine; painful urination; fever; chills.	Discontinue. Call doctor right away.
• Dizziness, headache, drowsiness, muscle cramps, dry skin, backache, unusual tiredness, decreased sex drive.	Continue. Call doctor when convenient.

WARNINGS & PRECAUTIONS

Don't take if:
You are allergic to any antihyperlipidemic.

Before you start, consult your doctor:
- If you have had liver or kidney disease.
- If you have had peptic-ulcer disease.
- If you have diabetes.

Over age 60:
Adverse reactions and side effects may be more frequent and severe than in younger persons.

Pregnancy:
Risk to unborn child outweighs drug benefits. Don't use.

Breast-feeding:
May harm child. Avoid.

Infants & children:
Not recommended.

Prolonged use:
Periodic blood-cell counts and liver-function studies recommended if you take gemfibrozil for a long time.

Skin & sunlight:
No problems expected.

Driving, piloting or hazardous work:
Avoid if you feel drowsy or dizzy. Otherwise, no problems expected.

Discontinuing:
Don't discontinue without doctor's advice until you complete prescribed dose, even though symptoms diminish or disappear.

Others:
Some studies question effectiveness. Many studies warn against toxicity.

POSSIBLE INTERACTION WITH OTHER DRUGS

GENERIC NAME OR DRUG CLASS	COMBINED EFFECT
Anticoagulants, oral*	Increased anti-coagulant effect. Dose reduction of anticoagulant necessary.
Antidiabetics, oral*	Increased antidiabetic effect.
Contraceptives, oral*	Decreased gemfibrozil effect.
Estrogens*	Decreased gemfibrozil effect.
Furosemide	Possible toxicity of both drugs.
Insulin	Increased insulin effect.
Thyroid hormones*	Increased gemfibrozil effect.

POSSIBLE INTERACTION WITH OTHER SUBSTANCES

INTERACTS WITH	COMBINED EFFECT
Alcohol:	None expected.
Beverages:	None expected.
Cocaine:	Decreased effect of gemfibrozil. Avoid.
Foods: Fatty foods.	Decreased gemfibrozil effect.
Marijuana:	None expected.
Tobacco:	Decreased gemfibrozil absorption. Avoid.

GLUCAGON

BRAND NAMES

Glucagon for Injection

BASIC INFORMATION

Habit forming? No
Prescription needed? Yes
Available as generic? Yes
Drug class: Antihypoglycemic, diagnostic aid

USES

- Treats low blood sugar in diabetics.
- Used as antidote for overdose of beta-adrenergic blockers, quinidine and tricyclic antidepressants.

DOSAGE & USAGE INFORMATION

How to take:
Injection—Given under doctor's supervision.

When to take:
When there are signs of low blood sugar (anxiety; chills; cool, pale skin; hunger; nausea; tremors; sweating; weakness; unconsciousness) in diabetics who don't respond to eating some form of sugar.

If you forget a dose:
Single dose only.

What drug does:
Forces liver to make more sugar and release it into the bloodstream.

Time lapse before drug works:
- For hypoglycemic condition—5 to 20 minutes.
- For muscle relaxant—1 to 10 minutes.

Don't take with:
Any other medicines (including over-the-counter drugs such as cough and cold medicines, laxatives, antacids, diet pills, caffeine, nose drops or vitamins) without consulting your doctor.

OVERDOSE

SYMPTOMS:
Nausea, vomiting, severe weakness, irregular heartbeat, hoarseness, cramps.
WHAT TO DO:
- **Dial 0 (operator) or 911 (emergency) for an ambulance or medical help. Then give first aid immediately.**
- **See emergency information on inside covers.**

POSSIBLE ADVERSE REACTIONS OR SIDE EFFECTS

SYMPTOMS	WHAT TO DO
Life-threatening:	
Unconsciousness.	Seek emergency treatment immediately.
Common:	
Nausea.	Continue. Call doctor when convenient.
Infrequent:	
Lightheadedness, breathing difficulty.	Discontinue. Call doctor right away.
Rare:	
Skin rash.	Discontinue. Call doctor right away.

WARNINGS & PRECAUTIONS

Don't take if:
You can't tolerate glucagon.

Before you start, consult your doctor:
- If you are allergic to beef or pork.
- If you have pheochromocytoma.*

Over age 60:
No special problems expected.

Pregnancy:
No proven harm to unborn child, but avoid if possible.

Breast-feeding:
No special problems expected.

Infants & children:
No special problems expected.

Prolonged use:
To be used intermittently and not for prolonged periods.

Skin & sunlight:
No problems expected.

Driving, piloting or hazardous work:
Don't drive or pilot aircraft until you learn how medicine affects you. Don't work around dangerous machinery. Don't climb ladders or work in high places. Danger increases if you drink alcohol or take medicine affecting alertness and reflexes.

Discontinuing:
No special problems expected.

Others:
- May affect results in some medical tests.
- Explain to other family members how to inject glucagon.
- Before injecting, try to eat some form of sugar, such as glucose tablets, corn syrup, honey, orange juice, hard candy or sugar cubes.
- Store glucagon in refrigerator, but don't freeze.

POSSIBLE INTERACTION WITH OTHER DRUGS

GENERIC NAME OR DRUG CLASS	COMBINED EFFECT
Anticoagulants*	Increased anticoagulant effect.

POSSIBLE INTERACTION WITH OTHER SUBSTANCES

INTERACTS WITH	COMBINED EFFECT
Alcohol:	Decreased glucagon effect.
Beverages:	No special problems expected.
Cocaine:	Increased adverse reactions.
Foods: Sugar, fruit juice, candy.	Enhances glucagon effect.
Marijuana:	Increased adverse reactions.
Tobacco:	No special problems expected.

GLYCOPYRROLATE

BRAND NAMES

Robinul   Robinul Forte

BASIC INFORMATION

Habit forming? No
Prescription needed? Yes
Available as generic? Yes
Drug class: Antispasmodic, anticholinergic

 USES

- Reduces spasms of digestive system.
- Reduces production of saliva during dental procedures.

 DOSAGE & USAGE INFORMATION

How to take:
Tablet—Swallow with liquid. If you can't swallow whole, crumble tablet and take with small amount of liquid or food.

When to take:
30 minutes before meals (unless directed otherwise by doctor).

If you forget a dose:
Wait for next scheduled dose (don't double this dose).

What drug does:
Blocks nerve impulses at parasympathetic nerve endings, preventing smooth (involuntary) muscle contractions and gland secretions of organs involved.

Time lapse before drug works:
15 to 30 minutes.

Don't take with:
Any other medicine without consulting your doctor or pharmacist.

 OVERDOSE

SYMPTOMS:
Dry mouth, blurred vision, low blood pressure, decreased breathing rate, rapid heartbeat, flushed skin, drowsiness.
WHAT TO DO:
- **Dial 0 (operator) or 911 (emergency) for an ambulance or medical help. Then give first aid immediately.**
- **See emergency information on inside covers.**

 POSSIBLE ADVERSE REACTIONS OR SIDE EFFECTS

SYMPTOMS	WHAT TO DO
Life-threatening:	
Hives, rash, intense itching, faintness soon after a dose (anaphylaxis).	Seek emergency treatment immediately.
Common:	
Dry mouth, loss of taste, constipation, difficult urination.	Continue. Call doctor when convenient.
Infrequent:	
• Confusion; dizziness; drowsiness; eye pain; headache; rash; sleep disturbance such as nightmares, frequent waking; nausea; vomiting; rapid heartbeat; lightheadedness.	Discontinue. Call doctor right away.
• Insomnia, blurred vision, diminished sex drive, decreased sweating, nasal congestion, altered taste.	Continue. Call doctor when convenient.
Rare:	
Rash, hives.	Discontinue. Call doctor right away.

 WARNINGS & PRECAUTIONS

Don't take if:
- You are allergic to any anticholinergic.
- You have trouble with stomach bloating.
- You have difficulty emptying your bladder completely.
- You have narrow-angle glaucoma.
- You have severe ulcerative colitis.

Before you start, consult your doctor:
- If you have open-angle glaucoma.
- If you have angina, chronic bronchitis or asthma, liver disease, hiatal hernia, enlarged prostate, myasthenia gravis, peptic ulcer, kidney or thyroid disease.
- If you will have surgery within 2 months, including dental surgery, requiring general or spinal anesthesia.

Over age 60:
Adverse reactions and side effects may be more frequent and severe than in younger persons.

Pregnancy:
Studies inconclusive on harm to unborn child. Animal studies show fetal abnormalities. Decide with your doctor whether drug benefits justify risk to unborn child.

Breast-feeding:
Drug passes into milk and decreases milk flow. Avoid drug or discontinue nursing until you finish medicine. Consult doctor for advice on maintaining milk supply.

Infants & children:
Use only under medical supervision.

Prolonged use:
Chronic constipation, possible fecal impaction. Consult doctor immediately.

Skin & sunlight:
No problems expected.

Driving, piloting or hazardous work:
Use disqualifies you for piloting aircraft. Otherwise, no problems expected.

Discontinuing:
May be unnecessary to finish medicine. Follow doctor's instructions.

Others:
- Heatstroke more likely if you become overheated during exertion.
- Advise any doctor or dentist whom you consult that you take this medicine.

POSSIBLE INTERACTION WITH OTHER DRUGS

GENERIC NAME OR DRUG CLASS	COMBINED EFFECT
Antacids*	Decreased glycopyrrolate absorption effect.
Amantadine	Increased glycopyrrolate effect.
Anticholinergics, other*	Increased glycopyrrolate effect.
Antidepressants, tricyclics (TCA)*	Increased glycopyrrolate effect.
Antidiarrheals*	Decreased glycoprrolate absorption effect.
Attapulgite	Decreased effect of anticholinergic.
Buclizine	Increased glycopyrrolate effect.
Cortisone drugs*	Increased internal-eye pressure.
Digitalis	Possible decreased absorption of digitalis.
Haloperidol	Increased internal eye pressure.

Ketoconazole	Decreased ketoconazole effect.
MAO inhibitors*	Increased glycopyrrolate effect.
Meperidine	Increased glycopyrrolate effect.
Methylphenidate	Increased anticholinergic effect.
Molindone	Increased nizatidine effect.
Orphenadrine	Increased glycopyrrolate effect
Phenothiazines	Increased glycopyrrolate effect.
Pilocarpine	Increased glycopyrrolate effect. Loss of pilocarpine effect in glaucoma treatment.
Potassium chloride tabs	Increased side effects of potassium tablets.
Quinidine	Increased glycopyrrolate effect.
Retocunazole	Decreased absorption of both.
Sedatives* or central nervous system depressants*	Increased sedative effect of both drugs.
Vitamin C	Increased glcopyrrolate effect. Avoid large vitamin C doses.

POSSIBLE INTERACTION WITH OTHER SUBSTANCES

INTERACTS WITH	COMBINED EFFECT
Alcohol:	None expected.
Beverages	None expected.
Cocaine	Excessively rapid heartbeat.
Foods	None exected.
Marijuana	Drowsiness and dry mouth.
Tobacco	None expected.

*See Glossary

GOLD COMPOUNDS

BRAND AND GENERIC NAMES

AURANOFIN
AUROTHIOGLUCOSE
Gold Sodium
  Thiomalate
Myochrysine—
  injection

Myocrisin
Ridaura—oral
SODIUM
  AUROTHIO-
  MALATE

BASIC INFORMATION

Habit forming? No
Prescription needed? Yes
Available as generic? No
Drug class: Gold compounds

 ## USES

Treatment for rheumatoid arthritis.

 ## DOSAGE & USAGE INFORMATION

How to take:
- Capsules—Swallow with full glass of fluid. Follow prescription directions. Taking too much can cause serious adverse reactions.
- Injections—Under medical supervision.

When to take:
Once or twice daily, morning and night.

If you forget a dose:
Take as soon as you remember up to 6 hours late, then go back to usual schedule.

What drug does:
Modifies disease activity of rheumatoid arthritis by mechanisms not yet understood.

Time lapse before drug works:
3 to 6 months.

Don't take with:
Any other medicine without consulting your doctor or pharmacist.

 ## OVERDOSE

SYMPTOMS:
Confusion, delirium, numbness and tingling in feet and hands.
WHAT TO DO:
- **Induce vomiting with syrup of ipecac if available.**
- **Dial 0 (operator) or 911 (emergency) for an ambulance or medical help. Then give first aid immediately.**
- **See emergency information on inside covers.**

 ## POSSIBLE ADVERSE REACTIONS OR SIDE EFFECTS

SYMPTOMS	WHAT TO DO
Life-threatening:	
Hives, rash, intense itching, faintness soon after a dose (anaphylaxis).	Seek emergency treatment immediately.
Common:	
• Itch; hives; sores or white spots in mouth, throat; appetite loss; diarrhea; vomiting; skin rashes; fever.	Discontinue. Call doctor right away.
• Abdominal cramps, indigestion, constipation.	Continue. Call doctor when convenient.
Infrequent:	
• Excessive fatigue; sore tongue, mouth or gums; metallic or odd taste; unusual bleeding or bruising; blood in urine; vaginal discharge; flushing; fainting; dizziness; sweating after injection.	Discontinue. Call doctor right away.
• Hair loss; pain in muscles, bones and joints (with injections).	Continue. Call doctor when convenient.
Rare:	
• Blood in stool, difficult breathing, coughing, seizures.	Discontinue. Seek emergency treatment.
• Abdominal pain, jaundice, numbness or tingling in hands or feet, muscle weakness.	Discontinue. Call doctor right away.
• "Pink eye."	Continue. Call doctor when convenient.

WARNINGS & PRECAUTIONS

Don't take if:
- You have history of allergy to gold or other metals.
- You have any blood disorder.
- You have kidney disease.

Before you start, consult your doctor:
- If you are pregnant or may become pregnant.
- If you have lupus erythematosus.
- If you have Schogren's syndrome.
- If you have chronic skin disease.

Over age 60:
Adverse reactions and side effects may be more frequent and severe than in younger persons.

Pregnancy:
Avoid if possible. Animal studies show that gold compounds can cause birth defects.

Breast-feeding:
Drug may filter into milk, causing side effects in infants. Avoid.

Infants & children:
Not recommended. Safety and dosage have not been established.

Prolonged use:
Request periodic laboratory studies of blood counts, urine and liver function. These should be done before use and at least once a month during treatment.

Skin & sunlight:
- Skin rash may be aggravated by sunlight.
- Blue-gray pigmentation in skin exposed to sunlight.

Driving, piloting or hazardous work:
Avoid if you have serious adverse reactions or side effects. Otherwise, no problems expected.

Discontinuing:
Don't discontinue without doctor's advice until you complete prescribed dose.

Others:
- Side effects and adverse reactions may appear during treatment or for many months after discontinuing.
- Gold has been shown to cause kidney tumors and kidney cancer in animals given excessive doses.
- May interfere with the accuracy of some medical tests.

POSSIBLE INTERACTION WITH OTHER DRUGS

GENERIC NAME OR DRUG CLASS	COMBINED EFFECT
Cyclosporine	May increase risk of kidney toxicity.
Non-steroidal anti-inflammatory drugs (NSAIDs) *	Possible increased likelihood of kidney damage.
Penicillamine	Increased likelihood of kidney damage.
Phenytoin	Increased phenytoin blood levels. Phenytoin dosage may require adjustment.
Isoniazid	Increased risk of liver damage
Tiopronin	Increased risk of toxicity to kidneys.

POSSIBLE INTERACTION WITH OTHER SUBSTANCES

INTERACTS WITH	COMBINED EFFECT
Alcohol:	None expected.
Beverages:	None expected.
Cocaine:	None expected.
Foods:	None expected.
Marijuana:	None expected.
Tobacco:	None expected.

*See Glossary

GRISEOFULVIN

BRAND NAMES

Fulvicin P/G
Fulvicin U/F
Grifulvin V
Gris-PEG

Grisactin
Grisactin Ultra
Grisovin-FP
grisOwen

BASIC INFORMATION

Habit forming? No
Prescription needed? Yes
Available as generic? Yes
Drug class: Antibiotic (antifungal)

 USES

Treatment for fungal infections susceptible to griseofulvin.

 DOSAGE & USAGE INFORMATION

How to take:
* Tablet or capsule—Swallow with liquid or food to lessen stomach irritation. If you can't swallow whole, crumble tablet or open capsule and take with liquid or food.
* Liquid—Follow label instructions.

When to take:
With or immediately after meals.

If you forget a dose:
Take as soon as you remember up to 2 hours late. If more than 2 hours, wait for next scheduled dose (don't double this dose).

What drug does:
Prevents fungi from growing and reproducing.

Time lapse before drug works:
2 to 10 days for skin infections. 2 to 4 weeks for infections of fingernails or toenails. Complete cure of either may require several months.

Don't take with:
Any other medicine without consulting your doctor or pharmacist.

 OVERDOSE

SYMPTOMS:
Nausea, vomiting, diarrhea. In sensitive individuals, severe diarrhea may occur without overdosing.
WHAT TO DO:
Overdose unlikely to threaten life. If person takes much larger amount than prescribed, call doctor, poison-control center or hospital emergency room for instructions.

 POSSIBLE ADVERSE REACTIONS OR SIDE EFFECTS

SYMPTOMS	WHAT TO DO
Life-threatening:	
In case of overdose, see previous column.	
Common:	
Headache.	Continue. Tell doctor at next visit.
Infrequent:	
• Confusion; rash, hives, itch; mouth or tongue irritation; soreness; nausea; vomiting; diarrhea; stomach pain.	Discontinue. Call doctor right away.
• Insomnia, tiredness.	Continue. Call doctor when convenient.
Rare:	
Sore throat, fever, numbness or tingling in hands or feet, cloudy urine, sensitivity to sunlight, jaundice.	Discontinue. Call doctor right away.

WARNINGS & PRECAUTIONS

Don't take if:
- You are allergic to any antifungal medicine.
- You are allergic to penicillin.
- You have liver disease.
- You have porphyria.
- The infection is minor and will respond to less-potent drugs.

Before you start, consult your doctor:
- If you plan to become pregnant within medication period.
- If you have liver disease.
- If you have lupus.

Over age 60:
Adverse reactions and side effects may be more frequent and severe than in younger persons.

Pregnancy:
Risk to unborn child outweighs drug benefits. Don't use.

Breast-feeding:
No problems expected, but consult your doctor.

Infants & children:
Not recommended for children younger than 2.

Prolonged use:
- You may become susceptible to infections caused by germs not responsive to griseofulvin.
- Talk to your doctor about the need for follow-up medical examinations or laboratory studies to check complete blood counts (white blood cell count, platelet count, red blood cell count, hemoglobin, hematocrit), liver function, kidney function.

Skin & sunlight:
May cause rash or intensify sunburn in areas exposed to sun or sunlamp.

Driving, piloting or hazardous work:
- Don't drive if you feel dizzy or have vision problems.
- Don't pilot aircraft.

Discontinuing:
Don't discontinue without doctor's advice until you complete prescribed dose, even though symptoms diminish or disappear.

Others:
Periodic laboratory blood studies and liver- and kidney-function tests recommended.

 POSSIBLE INTERACTION WITH OTHER DRUGS

GENERIC NAME OR DRUG CLASS	COMBINED EFFECT
Anticoagulants, oral*	Decreased anti-anticoagulant effect.
Barbiturates*	Decreased griseofulvin effect.
Contraceptives, oral*	Decreased contraceptive effect.
Drugs that increase sensitivity to sunlight	Increased sun hazard.

 POSSIBLE INTERACTION WITH OTHER SUBSTANCES

INTERACTS WITH	COMBINED EFFECT
Alcohol:	Increased intoxication. Possible disulfiram reaction.*
Beverages:	None expected.
Cocaine:	None expected.
Foods:	None expected, but foods high in fat will improve drug absorption.
Marijuana:	None expected.
Tobacco:	None expected.

*See Glossary

GUAIFENESIN

BRAND NAMES

See complete list of brand names in the *Brand Name Directory*, page 920.

BASIC INFORMATION

Habit forming? No
Prescription needed? No
Available as generic? Yes
Drug class: Cough/cold preparation

 USES

Loosens mucus in respiratory passages from allergies and infections (hay fever, cough, cold).

 DOSAGE & USAGE INFORMATION

How to take:
- Tablet, capsule, extended-release tablet, extended-release capsule—Swallow with liquid. If you can't swallow whole, crumble tablet or open capsule and take with liquid or food.
- Syrup or lozenge—Take as directed on label. Follow with 8 oz. water.

When to take:
As needed, no more often than every 3 hours.

If you forget a dose:
Take as soon as you remember. Wait 3 hours for next dose.

What drug does:
Increases production of watery fluids to thin mucus so it can be coughed out or absorbed.

Time lapse before drug works:
15 to 30 minutes. Regular use for 5 to 7 days necessary for maximum benefit.

Don't take with:
Any other medicine without consulting your doctor or pharmacist.

 OVERDOSE

SYMPTOMS:
Drowsiness, mild weakness, nausea, vomiting.
WHAT TO DO:
Overdose unlikely to threaten life. If person takes much larger amount than prescribed, call doctor, poison-control center or hospital emergency room for instructions.

 POSSIBLE ADVERSE REACTIONS OR SIDE EFFECTS

SYMPTOMS	WHAT TO DO
Life-threatening:	
None expected.	
Common:	
None expected.	
Infrequent:	
• Rash, stomach pain, diarrhea, nausea, vomiting.	Discontinue. Call doctor right away.
• Drowsiness.	Continue. Call doctor when convenient.
Rare:	
None expected.	

WARNINGS & PRECAUTIONS

Don't take if:
You are allergic to any cough or cold preparation containing guaifenesin.

Before you start, consult your doctor:
See Interaction column and consult doctor.

Over age 60:
Adverse reactions and side effects may be more frequent and severe than in younger persons. For drug to work, you must drink 8 to 10 glasses of fluid per day.

Pregnancy:
No proven harm to unborn child. Avoid if possible.

Breast-feeding:
No proven problems. Consult your doctor.

Infants & children:
No problems expected.

Prolonged use:
No problems expected.

Skin & sunlight:
No problems expected.

Driving, piloting or hazardous work:
Avoid if you feel drowsy. Otherwise, no problems expected.

Discontinuing:
May be unnecessary to finish medicine. Discontinue when symptoms disappear. If symptoms persist more than 1 week, consult doctor.

Others:
No problems expected.

POSSIBLE INTERACTION WITH OTHER DRUGS

GENERIC NAME OR DRUG CLASS	COMBINED EFFECT
Anticoagulants*	Possible risk of bleeding.

POSSIBLE INTERACTION WITH OTHER SUBSTANCES

INTERACTS WITH	COMBINED EFFECT
Alcohol:	No proven problems.
Beverages:	You must drink 8 to 10 glasses of fluid per day for drug to work.
Cocaine:	No proven problems.
Foods:	None expected.
Marijuana:	No proven problems.
Tobacco:	No proven problems.

GUANABENZ

BRAND NAMES
Wytensin

BASIC INFORMATION

Habit forming? No
Prescription needed? Yes
Available as generic? No
Drug class: Antihypertensive

 USES

Controls, but doesn't cure, high blood pressure.

 DOSAGE & USAGE INFORMATION

How to take:
Tablet—Swallow with liquid or food to lessen stomach irritation. If you can't swallow whole, crumble tablet and take with liquid or food.

When to take:
At the same times each day.

If you forget a dose:
Take as soon as you remember up to 2 hours late. If more than 2 hours, wait for next scheduled dose (don't double this dose).

What drug does:
● Relaxes muscle cells of small arteries.
● Slows heartbeat.

Time lapse before drug works:
1 hour.

Don't take with:
Any other medicine without consulting your doctor or pharmacist.

 OVERDOSE

SYMPTOMS:
Severe dizziness, slow heartbeat, unusual tiredness or weakness, pinpoint pupils, fainting, coma.
WHAT TO DO:
● **Dial 0 (operator) or 911 (emergency) for an ambulance or medical help. Then give first aid immediately.**
● **If patient is unconscious and not breathing, give mouth-to-mouth breathing. If there is no heartbeat, use cardiac massage and mouth-to-mouth breathing (CPR). Don't try to make patient vomit. If you can't get help quickly, take patient to nearest emergency facility.**
● **See emergency information on inside covers.**

 POSSIBLE ADVERSE REACTIONS OR SIDE EFFECTS

SYMPTOMS	WHAT TO DO
Life-threatening:	
In case of overdose, see previous column.	
Common:	
● Nervousness, rapid heartbeat, paleness, dry mouth, drowsiness.	Continue. Call doctor when convenient.
● Insomnia, weakness.	Continue. Tell doctor at next visit.
Infrequent:	
● Irregular heartbeat, shakiness in hands.	Discontinue. Call doctor right away.
● Dizziness, appetite loss, nausea, vomiting, painful or difficult urination, headache.	Continue. Call doctor when convenient.
Rare:	
Decreased sex drive.	Continue. Call doctor when convenient.

WARNINGS & PRECAUTIONS

Don't take if:
You are allergic to any sympathomimetic drug.

Before you start, consult your doctor:
● If you have blood disease.
● If you have heart disease.
● If you have liver disease.
● If you have diabetes or overactive thyroid.
● If you will have surgery within 2 months, including dental surgery, requiring general or spinal anesthesia.

Over age 60:
Adverse reactions and side effects may be more frequent and severe than in younger persons. Hot weather may cause need to reduce dosage.

Pregnancy:
Risk to unborn child outweighs drug benefits. Don't use.

Breast-feeding:
Avoid nursing.

Infants & children:
Not recommended.

Prolonged use:
Side effects tend to diminish. Request uric-acid and kidney-function studies periodically.

Skin & sunlight:
No problems expected.

Driving, piloting or hazardous work:
Avoid if you feel dizzy; otherwise, no problems expected.

Discontinuing:
Don't discontinue without consulting doctor. Dose may require gradual reduction if you have taken drug for a long time. Doses of other drugs may also require adjustment. Abrupt discontinuing may cause anxiety, chest pain, salivation, headache, abdominal cramps, fast heartbeat, increased sweating, tremors, insomnia.

Others:
- Stay away from high-sodium foods. Lose weight if you are overweight.
- May interfere with the accuracy of some medical tests.

POSSIBLE INTERACTION WITH OTHER DRUGS

GENERIC NAME OR DRUG CLASS	COMBINED EFFECT
ACE inhibitors*: captopril, enalapril, lisinopril	Possible excessive potassium in blood.
Antihypertensives, other*	Decreases blood pressure more than either alone. May be beneficial, but requires dosage adjustment.
Beta-blockers*	Blood pressure control more difficult.
Central nervous system (CNS) depressants* (sedatives,* sleeping pills,* tranquilizers,* antidepressants,* narcotics*)	Increased brain depression. Avoid.
Clozapine	Toxic effect on the central nervous system.
Diuretics*	Decreases blood pressure more than either alone. May be beneficial, but requires dosage adjustment.
Ethinamate	Dangerous increased effects of ethinamate. Avoid combining.

Fluoxetine	Increased depressant effects of both drugs.
Guanfacine	May increase depressant effects of either drug.
Leucovorin	High alcohol content of leucovorin may cause adverse effects.
Methyprylon	Increased sedative effect, perhaps to dangerous level. Avoid.
Nabilone	Greater depression of central nervous system.
Nicardipine	Blood pressure drop. Dosages may require adjustment.
Nimodipine	Dangerous blood pressure drop.
Sertraline	Increased depressive effects of both drugs.

POSSIBLE INTERACTION WITH OTHER SUBSTANCES

INTERACTS WITH	COMBINED EFFECT
Alcohol:	Oversedation. Avoid.
Beverages: Caffeine.	Overstimulation. Avoid.
Cocaine:	Overstimulation. Avoid.
Foods: Salt.	Decrease salt intake to increase beneficial effects of guanabenz.
Marijuana:	Overstimulation. Avoid.
Tobacco:	Decreased guanabenz effect.

GUANADREL

BRAND NAMES

Hylorel

BASIC INFORMATION

Habit forming? No
Prescription needed? Yes
Available as generic? No
Drug class: Antihypertensive

USES

Controls, but doesn't cure, high blood pressure.

DOSAGE & USAGE INFORMATION

How to take:
Tablet—Swallow with liquid or food to lessen stomach irritation. If you can't swallow whole, crumble tablet and take with liquid or food.

When to take:
At the same time each day.

If you forget a dose:
Take as soon as you remember up to 2 hours late. If more than 2 hours, wait for next scheduled dose (don't double this dose).

What drug does:
Relaxes muscle cells of small arteries.

Time lapse before drug works:
4 to 6 hours. May need to take for lifetime.

Don't take with:
Any other medicine without consulting your doctor or pharmacist.

OVERDOSE

SYMPTOMS:
Severe blood-pressure drop; fainting; slow, weak pulse; cold, sweaty skin; loss of consciousness.
WHAT TO DO:
- **Dial 0 (operator) or 911 (emergency) for an ambulance or medical help. Then give first aid immediately.**
- **See emergency information on inside covers.**

POSSIBLE ADVERSE REACTIONS OR SIDE EFFECTS

SYMPTOMS	WHAT TO DO
Life-threatening:	
In case of overdose, see previous column.	
Common:	
• Diarrhea, more bowel movements, fatigue, weakness.	Continue. Call doctor when convenient.
• Dizziness, lower sex drive, feet and ankle swelling, drowsiness.	Continue. Tell doctor at next visit.
• Stuffy nose, dry mouth.	No action necessary.
Infrequent:	
• Rash, blurred vision, drooping eyelids, chest pain or shortness of breath, muscle pain or tremor.	Discontinue. Call doctor right away.
• Nausea or vomiting, headache.	Continue. Call doctor when convenient.
• Impotence, nighttime urination.	Continue. Tell doctor at next visit.
Rare:	
Decreased white blood cells causing sore throat, fever.	Discontinue. Call doctor right away.

WARNINGS & PRECAUTIONS

Don't take if:
- You are allergic to guanadrel.
- You have taken MAO inhibitors within 2 weeks.

Before you start, consult your doctor:
- If you have stroke or heart disease.
- If you have asthma.
- If you have had kidney disease.
- If you have peptic ulcer or chronic acid indigestion.
- If you will have surgery within 2 months, including dental surgery, requiring general or spinal anesthesia.

Over age 60:
Adverse reactions and side effects may be more frequent and severe than in younger persons. Start with small doses and monitor blood pressure frequently.

Pregnancy:
No proven harm to unborn child. Avoid if possible.

Breast-feeding:
No proven harm to nursing infant. Avoid if possible.

Infants & children:
Not recommended.

Prolonged use:
- Due to drug's cumulative effect, dose will require adjustment to prevent wide fluctuations in blood pressure.
- Talk to your doctor about the need for follow-up medical examinations or laboratory studies.

Skin & sunlight:
No problems expected.

Driving, piloting or hazardous work:
Don't drive or pilot aircraft until you learn how medicine affects you. Don't work around dangerous machinery. Don't climb ladders or work in high places. Danger increases if you drink alcohol or take medicine affecting alertness and reflexes, such as antihistamines, tranquilizers, sedatives, pain medicine, narcotics and mind-altering drugs.

Discontinuing:
Don't discontinue without consulting doctor. Dose may require gradual reduction if you have taken drug for a long time. Doses of other drugs may also require adjustment.

Others:
Hot weather further lowers blood pressure, particularly in patients over 60.

POSSIBLE INTERACTION WITH OTHER DRUGS

GENERIC NAME OR DRUG CLASS	COMBINED EFFECT
ACE inhibitors*: captopril, enalapril, lisinopril	Possible excessive potassium in blood.
Antidepressants, tricyclic (TCA)*	Decreased effect of guanadrel.
Antihypertensives, other*	Increased effect of guanadrel.
Beta-adrenergic blockers*	Increased likelihood of dizziness and fainting.
Carteolol	Increased antihypertensive effect.
Contraceptives, oral*	Increased side effects of oral contraceptives.
Central nervous system (CNS) depressants* (anticonvulsants,* antihistamines,* muscle relaxants,* narcotics,* sedatives,* tranquilizers*)	Decreased effect of guanadrel.
Diuretics*	Increased likelihood of dizziness and fainting.
Haloperidol	Decreased effect of guanadrel.
Insulin	Increased insulin effect.
Loxapine	Decreased effect of guanadrel.
MAO inhibitors*	Severe high blood pressure. Avoid.
Nicardipine	Blood pressure drop. Dosages may require adjustment.
Nimodipine	Dangerous blood pressure drop.
Phenothiazines*	Decreased effect of guanadrel.
Rauwolfia alkaloids*	Increased likelihood of dizziness and fainting.
Sotalol	Increased antihypertensive effect.
Sympathomimetics*	Decreased effect of guanadrel.
Terazosin	Decreases effectiveness of terazosin.

POSSIBLE INTERACTION WITH OTHER SUBSTANCES

INTERACTS WITH	COMBINED EFFECT
Alcohol:	Decreased effect of guanadrel. Avoid.
Beverages: Caffeine.	Decreased effect of guanadrel.
Cocaine:	Increased risk of heart block and high blood pressure.
Foods:	No problems expected.
Marijuana:	Higher blood pressure. Avoid.
Tobacco:	Higher blood pressure. Avoid.

*See Glossary

GUANETHIDINE

BRAND NAMES

Apo-Guanethidine   Ismelin

BASIC INFORMATION

Habit forming? No
Prescription needed? Yes
Available as generic? Yes
Drug class: Antihypertensive

 USES

Reduces high blood pressure.

 DOSAGE & USAGE INFORMATION

How to take:
Tablet—Swallow with liquid. If you can't swallow tablet whole, crumble and take with liquid or food.

When to take:
At the same time each day.

If you forget a dose:
Take as soon as you remember up to 2 hours late. If more than 2 hours, wait for next scheduled dose (don't double this dose).

What drug does:
Displaces norepinephrine—hormone necessary to maintain small blood-vessel tone. Blood vessels relax and high blood pressure drops.

Time lapse before drug works:
Regular use for several weeks may be necessary to determine effectiveness.

Don't take with:
- Non-prescription drugs containing alcohol without consulting doctor.
- Any other medicine without consulting your doctor or pharmacist.

 OVERDOSE

SYMPTOMS:
Severe blood-pressure drop; fainting; slow, weak pulse; cold, sweaty skin; loss of consciousness.
WHAT TO DO:
- **Dial 0 (operator) or 911 (emergency) for an ambulance or medical help. Then give first aid immediately.**
- **See emergency information on inside covers.**

 POSSIBLE ADVERSE REACTIONS OR SIDE EFFECTS

SYMPTOMS	WHAT TO DO
Life-threatening:	
In case of overdose, see previous column.	
Common:	
• Unusually slow heartbeat.	Discontinue. Call doctor right away.
• Diarrhea; more bowel movements; swollen feet, legs; fatigue, weakness.	Continue. Call doctor when convenient.
• Dizziness, lower sex drive.	Continue. Tell doctor at next visit.
• Stuffy nose, dry mouth.	No action necessary.
Infrequent:	
• Rash, blurred vision, drooping eyelids, chest pain or shortness of breath, muscle pain or tremor.	Discontinue. Call doctor right away.
• Nausea or vomiting, headache.	Continue. Call doctor when convenient.
• Impotence, nighttime urination, hair loss.	Continue. Tell doctor at next visit.
Rare:	
Decreased white blood cells causing sore throat, fever.	Discontinue. Call doctor right away.

 WARNINGS & PRECAUTIONS

Don't take if:
- You are allergic to guanethidine.
- You have taken MAO inhibitors within 2 weeks.

Before you start, consult your doctor:
- If you have had stroke or heart disease.
- If you have asthma.
- If you have had kidney disease.
- If you have peptic ulcer or chronic acid indigestion.
- If you will have surgery within 2 months, including dental surgery, requiring general or spinal anesthesia.

Over age 60:
Adverse reactions and side effects may be more frequent and severe than in younger persons. Start with small doses and monitor blood pressure frequently.

Pregnancy:
No proven harm to unborn child. Avoid if possible.

Breast-feeding:
No proven harm to nursing infant. Avoid if possible.

Infants & children:
Not recommended.

Prolonged use:
- Due to drug's cumulative effect, dose will require adjustment to prevent wide fluctuations in blood pressure.
- Talk to your doctor about the need for follow-up medical examinations or laboratory studies.

Skin & sunlight:
No problems expected.

Driving, piloting or hazardous work:
Don't drive or pilot aircraft until you learn how medicine affects you. Don't work around dangerous machinery. Don't climb ladders or work in high places. Danger increases if you drink alcohol or take medicine affecting alertness and reflexes, such as antihistamines, tranquilizers, sedatives, pain medicine, narcotics and mind-altering drugs.

Discontinuing:
Don't discontinue without consulting doctor. Dose may require gradual reduction if you have taken drug for a long time. Doses of other drugs may also require adjustment.

Others:
Hot weather further lowers blood pressure.

POSSIBLE INTERACTION WITH OTHER DRUGS

GENERIC NAME OR DRUG CLASS	COMBINED EFFECT
ACE inhibitors*: captopril, enalapril, lisinopril	Possible excessive potassium in blood.
Amphetamines*	Decreased guanethidine effect.
Antidepressants, tricyclic (TCA)*	Decreased guanethidine effect.
Antihistamines*	Decreased guanethidine effect.
Carteolol	Increased antihypertensive effect.
Contraceptives, oral*	Decreased guanethidine effect. Increased side effects of oral contraceptives.
Digitalis preparations*	Slower heartbeat.
Diuretics, thiazide*	Increased guanethidine effect.
Haloperidol	Decreased guanethidine effect.
Indapamide	Possible increased effects of both drugs. When monitored carefully, combination may be beneficial in controlling hypertension.

Insulin	Increased insulin effect.
Loxapine	Decreased effect of guanethidine.
MAO inhibitors*	Increased blood pressure.
Minoxidil	Dosage adjustments may be necessary to keep blood pressure at proper level.
Nicardipine	Blood pressure drop. Dosages may require adjustment.
Nimodipine	Dangerous blood pressure drop.
Phenothiazines*	Decreased guanethidine effect.
Rauwolfia alkaloids*	Excessively slow heartbeat. Weakness and faintness upon rising from chair or bed.
Sotalol	Increased antihypertensive effect.
Terazosin	Decreases effectiveness of terazosin.

POSSIBLE INTERACTION WITH OTHER SUBSTANCES

INTERACTS WITH	COMBINED EFFECT
Alcohol:	Use caution. Decreases blood pressure.
Beverages: Carbonated drinks.	Use sparingly. Sodium content increases blood pressure.
Cocaine:	Increased risk of heart block and high blood pressure.
Foods: Spicy or acid foods.	Avoid if subject to indigestion or peptic ulcer.
Marijuana:	Excessively low blood pressure. Avoid.
Tobacco:	Possible blood pressure rise. Avoid.

*See Glossary

GUANETHIDINE & HYDROCHLOROTHIAZIDE

BRAND NAMES

Esimil   **Ismelin-Esidrix**

BASIC INFORMATION

Habit forming? No
Prescription needed? Yes
Available as generic? No
Drug class: Antihypertensive, diuretic

 ## USES

- Controls, but doesn't cure, high blood pressure.
- Reduces fluid retention (edema).

 ## DOSAGE & USAGE INFORMATION

How to take:
Tablet—Swallow with liquid. If you can't swallow whole, crumble tablet and take with liquid or food.

When to take:
At the same time each day.

If you forget a dose:
Take as soon as you remember up to 2 hours late. If more than 2 hours, wait for next scheduled dose (don't double this dose).

What drug does:
- Forces sodium and water secretion, reducing body fluid.
- Displaces norepinephrine—hormone necessary to maintain small blood-vessel tone. Blood vessels relax and high blood pressure drops.

Time lapse before drug works:
Regular use for several weeks may be necessary to determine effectiveness.

Continued next column

 ## OVERDOSE

SYMPTOMS:
Cramps, weakness, drowsiness, weak pulse, severe blood-pressure drop, fainting, cold and sweaty skin, loss of consciousness, coma.
WHAT TO DO:
- **Dial 0 (operator) or 911 (emergency) for an ambulance or medical help. Then give first aid immediately.**
- **See emergency information on inside covers.**

Don't take with:
- Non-prescription drugs containing alcohol without consulting doctor.
- Any other medicine without consulting your doctor or pharmacist.

 ## POSSIBLE ADVERSE REACTIONS OR SIDE EFFECTS

SYMPTOMS	WHAT TO DO
Life-threatening:	
Chest pain, shortness of breath, irregular heartbeat.	Discontinue. Seek emergency treatment.
Common:	
• Slow heartbeat, swollen feet and ankles, fatigue, weakness.	Discontinue. Call doctor right away.
• Dizziness, stuffy nose, dry mouth, diarrhea, diminished sex drive.	Continue. Call doctor when convenient.
Infrequent:	
• Mood change, rash or hives, blurred vision, drooping eyelids, muscle pain or tremors.	Discontinue. Call doctor right away.
• Increased nighttime urination, abdominal pain, vomiting, nausea, headache, weakness.	Continue. Call doctor when convenient.
• Impotence, nighttime urination, hair loss.	Continue. Tell doctor at next visit.
Rare:	
• Decreased white blood cells causing sore throat, fever; jaundice.	Discontinue. Call doctor right away.
• Weight gain or loss.	Continue. Call doctor when convenient.

 ## WARNINGS & PRECAUTIONS

Don't take if:
- You are allergic to any thiazide diuretic drug or guanethidine.
- You have taken MAO inhibitors within 2 weeks.

Before you start, consult your doctor:
- If you are allergic to any sulfa drug.
- If you have gout, asthma, liver, pancreas or kidney disorder, peptic ulcer or chronic acid indigestion.
- If you have had stroke or heart disease.
- If you will have surgery within 2 months, including dental surgery, requiring general or spinal anesthesia.

Over age 60:
Adverse reactions and side effects may be more frequent and severe than in younger persons, especially dizziness and excessive potassium loss.

Pregnancy:
Risk to unborn child outweighs drug benefits. Don't use.

Breast-feeding:
Drug passes into milk. Avoid drug or discontinue nursing until you finish medicine. Consult doctor for advice on maintaining milk supply.

Infants & children:
Not recommended.

Prolonged use:
- Due to drug's cumulative effect, dose will require adjustment to prevent wide fluctuations in blood pressure.
- Talk to your doctor about the need for follow-up medical examinations or laboratory studies.

Skin & sunlight:
May cause rash or intensify sunburn in areas exposed to sun or sunlamp.

Driving, piloting or hazardous work:
Don't drive or pilot aircraft until you learn how medicine affects you. Don't work around dangerous machinery. Don't climb ladders or work in high places. Danger increases if you drink alcohol or take medicine affecting alertness and reflexes, such as antihistamines, tranquilizers, sedatives, pain medicine, narcotics and mind-altering drugs.

Discontinuing:
Don't discontinue without consulting doctor. Dose may require gradual reduction if you have taken drug for a long time. Doses of other drugs may also require adjustment.

Others:
- Hot weather and fever may cause dehydration and drop in blood pressure. Dose may require temporary adjustment. Weigh daily and report any unexpected weight decreases to your doctor.
- May cause rise in uric acid, leading to gout.
- May cause blood-sugar rise in diabetics.

POSSIBLE INTERACTION WITH OTHER DRUGS

GENERIC NAME OR DRUG CLASS	COMBINED EFFECT
Allopurinol	Decreased allopurinol effect.
Amphetamines*	Decreased guanethidine effect.
Antidepressants, tricyclic (TCA)*	Dangerous drop in blood pressure. Avoid combination unless under medical supervision.
Antihistamines*	Decreased guanethidine effect.
Barbiturates*	Increased hydrochlorothiazide effect.
Beta-adrenergic blockers*	Increased antihypertensive effect. Dosages of both drugs may require adjustments.
Carteolol	Increased antihypertensive effect.
Cholestyramine	Decreased hydrochlorothiazide effect.
Contraceptives, oral*	Decreased guanethidine effect.
Cortisone drugs*	Excessive potassium loss that causes dangerous heart rhythms.
Digitalis preparations*	Excessive potassium loss that causes dangerous heart rhythms.

Continued page 946

POSSIBLE INTERACTION WITH OTHER SUBSTANCES

INTERACTS WITH	COMBINED EFFECT
Alcohol:	Use caution. Decreases blood pressure.
Beverages: Carbonated drinks.	Use sparingly. Sodium content increases blood pressure.
Cocaine:	Raises blood pressure. Avoid.
Foods: Spicy or acid foods. Licorice.	Avoid if subject to indigestion or peptic ulcer. Excessive potassium loss that causes dangerous heart rhythms.
Marijuana:	Effect on blood pressure unpredictable.
Tobacco:	Possible blood pressure rise. Avoid.

*See Glossary

GUANFACINE

BRAND NAMES

Tenex

BASIC INFORMATION

Habit forming? No
Prescription needed? Yes
Available as generic? No
Drug class: Antihypertensive

 ## USES

Treats high blood pressure, usually in combination with a diuretic drug.

 ## DOSAGE & USAGE INFORMATION

How to take:
Tablets—Swallow with liquid or food to lessen stomach irritation. If you can't swallow whole, crumble tablet and take with liquid or food.

When to take:
Usually at bedtime.

If you forget a dose:
Take as soon as you remember up to 2 hours late. If more than 2 hours, wait for next scheduled dose (don't double this dose).

What drug does:
- Decreases stimulating effects of the sympathetic nervous system on the heart, kidneys and arteries throughout the body.
- Decreases both systolic and diastolic blood pressure.

Time lapse before drug works:
Within 1 week.

Don't take with:
Any other medicine without consulting your doctor or pharmacist.

 ## OVERDOSE

SYMPTOMS:
Difficulty breathing, loss of consciousness, dizziness, very slow heartbeat.
WHAT TO DO:
- **Dial 0 (operator) or 911 (emergency) for an ambulance or medical help. Then give first aid immediately.**
- **See emergency information on inside covers.**

 ## POSSIBLE ADVERSE REACTIONS OR SIDE EFFECTS

SYMPTOMS	WHAT TO DO
Life-threatening:	
Shortness of breath.	Seek emergency treatment immediately.
Common:	
• Constipation.	Discontinue. Call doctor right away.
• Decreased sexual function, drowsiness.	Continue. Call doctor when convenient.
• Increased dental problems because of dry mouth and less salivation.	Consult your dentist about a prevention program.
Infrequent:	
• Confusion, dizziness or fainting, slow heartbeat.	Discontinue. Call doctor right away.
• Mental depression, eye irritation, insomnia, tiredness or weakness, headache, nausea and/or vomiting.	Continue. Call doctor when convenient.
Rare:	
May occur if medicine is abruptly discontinued—Anxiety, chest pain, heartbeat irregularities, excess salivation, sleep problems, nervousness, sweating.	Seek emergency treatment.

 ## WARNINGS & PRECAUTIONS

Don't take if:
You have had a recent heart attack.

Before you start, consult your doctor:
- If you have heart disease or liver disease.
- If you have coronary insufficiency.
- If you have mental depression.

Over age 60:
None expected.

Pregnancy:
No proven harm to unborn child, but avoid if possible.

Breast-feeding:
Effect not documented. Consult your doctor.

Infants & children:
Effect not documented. Consult your pediatrician.

Prolonged use:
Talk to your doctor about the need for follow-up medical examinations or laboratory studies to check blood pressure.

Skin & sunlight:
No problems expected.

Driving, piloting or hazardous work:
Don't drive or pilot aircraft until you learn how medicine affects you. Don't work around dangerous machinery. Don't climb ladders or work in high places. Danger increases if you drink alcohol or take medicine affecting alertness and reflexes.

Discontinuing:
* Don't discontinue without consulting doctor. Dose may require gradual reduction if you have taken drug for a long time. Doses of other drugs may also require adjustment.
* May occur if medicine is discontinued abruptly: anxiety, chest pain, heartbeat irregularities, excess salivation, sleep problems, nervousness, sweating.

Others:
* This medication works better if you attempt to reduce your weight to normal, exercise regularly, restrict salt in your diet and reduce stress wherever possible. Continue taking medicine even when you feel good.
* Adverse reactions are usually dose-related and diminish when dosage is reduced.

POSSIBLE INTERACTION WITH OTHER DRUGS

GENERIC NAME OR DRUG CLASS	COMBINED EFFECT
Antihypertensives, other*	May increase effects of guanfacine and other medicines.
Carteolol	Increased antihypertensive effect.
Central nervous system (CNS) depressants*	Increases depressant effect of both drugs.
Clozapine	Toxic effect on the central nervous system.
Estrogens*	May decrease antihypertensive effects of guanfacine.
Ethinamate	Dangerous increased effects of ethinamate. Avoid combining.
Fluoxetine	Increased depressant effects of both drugs.

Leucovorin	High alcohol content of leucovorin may cause adverse effects.
Lisinopril	Increased antihypertensive effect. Dosage of each may require adjustment.
Methyprylon	Increased sedative effect, perhaps to dangerous level. Avoid.
Nabilone	Greater depression of central nervous system.
Nicardipine	Blood pressure drop. Dosages may require adjustment.
Nimodipine	Dangerous blood pressure drop.
Non-steroidal anti-inflammatory drugs (NSAIDs)*	May decrease antihypertensive effects of guanfacine.
Propafenone	Increased effect of both drugs and increased risk of toxicity.
Sertraline	Increased depressive effects of both drugs.
Sotalol	Increased antihypertensive effect.

Continued page 947

POSSIBLE INTERACTION WITH OTHER SUBSTANCES

INTERACTS WITH	COMBINED EFFECT
Alcohol:	Excess use may lead to dangerous drop in blood pressure.
Beverages: Any containing caffeine, such as coffee, tea or cocoa.	May decrease antihypertensive effect of guanfacine.
Cocaine:	Increased risk of heart block and high blood pressure.
Foods:	None expected.
Marijuana:	May decrease antihypertensive effect of guanfacine.
Tobacco:	May decrease antihypertensive effect of guanfacine.

HALOPERIDOL

BRAND NAMES

Apo-Haloperidol
Haldol
Haldol Decanoate
Haldol LA

Halperon
Novoperidol
Peridol

BASIC INFORMATION

Habit forming? No
Prescription needed? Yes
Available as generic? Yes
Drug class: Tranquilizer (antipsychotic)

USES

Reduces severe anxiety, agitation and psychotic behavior.

DOSAGE & USAGE INFORMATION

How to take:
- Tablet or extended-release capsule—Swallow with liquid. If you can't swallow whole, crumble tablet and take with liquid or food.
- Drops—Dilute dose in beverage before swallowing.

When to take:
At the same times each day.

If you forget a dose:
Take as soon as you remember up to 2 hours late. If more than 2 hours, wait for next scheduled dose (don't double this dose).

What drug does:
Corrects an imbalance in nerve impulses from brain.

Time lapse before drug works:
3 weeks to 2 months for maximum benefit.

Continued next column

OVERDOSE

SYMPTOMS:
Weak, rapid pulse; shallow, slow breathing; tremor or muscle weakness; very low blood pressure; convulsions; deep sleep ending in coma.
WHAT TO DO:
- **Dial 0 (operator) or 911 (emergency) for an ambulance or medical help. Then give first aid immediately.**
- **If patient is unconscious and not breathing, give mouth-to-mouth breathing. If there is no heartbeat, use cardiac massage and mouth-to-mouth breathing (CPR). Don't try to make patient vomit. If you can't get help quickly, take patient to nearest emergency facility.**
- **See emergency information on inside covers.**

Don't take with:
- Non-prescription drugs without consulting doctor.
- Any other medicine without consulting your doctor or pharmacist.

POSSIBLE ADVERSE REACTIONS OR SIDE EFFECTS

SYMPTOMS	WHAT TO DO
Life-threatening:	
Uncontrolled muscle movements of tongue, face and other muscles (neuroleptic malignant syndrome, rare).	Discontinue. Seek emergency treatment.
Common:	
• Blurred vision, loss of balance, muscle spasms, severe restlessness.	Discontinue. Call doctor right away.
• Shuffling, stiffness, jerkiness, shakiness, constipation, weight gain.	Continue. Call doctor when convenient.
• Dry mouth.	No action necessary.
Infrequent:	
• Rash, circling motions of tongue, hallucinations, lip smacking.	Discontinue. Call doctor right away.
• Dizziness, faintness, drowsiness, difficult urination, decreased sexual ability, nausea or vomiting.	Continue. Call doctor when convenient.
Rare:	
Sore throat; fever; jaundice; abdominal pain; dry, warm skin.	Discontinue. Call doctor right away.

WARNINGS & PRECAUTIONS

Don't take if:
- You have ever been allergic to haloperidol.
- You are depressed.
- You have Parkinson's disease.
- Patient is younger than 3 years old.

Before you start, consult your doctor:
- If you take sedatives, sleeping pills, tranquilizers, antidepressants, antihistamines, narcotics or mind-altering drugs.
- If you have a history of mental depression.
- If you have had kidney or liver problems.
- If you have diabetes, epilepsy, glaucoma, high blood pressure or heart disease, prostate trouble.
- If you drink alcoholic beverages frequently.

Over age 60:
Adverse reactions and side effects may be more frequent and severe than in younger persons.

Pregnancy:
Risk to unborn child outweighs drug benefits. Don't use.

Breast-feeding:
No proven harm to nursing infant. Avoid if possible.

Infants & children:
Not recommended.

Prolonged use:
- May develop tardive dyskinesia (involuntary movements of jaws, lips and tongue).
- Talk to your doctor about the need for follow-up medical examinations or laboratory studies to check blood pressure, liver function.

Skin & sunlight:
May cause rash or intensify sunburn in areas exposed to sun or sunlamp.

Driving, piloting or hazardous work:
Don't drive or pilot aircraft until you learn how medicine affects you. Don't work around dangerous machinery. Don't climb ladders or work in high places. Danger increases if you drink alcohol or take medicine affecting alertness and reflexes.

Discontinuing:
Don't discontinue without consulting doctor. Dose may require gradual reduction if you have taken drug for a long time. Doses of other drugs may also require adjustment.

Others:
No problems expected.

POSSIBLE INTERACTION WITH OTHER DRUGS

GENERIC NAME OR DRUG CLASS	COMBINED EFFECT
Anticholinergics*	Increased anti-cholinergic effect. May cause pressure within the eye.
Anticonvulsants*	Changed seizure pattern.
Antidepressants*	Excessive sedation.
Antihistamines*	Excessive sedation.
Antihypertensives*	May cause severe blood-pressure drop.
Barbiturates*	Excessive sedation.
Bupropion	Increased risk of major seizures.
Central nervous system (CNS) depressants*	Increased CNS depression; increased blood pressure drop.
Clozapine	Toxic effect on the central nervous system.
Dronabinol	Increased effects of both drugs. Avoid.
Ethinamate	Dangerous increased effects of ethinamate. Avoid combining.
Fluoxetine	Increased depressant effects of both drugs.
Guanethidine	Decreased guanethidine effect.
Guanfacine	May increase depressant effects of either drug.
Loxapine	May increase toxic effects of both drugs.
Leucovorin	High alcohol content of leucovorin may cause adverse effects.
Levodopa	Decreased levodopa effect.
Lithium	Increased toxicity.
Methyldopa	Possible psychosis.
Methyprylon	Increased sedative effect, perhaps to dangerous level. Avoid.
Nabilone	Greater depression of central nervous system.
Narcotics*	Excessive sedation.
Pergolide	Decreased pergolide effect.
Phenindione	Decreased anticoagulant effect.
Procarbazine	Increased sedation.
Sedatives*	Excessive sedation.
Sertraline	Increased depressive effects of both drugs.
Tranquilizers*	Excessive sedation.

POSSIBLE INTERACTION WITH OTHER SUBSTANCES

INTERACTS WITH	COMBINED EFFECT
Alcohol:	Excessive sedation and depressed brain function. Avoid.
Beverages:	None expected.
Cocaine:	Decreased effect of haloperidol. Avoid.
Foods:	None expected.
Marijuana:	Occasional use— Increased sedation. Frequent use—Possible toxic psychosis.
Tobacco:	None expected.

*See Glossary

BRAND NAMES

Apo-Cimetidine	Novocimetine
Axid	Pepcid
CIMETIDINE	Peptol
FAMOTIDINE	RANITIDINE
NIZATIDINE	Tagamet
	Zantac

BASIC INFORMATION

Habit forming? No
Prescription needed? Yes
Available as generic? No
Drug class: Histamine H₂ antagonist

USES

Treatment for duodenal ulcers and other conditions in which stomach produces excess hydrochloric acid.

DOSAGE & USAGE INFORMATION

How to take:
Tablet or liquid—Swallow with liquid.

When to take:
- 1 dose per day—Take at bedtime.
- 2 or more doses per day—Take at the same times each day.

If you forget a dose:
Take as soon as you remember up to 2 hours late. If more than 2 hours, wait for next scheduled dose (don't double this dose).

What drug does:
Blocks histamine release so stomach secretes less acid.

Time lapse before drug works:
Begins in 30 minutes. May require several days to relieve pain.

Don't take with:
Any other medicine without consulting your doctor or pharmacist.

OVERDOSE

SYMPTOMS:
Confusion, slurred speech, breathing difficulty, rapid heartbeat, delirium.
WHAT TO DO:
Overdose unlikely to threaten life. If person takes much larger amount than prescribed, call doctor, poison-control center or hospital emergency room for instructions.

POSSIBLE ADVERSE REACTIONS OR SIDE EFFECTS

SYMPTOMS	WHAT TO DO
Life-threatening:	
In case of overdose, see previous column.	
Common:	
None expected.	
Infrequent:	
• Dizziness or headache, diarrhea.	Continue. Call doctor when convenient.
• Diminished sex drive, unusual milk flow in females, hair loss.	Continue. Tell doctor at next visit.
Rare:	
• Confusion; rash, hives; sore throat, fever; slow, fast or irregular heartbeat; unusual bleeding or bruising; muscle cramps or pain; fatigue; weakness.	Discontinue. Call doctor right away.
• Constipation.	Continue. Call doctor when convenient.

WARNINGS & PRECAUTIONS

Don't take if:
You are allergic to any histamine H₂ antagonist.

Before you start, consult your doctor:
- If you plan to become pregnant while on medication.
- If you take aspirin. Aspirin may irritate stomach.

Over age 60:
Adverse reactions and side effects may be more frequent and severe than in younger persons.

Pregnancy:
No proven harm to unborn child. Avoid if possible.

Breast-feeding:
No problems expected.

Infants & children:
Not recommended.

Prolonged use:
- Possible liver damage.
- Talk to your doctor about the need for follow-up medical examinations or laboratory studies to check blood levels of vitamin B-12.

Skin & sunlight:
No problems expected.

HISTAMINE H₂ RECEPTOR ANTAGONISTS

Driving, piloting or hazardous work:
Don't drive or pilot aircraft until you learn how medicine affects you. Don't work around dangerous machinery. Don't climb ladders or work in high places. Danger increases if you drink alcohol or take medicine affecting alertness and reflexes, such as antihistamines, tranquilizers, sedatives, pain medicine, narcotics and mind-altering drugs.

Discontinuing:
Don't discontinue without consulting a doctor. Dose may require gradual reduction if you have taken drug for a long time. Doses of other drugs may also require adjustment.

Others:
- Patients on kidney dialysis—Take at end of dialysis treatment.
- May interfere with the accuracy of some medical tests.

POSSIBLE INTERACTION WITH OTHER DRUGS

GENERIC NAME OR DRUG CLASS	COMBINED EFFECT
Alprazolam	Increased effect and toxicity of alprazolam.
Antacids*	Decreased absorption of histamine H₂ receptor antagonist.
Anticoagulants, oral*	Increased anticoagulant effect.
Anticholinergics*	Increased histamine H₂ receptor antagonist effect.
Bupropion	Increased bupropion effect.
Carbamazepine	Increased effect and toxicity of carbamazepine.
Carmustine (BCNU)	Severe impairment of red blood cell production; some interference with white blood cell formation.
Chlordiazepoxide	Increased effect and toxicity of chlordiazepoxide.
Diazepam	Increased effect and toxicity of diazepam.
Digitalis preparations*	Increased digitalis effect.
Encainide	Increased effect of histamine H₂ receptor antagonist.

Flurazepam	Increased effect and toxicity of flurazepam.
Glipizide	Increased effect and toxicity of glipizide.
Ketoconazole	Decreased ketoconazole absorption.
Labetalol	Increased antihypertensive effects.
Methadone	Increased effect and toxicity of methadone.
Metoclopramide	Decreased absorption of histamine H₂ receptor antagonist.
Metoprolol	Increased effect and toxicity of metoprolol.

Continued on page 947

POSSIBLE INTERACTION WITH OTHER SUBSTANCES

INTERACTS WITH	COMBINED EFFECT
Alcohol:	No interactions expected, but alcohol may slow body's recovery. Avoid.
Beverages: Milk.	Enhanced effectiveness. Small amounts useful for taking medication.
Caffeine drinks.	May increase acid secretion and delay healing.
Cocaine:	Decreased effect of histamine H₂ receptor antagonist.
Foods:	Enhanced effectiveness. Protein-rich foods should be eaten in moderation to minimize secretion of stomach acid.
Marijuana:	Increased chance of low sperm count. Marijuana may slow body's recovery. Avoid.
Tobacco:	Reversed effect of histamine H₂ receptor antagonist. Tobacco may slow body's recovery. Avoid.

*See Glossary

HMG-CoA REDUCTASE INHIBITORS

BRAND AND GENERIC NAMES

Epistatin
Eptastatin
LOVASTATIN
Mevacor
Mevinolin

Pravachol
PRAVASTATIN
SIMVASTATIN
Synvinolin
Zocor

BASIC INFORMATION

Habit forming? No
Prescription needed? Yes
Available as generic? No
Drug class: Antihyperlipidemic

USES

Lowers blood cholesterol levels caused by low-density cholesterol (LDL) in persons who haven't improved by exercising, dieting or using other measures.

DOSAGE & USAGE INFORMATION

How to take:
Tablet—Swallow with liquid. If you can't swallow whole, crumble tablet and take with liquid or food.

When to take:
According to directions on prescription.

If you forget a dose:
Take as soon as you remember up to 2 hours late. If more than 2 hours, wait for next scheduled dose (don't double this dose).

What drug does:
Inhibits an enzyme in the liver.

Time lapse before drug works:
Within 2 weeks.

Don't take with:
- A high-fat diet.
- Any other medicine without consulting your doctor or pharmacist.

OVERDOSE

SYMPTOMS:
None expected.
WHAT TO DO:
Overdose not expected to threaten life. If person takes much larger amount than prescribed, call doctor, poison-control center or hospital emergency room for instructions.

POSSIBLE ADVERSE REACTIONS OR SIDE EFFECTS

SYMPTOMS	WHAT TO DO
Life-threatening: None expected.	
Common: None expected.	
Infrequent:	
• Aching muscles, fever, blurred vision.	Discontinue. Call doctor right away.
• Constipation, nausea, tiredness, weakness, dizziness, skin rash, headache.	Continue. Call doctor when convenient.
Rare:	
• Muscle pain.	Discontinue. Call doctor right away.
• Impotence (Lovastatin only).	Continue. Call doctor when convenient.
• Insomnia (Lovastatin only).	Continue. Call doctor when convenient.

WARNINGS & PRECAUTIONS

Don't take if:
You are allergic to lovastatin.

Before you start, consult your doctor:
- If you take immunosuppressive drugs, particularly following a heart transplant.
- If you have low blood pressure.
- If you have hormone abnormalities
- If you have an active infection.
- If you have active liver disease.
- If you have a seizure disorder.
- If you have had a recent major accident.

Over age 60:
Likely to be more sensitive to drug.

Pregnancy:
Studies inconclusive on harm to unborn child. Decide with your doctor whether drug benefits justify risk to unborn child.

Breast-feeding:
No proven problems, but avoid if possible or discontinue nursing until you finish medicine. Consult doctor for advice on maintaining milk supply.

Infants & children:
Not recommended for children.

Prolonged use:
Talk to your doctor about the need for follow-up medical examinations or laboratory studies to check liver function, serum cholesterol, eyes.

Skin & sunlight:
No problems expected.

Driving, piloting or hazardous work:
No special problems expected.

Discontinuing:
Don't discontinue without consulting doctor. Dose may require gradual reduction if you have taken drug for a long time. Doses of other drugs may also require adjustment.

Others:
Request liver function tests and eye examinations before beginning this medicine and repeat every 2 to 6 months.

POSSIBLE INTERACTION WITH OTHER DRUGS

GENERIC NAME OR DRUG CLASS	COMBINED EFFECT
Cyclosporine or other drugs to suppress the immune system such as prednisone, azathioprine and others	Increased heart and kidney damage.
Erythromycin	Increased heart and kidney damage.
Gemfibrozil	Increased heart and kidney damage.
Niacin	Increased heart and kidney damage.

POSSIBLE INTERACTION WITH OTHER SUBSTANCES

INTERACTS WITH	COMBINED EFFECT
Alcohol:	None expected.
Beverages:	None expected.
Cocaine:	None expected.
Foods:	None expected.
Marijuana:	None expected.
Tobacco:	None expected.

HYDRALAZINE

BRAND NAMES

Apresoline   Ser-Ap-Es
Novo-Hylazin

BASIC INFORMATION

Habit forming? No
Prescription needed? Yes
Available as generic? Yes
Drug class: Antihypertensive

USES

Treatment for high blood pressure and congestive heart failure.

DOSAGE & USAGE INFORMATION

How to take:
Tablet—Swallow with liquid. If you can't swallow whole, crumble tablet and take with liquid or food.

When to take:
At the same time each day.

If you forget a dose:
Take as soon as you remember up to 2 hours late. If more than 2 hours, wait for next scheduled dose (don't double this dose).

What drug does:
Relaxes and expands blood-vessel walls, lowering blood pressure.

Time lapse before drug works:
Regular use for several weeks may be necessary to determine drug's effectiveness.

Continued next column

OVERDOSE

SYMPTOMS:
Rapid and weak heartbeat, fainting, extreme weakness, cold and sweaty skin, flushing.
WHAT TO DO:
- **Dial 0 (operator) or 911 (emergency) for an ambulance or medical help. Then give first aid immediately.**
- **If patient is unconscious and not breathing, give mouth-to-mouth breathing. If there is no heartbeat, use cardiac massage and mouth-to-mouth breathing (CPR). Don't try to make patient vomit. If you can't get help quickly, take patient to nearest emergency facility.**
- **See emergency information on inside covers.**

Don't take with:
- Non-prescription drugs containing alcohol without consulting doctor.
- Any other medicine without consulting your doctor or pharmacist.

POSSIBLE ADVERSE REACTIONS OR SIDE EFFECTS

SYMPTOMS	WHAT TO DO
Life-threatening:	
In case of overdose, see previous column.	
Common:	
• Nausea or vomiting, rapid or irregular heartbeat.	Discontinue. Call doctor right away.
• Headache, diarrhea, appetite loss, painful or difficult urination.	Continue. Tell doctor at next visit.
Infrequent:	
• Hives or rash, flushed face, sore throat, fever, chest pain, swelling of lymph glands, skin blisters, swelling in feet or legs, joint pain.	Discontinue. Call doctor right away.
• Confusion, dizziness, anxiety, depression, joint pain, general discomfort or weakness, fever, muscle pain, chest pain.	Continue. Call doctor when convenient.
• Watery eyes and irritation, constipation.	Continue. Tell doctor at next visit.
Rare:	
• Weakness and faintness when arising from bed or chair, jaundice.	Discontinue. Call doctor right away.
• Numbness or tingling in hands or feet, nasal congestion, impotence.	Continue. Call doctor when convenient.

WARNINGS & PRECAUTIONS

Don't take if:
- You are allergic to hydralazine or tartrazine dye.
- You have history of coronary-artery disease or rheumatic heart disease.

Before you start, consult your doctor:
- If you feel pain in chest, neck or arms on physical exertion.
- If you have had lupus.
- If you have had a stroke.

- If you have had kidney disease or impaired kidney function.
- If you will have surgery within 2 months, including dental surgery, requiring general or spinal anesthesia.

Over age 60:
Adverse reactions and side effects may be more frequent and severe than in younger persons.

Pregnancy:
Risk to unborn child outweighs drug benefits. Don't use.

Breast-feeding:
Drug filters into milk. May harm child. Avoid.

Infants & children:
Not recommended.

Prolonged use:
- May cause lupus (arthritis-like illness).
- Possible psychosis.
- May cause numbness, tingling in hands or feet.
- Talk to your doctor about the need for follow-up medical examinations or laboratory studies to check blood pressure, complete blood counts (white blood cell count, platelet count, red blood cell count, hemoglobin, hematocrit), ANA titers*.

Skin & sunlight:
No problems expected.

Driving, piloting or hazardous work:
Don't drive or pilot aircraft until you learn how medicine affects you. Don't work around dangerous machinery. Don't climb ladders or work in high places. Danger increases if you drink alcohol or take medicine affecting alertness and reflexes, such as antihistamines, tranquilizers, sedatives, pain medicine, narcotics and mind-altering drugs.

Discontinuing:
Don't discontinue without doctor's advice until you complete prescribed dose, even though symptoms diminish or disappear.

Others:
- Vitamin B-6 diet supplement may be advisable. Consult doctor.
- Some products contain tartrazine dye. Avoid, especially if you are allergic to aspirin.
- May interfere with the accuracy of some medical tests.

 POSSIBLE INTERACTION WITH OTHER DRUGS

GENERIC NAME OR DRUG CLASS	COMBINED EFFECT
Amphetamines*	Decreased hydralazine effect.
Antihypertensives, other*	Increased antihypertensive effect.
Carteolol	Increased antihypertensive effect.
Diazoxide & other anti-hypertensive drugs	Increased antihypertensive effect.
Didanosine	Increased risk of peripheral neuropathy.
Diuretics, oral*	Increased effects of both drugs. When monitored carefully, combination may be beneficial in controlling hypertension.
Guanfacine	Increased effects of both drugs.
Lisinopril	Increased antihypertensive effect. Dosage of each may require adjustment.
MAO inhibitors*	Increased hydralazine effect.
Nicardipine	Blood pressure drop. Dosages may require adjustment.
Nimodipine	Dangerous blood pressure drop.
Non-steroidal anti-inflammatory drugs (NSAIDs)*	Decreased effect of hydralazine.
Sotalol	Increased antihypertensive effect.
Terazosin	Decreases effectiveness of terazosin.

 POSSIBLE INTERACTION WITH OTHER SUBSTANCES

INTERACTS WITH	COMBINED EFFECT
Alcohol:	May lower blood pressure excessively. Use extreme caution.
Beverages:	None expected.
Cocaine:	Increased risk of heart block and high blood pressure.
Foods:	Increased hydralazine absorption.
Marijuana:	Weakness on standing.
Tobacco:	Possible angina attacks.

HYDRALAZINE & HYDROCHLOROTHIAZIDE

BRAND NAMES

Apresazide	Aprozide
Apresoline-Esidrix	Hydra-zide

BASIC INFORMATION

Habit forming? No
Prescription needed? Yes
Available as generic? Yes
Drug class: Antihypertensive, diuretic

USES

- Controls, but doesn't cure, high blood pressure.
- Reduces fluid retention (edema).

DOSAGE & USAGE INFORMATION

How to take:
Tablet or capsule—Swallow with liquid. If you can't swallow whole, crumble tablet or open capsule and take with liquid or food.

When to take:
At the same time each day.

If you forget a dose:
Take as soon as you remember up to 2 hours late. If more than 2 hours, wait for next scheduled dose (don't double this dose).

What drug does:
- Forces sodium and water excretion, reducing body fluid.
- Relaxes and expands blood-vessel walls, lowering blood pressure.

Continued next column

OVERDOSE

SYMPTOMS:
Cramps, drowsiness, weak pulse, rapid and weak heartbeat, fainting, extreme weakness, cold and sweaty skin, coma.
WHAT TO DO:
- **Dial 0 (operator) or 911 (emergency) for an ambulance or medical help. Then give first aid immediately.**
- **If patient is unconscious and not breathing, give mouth-to-mouth breathing. If there is no heartbeat, use cardiac massage and mouth-to-mouth breathing (CPR). Don't try to make patient vomit. If you can't get help quickly, take patient to nearest emergency facility.**
- **See emergency information on inside covers.**

- Reduced body fluid and relaxed arteries lower blood pressure.

Time lapse before drug works:
Regular use for several weeks may be necessary to determine drug's effectiveness.

Don't take with:
- Non-prescription drugs containing alcohol without consulting doctor.
- Any other medicine without consulting your doctor or pharmacist.

POSSIBLE ADVERSE REACTIONS OR SIDE EFFECTS

SYMPTOMS	WHAT TO DO
Life-threatening:	
Chest pain, irregular and fast heartbeat, weak pulse.	Discontinue. Seek emergency treatment.
Common:	
• Nausea, vomiting.	Discontinue. Call doctor right away.
• Headache, diarrhea, appetite loss, frequent urination, dry mouth, thirst.	Continue. Call doctor when convenient.
Infrequent:	
• Rash; black, bloody or tarry stool; red or flushed face; sore throat, fever, mouth sores; constipation; lymph glands swelling; blurred vision; skin blisters; swelling in feet or legs.	Discontinue. Call doctor right away.
• Dizziness; confusion; watery eyes; weight gain or loss; joint, muscle or chest pain; depression; anxiety; fever.	Continue. Call doctor when convenient.
Rare:	
• Weakness and faintness when arising from bed or chair, jaundice.	Discontinue. Call doctor right away.
• Numbness or tingling in hands or feet, nasal congestion, impotence.	Continue. Call doctor when convenient.

WARNINGS & PRECAUTIONS

Don't take if:
- You are allergic to hydralazine, any thiazide diuretic drug or tartrazine dye.
- You have history of coronary-artery disease or rheumatic heart disease.

HYDRALAZINE & HYDROCHLOROTHIAZIDE

Before you start, consult your doctor:
- If you feel pain in chest, neck or arms on physical exertion.
- If you are allergic to any sulfa drug.
- If you have had lupus or a stroke.
- If you have gout, liver, pancreas or kidney disorder.
- If you will have surgery within 2 months, including dental surgery, requiring general or spinal anesthesia.

Over age 60:
Adverse reactions and side effects may be more frequent and severe than in younger persons, especially dizziness and excessive potassium loss.

Pregnancy:
Risk to unborn child outweighs drug benefits. Don't use.

Breast-feeding:
Drug passes into milk. Avoid drug or discontinue nursing until you finish medicine. Consult doctor for advice on maintaining milk supply.

Infants & children:
Not recommended.

Prolonged use:
- May cause lupus (arthritis-like illness).
- Possible psychosis.
- May cause numbness, tingling in hands or feet.
- Talk to your doctor about the need for follow-up medical examinations or laboratory studies to check blood pressure, complete blood counts (white blood cell count, platelet count, red blood cell count, hemoglobin, hematocrit), ANA titers*.

Skin & sunlight:
May cause rash or intensify sunburn in areas exposed to sun or sunlamp.

Driving, piloting or hazardous work:
Don't drive or pilot aircraft until you learn how medicine affects you. Don't work around dangerous machinery. Don't climb ladders or work in high places. Danger increases if you drink alcohol or take medicine affecting alertness and reflexes, such as antihistamines, tranquilizers, sedatives, pain medicine, narcotics and mind-altering drugs.

Discontinuing:
Don't discontinue without consulting doctor's advice until you complete prescribed dose, even though symptoms diminish or disappear.

Others:
- Vitamin B-6 diet supplement may be advisable. Consult doctor.
- Hot weather and fever may cause dehydration and drop in blood pressure. Dose may require temporary adjustment. Weigh daily and report any unexpected weight decreases to your doctor.
- May cause rise in uric acid, leading to gout.
- May cause blood-sugar rise in diabetics.

POSSIBLE INTERACTION WITH OTHER DRUGS

GENERIC NAME OR DRUG CLASS	COMBINED EFFECT
Acebutolol	Decreased antihypertensive effect of acebutolol.
Allopurinol	Decreased allopurinol effect.
Amphetamines*	Decreased hydralazine effect.
Antidepressants, tricyclic (TCA)*	Dangerous drop in blood pressure. Avoid combination unless under medical supervision.
Antihypertensives, other*	Increased antihypertensive effect.
Barbiturates*	Increased hydrochlorothiazide effect.
Carteolol	Decreased antihypertensive effect.
Cholestyramine	Decreased hydrochlorothiazide effect.
Cortisone drugs*	Excessive potassium loss that causes dangerous heart rhythms.

Continued page 947

POSSIBLE INTERACTION WITH OTHER SUBSTANCES

INTERACTS WITH	COMBINED EFFECT
Alcohol:	May lower blood pressure excessively. Use extreme caution.
Beverages:	None expected.
Cocaine:	Dangerous blood pressure rise. Avoid.
Foods: Licorice.	Excessive potassium loss that causes dangerous heart rhythms.
Marijuana:	Weakness on standing. May increase blood pressure.
Tobacco:	Possible angina attacks.

*See Glossary

HYDROCORTISONE (Cortisol)

BRAND NAMES

See complete list of brand names in the *Brand Name Directory*, page 921.

BASIC INFORMATION

Habit forming? No
Prescription needed? Yes
Available as generic? Yes
Drug class: Cortisone drug (adrenal corticosteroid)

USES

- Reduces inflammation caused by many different medical problems.
- Treatment for some allergic diseases, blood disorders, kidney diseases, asthma and emphysema.
- Replaces corticosteroid deficiencies.

DOSAGE & USAGE INFORMATION

How to take:
- Tablet or liquid—Swallow with liquid or food to lessen stomach irritation. If you can't swallow whole, crumble tablet.
- Other forms—Follow label instructions.

When to take:
At the same times each day. Take once-a-day or once-every-other-day doses in mornings.

If you forget a dose:
- Several-doses-per-day prescription—Take as soon as you remember up to 2 hours late. If more than 2 hours, wait for next scheduled dose (don't double this dose).
- Once-a-day dose or less—Wait for next dose. Double this dose.

What drug does:
- Decreases inflammatory responses.
- Replaces cortisone in patients with adrenal insufficiency.

Continued in next column

OVERDOSE

SYMPTOMS:
Headache, convulsions, fluid retention, heart failure.
WHAT TO DO:
- **Dial 0 (operator) or 911 (emergency) for an ambulance or medical help. Then give first aid immediately.**
- **See emergency information on inside covers.**

Time lapse before drug works:
2 to 4 days.

Don't take with:
Any other medicine without consulting your doctor or pharmacist.

POSSIBLE ADVERSE REACTIONS OR SIDE EFFECTS

SYMPTOMS	WHAT TO DO
Life-threatening:	
Hives, rash, intense itching, faintness soon after a dose (anaphylaxis).	Seek emergency treatment immediately.
Common:	
Acne, poor wound healing, thirst, indigestion, nausea, vomiting.	Continue. Call doctor when convenient.
Infrequent:	
• Black, bloody or tarry stools.	Discontinue. Seek emergency treatment.
• Blurred vision; halos around lights; sore throat; fever; muscle cramps; swollen legs, feet.	Discontinue. Call doctor right away.
• Mood change, insomnia, fatigue, restlessness, frequent urination, weight gain, round face, weakness, irregular menstrual periods.	Continue. Tell doctor at next visit.
Rare:	
• Irregular heartbeat.	Discontinue. Seek emergency treatment.
• Rash, hallucinations, thrombophlebitis, pancreatitis, numbness or tingling in hands or feet, pancreatitis, convulsions.	Discontinue. Call doctor right away.

WARNINGS & PRECAUTIONS

Don't take if:
- You are allergic to any cortisone drug.
- You have tuberculosis or fungus infection.
- You have herpes infection of eyes, lips or genitals.

Before you start, consult your doctor:
- If you have had tuberculosis.
- If you have congestive heart failure.
- If you have diabetes, peptic ulcer, glaucoma, underactive thyroid, high blood pressure, myasthenia gravis, blood clots in legs or lungs.

HYDROCORTISONE (Cortisol)

Over age 60:
- Adverse reactions and side effects may be more frequent and severe than in younger persons.
- Likely to aggravate edema, diabetes or ulcers.
- Likely to cause cataracts and osteoporosis (softening of the bones).

Pregnancy:
Risk to unborn child outweighs drug benefits. Don't use.

Breast-feeding:
Drug passes into milk. Avoid drug or discontinue nursing until you finish medicine. Consult doctor for advice on maintaining milk supply.

Infants & children:
Use only under medical supervision.

Prolonged use:
- Retards growth in children.
- Possible glaucoma, cataracts, diabetes, fragile bones and thin skin.
- Functional dependence.
- Talk to your doctor about the need for follow-up medical examinations or laboratory studies to check blood sugar, eyes, serum electrolytes, stools for blood.

Skin & sunlight:
No problems expected.

Driving, piloting or hazardous work:
No problems expected.

Discontinuing:
- Don't discontinue without doctor's advice until you complete prescribed dose, even though symptoms diminish or disappear.
- Drug affects your response to surgery, illness, injury or stress for 2 years after discontinuing. Tell anyone who takes medical care of you about the drug for up to 2 years after discontinuing.

Others:
- Avoid immunizations if possible.
- Your resistance to infection is less while taking this medicine.
- Those who have inactive or "cured" tuberculosis may be subjected to possible recurrence of active tuberculosis.
- Children who must take cortisone drugs may grow less well.

 POSSIBLE INTERACTION WITH OTHER DRUGS

GENERIC NAME OR DRUG CLASS	COMBINED EFFECT
Amphotericin B	Potassium depletion.
Anticholinergics*	Possible glaucoma.
Anticoagulants, oral*	Decreased anti-coagulant effect.
Anticonvulsants, hydantoin*	Decreased hydro-cortisone effect.
Antidiabetics, oral*	Decreased anti-diabetic effect.
Antihistamines*	Decreased hydro-cortisone effect.
Aspirin	Increased hydro-cortisone effect.
Attentuated virus vaccines*	Possible viral infection.
Barbiturates*	Decreased hydro-cortisone effect. Oversedation.
Chloral hydrate	Decreased hydro-cortisone effect.
Chlorthalidone	Potassium depletion.
Cholestyramine	Decreased hydro-cortisone absorption effect.
Cholinergics*	Decreased cholinergic effect.
Colestipol	Decreased hydro-cortisone absorption effect.
Contraceptives, oral*	Increased hydro-cortisone effect.
Cyclosporine	Increased risk of infection.
Digitalis preparations*	Dangerous potassium depletion. Possible digitalis toxicity.
Diuretics, thiazide*	Potassium depletion.
Ephedrine	Decreased hydro-cortisone effect.

Continued page 948

 POSSIBLE INTERACTION WITH OTHER SUBSTANCES

INTERACTS WITH	COMBINED EFFECT
Alcohol:	Risk of stomach ulcers.
Beverages:	No proven problems.
Cocaine:	Overstimulation. Avoid.
Foods:	No proven problems.
Marijuana:	Decreased immunity.
Tobacco:	Increased hydrocortisone effect. Possible toxicity.

HYDROCORTISONE (Rectal)

BRAND AND GENERIC NAMES

Anusol-H.C.   Dermolate
Cort-Done   Proctocort
Corticaine   Rectocort
Cortiment

BASIC INFORMATION

Habit forming? No
Prescription needed? Yes
Available as generic? No
**Drug class: Anti-inflammatory, steroidal
(rectal); anesthetic (rectal)**

 USES

In or around the rectum to relieve swelling,
itching and pain for hemorrhoids (piles) and
other rectal conditions. Frequently used after
hemorrhoid surgery.

 **DOSAGE & USAGE
INFORMATION**

How to use:
* Follow instructions in package.
* Rectal cream or ointment—Apply to surface
  of rectum with fingers. Insert applicator into
  rectum
  no farther than 1/2 and apply inside. Wash
  applicator with warm soapy water or discard.
* Suppository—Remove wrapper and moisten
  with water. Lie on side. Push blunt end of
  suppository into rectum with finger. If
  suppository is too soft, run cold water over it
  or put in refrigerator for 15 to 45 minutes
  before using.
* Aerosol foam—Read patient instructions.
  Don't insert into rectum. Use the special
  applicator and wash carefully after using.

When to use:
Follow instructions in package or when needed.

Continued next column

 OVERDOSE

SYMPTOMS:
None expected.
WHAT TO DO:
**Not intended for internal use. If child
accidentally swallows, call poison-control
center.**

If you forget a dose:
Use as soon as you remember.

What drug does:
* Reduces inflammation.
* Relieves pain and itching.

Time lapse before drug works:
5 to 15 minutes.

Don't use with:
Other rectal medicines without consulting your
doctor.

 **POSSIBLE
ADVERSE REACTIONS
OR SIDE EFFECTS**

SYMPTOMS	WHAT TO DO
Life-threatening None expected.	
Common None expected.	
Infrequent	
• Nervousness, trembling, hives, rash, itch, inflammation or tenderness not present before application, slow heartbeat.	Discontinue. Call doctor right away.
• Dizziness, blurred vision, swollen feet.	Continue. Call doctor when convenient.
Rare	
• Blood in urine.	Discontinue. Call doctor right away.
• Increased or painful urination.	Continue. Call doctor when convenient.

HYDROCORTISONE (Rectal)

 WARNINGS & PRECAUTIONS

Don't use if:
You are allergic to any topical anesthetic.

Before you start, consult your doctor:
- If you have skin infection at site of treatment.
- If you have had severe or extensive skin disorders such as eczema or psoriasis.
- If you have bleeding hemorrhoids.

Over age 60:
Adverse reactions and side effects may be more frequent and severe than in younger persons.

Pregnancy:
No proven harm to unborn child. Avoid if possible.

Breast-feeding:
No problems expected.

Infants & children:
Don't use without careful medical supervision. Too much may be absorbed into the blood stream and affect growth.

Prolonged use:
Possible excess absorption. Don't use longer than 3 days for any one problem.

Skin & sunlight:
No problems expected.

Driving, piloting or hazardous work:
No problems expected.

Discontinuing:
May be unnecessary to finish medicine. Follow doctor's instructions.

Others:
- Report any rectal bleeding to your doctor.
- Keep cool, but don't freeze.

 POSSIBLE INTERACTION WITH OTHER DRUGS

GENERIC NAME OR DRUG CLASS	COMBINED EFFECT
Sulfa drugs*	Decreased anti-infective effect of sulfa drugs.

 POSSIBLE INTERACTION WITH OTHER SUBSTANCES

INTERACTS WITH	COMBINED EFFECT
Alcohol:	None expected.
Beverages:	None expected.
Cocaine:	Possible nervous-system toxicity. Avoid.
Foods:	None expected.
Marijuana:	None expected.
Tobacco:	None expected.

*See Glossary

HYDROXYCHLOROQUINE

BRAND NAMES

Plaquenil

BASIC INFORMATION

Habit forming? No
Prescription needed? Yes
Available as generic? No
Drug class: Antiprotozoal, antirheumatic

 USES

- Treatment for protozoal infections, such as malaria and amebiasis.
- Treatment for some forms of arthritis and lupus.

 DOSAGE & USAGE INFORMATION

How to take:
Tablet—Swallow with food or milk to lessen stomach irritation.

When to take:
- Depends on condition. Is adjusted during treatment.
- Malaria prevention—Begin taking medicine 2 weeks before entering areas with malaria.

If you forget a dose:
- 1 or more doses a day—Take as soon as you remember up to 2 hours late. If more than 2 hours, wait for next scheduled dose (don't double this dose).
- 1 dose weekly—Take as soon as possible, then return to regular dosing schedule.

What drug does:
- Inhibits parasite multiplication.
- Decreases inflammatory response in diseased joint.

Time lapse before drug works:
1 to 2 hours.

Don't take with:
Any other medicine without consulting your doctor or pharmacist.

 OVERDOSE

SYMPTOMS:
Severe breathing difficulty, drowsiness, faintness, headache, seizures.
WHAT TO DO:
- **Dial 0 (operator) or 911 (emergency) for an ambulance or medical help. Then give first aid immediately.**
- **See emergency information on inside covers.**

 POSSIBLE ADVERSE REACTIONS OR SIDE EFFECTS

SYMPTOMS	WHAT TO DO
Life-threatening:	
In case of overdose, see previous column.	
Common:	
Headache, appetite loss, abdominal pain.	Continue. Tell doctor at next visit.
Infrequent:	
• Blurred vision, changes in vision.	Discontinue. Call doctor right away.
• Rash or itch, diarrhea, nausea, vomiting, hair loss, blue-black skin or mouth, dizziness, nervousness.	Continue. Call doctor when convenient.
Rare:	
• Mood or mental changes, seizures, sore throat, fever, unusual bleeding or bruising, muscle weakness, convulsions.	Discontinue. Call doctor right away.
• Ringing or buzzing in ears, hearing loss.	Continue. Call doctor when convenient.

HYDROXYCHLOROQUINE

 ## WARNINGS & PRECAUTIONS

Don't take if:
You are allergic to chloroquine or hydroxychloroquine.

Before you start, consult your doctor:
- If you plan to become pregnant within the medication period.
- If you have blood disease.
- If you have eye or vision problems.
- If you have a G6PD deficiency.
- If you have liver disease.
- If you have nerve or brain disease (including seizure disorders).
- If you have porphyria.
- If you have psoriasis.
- If you have stomach or intestinal disease.
- If you drink more than 3 oz. of alcohol daily.

Over age 60:
Adverse reactions and side effects may be more frequent and severe than in younger persons.

Pregnancy:
Risk to unborn child outweighs drug benefits. Don't use.

Breast-feeding:
Drug passes into milk. Avoid drug or discontinue nursing.

Infants & children:
Not recommended. Dangerous.

Prolonged use:
- Permanent damage to the retina (back part of the eye) or nerve deafness.
- Talk to your doctor about the need for follow-up medical examinations or laboratory studies to check complete blood counts (white blood cell count, platelet count, red blood cell count, hemoglobin, hematocrit), eyes.

Skin & sunlight:
May cause rash or intensify sunburn in areas exposed to sun or sunlamp.

Driving, piloting or hazardous work:
Don't drive or pilot aircraft until you learn how medicine affects you. Don't work around dangerous machinery. Don't climb ladders or work in high places. Danger increases if you drink alcohol or take medicine affecting alertness and reflexes.

Discontinuing:
Don't discontinue without doctor's advice until you complete prescribed dose, even though symptoms diminish or disappear.

Others:
- Periodic physical and blood examinations recommended.
- If you are in a malaria area for a long time, you may need to change to another preventive drug every 2 years.

 ## POSSIBLE INTERACTION WITH OTHER DRUGS

GENERIC NAME OR DRUG CLASS	COMBINED EFFECT
Estrogens*	Possible liver toxicity.
Gold compounds*	Risk of severe rash and itch.
Kaolin	Decreased absorption of hydroxychloroquine.
Magnesium trisilicate	Decreased absorption of hydroxychloroquine.
Penicillamine	Possible blood or kidney toxicity.

 ## POSSIBLE INTERACTION WITH OTHER SUBSTANCES

INTERACTS WITH	COMBINED EFFECT
Alcohol:	Possible liver toxicity. Avoid.
Beverages:	None expected.
Cocaine:	None expected.
Foods:	None expected.
Marijuana:	None expected.
Tobacco:	None expected.

*See Glossary

HYDROXYUREA

BRAND NAMES

Hydrea

BASIC INFORMATION

Habit forming? No
Prescription needed? Yes
Available as generic? No
Drug class: Antineoplastic

USES

- Treats head, neck, ovarian and cervical cancer.
- Treats leukemia, melanoma and polycythemia vera.

DOSAGE & USAGE INFORMATION

How to take:
Capsules—Swallow with liquid. If you can't swallow whole, open capsule and take with liquid or food. Instructions to take on empty stomach mean 1 hour before or 2 hours after eating.

When to take:
According to doctor's instructions.

If you forget a dose:
Skip this dose. Never double dose. Resume regular schedule.

What drug does:
Probably interferes with synthesis of DNA.

Time lapse before drug works:
2 hours.

Don't take with:
Any other medicines (including over-the-counter drugs such as cough and cold medicines, laxatives, antacids, diet pills, caffeine, nose drops or vitamins) without consulting your doctor.

OVERDOSE

SYMPTOMS:
Black, tarry stools; fainting; seizures.
WHAT TO DO:
- **Dial 0 (operator) or 911 (emergency) for an ambulance or medical help. Then give first aid immediately.**
- **See emergency information on inside covers.**

POSSIBLE ADVERSE REACTIONS OR SIDE EFFECTS

SYMPTOMS	WHAT TO DO
Life-threatening:	
In case of overdose, see previous column.	
Common:	
• Skin rash, fever, chills, cough, back pain.	Discontinue. Call doctor right away.
• Diarrhea, drowsiness, nausea, vomiting.	Continue. Call doctor when convenient.
Infrequent:	
Mouth sores, bruising, constipation, red skin.	Discontinue. Call doctor right away.
Rare:	
Confusion, hallucinations, headache, swollen feet.	Continue. Call doctor when convenient.

WARNINGS & PRECAUTIONS

Don't take if:
- You have chicken pox.
- You have shingles (herpes zoster).

Before you start, consult your doctor:
- If you have anemia.
- If you have gout.
- If you have an infection.
- If you have kidney disease.

Over age 60:
Adverse reactions and side effects may be more frequent and severe than in younger persons. You may need smaller doses for shorter periods of time.

Pregnancy:
Risk to unborn child outweighs drug benefits. Don't use.

Breast-feeding:
Drug passes into milk. Avoid drug or discontinue nursing until you finish medicine. Consult doctor for advice on maintaining milk supply.

Infants & children:
Effect not documented. Consult your pediatrician.

Prolonged use:
Talk to your doctor about the need for follow-up medical examinations or laboratory studies to check kidney function, complete blood counts (white blood cell count, platelet count, red blood cell count, hemoglobin, hematocrit) and serum uric acid.

Skin & sunlight:
No problems expected.

Driving, piloting or hazardous work:
Avoid if you feel confused, drowsy or dizzy.

Discontinuing:
May still experience symptoms of bone marrow depression, such as: blood in stools, fever or chills, blood spots under the skin, back pain, hoarseness, bloody urine. If any of these occur, call your doctor right away.

Others:
- Advise any doctor or dentist whom you consult that you take this medicine.
- May affect results in some medical tests.

POSSIBLE INTERACTION WITH OTHER DRUGS

GENERIC NAME OR DRUG CLASS	COMBINED EFFECT
Bone marrow depressants, other*	Dangerous suppression of bone marrow activity.
Clozapine	Toxic effect on bone marrow.
Levamisole	Increased risk of bone marrow depression.
Probenecid	May require increased dosage to treat gout.
Sulfinpyrazone	May require increased dosage to treat gout.
Tiopronin	Increased risk of toxicity to bone marrow.
Vaccines, live or killed virus	Increased danger from vaccines.

POSSIBLE INTERACTION WITH OTHER SUBSTANCES

INTERACTS WITH	COMBINED EFFECT
Alcohol:	No special problems expected.
Beverages:	No special problems expected.
Cocaine:	Increased confusion. Avoid.
Foods:	No special problems expected.
Marijuana:	Increased confusion. Avoid.
Tobacco:	No special problems expected.

*See Glossary

HYDROXYZINE

BRAND NAMES

See complete list of brand names in the *Brand Name Directory*, page 921.

BASIC INFORMATION

Habit forming? No
Prescription needed? Yes
Available as generic? Yes
Drug class: Tranquilizer, antihistamine

 ## USES

- Treatment for anxiety, tension and agitation.
- Relieves itching from allergic reactions.

 ## DOSAGE & USAGE INFORMATION

How to take:
- Tablet, syrup or capsule—Swallow with liquid. If you can't swallow whole, crumble tablet or open capsule and take with liquid or food.
- Liquid—If desired, dilute dose in beverage before swallowing.

When to take:
At the same times each day.

If you forget a dose:
Take as soon as you remember up to 2 hours late. If more than 2 hours, wait for next scheduled dose (don't double this dose).

What drug does:
May reduce activity in areas of the brain that influence emotional stability.

Time lapse before drug works:
15 to 30 minutes.

Don't take with:
- Non-prescription drugs without consulting doctor.
- Any other medicine without consulting your doctor or pharmacist.

 ## OVERDOSE

SYMPTOMS:
Drowsiness, unsteadiness, agitation, purposeless movements, tremor, convulsions.
WHAT TO DO:
- **Dial 0 (operator) or 911 (emergency) for an ambulance or medical help. Then give first aid immediately.**
- **See emergency information on inside covers.**

 ## POSSIBLE ADVERSE REACTIONS OR SIDE EFFECTS

SYMPTOMS	WHAT TO DO
Life-threatening:	
In case of overdose, see previous column.	
Common:	
Drowsiness, difficult urination, dry mouth.	Continue. Tell doctor at next visit.
Infrequent:	
Headache.	Continue. Tell doctor at next visit.
Rare:	
Tremor, rash.	Discontinue. Call doctor right away.

 ## WARNINGS & PRECAUTIONS

Don't take if:
You are allergic to any antihistamine.

Before you start, consult your doctor:
- If you have epilepsy.
- If you will have surgery within 2 months, including dental surgery, requiring general or spinal anesthesia.

Over age 60:
- Adverse reactions and side effects may be more frequent and severe than in younger persons.
- Drug likely to increase urination difficulty caused by enlarged prostate gland.

Pregnancy:
Studies inconclusive on harm to unborn child. Animal studies show fetal abnormalities. Decide with your doctor whether drug benefits justify risk to unborn child.

Breast-feeding:
Drug passes into milk. Avoid drug or discontinue nursing until you finish medicine. Consult doctor for advice on maintaining milk supply.

Infants & children:
Use only under medical supervision.

Prolonged use:
Tolerance develops and reduces effectiveness.

HYDROXYZINE

Skin & sunlight:
No problems expected.

Driving, piloting or hazardous work:
Don't drive or pilot aircraft until you learn how medicine affects you. Don't work around dangerous machinery. Don't climb ladders or work in high places. Danger increases if you drink alcohol or take medicine affecting alertness and reflexes, such as antihistamines, tranquilizers, sedatives, pain medicine, narcotics and mind-altering drugs.

Discontinuing:
Don't discontinue without consulting doctor. Dose may require gradual reduction if you have taken drug for a long time. Doses of other drugs may also require adjustment.

Others:
No problems expected.

POSSIBLE INTERACTION WITH OTHER DRUGS

GENERIC NAME OR DRUG CLASS	COMBINED EFFECT
Antidepressants, tricyclic (TCA)*	Increased effect of both drugs.
Antihistamines*	Increased hydroxyzine effect.
Attapulgite	Decreased hydroxyzine effect.
Carteolol	Decreased antihistamine effect.
Central nervous system (CNS) depressants*	Greater depression of central nervous system.
Clozapine	Toxic effect on the central nervous system.
Dronabinol	Increased effects of both drugs. Avoid.
Ethinamate	Dangerous increased effects of ethinamate. Avoid combining.
Fluoxetine	Increased depressant effects of both drugs.
Guanfacine	May increase depressant effects of either drug.
Leucovorin	High alcohol content of leucovorin may cause adverse effects.
Methyprylon	Increased sedative effect, perhaps to dangerous level. Avoid.
Nabilone	Greater depression of central nervous system.
Narcotics*	Increased effect of both drugs.
Pain relievers*	Increased effect of both drugs.
Sedatives*	Increased effect of both drugs.
Sertraline	Increased depressive effects of both drugs.
Sleep inducers*	Increased effect of both drugs.
Sotalol	Increased antihistamine effect.
Tranquilizers*	Increased effect of both drugs.

POSSIBLE INTERACTION WITH OTHER SUBSTANCES

INTERACTS WITH	COMBINED EFFECT
Alcohol:	Increased sedation and intoxication. Use with caution.
Beverages: Caffeine drinks.	Decreased tranquilizer effect of hydroxyzine.
Cocaine:	Decreased hydroxyzine effect. Avoid.
Foods:	None expected.
Marijuana:	None expected.
Tobacco:	None expected.

*See Glossary

439

HYOSCYAMINE

BRAND NAMES

See complete list of brand names in the *Brand Name Directory*, page 921.

BASIC INFORMATION

Habit forming? No
Prescription needed?
　Low strength: No
　High strength: Yes
Available as generic? No
Drug class: Antispasmodic, anticholinergic

USES

Reduces spasms of digestive system, bladder and urethra.

DOSAGE & USAGE INFORMATION

How to take:
- Tablet or liquid—Swallow with liquid or food to lessen stomach irritation. You may chew or crush tablets.
- Extended-release capsules—Swallow each dose whole.
- Drops—Dilute dose in beverage before swallowing.

When to take:
30 minutes before meals (unless directed otherwise by doctor).

If you forget a dose:
Take as soon as you remember up to 2 hours late. If more than 2 hours, wait for next scheduled dose (don't double this dose).

What drug does:
Blocks nerve impulses at parasympathetic nerve endings, preventing muscle contractions and gland secretions of organs involved.

Continued next column

OVERDOSE

SYMPTOMS:
Dilated pupils, rapid pulse and breathing, dizziness, fever, hallucinations, confusion, slurred speech, agitation, flushed face, convulsions, coma.
WHAT TO DO:
- **Dial 0 (operator) or 911 (emergency) for an ambulance or medical help. Then give first aid immediately.**
- **See emergency information on inside covers.**

Time lapse before drug works:
15 to 30 minutes.

Don't take with:
- Antacids* or antidiarrheals*.
- Any other medicine without consulting your doctor or pharmacist.

POSSIBLE ADVERSE REACTIONS OR SIDE EFFECTS

SYMPTOMS	WHAT TO DO
Life-threatening:	
In case of overdose, see previous column.	
Common:	
Confusion, delirium, rapid heartbeat.	Discontinue. Call doctor right away.
Nausea, vomiting, decreased sweating.	Continue. Call doctor when convenient.
Constipation.	Continue. Tell doctor at next visit.
Dryness in ears, nose, throat, mouth.	No action necessary.
Infrequent:	
Headache, painful or difficult urination, nasal congestion, altered taste.	Continue. Call doctor when convenient.
Lightheadedness.	Discontinue. Call doctor right away.
Rare:	
Rash or hives, eye pain, blurred vision.	Discontinue. Call doctor right away.

WARNINGS & PRECAUTIONS

Don't take if:
- You are allergic to any anticholinergic.
- You have trouble with stomach bloating.
- You have difficulty emptying your bladder completely.
- You have narrow-angle glaucoma.
- You have severe ulcerative colitis.

Before you start, consult your doctor:
- If you have open-angle glaucoma.
- If you have angina.
- If you have chronic bronchitis or asthma.
- If you have hiatal hernia.
- If you have liver, kidney or thyroid disease.
- If you have enlarged prostate.
- If you have myasthenia gravis.
- If you have peptic ulcer.
- If you will have surgery within 2 months, including dental surgery, requiring general or spinal anesthesia.

HYOSCYAMINE

Over age 60:
Adverse reactions and side effects may be more frequent and severe than in younger persons.

Pregnancy:
Studies inconclusive on harm to unborn child. Animal studies show fetal abnormalities. Decide with your doctor whether drug benefits justify risk to unborn child.

Breast-feeding:
Drug passes into milk and decreases milk flow. Avoid drug or discontinue nursing until you finish medicine. Consult doctor for advice on maintaining milk supply.

Infants & children:
Use only under medical supervision.

Prolonged use:
Chronic constipation, possible fecal impaction. Consult doctor immediately.

Skin & sunlight:
No problems expected.

Driving, piloting or hazardous work:
Use disqualifies you for piloting aircraft. Otherwise, no problems expected.

Discontinuing:
May be unnecessary to finish medicine. Follow doctor's instructions.

Others:
Advise any doctor or dentist whom you consult that you take this medicine.

 POSSIBLE INTERACTION WITH OTHER DRUGS

GENERIC NAME OR DRUG CLASS	COMBINED EFFECT
Amantadine	Increased hyoscyamine effect.
Anticholinergics, other*	Increased hyoscyamine effect.
Antidepressants, tricyclic (TCA)*	Increased hyoscyamine effect.
Antihistamines*	Increased hyoscyamine effect.
Cortisone drugs*	Increased internal-eye pressure.
Haloperidol	Increased internal-eye pressure.
Ketoconazole	Decreased ketoconazole effect.
MAO inhibitors*	Increased hyoscyamine effect.
Meperidine	Increased hyoscyamine effect.
Methylphenidate	Increased hyoscyamine effect.
Molindone	Increased anticholinergic effect.
Nizatidine	Increased nizatidine effect.
Orphenadrine	Increased hyoscyamine effect.
Phenothiazines*	Increased hyoscyamine effect.
Pilocarpine	Loss of pilocarpine effect in glaucoma treatment.
Sedatives or central nervous system (CNS) depressants*	Increased sedative effect of both drugs.
Vitamin C	Decreased hyoscyamine effect. Avoid large doses of vitamin C.

 POSSIBLE INTERACTION WITH OTHER SUBSTANCES

INTERACTS WITH	COMBINED EFFECT
Alcohol:	None expected.
Beverages:	None expected.
Cocaine:	Excessively rapid heartbeat. Avoid.
Foods:	None expected.
Marijuana:	Drowsiness and dry mouth.
Tobacco:	None expected.

*See Glossary

441

INDAPAMIDE

BRAND NAMES

Lozide   Lozol

BASIC INFORMATION

Habit forming? No
Prescription needed? Yes
Available as generic? No
Drug class: Antihypertensive, diuretic

USES

- Controls, but doesn't cure, high blood pressure.
- Reduces fluid retention (edema) caused by conditions such as heart disorders.

DOSAGE & USAGE INFORMATION

How to take:
Tablet—Swallow with liquid or food to lessen stomach irritation.

When to take:
At the same times each day, usually at bedtime.

If you forget a dose:
Bedtime dose—If you forget your once-a-day bedtime dose, don't take it more than 3 hours late. Never double dose.

What drug does:
Forces kidney to excrete more sodium and causes excess salt and fluid to be excreted.

Time lapse before drug works:
2 hours for effect to begin. May require 1 to 4 weeks for full effects.

Don't take with:
Any other medicine without consulting your doctor or pharmacist.

OVERDOSE

SYMPTOMS:
Nausea, vomiting, diarrhea, very dry mouth, thirst, weakness, excessive fatigue, very rapid heart rate, weak pulse.
WHAT TO DO:
- **Dial 0 (operator) or 911 (emergency) for an ambulance or medical help. Then give first aid immediately.**
- **If patient is unconscious and not breathing, give mouth-to-mouth breathing. If there is no heartbeat, use cardiac massage and mouth-to-mouth breathing (CPR). Don't try to make patient vomit. If you can't get help quickly, take patient to nearest emergency facility.**
- **See emergency information on inside covers.**

POSSIBLE ADVERSE REACTIONS OR SIDE EFFECTS

SYMPTOMS	WHAT TO DO
Life-threatening:	
In case of overdose, see previous column.	
Common:	
• Excessive tiredness or weakness, muscle cramps.	Discontinue. Call doctor right away.
• Frequent urination.	Continue. Tell doctor at next visit.
Infrequent:	
Insomnia, mood change, dizziness on changing position, headache, excessive thirst, diarrhea, appetite loss, nausea, dry mouth, decreased sex drive.	Continue. Call doctor when convenient.
Rare:	
• Weak pulse.	Discontinue. Seek emergency treatment.
• Itching, rash, hives, irregular heartbeat.	Discontinue. Call doctor right away.

WARNINGS & PRECAUTIONS

Don't take if:
- You are allergic to indapamide or to any sulfa drug or thiazide diuretic. *
- You have severe kidney disease.

Before you start, consult your doctor:
- If you have severe kidney disease.
- If you have diabetes.
- If you have gout.
- If you have liver disease.
- If you will have surgery within 2 months, including dental surgery, requiring general or spinal anesthesia.
- If you have lupus erythematosus.
- If you are pregnant or plan to become pregnant.

Over age 60:
Adverse reactions and side effects may be more frequent and severe than in younger persons.

Pregnancy:
Risk to unborn child outweighs drug benefits. Don't use.

Breast-feeding:
Unknown effect on child. Consult doctor.

Infants & children:
Use only under close medical supervision.

Prolonged use:
Request laboratory studies for blood sugar, BUN, uric acid and serum electrolytes (potassium and sodium).

Skin & sunlight:
May cause rash or intensify sunburn in areas exposed to sun or sunlamp.

Driving, piloting or hazardous work:
Don't drive or pilot aircraft until you learn how medicine affects you. Don't work around dangerous machinery. Don't climb ladders or work in high places. Danger increases if you drink alcohol or take medicine affecting alertness and reflexes, such as antihistamines, tranquilizers, sedatives, pain medicine, narcotics and mind-altering drugs.

Discontinuing:
Don't discontinue without consulting doctor. Dose may require gradual reduction if you have taken drug for a long time. Doses of other drugs may also require adjustment.

Others:
No problems expected.

POSSIBLE INTERACTION WITH OTHER DRUGS

GENERIC NAME OR DRUG CLASS	COMBINED EFFECT
ACE inhibitors*: captopril, enalapril, lisinopril	Decreased blood pressure. Possible excessive potassium in blood.
Allopurinol	Decreased allopurinol effect.
Amiodarone	Increased risk of heartbeat irregularity due to low potassium.
Amphotericin B	Increased potassium.
Antidepressants, tricyclic (TCA)*	Dangerous drop in blood pressure.
Antidiabetic agents, oral*	Increased blood sugar.
Antihypertensives, other*	Increased antihypertensive effect.
Barbiturates*	Increased indapamide effect.
Beta-adrenergic blockers*	Increased effect of indapamide.
Calcium supplements*	Increased calcium in blood.
Carteolol	Increased antihypertensive effect.
Cholestyramine	Decreased indapamide effect.
Colestipol	Decreased indapamide effect.

Cortisone drugs*	Excessive potassium loss that may cause dangerous heart rhythms.
Digitalis preparations*	Excessive potassium loss that may cause dangerous heart rhythms.
Diuretics, thiazide*	Increased effect of thiazide diuretics.
Indomethacin	Decreased indapamide effect.
Lithium	High risk of lithium toxicity.
MAO inhibitors*	Increased indapamide effect.
Nicardipine	Dangerous blood pressure drop. Dosages may require adjustment.
Nimodipine	Dangerous blood pressure drop.
Opiates*	Weakness and faintness when arising from bed or chair.
Probenecid	Decreased probenecid effect.
Sotalol	Increased antihypertensive effect.
Terazosin	Decreased effectiveness of terazosin.

POSSIBLE INTERACTION WITH OTHER SUBSTANCES

INTERACTS WITH	COMBINED EFFECT
Alcohol:	Dangerous blood pressure drop. Avoid.
Beverages:	No problems expected.
Cocaine:	Increased risk of heart block and high blood pressure.
Foods: Licorice.	Excessive potassium loss that may cause dangerous heart rhythms.
Marijuana:	Reduced effectiveness of indapamide. Avoid.
Tobacco:	Reduced effectiveness of indapamide. Avoid.

INSULIN

BRAND NAMES

See complete list of brand names in the *Brand Name Directory*, page 922.

BASIC INFORMATION

Habit forming? No
Prescription needed? No
Available as generic? No
Drug class: Antidiabetic

USES

Controls diabetes, a complex metabolic disorder, in which the body does not manufacture insulin.

DOSAGE & USAGE INFORMATION

How to take:
Must be taken by injection under the skin. Use disposable, sterile needles. Rotate injection sites.

When to take:
At the same time each day.

If you forget a dose:
Take as soon as you remember. Wait at least 4 hours for next dose. Resume regular schedule.

What drug does:
Facilitates passage of blood sugar through cell membranes so sugar is usable.

Continued next column

OVERDOSE

SYMPTOMS:
Low blood sugar (hypoglycemia)—Anxiety; chills, cold sweats, pale skin; drowsiness; excess hunger; headache; nausea; nervousness; fast heartbeat; shakiness; unusual tiredness or weakness.
WHAT TO DO:
● **Eat some type of sugar immediately, such as orange juice, honey, sugar cubes, crackers, sandwich.**
● **If patient loses consciousness, give glucagon if you have it and know how to use it.**
● **Otherwise, dial 0 (operator) or 911 (emergency) for an ambulance or medical help. Then give first aid immediately.**
● **See emergency information on inside covers.**

Time lapse before drug works:
30 minutes to 8 hours, depending on type of insulin used.

Don't take with:
Any other medicine without consulting your doctor or pharmacist.

POSSIBLE ADVERSE REACTIONS OR SIDE EFFECTS

SYMPTOMS	WHAT TO DO
Life-threatening: Hives, rash, intense itching, faintness soon after a dose (anaphylaxis).	Seek emergency treatment immediately.
Common: Symptoms of low blood sugar— Nervousness, hunger (excessive), cold sweats, rapid pulse, anxiety, cold skin, chills, confusion, concentration loss, drowsiness, headache, nausea, weakness, shakiness, vision changes.	Seek emergency treatment.
Infrequent: ● Hives.	Discontinue. Call doctor right away.
● Swelling, redness, itch at injection site.	Continue. Call doctor when convenient.
Rare: None expected.	

WARNINGS & PRECAUTIONS

Don't take if:
● Your diagnosis and dose schedule is not established.
● You don't know how to deal with overdose emergencies.

Before you start, consult your doctor:
● If you are allergic to insulin.
● If you take MAO inhibitors.
● If you have liver or kidney disease or low thyroid function.

Over age 60:
Guard against hypoglycemia. Repeated episodes can cause permanent confusion and abnormal behavior.

Pregnancy:
Possible drug benefits outweigh risk to unborn child. Adhere rigidly to diabetes treatment program.

Breast-feeding:
No problems expected.

Infants & children:
Use only under medical supervision.

Prolonged use:
Talk to your doctor about the need for follow-up medical examinations or laboratory studies to check blood sugar, serum potassium, urine.

Skin & sunlight:
No problems expected.

Driving, piloting or hazardous work:
No problems expected after dose is established.

Discontinuing:
Don't discontinue without doctor's advice until you complete prescribed dose, even though symptoms diminish or disappear.

Others:
- Diet and exercise affect how much insulin you need. Work with your doctor to determine accurate dose.
- Notify your doctor if you skip a dose, overeat, have fever or infection.
- Notify doctor if you develop symptoms of high blood sugar: drowsiness, dry skin, orange fruit-like odor to breath, increased urination, appetite loss, unusual thirst.
- Never freeze insulin.
- May interfere with the accuracy of some medical tests.

POSSIBLE INTERACTION WITH OTHER DRUGS

GENERIC NAME OR DRUG CLASS	COMBINED EFFECT
Anticonvulsants, hydantoin*	Decreased insulin effect.
Antidiabetics, oral*	Increased antibiabetic effect.
Beta-adrenergic blockers*	Possible increased difficulty in regulating blood-sugar levels.
Bismuth subsalicylate	Increased insulin effect. May require dosage adjustment.

Carteolol	Hypoglycemic effects may be prolonged.
Contraceptives, oral*	Decreased insulin effect.
Cortisone drugs*	Decreased insulin effect.
Diuretics*	Decreased insulin effect.
Furosemide	Decreased insulin effect.
MAO inhibitors*	Increased insulin effect.
Nicotine gum and other smoking deterrents	Increased insulin effect.
Oxyphenbutazone	Increased insulin effect.
Phenylbutazone	Increased insulin effect.
Salicylates*	Increased insulin effect.
Sotalol	Hypoglycemic effects may be prolonged.
Sulfa drugs*	Increased insulin effect.
Tetracyclines*	Increased insulin effect.
Thyroid hormones*	Decreased insulin effect.

POSSIBLE INTERACTION WITH OTHER SUBSTANCES

INTERACTS WITH	COMBINED EFFECT
Alcohol:	Increased insulin effect. May cause hypoglycemia and brain damage.
Beverages:	None expected.
Cocaine:	May cause brain damage.
Foods:	None expected.
Marijuana:	Possible increase in blood sugar.
Tobacco:	None expected.

IODINATED GLYCEROL

BRAND NAMES

Iophen
Iophen-C Liquid
Iotuss
Iotuss-DM
Organic-1
Organidin
Par Glycerol

Par Glycerol C
Par Glycerol DM
R-Gen
Tussi-Organidin DM
  Liquid
Tussi-Organidin
  Liquid

BASIC INFORMATION

Habit forming? No
Prescription needed? Yes
Available as generic? Yes
Drug class: Expectorant

USES

Loosens mucus in bronchial tubes.

DOSAGE & USAGE INFORMATION

How to take:
• Tablets—Swallow with liquid. If you can't swallow whole, crumble tablet and take with liquid or food. Instructions to take on empty stomach mean 1 hour before or 2 hours after eating.
• Oral solution—Swallow with liquid to lessen stomach irritation.
• Elixir—Swallow with liquid.
• Drink a glass of water after each dose.

When to take:
Usually 4 times a day—approximately every 4 hours while awake.

If you forget a dose:
Take as soon as you remember up to 2 hours late. If more than 2 hours, wait for next scheduled dose (don't double this dose).

What drug does:
Increases secretions in bronchial tubes and makes them thinner, which aids in coughing them up.

Continued in next column

OVERDOSE

SYMPTOMS:
None expected.
WHAT TO DO:
Overdose unlikely to threaten life. If person takes much larger amount than prescribed, call doctor, poison-control center or hospital emergency room for instructions.

Time lapse before drug works:
None. Works immediately.

Don't take with:
Any other medicines (including over-the-counter drugs such as cough and cold medicines, laxatives, antacids, diet pills, caffeine, nose drops or vitamins) without consulting your doctor.

POSSIBLE ADVERSE REACTIONS OR SIDE EFFECTS

SYMPTOMS	WHAT TO DO
Life-threatening: Allergic reaction with fever, joint pain, hives, rash, swollen face.	Seek emergency treatment immediately.
Common: Diarrhea, nausea and vomiting, abdominal pain.	Continue. Call doctor when convenient.
Infrequent: Swollen glands below the ears.	Discontinue. Call doctor right away.
Rare: Iodism (burning mouth, headache, eye irritation, metallic taste, rash, sore teeth and gums).	Discontinue. Call doctor right away.

IODINATED GLYCEROL

WARNINGS & PRECAUTIONS

Don't take if:
You are allergic to iodine or inorganic iodides.

Before you start, consult your doctor:
- If you have adolescent acne.
- If you have cystic fibrosis.
- If you have thyroid disease.

Over age 60:
No special problems expected.

Pregnancy:
Risk to unborn child outweighs drug benefits. Don't use.

Breast-feeding:
Drug passes into milk. Avoid drug or discontinue nursing until you finish medicine. Consult doctor for advice on maintaining milk supply.

Infants & children:
Effect not documented. Consult your pediatrician.

Prolonged use:
- May cause decreased thyroid function (hypothyroidism).
- Talk to your doctor about the need for follow-up medical examinations or laboratory studies to check thyroid function.

Skin & sunlight:
No problems expected.

Driving, piloting or hazardous work:
Avoid if you feel confused, drowsy or dizzy.

Discontinuing:
No special problems expected.

Others:
- Advise any doctor or dentist whom you consult that you take this medicine.
- May affect results in some medical tests.
- Do *not* use for prolonged periods of time.

POSSIBLE INTERACTION WITH OTHER DRUGS

GENERIC NAME OR DRUG CLASS	COMBINED EFFECT
Antithyroid drugs*	Increased likelihood of adversely affecting thyroid gland function.
Lithium	Increased likelihood of adversely affecting thyroid gland function.

POSSIBLE INTERACTION WITH OTHER SUBSTANCES

INTERACTS WITH	COMBINED EFFECT
Alcohol:	Decreased iodinated glycerol effect.
Beverages:	No special problems expected.
Cocaine:	No special problems expected.
Foods:	No special problems expected.
Marijuana:	No special problems expected.
Tobacco:	No special problems expected.

*See Glossary

447

IODOQUINOL

BRAND NAMES

Diiodohydroxyquin   Diquinol
Diodoquin   Yodoxin

BASIC INFORMATION

Habit forming? No
Prescription needed? Yes
Available as generic? Yes
Drug class: Antiprotozoal

USES

Treatment for intestinal amebiasis.

DOSAGE & USAGE INFORMATION

How to take:
Tablets—Mix with applesauce or chocolate syrup if unable to swallow tablets.

When to take:
Three times daily after meals for 20 days. Treatment may be repeated after 2 to 3 weeks.

If you forget a dose:
Take as soon as you remember up to 2 hours late. If more than 2 hours, wait for next scheduled dose (don't double this dose).

What drug does:
Kills amoeba (microscopic parasites) in intestinal tract.

Time lapse before drug works:
May require full course of treatment (20 days) to cure.

Don't take with:
Any other medication without consulting your doctor or pharmacist.

OVERDOSE

SYMPTOMS:
- **Prolonged dosing at high level may produce blurred vision, muscle pain, eye pain, numbness and tingling in hands or feet.**
- **Single overdosage unlikely to threaten life.**

WHAT TO DO:
If person takes much larger amount than prescribed, call doctor, poison-control center or hospital emergency room for instructions.

POSSIBLE ADVERSE REACTIONS OR SIDE EFFECTS

SYMPTOMS	WHAT TO DO
Life-threatening:	
In case of overdose, see previous column.	
Common:	
Diarrhea, nausea, vomiting, abdominal pain.	Discontinue. Call doctor right away.
Infrequent:	
• Clumsiness, rash, hives, itching, blurred vision, muscle pain, numbness or tingling in hands or feet, chills, fever, weakness.	Discontinue. Call doctor right away.
• Swelling of neck (thyroid gland).	Continue. Call doctor when convenient.
Rare:	
• Dizziness, headache.	Discontinue. Call doctor right away.
• Rectal itching.	Continue. Call doctor when convenient.

WARNINGS & PRECAUTIONS

Don't take if:
You have kidney or liver disease.

Before you start, consult your doctor:
If you have optic atrophy thyroid disease.

Over age 60:
Adverse reactions and side effects may be more frequent and severe than in younger persons.

Pregnancy:
No proven problems, but avoid if possible.

Breast-feeding:
No proven problems, but avoid if possible. Discontinue nursing until you finish medicine. Consult doctor for advice on maintaining milk supply.

Infants & children:
Not recommended. Safety and dosage has not been established.

Prolonged use:
Not recommended.

Skin & sunlight:
No problems expected.

Driving, piloting or hazardous work:
No problems expected.

Discontinuing:
Don't discontinue without consulting doctor.

Others:
- Thyroid tests may be inaccurate for as long as 6 months after discontinuing iodoquinol treatment.
- May interfere with the accuracy of some medical tests.

POSSIBLE INTERACTION WITH OTHER DRUGS

GENERIC NAME OR DRUG CLASS	COMBINED EFFECT
None expected.	

POSSIBLE INTERACTION WITH OTHER SUBSTANCES

INTERACTS WITH	COMBINED EFFECT
Alcohol:	None expected.
Beverages:	None expected.
Cocaine:	None expected.
Foods:	Taking with food may decrease gastrointestinal side effects.
Marijuana:	None expected.
Tobacco:	None expected.

IPECAC

BRAND NAMES

Ipecac Syrup   **Quelidrine Cough**

BASIC INFORMATION

Habit forming? No
Prescription needed? No
Available as generic? Yes
Drug class: Emetic

 USES

- Used in emergencies to induce vomiting after medication overdose and in some instances of poisoning.
- *Don't* use if suspected substance to be vomited is strychnine or a corrosive such as lye, kerosene, gasoline, bleach, strong acid or cleaning fluid.

 DOSAGE & USAGE INFORMATION

How to take:
- Call doctor, poison-control center or emergency room before giving ipecac to anyone.
- Don't give to an unconscious person.
- Syrup, undiluted—Carefully follow instructions on the bottle.
- Drink water immediately after taking ipecac.
- Place person in a head-down position to prevent aspiration of vomitus.

When to take:
- Upon discovery of accidental or intentional poisoning or overdose.
- May repeat in 30 minutes if vomiting doesn't occur with first ipecac dose.
- Don't give more than 2 doses.

If you forget a dose:
One-time use only.

Continued next column

 OVERDOSE

SYMPTOMS:
Watery diarrhea, breathing difficulty, stiff muscles.
WHAT TO DO:
- **Dial 0 (operator) or 911 (emergency) for an ambulance or medical help. Then give first aid immediately.**
- **See emergency information on inside covers.**

What drug does:
Irritates stomach lining and stimulates the vomiting center in the brain.

Time lapse before drug works:
20 minutes.

Don't take with:
Any other medicines (including over-the-counter drugs such as cough and cold medicines, laxatives, antacids, diet pills, caffeine, nose drops or vitamins) without consulting your doctor.

 POSSIBLE ADVERSE REACTIONS OR SIDE EFFECTS

SYMPTOMS	WHAT TO DO
Life-threatening:	
Heartbeat irregularity.	Seek emergency treatment immediately.
Common:	
None expected.	
Infrequent:	
None expected.	
Rare:	
None expected.	

WARNINGS & PRECAUTIONS

Don't take if:
You are drunk from any source.

Before you start, consult your doctor:
If you have heart disease (ipecac can be poisonous to a damaged heart).

Over age 60:
No special problems expected.

Pregnancy:
No proven harm to unborn child, but avoid if possible.

Breast-feeding:
Consult your doctor.

Infants & children:
Give only after consulting doctor or poison-control center.

Prolonged use:
Not intended for long-term use.

Skin & sunlight:
No problems expected.

Driving, piloting or hazardous work:
Don't drive or pilot aircraft until you learn how medicine affects you. Don't work around dangerous machinery. Don't climb ladders or work in high places. Danger increases if you drink alcohol or take medicine affecting alertness and reflexes.

Discontinuing:
No special problems expected.

Others:
- If you are instructed to also use activated charcoal, don't use until after ipecac has induced vomiting.
- Don't give more than 2 doses to anyone.

POSSIBLE INTERACTION WITH OTHER DRUGS

GENERIC NAME OR DRUG CLASS	COMBINED EFFECT
Charcoal, activated	Improves treatment. If taken for the same overdose, charcoal should follow vomiting induced by ipecac.
Other medicines or herbs to cause vomiting	Decreased ipecac effect.

POSSIBLE INTERACTION WITH OTHER SUBSTANCES

INTERACTS WITH	COMBINED EFFECT
Alcohol:	Avoid. Vomiting while drunk can be dangerous.
Beverages: Carbonated.	Stomach distention. Avoid.
Milk.	Decreased ipecac effect.
Cocaine:	Avoid.
Foods:	No problems expected.
Marijuana:	Avoid. Aspiration of vomitus could be fatal.
Tobacco:	No problems expected.

IPRATROPIUM

BRAND NAMES

Atrovent

BASIC INFORMATION

Habit forming? No
Prescription needed? Yes
Available as generic? No
Drug class: Bronchodilator

 ## USES

- Treats asthma, bronchitis and emphysema.
- Should not be used alone for acute asthma attacks. May be used with inhalation forms of albuterol or fenoterol.

 ## DOSAGE & USAGE INFORMATION

How to use:
- By inhalation. Follow printed instructions on package.
- Avoid contact with eyes.
- Allow 1 minute between inhalations.

When to take:
Follow your doctor's instructions.

If you forget a dose:
Take as soon as you remember up to 2 hours late. If more than 2 hours, wait for next scheduled dose (don't double this dose).

What drug does:
Dilates bronchial tubes by direct effect on them.

Time lapse before drug works:
None. Effect begins right away.

Don't take with:
Any other medicines (including over-the-counter drugs such as cough and cold medicines, laxatives, antacids, diet pills, caffeine, nose drops or vitamins) without consulting your doctor.

 ## OVERDOSE

SYMPTOMS:
None likely.
WHAT TO DO:
Overdose unlikely to threaten life. If person takes much larger amount than prescribed, call doctor, poison-control center or hospital emergency room for instructions.

 ## POSSIBLE ADVERSE REACTIONS OR SIDE EFFECTS

SYMPTOMS	WHAT TO DO
Life-threatening:	
Pounding heartbeat.	Discontinue. Call doctor right away.
Common:	
Cough, headache, dizziness, nervousness, nausea.	Continue. Call doctor when convenient.
Infrequent:	
Blurred vision, difficult urination, stuffy nose, insomnia, tremors, weakness.	Continue. Call doctor when convenient.
Rare:	
Skin rash, ulcers on lips or in mouth, hives.	Discontinue. Call doctor right away.

WARNINGS & PRECAUTIONS

Don't take if:
You are sensitive to belladonna or atropine.

Before you start, consult your doctor:
- If you have prostate trouble.
- If you have glaucoma.
- If you have severe dental problems.

Over age 60:
Adverse reactions and side effects may be more frequent and severe than in younger persons. You may need smaller doses for shorter periods of time.

Pregnancy:
Risk to unborn child outweighs drug benefits. Don't use.

Breast-feeding:
No special problems expected.

Infants & children:
Effect not documented. Consult your pediatrician.

Prolonged use:
Decreases saliva flow and may increase cavities, gum disease, thrush and discomfort.

Skin & sunlight:
No problems expected.

Driving, piloting or hazardous work:
Avoid if you feel confused, drowsy or dizzy.

Discontinuing:
No special problems expected.

Others:
- Advise any doctor or dentist whom you consult that you take this medicine.
- Allow 5-minute intervals between ipratropium inhalations and inhalations of cromolyn, cortisone or other inhalant medicines.
- Check with doctor if this medicine doesn't bring relief within 30 minutes.

POSSIBLE INTERACTION WITH OTHER DRUGS

GENERIC NAME OR DRUG CLASS	COMBINED EFFECT
Cromolyn	Decreased effectiveness of both drugs.

POSSIBLE INTERACTION WITH OTHER SUBSTANCES

INTERACTS WITH	COMBINED EFFECT
Alcohol:	No special problems expected.
Beverages:	No special problems expected.
Cocaine:	Excess central nervous system stimulation. Avoid.
Foods:	No special problems expected.
Marijuana:	Decreased ipratropium effect.
Tobacco:	Decreased ipratropium effect.

IRON SUPPLEMENTS

BRAND NAMES

See complete list of brand names in the *Brand Name Directory*, page 922

BASIC INFORMATION

Habit forming? No
Prescription needed?
  With folic acid: Yes
  Without folic acid: No
Available as generic? Yes
Drug class: Mineral supplement (iron)

 ## USES

Treatment for dietary iron deficiency or iron-deficiency anemia from other causes.

 ## DOSAGE & USAGE INFORMATION

How to take:
- Tablet, capsule or syrup—Swallow with liquid or food to lessen stomach irritation. If you can't swallow whole, crumble tablet or open capsule and take with liquid or food. Place medicine far back on tongue to avoid staining teeth.
- Elixir—Dilute dose in beverage before swallowing and drink through a straw.

When to take:
1 hour before or 2 hours after eating.

If you forget a dose:
Take up to 2 hours late. If more than 2 hours, wait for next dose (don't double this dose).

Continued next column

 ## OVERDOSE

SYMPTOMS:
- **Moderate overdose—Stomach pain, vomiting, diarrhea, black stools, lethargy.**
- **Serious overdose—Weakness and collapse; pallor, weak and rapid heartbeat; shallow breathing; convulsions and coma.**

WHAT TO DO:
- **Dial 0 (operator) or 911 (emergency) for an ambulance or medical help. Then give first aid immediately.**
- **See emergency information on inside covers.**

What drug does:
Stimulates bone marrow's production of hemoglobin (red blood cell pigment that carries oxygen to body cells).

Time lapse before drug works:
3 to 7 days. May require 3 weeks for maximum benefit.

Don't take with:
- Multiple vitamin and mineral supplements.
- Any other medicine without consulting your doctor or pharmacist.

 ## POSSIBLE ADVERSE REACTIONS OR SIDE EFFECTS

SYMPTOMS	WHAT TO DO
Life-threatening:	
Weak, rapid heartbeat.	Seek emergency treatment immediately.
Always:	
Gray or black stool.	No action necessary.
Common:	
• Stained teeth with liquid iron.	No action necessary.
• Abdominal pain.	Continue. Call doctor when convenient.
Infrequent:	
• Constipation or diarrhea, heartburn, nausea, vomiting.	Discontinue. Call doctor right away.
• Fatigue, weakness.	Continue. Call doctor when convenient.
Rare:	
• Blue lips, fingernails, palms of hands; pale, clammy skin.	Discontinue. Seek emergency treatment.
• Throat pain on swallowing, pain, cramps, blood in stool.	Discontinue. Call doctor right away.
• Drowsiness.	Continue. Call doctor when convenient.

 ## WARNINGS & PRECAUTIONS

Don't take if:
- You are allergic to any iron supplement or tartrazine dye.
- You take iron injections.
- You have acute hepatitis, hemosiderosis or hemochromatosis (conditions involving excess iron in body).
- You have hemolytic anemia.

Before you start, consult your doctor:
- If you plan to become pregnant while on medication.
- If you have had stomach surgery.
- If you have had peptic ulcer, enteritis or colitis.

Over age 60:
May cause hemochromatosis (iron storage disease) with bronze skin, liver damage, diabetes, heart problems and impotence.

Pregnancy:
No proven harm to unborn child. Avoid if possible. Take only if your doctor advises supplement during last half of pregnancy.

Breast-feeding:
No problems expected. Take only if your doctor confirms you have a dietary deficiency or an iron-deficiency anemia.

Infants & children:
Use only under medical supervision. Overdose common and dangerous. Keep out of children's reach.

Prolonged use:
- May cause hemochromatosis (iron storage disease) with bronze skin, liver damage, diabetes, heart problems and impotence.
- Talk to your doctor about the need for follow-up medical examinations or laboratory studies to check complete blood counts (white blood cell count, platelet count, red blood cell count, hemoglobin, hematocrit), serum iron, total iron-binding capacity.

Skin & sunlight:
No problems expected.

Driving, piloting or hazardous work:
No problems expected.

Discontinuing:
May be unnecessary to finish medicine. Follow doctor's instructions.

Others:
- Liquid form stains teeth. Mix with water or juice to lessen the effect. Brush with baking soda or hydrogen peroxide to help remove stain.
- Some products contain tartrazine dye. Avoid, especially if you are allergic to aspirin.
- May interfere with the accuracy of some medical tests.

POSSIBLE INTERACTION WITH OTHER DRUGS

GENERIC NAME OR DRUG CLASS	COMBINED EFFECT
Acetohydroxamic acid	Decreased effects of both drugs.
Allopurinol	Possible excess iron storage in liver.
Antacids*	Poor iron absorption.
Chloramphenicol	Decreased effect of iron. Interferes with formation of red blood cells and hemoglobin.
Cholestyramine	Decreased iron effect.
Iron supplements, other*	Possible excess iron storage in liver.
Tetracyclines*	Decreased tetracycline effect. Take iron 3 hours before or 2 hours after taking tetracycline.
Vitamin E	Decreased iron and vitamin E effect.
Zinc supplements	Increased need for zinc.

POSSIBLE INTERACTION WITH OTHER SUBSTANCES

INTERACTS WITH	COMBINED EFFECT
Alcohol:	Increased iron absorption. May cause organ damage. Avoid or use in moderation.
Beverages: Milk, tea.	Decreased iron effect.
Cocaine:	None expected.
Foods: Dairy foods, eggs, whole-grain bread and cereal.	Decreased iron effect.
Marijuana:	None expected.
Tobacco:	None expected.

*See Glossary

ISOMETHEPTENE, DICHLORALPHENAZONE & ACETAMINOPHEN

BRAND NAMES

Amidrin	Migratine
I.D.A.	Migrazone
Iso-Acetazone	Migrex
Isocom	Mitride
Midrin	

BASIC INFORMATION

Habit forming? No
Prescription needed? Yes
Available as generic? No
Drug class: Analgesic, sedative, vascular headache suppressant

 ## USES

Treatment of vascular (throbbing or migraine type) and tension headaches.

 ## DOSAGE & USAGE INFORMATION

How to take:
Capsules—Take with fluid. Usual dose—2 capsules at start, then 1 every hour until fully relieved. Don't exceed 5 capsules in 12 hours.

When to take:
At first sign of headache.

If you forget a dose:
Use as soon as you remember.

What drug does:
Causes blood vessels in head to constrict or become narrower. Acetaminophen relieves pain by effects on hypothalamus—the part of the brain that helps regulate body heat and receives body's pain messages.

Time lapse before drug works:
30-60 minutes.

Continued next column

 ## OVERDOSE

SYMPTOMS:
Stomach upsets, irritability, sweating, severe diarrhea, convulsions, coma.
WHAT TO DO:
* **Dial 0 (operator) or 911 (emergency) for an ambulance or medical help. Then give first aid immediately.**
* **See emergency information on inside covers.**

Don't take with:
* Any medicine that will decrease mental alertness or reflexes, such as alcohol, other mind-altering drugs, cough/cold medicines, antihistamines, allergy medicine, sedatives, tranquilizers (sleeping pills or "downers") barbiturates, seizure medicine, narcotics, other prescription medicine for pain, muscle relaxants, anesthetics.
* See Interaction column and consult doctor.

 ## POSSIBLE ADVERSE REACTIONS OR SIDE EFFECTS

SYMPTOMS	WHAT TO DO
Life-threatening:	
In case of overdose, see previous column.	
Common:	
Dizziness, drowsiness.	Continue. Call doctor when convenient.
Infrequent:	
Diarrhea, vomiting, nausea, abdominal cramps, upper abdominal pain.	Discontinue. Call doctor right away.
Rare:	
Rash; itchy skin; sore throat, fever, mouth sores; unusual bleeding or bruising; weakness; jaundice.	Discontinue. Call doctor right away.

ISOMETHEPTENE, DICHLORALPHENAZONE & ACETAMINOPHEN

 ## WARNINGS & PRECAUTIONS

Don't take if:
- You are allergic to acetaminophen or any other component of this combination medicine.
- Your symptoms don't improve after 2 days use. Call your doctor.

Before you start, consult your doctor:
If you have kidney disease, liver damage, glaucoma, heart or blood vessel disorder, hypertension.

Over age 60:
Don't exceed recommended dose. You can't eliminate drug as efficiently as younger persons.

Pregnancy:
No proven harm to unborn child. Avoid if possible.

Breast-feeding:
No proven harm to nursing infant.

Infants & children:
Give under careful medical supervision only.

Prolonged use:
- May affect blood system and cause anemia. Limit use to 5 days for children 12 and under, and 10 days for adults.
- Talk to your doctor about the need for follow-up medical examinations or laboratory studies to check complete blood counts (white blood cell count, platelet count, red blood cell count, hemoglobin, hematocrit), liver function.

Skin & sunlight:
No problems expected.

Driving, piloting or hazardous work:
Avoid if you feel drowsy. Otherwise, no restrictions.

Discontinuing:
Discontinue in 2 days if symptoms don't improve.

Others:
No problems expected.

 ## POSSIBLE INTERACTION WITH OTHER DRUGS

GENERIC NAME OR DRUG CLASS	COMBINED EFFECT
Anticoagulants, oral*	May increase anticoagulant effect. If combined frequently, prothrombin time should be monitored.
Aspirin or other salicylates*	Long-term combined effect (3 years or longer) increases chance of damage to kidney, including malignancy.
Beta-adrenergic blockers*	Narrowed arteries in heart if taken in large doses.
MAO inhibitors*	Sudden increase in blood pressure.
Non-steroidal anti-inflammatory drugs (NSAIDs)*	Long-term combined effect (3 years or longer) increases chance of damage to kidney, including malignancy.
Phenacetin	Long-term combined effect (3 years or longer) increases chance of damage to kidney, including malignancy.
Phenobarbital	Quicker elimination and decreased effect of acetaminophen.
Tetracyclines* (effervescent granules or tablets)	May slow tetracycline absorption. Space doses 2 hours apart.
Zidovudine (AZT)	Increased toxic effect of zidovudine.

 ## POSSIBLE INTERACTION WITH OTHER SUBSTANCES

INTERACTS WITH	COMBINED EFFECT
Alcohol:	Drowsiness. Toxicity to liver.
Beverages:	None expected.
Cocaine:	None expected. However, cocaine may slow body's recovery. Avoid.
Foods:	None expected.
Marijuana:	Increased pain relief. However, marijuana may slow body's recovery. Avoid.
Tobacco:	May decrease medicine's effectiveness.

*See Glossary

ISONIAZID

BRAND NAMES

INH
Isotamine
Laniazid
Nydrazid

PMS Isoniazid
Rifamate
Rimifon
Tubizid

BASIC INFORMATION

Habit forming? No
Prescription needed? Yes
Available as generic? Yes
Drug class: Antitubercular

 USES

Kills tuberculosis germs.

 DOSAGE & USAGE INFORMATION

How to take:
- Tablet—Swallow with liquid to lessen stomach irritation.
- Syrup—Follow label directions.

When to take:
At the same time each day.

If you forget a dose:
Take as soon as you remember up to 12 hours late. If more than 12 hours, wait for next scheduled dose (don't double this dose).

What drug does:
Interferes with TB germ metabolism. Eventually destroys the germ.

Continued next column

 OVERDOSE

SYMPTOMS:
Difficult breathing, convulsions, coma.
WHAT TO DO:
- **Dial 0 (operator) or 911 (emergency) for an ambulance or medical help. Then give first aid immediately.**
- **If patient is unconscious and not breathing, give mouth-to-mouth breathing. If there is no heartbeat, use cardiac massage and mouth-to-mouth breathing (CPR). Don't try to make patient vomit. If you can't get help quickly, take patient to nearest emergency facility.**
- **See emergency information on inside covers.**

Time lapse before drug works:
3 to 6 months. You may need to take drug as long as 2 years.

Don't take with:
Any other medication without consulting your doctor or pharmacist.

 POSSIBLE ADVERSE REACTIONS OR SIDE EFFECTS

SYMPTOMS	WHAT TO DO
Life-threatening:	
In case of overdose, see previous column.	
Common:	
• Muscle pain and pain in joints, tingling or numbness in extremities, jaundice.	Discontinue. Call doctor right away.
• Confusion, unsteady walk.	Continue. Call doctor when convenient.
Infrequent:	
• Swollen glands, nausea, indigestion, diarrhea, vomiting, appetite loss.	Discontinue. Call doctor right away.
• Dizziness.	Continue. Call doctor when convenient.
Rare:	
• Rash, fever, impaired vision, anemia with fatigue, weakness, fever, sore throat, unusual bleeding or bruising.	Discontinue. Call doctor right away.
• Breast enlargement or discomfort.	Continue. Tell doctor at next visit.

 WARNINGS & PRECAUTIONS

Don't take if:
You are allergic to isoniazid.

Before you start, consult your doctor:
- If you plan to become pregnant within medication period.
- If you are allergic to athionamide, pyrazinamide or nicotinic acid.
- If you drink alcohol.
- If you have liver or kidney disease.
- If you have epilepsy, diabetes or lupus.

Over age 60:
Adverse reactions and side effects, especially jaundice, may be more frequent and severe than in younger persons. Kidneys may be less efficient.

Pregnancy:
No proven harm to unborn child. Avoid if possible, especially in the first 6 months of pregnancy. Consult doctor about use in last 3 months.

Breast-feeding:
Drug passes into milk. Avoid drug or discontinue nursing until you finish medicine. Consult doctor for advice on maintaining milk supply.

Infants & children:
Use only under medical supervision.

Prolonged use:
- Numbness and tingling of hands and feet.
- Talk to your doctor about the need for follow-up medical examinations or laboratory studies to check liver function, eyes.

Skin & sunlight:
No problems expected.

Driving, piloting or hazardous work:
Avoid if you feel dizzy. Otherwise, no problems expected.

Discontinuing:
Don't discontinue without doctor's advice until you complete prescribed dose, even though symptoms diminish or disappear.

Others:
- Diabetic patients may have false blood-sugar tests.
- Periodic liver-function tests and laboratory blood studies recommended.
- Prescription for vitamin B-6 (pyridoxine) recommended to prevent nerve damage.

POSSIBLE INTERACTION WITH OTHER DRUGS

GENERIC NAME OR DRUG CLASS	COMBINED EFFECT
Acetaminophen	Increased risk of liver damage.
Alfentanil	Prolonged duration of alfentanil effect (undesirable).
Antacids* (aluminum-containing)	Decreased absorption of isoniazid.
Anticholinergics*	May increase pressure within eyeball.
Anticoagulants*	Increased anticoagulant effect.
Antidiabetics*	Increased antidiabetic effect.
Antihypertensives*	Increased antihypertensive effect.
Carbamazepine	Increased risk of liver damage.

Cycloserine	Increased risk of central nervous system effects.
Didanosine	Increased risk of peripheral neuropathy.
Disulfiram	Increased effect of disulfiram.
Laxatives*	Decreased absorption and effect of isoniazid.
Hepatotoxics*	Increased risk of liver damage.
Ketoconazole	Increased risk of liver damage
Narcotics*	Increased narcotic effect.
Niacin	Decreased niacin effect.
Phenytoin	Increased phenytoin effect.
Pyridoxine (Vitamin B-6)	Decreased chance of nerve damage in extremities.
Rifampin	Increased isoniazid toxicity to liver.
Sedatives*	Increased sedative effect.
Stimulants*	Increased stimulant effect.

POSSIBLE INTERACTION WITH OTHER SUBSTANCES

INTERACTS WITH	COMBINED EFFECT
Alcohol:	Increased incidence of liver disease.
Beverages:	None expected.
Cocaine:	None expected.
Foods: Swiss or Cheshire cheese, fish.	Red or itching skin, fast heartbeat. Seek emergency treatment.
Marijuana:	No interactions expected, but marijuana may slow body's recovery.
Tobacco:	No interactions expected, but tobacco may slow body's recovery.

*See Glossary

ISOPROTERENOL & PHENYLEPHRINE

BRAND NAMES

Duo-Medihaler

BASIC INFORMATION

Habit forming? No
Prescription needed? Yes
Available as generic? No
Drug class: Sympathomimetic,
bronchodilator

USES

- Temporary relief of congestion of nose, sinuses and throat caused by allergies, colds or sinusitis.
- Treatment for breathing difficulty from acute asthma, bronchitis and emphysema.

DOSAGE & USAGE INFORMATION

How to take:
Aerosol inhaler—Don't inhale more than twice per dose. Follow package instructions.

When to take:
As needed, no more often than every 4 hours.

If you forget a dose:
Take as soon as you remember. Wait 4 hours for next dose. Don't double this dose.

What drug does:
- Dilates constricted bronchial tubes, improving air flow.
- Stimulates heart muscle and dilates blood vessels.

Time lapse before drug works:
2 to 4 minutes.

Continued next column

OVERDOSE

SYMPTOMS:
Headache, blood-pressure rise, slow and forceful pulse, nervousness, rapid or irregular heartbeat, fainting, sweating, tremor, vomiting, chest pain, convulsions, coma.
WHAT TO DO:
- **Dial 0 (operator) or 911 (emergency) for an ambulance or medical help. Then give first aid immediately.**
- **See emergency information on inside covers.**

Don't take with:
Non-prescription drugs for asthma, cough, cold, allergy, appetite suppressants, sleeping pills or drugs containing caffeine without consulting doctor.

POSSIBLE ADVERSE REACTIONS OR SIDE EFFECTS

SYMPTOMS	WHAT TO DO
Life-threatening:	
In case of overdose, see previous column.	
Common:	
Chest pain; irregular, fast heartbeat; dry mouth.	Discontinue. Call doctor right away.
Infrequent:	
• Increased sweating.	Discontinue. Call doctor right away.
• Nervousness, insomnia, dizziness, headache, shakiness, weakness, red or flushed face, vomiting, nausea, pale skin.	Continue. Call doctor when convenient.
Rare:	
Tingling hands or feet.	Discontinue. Call doctor right away.

WARNINGS & PRECAUTIONS

Don't take if:
- You are allergic to any sympathomimetic, including some diet pills.
- You have serious heart-rhythm disorder.
- You have taken MAO inhibitors in past 2 weeks.

Before you start, consult your doctor:
- If you have high blood pressure, heart disease, or take a digitalis preparation.
- If you have diabetes or overactive thyroid.
- If you have taken MAO inhibitors in past 2 weeks.
- If you are sensitive to sympathomimetics.
- If you use epinephrine.
- If your heartbeat is faster than 100 beats per minute.

Over age 60:
You may be more sensitive to drug's stimulant effects. Use with caution if you have hardening of the arteries.

ISOPROTERENOL & PHENYLEPHRINE

Pregnancy:
Risk to unborn child outweighs drug benefits. Don't use.

Breast-feeding:
Drug passes into milk. Avoid drug or discontinue nursing until you finish medicine. Consult doctor for advice on maintaining milk supply.

Infants & children:
Use only under close supervision.

Prolonged use:
● May cause functional dependence.
● Salivary glands may swell.

Skin & sunlight:
No problems expected.

Driving, piloting or hazardous work:
Use caution if you feel dizzy or nervous.

Discontinuing:
Discontinue if drug fails to provide relief after 2 or 3 days. Consult doctor.

Others:
No problems expected.

POSSIBLE INTERACTION WITH OTHER DRUGS

GENERIC NAME OR DRUG CLASS	COMBINED EFFECT
Acebutolol	Decreased effect of both drugs.
Amphetamines*	Increased nervousness.
Antiasthmatics*	Nervous stimulation.
Antidepressants*	Increased effect of both drugs.
Antihypertensives*	Increased antihypertensive effect.
Beta-adrenergic blockers*	Decreased effect of both drugs.
Ephedrine	Increased ephedrine effect.
Epinephrine	Increased chance of serious heart disturbances.
Furazolidine	Sudden, severe increase in blood pressure.

MAO inhibitors*	Dangerous blood-pressure rise.
Nitrates*	Possible decreased effect of both drugs.
Oxprenolol	Decreased effect of both drugs.
Sedatives*	Decreased sedative effect.
Sympathomimetics, other*	Increased effect of both drugs, especially harmful side effects.
Terazosin	Decreases effectiveness of terazosin.
Theophylline	Possible increased effect and toxicity of both drugs.
Tranquilizers*	Decreased tranquilizer effect.

POSSIBLE INTERACTION WITH OTHER SUBSTANCES

INTERACTS WITH	COMBINED EFFECT
Alcohol:	Decreased isoproterenol effect.
Beverages: Caffeine drinks.	Overstimulation. Avoid.
Cocaine:	High risk of heartbeat irregularities and high blood pressure. Overstimulation of brain. Avoid.
Foods:	None expected.
Marijuana:	Increased antiasthmatic effect of isoproterenol.
Tobacco:	None expected.

ISOTRETINOIN

BRAND NAMES

Accutane

BASIC INFORMATION

Habit forming? No
Prescription needed? Yes
Available as generic? No
Drug classification: Anti-acne (topical)

 USES

- Decreases cystic acne formation in severe cases.
- Certain other skin disorders involving an overabundance of outer skin layer.

 DOSAGE & USAGE INFORMATION

How to take:
Capsule—Swallow with liquid or food to lessen stomach irritation. If you can't swallow whole, open capsule and take with liquid or food.

When to take:
Twice a day. Follow prescription directions.

If you forget a dose:
Take as soon as you remember up to 2 hours late. If more than 2 hours, wait for next scheduled dose and double dose.

What drug does:
Reduces sebaceous gland activity and size.

Time lapse before drug works:
May require 15 to 20 weeks to experience full benefit.

Don't take with:
- Vitamin A or supplements containing Vitamin A.
- Any other medication without consulting your doctor or pharmacist.

 OVERDOSE

SYMPTOMS:
None reported.
WHAT TO DO:
Overdose unlikely to threaten life. If person takes much larger amount than prescribed, call doctor, poison-control center or hospital emergency room for instructions.

 POSSIBLE ADVERSE REACTIONS OR SIDE EFFECTS

SYMPTOMS	WHAT TO DO
Life-threatening: None expected.	
Common:	
• Burning, red, itching eyes; lip scaling; burning pain; nosebleeds.	Discontinue. Call doctor right away.
• Itchy skin.	Continue. Call doctor when convenient.
• Dry mouth.	Continue. Tell doctor at next visit. (Suck ice or chew gum.)
Infrequent:	
• Rash, infection, nausea, vomiting.	Discontinue. Call doctor right away.
• Pain in muscles, bones, joints; hair thinning; tiredness.	Continue. Call doctor when convenient.
Rare:	
Abdominal pain, bleeding gums, blurred vision, diarrhea, headache, moodiness, vomiting, eye pain, rectal bleeding, yellow skin or eyes.	Discontinue. Call doctor right away.

ISOTRETINOIN

WARNINGS & PRECAUTIONS

Don't take if:
- You are allergic to isotretinoin.
- You are pregnant or plan pregnancy.
- *You are even able to bear children. Read, understand and follow the patient information enclosure with your prescription.*

Before you start, consult your doctor:
- If you have diabetes.
- If you or any member of family have high triglyceride levels in blood.

Over age 60:
Adverse reactions and side effects may be more frequent and severe than in younger persons.

Pregnancy:
Causes birth defects in fetus. Don't use.

Breast-feeding:
Drug filters into milk. May harm child. Avoid.

Infants & children:
Not recommended.

Prolonged use:
- Possible damage to cornea.
- Talk to your doctor about the need for follow-up medical examinations or laboratory studies to check complete blood counts (white blood cell count, platelet count, red blood cell count, hemoglobin, hematocrit), liver function, blood lipids, blood sugar.

Skin & sunlight:
May cause rash or intensify sunburn in areas exposed to sun or sunlamp.

Driving, piloting or hazardous work:
No problems expected.

Discontinuing:
Single course of treatment is usually all that's needed. If second course required, wait 8 weeks after completing first course.

Others:
- Use only for severe cases of cystic acne that have not responded to less hazardous forms of acne treatment.
- May interfere with the accuracy of some medical tests.
- Don't donate blood for at least 30 days after discontinuing medicine.
- **If you are planning pregnancy or at risk of pregancy, don't take this drug.**

POSSIBLE INTERACTION WITH OTHER DRUGS

GENERIC NAME OR DRUG CLASS	COMBINED EFFECT
Etretinate	Increased chance of toxicity of each drug.
Tetracyclines*	Increased risk of developing pseudotumor cerebri.*
Vitamin A	Additive toxic effect of each. Avoid.

POSSIBLE INTERACTION WITH OTHER SUBSTANCES

INTERACTS WITH	COMBINED EFFECT
Alcohol:	Significant increase in triglycerides in blood. Avoid.
Beverages:	No problems expected.
Cocaine:	Increased chance of toxicity of isotretinoin. Avoid.
Foods:	No problems expected.
Marijuana:	Increased chance of toxicity of isotretinoin. Avoid.
Tobacco:	May decrease absorption of medicine. Avoid tobacco while in treatment.

ISOXSUPRINE

BRAND NAMES

Vasodilan   Vasoprine

BASIC INFORMATION

Habit forming? No
Prescription needed? Yes
Available as generic? Yes
Drug class: Vasodilator

 USES

- May improve poor blood circulation.
- Management of premature labor.

 DOSAGE & USAGE INFORMATION

How to take:
Tablet—Swallow with liquid or food to lessen
stomach irritation. If you can't swallow whole,
crumble tablet and take with liquid or food.

When to take:
At the same times each day.

If you forget a dose:
Take as soon as you remember up to 2 hours
late. If more than 2 hours, wait for next
scheduled dose (don't double this dose).

What drug does:
Expands blood vessels, increasing flow and
permitting distribution of oxygen and nutrients.

Time lapse before drug works:
1 hour.

Don't take with:
Any other medication without consulting your
doctor or pharmacist.

 OVERDOSE

SYMPTOMS:
Headache, dizziness, flush, vomiting,
weakness, sweating, fainting, shortness of
breath, coma.
WHAT TO DO:
- Dial 0 (operator) or 911 (emergency) for
  an ambulance or medical help. Then give
  first aid immediately.
- If patient is unconscious and not
  breathing, give mouth-to-mouth
  breathing. If there is no heartbeat, use
  cardiac massage and mouth-to-mouth
  breathing (CPR). Don't try to make patient
  vomit. If you can't get help quickly, take
  patient to nearest emergency facility.
- See emergency information on inside covers.

 POSSIBLE ADVERSE REACTIONS OR SIDE EFFECTS

SYMPTOMS	WHAT TO DO
Life-threatening:	
In case of overdose, see previous column.	
Common:	
• Appetite loss, nausea, vomiting.	Discontinue. Call doctor right away.
• Dizziness, faintness, flushing.	Continue. Call doctor when convenient.
• Weakness, lethargy.	Continue. Tell doctor at next visit.
Infrequent:	
Rash, chest pain, shortness of breath.	Discontinue. Call doctor right away.
Rare:	
Rapid or irregular heartbeat.	Discontinue. Call doctor right away.

WARNINGS & PRECAUTIONS

Don't take if:
- You are allergic to any vasodilator.
- You have any bleeding disease.

Before you start, consult your doctor:
- If you have high blood pressure, hardening of the arteries or heart disease.
- If you plan to become pregnant within medication period.
- If you have glaucoma.

Over age 60:
Adverse reactions and side effects may be more frequent and severe than in younger persons.

Pregnancy:
Studies inconclusive on harm to unborn child. Decide with your doctor whether drug benefits justify risk to unborn child.

Breast-feeding:
No problems expected, but consult doctor.

Infants & children:
Not recommended.

Prolonged use:
Talk to your doctor about the need for follow-up medical examinations or laboratory studies.

Skin & sunlight:
No problems expected.

Driving, piloting or hazardous work:
Avoid if you feel dizzy or faint. Otherwise, no problems expected.

Discontinuing:
Don't discontinue without doctor's advice until you complete prescribed dose, even though symptoms diminish or disappear.

Others:
- Be cautious when arising from lying or sitting position, when climbing stairs, or if dizziness occurs.
- May interfere with the accuracy of some medical tests.

POSSIBLE INTERACTION WITH OTHER DRUGS

GENERIC NAME OR DRUG CLASS	COMBINED EFFECT
None expected.	

POSSIBLE INTERACTION WITH OTHER SUBSTANCES

INTERACTS WITH	COMBINED EFFECT
Alcohol:	None expected.
Beverages: Milk.	Decreased stomach irritation.
Cocaine:	Decreased blood circulation to extremities. Avoid.
Foods:	None expected.
Marijuana:	Rapid heartbeat.
Tobacco:	Decreased isoxsuprine effect; nicotine constricts blood vessels.

KANAMYCIN

BRAND NAMES

Kantrex

BASIC INFORMATION

Habit forming? No
Prescription needed? Yes
Available as generic? No
Drug class: Bowel preparation

 ## USES

- To cleanse bowel of bacteria prior to intestinal surgery.
- Treats hepatic coma.

 ## DOSAGE & USAGE INFORMATION

How to take:
Capsules—Swallow with liquid. If you can't swallow whole, open capsule and take with liquid or food. Instructions to take on empty stomach mean 1 hour before or 2 hours after eating.

When to take:
At the same time each day, according to instructions on prescription label.

If you forget a dose:
Take as soon as you remember up to 2 hours late. If more than 2 hours, wait for next scheduled dose (don't double this dose).

What drug does:
Kills susceptible bacteria in the intestines.

Time lapse before drug works:
15 to 30 minutes.

Don't take with:
Any other medication without consulting your doctor or pharmacist.

 ## OVERDOSE

SYMPTOMS:
Clumsiness, dizziness, seizures, coma.
WHAT TO DO:
- **Dial 0 (operator) or 911 (emergency) for an ambulance or medical help. Then give first aid immediately.**
- **See emergency information on inside covers.**

 ## POSSIBLE ADVERSE REACTIONS OR SIDE EFFECTS

SYMPTOMS	WHAT TO DO
Life-threatening:	
In case of overdose, see previous column.	
Common:	
Mouth irritation or soreness, nausea.	Continue. Call doctor when convenient.
Infrequent:	
Vomiting.	Discontinue. Call doctor right away.
Rare:	
Decreased urine, hearing loss, ringing in ears, clumsiness, unsteadiness, skin rash.	Discontinue. Call doctor right away.

WARNINGS & PRECAUTIONS

Don't take if:
- You are allergic to kanamycin.
- You can't tolerate any aminoglycoside.

Before you start, consult your doctor:
- If you have hearing difficulty.
- If you have intestinal obstruction.
- If you have severe kidney disease.
- If you have ulcerative colitis.

Over age 60:
Adverse reactions and side effects may be more frequent and severe than in younger persons. You may need smaller doses for shorter periods of time.

Pregnancy:
No special problems expected.

Breast-feeding:
No special problems expected.

Infants & children:
Not recommended for prolonged use.

Prolonged use:
Not recommended for prolonged use.

Skin & sunlight:
No problems expected.

Driving, piloting or hazardous work:
Avoid if you feel confused, drowsy or dizzy.

Discontinuing:
Not recommended for prolonged use.

Others:
No problems expected.

POSSIBLE INTERACTION WITH OTHER DRUGS

GENERIC NAME OR DRUG CLASS	COMBINED EFFECT
None expected.	

POSSIBLE INTERACTION WITH OTHER SUBSTANCES

INTERACTS WITH	COMBINED EFFECT
Alcohol:	No special problems expected.
Beverages:	No special problems expected.
Cocaine:	No special problems expected.
Foods:	No special problems expected.
Marijuana:	No special problems expected.
Tobacco:	No special problems expected.

*See Glossary

KAOLIN & PECTIN

BRAND NAMES

Donnagel-MB	Kaypectol
Donnagel-PG	K-C
Kao-Con	K-P
Kaopectate	K-Pek
Kaotin	Parepectolin
Kapectolin	Pecto Kay

BASIC INFORMATION

Habit forming? No
Prescription needed? No
Available as generic? No
Drug class: Antidiarrheal

 USES

Reduces intestinal cramps and diarrhea.

 DOSAGE & USAGE INFORMATION

How to take:
Liquid—Swallow prescribed dosage (without diluting) after each loose bowel movement.

When to take:
After each loose bowel movement.

If you forget a dose:
Take when you remember.

What drug does:
Makes loose stools less watery, but may not prevent loss of fluids.

Time lapse before drug works:
15 to 30 minutes.

Don't take with:
Any other medication without consulting your doctor or pharmacist.

 OVERDOSE

SYMPTOMS:
Fecal impaction.
WHAT TO DO:
Overdose unlikely to threaten life. If person takes much larger amount than prescribed, call doctor, poison-control center or hospital emergency room for instructions.

 POSSIBLE ADVERSE REACTIONS OR SIDE EFFECTS

SYMPTOMS	WHAT TO DO
Life-threatening: None expected.	
Common: None expected.	
Infrequent: None expected.	
Rare: Constipation (mild).	Continue. Call doctor when convenient.

WARNINGS & PRECAUTIONS

Don't take if:
You are allergic to kaolin or pectin.

Before you start, consult your doctor:
- If patient is child or infant.
- If you have any chronic medical problem with heart disease, peptic ulcer, asthma or others.
- If you have fever over 101F.

Over age 60:
Fluid loss caused by diarrhea, especially if taking other medicines, may lead to serious disability. Consult doctor.

Pregnancy:
No problems expected.

Breast-feeding:
No problems expected.

Infants & children:
Fluid loss caused by diarrhea in infants and children can cause serious dehydration. Consult doctor before giving any medicine for diarrhea.

Prolonged use:
Not recommended.

Skin & sunlight:
No problems expected.

Driving, piloting or hazardous work:
No problems expected.

Discontinuing:
May be unnecessary to finish medicine. Follow doctor's instructions.

Others:
Consult doctor about fluids, diet and rest.

POSSIBLE INTERACTION WITH OTHER DRUGS

GENERIC NAME OR DRUG CLASS	COMBINED EFFECT
Digoxin	Decreases absorption of digoxin. Separate doses by at least 2 hours.
Lincomycins*	Decreases absorption of lincomycin. Separate doses by at least 2 hours.
All other oral medicines	May decrease absorption of other medicines. Separate doses by at least 2 hours.

POSSIBLE INTERACTION WITH OTHER SUBSTANCES

INTERACTS WITH	COMBINED EFFECT
Alcohol:	Increased diarrhea. Prevents action of kaolin and pectin.
Beverages:	No problems expected.
Cocaine:	Aggravates underlying disease. Avoid.
Foods:	No problems expected.
Marijuana:	Aggravates underlying disease. Avoid.
Tobacco:	Aggravates underlying disease. Avoid.

KAOLIN, PECTIN, BELLADONNA & OPIUM

BRAND NAMES

Amogel PG
Donnachem-PG
Donnagel-PG
Donnapectolin-PG
Kaodene with
  Paregoric

Kaodonna-PG
Kapectolin PG
Quiagel PG

BASIC INFORMATION

Habit forming? Yes
Prescription needed? Yes
Available as generic? No
Drug class: Narcotic, antidiarrheal,
  antispasmodic

 USES

Reduces intestinal cramps and diarrhea.

 DOSAGE & USAGE INFORMATION

How to take:
Liquid—Swallow prescribed dosage (without diluting) after each loose bowel movement.

When to take:
As needed for diarrhea, no more often than every 4 hours.

If you forget a dose:
Take when you remember.

What drug does:
- Blocks nerve impulses at parasympathetic nerve endings, preventing muscle contractions and gland secretions of organs involved.
Continued next column

 OVERDOSE

SYMPTOMS:
Fecal impaction, rapid pulse, dizziness, fever, hallucinations, confusion, slurred speech, agitation, flushed face, convulsions, deep sleep, slow breathing, slow pulse, warm skin, constricted pupils, coma.
WHAT TO DO:
- **Dial 0 (operator) or 911 (emergency) for an ambulance or medical help. Then give first aid immediately.**
- **If patient is unconscious and not breathing, give mouth-to-mouth breathing. If there is no heartbeat, use cardiac massage and mouth-to-mouth breathing (CPR). Don't try to make patient vomit. If you can't get help quickly, take patient to nearest emergency facility.**
- **See emergency information on inside covers.**

- Makes loose stools less watery, but may not prevent loss of fluids.
- Anesthetizes surface membranes of intestines and blocks nerve impulses.

Time lapse before drug works:
15 to 30 minutes.

Don't take with:
Any other medication without consulting your doctor or pharmacist.

 POSSIBLE ADVERSE REACTIONS OR SIDE EFFECTS

SYMPTOMS	WHAT TO DO
Life-threatening: Unusually rapid heartbeat (over 100), difficult breathing, slow heartbeat (under 50/minute).	Discontinue. Seek emergency treatment.
Common: (with large dosage) Weakness, increased sweating, red or flushed face, lightheadedness, headache, dry mouth, dry skin, drowsiness, dizziness, frequent urination, decreased sweating, constipation, confusion, tiredness.	Continue. Call doctor when convenient.
Infrequent: • Taste sense reduced, nervousness, sunlight hurts eyes, blurred vision.	Discontinue. Call doctor right away.
• Diminished sex drive, memory loss.	Continue. Call doctor when convenient.
Rare: Bloating, abdominal cramps and vomiting, eye pain, hallucinations, shortness of breath, rash, itchy skin, slow heartbeat.	Discontinue. Call doctor right away.

 WARNINGS & PRECAUTIONS

Don't take if:
- You are allergic to any anticholinergic, narcotic, kaolin or pectin.
- You have trouble with stomach bloating, difficulty emptying your bladder completely, narrow-angle glaucoma, severe ulcerative colitis.

KAOLIN, PECTIN, BELLADONNA & OPIUM

Before you start, consult your doctor:
- If you have open-angle glaucoma, angina, chronic bronchitis or asthma, hiatal hernia, liver disease, enlarged prostate, myasthenia gravis, peptic ulcer, impaired liver or kidney function, fever over 101F, any chronic medical problem with heart disease, peptic ulcer, asthma or others.
- If patient is child or infant.
- If you will have surgery within 2 months, including dental surgery, requiring general or spinal anesthesia.

Over age 60:
- Adverse reactions and side effects may be more frequent and severe than in younger persons.
- More likely to be drowsy, dizzy, unsteady or constipated.
- Fluid loss caused by diarrhea, especially if taking other medicines, may lead to serious disability. Consult doctor.

Pregnancy:
No proven harm to unborn child. Avoid if possible.

Breast-feeding:
Drug passes into milk. Avoid drug or discontinue nursing until you finish medicine. Consult doctor for advice on maintaining milk supply.

Infants & children:
Fluid loss caused by diarrhea in infants and children can cause serious dehydration. Consult doctor before giving any medicine for diarrhea.

Prolonged use:
- Causes psychological and physical dependence. Not recommended.
- Talk to your doctor about the need for follow-up medical examinations or laboratory studies to check liver function, kidney function.

Skin & sunlight:
May cause rash or intensify sunburn in areas exposed to sun or sunlamp.

Driving, piloting or hazardous work:
Don't drive or pilot aircraft until you learn how medicine affects you. Don't work around dangerous machinery. Don't climb ladders or work in high places. Danger increases if you drink alcohol or take medicine affecting alertness and reflexes, such as antihistamines, tranquilizers, sedatives, pain medicine, narcotics and mind-altering drugs.

Discontinuing:
May be unnecessary to finish medicine. Follow doctor's instructions.

Others:
- Great potential for abuse.
- Consult doctor about fluids, diet and rest.

POSSIBLE INTERACTION WITH OTHER DRUGS

GENERIC NAME OR DRUG CLASS	COMBINED EFFECT
Amantadine	Increased belladonna effect.
Analgesics*	Increased analgesic effect.
Antidepressants*	Increased sedative effect.
Antihistamines*	Increased sedative effect.
Carteolol	Increased narcotic effect. Dangerous sedation.
Central nervous system (CNS) depressants*	Increased depressant effect of both.
Cortisone drugs*	Increased internal-eye pressure.
Digoxin	Decreases absorption of digoxin. Separate doses by at least 2 hours.
Haloperidol	Increased internal-eye pressure.

Continued page 948

POSSIBLE INTERACTION WITH OTHER SUBSTANCES

INTERACTS WITH	COMBINED EFFECT
Alcohol:	Increases alcohol's intoxicating effect, increased diarrhea, prevents action of kaolin and pectin. Avoid.
Beverages:	No problems expected.
Cocaine:	Aggravates underlying disease. Avoid.
Foods:	No problems expected.
Marijuana:	Impairs physical and mental performance, aggravates underlying disease. Avoid.
Tobacco:	Aggravates underlying disease. Avoid.

*See Glossary

KAOLIN, PECTIN & PAREGORIC

BRAND NAMES

Donnagel-PG   Parepectolin
Kapectolin with
  Paregoric

BASIC INFORMATION

Habit forming? Yes
Prescription needed? Yes
Available as generic? No
Drug class: Narcotic, antidiarrheal,
  antispasmodic

 USES

- Reduces intestinal cramps and diarrhea.
- Relieves pain.

 DOSAGE & USAGE INFORMATION

How to take:
Liquid—Swallow prescribed dosage (without diluting) after each loose bowel movement.

When to take:
After each loose bowel movement. No more often then every 4 hours.

If you forget a dose:
Take when you remember.

What drug does:
Makes loose stools less watery, but may not prevent loss of fluids.

Time lapse before drug works:
15 to 30 minutes.

Don't take with:
Any other medication without consulting your doctor or pharmacist.

 OVERDOSE

SYMPTOMS:
Deep sleep; slow breathing; slow pulse; flushed, warm skin.
WHAT TO DO:
- **Dial 0 (operator) or 911 (emergency) for an ambulance or medical help. Then give first aid immediately.**
- **If patient is unconscious and not breathing, give mouth-to-mouth breathing. If there is no heartbeat, use cardiac massage and mouth-to-mouth breathing (CPR). Don't try to make patient vomit. If you can't get help quickly, take patient to nearest emergency facility.**
- **See emergency information on inside covers.**

 POSSIBLE ADVERSE REACTIONS OR SIDE EFFECTS

SYMPTOMS	WHAT TO DO
Life-threatening:	
Unusually rapid heartbeat (over 100), difficult breathing, slow heartbeat (under 50/minute).	Discontinue. Seek emergency treatment.
Common:	
(with large dosage) Weakness, increased sweating, red or flushed face, lightheadedness, headache, dry mouth, dry skin, drowsiness, dizziness, frequent urination, decreased sweating, constipation, confusion, tiredness.	Continue. Call doctor when convenient.
Infrequent:	
• Taste sense reduced, nervousness, sunlight hurts eyes, blurred vision.	Discontinue. Call doctor right away.
• Diminished sex drive, memory loss.	Continue. Call doctor when convenient.
Rare:	
Bloating, abdominal cramps and vomiting, eye pain, hallucinations, shortness of breath, rash, itchy skin, slow heartbeat.	Discontinue. Call doctor right away.

 WARNINGS & PRECAUTIONS

Don't take if:
You are allergic to any narcotic, kaolin or pectin.

Before you start, consult your doctor:
- If you have impaired liver or kidney function, chronic medical problem with heart disease, peptic ulcer, asthma or others, fever over 101F.
- If patient is child or infant.
- If you will have surgery within 2 months, including dental surgery, requiring general or spinal anesthesia.

Over age 60:
Fluid loss caused by diarrhea, especially if taking other medicines, may lead to serious disability. Consult doctor.

Pregnancy:
Abuse by pregnant woman will result in addicted newborn. Withdrawal of newborn can be life-threatening.

Breast-feeding:
Drug filters into milk. May harm child. Avoid.

Infants & children:
Fluid loss caused by diarrhea in infants and children can cause serious dehydration. Consult doctor before giving any medicine for diarrhea.

Prolonged use:
- Causes psychological and physical dependence. Not recommended.
- Talk to your doctor about the need for follow-up medical examinations or laboratory studies to check liver function, kidney function.

Skin & sunlight:
May cause rash or intensify sunburn in areas exposed to sun or sunlamp.

Driving, piloting or hazardous work:
Don't drive or pilot aircraft until you learn how medicine affects you. Don't work around dangerous machinery. Don't climb ladders or work in high places. Danger increases if you drink alcohol or take medicine affecting alertness and reflexes, such as antihistamines, tranquilizers, sedatives, pain medicine, narcotics and mind-altering drugs.

Discontinuing:
May be unnecessary to finish medicine. Follow doctor's instructions.

Others:
Consult doctor about fluids, diet and rest.

POSSIBLE INTERACTION WITH OTHER DRUGS

GENERIC NAME OR DRUG CLASS	COMBINED EFFECT
Analgesics, other*	Increased analgesic effect.
Antidepressants*	Increased sedative effect.
Antihistamines*	Increased sedative effect.
Carteolol	Increased narcotic effect. Dangerous sedation.
Digoxin	Decreases absorption of digoxin. Separate doses by at least 2 hours.
Lincomycins*	Decreases absorption of lincomycin. Separate doses by at least 2 hours.
Mind-altering drugs*	Increased sedative effect.

Narcotics, other*	Increased narcotic effect.
Phenothiazines*	Increased phenothiazine effect.
Sedatives*	Increased sedative effect.
Sleep inducers*	Increased sedative effect.
Sotalol	Increased narcotic effect. Dangerous sedation.
Tranquilizers*	Increased sedative effect.
All other oral medicines	Decreases absorption of other medicines. Separate doses by at least 2 hours.

POSSIBLE INTERACTION WITH OTHER SUBSTANCES

INTERACTS WITH	COMBINED EFFECT
Alcohol:	Increases alcohol's intoxicating effect, increased diarrhea, prevents action of kaolin and pectin. Avoid.
Beverages:	No problems expected.
Cocaine:	Increased cocaine toxic effects, aggravates underlying disease. Avoid.
Foods:	No problems expected.
Marijuana:	Aggravates underlying disease. Avoid.
Tobacco:	Aggravates underlying disease. Avoid.

KETOCONAZOLE

BRAND NAMES

Nizoral

BASIC INFORMATION

Habit forming? No
Prescription needed? Yes
Available as generic? No
Drug class: Antifungal

USES

Treatment of fungus infections susceptible to ketoconazole.

DOSAGE & USAGE INFORMATION

How to take:
Tablet or oral suspension—Swallow with liquid or food to lessen stomach irritation. If you can't swallow whole, crumble tablet and take with liquid or food.

When to take:
At same time once a day.

If you forget a dose:
Take as soon as you remember up to 2 hours late. If more than 2 hours, wait for next scheduled dose (don't double this dose).

What drug does:
Prevents fungi from growing and reproducing.

Time lapse before drug works:
8 to 10 months or longer.

Don't take with:
Any other medication without consulting your doctor or pharmacist.

OVERDOSE

SYMPTOMS:
Nausea, vomiting, diarrhea.
WHAT TO DO:
Overdose unlikely to threaten life. If person takes much larger amount than prescribed, call doctor, poison-control center or hospital emergency room for instructions.

POSSIBLE ADVERSE REACTIONS OR SIDE EFFECTS

SYMPTOMS	WHAT TO DO
Life-threatening:	
None expected.	
Common:	
Nausea or vomiting.	Discontinue. Call doctor right away.
Infrequent:	
• Rash or itchy skin, increased sensitivity to light.	Discontinue. Call doctor right away.
• Drowsiness, dizziness, headache, insomnia, diarrhea.	Continue. Call doctor when convenient.
Rare:	
• Pale stools, abdominal pain, dark or amber urine, jaundice.	Discontinue. Call doctor right away.
• Diminished sex drive in males, swollen breasts in males, tiredness, weakness, appetite loss.	Continue. Call doctor when convenient.

WARNINGS & PRECAUTIONS

Don't take if:
You are allergic to ketoconazole.

Before you start, consult your doctor:
• If you have absence of stomach acid (achlorhydria).
• If you have liver disease.

Over age 60:
Adverse reactions and side effects may be more frequent and severe than in younger persons.

Pregnancy:
Risk to unborn child outweighs drug benefits. Don't use.

Breast-feeding:
Drug passes into milk. Avoid drug or discontinue nursing until you finish medicine. Consult doctor for advice on maintaining milk supply.

Infants & children:
Only under close medical supervision.

Prolonged use:
Request liver-function studies.

Skin & sunlight:
Increased sensitivity to sunlight.

Driving, piloting or hazardous work:
Don't drive or pilot aircraft until you learn how medicine affects you. Don't work around dangerous machinery. Don't climb ladders or work in high places. Danger increases if you drink alcohol or take medicine affecting alertness and reflexes, such as antihistamines, tranquilizers, sedatives, pain medicine, narcotics and mind-altering drugs.

Discontinuing:
May be unnecessary to finish medicine. Follow doctor's instructions.

Others:
No problems expected.

POSSIBLE INTERACTION WITH OTHER DRUGS

GENERIC NAME OR DRUG CLASS	COMBINED EFFECT
Antacids*	Decreased absorption of ketoconazole.
Anticoagulants*	Increased anticoagulant effect.
Anticholinergics*	Decreased absorption of ketoconazole.
Atropine	Decreased absorption of ketoconazole.
Belladonna	Decreased absorption of ketoconazole.
Cimetidine	Decreased absorption of ketoconazole.
Clidinium	Decreased absorption of ketoconazole.
Cyclosporine	Increased risk of toxicity to kidney.
Didanosine	Reduced absorption of both drugs. Increased risk of pancreatitis.
Famotidine	Reduced absorption of ketoconazole. Take famatidine at least 2 hours after any dose of ketoconazole.
Glycopyrrolate	Decreased absorption of ketoconazole.
Hyoscyamine	Decreased absorption of ketoconazole.
Hypoglycemics, oral*	Increased effect of oral hypoglycemics.
Isoniazid	Decreased effect of ketoconazole.
Methscopolamine	Decreased absorption of ketoconazole.
Methylprednisolone	Increased effect of methylprednisolone.
Nizatidine	Decreased absorption of ketoconazole.
Phenytoin	May alter effect of both drugs.
Propantheline	Decreased absorption of ketoconazole.
Ranitidine	Decreased absorption of ketoconazole.
Rifampin	Decreased effect of ketoconazole.
Scopolamine	Decreased absorption of ketoconazole.
Sodium bicarbonate	Decreased absorption of ketoconazole.
Terfenadine	Life-threatening heartbeat irregularity. Avoid.

POSSIBLE INTERACTION WITH OTHER SUBSTANCES

INTERACTS WITH	COMBINED EFFECT
Alcohol:	Increased chance of liver damage and disulfiram reaction.*
Beverages:	No problems expected.
Cocaine:	Decreased ketoconazole effect. Avoid.
Foods:	No problems expected.
Marijuana:	Decreased ketoconazole effect. Avoid.
Tobacco:	Decreased ketoconazole effect. Avoid.

*See Glossary

LACTULOSE

BRAND NAMES

Cholac
Chronulac
Constilac
Duphalac

Enulose
Generlac
Portalac

BASIC INFORMATION

Habit forming? No
Prescription needed? No
Available as generic? No
Drug class: Laxative (hyperosmotic)

USES

- Constipation relief.
- Treats brain changes caused by liver disease.

DOSAGE & USAGE INFORMATION

How to take:
Liquid—Dilute dose in beverage before swallowing.

When to take:
Usually once a day, preferably in the morning.

If you forget a dose:
Take as soon as you remember up to 8 hours before bedtime. If later, wait for next scheduled dose (don't double this dose). Don't take at bedtime.

What drug does:
Draws water into bowel from other body tissues. Causes distention through fluid accumulation, which promotes soft stool and accelerates bowel motion.

Time lapse before drug works:
30 minutes to 3 hours.

Don't take with:
Another medicine. Space 2 hours apart.

OVERDOSE

SYMPTOMS:
Fluid depletion, weakness, vomiting, fainting.
WHAT TO DO:
Overdose unlikely to threaten life. If person takes much larger amount than prescribed, call doctor, poison-control center or hospital emergency room for instructions.

POSSIBLE ADVERSE REACTIONS OR SIDE EFFECTS

SYMPTOMS	WHAT TO DO
Life-threatening: None expected.	
Common: Increased thirst, cramps, nausea, diarrhea, gaseousness.	Continue. Tell doctor at next visit.
Infrequent: Irregular heartbeat, muscle cramps.	Discontinue. Call doctor right away.
Rare: Dizziness, confusion, fatigue, weakness.	Continue. Call doctor when convenient.

WARNINGS & PRECAUTIONS

Don't take if:
- You are allergic to any hyperosmotic laxative.
- You have symptoms of appendicitis, inflamed bowel or intestinal blockage.
- You have missed a bowel movement for only 1 or 2 days.

Before you start, consult your doctor:
- If you have congestive heart disease.
- If you have diabetes.
- If you have high blood pressure.
- If you have a colostomy or ileostomy.
- If you have kidney disease.
- If you have a laxative habit.
- If you have rectal bleeding.
- If you take another laxative.
- If you require a low-galactose diet.

Over age 60:
Adverse reactions and side effects may be more frequent and severe than in younger persons.

Pregnancy:
No proven problems. Avoid if possible.

Breast-feeding:
No problems expected.

Infants & children:
Use only under medical supervision.

Prolonged use:
Don't take for more than 1 week unless under a doctor's supervision. May cause laxative dependence.

Skin & sunlight:
No problems expected.

Driving, piloting or hazardous work:
No problems expected.

Discontinuing:
May be unnecessary to finish medicine. Follow doctor's instructions.

Others:
Don't take to ''flush out'' your system or as a ''tonic.''

POSSIBLE INTERACTION WITH OTHER DRUGS

GENERIC NAME OR DRUG CLASS	COMBINED EFFECT
Laxatives, other*	Diarrhea.
Neomycin	Increased effect of both in brain changes caused by liver disease.

POSSIBLE INTERACTION WITH OTHER SUBSTANCES

INTERACTS WITH	COMBINED EFFECT
Alcohol:	None expected.
Beverages:	None expected.
Cocaine:	None expected.
Foods:	None expected.
Marijuana:	None expected.
Tobacco:	None expected.

*See Glossary

LEUCOVORIN

BRAND NAMES

Citrocovorin Calcium   Folinic Acid
Citrovorum Factor   Wellcoverin

BASIC INFORMATION

Habit forming? No
Prescription needed? Yes
Available as generic? Yes
Drug class: Antianemic

USES

- Antidote to folic acid antagonists.
- Treats anemia.

DOSAGE & USAGE INFORMATION

How to take:
- Oral solution—Take after meals with liquid to decrease stomach irritation.
- Tablets—Swallow with liquid or food to lessen stomach irritation. If you can't swallow whole, crumble tablet and take with liquid or food.

When to take:
At the same time each day, according to instructions on prescription label.

If you forget a dose:
Take as soon as you remember up to 2 hours late. If more than 2 hours, wait for next scheduled dose (don't double this dose).

What drug does:
Favors development of DNA, RNA and protein synthesis.

Time lapse before drug works:
20 to 30 minutes.

Don't take with:
Any other medicine without consulting your doctor or pharmacist.

OVERDOSE

SYMPTOMS:
Unlikely to threaten life. If overdose is suspected, follow instructions below.
WHAT TO DO:
- **Dial 0 (operator) or 911 (emergency) for an ambulance or medical help. Then give first aid immediately.**
- **See emergency information on inside covers.**

POSSIBLE ADVERSE REACTIONS OR SIDE EFFECTS

SYMPTOMS	WHAT TO DO
Life-threatening: Wheezing.	Seek emergency treatment immediately.
Common: None expected.	
Infrequent: None expected.	
Rare: Skin rash, hives.	Discontinue. Call doctor right away.

WARNINGS & PRECAUTIONS

Don't take if:
- You have pernicious anemia.
- You have vitamin B-12 deficiency.

Before you start, consult your doctor:
- If you have acid urine, acites, dehydration.
- If you have kidney function impairment.

Over age 60:
Adverse reactions and side effects may be more frequent and severe than in younger persons. You may need smaller doses for shorter periods of time.

Pregnancy:
Recommended for treatment of megaloblastic anemia caused by pregnancy.

Breast-feeding:
No problems expected.

Infants & children:
May increase frequency of seizures. Avoid if possible.

Prolonged use:
No problems expected.

Skin & sunlight:
No problems expected.

Driving, piloting or hazardous work:
Don't drive or pilot aircraft until you learn how medicine affects you. Don't work around dangerous machinery. Don't climb ladders or work in high places. Danger increases if you drink alcohol or take medicine affecting alertness and reflexes.

Discontinuing:
Don't discontinue without consulting doctor. Dose may require gradual reduction if you have taken drug for a long time. Doses of other drugs may also require adjustment.

Others:
No problems expected.

 ## POSSIBLE INTERACTION WITH OTHER DRUGS

GENERIC NAME OR DRUG CLASS	COMBINED EFFECT
Anticonvulsants, barbiturate and hydantoin*	Large doses of leucovorin may counteract the effects of these medicines.
Central nervous system (CNS) depressants*	High alcohol content of leucovorin may cause adverse effects.
Primidone	Large doses of leucovorin may counteract the effects of both drugs.

 ## POSSIBLE INTERACTION WITH OTHER SUBSTANCES

INTERACTS WITH	COMBINED EFFECT
Alcohol:	Increased adverse reactions of both.
Beverages:	None expected.
Cocaine:	Increased adverse reactions of both drugs.
Foods:	None expected.
Marijuana:	Increased adverse reactions of both drugs.
Tobacco:	Increased adverse reactions of both.

*See Glossary

LEVAMISOLE

BRAND NAMES

Ergamisol

BASIC INFORMATION

Habit forming? No
Prescription needed? Yes
Available as generic? No
Drug class: Anticancer treatment adjunct

 USES

- Treats colorectal cancer when used in combination with fluorouracil.
- Treats malignant melanoma after surgical removal when there is no evidence of spread to organs other than the skin.

 DOSAGE & USAGE INFORMATION

How to take:
Tablet—Swallow with liquid or food to lessen stomach irritation. If you can't swallow whole, crumble tablet and take with liquid or food.

When to take:
At the same time each day, according to instructions on prescription label.

If you forget a dose:
Don't take until you notify your doctor.

What drug does:
Acts to help restore the immune system. May activate T-cell lymphocytes and other white cells. Also elevates mood.

Time lapse before drug works:
1-1/2 to 2 hours.

Don't take with:
Any other medicine without consulting your doctor or pharmacist.

 OVERDOSE

SYMPTOMS:
None expected.
WHAT TO DO:
Overdose unlikely to threaten life. If person takes much larger amount than prescribed, call doctor, poison-control center or hospital emergency room for instructions.

 POSSIBLE ADVERSE REACTIONS OR SIDE EFFECTS

SYMPTOMS	WHAT TO DO
Life-threatening:	
Fever, muscle aches, headache, cough, hoarseness, sore throat, painful or difficult urination, low back or side pain.	Seek emergency treatment.
Common:	
• Diarrhea, metallic taste, nausea, joint or muscle pain, skin rash, insomnia, mental depression, night-mares, sleepiness or tiredness, increased dental problems.	Continue. Call doctor when convenient.
• Hair loss.	No action necessary.
Infrequent:	
Mouth, tongue and lip sores.	Call doctor right away.
Rare:	
Unsteady gait while walking; blurred vision; confusion; tremors; tingling or numbness in hands, feet or face; seizures; smacking and puckering of lips; uncontrolled tongue movements.	Call doctor right away.

LEVAMISOLE

 ## WARNINGS & PRECAUTIONS

Don't take if:
You are allergic to levamisole.

Before you start, consult your doctor:
- If you take other drugs for cancer.
- If you have an active infection.
- If you have a seizure disorder.
- If you have allergies to other medications.

Over age 60:
No special problems expected.

Pregnancy:
Adequate studies not yet done. Consult your doctor.

Breast-feeding:
Delay breast feeding until you no longer take levamisole.

Infants & children:
Effect not documented. Consult your family doctor or pediatrician.

Prolonged use:
No special problems expected.

Skin & sunlight:
No special problems expected.

Driving, piloting or hazardous work:
No special problems expected.

Discontinuing:
Don't discontinue without consulting doctor. Dose may require gradual reduction if you have taken drug for a long time. Doses of other drugs may also require adjustment.

Others:
- Advise any doctor or dentist whom you consult that you take this medicine.
- Defer dental treatments until your blood count is normal. Pay particular attention to dental hygiene. You may be subject to additional risk of oral infection, delayed healing and bleeding.
- Avoid aspirin. May increase risk of internal bleeding.
- Avoid constipation. May increase risk of internal bleeding.

 ## POSSIBLE INTERACTION WITH OTHER DRUGS

GENERIC NAME OR DRUG CLASS	COMBINED EFFECT
Anticoagulants*	Increased risk of bleeding.
Aspirin	Increased risk of bleeding.
Bone marrow depressants*	Increased risk of bone marrow depression.

 ## POSSIBLE INTERACTION WITH OTHER SUBSTANCES

INTERACTS WITH	COMBINED EFFECT
Alcohol:	Increased risk of gastritis and internal bleeding.
Beverages:	None expected.
Cocaine:	Increased risk of mental disturbances. Avoid.
Foods:	None expected.
Marijuana:	None expected.
Tobacco:	None expected.

*See Glossary

481

LEVOCARNITINE

BRAND NAMES

Carnitor
Vita Carn
L-Carnitine

BASIC INFORMATION

Habit forming? No
Prescription needed? Yes
Available as generic? No
Drug class: Nutritional supplement

USES

Treats carnitine deficiency, a genetic impairment preventing normal utilization from diet.

DOSAGE & USAGE INFORMATION

How to take:
- Oral solution—Take after meals with liquid to decrease stomach irritation.
- Tablets—Swallow with liquid or food to lessen stomach irritation. If you can't swallow whole, crumble tablet and take with liquid or food.

When to take:
Immediately following or during meals to reduce stomach irritation.

If you forget a dose:
Take as soon as you remember up to 2 hours late. If more than 2 hours, wait for next scheduled dose (don't double this dose).

What drug does:
Facilitates normal use of fat to produce energy. Dietary source is meat and milk.

Time lapse before drug works:
Immediate action.

Don't take with:
Any other medicine without consulting your doctor or pharmacist.

OVERDOSE

SYMPTOMS:
Severe muscle weakness.
WHAT TO DO:
- **Dial 0 (operator) or 911 (emergency) for an ambulance or medical help. Then give first aid immediately.**
- **See emergency information on inside covers.**

POSSIBLE ADVERSE REACTIONS OR SIDE EFFECTS

SYMPTOMS	WHAT TO DO
Life-threatening: None expected.	
Common: Changed body odor.	Continue. Call doctor when convenient.
Infrequent: Diarrhea, abdominal pain, nausea, vomiting.	Discontinue. Call doctor right away.
Rare: None expected.	

WARNINGS & PRECAUTIONS

Don't take if:
No contraindications.

Before you start, consult your doctor:
No documented reasons not to take.

Over age 60:
No problems expected.

Pregnancy:
No proven harm to unborn child, but avoid if possible.

Breast-feeding:
No problems expected.

Infants & children:
No problems expected. Deficiency can cause impaired growth and development.

Prolonged use:
Talk to your doctor about the need for follow-up medical examinations or laboratory studies to check triglycerides.

Skin & sunlight:
No problems expected.

Driving, piloting or hazardous work:
No problems expected.

Discontinuing:
Don't discontinue without consulting doctor. Dose may require gradual reduction if you have taken drug for a long time. Doses of other drugs may also require adjustment.

Others:
Health food store "vitamin B-T" contains dextro- and levo-carnitine which completely negates the effectiveness of levocarnitine (L-carnitine). Only the L-carnitine form is effective in levocarnitine deficiency.

POSSIBLE INTERACTION WITH OTHER DRUGS

GENERIC NAME OR DRUG CLASS	COMBINED EFFECT
Valproic acid	Decreased levocarnitine effect. Patients taking valproic acid may need to take the supplement levocarnitine.

POSSIBLE INTERACTION WITH OTHER SUBSTANCES

INTERACTS WITH	COMBINED EFFECT
Alcohol:	None expected.
Beverages:	None expected.
Cocaine:	None expected.
Foods:	None expected.
Marijuana:	None expected.
Tobacco:	None expected.

LEVODOPA

BRAND NAMES

Dopar   **Larodopa**

BASIC INFORMATION

Habit forming? No
Prescription needed? Yes
Available as generic? Yes
Drug class: Antiparkinsonism

 ## USES

Controls Parkinson's disease symptoms such as rigidity, tremor and unsteady gait.

 ## DOSAGE & USAGE INFORMATION

How to take:
Tablet or capsule—Swallow with liquid or food to lessen stomach irritation. If you can't swallow whole, crumble tablet or open capsule and take with liquid or food.

When to take:
At the same times each day.

If you forget a dose:
Take as soon as you remember up to 2 hours late. If more than 2 hours, wait for next scheduled dose (don't double this dose).

What drug does:
Restores chemical balance necessary for normal nerve impulses.

Continued next column

 ## OVERDOSE

SYMPTOMS:
Muscle twitch, spastic eyelid closure, nausea, vomiting, diarrhea, irregular and rapid pulse, weakness, fainting, confusion, agitation, hallucination, coma.
WHAT TO DO:
- **Dial 0 (operator) or 911 (emergency) for an ambulance or medical help. Then give first aid immediately.**
- **If patient is unconscious and not breathing, give mouth-to-mouth breathing. If there is no heartbeat, use cardiac massage and mouth-to-mouth breathing (CPR). Don't try to make patient vomit. If you can't get help quickly, take patient to nearest emergency facility.**
- **See emergency information on inside covers.**

Time lapse before drug works:
2 to 3 weeks to improve; 6 weeks or longer for maximum benefit.

Don't take with:
Any other medication without consulting your doctor or pharmacist.

 ## POSSIBLE ADVERSE REACTIONS OR SIDE EFFECTS

SYMPTOMS	WHAT TO DO
Life-threatening:	
In case of overdose, see previous column.	
Common:	
• Mood change, diarrhea, depression, anxiety.	Continue. Call doctor when convenient.
• Dry mouth, body odor.	No action necessary.
• Uncontrollable body movements.	Discontinue. Call doctor right away.
Infrequent:	
• Fainting, severe dizziness, headache, insomnia, nightmares, itchy skin, rash, nausea, vomiting, irregular heartbeat, eyelid spasm.	Discontinue. Call doctor right away.
• Flushed face, muscle twitching, discolored or dark urine, difficult urination, blurred vision, appetite loss.	Continue. Call doctor when convenient.
• Constipation, tiredness.	Continue. Tell doctor at next visit.
Rare:	
• High blood pressure.	Discontinue. Call doctor right away.
• Upper abdominal pain, anemia, increased sex drive.	Continue. Call doctor when convenient.

 ## WARNINGS & PRECAUTIONS

Don't take if:
- You are allergic to levodopa or carbidopa.
- You have taken MAO inhibitors in past 2 weeks.
- You have glaucoma (narrow-angle type).

Before you start, consult your doctor:
- If you have diabetes or epilepsy.
- If you have had high blood pressure, heart or lung disease.
- If you have had liver or kidney disease.
- If you have a peptic ulcer.
- If you have malignant melanoma.
- If you will have surgery within 2 months, including dental surgery, requiring general or spinal anesthesia.

Over age 60:
Adverse reactions and side effects may be more frequent and severe than in younger persons.

Pregnancy:
Risk to unborn child outweighs drug benefits. Don't use.

Breast-feeding:
Drug filters into milk. May harm child. Avoid.

Infants & children:
Not recommended.

Prolonged use:
- May lead to uncontrolled movements of head, face, mouth, tongue, arms or legs.
- Talk to your doctor about the need for follow-up medical examinations or laboratory studies to check complete blood counts (white blood cell count, platelet count, red blood cell count, hemoglobin, hematocrit), kidney function, liver function.

Skin & sunlight:
No problems expected.

Driving, piloting or hazardous work:
Don't drive or pilot aircraft until you learn how medicine affects you. Don't work around dangerous machinery. Don't climb ladders or work in high places. Danger increases if you drink alcohol or take medicine affecting alertness and reflexes, such as antihistamines, tranquilizers, sedatives, pain medicine, narcotics and mind-altering drugs.

Discontinuing:
Don't discontinue without doctor's advice until you complete prescribed dose, even though symptoms diminish or disappear.

Others:
Expect to start with small dose and increase gradually to lessen frequency and severity of adverse reactions.

POSSIBLE INTERACTION WITH OTHER DRUGS

GENERIC NAME OR DRUG CLASS	COMBINED EFFECT
Albuterol	Increased risk of heartbeat irregularity.
Antidepressants, tricyclic (TCA)*	Decreased blood pressure. Weakness and faintness when arising from bed or chair.
Anticonvulsants*	Decreased levodopa effect.
Antihypertensives*	Decreased blood pressure and levodopa effect.
Antiparkinsonism drugs, other*	Increased levodopa effect.
Guanfacine	Increased effects of both drugs.
Haloperidol	Decreased levodopa effect.
MAO inhibitors*	Dangerous rise in blood pressure.
Methyldopa	Decreased levodopa effect.
Molindone	Decreased levodopa effect.
Papaverine	Decreased levodopa effect.
Phenothiazines*	Decreased levodopa effect.
Phenytoin	Decreased levodopa effect.
Pyridoxine (Vitamin B-6)	Decreased levodopa effect.
Rauwolfia alkaloids*	Decreased levodopa effect.

POSSIBLE INTERACTION WITH OTHER SUBSTANCES

INTERACTS WITH	COMBINED EFFECT
Alcohol:	None expected.
Beverages:	None expected.
Cocaine:	Increased risk of heartbeat irregularity.
Foods: High-protein diet.	Decreased levodopa effect.
Marijuana:	Increased fatigue, lethargy, fainting.
Tobacco:	None expected.

LEVONORGESTREL

BRAND NAMES

Norplant

BASIC INFORMATION

Habit forming? No
Prescription needed? Yes
Available as generic? No
Drug class: Female sex hormone (progestin)

 USES

Highly effective long-term reversible contraceptive method.

 DOSAGE & USAGE INFORMATION

How to take:
Administered by means of implants consisting of six flexible closed capsules (about the size of matchsticks) that are inserted beneath the skin on the inside of the upper arm. Implantation is done by a health-care professional within seven days of the start of the last menstrual period. The drug slowly diffuses into the bloodstream, delivering a nearly constant level of levonorgestrel to the body for up to 5 years.

When to take:
Implanted when long-term (up to 5 years) contraception is desired.

If you forget a dose:
Not a concern.

What drug does:
Inhibits ovulation in some women so that eggs are not produced regularly. Causes the mucus of the cervix to thicken, preventing the sperm from reaching the egg if one is produced.

Time lapse before drug works:
24 hours

Don't take with:
Any other medicine without consulting your doctor or pharmacist.

 OVERDOSE

SYMPTOMS:
None expected.

 POSSIBLE ADVERSE REACTIONS OR SIDE EFFECTS

SYMPTOMS	WHAT TO DO
Life-threatening: None expected.	
Common: Increased, decreased, irregular or prolonged menstruation; spotting between periods.	Call doctor when convenient.
Infrequent: Headache, acne.	Call doctor when convenient.
Rare: • Severe bleeding, infection with pus at implant site, vaginal infection.	Call doctor right away.
• Swelling, numbness, discoloration or tenderness at implant site; breast discharge or tenderness; weight gain or loss; excess hair growth; hair loss from scalp; nausea; dizziness; muscle or abdominal pain; appetite changes; nervousness; depression.	Call doctor when convenient.

WARNINGS & PRECAUTIONS

Don't take if:
• You are allergic to any progestin hormone.
• You are or suspect you might be pregnant.
• You have liver disease or liver tumors.
• You have unexplained vaginal bleeding.
• You have breast cancer.
• You have now, or have a history of, blood clots in the legs, lungs or eyes.

Before you start, consult your doctor:
If you have a condition that could be aggravated by fluid retention.

Over age 60:
Not recommended.

Pregnancy:
If pregnancy occurs, the capsules should be removed.

Breast-feeding:
Drug passes into milk. Consult your doctor about the advisability of breast-feeding.

Infants & children:
Not recommended.

Prolonged use:
• No problems expected.
• Capsules should be removed at end of five years. New capsules may be implanted if continuing contraception is desired.

Skin & sunlight:
No problems expected.

Driving, piloting or hazardous work:
No problems expected.

Discontinuing:
• Must be removed by a health-care professional.
• May be removed at your request at any time for any reason.
• Removal should be considered if you will be immobile for a long time due to illness or surgery.

Others:
• May affect results of some medical tests.
• Does not protect against sexually transmitted diseases. For additional protection, couples may also use condoms and/or spermicidal agents.
• Fertility returns shortly after implants are removed, usually within two weeks.
• Have blood pressure checked by your doctor 3 months after implant.

POSSIBLE INTERACTION WITH OTHER DRUGS

GENERIC NAME OR DRUG CLASS	COMBINED EFFECT
Phenytoin	Decreased contraceptive effect.
Carbamazepine	Decreased contraceptive effect.
Barbiturates*	Decreased contraceptive effect.
Phenylbutazone	Decreased contraceptive effect.
Isoniazid	Decreased contraceptive effect.
Rifampin	Decreased contraceptive effect.

POSSIBLE INTERACTION WITH OTHER SUBSTANCES

INTERACTS WITH	COMBINED EFFECT
Alcohol:	None expected.
Beverages:	None expected.
Cocaine:	None expected.
Foods:	None expected.
Marijuana:	None expected.
Tobacco:	None expected, but consult doctor.

LINCOMYCIN

BRAND NAMES

Lincocin

BASIC INFORMATION

Habit forming? No
Prescription needed? Yes
Available as generic? Yes
Drug class: Antibiotic (lincomycin)

USES

Treatment of bacterial infections that are susceptible to lincomycin.

DOSAGE & USAGE INFORMATION

How to take:
Capsule—Swallow with liquid 1 hour before or 2 hours after eating.

When to take:
At the same times each day.

If you forget a dose:
Take as soon as you remember up to 2 hours late. If more than 2 hours, wait for next scheduled dose (don't double this dose).

What drug does:
Destroys susceptible bacteria. Does not kill viruses.

Time lapse before drug works:
3 to 5 days.

Don't take with:
Any other medication without consulting your doctor or pharmacist.

OVERDOSE

SYMPTOMS:
Severe nausea, vomiting, diarrhea.
WHAT TO DO:
Overdose unlikely to threaten life. If person takes much larger amount than prescribed, call doctor, poison-control center or hospital emergency room for instructions.

POSSIBLE ADVERSE REACTIONS OR SIDE EFFECTS

SYMPTOMS	WHAT TO DO
Life-threatening:	
Hives, wheezing, faintness, itching, coma.	Seek emergency treatment.
Common:	
Bloating	Discontinue. Call doctor right away.
Infrequent:	
• Unusual thirst; vomiting; stomach cramps; severe and watery diarrhea with blood or mucus; painful, swollen joints; jaundice; fever; tiredness; weakness; weight loss.	Discontinue. Call doctor right away.
• Rash; itch around groin, rectum or armpits; white patches in mouth; vaginal discharge, itching.	Continue. Call doctor when convenient.
Rare:	
Skin rash.	Discontinue. Call doctor right away.

WARNINGS & PRECAUTIONS

Don't take if:
- You are allergic to lincomycins.
- You have had ulcerative colitis.
- Prescribed for infant under 1 month old.

Before you start, consult your doctor:
- If you have had yeast infections of mouth, skin or vagina.
- If you will have surgery within 2 months, including dental surgery, requiring general or spinal anesthesia.
- If you have kidney or liver disease.
- If you have allergies of any kind.

Over age 60:
Adverse reactions and side effects may be more frequent and severe than in younger persons.

Pregnancy:
Risk to unborn child outweighs drug benefits. Don't use.

Breast-feeding:
Drug passes into milk. Avoid drug or discontinue nursing until you finish medicine. Consult doctor for advice on maintaining milk supply.

Infants & children:
Don't give to infants younger than 1 month. Use for children only under medical supervision.

Prolonged use:
- Severe colitis with diarrhea and bleeding.
- You may become more susceptible to infections caused by germs not responsive to lincomycin.
- Talk to your doctor about the need for follow-up medical examinations or laboratory studies to check proctosigmoidoscopy.

Skin & sunlight:
No problems expected.

Driving, piloting or hazardous work:
No problems expected.

Discontinuing:
Don't discontinue without doctor's advice until you complete prescribed dose, even though symptoms diminish or disappear.

Others:
May interfere with the accuracy of some medical tests.

 ## POSSIBLE INTERACTION WITH OTHER DRUGS

GENERIC NAME OR DRUG CLASS	COMBINED EFFECT
Antidiarrheal preparations*	Decreased lincomycin effect.
Attapulgite	May decrease effectiveness of lincomycin.
Chloramphenicol	Decreased lincomycin effect.
Diphenoxylate	May delay removal of toxins from colon in cases of diarrhea caused by side effects of lincomycin.
Erythromycins*	Decreased lincomycin effect.
Loperamide	May delay removal of toxins from colon in cases of diarrhea caused by side effects of lincomycin.

 ## POSSIBLE INTERACTION WITH OTHER SUBSTANCES

INTERACTS WITH	COMBINED EFFECT
Alcohol:	None expected.
Beverages:	None expected.
Cocaine:	None expected.
Foods:	None expected.
Marijuana:	None expected.
Tobacco:	None expected.

LITHIUM

BRAND NAMES

Carbolith	Lithizine
Cibalith-S	Lithobid
Duralith	Lithonate
Eskalith	Lithotabs
Eskalith CR	Pfi-Lithium
Lithane	

BASIC INFORMATION

Habit forming? No
Prescription needed? Yes
Available as generic? Yes
Drug class: Tranquilizer

USES

- Normalizes mood and behavior in manic-depressive illness.
- Treats alcohol toxicity and addiction.
- Treats schizoid personality disorders.

DOSAGE & USAGE INFORMATION

How to take:
- Tablet or capsule—Swallow with liquid or food to lessen stomach irritation. If you can't swallow whole, crumble tablet or open capsule and take with liquid or food. Drink 2 or 3 quarts liquid per day.
- Extended-release tablets—Swallow each dose whole.
- Syrup—Take at mealtime. Follow with 8 oz. water.

When to take:
At the same times each day, preferably mealtime.

If you forget a dose:
Take as soon as you remember up to 2 hours late. If more than 2 hours, wait for next scheduled dose (don't double this dose).

Continued next column

OVERDOSE

SYMPTOMS:
Moderate overdose increases some side effects and may cause diarrhea, nausea. Large overdose may cause vomiting, muscle weakness, convulsions, stupor and coma.
WHAT TO DO:
- **Dial 0 (operator) or 911 (emergency) for an ambulance or medical help. Then give first aid immediately.**
- **See emergency information on inside covers.**

What drug does:
May correct chemical imbalance in brain's transmission of nerve impulses that influence mood and behavior.

Time lapse before drug works:
1 to 3 weeks. May require 3 months before depressive phase of illness improves.

Don't take with:
Any other medication without consulting your doctor or pharmacist.

POSSIBLE ADVERSE REACTIONS OR SIDE EFFECTS

SYMPTOMS	WHAT TO DO
Life-threatening: In case of overdose, see previous column.	
Common:	
• Dizziness, diarrhea, nausea, vomiting, shakiness, tremor.	Continue. Call doctor when convenient.
• Dry mouth, thirst, decreased sexual ability, increased urination, anorexia.	Continue. Tell doctor at next visit.
Infrequent:	
• Rash, stomach pain, fainting, heartbeat irregularities, shortness of breath, ear noises.	Discontinue. Call doctor right away.
• Swollen hands, feet; slurred speech; thyroid impairment (coldness, dry, puffy skin); muscle aches; headache; weight gain; fatigue; menstrual irregularities, acne-like eruptions.	Continue. Call doctor when convenient.
• Drowsiness, confusion, weakness.	Continue. Tell doctor at next visit.
Rare:	
• Blurred vision, eye pain.	Discontinue. Call doctor right away.
• Jerking of arms and legs, worsening of psoriasis, hair loss.	Continue. Call doctor when convenient.

WARNINGS & PRECAUTIONS

Don't take if:
- You are allergic to lithium or tartrazine dye.
- You have kidney or heart disease.
- Patient is younger than 12.

Before you start, consult your doctor:
- About all medications you take.
- If you plan to become pregnant within medication period.

- If you have diabetes, low thyroid function, epilepsy or any significant medical problem.
- If you are on a low-salt diet or drink more than 4 cups of coffee per day.
- If you plan surgery within 2 months.

Over age 60:
Adverse reactions and side effects may be more frequent and severe than in younger persons.

Pregnancy:
Risk to unborn child outweighs drug benefits. Don't use.

Breast-feeding:
Drug passes into milk. Avoid drug or discontinue nursing until you finish medicine. Consult doctor for advice on maintaining milk supply.

Infants & children:
Don't give to children younger than 12.

Prolonged use:
- Enlarged thyroid with possible impaired function.
- Talk to your doctor about the need for follow-up medical examinations or laboratory studies to check lithium levels, ECG*, kidney function, thyroid, complete blood counts (white blood cell count, platelet count, red blood cell count, hemoglobin, hematocrit).

Skin & sunlight:
No problems expected.

Driving, piloting or hazardous work:
Don't drive or pilot aircraft until you learn how medicine affects you. Don't work around dangerous machinery. Don't climb ladders or work in high places. Danger increases if you drink alcohol or take medicine affecting alertness and reflexes.

Discontinuing:
Don't discontinue without consulting doctor. Dose may require gradual reduction if you have taken drug for a long time. Doses of other drugs may also require adjustment.

Others:
- Regular checkups, periodic blood tests, and tests of lithium levels and thyroid function recommended.
- Avoid exercise in hot weather and other activities that cause heavy sweating. This contributes to lithium poisoning.
- Some products contain tartrazine dye. Avoid, especially if allergic to aspirin.

POSSIBLE INTERACTION WITH OTHER DRUGS

GENERIC NAME OR DRUG CLASS	COMBINED EFFECT
Acetazolamide	Decreased lithium effect.
Antihistamines*	Possible excessive sedation.
Bupropion	Increased risk of major seizures.
Carbamazepine	Increased lithium effect.
Desmopressin	Possible decreased desmopressin effect.
Diazepam	Possible hypothermia.
Diclofenac	Possible increase in effect and toxicity.
Didanosine	Increased risk of peripheral neuropathy.
Diuretics*	Increased lithium effect.
Dronabinol	Increased effects of both drugs. Avoid.
Haloperidol	Increased toxicity of both drugs.
Indomethacin	Increased lithium effect.
Iodide salts	Increased lithium effects on thyroid function.
Ketoprofen	May increase lithium in blood.
Methyldopa	Increased lithium effect.
Molindone	Brain changes.
Muscle relaxants, skeletal*	Increased skeletal-muscle relaxation.
Nicardipine	Possible decreased lithium effect.

Continued on page 949

POSSIBLE INTERACTION WITH OTHER SUBSTANCES

INTERACTS WITH	COMBINED EFFECT
Alcohol:	Possible lithium poisoning.
Beverages: Caffeine drinks.	Decreased lithium effect.
Cocaine:	Possible psychosis.
Foods: Salt.	High intake could decrease lithium effect. Low intake could increase lithium effect. *Don't* restrict intake.
Marijuana:	Increased tremor and possible psychosis.
Tobacco:	None expected.

*See Glossary

LOMUSTINE

BRAND NAMES

CeeNU   **CCNU**

BASIC INFORMATION

Habit forming? No
Prescription needed? Yes
Available as generic? No
Drug class: Antineoplastic

 USES

- Treats brain cancer and Hodgkin's lymphoma.
- Sometimes used to treat breast, lung, skin and gastrointestinal cancer.

 DOSAGE & USAGE INFORMATION

How to take:
Capsules—Swallow with liquid. If you can't swallow whole, open capsule and take with liquid or food. Instructions to take on empty stomach mean 1 hour before or 2 hours after eating. *Note:* There may be two or more different types of capsules in the container. This is not an error.

When to take:
According to doctor's instructions. Usual course of treatment requires single dosage repeated every 6 weeks.

If you forget a dose:
Take as soon as you remember. Don't ever double doses.

What drug does:
Interferes with growth of cancer cells.

Time lapse before drug works:
None. Works immediately.

Don't take with:
Any other medicines (including over-the-counter drugs such as cough and cold medicines, laxatives, antacids, diet pills, caffeine, nose drops or vitamins) without consulting your doctor.

 OVERDOSE

SYMPTOMS:
Decreased urine (kidney failure); high fever, chills (infection); bloody or black stools (bleeding).
WHAT TO DO:
- **Dial 0 (operator) or 911 (emergency) for an ambulance or medical help. Then give first aid immediately.**
- **See emergency information on inside covers.**

 POSSIBLE ADVERSE REACTIONS OR SIDE EFFECTS

SYMPTOMS	WHAT TO DO
Life-threatening:	
In case of overdose, see previous column.	
Common:	
• Fever, chills, difficult urination, unusual bleeding.	Continue. Call doctor when convenient.
• Appetite loss, nausea, hair loss.	No action necessary.
Infrequent:	
• Anemia, confusion, slurred speech, mouth sores, skin rash.	Continue. Call doctor when convenient.
• Darkened skin.	No action necessary.
Rare:	
• Jaundice (yellow skin and eyes), cough.	Continue. Call doctor when convenient.
• Shortness of breath.	Discontinue. Call doctor right away.

WARNINGS & PRECAUTIONS

Don't take if:
- You have chicken pox.
- You have shingles (herpes zoster).

Before you start, consult your doctor:
- If you have an infection.
- If you have kidney disease.
- If you have had previous cancer chemotherapy or radiation treatment.

Over age 60:
Adverse reactions and side effects may be more frequent and severe than in younger persons. You may need smaller doses for shorter periods of time.

Pregnancy:
Risk to unborn child outweighs drug benefits. Don't use.

Breast-feeding:
Drug passes into milk. Avoid drug or discontinue nursing until you finish medicine. Consult doctor for advice on maintaining milk supply.

Infants & children:
Effect not documented. Consult your doctor.

Prolonged use:
Talk to your doctor about the need for follow-up medical examinations or laboratory studies to check kidney function, liver function and complete blood counts (white blood cell count, platelet count, red blood cell count, hemoglobin, hematocrit).

Skin & sunlight:
No problems expected.

Driving, piloting or hazardous work:
Don't drive or pilot aircraft until you learn how medicine affects you. Don't work around dangerous machinery. Don't climb ladders or work in high places. Danger increases if you drink alcohol or take medicine affecting alertness and reflexes.

Discontinuing:
Call doctor if any of these occur after discontinuing: black or tarry stools, bloody urine, hoarseness, bleeding or bruising, fever or chills.

Others:
- Advise any doctor or dentist whom you consult that you take this medicine.
- May affect results in some medical tests.
- Most adverse reactions and side effects are unavoidable.
- Avoid immunizations, if possible.
- Avoid persons with infections.
- Check with doctor about brushing or flossing teeth.
- Avoid contact sports.

POSSIBLE INTERACTION WITH OTHER DRUGS

GENERIC NAME OR DRUG CLASS	COMBINED EFFECT
Antineoplastic drugs, other*	Increased chance of drug toxicity.
Blood dyscrasia-causing medicines*	Adverse effect on bone marrow, causing decreased white cells and platelets.
Clozapine	Toxic effect on bone marrow.
Levamisole	Increased risk of bone marrow depression.
Tiopronin	Increased risk of toxicity to bone marrow.
Vaccines, live or killed virus	Increased chance of toxicity or reduced effectiveness of vaccine. Wait 3 to 12 months after lomustine treatment before getting vaccination.

POSSIBLE INTERACTION WITH OTHER SUBSTANCES

INTERACTS WITH	COMBINED EFFECT
Alcohol:	Increased chance of liver damage.
Beverages:	No special problems expected.
Cocaine:	Increased chance of central nervous system toxicity.
Foods:	No special problems expected.
Marijuana:	No special problems expected.
Tobacco:	No special problems expected.

*See Glossary

LOPERAMIDE

BRAND NAMES

Imodium   Imodium A-D

BASIC INFORMATION

**Habit forming? No, unless taken in high
doses for long periods.
Prescription needed? No
Available as generic? Yes
Drug class: Antidiarrheal**

 ## USES

Relieves diarrhea and reduces volume of
discharge from ileostomies and colostomies.

 ## DOSAGE & USAGE INFORMATION

How to take:
- Capsule—Swallow with food to lessen
  stomach irritation.
- Liquid—Follow label instructions and use
  marked dropper.

When to take:
No more often than directed on label.

If you forget a dose:
Take as soon as you remember up to 2 hours
late. If more than 2 hours, wait for next
scheduled dose (don't double this dose).

What drug does:
Blocks digestive tract's nerve supply, which
reduces irritability and contractions in intestinal
tract.

Time lapse before drug works:
1 to 2 hours.

Don't take with:
Any other medication without consulting your
doctor or pharmacist.

 ## OVERDOSE

**SYMPTOMS:
Constipation, lethargy, drowsiness or
unconsciousness.
WHAT TO DO:
Overdose unlikely to threaten life. If person
takes much larger amount than prescribed,
call doctor, poison-control center or
hospital emergency room for instructions.**

 ## POSSIBLE ADVERSE REACTIONS OR SIDE EFFECTS

SYMPTOMS	WHAT TO DO
Life-threatening:	
Unconsciousness.	Seek emergency treatment.
Common:	
None expected.	
Infrequent:	
• Rash.	Discontinue. Call doctor right away.
• Drowsiness, dizziness, dry mouth, bloating, constipation, appetite loss, abdominal pain.	Continue. Call doctor when convenient.
Rare:	
Unexplained fever, nausea, vomiting.	Discontinue. Call doctor right away.

WARNINGS & PRECAUTIONS

Don't take if:
- You have severe colitis.
- You have colitis resulting from antibiotic treatment or infection.

Before you start, consult your doctor:
- If you are dehydrated from fluid loss caused by diarrhea.
- If you have liver disease.

Over age 60:
Adverse reactions and side effects may be more frequent and severe than in younger persons.

Pregnancy:
No proven harm. Avoid if possible.

Breast-feeding:
No proven problems, but avoid if possible or discontinue nursing until you finish medicine. Consult doctor for advice on maintaining milk supply.

Infants & children:
Don't give to infants or toddlers. Use only under doctor's supervision for children older than 2.

Prolonged use:
Habit forming at high dose.

Skin & sunlight:
No problems expected.

Driving, piloting or hazardous work:
Don't drive or pilot aircraft until you learn how medicine affects you. Don't work around dangerous machinery. Don't climb ladders or work in high places. Danger increases if you drink alcohol or take medicine affecting alertness and reflexes.

Discontinuing:
- May be unnecessary to finish medicine. Follow doctor's instructions.
- After discontinuing, consult doctor if you experience muscle cramps, nausea, vomiting, trembling, stomach cramps or unusual sweating.

Others:
If acute diarrhea lasts longer than 48 hours, discontinue and call doctor. In chronic diarrhea, loperamide is unlikely to be effective if diarrhea doesn't improve in 10 days.

POSSIBLE INTERACTION WITH OTHER DRUGS

GENERIC NAME OR DRUG CLASS	COMBINED EFFECT
Antibiotics* **(cephalosporins, clindamycin, lincomycins, penicillins)**	May delay removal of toxins from colon in cases of diarrhea caused by side effects of these antibiotics.

POSSIBLE INTERACTION WITH OTHER SUBSTANCES

INTERACTS WITH	COMBINED EFFECT
Alcohol:	Depressed brain function. Avoid.
Beverages:	None expected.
Cocaine:	Decreased loperamide effect.
Foods:	None expected.
Marijuana:	None expected.
Tobacco:	None expected.

LOXAPINE

BRAND NAMES

Loxapac
Loxitane

Loxitane C
Loxitane IM

BASIC INFORMATION

Habit forming? No
Prescription needed? Yes
Available as generic? No
Drug class: Tranquilizer, antidepressant

 USES

- Treats serious mental illness.
- Treats anxiety and depression.

 DOSAGE & USAGE INFORMATION

How to take:
- Oral solution—Take after meals with liquid to decrease stomach irritation.
- Tablets—Swallow with liquid or food to lessen stomach irritation. If you can't swallow whole, crumble tablet and take with liquid or food.
- Capsules—Swallow with liquid or food to lessen stomach irritation. If you can't swallow whole, open capsule and take with liquid or food.

When to take:
At the same time each day, according to instructions on prescription label.

If you forget a dose:
Take as soon as you remember up to 2 hours late. If more than 2 hours, wait for next scheduled dose (don't double this dose).

What drug does:
Probably blocks the effects of dopamine in the brain.

Time lapse before drug works:
1/2 to 3 hours.

Don't take with:
Any other medicine without consulting your doctor or pharmacist.

 OVERDOSE

SYMPTOMS:
Dizziness, drowsiness, severe shortness of breath, muscle spasms, coma.
WHAT TO DO:
- **Dial 0 (operator) or 911 (emergency) for an ambulance or medical help. Then give first aid immediately.**
  See emergency information on inside covers.

 POSSIBLE ADVERSE REACTIONS OR SIDE EFFECTS

SYMPTOMS	WHAT TO DO
Life-threatening:	
Severe shortness of breath, skin rash, heartbeat irregularities, profuse sweating, fever, convulsions (rare).	Seek emergency treatment immediately.
Common:	
• Increased dental problems because of dry mouth and less salivation.	Consult your dentist about a prevention program.
• Swallowing difficulty, face expressionless, arms and legs stiff, dizziness.	Discontinue. Call doctor right away.
Infrequent:	
• Chewing movements with lip smacking, loss of balance, shuffling walk, tremor of fingers and hands, uncontrolled tongue movements.	Discontinue. Call doctor right away.
• Constipation, difficult urination, blurred vision, confusion, loss of sex drive, headache, insomnia, menstrual irregularities, weight gain, light sensitivity, nausea.	Continue. Call doctor when convenient.
Rare:	
Rapid heartbeat, fever, sore throat, jaundice, unusual bleeding.	Discontinue. Call doctor right away.

 WARNINGS & PRECAUTIONS

Don't take if:
- You are an alcoholic.
- You have liver disease.

Before you start, consult your doctor:
- If you have a seizure disorder.
- If you have an enlarged prostate, glaucoma, Parkinson's disease, heart disease.

Over age 60:
Adverse reactions and side effects may be more frequent and severe than in younger persons. You may need smaller doses for shorter periods of time.

Pregnancy:
Risk to unborn child outweighs drug benefits. Don't use.

Breast-feeding:
Drug passes into milk. Avoid drug or discontinue nursing until you finish medicine. Consult doctor for advice on maintaining milk supply.

Infants & children:
Not recommended.

Prolonged use:
Talk to your doctor about the need for follow-up medical examinations or laboratory studies to check complete blood counts (white blood cell count, platelet count, red blood cell count, hemoglobin, hematocrit), liver function, eyes.

Skin & sunlight:
Increased sensitivity to sunlight.

Driving, piloting or hazardous work:
Don't drive or pilot aircraft until you learn how medicine affects you. Don't work around dangerous machinery. Don't climb ladders or work in high places. Danger increases if you drink alcohol or take medicine affecting alertness and reflexes.

Discontinuing:
- Don't discontinue without consulting doctor. Dose may require gradual reduction if you have taken drug for a long time. Doses of other drugs may also require adjustment.
- These symptoms may occur after medicine has been discontinued: dizziness; nausea; abdominal pain; uncontrolled movements of mouth, tongue and jaw.

Others:
Use careful oral hygiene.

 POSSIBLE INTERACTION WITH OTHER DRUGS

GENERIC NAME OR DRUG CLASS	COMBINED EFFECT
Anticonvulsants*	Decreased effect of anticonvulsants.
Antidepressants, tricyclic (TCA)*	May increase toxic effects of both drugs.
Bupropion	Increased risk of major seizures.
Central nervous system (CNS) depressants*	Increased sedative effect of both drugs.
Clozapine	Toxic effect on the central nervous system.
Epinephrine	Rapid heart rate and severe drop in blood pressure.
Ethinamate	Dangerous increased effects of ethinamate. Avoid combining.
Fluoxetine	Increased depressant effects of both drugs.
Guanadrel	Decreased effect of guanadrel.
Guanethidine	Decreased effect of guanethidine.
Guanfacine	Increased effect of both drugs.
Haloperidol	May increase toxic effects of both drugs.
Leucovorin	High alcohol content of leucovorin may cause adverse effects.
Methyldopa	May increase toxic effects of both drugs.
Methyprylon	Increased sedative effect, perhaps to dangerous level. Avoid.
Metoclopramide	May increase toxic effects of both drugs.
Metyrosine	May increase toxic effects of both drugs.
Molindone	May increase toxic effects of both drugs.
Nabilone	Greater depression of central nervous system.
Pemoline	May increase toxic effects of both drugs.
Pergolide	Decreased pergolide effect.
Phenothiazines*	May increase toxic effects of both drugs.
Pimozide	May increase toxic effects of both drugs.
Rauwolfia	May increase toxic effects of both drugs.
Sertraline	Increased depressive effects of both drugs.
Thioxanthenes*	May increase toxic effects of both drugs.

 POSSIBLE INTERACTION WITH OTHER SUBSTANCES

INTERACTS WITH	COMBINED EFFECT
Alcohol:	May decrease effect of loxapine. Avoid.
Beverages:	None expected.
Cocaine:	May increase toxicity of both drugs. Avoid.
Foods:	None expected.
Marijuana:	May increase toxicity of both drugs. Avoid
Tobacco:	May increase toxici of both drugs. Avo

MAGNESIUM CITRATE

BRAND NAMES

Citrate of Magnesia   Citro-Nesia
Citro-Mag   Citroma

BASIC INFORMATION

Habit forming? No
Prescription needed? No
Available as generic? Yes
Drug class: Laxative (hyperosmotic)

 ## USES

Constipation relief.

 ## DOSAGE & USAGE INFORMATION

How to take:
Liquid—Dilute dose in beverage before swallowing.

When to take:
Usually once a day, preferably in the morning.

If you forget a dose:
Take as soon as you remember up to 8 hours before bedtime. If later, wait for next scheduled dose (don't double this dose). Don't take at bedtime.

What drug does:
Draws water into bowel from other body tissues. Causes distention through fluid accumulation, which promotes soft stool and accelerates bowel motion.

Time lapse before drug works:
30 minutes to 3 hours.

Don't take with:
Any other medicine without consulting your doctor or pharmacist.

 ## OVERDOSE

SYMPTOMS:
Fluid depletion, weakness, vomiting, fainting.
WHAT TO DO:
- Dial O (operator) or 911 (emergency) for an ambulance or medical help. Then give first aid immediately.
- See emergency information on inside cover.

 ## POSSIBLE ADVERSE REACTIONS OR SIDE EFFECTS

SYMPTOMS	WHAT TO DO
Life-threatening: In case of overdose, see previous column.	
Common: None expected.	
Infrequent:	
• Irregular heartbeat.	Discontinue. Call doctor right away.
• Increased thirst, cramps, nausea, diarrhea, gaseousness.	Continue. Tell doctor at next visit.
Rare: Dizziness, confusion, tiredness or weakness.	Continue. Call doctor when convenient.

WARNINGS & PRECAUTIONS

Don't take if:
- You are allergic to any hyperosmotic laxative.
- You have symptoms of appendicitis, inflamed bowel or intestinal blockage.
- You have missed a bowel movement for only 1 or 2 days.

Before you start, consult your doctor:
- If you have congestive heart disease.
- If you have diabetes.
- If you have high blood pressure.
- If you have a colostomy or ileostomy.
- If you have kidney disease.
- If you have a laxative habit.
- If you have rectal bleeding.
- If you take another laxative.

Over age 60:
Adverse reactions and side effects may be more frequent and severe than in younger persons.

Pregnancy:
Salt content may cause fluid retention and swelling. Avoid if possible.

Breast-feeding:
No problems expected.

Infants & children:
Use only under medical supervision.

Prolonged use:
Don't take for more than 1 week unless under a doctor's supervision. May cause laxative dependence.

Skin & sunlight:
No problems expected.

Driving, piloting or hazardous work:
No problems expected.

Discontinuing:
May be unnecessary to finish medicine. Follow doctor's instructions.

Others:
- Don't take to "flush out" your system or as a "tonic."
- Don't take within 2 hours of taking another medicine.

POSSIBLE INTERACTION WITH OTHER DRUGS

GENERIC NAME OR DRUG CLASS	COMBINED EFFECT
Antidepressants, tricyclic (TCA)*	Decreased TCA effect.
Chlordiazepoxide	Decreased chlordiazepoxide effect.
Chlorpromazine	Decreased chlorpromazine effect.
Dicumarol	Decreased dicumarol effect.
Digoxin	Decreased digoxin effect.
Isoniazid	Decreased isoniazid effect.
Mexiletine	May slow elimination of mexiletine and cause need to adjust dosage.
Tetracyclines*	Possible intestinal blockage.

POSSIBLE INTERACTION WITH OTHER SUBSTANCES

INTERACTS WITH	COMBINED EFFECT
Alcohol:	None expected.
Beverages:	None expected.
Cocaine:	None expected.
Foods:	None expected.
Marijuana:	None expected.
Tobacco:	None expected.

MAGNESIUM SULFATE

BRAND NAMES

Bilagog   **Epsom Salts**

BASIC INFORMATION

Habit forming? No
Prescription needed? No
Available as generic? Yes
Drug class: Laxative (hyperosmotic)

 ## USES

Constipation relief.

 ## DOSAGE & USAGE INFORMATION

How to take:
- Tablet—Swallow with liquid.
- Powder or solid form—Dilute dose in beverage before swallowing. Solid form must be dissolved.

When to take:
Usually once a day, preferably in the morning.

If you forget a dose:
Take as soon as you remember up to 8 hours before bedtime. If later, wait for next scheduled dose (don't double this dose). Don't take at bedtime.

What drug does:
Draws water into bowel from other body tissues. Causes distention through fluid accumulation, which promotes soft stool and accelerates bowel motion.

Time lapse before drug works:
30 minutes to 3 hours.

Don't take with:
Any other medicine without consulting your doctor or pharmacist.

 ## OVERDOSE

SYMPTOMS:
Fluid depletion, weakness, vomiting, fainting.
WHAT TO DO:
- **Dial O (operator) or 911 (emergency) for an ambulance or medical help. Then give first aid immediately.**
- **See emergency information on inside cover.**

 ## POSSIBLE ADVERSE REACTIONS OR SIDE EFFECTS

SYMPTOMS	WHAT TO DO
Life-threatening:	
In case of overdose, see previous column.	
Common:	
Nausea.	Continue. Call doctor when convenient.
Infrequent:	
• Irregular heartbeat.	Discontinue. Call doctor right away.
• Increased thirst, cramps, diarrhea, gaseousness.	Continue. Tell doctor at next visit.
Rare:	
Dizziness, confusion, tiredness or weakness.	Continue. Call doctor when convenient.

MAGNESIUM SULFATE

WARNINGS & PRECAUTIONS

Don't take if:
- You are allergic to any hyperosmotic laxative.
- You have symptoms of appendicitis, inflamed bowel or intestinal blockage.
- You have missed a bowel movement for only 1 or 2 days.

Before you start, consult your doctor:
- If you have congestive heart disease.
- If you have diabetes.
- If you have high blood pressure.
- If you have a colostomy or ileostomy.
- If you have kidney disease.
- If you have a laxative habit.
- If you have rectal bleeding.
- If you take another laxative.

Over age 60:
Adverse reactions and side effects may be more frequent and severe than in younger persons.

Pregnancy:
Salt content may cause fluid retention and swelling. Avoid if possible.

Breast-feeding:
No problems expected.

Infants & children:
Use only under medical supervision.

Prolonged use:
Don't take for more than 1 week unless under a doctor's supervision. May cause laxative dependence.

Skin & sunlight:
No problems expected.

Driving, piloting or hazardous work:
No problems expected.

Discontinuing:
May be unnecessary to finish medicine. Follow doctor's instructions.

Others:
- Don't take to "flush out" your system or as a "tonic."
- Don't take within 2 hours of taking another medicine.

POSSIBLE INTERACTION WITH OTHER DRUGS

GENERIC NAME OR DRUG CLASS	COMBINED EFFECT
Antidepressants, tricyclic (TCA)*	Decreased antidepressant effect.
Chlordiazepoxide	Decreased chlordiazepoxide effect.
Chlorpromazine	Decreased chlorpromazine effect.
Clozapine	Toxic effect on the central nervous system.
Dicumarol	Decreased dicumarol effect.
Digoxin	Decreased digoxin effect.
Isoniazid	Decreased isoniazid effect.
Mexiletine	May slow elimination of mexiletine and cause need to adjust dosage.
Propafenone	Increased effect of both drugs and increased risk of toxicity.
Tetracyclines*	Possible intestinal blockage.

POSSIBLE INTERACTION WITH OTHER SUBSTANCES

INTERACTS WITH	COMBINED EFFECT
Alcohol:	None expected.
Beverages:	None expected.
Cocaine:	None expected.
Foods:	None expected.
Marijuana:	None expected.
Tobacco:	None expected.

MALT SOUP EXTRACT

BRAND NAMES

Maltsupex

BASIC INFORMATION

Habit forming? No
Prescription needed? No
Available as generic? No
Drug class: Laxative (bulk-forming)

 USES

Relieves constipation and prevents straining for bowel movement.

 DOSAGE & USAGE INFORMATION

How to take:
- Liquid or powder—Dilute dose in 8 oz. cold water or fruit juice.
- Tablets—Swallow with 8 oz. cold liquid. Drink 6 to 8 glasses of water each day in addition to the one with each dose.

When to take:
At the same time each day, preferably morning.

If you forget a dose:
Take as soon as you remember. Resume regular schedule.

What drug does:
Absorbs water, stimulating the bowel to form a soft, bulky stool.

Time lapse before drug works:
May require 2 or 3 days to begin, then works in 12 to 24 hours.

Don't take with:
- Don't take within 2 hours of taking another medicine.
- Any other medicine without consulting your doctor or pharmacist.

 OVERDOSE

SYMPTOMS:
Wheezing.
WHAT TO DO:
Overdose unlikely to threaten life. If person takes much larger amount than prescribed, call doctor, poison-control center or hospital emergency room for instructions.

 POSSIBLE ADVERSE REACTIONS OR SIDE EFFECTS

SYMPTOMS	WHAT TO DO
Life-threatening: None expected.	
Common: None expected.	
Infrequent: Swallowing difficulty, "lump in throat" sensation, nausea, vomiting, diarrhea.	Continue. Call doctor when convenient.
Rare: Itchy skin, rash, asthma, intestinal blockage.	Discontinue. Call doctor right away.

WARNINGS & PRECAUTIONS

Don't take if:
- You are allergic to any bulk-forming laxative.
- You have symptoms of appendicitis, inflamed bowel or intestinal blockage.
- You have missed a bowel movement for only 1 or 2 days.

Before you start, consult your doctor:
- If you have diabetes.
- If you have a laxative habit.
- If you have rectal bleeding.
- If you have difficulty swallowing.
- If you take other laxatives.

Over age 60:
Adverse reactions and side effects may be more frequent and severe than in younger persons.

Pregnancy:
Most bulk-forming laxatives contain sodium or sugars which may cause fluid retention. Avoid if possible.

Breast-feeding:
No problems expected.

Infants & children:
Use only under medical supervision.

Prolonged use:
Don't take for more than 1 week unless under a doctor's supervision. May cause laxative dependence.

Skin & sunlight:
No problems expected.

Driving, piloting or hazardous work:
No problems expected.

Discontinuing:
May be unnecessary to finish medicine. Follow doctor's instructions.

Others:
Don't take to "flush out" your system or as a "tonic."

POSSIBLE INTERACTION WITH OTHER DRUGS

GENERIC NAME OR DRUG CLASS	COMBINED EFFECT
Antibiotics*	Possible decreased antibiotic effect.
Digitalis preparations*	Decreased digitalis effect.
Salicylates* (including aspirin)	Decreased salicylate effect.

POSSIBLE INTERACTION WITH OTHER SUBSTANCES

INTERACTS WITH	COMBINED EFFECT
Alcohol:	None expected.
Beverages:	None expected.
Cocaine:	None expected.
Foods:	None expected.
Marijuana:	None expected.
Tobacco:	None expected.

*See Glossary

MAPROTILINE

BRAND NAMES

Ludiomil

BASIC INFORMATION

Habit forming? No
Prescription needed? Yes
Available as generic? Yes
Drug class: Antidepressant

 ## USES

Treatment for depression or anxiety associated
with depression.

 ## DOSAGE & USAGE INFORMATION

How to take:
Tablet—Swallow with liquid.

When to take:
At the same time each day, usually bedtime.

If you forget a dose:
Bedtime dose—If you forget your once-a-day
bedtime dose, don't take it more than 3 hours
late. If more than 3 hours, wait for next
scheduled dose. Don't double this dose.

What drug does:
Probably affects part of brain that controls
messages between nerve cells.

Time lapse before drug works:
Begins in 1 to 2 weeks. May require 4 to 6
weeks for maximum benefit.

Don't take with:
- Non-prescription drugs without consulting
  doctor.
- See Interaction column and consult doctor.

 ## OVERDOSE

SYMPTOMS:
**Respiratory failure, fever, cardiac arrhythmia,
muscle stiffness, drowsiness, hallucinations, convulsions, coma.**
WHAT TO DO:
- **Dial 0 (operator) or 911 (emergency) for
  an ambulance or medical help. Then give
  first aid immediately.**
- **If patient is unconscious and not
  breathing, give mouth-to-mouth breathing.
  If there is no heartbeat, use cardiac
  massage and mouth-to-mouth breathing
  (CPR). Don't try to make patient vomit. If
  you can't get help quickly, take patient to
  nearest emergency facility.**
- **See emergency information on inside covers.**

 ## POSSIBLE ADVERSE REACTIONS OR SIDE EFFECTS

SYMPTOMS	WHAT TO DO
Life-threatening:	
Seizures.	Seek emergency treatment immediately.
Common:	
• Tremor.	Discontinue. Call doctor right away.
• Headache, dry mouth or unpleasant taste, constipation or diarrhea, nausea, indigestion, fatigue, weakness, drowsiness, nervousness, anxiety, excessive sweating.	Continue. Call doctor when convenient.
• Insomnia, craving sweets.	Continue. Tell doctor at next visit.
Infrequent:	
• Convulsions.	Discontinue. Seek emergency treatment.
• Hallucinations, shakiness, dizziness, fainting, blurred vision, eye pain, vomiting, irregular heartbeat or slow pulse, inflamed tongue, abdominal pain, jaundice, hair loss, rash, chills, joint pain, palpitations, hiccups, vision changes.	Discontinue. Call doctor right away.
• Painful or difficult urination; fatigue; decreased sex drive; abnormal dreams; nasal congestion; back pain; muscle aches; frequent urination; painful, absent or irregular menstruation.	Continue. Call doctor when convenient.
Rare:	
Itchy skin; sore throat; jaundice; fever; involuntary movements of jaw, lips and tongue; nightmares; confusion; swollen breasts in men.	Discontinue. Call doctor right away.

WARNINGS & PRECAUTIONS

Don't take if:
- You are allergic to any tricyclic antidepressant.
- You drink alcohol.
- You have had a heart attack within 6 weeks.
- You have glaucoma.
- You have taken MAO inhibitors within 2 weeks.
- Patient is younger than 12.

Before you start, consult your doctor:
- If you will have surgery within 2 months, including dental surgery, requiring general or spinal anesthesia.
- If you have an enlarged prostate, heart disease or high blood pressure, stomach or intestinal problems, overactive thyroid, asthma, liver disease.

Over age 60:
More likely to develop urination difficulty and side effects such as hallucinations, shakiness, dizziness, fainting, headache or insomnia.

Pregnancy:
Studies inconclusive on harm to unborn child. Animal studies show fetal abnormalities. Decide with your doctor whether drug benefits justify risk to unborn child.

Breast-feeding:
Drug passes into milk. Avoid drug or discontinue nursing until you finish medicine. Consult doctor for advice on maintaining milk supply.

Infants & children:
Don't give to children younger than 12.

Prolonged use:
Request blood cell counts, liver-function studies, monitor blood pressure closely.

Skin & sunlight:
May cause rash or intensify sunburn in areas exposed to sun or sunlamp.

Driving, piloting or hazardous work:
Don't drive or pilot aircraft until you learn how medicine affects you. Don't work around dangerous machinery. Don't climb ladders or work in high places. Danger increases if you drink alcohol or take medicine affecting alertness and reflexes.

Discontinuing:
Don't discontinue without consulting doctor. Dose may require gradual reduction if you have taken drug for a long time. Doses of other drugs may also require adjustment.

Others:
No problems expected.

POSSIBLE INTERACTION WITH OTHER DRUGS

GENERIC NAME OR DRUG CLASS	COMBINED EFFECT
Anticoagulants*	Increased anticoagulant effect.
Anticholinergics*	Increased sedation.
Antihistamines*	Increased antihistamine effect.
Barbiturates*	Decreased anti-depressant effect.
Benzodiazepine	Increased sedation.
Central nervous system (CNS) depressants*	Increased sedation.
Cimetidine	Possible increased antidepressant effect and toxicity.
Clonidine	Decreased clonidine effect.
Clozapine	Toxic effect on the central nervous system.
Disulfiram	Delirium.
Diuretics, thiazide*	Increased maprotiline effect.
Ethchlorvynol	Delirium.
Ethinamate	Dangerous increased effects of ethinamate. Avoid combining.

Continued page 949

POSSIBLE INTERACTION WITH OTHER SUBSTANCES

INTERACTS WITH	COMBINED EFFECT
Alcohol: Beverages or medicines with alcohol.	Excessive intoxication. Avoid.
Beverages:	None expected.
Cocaine:	Excessive intoxication. Avoid.
Foods:	None expected.
Marijuana:	Excessive drowsiness. Avoid.
Tobacco:	May decrease absorption of maprotiline. Avoid.

MEBENDAZOLE

BRAND NAMES

Mebendacin   Nemasole
Mebutar   Vermox

BASIC INFORMATION

Habit forming? No
Prescription needed? Yes
Available as generic? No
Drug class: Antihelminthic

 USES

Treatment of roundworms, pinworms, whipworms, hookworms and other intestinal parasites.

 DOSAGE & USAGE INFORMATION

How to take:
Chewable tablets—May be chewed, swallowed whole or mixed with food.

When to take:
Morning and evening with food to increase uptake.

If you forget a dose:
Skip dose and begin treatment again.

What drug does:
Kills parasites by blocking their uptake of glucose.

Time lapse before drug works:
2 to 5 hours.

Don't take with:
Any other medicine without consulting your doctor or pharmacist.

 OVERDOSE

SYMPTOMS:
None expected.
WHAT TO DO:
Overdose unlikely to threaten life.

 POSSIBLE ADVERSE REACTIONS OR SIDE EFFECTS

SYMPTOMS	WHAT TO DO
Life-threatening: None expected.	
Common: None expected.	
Infrequent: Abdominal pain, diarrhea, dizziness, fever, nausea.	Continue. Call doctor when convenient.
Rare: Skin rash, itching, sore throat and fever, weakness (severe), hair loss, headache.	Discontinue. Call doctor right away.

WARNINGS & PRECAUTIONS

Don't take if:
- You have Crohn's disease.
- You have ulcerative colitis.

Before you start, consult your doctor:
If you have liver disease.

Over age 60:
Adverse reactions and side effects may be more frequent and severe than in younger persons. You may need smaller doses for shorter periods of time.

Pregnancy:
High dose may cause slight maternal toxicity. Avoid if possible.

Breast-feeding:
No problems expected.

Infants & children:
No problems expected.

Prolonged use:
- Not intended for long-term use.
- Talk to your doctor about the need for follow-up medical examinations or laboratory studies to check stools, cellophane tape swabs pressed against rectal area to check for parasite eggs, complete blood counts (white blood cell count, platelet count, red blood cell count, hemoglobin, hematocrit).

Skin & sunlight:
No problems expected.

Driving, piloting or hazardous work:
No problems expected.

Discontinuing:
No problems expected.

Others:
- Take full course of treatment. Repeat course may be necessary if follow-up examinations reveal persistent infection.
- Wash all bedding after treatment to prevent re-infection.

POSSIBLE INTERACTION WITH OTHER DRUGS

GENERIC NAME OR DRUG CLASS	COMBINED EFFECT
Carbamazapine	Decreased effect of mebendazole.

POSSIBLE INTERACTION WITH OTHER SUBSTANCES

INTERACTS WITH	COMBINED EFFECT
Alcohol:	Decreased mebendazole effect. Avoid.
Beverages:	None expected.
Cocaine:	None expected.
Foods:	None expected.
Marijuana:	None expected.
Tobacco:	None expected.

MECAMYLAMINE

BRAND NAMES

Inversine

BASIC INFORMATION

Habit forming? No
Prescription needed? Yes
Available as generic? No
Drug class: Antihypertensive

 USES

Helps control, but doesn't cure, high blood pressure.

 DOSAGE & USAGE INFORMATION

How to take:
Tablets—Swallow with liquid. If you can't swallow whole, crumble tablet and take with liquid or food. Instructions to take on empty stomach mean 1 hour before or 2 hours after eating.

When to take:
- At the same time each day, according to instructions on prescription label.
- Usually twice a day, every 8 or 12 hours apart. Follow label directions.

If you forget a dose:
Take as soon as you remember up to 2 hours late. If more than 2 hours, wait for next scheduled dose (don't double this dose).

What drug does:
Blocks transmission of electrical impulse where two nerve cells connect. Causes constricted blood vessels to relax.

Time lapse before drug works:
30 minutes to 2 hours.

Don't take with:
Any other medicines (including over-the-counter drugs such as cough and cold medicines, laxatives, antacids, diet pills, caffeine, nose drops or vitamins) without consulting your doctor.

 OVERDOSE

SYMPTOMS:
Confusion, excitement, seizures, coma.
WHAT TO DO:
- Dial 0 (operator) or 911 (emergency) for an ambulance or medical help. Then give first aid immediately.
- See emergency information on inside covers.

 POSSIBLE ADVERSE REACTIONS OR SIDE EFFECTS

SYMPTOMS	WHAT TO DO
Life-threatening:	
In case of overdose, see previous column.	
Common:	
Dizziness upon arising from chair or bed, blurred vision, decreased sex drive, dry mouth, enlarged pupils, constipation.	Continue. Call doctor when convenient.
Infrequent:	
• Confusion, depression, tremors, shortness of breath.	Discontinue. Call doctor right away.
• Difficult urination, tiredness.	Continue. Tell doctor at next visit.
Rare:	
Appetite loss, nausea and vomiting.	Continue. Tell doctor at next visit.

WARNINGS & PRECAUTIONS

Don't take if:
You are allergic to mecamylamine.

Before you start, consult your doctor:
- If you have heart disease.
- If you had a recent heart attack.
- If you have glaucoma or gout.
- If you have kidney disease.

Over age 60:
Adverse reactions and side effects may be more frequent and severe than in younger persons. You may need smaller doses for shorter periods of time.

Pregnancy:
Risk to unborn child outweighs drug benefits. Don't use.

Breast-feeding:
Drug passes into milk. Avoid drug or discontinue nursing until you finish medicine. Consult doctor for advice on maintaining milk supply.

Infants & children:
Effect not documented. Consult your pediatrician.

Prolonged use:
Talk to your doctor about the need for follow-up medical examinations or laboratory studies to check blood pressure, kidney function and heart function.

Skin & sunlight:
No problems expected.

Driving, piloting or hazardous work:
Avoid if you feel confused, drowsy or dizzy.

Discontinuing:
Don't discontinue without consulting doctor. Dose may require gradual reduction if you have taken drug for a long time. Doses of other drugs may also require adjustment.

Others:
- Advise any doctor or dentist whom you consult that you take this medicine.
- May affect results in some medical tests.
- Get up slowly from chair or bed.
- Dosage may need to be adjusted for hot weather or heavy exercise.

POSSIBLE INTERACTION WITH OTHER DRUGS

GENERIC NAME OR DRUG CLASS	COMBINED EFFECT
Ambenonium	Swallowing difficulty.
Antacids*	Prolonged effect of mecamylamine.
Antibiotics*	Decreased antibiotic effect.
Alkalizers, urine*	Prolonged effect of mecamylamine.
Neostigmine	Swallowing difficulty.
Nimodipine	Dangerous blood pressure drop.
Pyridostigmine	Swallowing difficulty.
Sodium bicarbonate	Reduced mecamylamine effect.
Sulfa drugs*	Decreased antibiotic effect.

POSSIBLE INTERACTION WITH OTHER SUBSTANCES

INTERACTS WITH	COMBINED EFFECT
Alcohol:	Increased likelihood of fainting.
Beverages:	No special problems expected.
Cocaine:	Increased central nervous system stimulation. Avoid.
Foods: Food with high salt or sodium.	Decreased effectiveness of mecamylamine.
Marijuana:	Increased central nervous system stimulation. Avoid.
Tobacco:	No special problems expected.

MECHLORETHAMINE (Topical)

BRAND NAMES

Mustargen

BASIC INFORMATION

Habit forming? No
Prescription needed? Yes
Available as generic? No
Drug class: Antineoplastic (topical)

 ## USES

- Treats mycosis fungoides.
- Treats other malignancies (by injection).

 ## DOSAGE & USAGE INFORMATION

How to use:
- Solution—Mix according to doctor's instructions. Don't inhale vapors or powder.
- Shower and rinse before treatment.
- Use rubber gloves to apply over entire body.
- Avoid contact with eyes, nose and mouth.
- Ointment—Use according to doctor's instructions.

When to use:
Usually once a day.

If you forget a dose:
Notify your doctor.

What drug does:
Destroys cells that produce mycosis fungoides.

Time lapse before drug works:
None. Works immediately.

Don't use with:
Any other medicines (including over-the-counter drugs such as cough and cold medicines, laxatives, antacids, diet pills, caffeine, nose drops or vitamins) without consulting your doctor.

 ## OVERDOSE

SYMPTOMS:
None expected for topical solutions.
WHAT TO DO:
Not intended for internal use. If child accidentally swallows, call poison-control center.

 ## POSSIBLE ADVERSE REACTIONS OR SIDE EFFECTS

SYMPTOMS	WHAT TO DO
Life-threatening: Immediate hives, shortness of breath.	Seek emergency treatment immediately.
Common: Darkening, dry skin.	Continue. Tell doctor at next visit.
Infrequent: Allergic reaction with rash, itching, hives.	Seek emergency treatment immediately.
Rare: None expected.	

WARNINGS & PRECAUTIONS

Don't use if:
You are allergic to mechlorethamine.

Before you start, consult your doctor:
- If you have chicken pox.
- If you have shingles (herpes zoster).
- If you have skin infection.

Over age 60:
No special problems expected.

Pregnancy:
Risk to unborn child outweighs drug benefits. Don't use.

Breast-feeding:
Drug passes into milk. Avoid drug or discontinue nursing until you finish medicine. Consult doctor for advice on maintaining milk supply.

Infants & children:
No special problems expected.

Prolonged use:
- Allergic or hypersensitive reactions more likely.
- Talk to your doctor about the need for follow-up medical examinations or laboratory studies to check liver function, complete blood counts (white blood cell count, platelet count, red blood cell count, hemoglobin, hematocrit) and hearing tests.

Skin & sunlight:
No problems expected.

Driving, piloting or hazardous work:
Don't drive or pilot aircraft until you learn how medicine affects you. Don't work around dangerous machinery. Don't climb ladders or work in high places. Danger increases if you drink alcohol or take medicine affecting alertness and reflexes.

Discontinuing:
No special problems expected.

Others:
- Advise any doctor or dentist whom you consult that you take this medicine.
- May affect results in some medical tests.
- Don't use if solution is discolored.

POSSIBLE INTERACTION WITH OTHER DRUGS

GENERIC NAME OR DRUG CLASS	COMBINED EFFECT
None expected.	

POSSIBLE INTERACTION WITH OTHER SUBSTANCES

INTERACTS WITH	COMBINED EFFECT
Alcohol:	None expected.
Beverages:	None expected.
Cocaine:	None expected.
Foods:	None expected.
Marijuana:	None expected.
Tobacco:	None expected.

MECLIZINE

BRAND NAMES

Antivert
Antrizine
Bonamine
Bonine

Dizmiss
Meni-D
Ru-Vert-M

BASIC INFORMATION

Habit forming? No
Prescription needed?
  U.S.—Tablets: No
      Liquid: Yes
  Canada: Yes
Available as generic? Yes
Drug class: Antihistamine, antiemetic, anti-motion sickness

 USES

Prevents motion sickness.

 DOSAGE & USAGE INFORMATION

How to take:
Tablet—Swallow with liquid or food to lessen stomach irritation. If you can't swallow whole, crumble tablet and chew or take with liquid or food.

When to take:
30 minutes to 1 hour before traveling.

If you forget a dose:
Take as soon as you remember. Wait 4 hours for next dose.

What drug does:
Reduces sensitivity of nerve endings in inner ear, blocking messages to brain's vomiting center.

Time lapse before drug works:
30 to 60 minutes.

Don't take with:
Any other medicine without consulting your doctor or pharmacist.

 OVERDOSE

SYMPTOMS:
Drowsiness, confusion, incoordination, stupor, coma, weak pulse, shallow breathing, hallucinations.
WHAT TO DO:
- **Dial 0 (operator) or 911 (emergency) for an ambulance or medical help. Then give first aid immediately.**
- **See emergency information on inside covers.**

 POSSIBLE ADVERSE REACTIONS OR SIDE EFFECTS

SYMPTOMS	WHAT TO DO
Life-threatening: In case of overdose, see previous column.	
Common: Drowsiness.	Continue. Tell doctor at next visit.
Infrequent: • Headache, diarrhea or constipation, fast heartbeat.	Continue. Call doctor when convenient.
• Dry mouth, nose, throat.	Continue. Tell doctor at next visit.
Rare: • Rash, hives.	Discontinue. Call doctor right away.
• Restlessness, excitement, insomnia, blurred vision, frequent and difficult urination, hallucinations.	Continue. Call doctor when convenient.
• Appetite loss, nausea.	Continue. Tell doctor at next visit.

 WARNINGS & PRECAUTIONS

Don't take if:
- You are allergic to meclizine, buclizine or cyclizine.
- You have taken MAO inhibitors in the past 2 weeks.

Before you start, consult your doctor:
- If you have glaucoma.
- If you have prostate enlargement.
- If you have reacted badly to any antihistamine.

Over age 60:
Adverse reactions and side effects may be more frequent and severe than in younger persons, especially impaired urination from enlarged prostate gland.

Pregnancy:
Studies inconclusive on harm to unborn child. Animal studies show fetal abnormalities. Decide with your doctor whether drug benefits justify risk to unborn child.

Breast-feeding:
Drug passes into milk. Avoid drug or discontinue nursing until you finish medicine. Consult doctor for advice on maintaining milk supply.

Infants & children:
Safety not established. Avoid if under age 12.

Prolonged use:
No problems expected.

Skin & sunlight:
No problems expected.

Driving, piloting or hazardous work:
Don't fly aircraft. Don't drive until you learn how medicine affects you. Don't work around dangerous machinery. Don't climb ladders or work in high places. Danger increases if you drink alcohol or take medicine affecting alertness and reflexes, such as antihistamines, tranquilizers, sedatives, pain medicine, narcotics and mind-altering drugs.

Discontinuing:
No problems expected.

Others:
Some products contain tartrazine dye. Avoid, especially if you are allergic to aspirin.

POSSIBLE INTERACTION WITH OTHER DRUGS

GENERIC NAME OR DRUG CLASS	COMBINED EFFECT
Amphetamines*	May decrease drowsiness caused by meclizine.
Anticholinergics*	Increased effect of both drugs.
Antidepressants, tricyclic (TCA)*	Increased effect of both drugs.
Carteolol	Decreased antihistamine effect.
Clozapine	Toxic effect on the central nervous system.
Dronabinol	Increases meclizine effect.
Ethinamate	Dangerous increased effects of ethinamate. Avoid combining.
Fluoxetine	Increased depressant effects of both drugs.
Guanfacine	May increase depressant effects of either drug.
Leucovorin	High alcohol content of leucovorin may cause adverse effects.

MAO inhibitors*	Increased meclizine effect.
Methyprylon	Increased sedative effect, perhaps to dangerous level. Avoid.
Nabilone	Greater depression of central nervous system.
Narcotics*	Increased effect of both drugs.
Pain relievers*	Increased effect of both drugs.
Sedatives*	Increased effect of both drugs.
Sertraline	Increased depressive effects of both drugs.
Sleep inducers*	Increased effect of both drugs.
Sotalol	Increased antihistamine effect.
Tranquilizers*	Increased effect of both drugs.

POSSIBLE INTERACTION WITH OTHER SUBSTANCES

INTERACTS WITH	COMBINED EFFECT
Alcohol:	Increased sedation. Avoid.
Beverages: Caffeine drinks.	May decrease drowsiness.
Cocaine:	None expected.
Foods:	None expected.
Marijuana:	Increased drowsiness, dry mouth.
Tobacco:	None expected.

MEFLOQUINE

BRAND NAMES

Lariam

BASIC INFORMATION

Habit forming? No
Prescription needed? Yes
Available as generic? No
Drug class: Antiprotozoal, antimalarial

 ## USES

- Treats malaria caused by *plasmodium falciparum* (either chloroquine-sensitive or chloroquine-resistant).
- Treats malaria caused by *plasmodium vivax.*
- Helps prevent malaria in people traveling into areas where malaria is prevalent.

 ## DOSAGE & USAGE INFORMATION

How to take:
Tablet—Swallow with food, milk or 8 oz. of water to lessen stomach irritation.

When to take:
- Treatment—Usually given as 5 tablets in a single dose. Follow your doctor's instructions.
- Prevention—Start one week prior to traveling to an area where malaria is endemic. Continue during travel and for 4 weeks after return.

If you forget a dose:
Take as soon as you remember, then return to regular dosing schedule.

What drug does:
Exact mechanism unknown. Kills parasite in one of its developmental stages.

Continued in next column

 ## OVERDOSE

SYMPTOMS:
Seizures, heart rhythm disturbances.
WHAT TO DO:
- **Dial 0 (operator) or 911 (emergency) for an ambulance or medical help. Then give first aid immediately.**
- **Induce vomiting and see a doctor immediately because of the potential cardiotoxic effect. Treat vomiting or diarrhea with standard fluid therapy.**
- **See emergency information on inside covers.**

Time lapse before drug works:
7 to 24 hours.

Don't take with:
- Sulfadoxine and pyrimethamine combination (Fansidar).
- Any other medicines (including over-the-counter drugs such as cough and cold medicines, laxatives, antacids, diet pills, caffeine, nose drops or vitamins) without consulting your doctor.
- See Interaction column and consult doctor.

 ## POSSIRLE ADVERSE REACTIONS OR SIDE EFFECTS

SYMPTOMS	WHAT TO DO
Life-threatening:	
Seizures.	Seek emergency treatment immediately.
Common:	
Dizziness, headache, insomnia, lightheadedness, abdominal pain, diarrhea, appetite loss, nausea or vomiting, visual disturbances.	Discontinue. Call doctor right away.
Infrequent:	
None expected.	
Rare:	
Slow heart rate, confusion, anxiety, depression, hallucinations, psychosis.	Discontinue. Call doctor right away.

WARNINGS & PRECAUTIONS

Don't take if:
You are allergic to mefloquine, quinine, quinidine or related medications.

Before you start, consult your doctor:
- If you plan to become pregnant within the medication period or 2 months after.
- If you have heart trouble, especially heart block.
- If you have depression or other emotional problems.
- If you are giving this to a child under 40 pounds of body weight.
- If you have epilepsy or a seizure disorder.

Over age 60:
Adverse reactions and side effects may be more frequent and severe than in younger persons.

Pregnancy:
Not recommended. If traveling to an area where malaria is endemic, consult your doctor about prophylaxis.

Breast-feeding:
Mefloquine passes into mother's milk. Avoid drug or discontinue nursing.

Infants & children:
Not recommended for children under 2.

Prolonged use:
Not recommended.

Skin & sunlight:
No problems expected.

Driving, piloting or hazardous work:
Don't drive or pilot aircraft until you learn how medicine affects you. Don't work around dangerous machinery. Don't climb ladders or work in high places. Danger increases if you drink alcohol or take medicine affecting alertness and reflexes.

Discontinuing:
Don't discontinue without doctor's advice until you complete the prescribed dosage.

Others:
- Periodic physical and blood examinations recommended.
- Resistance to mefloquine by some strains of malaria have been reported, so prevention and treatment of malaria may not be uniformly effective.

POSSIBLE INTERACTION WITH OTHER DRUGS

GENERIC NAME OR DRUG CLASS	COMBINED EFFECT
Antiseizure medications	Possible lowered seizure control.
Beta-blockers*	Heartbeat irregularities or cardiac arrest. Avoid.
Calcium channel blockers*	Heartbeat irregularities.
Chloroquine	Increased chance of seizures. Avoid.
Divalproex	Increased risk of seizures.
Propranolol	Heartbeat irregularities.
Quinidine	Increased chance of seizures and heart rhythm disturbances.
Quinine	Increased chance of seizures and heart rhythm disturbances.
Typhoid vaccine (oral)	Concurrent use may decrease effectiveness of vaccine.
Valproic acid	Decreased valproic acid effect.

POSSIBLE INTERACTION WITH OTHER SUBSTANCES

INTERACTS WITH	COMBINED EFFECT
Alcohol:	Possible liver toxicity. Avoid.
Beverages: Any alcoholic beverage.	Possible liver toxicity. Avoid.
Cocaine:	No problems expected.
Foods:	No problems expected.
Marijuana:	No problems expected.
Tobacco:	No problems expected.

MELPHALAN (PAM, L-PAM, Phenylalanine Mustard)

BRAND NAMES

Alkeran
L-PAM

Phenylalanine
Mustard

BASIC INFORMATION

Habit forming? No
Prescription needed? Yes
Available as generic? No
Drug class: Antineoplastic

USES

- Treatment for some kinds of cancer.
- Suppresses immune response after transplant and in immune disorders.

DOSAGE & USAGE INFORMATION

How to take:
Tablet—Swallow with liquid after light meal. Don't drink fluids with meals. Drink extra fluids between meals. Avoid sweet or fatty foods.

When to take:
At the same time each day.

If you forget a dose:
Take as soon as you remember. Don't ever double dose.

What drug does:
Inhibits abnormal cell reproduction. May suppress immune system.

Continued next column

OVERDOSE

SYMPTOMS:
Bleeding, chills, fever, collapse, stupor, seizure.
WHAT TO DO:
- **Dial 0 (operator) or 911 (emergency) for an ambulance or medical help. Then give first aid immediately.**
- **If patient is unconscious and not breathing, give mouth-to-mouth breathing. If there is no heartbeat, use cardiac massage and mouth-to-mouth breathing (CPR). Don't try to make patient vomit. If you can't get help quickly, take patient to nearest emergency facility.**
- **See emergency information on inside covers.**

Time lapse before drug works:
Up to 6 weeks for full effect.

Don't take with:
Any other medicine without consulting your doctor or pharmacist.

POSSIBLE ADVERSE REACTIONS OR SIDE EFFECTS

SYMPTOMS	WHAT TO DO
Life-threatening:	
In case of overdose, see previous column.	
Common:	
• Unusual bleeding or bruising, mouth sores with sore throat, chills and fever, black stools, sores in mouth and lips, menstrual irregularities, back pain.	Discontinue. Call doctor right away.
• Hair loss, joint pain.	Continue. Call doctor when convenient.
• Nausea, vomiting, diarrhea (unavoidable), tiredness, weakness.	Continue. Tell doctor at next visit.
Infrequent:	
• Skin rash.	Discontinue. Call doctor right away.
• Mental confusion, shortness of breath.	Continue. Call doctor when convenient.
• Cough.	Continue. Tell doctor at next visit.
Rare:	
Jaundice, swelling in feet or legs.	Discontinue. Call doctor right away.

MELPHALAN (PAM, L-PAM, Phenylalanine Mustard)

 WARNINGS & PRECAUTIONS

Don't take if:
- You have had hypersensitivity to alkylating antineoplastic drugs.
- Your physician has not explained serious nature of your medical problem and risks of taking this medicine.

Before you start, consult your doctor:
- If you have gout.
- If you have had kidney stones.
- If you have active infection.
- If you have impaired kidney or liver function.
- If you have taken other antineoplastic drugs or had radiation treatment in last 3 weeks.

Over age 60:
Adverse reactions and side effects may be more frequent and severe than in younger persons.

Pregnancy:
Consult doctor. Risk to child is significant.

Breast-feeding:
Drug passes into milk. Don't nurse.

Infants & children:
Use only under special medical supervision at center experienced in anticancer drugs.

Prolonged use:
- Adverse reactions more likely the longer drug is required.
- Talk to your doctor about the need for follow-up medical examinations or laboratory studies to check complete blood counts (white blood cell count, platelet count, red blood cell count, hemoglobin, hematocrit), kidney function.

Skin & sunlight:
No problems expected.

Driving, piloting or hazardous work:
No problems expected.

Discontinuing:
Don't discontinue without doctor's advice until you complete prescribed dose, even though symptoms diminish or disappear. Some side effects may follow discontinuing. Report to doctor blurred vision, convulsions, confusion, persistent headache, fever or chills, blood in urine, unusual bleeding.

Others:
- May cause sterility.
- May increase chance of developing leukemia.

 POSSIBLE INTERACTION WITH OTHER DRUGS

GENERIC NAME OR DRUG CLASS	COMBINED EFFECT
Antigout drugs*	Decreased antigout effect.
Antineoplastic drugs, other*	Increased effect of all drugs (may be beneficial).
Chloramphenicol	Increased likelihood of toxic effects of both drugs.
Clozapine	Toxic effect on bone marrow.
Lovastatin	Increased heart and kidney damage.
Probenecid	Increased likelihood of bone marrow toxicity.
Sulfinpyrazone	Increased likelihood of bone marrow toxicity.
Tiopronin	Increased risk of toxicity to bone marrow.

 POSSIBLE INTERACTION WITH OTHER SUBSTANCES

INTERACTS WITH	COMBINED EFFECT
Alcohol:	May increase chance of intestinal bleeding.
Beverages:	No problems expected.
Cocaine:	Increases chance of toxicity.
Foods:	Reduces irritation in stomach.
Marijuana:	No problems expected.
Tobacco:	Increases lung toxicity.

*See Glossary

MEPHENYTOIN

BRAND NAMES

Mesantoin

BASIC INFORMATION

Habit forming? No
Prescription needed? Yes
Available as generic? No
Drug class: Anticonvulsant (hydantoin)

 USES

- Prevents epileptic seizures.
- Stabilizes irregular heartbeat.

 DOSAGE & USAGE INFORMATION

How to take:
- Tablet—Swallow with liquid.
- Chewable tablets—Chew well before swallowing.
- Suspension—Shake well before taking with liquid.

When to take:
At the same time each day.

If you forget a dose:
- If drug taken 1 time per day—Take as soon as you remember up to 12 hours late. If more than 12 hours, wait for next scheduled dose (don't double this dose).
- If taken several times per day—Take as soon as possible, then return to regular schedule.

What drug does:
Promotes sodium loss from nerve fibers. This lessens excitability and inhibits spread of nerve impulses.

Time lapse before drug works:
7 to 10 days continual use.

Don't take with:
Any other medicine without consulting your doctor or pharmacist.

 OVERDOSE

SYMPTOMS:
Jerky eye movements; stagger; slurred speech; imbalance; drowsiness; blood-pressure drop; slow, shallow breathing; coma.
WHAT TO DO:
- **Dial 0 (operator) or 911 (emergency) for an ambulance or medical help. Then give first aid immediately.**
- **See emergency information on inside covers.**

 POSSIBLE ADVERSE REACTIONS OR SIDE EFFECTS

SYMPTOMS	WHAT TO DO
Life-threatening: In case of overdose, see previous column.	
Common: Mild dizziness; drowsiness; nausea; constipation; vomiting; bleeding, swollen or tender gums.	Continue. Call doctor when convenient.
Infrequent: • Hallucinations, confusion, slurred speech, stagger, rash, change in vision, agitation.	Discontinue. Call doctor right away.
• Headache, diarrhea, muscle twitching.	Continue. Call doctor when convenient.
• Increased body and facial hair, breast swelling, insomnia.	Continue. Tell doctor at next visit.
Rare: Sore throat, fever, abdominal pain, unusual bleeding or bruising, jaundice, swollen lymph glands.	Discontinue. Call doctor right away.

 WARNINGS & PRECAUTIONS

Don't take if:
You are allergic to any hydantoin anticonvulsant.

Before you start, consult your doctor:
- If you have had impaired liver function or disease.
- If you will have surgery within 2 months, including dental surgery, requiring general or spinal anesthesia.

Over age 60:
Adverse reactions and side effects may be more frequent and severe than in younger persons.

Pregnancy:
Risk to unborn child outweighs drug benefits. Don't use.

Breast-feeding:
Drug passes into milk. Avoid drug or discontinue nursing until you finish medicine. Consult doctor for advice on maintaining milk supply.

Infants & children:
Use only under medical supervision.

Prolonged use:
- Weakened bones.
- Lymph gland enlargement.
- Possible liver damage.
- Numbness and tingling of hands and feet.

- Continual back-and-forth eye movements.
- Bleeding, swollen or tender gums.
- Talk to your doctor about the need for follow-up medical examinations or laboratory studies to check complete blood counts (white blood cell count, platelet count, red blood cell count, hemoglobin, hematocrit), liver function, EEG*

Skin & sunlight:
May cause rash or intensify sunburn in areas exposed to sun or sunlamp.

Driving, piloting or hazardous work:
Don't drive or pilot aircraft until you learn how medicine affects you. Don't work around dangerous machinery. Don't climb ladders or work in high places. Danger increases if you drink alcohol or take medicine affecting alertness and reflexes.

Discontinuing:
Don't discontinue without consulting doctor. Dose may require gradual reduction if you have taken drug for a long time. Doses of other drugs may also require adjustment.

Others:
May cause learning disability.

 ## POSSIBLE INTERACTION WITH OTHER DRUGS

GENERIC NAME OR DRUG CLASS	COMBINED EFFECT
Anticoagulants*	Increased effect of both drugs.
Antidepressants, tricyclic (TCA)*	Need to adjust mephenytoin dose.
Barbiturates*	Changed seizure pattern.
Carbamazepine	Possible increased mephenytoin metabolism.
Carbonic anhydrase inhibitors*	Increased chance of bone disease.
Central nervous system (CNS) depressants*	Oversedation.
Chloramphenicol	Increased mephenytoin effect.
Cimetidine	Increased mephenytoin toxicity.
Contraceptives, oral*	Increased seizures.
Cortisone drugs*	Decreased cortisone effect.
Cyclosporine	May decrease cyclosporine effect.
Digitalis preparations*	Decreased digitalis effect.

Disopyramide	Decreased disopyramide effect.
Disulfiram	Increased mephenytoin effect.
Estrogens*	Increased estrogen effect.
Furosemide	Decreased furosemide effect.
Glutethimide	Decreased mephenytoin effect.
Griseofulvin	Increased griseofulvin effect.
Hypoglycemics, other*	Possible decreased hypoglycemic effect.
Isoniazid	Increased mephenytoin effect.
Methadone	Decreased methadone effect.
Methotrexate	Increased methotrexate effect.
Methylphenidate	Increased mephenytoin effect.
Nicardipine	Increased anti-convulsant effect.
Nimodipine	Increased anticonvulsant effect.
Oxyphenbutazone	Increased mephenytoin effect.
Para-aminosalicylic acid (PAS)	Increased mephenytoin effect.
Phenothiazines*	Increased mephenytoin effect.
Phenylbutazone	Increased mephenytoin effect.

Continued page 949

 ## POSSIBLE INTERACTION WITH OTHER SUBSTANCES

INTERACTS WITH	COMBINED EFFECT
Alcohol:	Possible decreased anticonvulsant effect. Use with caution.
Beverages:	None expected.
Cocaine:	Possible seizures.
Foods:	None expected.
Marijuana:	Drowsiness, unsteadiness, decreased anticonvulsant effect.
Tobacco:	None expected.

*See Glossary

MEPROBAMATE

BRAND NAMES

See complete list of brand names in the *Brand Name Directory,* page 922.

BASIC INFORMATION

Habit forming? Yes
Prescription needed? Yes
Available as generic? Yes
Drug class: Tranquilizer

 ## USES

Reduces mild anxiety, tension and insomnia.

 ## DOSAGE & USAGE INFORMATION

How to take:
• Tablet—Swallow with liquid.
• Extended-release capsules—Swallow each dose whole.

When to take:
At the same time each day.

If you forget a dose:
Take as soon as you remember up to 2 hours late. If more than 2 hours, wait for next scheduled dose (don't double this dose).

What drug does:
Sedates brain centers which control behavior and emotions.

Time lapse before drug works:
1 to 2 hours.

Don't take with:
• Non-prescription drugs containing alcohol or caffeine without consulting doctor.
• Any other medicine without consulting your doctor or pharmacist.

 ## OVERDOSE

SYMPTOMS:
Dizziness, slurred speech, stagger, confusion, depressed breathing and heart function, stupor, coma.
WHAT TO DO:
• **Dial 0 (operator) or 911 (emergency) for an ambulance or medical help. Then give first aid immediately.**
• **See emergency information on inside covers.**

 ## POSSIBLE ADVERSE REACTIONS OR SIDE EFFECTS

SYMPTOMS	WHAT TO DO
Life-threatening:	
Hives, rash, intense itching, faintness soon after a dose, wheezing (anaphylaxis).	Seek emergency treatment immediately.
Common:	
Dizziness, confusion, agitation, drowsiness, unsteadiness, fatigue, weakness.	Continue. Tell doctor at next visit.
Infrequent:	
• Rash, hives, itchy skin; change in vision; diarrhea, nausea or vomiting.	Discontinue. Call doctor right away.
• False sense of well-being, headache, slurred speech, blurred vision.	Continue. Call doctor when convenient.
Rare:	
Sore throat; fever; rapid, pounding, unusually slow or irregular heartbeat; difficult breathing; unusual bleeding or bruising.	Discontinue. Call doctor right away.

 ## WARNINGS & PRECAUTIONS

Don't take if:
• You are allergic to meprobamate, tybamate, carbromal or carisoprodol.
• You have had porphyria.
• Patient is younger than 6.

Before you start, consult your doctor:
• If you have epilepsy.
• If you have impaired liver or kidney function.
• If you have tartrazine dye allergy.

Over age 60:
Adverse reactions and side effects may be more frequent and severe than in younger persons.

Pregnancy:
Risk to unborn child outweighs drug benefits. Don't use.

Breast-feeding:
Drug filters into milk. May harm child. Avoid.

Infants & children:
Not recommended.

Prolonged use:
- Habit forming.
- May impair blood-cell production.

Skin & sunlight:
No problems expected.

Driving, piloting or hazardous work:
Don't drive or pilot aircraft until you learn how medicine affects you. Don't work around dangerous machinery. Don't climb ladders or work in high places. Danger increases if you drink alcohol or take medicine affecting alertness and reflexes, such as antihistamines, tranquilizers, sedatives, pain medicine, narcotics and mind-altering drugs.

Discontinuing:
Don't discontinue without consulting doctor. Dose may require gradual reduction if you have taken drug for a long time. Doses of other drugs may also require adjustment. Report to your doctor any unusual symptom that begins in the first week you discontinue this medicine. These symptoms may include convulsions, confusion, nightmares, insomnia.

Others:
No problems expected.

 POSSIBLE INTERACTION WITH OTHER DRUGS

GENERIC NAME OR DRUG CLASS	COMBINED EFFECT
Anticoagulants*	Decreased anticoagulant effect.
Anticonvulsants*	Change in seizure pattern.
Antidepressants, tricyclic (TCA)*	Increased anti-depressant effect.
Antihistamines*	Possible excessive sedation.
Clozapine	Toxic effect on the central nervous system.
Contraceptives, oral*	Decreased contra-ceptive effect.
Dronabinol	Increased effects of both drugs. Avoid.
Estrogens*	Decreased estrogen effect.
Ethinamate	Dangerous increased effects of ethinamate. Avoid combining.
Fluoxetine	Increased depressant effects of both drugs.
Guanfacine	May increase depressant effects of either drug.
Leucovorin	High alcohol content of leucovorin may cause adverse effects.
MAO inhibitors*	Increased meprobamate effect.
Methyprylon	Increased sedative effect, perhaps to dangerous level. Avoid.
Molindone	Increased tranquilizer effect.
Nabilone	Greater depression of central nervous system.
Narcotics*	Increased narcotic effect.
Sedatives*	Increased sedative effect.
Sertraline	Increased depressive effects of both drugs.
Sleep inducers*	Increased effect of sleep inducer.
Tranquilizers*	Increased tranquilizer effect.

 POSSIBLE INTERACTION WITH OTHER SUBSTANCES

INTERACTS WITH	COMBINED EFFECT
Alcohol:	Dangerous increased effect of meprobamate.
Beverages: Caffeine drinks.	Decreased calming effect of meprobamate.
Cocaine:	Decreased meprobamate effect.
Foods:	None expected.
Marijuana:	Increased sedative effect of meprobamate.
Tobacco:	None expected.

MEPROBAMATE & ASPIRIN

BRAND NAMES

Epromate-M	Meprogesic
Equagesic	Meprogesic Q
Equazine-M	Micrainin
Heptogesic	Q-gesic
Mepro Analgesic	Tranquigesic
Meprogese	

BASIC INFORMATION

Habit forming? Yes
Prescription needed? Yes
Available as generic? No
Drug class: Anti-inflammatory (non-steroidal), analgesic, tranquilizer

USES

- Reduces mild anxiety, tension and insomnia.
- Reduces pain, fever, inflammation.
- Relieves swelling, stiffness, joint pain.
- Antiplatelet effect.

DOSAGE & USAGE INFORMATION

How to take:
- Tablet—Swallow with liquid.
- Effervescent tablets—Dissolve in water.

When to take:
Pain, fever, inflammation—As needed, no more often than every 4 hours.

If you forget a dose:
Take as soon as you remember up to 2 hours late. If more than 2 hours, wait for next scheduled dose (don't double this dose).

What drug does:
- Sedates brain centers which control behavior and emotions.
- Affects hypothalamus, the part of the brain which regulates temperature by dilating small blood vessels in skin.

Continued next column

OVERDOSE

SYMPTOMS:
Dizziness; slurred speech; stagger; depressed heart function; ringing in ears; nausea; vomiting; fever; deep, rapid breathing; hallucinations; convulsions; stupor; coma.
WHAT TO DO:
- **Dial 0 (operator) or 911 (emergency) for an ambulance or medical help. Then give first aid immediately.**
- **See emergency information on inside covers.**

- Prevents clumping of platelets (small blood cells) so blood vessels remain open.
- Decreases prostaglandin effect.
- Suppresses body's pain messages.

Time lapse before drug works:
1 to 2 hours.

Don't take with:
- Tetracyclines.
- Non-prescription drugs containing alcohol or caffeine without consulting doctor.
- Any other medicine without consulting your doctor or pharmacist.

POSSIBLE ADVERSE REACTIONS OR SIDE EFFECTS

SYMPTOMS	WHAT TO DO
Life-threatening:	
Hives, rash, intense itching, faintness soon after a dose (anaphylaxis); difficulty breathing.	Seek emergency treatment immediately.
Common:	
• Nausea, vomiting.	Discontinue. Call doctor right away.
• Dizziness, confusion, agitation, drowsiness, unsteadiness, fatigue, weakness, ears ringing, heartburn, indigestion, abdominal pain.	Continue. Call doctor when convenient.
Infrequent:	
Blurred vision, headache.	Continue. Call doctor when convenient.
Rare:	
• Black, bloody or tarry stool; vomiting blood or black material; blood in urine.	Discontinue. Seek emergency treatment.
• Rash, hives, itchy skin, change in vision, fever, jaundice, mental confusion.	Discontinue. Call doctor right away.

WARNINGS & PRECAUTIONS

Don't take if:
- You are allergic to meprobamate, tybamate, carbromal or carisoprodol.
- You are sensitive to aspirin.
- You have had porphyria.
- You have a peptic ulcer of stomach or duodenum or a bleeding disorder.
- Patient is younger than 6.

Before you start, consult your doctor:
- If you have epilepsy, impaired liver or kidney function, asthma or nasal polyps.

- If you are allergic to tartrazine.
- If you have had gout, stomach or duodenal ulcers.

Over age 60:
Adverse reactions and side effects may be more frequent and severe than in younger persons. More likely to cause hidden bleeding in stomach or intestines. Watch for dark stools.

Pregnancy:
Risk to unborn child outweighs drug benefits. Don't use.

Breast-feeding:
Drug passes into milk. Avoid drug or discontinue nursing until you finish medicine. Consult doctor for advice on maintaining milk supply.

Infants & children:
Not recommended.

Prolonged use:
- Habit forming.
- May impair blood-cell production.
- Kidney damage. Periodic kidney-function test recommended.

Skin & sunlight:
Aspirin combined with sunscreen may decrease sunburn.

Driving, piloting or hazardous work:
Don't drive or pilot aircraft until you learn how medicine affects you. Don't work around dangerous machinery. Don't climb ladders or work in high places. Danger increases if you drink alcohol or take medicine affecting alertness and reflexes, such as antihistamines, tranquilizers, sedatives, pain medicine, narcotics and mind-altering drugs.

Discontinuing:
Don't discontinue without consulting doctor. Dose may require gradual reduction if you have taken drug for a long time. Doses of other drugs may also require adjustment.

Others:
- Aspirin can complicate surgery; illness; pregnancy, labor and delivery.
- Urine tests for blood sugar may be inaccurate.

 ## POSSIBLE INTERACTION WITH OTHER DRUGS

GENERIC NAME OR DRUG CLASS	COMBINED EFFECT
Acebutolol	Decreased antihypertensive effect of acebutolol.
ACE inhibitors*: captopril, enalapril, lisinopril	Decreased effect of inhibitors.
Allopurinol	Decreased allopurinol effect.

Antacids*	Decreased aspirin effect.
Anticoagulants*	Increased anticoagulant effect. Abnormal bleeding.
Anticonvulsants*	Change in seizure pattern.
Antidepressants, tricyclic (TCA)*	Increased antidepressant effect.
Antidiabetics, oral*	Low blood sugar.
Aspirin, other	Likely aspirin toxicity.
Bumetanide	Possible aspirin toxicity.
Contraceptives, oral*	Decreased contraceptive effect.
Cortisone drugs*	Increased cortisone effect. Risk of ulcers and stomach bleeding.
Dronabinol	Increased effect of both drugs.
Estrogens*	Decreased estrogen effect.
Ethacrynic acid	Possible aspirin toxicity.
Furosemide	Possible aspirin toxicity. May decrease furosemide effect.
Gold compounds*	Increased likelihood of kidney damage.
Indomethacin	Risk of stomach bleeding and ulcers.

Continued page 950

 ## POSSIBLE INTERACTION WITH OTHER SUBSTANCES

INTERACTS WITH	COMBINED EFFECT
Alcohol:	Possible stomach irritation and bleeding. Dangerous increased effect of meprobamate. Avoid.
Beverages: Caffeine drinks.	Decreased calming effect of meprobamate.
Cocaine:	Decreased meprobamate effect.
Foods:	None expected.
Marijuana:	Possible increased pain relief, but marijuana may slow body's recovery. Avoid.
Tobacco:	None expected.

MERCAPTOPURINE

BRAND NAMES

Purinethol   6-MP

BASIC INFORMATION

Habit forming? No
Prescription needed? Yes
Available as generic? No
Drug class: Antineoplastic,
   immunosuppressant

USES

- Treatment for some kinds of cancer.
- Treatment for regional enteritis and ulcerative colitis and other immune disorders.

DOSAGE & USAGE INFORMATION

How to take:
Tablet—Swallow with liquid.

When to take:
At the same time each day.

If you forget a dose:
Skip the missed dose. Don't double the next dose.

What drug does:
Inhibits abnormal-cell reproduction.

Time lapse before drug works:
May require 6 weeks for maximum effect.

Don't take with:
Any other medicine without consulting your doctor or pharmacist.

OVERDOSE

SYMPTOMS:
Headache, stupor, seizures.
WHAT TO DO:
- **Dial 0 (operator) or 911 (emergency) for an ambulance or medical help. Then give first aid immediately.**
- **If patient is unconscious and not breathing, give mouth-to-mouth breathing. If there is no heartbeat, use cardiac massage and mouth-to-mouth breathing (CPR). Don't try to make patient vomit. If you can't get help quickly, take patient to nearest emergency facility.**
- **See emergency information on inside covers.**

POSSIBLE ADVERSE REACTIONS OR SIDE EFFECTS

SYMPTOMS	WHAT TO DO
Life-threatening:	
In case of overdose, see previous column.	
Common:	
• Black stools or bloody vomit.	Discontinue. Seek emergency treatment.
• Mouth sores, sore throat, unusual bleeding or bruising.	Discontinue. Call doctor right away.
• Abdominal pain, nausea, vomiting, weakness, tiredness.	Continue. Call doctor when convenient.
Infrequent:	
• Seizures.	Discontinue. Seek emergency treatment.
• Diarrhea, headache, confusion, blurred vision, shortness of breath, joint pain, blood in urine, jaundice, back pain, appetite loss, feet and leg swelling.	Discontinue. Call doctor right away.
• Cough.	Continue. Call doctor when convenient.
• Acne, boils, hair loss, itchy skin.	Continue. Tell doctor at next visit.
Rare:	
Fever and chills.	Discontinue. Call doctor right away.

WARNINGS & PRECAUTIONS

Don't take if:
You are allergic to any antineoplastic.

Before you start, consult your doctor:
- If you are alcoholic.
- If you have blood, liver or kidney disease.
- If you have colitis or peptic ulcer.
- If you have gout.
- If you have an infection.
- If you plan to become pregnant within 3 months.

Over age 60:
Adverse reactions and side effects may be more frequent and severe than in younger persons.

Pregnancy:
Consult doctor.

Breast-feeding:
Drug passes into milk. Avoid drug or discontinue nursing.

Infants & children:
Use only under special medical supervision.

Prolonged use:
- Adverse reactions more likely the longer drug is required.
- Talk to your doctor about the need for follow-up medical examinations or laboratory studies to check complete blood counts (white blood cell count, platelet count, red blood cell count, hemoglobin, hematocrit), liver function, kidney function, uric acid.

Skin & sunlight:
No problems expected.

Driving, piloting or hazardous work:
Avoid if you feel dizzy, drowsy or confused. Otherwise, no problems expected.

Discontinuing:
Don't discontinue without doctor's advice until you complete prescribed dose, even though symptoms diminish or disappear. Some side effects may follow discontinuing. Report to doctor blurred vision, convulsions, confusion, persistent headache, chills or fever, bloody urine or stools, back pain, jaundice.

Others:
- Drink more water than usual to cause frequent urination.
- Don't give this medicine to anyone else for any purpose. It is a strong drug that requires close medical supervision.
- Report for frequent medical follow-up and laboratory studies.

POSSIBLE INTERACTION WITH OTHER DRUGS

GENERIC NAME OR DRUG CLASS	COMBINED EFFECT
Acetaminophen	Increased likelihood of liver toxicity.
Allopurinol	Increased toxic effect of mercaptopurine.
Anticoagulants, oral*	May increase or decrease anticoagulant effect.
Antineoplastic drugs, other*	Increased effect of both (may be desirable) or increased toxicity of each.
Chloramphenicol	Increased toxicity of each.
Clozapine	Toxic effect on bone marrow.

Cyclosporine	May increase risk of infection.
Immunosuppresants, other*	Increased risk of infections and neoplasms*.
Isoniazid	Increased risk of liver damage.
Levamisole	Increased risk of bone marrow depression.
Lovastatin	Increased heart and kidney damage.
Sulfinpyrazone	Increased toxic effect of mercaptopurine.
Tiopronin	Increased risk of toxicity to bone marrow.

POSSIBLE INTERACTION WITH OTHER SUBSTANCES

INTERACTS WITH	COMBINED EFFECT
Alcohol:	May increase chance of intestinal bleeding.
Beverages:	No problems expected.
Cocaine:	Increases chance of toxicity.
Foods:	Reduced irritation in stomach.
Marijuana:	No problems expected.
Tobacco:	Increases lung toxicity.

MESALAMINE (Rectal)

BRAND NAMES

Mesalazine	Salofalk
Rowasa	5-ASA

BASIC INFORMATION

Habit forming? No
Prescription needed? Yes
Available as generic? No
Drug class: Anti-inflammatory (non-steroidal)

USES

- Treats ulcerative colitis.
- Reduces inflammatory conditions of the lower colon and rectum.

DOSAGE & USAGE INFORMATION

How to use:
Use as an enema. Insert the tip of the pre-packaged medicine container into the rectum. Squeeze container to empty contents. Retain in rectum all night or as long as possible.

When to use:
Each night, preferably after a bowel movement. Continue for 3 to 6 weeks according to your doctor's instructions.

If you forget a dose:
Take as soon as you remember up to 2 hours late. If more than 2 hours, wait for next scheduled dose (don't double this dose).

What drug does:
Decreases production of arachidonic acid forms which are increased in patients with chronic inflammatory bowel disease.

Time lapse before drug works:
3 to 21 days.

Don't take with:
- Oral sulfasalazine concurrently. To do so may increase chances of kidney damage.
- Any other medicine without consulting your doctor or pharmacist.

OVERDOSE

SYMPTOMS:
None expected.
WHAT TO DO:
No action needed.

POSSIBLE ADVERSE REACTIONS OR SIDE EFFECTS

SYMPTOMS	WHAT TO DO
Life-threatening: None expected.	
Common: None expected.	
Infrequent: Hair loss.	Continue. Call doctor when convenient.
Rare:	
• Abdominal pain, bloody diarrhea, fever, skin rash.	Discontinue. Call doctor right away.
• Gaseousness, nausea, headache.	Continue. Call doctor when convenient.

WARNINGS & PRECAUTIONS

Don't take if:
You are allergic to any medication containing sulfasalazine (such as Azulfidine) or mesalamine.

Before you start, consult your doctor:
If you have had chronic kidney disease.

Over age 60:
More sensitive to drug. Aggravates symptoms of enlarged prostate. Causes impaired thinking, hallucinations, nightmares. Consult doctor about any of these.

Pregnancy:
Studies inconclusive on harm to unborn child. Decide with your doctor whether drug benefits justify risk to unborn child.

Breast-feeding:
No problems expected. Consult your doctor.

Infants & children:
Not recommended for children 3 and younger. Use for older children only under doctor's supervision.

Prolonged use:
Talk to your doctor about the need for follow-up medical examinations or laboratory studies to check urine.

Skin & sunlight:
No problems expected.

Driving, piloting or hazardous work:
Don't drive or pilot aircraft until you learn how medicine affects you. Don't work around dangerous machinery. Don't climb ladders or work in high places. Danger increases if you drink alcohol or take medicine affecting alertness and reflexes.

Discontinuing:
Don't discontinue without consulting doctor. Dose may require gradual reduction if you have taken drug for a long time. Doses of other drugs may also require adjustment.

Others:
- Internal eye pressure should be measured regularly.
- Avoid becoming overheated.

POSSIBLE INTERACTION WITH OTHER DRUGS

GENERIC NAME OR DRUG CLASS	COMBINED EFFECT
None expected.	

POSSIBLE INTERACTION WITH OTHER SUBSTANCES

INTERACTS WITH	COMBINED EFFECT
Alcohol:	None expected.
Beverages:	None expected.
Cocaine:	None expected.
Foods:	None expected.
Marijuana:	None expected.
Tobacco:	None expected.

METHENAMINE

BRAND NAMES

Azo-Mandelamine	Prov-U-Sep
Deltamine	Renalgin
Hexamine	Sterine
Hip-Rex	Trac 2X
Hiprex	Urex
Mandelamine	Urised
Mandelets	Uro-phosphate
Methandine	Uroblue
Methendelate	Uroquid-Acid

BASIC INFORMATION

Habit forming? No
Prescription needed? Yes
Available as generic? Yes
Drug class: Anti-infective (urinary)

 ## USES

Suppresses chronic urinary-tract infections.

 ## DOSAGE & USAGE INFORMATION

How to take:
- Tablet—Swallow with liquid or food to lessen stomach irritation. If you can't swallow whole, crumble tablet and take with liquid or food.
- Liquid form—Use a measuring spoon to ensure correct dose.
- Granules—Dissolve dose in 4 oz. of water. Drink all the liquid.

When to take:
At the same times each day.

If you forget a dose:
Take as soon as you remember up to 8 hours late. If more than 8 hours, wait for next scheduled dose (don't double this dose).

What drug does:
A chemical reaction in the urine changes methenamine into formaldehyde, which destroys certain bacteria.

Continued next column

 ## OVERDOSE

SYMPTOMS:
Bloody urine, weakness, deep breathing, stupor, coma.
WHAT TO DO:
- **Dial 0 (operator) or 911 (emergency) for an ambulance or medical help. Then give first aid immediately.**
- **See emergency information on inside covers.**

Time lapse before drug works:
Continual use for 3 to 6 months.

Don't take with:
Any other medicine without consulting your doctor or pharmacist.

 ## POSSIBLE ADVERSE REACTIONS OR SIDE EFFECTS

SYMPTOMS	WHAT TO DO
Life-threatening:	
In case of overdose, see previous column.	
Common:	
• Rash.	Discontinue. Call doctor right away.
• Nausea, difficult urination.	Continue. Call doctor when convenient.
Infrequent:	
• Blood in urine.	Discontinue. Call doctor right away.
• Burning on urination, lower back pain.	Continue. Call doctor when convenient.
Rare:	
None expected.	

WARNINGS & PRECAUTIONS

Don't take if:
- You are allergic to methenamine.
- You have a severe impairment of kidney or liver function.
- The urine cannot or should not be acidified (check with your doctor).

Before you start, consult your doctor:
- If you have had kidney or liver disease.
- If you plan to become pregnant within medication period.
- If you have had gout.

Over age 60:
Don't exceed recommended dose.

Pregnancy:
Studies inconclusive on harm to unborn child. Avoid if possible, especially first 3 months.

Breast-feeding:
Drug passes into milk in small amounts. Consult doctor.

Infants & children:
Use only under medical supervision.

Prolonged use:
No problems expected.

Skin & sunlight:
No problems expected.

Driving, piloting or hazardous work:
No problems expected.

Discontinuing:
Don't discontinue without doctor's advice until you complete prescribed dose, even though symptoms diminish or disappear.

Others:
Requires an acid urine to be effective. Eat more protein foods, cranberries, cranberry juice with vitamin C, plums, prunes.

POSSIBLE INTERACTION WITH OTHER DRUGS

GENERIC NAME OR DRUG CLASS	COMBINED EFFECT
Antacids*	Decreased methenamine effect.
Carbonic anhydrase inhibitors*	Decreased methenamine effect.
Citrates*	Decreases effects of methenamine.
Diuretics, thiazide*	Decreased urine acidity.
Sodium bicarbonate	Decreased methenamine effect.
Sulfadoxine and pyrimethamine	Increased risk of kidney toxiclty.
Sulfa drugs*	Possible kidney damage.
Vitamin C (1 to 4 grams per day)	Increased effect of methenamine, contributing to urine's acidity.

POSSIBLE INTERACTION WITH OTHER SUBSTANCES

INTERACTS WITH	COMBINED EFFECT
Alcohol:	Possible brain depression. Avoid or use with caution.
Beverages: Milk and other dairy products.	Decreased methenamine effect.
Cocaine:	None expected.
Foods: Citrus, cranberries, plums, prunes.	Increased methenamine effect.
Marijuana:	Drowsiness, muscle weakness or blood-pressure drop.
Tobacco:	None expected.

METHICILLIN

BRAND NAMES

Staphcillin

BASIC INFORMATION

Habit forming? No
Prescription needed? Yes
Available as generic? No
Drug class: Antibiotic (penicillin)

 USES

Treatment of bacterial infections that are susceptible to methicillin.

 DOSAGE & USAGE INFORMATION

How to take:
By injection only.

When to take:
Follow doctor's instructions.

If you forget a dose:
Consult doctor.

What drug does:
Destroys susceptible bacteria. Does not kill viruses.

Time lapse before drug works:
May be several days before medicine affects infection.

Don't take with:
Any other medicine without consulting your doctor or pharmacist.

 OVERDOSE

SYMPTOMS:
Severe diarrhea, nausea or vomiting.
WHAT TO DO:
Overdose unlikely to threaten life. If person takes much larger amount than prescribed, call doctor, poison-control center or hospital emergency room for instructions.

 POSSIBLE ADVERSE REACTIONS OR SIDE EFFECTS

SYMPTOMS	WHAT TO DO
Life-threatening:	
Hives, rash, intense itching, faintness soon after a dose (anaphylaxis).	Seek emergency treatment immediately.
Common:	
Dark or discolored tongue.	Continue. Tell doctor at next visit.
Infrequent:	
• Mild nausea, vomiting, diarrhea.	Continue. Call doctor when convenient.
• Bloody urine, face and ankle swelling.	Discontinue. Call doctor right away.
Rare:	
Unexplained bleeding or bruising, weakness, sore throat, fever, abdominal cramps, convulsions.	Discontinue. Call doctor right away.

WARNINGS & PRECAUTIONS

Don't take if:
You are allergic to methicillin, cephalosporin antibiotics, other penicillins or penicillamine. Life-threatening reaction may occur.

Before you start, consult your doctor:
- If you are allergic to any substance or drug.
- If you take birth control pills.

Over age 60:
You may have skin reactions, particularly around genitals and anus.

Pregnancy:
Studies inconclusive on harm to unborn child. Animal studies show fetal abnormalities. Decide with your doctor whether drug benefits justify risk to unborn child.

Breast-feeding:
Drug passes into milk. Child may become sensitive to penicillins and have allergic reactions to penicillin drugs. Avoid methicillin or discontinue nursing until you finish medicine. Consult doctor for advice on maintaining milk supply.

Infants & children:
No problems expected.

Prolonged use:
- You may become more susceptible to infections caused by germs not responsive to methicillin.
- Talk to your doctor about the need for follow-up medical examinations or laboratory studies to check SGPT*, SGOT*.

Skin & sunlight:
No problems expected.

Driving, piloting or hazardous work:
Usually not dangerous. Most hazardous reactions likely to occur a few minutes after taking methicillin.

Discontinuing:
Don't discontinue without doctor's advice until you complete prescribed dose, even though symptoms diminish or disappear.

Others:
- May interfere with the accuracy of some medical tests.
- Birth control pills may not be effective. Use additional birth-control methods.

POSSIBLE INTERACTION WITH OTHER DRUGS

GENERIC NAME OR DRUG CLASS	COMBINED EFFECT
Beta-adrenergic blockers*	Increased chance of anaphylaxis (see emergency information on inside front cover).
Birth control pills	Impaired contraceptive efficiency.
Chloramphenicol	Decreased effect of both drugs.
Erythromycins*	Decreased effect of both drugs.
Loperamide	Decreased methicillin effect.
Paromomycin	Decreased effect of both drugs.
Probenecid	Increased effect of all penicillins.
Tetracyclines*	Decreased effect of both drugs.
Troleandomycin	Decreased effect of both drugs.

POSSIBLE INTERACTION WITH OTHER SUBSTANCES

INTERACTS WITH	COMBINED EFFECT
Alcohol:	Occasional stomach irritation.
Beverages: Acidic fruits or juices, aged cheese, wines, syrups (if taken with).	Decreased antibiotic effect.
Cocaine:	No proven problems.
Foods:	None expected.
Marijuana:	No proven problems.
Tobacco:	None expected.

METHOTREXATE

BRAND NAMES

Amethopterin	Mexate
Folex	Mexate AQ
Folex PFS	Rheumatrex

BASIC INFORMATION

Habit forming? No
Prescription needed? Yes
Available as generic? Yes
Drug class: Antimetabolite, antipsoriatic

USES

- Treatment for some kinds of cancer.
- Treatment for psoriasis in patients with severe problems.
- Treatment for severe rheumatoid arthritis.

DOSAGE & USAGE INFORMATION

How to take:
Tablet—Swallow with liquid.

When to take:
At the same time each day.

If you forget a dose:
Skip the missed dose. Don't double the next dose.

What drug does:
Inhibits abnormal-cell reproduction.

Time lapse before drug works:
May require 6 weeks for maximum effect.

Don't take with:
Any other medicine without consulting your doctor or pharmacist.

OVERDOSE

SYMPTOMS:
Headache, stupor, seizures.
WHAT TO DO:
- **Dial 0 (operator) or 911 (emergency) for an ambulance or medical help. Then give first aid immediately.**
- **If patient is unconscious and not breathing, give mouth-to-mouth breathing. If there is no heartbeat, use cardiac massage and mouth-to-mouth breathing (CPR). Don't try to make patient vomit. If you can't get help quickly, take patient to nearest emergency facility.**
- **See emergency information on inside covers.**

POSSIBLE ADVERSE REACTIONS OR SIDE EFFECTS

SYMPTOMS	WHAT TO DO
Life-threatening:	
Hives, rash, intense itching, faintness soon after a dose (anaphylaxis).	Seek emergency treatment immediately.
Common:	
• Black stools or bloody vomit.	Discontinue. Seek emergency treatment.
• Sore throat, fever, mouth sores; chills; unusual bleeding or bruising.	Discontinue. Call doctor right away.
• Abdominal pain, nausea, vomiting.	Continue. Call doctor when convenient.
Infrequent:	
• Seizures.	Discontinue. Seek emergency treatment.
• Dizziness when standing after sitting or lying, drowsiness, headache, confusion, blurred vision, shortness of breath, joint pain, blood in urine, jaundice, diarrhea, red skin, back pain.	Discontinue. Call doctor right away.
• Cough, rash, sexual difficulties in males.	Continue. Call doctor when convenient.
• Acne, boils, hair loss, itchy skin.	Continue. Tell doctor at next visit.
Rare:	
• Convulsions.	Seek emergency treatment.
• Painful urination.	Discontinue. Seek emergency treatment.

WARNINGS & PRECAUTIONS

Don't take if:
You are allergic to any antimetabolite.

Before you start, consult your doctor:
- If you are alcoholic.
- If you have blood, liver or kidney disease.
- If you have colitis or peptic ulcer.
- If you have gout.
- If you have an infection.
- If you plan to become pregnant within 3 months.

Over age 60:
Adverse reactions and side effects may be more frequent and severe than in younger persons.

Pregnancy:
- Psoriasis—Risk to unborn child outweighs drug benefits. Don't use.
- Cancer—Consult doctor.

Breast-feeding:
Drug passes into milk. Avoid drug or discontinue nursing.

Infants & children:
Use only under special medical supervision.

Prolonged use:
- Adverse reactions more likely the longer drug is required.
- Talk to your doctor about the need for follow-up medical examinations or laboratory studies to check liver function, kidney function, complete blood counts (white blood cell count, platelet count, red blood cell count, hemoglobin, hematocrit).

Skin & sunlight:
Increased sensitivity to sunlight.

Driving, piloting or hazardous work:
Avoid if you feel dizzy, drowsy or confused. Otherwise, no problems expected.

Discontinuing:
Don't discontinue without doctor's advice until you complete prescribed dose, even though symptoms diminish or disappear. Some side effects may follow discontinuing. Report to doctor blurred vision, convulsions, confusion, persistent headache.

Others:
- Drink more water than usual to cause frequent urination.
- Don't give this medicine to anyone else for any purpose. It is a strong drug that requires close medical supervision.
- Report for frequent medical follow-up and laboratory studies.

 POSSIBLE INTERACTION WITH OTHER DRUGS

GENERIC NAME OR DRUG CLASS	COMBINED EFFECT
Anticoagulants, oral*	Increased anticoagulant effect.
Anticonvulsants, hydantoin*	Possible methotrexate toxicity.
Antigout drugs*	Decreased antigout effect. Toxic levels of methotrexate.
Asparaginase	Decreased methotrexate effect.
Clozapine	Toxic effect on bone marrow.
Diclofenac	May increase toxicity.
Etretinate	Increased chance of toxicity to liver.
Flurouracil	Decreased methotrexate effect.
Folic acid	Possible decreased methotrexate effect.
Isoniazid	Increased risk of liver damage.
Leukovorin calcium	Decreased methotrexate toxicity.
Levamisole	Increased risk of bone marrow depression.
Non-steroidal anti-inflammatory drugs (NSAIDs)*	Possible increased methotrexate toxicity.
Oxyphenbutazone	Possible methotrexate toxicity.
Phenylbutazone	Possible methotrexate toxicity.
Phenytoin	Possible increased methotrexate toxicity.
Probenecid	Possible methotrexate toxicity.
Pyrimethamine	Increased toxic effect of methotrexate.
Salicylates* (including aspirin)	Possible methotrexate toxicity.
Sulfadoxine and pyrimethamine	Increased risk of toxicity.
Sulfa drugs*	Possible methotrexate toxicity.
Tetracyclines*	Possible methotrexate toxicity.
Tiopronin	Increased risk of toxicity to bone marrow and kidneys.

 POSSIBLE INTERACTION WITH OTHER SUBSTANCES

INTERACTS WITH	COMBINED EFFECT
Alcohol:	Likely liver damage. Avoid.
Beverages:	Extra fluid intake decreases chance of methotrexate toxicity.
Cocaine:	Increased chance of methotrexate adverse reactions. Avoid.
Foods:	None expected.
Marijuana:	None expected.
Tobacco:	None expected.

*See Glossary

METHSUXIMIDE

BRAND NAMES

Celontin

BASIC INFORMATION

Habit forming? No
Prescription needed? Yes
Available as generic? No
Drug class: Anticonvulsant (succinimide)

 USES

Controls seizures in treatment of epilepsy.

 DOSAGE & USAGE INFORMATION

How to take:
Capsule—Swallow with liquid or food to lessen stomach irritation.

When to take:
Every day in regularly spaced doses, according to prescription.

If you forget a dose:
Take as soon as you remember up to 2 hours late. If more than 2 hours, wait for next scheduled dose (don't double this dose).

What drug does:
Depresses nerve transmissions in part of brain that controls muscles.

Time lapse before drug works:
3 hours.

Don't take with:
Any other medicine without consulting your doctor or pharmacist.

 OVERDOSE

SYMPTOMS:
Coma
WHAT TO DO:
- Dial 0 (operator) or 911 (emergency) for an ambulance or medical help. Then give first aid immediately.
- If patient is unconscious and not breathing, give mouth-to-mouth breathing. If there is no heartbeat, use cardiac massage and mouth-to-mouth breathing (CPR). Don't try to make patient vomit. If you can't get help quickly, take patient to nearest emergency facility.
- See emergency information on inside covers.

 POSSIBLE ADVERSE REACTIONS OR SIDE EFFECTS

SYMPTOMS	WHAT TO DO
Life-threatening:	
In case of overdose, see previous column.	
Common:	
Nausea, vomiting, appetite loss, dizziness, drowsiness, hiccups, abdominal pain.	Continue. Call doctor when convenient.
Infrequent:	
Headache, irritability, mood change, tiredness.	Continue. Call doctor when convenient.
Rare:	
• Rash, sore throat, fever, unusual bleeding or bruising, depression, confusion, eye or gum swelling, blood in urine, vaginal bleeding.	Discontinue. Call doctor right away.
• Swollen lymph glands.	Continue. Call doctor when convenient.

WARNINGS & PRECAUTIONS

Don't take if:
You are allergic to any succinimide anticonvulsant.

Before you start, consult your doctor:
- If you plan to become pregnant within medication period.
- If you take other anticonvulsants.
- If you have blood disease.
- If you have kidney or liver disease.

Over age 60:
Adverse reactions and side effects may be more frequent and severe than in younger persons.

Pregnancy:
Risk to unborn child outweighs drug benefits. Don't use.

Breast-feeding:
Drug passes into milk. Avoid drug or discontinue nursing.

Infants & children:
Use only under medical supervision.

Prolonged use:
Talk to your doctor about the need for follow-up medical examinations or laboratory studies to check complete blood counts (white blood cell count, platelet count, red blood cell count, hemoglobin, hematocrit), liver function, kidney function, urine.

Skin & sunlight:
No problems expected.

Driving, piloting or hazardous work:
Don't drive or pilot aircraft until you learn how medicine affects you. Don't work around dangerous machinery. Don't climb ladders or work in high places. Danger increases if you drink alcohol or take medicine affecting alertness and reflexes, such as antihistamines, tranquilizers, sedatives, pain medicine, narcotics and mind-altering drugs.

Discontinuing:
Don't discontinue without doctor's advice until you complete prescribed dose, even though symptoms diminish or disappear.

Others:
- Your response to medicine should be checked regularly by your doctor. Dose and schedule may have to be altered frequently to fit individual needs.
- Periodic blood-cell counts, kidney- and liver-function studies recommended.
- May discolor urine pink to red-brown. No action necessary.

POSSIBLE INTERACTION WITH OTHER DRUGS

GENERIC NAME OR DRUG CLASS	COMBINED EFFECT
Anticonvulsants, other*	Increased effect of both drugs.
Antidepressants, tricyclic (TCA)*	May provoke seizures.
Antipsychotics*	May provoke seizures.
Haloperidol	Decreased haloperidol effect; changed seizure pattern.

POSSIBLE INTERACTION WITH OTHER SUBSTANCES

INTERACTS WITH	COMBINED EFFECT
Alcohol:	May provoke seizures.
Beverages:	None expected.
Cocaine:	May provoke seizures.
Foods:	None expected.
Marijuana:	May provoke seizures.
Tobacco:	None expected.

*See Glossary

METHYLCELLULOSE

BRAND NAMES

Cellothyl   Cologel
Citrucel

BASIC INFORMATION

Habit forming? No
Prescription needed? No
Available as generic? Yes
Drug class: Laxative (bulk-forming)

 ## USES

Relieves constipation and prevents straining for
bowel movement.

 ## DOSAGE & USAGE INFORMATION

How to take:
Tablet, liquid, powder, flakes, granules—Dilute
dose in 8 oz. cold water or fruit juice. Drink 6 to
8 glasses of water each day in addition to the
one with each dose.

When to take:
At the same time each day, preferably morning.

If you forget a dose:
Take as soon as you remember. Resume
regular schedule.

What drug does:
Absorbs water, stimulating the bowel to form a
soft, bulky stool.

Time lapse before drug works:
May require 2 or 3 days to begin, then works in
12 to 24 hours.

Don't take with:
- Any other medicine without consulting your
  doctor or pharmacist.
- Don't take within 2 hours of taking another
  medicine. Laxative interferes with medicine
  absorption.

 ## OVERDOSE

SYMPTOMS:
None expected.
WHAT TO DO:
**Overdose unlikely to threaten life. If person
takes much larger amount than prescribed,
call doctor, poison-control center or
hospital emergency room for instructions.**

 ## POSSIBLE ADVERSE REACTIONS OR SIDE EFFECTS

SYMPTOMS	WHAT TO DO
Life-threatening:	
None expected.	
Common:	
None expected.	
Infrequent:	
Swallowing difficulty, "lump in throat" sensation, nausea, vomiting, diarrhea.	Continue. Call doctor when convenient.
Rare:	
Itchy skin, rash, intestinal blockage, asthma.	Discontinue. Call doctor right away.

WARNINGS & PRECAUTIONS

Don't take if:
- You are allergic to any bulk-forming laxative.
- You have symptoms of appendicitis, inflamed bowel or intestinal blockage.
- You have missed a bowel movement for only 1 or 2 days.

Before you start, consult your doctor:
- If you have diabetes.
- If you have a laxative habit.
- If you have rectal bleeding.
- If you have difficulty swallowing.
- If you take other laxatives.

Over age 60:
Adverse reactions and side effects may be more frequent and severe than in younger persons.

Pregnancy:
Most bulk-forming laxatives contain sodium or sugars which may cause fluid retention. Avoid if possible.

Breast-feeding:
No problems expected.

Infants & children:
Use only under medical supervision.

Prolonged use:
Don't take for more than 1 week unless under a doctor's supervision. May cause laxative dependence.

Skin & sunlight:
No problems expected.

Driving, piloting or hazardous work:
No problems expected.

Discontinuing:
May be unnecessary to finish medicine. Follow doctor's instructions.

Others:
Don't take to "flush out" your system or as a "tonic."

POSSIBLE INTERACTION WITH OTHER DRUGS

GENERIC NAME OR DRUG CLASS	COMBINED EFFECT
Digitalis preparations*	Decreased digitalis effect.
Salicylates* (including aspirin)	Decreased salicylate effect.

POSSIBLE INTERACTION WITH OTHER SUBSTANCES

INTERACTS WITH	COMBINED EFFECT
Alcohol:	None expected.
Beverages:	None expected.
Cocaine:	None expected.
Foods:	None expected.
Marijuana:	None expected.
Tobacco:	None expected.

METHYLDOPA

BRAND NAMES

Aldoclor
Aldomet
Aldoril
Apo-Methyldopa

Dopamet
Novomedopa
Nu-Medopa
PMS Dopazide

BASIC INFORMATION

Habit forming? No
Prescription needed? Yes
Available as generic? Yes
Drug class: Antihypertensive

 USES

Reduces high blood pressure.

 DOSAGE & USAGE INFORMATION

How to take:
Liquid or tablet—Swallow with liquid. If you can't swallow whole, crumble tablet and take with liquid or food.

When to take:
At the same times each day.

If you forget a dose:
Take as soon as you remember up to 2 hours late. If more than 2 hours, wait for next scheduled dose (don't double this dose).

What drug does:
Relaxes walls of small arteries to decrease blood pressure.

Time lapse before drug works:
Continual use for 2 to 4 weeks may be necessary to determine effectiveness.

Continued next column

 OVERDOSE

SYMPTOMS:
Drowsiness; exhaustion; stupor; confusion; slow, weak pulse.
WHAT TO DO:
- **Dial 0 (operator) or 911 (emergency) for an ambulance or medical help. Then give first aid immediately.**
- **If patient is unconscious and not breathing, give mouth-to-mouth breathing. If there is no heartbeat, use cardiac massage and mouth-to-mouth breathing (CPR). Don't try to make patient vomit. If you can't get help quickly, take patient to nearest emergency facility.**
- **See emergency information on inside covers.**

Don't take with:
Any other medicine without consulting your doctor or pharmacist.

 POSSIBLE ADVERSE REACTIONS OR SIDE EFFECTS

SYMPTOMS	WHAT TO DO
Life-threatening: In case of overdose, see previous column.	
Common: Depression, sedation, nightmares, headache, drowsiness, weakness, stuffy nose, dry mouth, fluid retention, swollen feet or legs.	Continue. Call doctor when convenient.
Infrequent: • Fast heartbeat, fainting.	Discontinue. Call doctor right away.
• Insomnia, nausea, vomiting, diarrhea, constipation, foot and hand numbness and tingling.	Continue. Call doctor when convenient.
• Swollen breasts, diminished sex drive.	Continue. Tell doctor at next visit.
Rare: Rash, jaundice, dark urine, chills, breathing difficulty, unexplained fever, sore or "black" tongue, severe abdominal pain, decreased mental activity and memory impairment, facial paralysis, slow heartbeat, chest pain, swollen abdomen.	Discontinue. Call doctor right away.

 WARNINGS & PRECAUTIONS

Don't take if:
You will have surgery within 2 months, including dental surgery, requiring general or spinal anesthesia.

Before you start, consult your doctor:
If you have liver disease.

Over age 60:
- Increased susceptibility to dizziness, unsteadiness, fainting, falling.
- Drug can produce or intensify Parkinson's disease.

Pregnancy:
No proven problems. Consult doctor.

Breast-feeding:
No proven problems. Consult doctor.

Infants & children:
Not used.

Prolonged use:
- May cause anemia.
- Severe edema (fluid retention).
- Talk to your doctor about the need for follow-up medical examinations or laboratory studies to check complete blood counts (white blood cell count, platelet count, red blood cell count, hemoglobin, hematocrit), blood pressure, liver function.

Skin & sunlight:
No problems expected.

Driving, piloting or hazardous work:
Don't drive or pilot aircraft until you learn how medicine affects you. Don't work around dangerous machinery. Don't climb ladders or work in high places. Danger increases if you drink alcohol or take medicine affecting alertness and reflexes, such as antihistamines, tranquilizers, sedatives, pain medicine, narcotics and mind-altering drugs.

Discontinuing:
Don't discontinue without consulting doctor. Dose may require gradual reduction if you have taken drug for a long time. Doses of other drugs may also require adjustment.

Others:
Avoid heavy exercise, exertion, sweating.

POSSIBLE INTERACTION WITH OTHER DRUGS

GENERIC NAME OR DRUG CLASS	COMBINED EFFECT
ACE inhibitors*: captopril, enalapril, lisinopril	Possible excessive potassium in blood.
Amphetamines*	Decreased methyldopa effect.
Anticoagulants, oral*	Increased anticoagulant effect.
Antidepressants, tricyclic (TCA)*	Dangerous blood pressure rise. Decreased methyldopa effect.
Antihypertensives*	Increased antihypertensive effect.
Carteolol	Increased antihypertensive effect.
Clozapine	Toxic effect on the central nervous system.
Dapsone	Increased risk of adverse effect on blood cells.
Didanosine	Increased risk of pancreatitis.

Digitalis preparations*	Excessively slow heartbeat.
Diuretics, thiazide*	Increased methyldopa effect.
Ethinamate	Dangerous increased effects of ethinamate. Avoid combining.
Fluoxetine	Increased depressant effects of both drugs.
Guanfacine	May increase depressant effects of either drug.
Haloperidol	Increased sedation. Possibly dementia.
Isoniazid	Increased risk of liver damage.
Leucovorin	High alcohol content of leucovorin may cause adverse effects.
Levodopa	Increased effect of both drugs.
Loxapine	May increase toxic effects of both drugs.
MAO inhibitors*	Dangerous blood pressure rise.
Methyprylon	Increased sedative effect, perhaps to dangerous level. Avoid.
Nabilone	Greater depression of central nervous system.
Nicardipine	Blood pressure drop. Dosages may require adjustment.

Continued on page 950

POSSIBLE INTERACTION WITH OTHER SUBSTANCES

INTERACTS WITH	COMBINED EFFECT
Alcohol:	Increased sedation. Excessive blood pressure drop. Avoid.
Beverages:	None expected.
Cocaine:	Increased risk of heart block and high blood pressure.
Foods:	None expected.
Marijuana:	Possible fainting.
Tobacco:	Possible increased blood pressure.

METHYLDOPA & THIAZIDE DIURETICS

BRAND AND GENERIC NAMES

Aldoclor
Aldoril
METHYLDOPA &
   CHLOROTHIAZIDE

METHYLDOPA &
HYDROCHLORO-
THIAZIDE
Novodoparil
Novomedopa
PMS Dopazide

BASIC INFORMATION

Habit forming? No
Prescription needed? Yes
Available as generic? Yes
Drug class: Antihypertensive, diuretic (thiazide)

USES

* Controls, but doesn't cure, high blood pressure.
* Reduces fluid retention (edema).

DOSAGE & USAGE INFORMATION

How to take:
Tablet—Swallow with liquid. If you can't swallow whole, crumble tablet and take with liquid or food.

When to take:
At the same times each day.

If you forget a dose:
Take as soon as you remember up to 2 hours late. If more than 2 hours, wait for next scheduled dose (don't double this dose).

What drug does:
* Relaxes walls of small arteries to decrease blood pressure.
* Forces sodium and water excretion, reducing body fluid.

Continued next column

OVERDOSE

SYMPTOMS:
Drowsiness; exhaustion; cramps; weakness; stupor; confusion; slow, weak pulse; coma.
WHAT TO DO:
* **Dial 0 (operator) or 911 (emergency) for an ambulance or medical help. Then give first aid immediately.**
* **If patient is unconscious and not breathing, give mouth-to-mouth breathing. If there is no heartbeat, use cardiac massage and mouth-to-mouth breathing (CPR). Don't try to make patient vomit. If you can't get help quickly, take patient to nearest emergency facility.**
* **See emergency information on inside covers.**

* Reduced body fluid and relaxed arteries lower blood pressure.

Time lapse before drug works:
Continual use for 2 to 4 weeks may be necessary to determine effectiveness.

Don't take with:
* Non-prescription drugs without consulting doctor.
* Any other medicine without consulting your doctor or pharmacist.

POSSIBLE ADVERSE REACTIONS OR SIDE EFFECTS

SYMPTOMS	WHAT TO DO
Life-threatening: Irregular heartbeat, weak pulse.	Discontinue. Seek emergency treatment.
Common: Depression, nightmares, drowsiness, weakness, stuffy nose, dry mouth, swollen feet and ankles, dizziness, sedation, increased thirst, muscle cramps.	Continue. Call doctor when convenient.
Infrequent: • Fast heartbeat, change in vision, abdominal pain, nervousness.	Discontinue. Call doctor right away.
• Insomnia, nausea, vomiting, diarrhea, headache, constipation.	Continue. Call doctor when convenient.
Rare: Rash, jaundice, dark urine, chills, breathing difficulty, hives, sore throat, fever, mouth sores, sore or "black" tongue, severe abdominal pain, decreased mental activity, memory impairment, facial paralysis, slow heartbeat, chest pain.	Discontinue. Call doctor right away.

WARNINGS & PRECAUTIONS

Don't take if:
* You are allergic to any thiazide diuretic drug.
* If you will have surgery within 2 months, including dental surgery, requiring general or spinal anesthesia.

Before you start, consult your doctor:
* If you are allergic to any sulfa drug.
* If you have gout, liver, pancreas or kidney disorder.

Over age 60:
- Increased susceptibility to dizziness, unsteadiness, fainting, falling.
- Drug can produce or intensify Parkinson's disease.

Pregnancy:
Risk to unborn child outweighs drug benefits. Don't use.

Breast-feeding:
Drug passes into milk. Avoid drug or discontinue nursing until you finish medicine. Consult doctor for advice on maintaining milk supply.

Infants & children:
Not recommended.

Prolonged use:
- May cause anemia.
- Severe edema (fluid retention).
- Talk to your doctor about the need for follow-up medical examinations or laboratory studies to check complete blood counts (white blood cell count, platelet count, red blood cell count, hemoglobin, hematocrit), blood pressure, liver function.

Skin & sunlight:
May cause rash or intensify sunburn in areas exposed to sun or sunlamp.

Driving, piloting or hazardous work:
Don't drive or pilot aircraft until you learn how medicine affects you. Don't work around dangerous machinery. Don't climb ladders or work in high places. Danger increases if you drink alcohol or take medicine affecting alertness and reflexes, such as antihistamines, tranquilizers, sedatives, pain medicine, narcotics and mind-altering drugs.

Discontinuing:
Don't discontinue without consulting doctor. Dose may require gradual reduction if you have taken drug for a long time. Doses of other drugs may also require adjustment.

Others:
- Hot weather and fever may cause dehydration and drop in blood pressure. Dose may require temporary adjustment. Weigh daily and report any unexpected weight decreases to your doctor.
- May cause rise in uric acid, leading to gout.
- May cause blood-sugar rise in diabetics.
- Avoid heavy exercise, exertion, sweating.

POSSIBLE INTERACTION WITH OTHER DRUGS

GENERIC NAME OR DRUG CLASS	COMBINED EFFECT
Acebutolol	Increased antihypertensive effect. Dosages of both drugs may require adjustments.
ACE inhibitors*: captopril, enalapril, lisinopril	Possible excessive potassium in blood.
Allopurinol	Decreased allopurinol effect.
Amphetamines*	Decreased methyldopa effect.
Anticoagulants, oral*	Increased anticoagulant effect.
Antidepressants, tricyclic (TCA)*	Dangerous changes in blood pressure. Avoid combination unless under medical supervision.
Antihypertensives*	Increased antihypertensive effect.
Barbiturates*	Increased hydrochlorothiazide effect.
Carteolol	Increased antihypertensive effect.
Cholestyamine	Decreased hydrochlorothiazide effect.

Continued page 950

POSSIBLE INTERACTION WITH OTHER SUBSTANCES

INTERACTS WITH	COMBINED EFFECT
Alcohol:	Increased sedation. Excessive blood pressure drop. Avoid.
Beverages:	None expected.
Cocaine:	Increased risk of heart block and high blood pressure.
Foods: Licorice.	Excessive potassium loss that causes dangerous heart rhythms.
Marijuana:	May increase blood pressure.
Tobacco:	Possible increased blood pressure.

*See Glossary

METHYLERGONOVINE

BRAND NAMES

Methergine   Methylergometrine

BASIC INFORMATION

Habit forming? No
Prescription needed? Yes
Available as generic? No
Drug class: Ergot preparation (uterine stimulant)

 ## USES

Retards excessive post-delivery bleeding.

 ## DOSAGE & USAGE INFORMATION

How to take:
Tablet—Swallow with liquid or food to lessen stomach irritation.

When to take:
At the same times each day.

If you forget a dose:
Don't take missed dose and don't double next one. Wait for next scheduled dose.

What drug does:
Causes smooth-muscle cells of uterine wall to contract and surround bleeding blood vessels of relaxed uterus.

Time lapse before drug works:
Tablets—20 to 30 minutes.

Don't take with:
Any other medicine without consulting your doctor or pharmacist.

 ## OVERDOSE

SYMPTOMS:
Vomiting, diarrhea, weak pulse, low blood pressure, dyspnea, angina, convulsions.
WHAT TO DO:
- **Dial 0 (operator) or 911 (emergency) for an ambulance or medical help. Then give first aid immediately.**
- **If patient is unconscious and not breathing, give mouth-to-mouth breathing. If there is no heartbeat, use cardiac massage and mouth-to-mouth breathing (CPR). Don't try to make patient vomit. If you can't get help quickly, take patient to nearest emergency facility.**
- **See emergency information on inside covers.**

 ## POSSIBLE ADVERSE REACTIONS OR SIDE EFFECTS

SYMPTOMS	WHAT TO DO
Life-threatening:	
In case of overdose, see previous column.	
Common:	
Nausea, vomiting, severe lower abdominal menstrual-like cramps.	Discontinue. Call doctor right away.
Infrequent:	
• Confusion, ringing in ears, diarrhea, muscle cramps.	Discontinue. Call doctor right away.
• Unusual sweating.	Continue. Call doctor when convenient.
Rare:	
Sudden, severe headache; shortness of breath; chest pain; numb, cold hands and feet.	Discontinue. Seek emergency treatment.

METHYLERGONOVINE

WARNINGS & PRECAUTIONS

Don't take if:
You are allergic to any ergot preparation.

Before you start, consult your doctor:
- If you have coronary-artery or blood-vessel disease.
- If you have liver or kidney disease.
- If you have high blood pressure.
- If you have postpartum infection.

Over age 60:
Not recommended.

Pregnancy:
Risk to unborn child outweighs drug benefits. Don't use.

Breast-feeding:
Drug passes into milk. Avoid drug or discontinue nursing until you finish medicine. Consult doctor for advice on maintaining milk supply.

Infants & children:
Not recommended.

Prolonged use:
Talk to your doctor about the need for follow-up medical examinations or laboratory studies to check blood pressure, ECG*.

Skin & sunlight:
No problems expected.

Driving, piloting or hazardous work:
No problems expected.

Discontinuing:
May be unnecessary to finish medicine. Follow doctor's instructions.

Others:
Drug should be used for short time only following childbirth or miscarriage.

POSSIBLE INTERACTION WITH OTHER DRUGS

GENERIC NAME OR DRUG CLASS	COMBINED EFFECT
Beta-adrenergic blockers*	Possible vasospasm (peripheral and cardiac)
Ergot preparations, other*	Increased methyl-ergonovine effect.

POSSIBLE INTERACTION WITH OTHER SUBSTANCES

INTERACTS WITH	COMBINED EFFECT
Alcohol:	None expected.
Beverages:	None expected.
Cocaine:	None expected.
Foods:	None expected.
Marijuana:	None expected.
Tobacco:	Decreased methylergonovine effect. Don't smoke.

METHYLPHENIDATE

BRAND NAMES

Ritalin   Ritalin SR

BASIC INFORMATION

Habit forming? Yes
Available as generic? Yes
Prescription needed? Yes
Drug class: Sympathomimetic

 USES

- Treatment for hyperactive children.
- Treatment for narcolepsy (uncontrollable attacks of sleepiness).

 DOSAGE & USAGE INFORMATION

How to take:
Tablet or extended-release tablet—Swallow with liquid or food to lessen stomach irritation. If you can't swallow whole, crumble tablet and take with liquid or food.

When to take:
At the same times each day, preferably on an empty stomach.

If you forget a dose:
Take as soon as you remember up to 2 hours late. If more than 2 hours, wait for next scheduled dose (don't double this dose).

Continued next column

 OVERDOSE

SYMPTOMS:
Rapid heartbeat, fever, confusion, vomiting, agitation, hallucinations, convulsions, coma.
WHAT TO DO:
- **Dial 0 (operator) or 911 (emergency) for an ambulance or medical help. Then give first aid immediately.**
- **If patient is unconscious and not breathing, give mouth-to-mouth breathing. If there is no heartbeat, use cardiac massage and mouth-to-mouth breathing (CPR). Don't try to make patient vomit. If you can't get help quickly, take patient to nearest emergency facility.**
- **See emergency information on inside covers.**

What drug does:
Stimulates brain to improve alertness, concentration and attention span. Calms the hyperactive child.

Time lapse before drug works:
- 1 month or more for maximum effect on child.
- 30 minutes to stimulate adults.

Don't take with:
Any other medicine without consulting your doctor or pharmacist.

 POSSIBLE ADVERSE REACTIONS OR SIDE EFFECTS

SYMPTOMS	WHAT TO DO
Life-threatening:	
In case of overdose, see previous column.	
Common:	
• Mood change.	Continue. Call doctor when convenient.
• Nervousness, insomnia, dizziness, headache, appetite loss.	Continue. Tell doctor at next visit.
Infrequent:	
• Rash or hives; chest pain; fast, irregular heartbeat; unusual bruising; joint pain; psychosis; uncontrollable movements; unexplained fever.	Discontinue. Call doctor right away.
• Nausea, abdominal pain.	Continue. Call doctor when convenient.
Rare:	
• Blurred vision, sore throat, red spots under skin, convulsions.	Discontinue. Call doctor right away.
• Unusual tiredness.	Continue. Call doctor when convenient.

 WARNINGS & PRECAUTIONS

Don't take if:
- You are allergic to methylphenidate.
- You have glaucoma.
- Patient is younger than 6.

Before you start, consult your doctor:
- If you have epilepsy.
- If you have high blood pressure.
- If you take MAO inhibitors.

Over age 60:
Adverse reactions and side effects may be more frequent and severe than in younger persons.

Pregnancy:
No proven harm to unborn child. Avoid if possible.

Breast-feeding:
No proven problems. Consult doctor.

Infants & children:
Use only under medical supervision for children 6 or older.

Prolonged use:
- Rare possibility of physical growth retardation.
- Talk to your doctor about the need for follow-up medical examinations or laboratory studies to check blood pressure, complete blood counts (white blood cell count, platelet count, red blood cell count, hemoglobin, hematocrit), growth charts.

Skin & sunlight:
No problems expected.

Driving, piloting or hazardous work:
No problems expected.

Discontinuing:
Don't discontinue abruptly. Don't discontinue without doctor's advice until you complete prescribed dose, even though symptoms diminish or disappear. Report to your doctor any new symptoms of depression, unusual behavior, unusual weakness or tiredness.

Others:
Dose must be carefully adjusted by doctor.

POSSIBLE INTERACTION WITH OTHER DRUGS

GENERIC NAME OR DRUG CLASS	COMBINED EFFECT
Acebutolol	Decreased effects of both drugs.
Anticholinergics*	Increased anticholinergic effect.
Anticoagulants, oral*	Increased anticoagulant effect.
Anticonvulsants*	Increased anticonvulsant effect.
Antidepressants, tricyclic (TCA)*	Increased antidepressant effect. Decreased methylphenidate effect.
Antihypertensives*	Decreased antihypertensive effect.

Central nervous system (CNS) depressants*	Decreased effect of CNS depressant.
Dextrothyroxine	Increased methylphenidate effect.
Guanadrel	Decreased guanadrel effect.
Guanethidine	Decreased guanethidine effect.
MAO inhibitors*	Dangerous rise in blood pressure.
Minoxidil	Decreased minoxidil effect.
Nitrates*	Possible decreased effects of both drugs.
Oxprenolol	Decreased effects of both drugs.
Oxyphenbutazone	Increased oxyphenbutazone effect.
Phenylbutazone	Increased phenylbutazone effect.
Terazosin	Decreases effectiveness of terazosin.

POSSIBLE INTERACTION WITH OTHER SUBSTANCES

INTERACTS WITH	COMBINED EFFECT
Alcohol:	None expected.
Beverages: Caffeine drinks.	May raise blood pressure.
Cocaine:	High risk of heartbeat irregularities and high blood pressure.
Foods: Foods containing tyramine*	May raise blood pressure.
Marijuana:	None expected.
Tobacco:	None expected.

METHYLPRENISOLONE

BRAND NAMES

See complete list of brand names in the *Brand Name Directory*, page 922.

BASIC INFORMATION

Habit forming? No
Prescription needed? Yes
Available as generic? Yes
Drug class: Cortisone drug (adrenal corticosteroid)

USES

- Reduces inflammation caused by many different medical problems.
- Treatment for some allergic diseases, blood disorders, kidney diseases, asthma and emphysema.
- Replaces corticosteroid deficiencies.

DOSAGE & USAGE INFORMATION

How to take:
- Tablet—Swallow with liquid or food to lessen stomach irritation. If you can't swallow whole, crumble tablet and take with liquid or food.
- Injection—Take under doctor's supervision.

When to take:
At the same times each day. Take once-a-day or once-every-other-day doses in mornings.

If you forget a dose:
- Several-doses-per-day prescription—Take as soon as you remember up to 2 hours late. If more than 2 hours, wait for next scheduled dose (don't double this dose).
- Once-a-day dose or less—Wait for next dose. Double this dose.

What drug does:
Decreases inflammatory responses.

Time lapse before drug works:
2 to 4 days.

Don't take with:
Any other medicine without consulting your doctor or pharmacist.

OVERDOSE

SYMPTOMS:
Headache, convulsions, heart failure.
WHAT TO DO:
- Dial 0 (operator) or 911 (emergency) for an ambulance or medical help. Then give first aid immediately.
- See emergency information on inside covers.

POSSIBLE ADVERSE REACTIONS OR SIDE EFFECTS

SYMPTOMS	WHAT TO DO
Life-threatening:	
Hives, rash, intense itching, faintness soon after a dose (anaphylaxis).	Seek emergency treatment immediately.
Common:	
Acne, poor wound healing, thirst, indigestion, nausea, vomiting, constipation, gaseousness, unpleasant taste, diarrhea, headache, cough, dizziness, hoarseness, appetite gain or loss.	Continue. Call doctor when convenient.
Infrequent:	
• Black, bloody or tarry stools; various infections; swallowing difficulty.	Discontinue. Seek emergency treatment.
• Blurred vision, halos around lights, sore throat, fever, muscle cramps, swollen legs or feet.	Discontinue. Call doctor right away.
• Mood change, insomnia, fatigue, restlessness, frequent urination, weight gain, round face, weakness, irregular menstrual periods, dry mouth, euphoria, nosebleeds.	Continue. Call doctor when convenient.
Rare:	
• Irregular heartbeat.	Discontinue. Seek emergency treatment.
• Rash, numbness or tingling in hands or feet, pancreatitis, thrombophlebitis, hallucinations, convulsions.	Discontinue. Call doctor right away.

WARNINGS & PRECAUTIONS

Don't take if:
- You are allergic to any cortisone drug.
- You have tuberculosis or fungus infection.
- You have herpes infection of eyes, lips or genitals.
- You have bone disease, thyroid disease, colitis, peptic ulcer, diabetes, myasthenia gravis, liver or kidney disease, diverticulitis, glaucoma, heart disease.

Before you start, consult your doctor:
- If you have had tuberculosis.
- If you have congestive heart failure.
- If you have diabetes, peptic ulcer, glaucoma, underactive thyroid, high blood pressure, myasthenia gravis, blood clots in legs or lungs.

Over age 60:
Adverse reactions and side effects may be more frequent and severe than in younger persons. Likely to aggravate edema, diabetes or ulcers. Likely to cause cataracts and osteoporosis (softening of the bones).

Pregnancy:
Risk to unborn child outweighs drug benefits. Don't use.

Breast-feeding:
Drug passes into milk. Avoid drug or discontinue nursing until you finish medicine. Consult doctor for advice on maintaining milk supply.

Infants & children:
Use only under medical supervision.

Prolonged use:
- Retards growth in children.
- Possible glaucoma, cataracts, diabetes, fragile bones and thin skin.
- Functional dependence.
- Talk to your doctor about the need for follow-up medical examinations or laboratory studies to check blood pressure, serum electrolytes, stools for blood.

Skin & sunlight:
No problems expected.

Driving, piloting or hazardous work:
No problems expected.

Discontinuing:
- Don't discontinue without doctor's advice until you complete prescribed dose, even though symptoms diminish or disappear.
- Drug affects your response to surgery, illness, injury or stress for 2 years after discontinuing. Tell anyone who takes medical care of you within 2 years about drug.

Others:
- Avoid immunizations if possible.
- Your resistance to infection is less while taking this drug.
- Advise any doctor or dentist whom you consult that you take this medicine.
- Those who have inactive or "cured" tuberculosis may be subjected to a possible recurrence of active tuberculosis.
- Children who must take cortisone drugs may grow less well.

POSSIBLE INTERACTION WITH OTHER DRUGS

GENERIC NAME OR DRUG CLASS	COMBINED EFFECT
Amphotericin B	Potassium depletion.
Anticholinergics*	Possible glaucoma.
Anticoagulants, oral*	Decreased anticoagulant effect.
Anticonvulsants, hydantoin*	Decreased methylprednisolone effect.
Antidiabetics, oral*	Decreased antidiabetic effect.
Antihistamines*	Decreased methylprednisolone effect.
Aspirin	Increased methylprednisolone effect.
Attentuated virus vaccines*	Possible viral infection.
Barbiturates*	Decreased methylprednisolone effect. Oversedation.
Chloral hydrate	Decreased methylprednisolone effect.
Chlorthalidone	Potassium depletion.
Cholestyramine	Decreased methylprednisolone absorption.
Cholinergics*	Decreased cholinergic effect.
Colestipol	Decreased methylprednisolone absorption.
Contraceptives, oral*	Increased methylprednisolone effect.

Continued page 951

POSSIBLE INTERACTION WITH OTHER SUBSTANCES

INTERACTS WITH	COMBINED EFFECT
Alcohol:	Risk of stomach ulcers.
Beverages:	No proven problems.
Cocaine:	Overstimulation. Avoid.
Foods:	No proven problems.
Marijuana:	Decreased immunity.
Tobacco:	Increased methylprednisolone effect. Possible toxicity.

*See Glossary

METHYPRYLON

BRAND NAMES

Noludar

BASIC INFORMATION

Habit forming? Yes
Prescription needed? Yes
Available as generic? No
Drug class: Sedative (hypnotic)

 ## USES

Treats insomnia.

 ## DOSAGE & USAGE INFORMATION

How to take:
Capsules or tablets—Swallow with liquid or food to lessen stomach irritation. If you can't swallow whole, open capsule and take with liquid or food.

When to take:
At bedtime.

If you forget a dose:
Take as soon as you remember up to 2 hours late. If more than 2 hours, wait for next scheduled dose (don't double this dose).

What drug does:
Increases threshold of arousal centers in the midbrain.

Time lapse before drug works:
Within 45 minutes.

Don't take with:
- Any other medicine that will affect alertness or reflexes.
- Any other medicine without consulting your doctor or pharmacist.

 ## OVERDOSE

SYMPTOMS:
Confusion, difficulty breathing, slow heartbeat, staggering, severe weakness, convulsions, coma.
WHAT TO DO:
- **Dial 0 (operator) or 911 (emergency) for an ambulance or medical help. Then give first aid immediately.**
- **See emergency information on inside covers.**

 ## POSSIBLE ADVERSE REACTIONS OR SIDE EFFECTS

SYMPTOMS	WHAT TO DO
Life-threatening:	
Coma.	Seek emergency treatment immediately.
Common:	
Dizziness, headache, daytime drowsiness.	Continue. Call doctor when convenient.
Infrequent:	
Diarrhea, nausea, vomiting, skin rash, unusual excitement, blurred vision, constipation.	Discontinue. Call doctor right away.
Rare:	
Mouth ulcers, unusual bleeding or bruising, depression, fever.	Discontinue. Call doctor right away.

WARNINGS & PRECAUTIONS

Don't take if:
You have a history of drug abuse.

Before you start, consult your doctor:
• If you have liver disease.
• If you have intermittent porphyria.
• If you have significant kidney disease.

Over age 60:
Adverse reactions and side effects may be more frequent and severe than in younger persons. You may need smaller doses for shorter periods of time.

Pregnancy:
Risk to unborn child outweighs drug benefits. Don't use.

Breast-feeding:
Drug passes into milk. Avoid drug or discontinue nursing until you finish medicine. Consult doctor for advice on maintaining milk supply.

Infants & children:
Not recommended. Avoid.

Prolonged use:
• Not intended for prolonged use.
• Talk to your doctor about the need for follow-up medical examinations or laboratory studies to check complete blood counts (white blood cell count, platelet count, red blood cell count, hemoglobin, hematocrit).

Skin & sunlight:
No problems expected.

Driving, piloting or hazardous work:
Don't drive or pilot aircraft until you learn how medicine affects you. Don't work around dangerous machinery. Don't climb ladders or work in high places. Danger increases if you drink alcohol or take medicine affecting alertness and reflexes.

Discontinuing:
These symptoms may occur after medicine has been discontinued: confusion, seizures, hallucinations, increased dreaming, vomiting, nightmares, restlessness, trembling, insomnia, weakness.

Others:
No problems expected.

POSSIBLE INTERACTION WITH OTHER DRUGS

GENERIC NAME OR DRUG CLASS	COMBINED EFFECT
Central nervous system (CNS) depressants*	Increased sedative effect, perhaps to dangerous level. Avoid.
Clozapine	Toxic effect on the central nervous system.
Ethinamate	Dangerous increased effects of ethinamate. Avoid combining.
Fluoxetine	Increased depressant effects of both drugs.
Guanfacine	May increase depressant effects of either drug.
Leucovorin	High alcohol content of leucovorin may cause adverse effects.
Nabilone	Greater depression of central nervous system.
Other addictive drugs*	Increased risk of habituation.
Sertraline	Increased depressive effects of both drugs.

POSSIBLE INTERACTION WITH OTHER SUBSTANCES

INTERACTS WITH	COMBINED EFFECT
Alcohol:	Excess sedation. Avoid.
Beverages: Caffeine drinks.	Decreased methyprylon effect. Avoid.
Cocaine:	Decreased methyprylon effect.
Foods:	None expected.
Marijuana:	Decreased methyprylon effect.
Tobacco:	None expected.

METHYSERGIDE

BRAND NAMES

Sansert

BASIC INFORMATION

Habit forming? Yes
Prescription needed? Yes
Available as generic? No
Drug class: Vasoconstrictor

 USES

Prevents migraine and other recurring vascular headaches. Not for acute attack.

 DOSAGE & USAGE INFORMATION

How to take:
Tablet—Swallow with liquid or with food to lessen stomach irritation. If you can't swallow whole, crumble tablet and take with liquid or food.

When to take:
At the same times each day.

If you forget a dose:
Don't take missed dose. Wait for next scheduled dose (don't double this dose).

What drug does:
Blocks the action of serotonin, a chemical that constricts blood vessels.

Time lapse before drug works:
About 3 weeks.

Don't take with:
Any other medicine without consulting your doctor or pharmacist.

 OVERDOSE

SYMPTOMS:
Nausea, vomiting, abdominal pain, severe diarrhea, lack of coordination, extreme thirst.
WHAT TO DO:
Overdose unlikely to threaten life. If person takes much larger amount than prescribed, call doctor, poison-control center or hospital emergency room for instructions.

 POSSIBLE ADVERSE REACTIONS OR SIDE EFFECTS

SYMPTOMS	WHAT TO DO
Life-threatening:	
In case of overdose, see previous column.	
Common:	
• Itchy skin.	Discontinue. Call doctor right away.
• Nausea, vomiting, diarrhea, numbness or tingling of extremities, leg weakness, abdominal pain.	Continue. Call doctor when convenient.
• Drowsiness, constipation.	Continue. Tell doctor at next visit.
Infrequent:	
• Anxiety, agitation, hallucinations, unusually fast or slow heartbeat, dizziness.	Discontinue. Call doctor right away.
• Change in vision, nightmares, insomnia.	Continue. Call doctor when convenient.
Rare:	
• Extreme thirst, chest pain, shortness of breath, fever, pale or swollen extremities, leg cramps, lower back pain, side or groin pain, appetite loss, joint and muscle pain, rash, facial flush.	Discontinue. Call doctor right away.
• Painful or difficult urination.	Continue. Call doctor when convenient.
• Weight change, hair loss.	Continue. Tell doctor at next visit.

 WARNINGS & PRECAUTIONS

Don't take if:
• You are allergic to any antiserotonin.
• You plan to become pregnant within medication period.
• You have an infection.
• You have a heart or blood-vessel disease.
• You have a chronic lung disease.
• You have a collagen (connective tissue) disorder.
• You have impaired liver or kidney function.

Before you start, consult your doctor:
- If you have been allergic to any ergot preparation.
- If you have had a peptic ulcer.

Over age 60:
Adverse reactions and side effects may be more frequent and severe than in younger persons.

Pregnancy:
Manufacturer suggests risk to unborn child outweighs drug benefits, even though studies are inconclusive.

Breast-feeding:
Drug probably passes into milk. Avoid drug or discontinue nursing until you finish medicine. Consult doctor for advice on maintaining milk supply.

Infants & children:
Not recommended.

Prolonged use:
- May cause fibrosis, a condition in which scar tissue is deposited on heart valves, in lung tissue, blood vessels and internal organs. After 6 months, decrease dose over 2 to 3 weeks. Then discontinue for at least 2 months for re-evaluation.
- Talk to your doctor about the need for follow-up medical examinations or laboratory studies to check retroperitoneal imaging.

Skin & sunlight:
No problems expected.

Driving, piloting or hazardous work:
Avoid if you feel drowsy or dizzy. Otherwise, no problems expected.

Discontinuing:
- Don't discontinue without consulting doctor. Dose may require gradual reduction if you have taken drug for a long time. Doses of other drugs may also require adjustment.
- Probably should discontinue drug if you don't improve after 3 weeks use.

Others:
- Periodic laboratory tests for liver function and blood counts recommended.
- Potential for abuse.
- Some products contain tartrazine dye. Avoid, especially if you are allergic to aspirin.

 POSSIBLE INTERACTION WITH OTHER DRUGS

GENERIC NAME OR DRUG CLASS	COMBINED EFFECT
Ergot preparations*	Unpredictable increased or decreased effect of either drug.
Narcotics*	Decreased narcotic effect.

 POSSIBLE INTERACTION WITH OTHER SUBSTANCES

INTERACTS WITH	COMBINED EFFECT
Alcohol:	None expected. However, alcohol may trigger a migraine headache.
Beverages: Caffeine drinks.	Decreased methysergide effect.
Cocaine:	May make headache worse.
Foods:	None expected. Avoid foods to which you are allergic.
Marijuana:	No proven problems.
Tobacco:	Blood-vessel constriction. Makes headache worse.

METOCLOPRAMIDE

BRAND NAMES

Clora	Maxolon
Emex	Reclomide
Maxeran	Reglan

BASIC INFORMATION

Habit forming? No
Prescription needed? Yes
Available as generic? Yes
Drug class: Antiemetic, dopaminergic blocker

 USES

- Relieves nausea and vomiting caused by chemotherapy and drug related postoperative factors.
- Relieves symptoms of esophagitis and stomach swelling in people with diabetes.

 DOSAGE & USAGE INFORMATION

How to take:
Tablet or syrup—Swallow with liquid or food to lessen stomach irritation.

When to take:
30 minutes before symptoms expected, up to 4 times a day.

If you forget a dose:
Take as soon as you remember up to 2 hours late. If more than 2 hours, wait for next scheduled dose (don't double this dose).

What drug does:
- Prevents smooth muscle in stomach from relaxing.
- Affects vomiting center in brain.

Continued next column

 OVERDOSE

SYMPTOMS:
Severe drowsiness, muscle spasms, mental confusion, trembling, seizure, coma.
WHAT TO DO:
- **Dial 0 (operator) or 911 (emergency) for an ambulance or medical help. Then give first aid immediately.**
- **If patient is unconscious and not breathing, give mouth-to-mouth breathing. If there is no heartbeat, use cardiac massage and mouth-to-mouth breathing (CPR). Don't try to make patient vomit. If you can't get help quickly, take patient to nearest emergency facility.**
- **See emergency information on inside covers.**

Time lapse before drug works:
30 to 60 minutes.

Don't take with:
Any other medicine without consulting your doctor or pharmacist.

 POSSIBLE ADVERSE REACTIONS OR SIDE EFFECTS

SYMPTOMS	WHAT TO DO
Life-threatening:	
In case of overdose, see previous column.	
Common:	
Drowsiness, restlessness.	Continue. Call doctor when convenient.
Frequent	
Rash.	Continue. Call doctor when convenient.
Infrequent:	
• Wheezing, shortness of breath.	Discontinue. Call doctor right away.
• Dizziness; headache; insomnia; tender, swollen breasts; increased milk flow; menstrual changes; decreased sex drive.	Continue. Call doctor when convenient.
Rare:	
• Abnormal, involuntary movements of jaw, lips and tongue; depression; Parkinson* syndrome.	Discontinue. Call doctor right away.
• Constipation, nausea, diarrhea, dry mouth.	Continue. Call doctor when convenient.

 WARNINGS & PRECAUTIONS

Don't take if:
You are allergic to procaine, procainamide or metoclopramide.

Before you start, consult your doctor:
- If you have Parkinson's disease.
- If you have liver or kidney disease.
- If you have epilepsy.
- If you have bleeding from gastrointestinal tract or intestinal obstruction.
- If you will have surgery within 2 months, including dental surgery, requiring general or spinal anesthesia.

Over age 60:
Adverse reactions and side effects may be more frequent and severe than in younger persons.

Pregnancy:
No proven harm to unborn child. Avoid if possible.

Breast-feeding:
Unknown effect.

Infants & children:
Adverse reactions more likely to occur than in adults.

Prolonged use:
Adverse reactions including muscle spasms and trembling hands more likely to occur.

Skin & sunlight:
No problems expected.

Driving, piloting or hazardous work:
Don't drive or pilot aircraft until you learn how medicine affects you. Don't work around dangerous machinery. Don't climb ladders or work in high places. Danger increases if you drink alcohol or take medicine affecting alertness and reflexes, such as antihistamines, tranquilizers, sedatives, pain medicine, narcotics and mind-altering drugs.

Discontinuing:
May be unnecessary to finish medicine. Follow doctor's instructions.

Others:
No problems expected.

WARNINGS & PRECAUTIONS

GENERIC NAME OR DRUG CLASS	COMBINED EFFECT
Acetaminophen	Increased absorption of acetaminophen.
Anticholinergics*	Decreased metoclopramide effect.
Aspirin	Increased absorption of aspirin.
Bromocriptine	Decreased bromocriptine effect.
Butyophenone	Increased chance of muscle spasm and trembling.
Central nervous system (CNS) depressants*	Excess sedation.
Clozapine	Toxic effect on the central nervous system.
Digitalis preparations*	Decreased absorption of digitalis.
Ethinamate	Dangerous increased effects of ethinamate. Avoid combining.
Fluoxetine	Increased depressant effects of both drugs.
Guanfacine	May increase depressant effects of either drug.
Insulin	Unpredictable changes in blood glucose. Dosages may require adjustment.
Leucovorin	High alcohol content of leucovorin may cause adverse effects.
Levodopa	Increased absorption of levodopa.
Lithium	Increased absorption of lithium.
Loxapine	May increase toxic effects of both drugs.
Methyprylon	Increased sedative effect, perhaps to dangerous level. Avoid.
Nabilone	Greater depression of central nervous system.
Narcotics*	Decreased metoclopramide effect.
Nizatidine	Decreased nizatidine absorption.
Pergolide	Decreased pergolide effect.
Phenothiazines*	Increased chance of muscle spasm and trembling.
Sertraline	Increased depressive effects of both drugs.
Tetracyclines*	Slow stomach emptying.
Thiothixines*	Increased chance of muscle spasm and trembling.

POSSIBLE INTERACTION WITH OTHER SUBSTANCES

INTERACTS WITH	COMBINED EFFECT
Alcohol:	Excess sedation. Avoid.
Beverages: Coffee.	Decreased metoclopramide effect.
Cocaine:	Decreased metoclopramide effect.
Foods:	No problems expected.
Marijuana:	Decreased metoclopramide effect.
Tobacco:	Decreased metoclopramide effect.

*See Glossary

METRONIDAZOLE

BRAND NAMES

Apo-Metronidazole
Flagyl
Flagyl I.V.
Flagyl I.V. RTU
Metizol
Metric 21
Metrogel
Metrogel-Vaginal
Metro I.V.
Metronid

Metryl
Metryl IV
Neo-Metric
Neo-Tric
Novonidazol
PMS Metronidazole
Protostat
Satric
Trikacide

BASIC INFORMATION

Habit forming? No
Prescription needed? Yes
Available as generic? Yes
Drug class: Antiprotozoal

USES

- Treatment for infections susceptible to metronidazole, such as trichomoniasis and amebiasis.
- Topical—Treats acne rosacea (adult acne).
- Vaginal—Treats vaginal infections.

DOSAGE & USAGE INFORMATION

How to take:
- Tablet—Swallow with liquid or food to lessen stomach irritation. If you can't swallow whole, crumble tablet and take with liquid or food.
- Topical gel—Apply thin layer to involved area.

When to take:
- At the same times each day.
- Gel—Apply twice a day.

If you forget a dose:
Take as soon as you remember up to 2 hours late. If more than 2 hours, wait for next scheduled dose (don't double this dose).

What drug does:
Kills organisms causing the infection.

Continued next column

OVERDOSE

SYMPTOMS:
Weakness, nausea, vomiting, diarrhea, confusion, seizures.
WHAT TO DO:
Overdose unlikely to threaten life. If person takes much larger amount than prescribed, call doctor, poison-control center or hospital emergency room for instructions.

Time lapse before drug works:
Begins in 1 hour. May require regular use for 10 days to cure infection.

Don't take with:
- Non-prescription medicines containing alcohol.
- Any other medicine without consulting your doctor or pharmacist.

POSSIBLE ADVERSE REACTIONS OR SIDE EFFECTS

SYMPTOMS	WHAT TO DO
Life-threatening:	
In case of overdose, see previous column.	
Common:	
• Appetite loss, nausea, abdominal pain, diarrhea, vomiting.	Discontinue. Call doctor right away.
• Unpleasant taste.	Continue. Tell doctor at next visit.
Infrequent:	
• Dizziness; headache; rash; hives; skin redness; itchy skin; mouth irritation, soreness or infection; sore throat; fever.	Discontinue. Call doctor right away.
• Vaginal irritation, discharge, dryness; fatigue; weakness.	Continue. Call doctor when convenient.
• Constipation.	Continue. Tell doctor at next visit.
Rare:	
• Mood change; unsteadiness; numbness, tingling, weakness or pain in hands or feet.	Discontinue. Call doctor right away.
• Metallic taste.	Continue. Call doctor when convenient.

WARNINGS & PRECAUTIONS

Don't take if:
- You are allergic to metronidazole.
- You have had a blood-cell or bone-marrow disorder.

Before you start, consult your doctor:
- If you plan to become pregnant within medication period.
- If you have a brain or nervous-system disorder.
- If you have liver or heart disease.
- If you drink alcohol.

Over age 60:
Adverse reactions and side effects may be more frequent and severe than in younger persons.

Pregnancy:
Risk to unborn child outweighs drug benefits. Manufacturer advises against use during first 3 months and only limited use after that. Don't use.

Breast-feeding:
Drug passes into milk. Avoid drug or discontinue nursing until you finish medicine. Consult doctor for advice on maintaining milk supply.

Infants & children:
Use in children for amoeba infection only under close medical supervision.

Prolonged use:
Talk to your doctor about the need for follow-up medical examinations or laboratory studies to check for giardiasis in stools.

Skin & sunlight:
No problems expected.

Driving, piloting or hazardous work:
Avoid if you feel dizzy or unsteady. Otherwise, no problems expected.

Discontinuing:
Don't discontinue without doctor's advice until you complete prescribed dose, even though symptoms diminish or disappear.

Others:
Avoid alcohol 12 hours before and *at least* 24 hours after treatment period with metronidazole.

POSSIBLE INTERACTION WITH OTHER DRUGS

GENERIC NAME OR DRUG CLASS	COMBINED EFFECT
Anticoagulants, oral*	Increased anti-coagulant effect. Possible bleeding or bruising.
Cimetidine	Prolongs increased serum levels.
Didanosine	Increased risk of peripheral neuropathy.
Disulfiram	Disulfiram reaction.* Avoid.
Nizatidine	Increased effect and toxicity of metoprolol.
Oxytetracycline	Decreased metronidazole effect.
Phenobarbital	Decreased effect of metronidazole.
Phenytoin	Decreased effect of metronidazole.

POSSIBLE INTERACTION WITH OTHER SUBSTANCES

INTERACTS WITH	COMBINED EFFECT
Alcohol:	Possible disulfiram reaction.* Avoid alcohol in *any* form or amount.
Beverages:	None expected.
Cocaine:	Decreased metronidazole effect. Avoid.
Foods:	None expected.
Marijuana:	None expected.
Tobacco:	None expected.

*See Glossary

METYRAPONE

BRAND NAMES

Metopirone

BASIC INFORMATION

Habit forming? No
Prescription needed? Yes
Available as generic? No
Drug class: Antiadrenal

 USES

- To diagnose the function of the pituitary gland.
- Treats Cushing's disease, a disorder characterized by higher-than-normal concentrations of cortisol (one of the hormones secreted by the adrenal glands) in the blood.

 DOSAGE & USAGE INFORMATION

How to take:
- For medical testing purposes—Take the prescribed number of tablets with milk or food on the day before the scheduled test. On the day of the test, blood and urine studies will show the amount of hormones in your blood. Results of the test will help establish your diagnosis.
- For treatment of Cushing's syndrome— Swallow tablet with liquid. If you can't swallow whole, crumble tablet and take with liquid or food.

When to take:
- For medical testing—Take the prescribed number of tablets on the day before the scheduled test.
- For treatment of Cushing's disease—Take total daily amount in divided doses. Follow prescription directions carefully.

Continued next column

 OVERDOSE

SYMPTOMS:
Nausea (severe), vomiting, diarrhea, abdominal pain, sudden weakness, irregular heartbeat.
WHAT TO DO:
- **Dial 0 (operator) or 911 (emergency) for an ambulance or medical help. Then give first aid immediately.**
- **See emergency information on inside covers.**

If you forget a dose:
Take as soon as you remember up to 2 hours late. If more than 2 hours, wait for next scheduled dose (don't double this dose).

What drug does:
Prevents one of the chemical reactions in the production of cortisol by the adrenal glands.

Time lapse before drug works:
Approximately 1 hour.

Don't take with:
Cortisone*-like medicines for 48 hours prior to testing.

 POSSIBLE ADVERSE REACTIONS OR SIDE EFFECTS

SYMPTOMS	WHAT TO DO?
Life-threatening: In case of overdose, see previous column.	
Common: Dizziness, headache, nausea.	Continue. Call doctor when convenient.
Infrequent: Drowsiness.	Continue. Call doctor when convenient.
Rare: Hair loss or excess growth, decreased appetite, confusion, acne (may begin or may worsen if already present).	Continue. Call doctor when convenient.

WARNINGS & PRECAUTIONS

Don't take if:
- You have adrenal insufficiency (Addison's disease).
- You have decreased pituitary function.

Before you start, consult your doctor:
- If you are allergic to metyrapone.
- If you have porphyria.

Over age 60:
No special problems expected.

Pregnancy:
Safety not established. Take only under careful supervision of medical professional.

Breast-feeding:
Drug may pass into milk, although controlled studies in humans have not been performed. Since the possibility exists, avoid nursing until you finish the medicine.

Infants & children:
No special problems expected.

Prolonged use:
No special problems expected.

Skin & sunlight:
No special problems expected.

Driving, piloting or hazardous work:
Don't drive or pilot aircraft until you learn how medicine affects you. Don't work around dangerous machinery. Don't climb ladders or work in high places. Danger increases if you drink alcohol or take medicine affecting alertness and reflexes.

Discontinuing:
No special problems expected.

Others:
Advise any doctor or dentist whom you consult that you take this medicine.

POSSIBLE INTERACTION WITH OTHER DRUGS

GENERIC NAME OR DRUG CLASS	COMBINED EFFECT
Estrogens	Possible inaccurate test results.
Oral contraceptives	Possible inaccurate test results.
Phenytoin	Possible inaccurate test results.

POSSIBLE INTERACTION WITH OTHER SUBSTANCES

INTERACTS WITH	COMBINED EFFECT
Alcohol:	None expected.
Beverages:	None expected.
Cocaine:	None expected.
Foods:	Increased appetite and absorption of nutrients, causing difficulty with weight control.
Marijuana:	None expected.
Tobacco:	None expected.

METYROSINE

BRAND NAMES

Demser

BASIC INFORMATION

Habit forming? No
Prescription needed? Yes
Available as generic? No
Drug class: Antihypertensive

USES

- Treatment of pheochromocytoma* (adrenal gland tumor) that causes high blood pressure.
- Preoperative medication for removal of the tumor.

DOSAGE & USAGE INFORMATION

How to take:
Capsules—Swallow with liquid. If you can't swallow whole, open capsule and take with liquid or food. Instructions to take on empty stomach mean 1 hour before or 2 hours after eating.

When to take:
- Usually 4 times a day, approximately 6 hours apart.
- If used before surgery, take for at least 5 to 7 days.

If you forget a dose:
Take as soon as you remember up to 2 hours late. If more than 2 hours, wait for next scheduled dose (don't double this dose).

What drug does:
Reduces blood pressure in patients with pheochromocytoma* by reducing synthesis of catecholamines.

Time lapse before drug works:
2 to 3 days.

Don't take with:
Any other medicines (including over-the-counter drugs such as cough and cold medicines, laxatives, antacids, diet pills, caffeine, nose drops or vitamins) without consulting your doctor.

OVERDOSE

SYMPTOMS:
Confusion, sudden shortness of breath, hallucinations, seizures, coma.
WHAT TO DO:
- **Dial 0 (operator) or 911 (emergency) for an ambulance or medical help. Then give first aid immediately.**
- **See emergency information on inside covers.**

POSSIBLE ADVERSE REACTIONS OR SIDE EFFECTS

SYMPTOMS	WHAT TO DO
Life-threatening:	
In case of overdose, see previous column.	
Common:	
• Severe diarrhea, tremors, drooling, speech difficulties.	Continue. Call doctor when convenient.
• Drowsiness.	Continue. Tell doctor at next visit.
Infrequent:	
Skin rash, sexual difficulties in males.	Continue. Call doctor when convenient.
Rare:	
• Shortness of breath, itching, bloody urine, muscle spasms, swollen feet.	Discontinue. Call doctor right away.
• Depression.	Continue. Call doctor when convenient.

WARNINGS & PRECAUTIONS

Don't take if:
You are allergic to metyrosine.

Before you start, consult your doctor:
• If you have liver disease.
• If you have mental depression.
• If you have Parkinson's disease.
• If you have kidney disease.

Over age 60:
Adverse reactions and side effects may be more frequent and severe than in younger persons. You may need smaller doses for shorter periods of time.

Pregnancy:
No proven harm to unborn child, but avoid if possible.

Breast-feeding:
No proven problems.

Infants & children:
No proven problems.

Prolonged use:
Talk to your doctor about the need for follow-up medical examinations or laboratory studies to check blood pressure, heart function, ECG*, kidney function and urinary catecholamine measurements.

Skin & sunlight:
No problems expected.

Driving, piloting or hazardous work:
Don't drive or pilot aircraft until you learn how medicine affects you. Don't work around dangerous machinery. Don't climb ladders or work in high places. Danger increases if you drink alcohol or take medicine affecting alertness and reflexes.

Discontinuing:
May experience increased energy and insomnia for a short period (2 to 7 days).

Others:
• Advise any doctor or dentist whom you consult that you take this medicine.
• May affect results in some medical tests.

POSSIBLE INTERACTION WITH OTHER DRUGS

GENERIC NAME OR DRUG CLASS	COMBINED EFFECT
Antidepressants, tricyclic (TCA)*	Increased sedative effect of each.
Clozapine	Toxic effect on the central nervous system.
Phenothiazines*	Increased likelihood of toxic symptoms of each.
Sertraline	Increased depressive effects of both drugs.
Trimeprazine	Increased likelihood of toxic symptoms of each.

POSSIBLE INTERACTION WITH OTHER SUBSTANCES

INTERACTS WITH	COMBINED EFFECT
Alcohol:	May cause Parkinson's-like disorder. Don't mix.
Beverages:	No special problems expected.
Cocaine:	No special problems expected.
Foods:	No special problems expected.
Marijuana:	No special problems expected.
Tobacco:	No special problems expected.

MEXILETINE

BRAND NAMES

Mexitil

BASIC INFORMATION

Habit forming? No
Prescription needed? Yes
Available as generic? No
Drug class: Antiarrhythmic

 USES

Stabilizes irregular heartbeat.

 DOSAGE & USAGE INFORMATION

How to take:
Capsules—Swallow whole with food, milk or antacid to lessen stomach irritation.

When to take:
At the same times each day as directed by your doctor.

If you forget a dose:
Take as soon as you remember up to 4 hours late. If more than 4 hours, wait for next scheduled dose (don't double this dose).

What drug does:
Blocks the fast sodium channel in heart tissue.

Time lapse before drug works:
30 minutes to 2 hours.

Don't take with:
Any other medicine without consulting your doctor or pharmacist.

 OVERDOSE

SYMPTOMS:
Nausea, vomiting, seizures, convulsions, cardiac arrest.
WHAT TO DO:
- **Dial 0 (operator) or 911 (emergency) for an ambulance or medical help. Then give first aid immediately.**
- **See emergency information on inside covers.**

 POSSIBLE ADVERSE REACTIONS OR SIDE EFFECTS

SYMPTOMS	WHAT TO DO
Life-threatening: Chest pain, shortness of breath, irregular or fast heartbeat.	Discontinue. Seek emergency treatment.
Common: Dizziness, anxiety, shakiness, unsteadiness when walking, heartburn, nausea, vomiting.	Discontinue. Call doctor right away.
Infrequent: • Sore throat, fever, mouth sores; blurred vision; confusion; constipation; diarrhea; headache; numbness or tingling in hands or feet; ringing in ears; unexplained bleeding or bruising; rash; slurred speech; insomnia; weakness; difficult swallowing.	Discontinue. Call doctor right away.
• Loss of taste.	Continue. Call doctor when convenient.
Rare: • Seizures.	Discontinue. Seek emergency treatment.
• Hallucinations, psychosis, memory loss, difficult breathing, swollen feet and ankles, hiccups, jaundice.	Discontinue. Call doctor right away.
• Hair loss, impotence.	Continue. Call doctor when convenient.

 WARNINGS & PRECAUTIONS

Don't take if:
- If you are allergic to mexiletine, lidocaine or tocainide.
- If you take other heart medicine such as digitalis.

Before you start, consult your doctor:
- If you have had liver or kidney disease or impaired kidney function.
- If you have had lupus.
- If you have a history of seizures.
- If you will have surgery within 2 months, including dental surgery, requiring general or spinal anesthesia.

Over age 60:
Adverse reactions and side effects may be more frequent and severe than in younger persons. Ask doctor about smaller doses.

Pregnancy:
Risk to unborn child outweighs drug benefits. Don't use.

Breast-feeding:
Drug passes into milk. Avoid drug or discontinue nursing until you finish medicine. Consult doctor for advice on maintaining milk supply.

Infants & children:
Use only under close medical supervision.

Prolonged use:
- May cause lupus-like illness.
- Talk to your doctor about the need for follow-up medical examinations or laboratory studies to check ECG*, liver function.

Skin & sunlight:
No problems expected.

Driving, piloting or hazardous work:
Use caution if you feel dizzy or weak. Otherwise, no problems expected.

Discontinuing:
Don't discontinue without consulting doctor. Dose may require gradual reduction if you have taken drug for a long time. Doses of other drugs may also require adjustment.

Others:
No problems expected.

POSSIBLE INTERACTION WITH OTHER DRUGS

GENERIC NAME OR DRUG CLASS	COMBINED EFFECT
Cimetidine	Increased mexiletine effect and toxicity.
Encainide	Increased effect of toxicity on the heart muscle.
Nicardipine	Possible increased effect and toxicity of each drug.
Phenobarbital	Decreased mexiletine effect.
Phenytoin	Decreased mexiletine effect.
Propafenone	Increased effect of both drugs and increased risk of toxicity.
Rifampin	Decreased mexiletine effect.
Urinary acidifiers* (ammonium chloride, ascorbic acid, potassium or sodium phosphate)	May decrease effectiveness of medicine.
Urinary alkalizers* (acetazolamide, antacids with calcium or magnesium, citric acid, dichlorphenamide, methazolamide, potassium citrate, sodium bicarbonate, sodium citrate)	May slow elimination of mexiletine and cause need to adjust dosage.

POSSIBLE INTERACTION WITH OTHER SUBSTANCES

INTERACTS WITH	COMBINED EFFECT
Alcohol:	Causes irregular effectiveness of mexiletine. Avoid.
Beverages: Caffeine drinks, iced drinks.	Irregular heartbeat.
Cocaine:	Decreased mexiletine effect.
Foods:	None expected.
Marijuana:	Irregular heartbeat. Avoid.
Tobacco:	Dangerous combination. May lead to liver problems and reduce excretion of mexiletine.

MINERAL OIL

BRAND NAMES

Agoral	Liqui-Doss
Fleet Enema	Milkinol
Mineral Oil	Neo-Cultol
Kondremul	Nujol
Kondremul with	Petrogalar
Cascara	Zymenol
Lansoyl	

BASIC INFORMATION

Habit forming? Yes
Prescription needed? No
Available as generic? Yes
Drug class: Laxative (lubricant)

 USES

Treats the temporary symptoms of constipation.

 DOSAGE & USAGE INFORMATION

How to take:
Follow package instructions.

When to take:
According to instructions provided.

If you forget a dose:
No set dosage schedule. Use only when needed.

What drug does:
Coats the stool and the surface of the intestine with lubricant to make the passage of the stool easier.

Time lapse before drug works:
None.

Don't take with:
Other drugs without talking to your doctor or pharmacist.

 OVERDOSE

SYMPTOMS:
Loose stools.
WHAT TO DO:
Overdose unlikely to threaten life. If person takes much larger amount than prescribed, call doctor, poison-control center or hospital emergency room for instructions.

 POSSIBLE ADVERSE REACTIONS OR SIDE EFFECTS

SYMPTOMS	WHAT TO DO
Life-threatening: None expected.	
Common: Skin irritation around rectum.	Continue. Call doctor when convenient.
Infrequent: None expected.	
Rare: None expected.	

WARNINGS & PRECAUTIONS

Don't take if:
- You have abdominal pain, bloating or suspected appendicitis.
- You have undiagnosed rectal bleeding.

Before you start, consult your doctor:
- If you have difficulty swallowing.
- If you are bed-ridden.

Over age 60:
More susceptible to adverse effects.

Pregnancy:
Risk to unborn child outweighs benefits. May produce a bleeding disease in a newborn.

Breast-feeding:
No problems expected, but consult doctor.

Infants & children:
Use only under close medical supervision, particularly up to 6 years of age.

Prolonged use:
- Not intended for prolonged use. May interfere with absorption of essential nutrients.
- Don't take for longer than 1 week unless under a doctor's supervision. May cause laxative dependence.

Skin & sunlight:
No special problems expected.

Driving, piloting or hazardous work:
No special problems expected.

Discontinuing:
May be unnecessary to finish medicine. Follow doctor's instructions.

Others:
- May affect results of some medical tests.
- Don't take to "flush out" your system or as a tonic.

POSSIBLE INTERACTION WITH OTHER DRUGS

GENERIC NAME OR DRUG CLASS	COMBINED EFFECT
Anticoagulants*	Decreased absorption of anticoagulants.
Contraceptives, oral*	Decreased effect of contraceptive drug.
Digitalis	Decreased effect of digitalis.
Laxatives*, stool-softening	May cause tumor-like deposits in tissues.
Medications, other	Decreased absorption of many medicines taken with mineral oil.
Vitamins A,D,E and K	Decreased absorption of vitamins.

POSSIBLE INTERACTION WITH OTHER SUBSTANCES

INTERACTS WITH	COMBINED EFFECT
Alcohol:	No proven problems.
Beverages:	No proven problems.
Cocaine:	No proven problems.
Foods:	Decreased absorption of foods and fat-soluble vitamins (A, D, E and K).
Marijuana:	No proven problems.
Tobacco:	Possible increased laxative effect.

MINOXIDIL

BRAND NAMES

Loniten

BASIC INFORMATION

Habit forming? No
Prescription needed? Yes
Available as generic? Yes
Drug class: Antihypertensive

 USES

- Treatment for high blood pressure in conjunction with other drugs, such as beta-adrenergic blockers and diuretics.
- Treatment for congestive heart failure.
- Can stimulate hair growth.

 DOSAGE & USAGE INFORMATION

How to take:
Tablet—Swallow with liquid. If you can't swallow whole, crumble tablet and take with liquid or food.

When to take:
At the same time each day, according to instructions on prescription label.

If you forget a dose:
Take as soon as you remember up to 2 hours late. If more than 2 hours, wait for next scheduled dose (don't double this dose).

What drug does:
Relaxes small blood vessels (arterioles) so blood can pass through more easily.

Time lapse before drug works:
2 to 3 hours for effect to begin; 3 to 7 days of continuous use may be necessary for maximum blood-pressure response.

Don't take with:
Any other medicine without consulting your doctor or pharmacist.

 OVERDOSE

SYMPTOMS:
Low blood pressure, fainting, chest pain, shortness of breath, coma.
WHAT TO DO:
- **Dial 0 (operator) or 911 (emergency) for an ambulance or medical help. Then give first aid immediately.**
- **See emergency information on inside covers.**

 POSSIBLE ADVERSE REACTIONS OR SIDE EFFECTS

SYMPTOMS	WHAT TO DO
Life-threatening:	
In case of overdose, see previous column.	
Common:	
• Excessive hair growth, flushed skin or redness.	Continue. Call doctor when convenient.
• Bloating.	Discontinue. Call doctor right away.
Infrequent:	
• Chest pain, irregular or slow heartbeat, shortness of breath, swollen feet or legs, rapid weight gain.	Discontinue. Call doctor right away.
• Numbness of hands, feet, or face; headache; tender breasts; darkening of skin.	Continue. Call doctor when convenient.
Rare:	
Rash.	Discontinue. Call doctor right away.

WARNINGS & PRECAUTIONS

Don't take if:
You are allergic to minoxidil.

Before you start, consult your doctor:
- If you have had recent stroke, heart attack or angina pectoris in past 3 weeks.
- If you have impaired kidney function.

Over age 60:
Adverse reactions and side effects may be more frequent and severe than in younger persons.

Pregnancy:
Human studies not available. Avoid if possible.

Breast-feeding:
Human studies not available. Avoid if possible.

Infants & children:
Not recommended. Safety and dosage have not been established.

Prolonged use:
Request periodic blood examinations that include potassium levels.

Skin & sunlight:
No problems expected.

Driving, piloting or hazardous work:
Avoid if you become dizzy or faint. Otherwise, no problems expected.

Discontinuing:
Don't discontinue without consulting doctor. Dose may require gradual reduction if you have taken drug for a long time. Doses of other drugs may also require adjustment.

Others:
- Check pulse regularly. If it exceeds 20 or more beats per minute over your normal rate, consult doctor immediately.
- Check blood pressure frequently.

POSSIBLE INTERACTION WITH OTHER DRUGS

GENERIC NAME OR DRUG CLASS	COMBINED EFFECT
Anesthesia	Drastic blood pressure drop.
Antihypertensives, other*	Dosage adjustments may be necessary to keep blood pressure at desired level.
Carteolol	Increased antihypertensive effect.
Diuretics*	Dosage adjustments may be necessary to keep blood pressure at desired level.
Guanadrel	Weakness and faintness when arising from bed or chair.
Guanethidine	Weakness and faintness when arising from bed or chair.
Lisinopril	Increased antihypertensive effect. Dosage of each may require adjustment.
Nicardipine	Blood pressure drop. Dosages may require adjustment.
Nimodipine	Dangerous blood pressure drop.
Nitrates*	Drastic blood pressure drop.
Sotalol	Increased antihypertensive effect.
Sympathomimetics*	Possible decreased minoxidil effect.
Terazosin	Decreases effectiveness of terazosin.

POSSIBLE INTERACTION WITH OTHER SUBSTANCES

INTERACTS WITH	COMBINED EFFECT
Alcohol:	Possible excessive blood pressure drop.
Beverages:	None expected.
Cocaine:	Increased risk of heart block and high blood pressure.
Foods: Salt substitutes.	Possible excessive potassium levels in blood.
Marijuana:	Increased dizziness.
Tobacco:	May decrease minoxidil effect. Avoid.

MINOXIDIL (Topical)

BRAND NAMES

Rogaine

BASIC INFORMATION

Habit forming? No
Prescription needed? Yes
Available as generic? No
Drug class: Hair growth stimulant

 ## USES

Hair loss on scalp from male and female pattern baldness (alopecia androgenetica).

 ## DOSAGE & USAGE INFORMATION

How to use:
- Topical solution—Apply only to dry hair and scalp. With the provided applicator, apply the amount prescribed to the scalp area being treated. Begin in center of the treated area.
- Wash hands immediately after use.
- Don't use a blow dryer.
- If you are using at bedtime, wait 30 minutes after applying before retiring.

When to use:
Twice a day or as directed.

If you forget a dose:
Use as soon as you remember. No need to ever double the dose.

What drug does:
Stimulates hair growth by possibly dilating small blood capillaries, thereby providing more blood to hair follicles.

Time lapse before drug works:
Varies with individuals.

Don't use with:
Any other medicine without consulting your doctor or pharmacist.

Continued next column

 ## OVERDOSE

SYMPTOMS:
None expected.
WHAT TO DO:
Not for internal use. If child accidentally swallows, call poison-control center.

 ## POSSIBLE ADVERSE REACTIONS OR SIDE EFFECTS

SYMPTOMS	WHAT TO DO
Life-threatening Fast, irregular heartbeat (rare; represents too much absorbed into body).	Discontinue. Seek emergency treatment.
Common None expected.	
Infrequent Itching scalp; flaking, reddened skin.	Continue. Call doctor when convenient.
Rare Burning scalp, skin rash, swollen face, headache, dizziness or fainting, hands and feet numb or tingling, rapid weight gain.	Discontinue. Call doctor right away.

MINOXIDIL (Topical)

WARNINGS & PRECAUTIONS

Don't use if:
You are allergic to minoxidil.

Before you start, consult your doctor:
If you are allergic to anything.

Over age 60:
No problems expected.

Pregnancy:
Don't use.

Breast-feeding:
Don't use.

Infants & children:
Don't use.

Prolonged use:
No problems expected.

Skin & sunlight:
No problems expected.

Driving, piloting or hazardous work:
No problems expected.

Discontinuing:
No problems expected.

Others:
- Keep away from eyes, nose and mouth. Flush with plain water if accident occurs.
- New hair will drop out when you stop using minoxidil.
- Keep cool, but don't freeze.

POSSIBLE INTERACTION WITH OTHER DRUGS

GENERIC NAME OR DRUG CLASS	COMBINED EFFECT
Adrenocorticoids, topical	May cause undesirable absorption of minoxidil.
Petrolatum, topical	May cause undesirable absorption of minoxidil.
Retinoids, topical	May cause undesirable absorption of minoxidil.

POSSIBLE INTERACTION WITH OTHER SUBSTANCES

INTERACTS WITH	COMBINED EFFECT
Alcohol:	None expected.
Beverages:	None expected.
Cocaine:	None expected.
Foods:	None expected.
Marijuana:	None expected.
Tobacco:	None expected.

MISOPROSTOL

BRAND NAMES

Cytotec

BASIC INFORMATION

Habit forming? No
Prescription needed? Yes
Available as generic? No
Drug class: Antiulcer

 ## USES

Prevents development of stomach ulcers in persons taking non-steroidal, anti-inflammatory drugs (NSAIDs), including aspirin.

 ## DOSAGE & USAGE INFORMATION

How to take:
Tablets—Swallow with liquid. If you can't swallow whole, crumble tablet and take with liquid or food. Instructions to take on empty stomach mean 1 hour before or 2 hours after eating.

When to take:
Usually 4 times a day while awake, with or after meals and at bedtime.

If you forget a dose:
Take as soon as you remember up to 2 hours late. If more than 2 hours, wait for next scheduled dose (don't double this dose).

What drug does:
- Improves defense against peptic ulcers by strengthening natural defenses of the stomach lining.
- Decreases stomach acid production.

Time lapse before drug works:
10 to 15 minutes.

Don't take with:
Any other medicines (including over-the-counter drugs such as cough and cold medicines, laxatives, antacids, diet pills, caffeine, nose drops or vitamins) without consulting your doctor or pharmacist.

 ## OVERDOSE

SYMPTOMS:
None expected.
WHAT TO DO:
Overdose unlikely to threaten life. If person takes much larger amount than prescribed, call doctor, poison-control center or hospital emergency room for instructions.

 ## POSSIBLE ADVERSE REACTIONS OR SIDE EFFECTS

SYMPTOMS	WHAT TO DO
Life-threatening: None expected.	
Common: Abdominal pain, diarrhea.	Discontinue. Call doctor right away.
Infrequent: • Nausea or vomiting.	Continue. Call doctor when convenient.
• Constipation, headache.	Continue. Tell doctor at next visit.
Rare: Gaseousness.	Continue. Tell doctor at next visit.

WARNINGS & PRECAUTIONS

Don't take if:
- You are allergic to any prostaglandin.
- You are pregnant or of child-bearing age.

Before you start, consult your doctor:
- If you have epilepsy.
- If you have heart disease.
- If you have blood vessel disease of any kind.

Over age 60:
No special problems expected.

Pregnancy:
- Risk to unborn child outweighs drug benefits. Don't use.
- May also lead to serious complications in pregnant women, including excessive bleeding and future infertility.

Breast-feeding:
Drug passes into milk. Avoid drug or discontinue nursing until you finish medicine. Consult doctor for advice on maintaining milk supply.

Infants & children:
Not recommended for children under 18.

Prolonged use:
Talk to your doctor about the need for follow-up medical examinations or laboratory studies to check gastric analysis.

Skin & sunlight:
No problems expected.

Driving, piloting or hazardous work:
Avoid if you feel confused, drowsy or dizzy.

Discontinuing:
No special problems expected.

Others:
Advise any doctor or dentist whom you consult that you take this medicine.

POSSIBLE INTERACTION WITH OTHER DRUGS

GENERIC NAME OR DRUG CLASS	COMBINED EFFECT
Antacids*, magnesium-containing	Severe diarrhea.

POSSIBLE INTERACTION WITH OTHER SUBSTANCES

INTERACTS WITH	COMBINED EFFECT
Alcohol:	Decreases misoprostol effect. Avoid.
Beverages: Caffeine-containing.	Decreases misoprostol effect. Avoid.
Cocaine:	Decreases misoprostol effect. Avoid.
Foods:	No special problems expected.
Marijuana:	Decreases misoprostol effect. Avoid.
Tobacco:	Decreases misoprostol effect. Avoid.

MITOTANE

BRAND NAMES

Lysodren   o,p'-DDD

BASIC INFORMATION

Habit forming? No
Prescription needed? Yes
Available as generic? No
Drug class: Antineoplastic, antiadrenal

USES

- Treatment for some kinds of cancer.
- Treatment of Cushing's disease.

DOSAGE & USAGE INFORMATION

How to take:
Tablet—Take with liquid after light meal. Don't drink fluid with meals. Drink extra fluids between meals. Avoid sweet and fatty foods.

When to take:
At the same time each day.

If you forget a dose:
Take as soon as you remember. Don't ever double dose.

What drug does:
Suppresses adrenal cortex to prevent manufacture of excess cortisone.

Time lapse before drug works:
2 to 3 weeks for full effect.

Don't take with:
Any other medicine without consulting your doctor or pharmacist.

OVERDOSE

SYMPTOMS:
Headache, vomiting blood, stupor, seizure.
WHAT TO DO:
- **Dial 0 (operator) or 911 (emergency) for an ambulance or medical help. Then give first aid immediately.**
- **If patient is unconscious and not breathing, give mouth-to-mouth breathing. If there is no heartbeat, use cardiac massage and mouth-to-mouth breathing (CPR). Don't try to make patient vomit. If you can't get help quickly, take patient to nearest emergency facility.**
- **See emergency information on inside covers.**

POSSIBLE ADVERSE REACTIONS OR SIDE EFFECTS

SYMPTOMS	WHAT TO DO
Life-threatening:	
In case of overdose, see previous column.	
Common:	
• Darkened skin, appetite loss, nausea, vomiting.	Continue. Call doctor when convenient.
• Mental depression. drowsiness.	Continue. Tell doctor at next visit.
Infrequent:	
• Fever, chills, sore throat.	Discontinue. Seek emergency treatment.
• Unusual bleeding or bruising, difficult breathing.	Discontinue. Call doctor right away.
• Rash, hair loss, blurred vision, seeing double, cough, tiredness, weakness, dizziness when standing after sitting or lying down.	Continue. Call doctor when convenient.
Rare:	
Blood in urine.	Continue. Call doctor when convenient.

WARNINGS & PRECAUTIONS

Don't take if:
You are allergic to mitotane, adrenocorticosteroids or any antineoplastic drug.

Before you start, consult your doctor:
- If you have liver disease.
- If you have infection.

Over age 60:
Adverse reactions and side effects may be more frequent and severe than in younger persons.

Pregnancy:
Consult doctor. Risk to child is significant.

Breast-feeding:
Drug passes into milk. Don't nurse.

Infants & children:
Use only under care of medical supervisors who are experienced in anticancer drugs.

Prolonged use:
Adverse reactions more likely the longer drug is required.

Skin & sunlight:
No problems expected.

Driving, piloting or hazardous work:
No problems expected.

Discontinuing:
- Don't discontinue without consulting doctor. Dose may require gradual reduction if you have taken drug for a long time. Doses of other drugs may also require adjustment.
- Some side effects may follow discontinuing. Report any new symptoms.

Others:
No problems expected.

POSSIBLE INTERACTION WITH OTHER DRUGS

GENERIC NAME OR DRUG CLASS	COMBINED EFFECT
Antidepressants*	Increased central nervous system depression.
Antihistamines*	Increased central nervous system depression.
Central nervous system (CNS) depressants*	Increased sedation.
Clozapine	Toxic effect on the central nervous system.
Corticosteroids*	Decreased effect of corticosteroid.
Ethinamate	Dangerous increased effects of ethinamate. Avoid combining.
Fluoxetine	Increased depressant effects of both drugs.
Guanfacine	May increase depressant effects of either drug.
Leucovorin	High alcohol content of leucovorin may cause adverse effects.
Methyprylon	Increased sedative effect, perhaps to dangerous level. Avoid.
Mind-altering drugs*	Increased central nervous system depression.
Nabilone	Greater depression of central nervous system.
Narcotics*	Increased central nervous system depression.
Phenytoin	Possible increased metabolism.
Sedatives*	Increased central nervous system depression.
Sertraline	Increased depressive effects of both drugs.
Sleeping pills*	Increased central nervous system depression.
Spironolactone	Decreased mitotane effect.
Tranquilizers*	Increased central nervous system depression.
Trilostane	Too much decrease in adrenal function.
Warfarin	Possible increased metabolism.

POSSIBLE INTERACTION WITH OTHER SUBSTANCES

INTERACTS WITH	COMBINED EFFECT
Alcohol:	Increased depression. Avoid.
Beverages:	No problems expected.
Cocaine:	Increased toxicity. Avoid.
Foods:	Reduced irritation in stomach.
Marijuana:	No problems expected.
Tobacco:	Increased possibility of lung toxicity.

MOLINDONE

BRAND NAMES

Moban

BASIC INFORMATION

Habit forming? No
Prescription needed? Yes
Available as generic? No
Drug class: Antipsychotic

 ## USES

Treats severe emotional, mental or nervous problems.

 ## DOSAGE & USAGE INFORMATION

How to take:
Tablet or solution—Swallow with liquid or food to lessen stomach irritation. If you can't swallow tablet whole, crumble and take with food or liquid.

When to take:
Follow instructions on prescription label or side of package. Doses should be evenly spaced. For example, 4 times a day means every 6 hours.

If you forget a dose:
Take as soon as you remember up to 2 hours late. If more than 2 hours, wait for next scheduled dose (don't double this dose).

What drug does:
Corrects an imbalance in nerve impulses from the brain.

Time lapse before drug works:
- Nausea and vomiting—1 hour or less.
- Nervous and mental disorders—4 to 6 weeks.

Don't take with:
- Antacid or medicine for diarrhea.
- Non-prescription drugs for cough, cold or allergy.
- See Interaction column and consult doctor.

 ## OVERDOSE

SYMPTOMS:
Stupor, convulsions, coma.
WHAT TO DO:
- Dial 0 (operator) or 911 (emergency) for an ambulance or medical help. Then give first aid immediately.
- See emergency information on inside covers.

 ## POSSIBLE ADVERSE REACTIONS OR SIDE EFFECTS

SYMPTOMS	WHAT TO DO
Life-threatening:	
Uncontrolled muscle movements of tongue, face and other muscles (neuroleptic malignant syndrome, rare); unsteady gait; difficult breathing; fever; muscle stiffness.	Discontinue. Seek emergency treatment.
Common:	
• Muscle spasms of face and neck, unsteady gait.	Discontinue. Seek emergency treatment.
• Restlessness, tremor, drowsiness, swallowing difficulty.	Discontinue. Call doctor right away.
• Decreased sweating, dry mouth, runny nose, constipation, headache.	Continue. Call doctor when convenient.
Infrequent:	
• Fainting.	Discontinue. Seek emergency treatment.
• Rash.	Discontinue. Call doctor right away.
• Frequent urination, diminished sex drive, swollen breasts, menstrual irregularities, depression.	Continue. Call doctor when convenient.
Rare:	
Change in vision, sore throat, fever, jaundice, abdominal pain, confusion.	Discontinue. Call doctor right away.

 ## WARNINGS & PRECAUTIONS

Don't take if:
- You are allergic to any phenothiazine.
- You have a blood or bone-marrow disease.

Before you start, consult your doctor:
- If you will have surgery within 2 months, including dental surgery, requiring general or spinal anesthesia.
- If you have asthma, emphysema or other lung disorder, glaucoma, prostate trouble.
- If you take non-prescription ulcer medicine, asthma medicine or amphetamines.

Over age 60:
Adverse reactions and side effects may be more frequent and severe than in younger persons. More likely to develop involuntary movement of jaws, lips, tongue, chewing. Report this to your doctor immediately. Early treatment can help.

Pregnancy:
Risk to unborn child outweighs drug benefits. Don't use.

Breast-feeding:
Safety not established. Consult doctor.

Infants & children:
Don't give to children younger than 2.

Prolonged use:
• May lead to tardive dyskinesia (involuntary movement of jaws, lips, tongue, chewing).
• Talk to your doctor about the need for follow-up medical examinations or laboratory studies to check kidney function, eyes.

Skin & sunlight:
May cause rash or intensify sunburn in areas exposed to sun or sunlamp. Skin may remain sensitive for 3 months after discontinuing.

Driving, piloting or hazardous work:
Don't drive or pilot aircraft until you learn how medicine affects you. Don't work around dangerous machinery. Don't climb ladders or work in high places. Danger increases if you drink alcohol or take medicine affecting alertness and reflexes.

Discontinuing:
• Nervous and mental disorders—Don't discontinue without doctor's advice until you complete prescribed dose, even though symptoms diminish or disappear.
• Notify your doctor if any of the following occurs: uncontrollable movements of tongue, arms and legs; lip smacking.

Others:
No problems expected.

 POSSIBLE INTERACTION WITH OTHER DRUGS

GENERIC NAME OR DRUG CLASS	COMBINED EFFECT
Anticholinergics*	Increased anti-cholinergic effect.
Antidepressants, tricyclic (TCA)*	Increased molindone effect.
Antihistamines*	Increased antihistamine effect.
Appetite suppressants*	Decreased suppressant effect.
Bupropion	Increased risk of major seizures.

Carteolol	Increased tranquilizer effect.
Clozapine	Toxic effect on the central nervous system.
Dronabinol	Increased effects of both drugs. Avoid.
Ethinamate	Dangerous increased effects of ethinamate. Avoid combining.
Extrapyramidal reaction-causing medications*	Increased frequency and severity of extrapyramidal effects.
Fluoxetine	Increased depressant effects of both drugs.
Guanethidine	Decreased guanethidine effect.
Guanfacine	May increase depressant effects of either drug.
Leucovorin	High alcohol content of leucovorin may cause adverse effects.
Levodopa	Decreased levodopa effect.
Loxapine	May increase toxic effects of both drugs.
Methyprylon	Increased sedative effect, perhaps to dangerous level. Avoid.
Mind-altering drugs*	Increased effect of mind-altering drugs.

Continued on page 951

 POSSIBLE INTERACTION WITH OTHER SUBSTANCES

INTERACTS WITH	COMBINED EFFECT
Alcohol:	Dangerous oversedation.
Beverages:	None expected.
Cocaine:	Decreased molindone effect. Avoid.
Foods:	None expected.
Marijuana:	Drowsiness. May increase antinausea effect.
Tobacco:	None expected.

*See Glossary

MONOAMINE OXIDASE (MAO) INHIBITORS

BRAND AND GENERIC NAMES

ISOCARBOXAZID
Marplan
Nardil
PARGYLINE

Parnate
PHENELZINE
TRANYLCYPROMINE

BASIC INFORMATION

Habit forming? No
Prescription needed? Yes
Available as generic? No
Drug class: MAO (monoamine oxidase)
inhibitor, antidepressant

USES

- Treatment for depression.
- Pargyline sometimes used to lower blood pressure.

DOSAGE & USAGE INFORMATION

How to take:
Tablet—Swallow with liquid. If you can't swallow whole, crumble tablet and take with liquid or food.

When to take:
At the same times each day.

If you forget a dose:
Take as soon as you remember up to 2 hours late. If more than 2 hours, wait for next scheduled dose (don't double this dose).

What drug does:
Inhibits nerve transmissions in brain that may cause depression.

Time lapse before drug works:
4 to 6 weeks for maximum effect.

Continued next column

OVERDOSE

SYMPTOMS:
Restlessness, agitation, excitement, fever, confusion, dizziness, heartbeat irregularities, hallucinations, sweating, breathing difficulties, insomnia, irritability, convulsions, coma.
WHAT TO DO:
- **Dial 0 (operator) or 911 (emergency) for an ambulance or medical help. Then give first aid immediately.**
- **See emergency information on inside covers.**

Don't take with:
- Non-prescription diet pills, nose drops, medicine for asthma, cough, cold or allergy, or medicine containing caffeine or alcohol.
- Foods containing tyramine*.
- Any other medicine without consulting your doctor or pharmacist.

POSSIBLE ADVERSE REACTIONS OR SIDE EFFECTS

SYMPTOMS	WHAT TO DO
Life-threatening:	
In case of overdose, see previous column.	
Common:	
Fatigue, weakness.	Continue. Call doctor when convenient.
Dizziness when changing position, restlessness, tremors, dry mouth, constipation, difficult urination, blurred vision, "sweet tooth."	Continue. Tell doctor at next visit.
Infrequent:	
Fainting, enlarged pupils.	Discontinue. Seek emergency treatment.
Severe headache, chest pain.	Discontinue. Call doctor right away.
Hallucinations, insomnia, nightmares, diarrhea, rapid or pounding heartbeat, swollen feet or legs, joint pain.	Continue. Call doctor when convenient.
Diminished sex drive.	Continue. Tell doctor at next visit.
Rare:	
Rash, nausea, vomiting, stiff neck, jaundice, fever, increased sweating, dark urine, slurred speech.	Discontinue. Call doctor right away.

WARNINGS & PRECAUTIONS

Don't take if:
- You are allergic to any MAO inhibitor.
- You have heart disease, congestive heart failure, heart-rhythm irregularities or high blood pressure.
- You have liver or kidney disease.

Before you start, consult your doctor:
- If you are alcoholic.
- If you have had a stroke.
- If you have diabetes, epilepsy, asthma, overactive thyroid, schizophrenia, Parkinson's disease, adrenal-gland tumor.
- If you will have surgery within 2 months, including dental surgery, requiring general or spinal anesthesia.

MONOAMINE OXIDASE (MAO) INHIBITORS

Over age 60:
Not recommended.

Pregnancy:
Risk to unborn child outweighs benefits. Don't use, especially during first 3 months.

Breast-feeding:
Safety not established. Consult doctor.

Infants & children:
Not recommended.

Prolonged use:
- May be toxic to liver.
- Talk to your doctor about the need for follow-up medical examinations or laboratory studies to check blood pressure, liver function.

Skin & sunlight:
May cause rash or intensify sunburn in areas exposed to sun or sunlamp.

Driving, piloting or hazardous work:
Don't drive or pilot aircraft until you learn how medicine affects you. Don't work around dangerous machinery. Don't climb ladders or work in high places. Danger increases if you drink alcohol or take medicine affecting alertness and reflexes.

Discontinuing:
- Don't discontinue without doctor's advice until you complete prescribed dose, even though symptoms diminish or disappear.
- Follow precautions regarding foods, drinks and other medicines for 2 weeks after discontinuing.
- Adverse symtoms caused by this medicine may occur even after discontinuation. If you develop any of the symptoms listed under Overdose, notify your doctor immediately.

Others:
- May affect blood-sugar levels in patients with diabetes.
- Fever may indicate that MAO inhibitor dose requires adjustment.

 POSSIBLE INTERACTION WITH OTHER DRUGS

GENERIC NAME OR DRUG CLASS	COMBINED EFFECT
Amphetamines*	Blood pressure rise to life-threatening level.
Anticholinergics*	Increased anti-cholinergic effect.
Anticonvulsants*	Changed seizure pattern.
Antidepressants, tricyclic (TCA)*	Blood pressure rise to life-threatening level. Possible fever, convulsions, delirium.

Antidiabetics, oral and insulin*	Excessively low blood sugar.
Antihypertensives*	Excessively low blood pressure.
Beta-adrenergic blockers*	Possible blood pressure rise if MAO inhibitor is discontinued after simultaneous use with acebutolol.
Bupropion	Increased risk of bupropion toxicity.
Buspirone	Very high blood pressure.
Caffeine	Irregular heartbeat or high blood pressure.
Carbamazepine	Fever, seizures. Avoid.
Central nervous system (CNS) depressants*	Excessive depressant action.
Clozapine	Toxic effect on the central nervous system.
Cyclobenzaprine	Fever, seizures. Avoid.
Dextromethorphan	Very high blood pressure.
Diuretics*	Excessively low blood pressure.
Ephedrine	Increased blood pressure.

Continued page 952

 POSSIBLE INTERACTION WITH OTHER SUBSTANCES

INTERACTS WITH	COMBINED EFFECT
Alcohol:	Increased sedation to dangerous level.
Beverages: Caffeine drinks.	Irregular heartbeat or high blood pressure.
Drinks containing tyramine*.	Blood pressure rise to life-threatening level.
Cocaine:	Overstimulation. Possibly fatal.
Foods: Foods containing tyramine*.	Blood pressure rise to life-threatening level.
Marijuana:	Overstimulation. Avoid.
Tobacco:	No proven problems.

*See Glossary

MORICIZINE

BRAND NAMES

Ethmozine

BASIC INFORMATION

Habit forming? No
Prescription needed? Yes
Available as generic? No
Drug class: Antiarrhythmic

USES

Treats severe heartbeat irregularities, primarily life-threatening ventricular tachycardia.

DOSAGE & USAGE INFORMATION

How to take:
Tablets—As directed, by mouth with water.

When to take:
When directed. The first dose of this medicine is usually given in an emergency room or in the hospital under continuous monitoring.

If you forget a dose:
Report to your doctor right away.

What drug does:
Affects the electrical conduction system inside the heart.

Time lapse before drug works:
Promptly, but may require up to 2 hours for full effect.

Don't take with:
Any other medicine without consulting your doctor or pharmacist.

OVERDOSE

SYMPTOMS:
Fainting, chest pain, vomiting, lethargy, coma.
WHAT TO DO:
- **Dial 0 (operator) or 911 (emergency) for an ambulance or medical help. Then give first aid immediately.**
- **See emergency information on inside covers.**

POSSIBLE ADVERSE REACTIONS OR SIDE EFFECTS

SYMPTOMS	WHAT TO DO
Life-threatening:	
In case of overdose, see previous column.	
Common:	
Dizziness.	Discontinue. Call doctor right away.
Infrequent:	
Chest pain; blurred vision; diarrhea; dry mouth; headache; numbness and tingling in arms, legs; nausea; abdominal pain.	Discontinue. Call doctor right away.
Rare:	
Sudden high fever.	Discontinue. Call doctor right away.

WARNINGS & PRECAUTIONS

Don't take if:
- You have pre-existing heart block.
- You have right bundle branch block.

Before you start, consult your doctor:
- If you take any other prescription or non-prescription medicine.
- If you have liver or kidney disease.

Over age 60:
No age-related adverse effects expected.

Pregnancy:
Adequate human studies not yet done.

Breast-feeding:
No documented problems.

Infants & children:
No special problems expected.

Prolonged use:
No special problems expected.

Skin & sunlight:
No special problems expected.

Driving, piloting or hazardous work:
Don't drive or pilot aircraft until you learn how medicine affects you. Don't work around dangerous machinery. Don't climb ladders or work in high places. Danger increases if you drink alcohol or take medicine affecting alertness and reflexes.

Discontinuing:
No special problems expected.

Others:
The first dose of this medication is usually given while the patient is being closely monitored in an intensive care setting with cardiac monitoring or in an emergency room.

 POSSIBLE INTERACTION WITH OTHER DRUGS

GENERIC NAME OR DRUG CLASS	COMBINED EFFECT
Antiarrhythmics*, other	Possible increased effects of both drugs.
Cimetidine	Increased concentration of cimetidine in the blood.
Theophylline	Decreased effect of theophylline.

 POSSIBLE INTERACTION WITH OTHER SUBSTANCES

INTERACTS WITH	COMBINED EFFECT
Alcohol:	Avoid.
Beverages:	None expected.
Cocaine:	Increased irregular heartbeat. Avoid.
Foods:	None expected.
Marijuana:	Possible increased irregular heartbeat. Avoid.
Tobacco:	Possible increased irregular heartbeat. Avoid.

BRAND AND GENERIC NAMES

See complete list of brand and generic names in the *Brand Names Directory,* page 922.

BASIC INFORMATION

Habit forming? Possibly
Prescription needed? Yes
Available as generic? Yes, for some.
Drug class: Muscle relaxant

 ## USES

Adjunctive treatment to rest, analgesics, and physical therapy for muscle spasms.

 ## DOSAGE & USAGE INFORMATION

How to take:
Tablets—Swallow with liquid. If you can't swallow whole, crumble tablet and take with liquid or food. Instructions to take on empty stomach mean 1 hour before or 2 hours after eating.

When to take:
As needed, no more often than every 4 hours.

If you forget a dose:
Take as soon as you remember. Wait 4 hours for next dose.

What drug does:
Blocks body's pain messages to brain. Also causes sedation.

Time lapse before drug works:
60 minutes.

Don't take with:
Any other medicine without consulting your doctor or pharmacist.

 ## OVERDOSE

SYMPTOMS:
Nausea, vomiting, diarrhea, convulsions, headache. May progress to severe weakness, difficult breathing, sensation of paralysis, coma.
WHAT TO DO:
● **Dial 0 (operator) or 911 (emergency) for an ambulance or medical help. Then give first aid immediately.**
● **See emergency information on inside covers.**

 ## POSSIBLE ADVERSE REACTIONS OR SIDE EFFECTS

SYMPTOMS	WHAT TO DO
Life-threatening:	
Hives, rash, intense itching, faintness soon after a dose (anaphylaxis); extreme weakness, transient paralysis, temporary vision loss.	Seek emergency treatment immediately.
Common:	
● Drowsiness, fainting, dizziness.	Continue. Call doctor when convenient.
● Orange or red-purple urine.	No action necessary.
Infrequent:	
● Agitation, constipation or diarrhea, nausea, cramps, vomiting, wheezing, shortness of breath, headache, depression, muscle weakness, trembling, insomnia, uncontrolled eye movements.	Discontinue. Call doctor right away.
● Blurred vision.	Continue. Call Doctor when convenient.
Rare:	
● Black, tarry or bloody stool; convulsions.	Discontinue. Seek emergency treatment.
● Rash, hives, or itch; sore throat; fever; jaundice; tiredness; weakness; hiccups.	Discontinue. Call doctor right away.

WARNINGS & PRECAUTIONS

Don't take if:
- You are allergic to any skeletal-muscle relaxant.
- You have porphyria.

Before you start, consult your doctor:
- If you have had liver or kidney disease.
- If you plan pregnancy within medication period.
- If you are allergic to tartrazine dye.

Over age 60:
Adverse reactions and side effects may be more frequent and severe than in younger persons.

Pregnancy:
Safety not proven. Avoid if possible.

Breast-feeding:
Drug passes into milk. Avoid drug or discontinue nursing until you finish medicine. Consult doctor for advice on maintaining milk supply.

Infants & children:
Not recommended.

Prolonged use:
- Talk to your doctor about the need for follow-up medical examinations or laboratory studies to check liver function, kidney function, complete blood counts (white blood cell count, platelet count, red blood cell count, hemoglobin, hematocrit).
- Safety beyond 8 weeks of treatment not established.

Skin & sunlight:
No problems expected.

Driving, piloting or hazardous work:
Don't drive or pilot aircraft until you learn how medicine affects you. Don't work around dangerous machinery. Don't climb ladders or work in high places. Danger increases if you drink alcohol or take medicine affecting alertness and reflexes, such as antihistamines, tranquilizers, sedatives, pain medicine, narcotics and mind-altering drugs.

Discontinuing:
Don't discontinue without doctor's advice until you complete prescribed dose, even though symptoms diminish or disappear.

Others:
- May affect results in some medical tests.
- Advise any doctor or dentist whom you consult that you take this medicine.

POSSIBLE INTERACTION WITH OTHER DRUGS

GENERIC NAME OR DRUG CLASS	COMBINED EFFECT
Antidepressants*	Increased sedation.
Antihistamines*	Increased sedation.
Clozapine	Toxic effect on the central nervous system.
Dronabinol	Increased effect of dronabinol on central nervous system. Avoid combination.
Mind-altering drugs*	Increased sedation.
Muscle relaxants, others*	Increased sedation.
Narcotics*	Increased sedation.
Sedatives*	Increased sedation.
Sertraline	Increased depressive effects of both drugs.
Sleep inducers*	Increased sedation.
Tranquilizers*	Increased sedation.

POSSIBLE INTERACTION WITH OTHER SUBSTANCES

INTERACTS WITH	COMBINED EFFECT
Alcohol:	Increased sedation.
Beverages:	None expected.
Cocaine:	Lack of coordination, increased sedation.
Foods:	None expected.
Marijuana:	Lack of coordination, drowsiness, fainting.
Tobacco:	None expected.

NABILONE

BRAND NAMES

Cesamet

BASIC INFORMATION

Habit forming? No
Prescription needed? Yes
Available as generic? No
Drug class: Antiemetic

 USES

- Treats nausea and vomiting.
- Prevents nausea and vomiting in patients receiving cancer chemotherapy.

 DOSAGE & USAGE INFORMATION

How to take:
Capsule—Swallow with liquid. If you can't swallow whole, open capsule and take with liquid or food.

When to take:
At the same each day, according to instructions on prescription label.

If you forget a dose:
Take as soon as you remember up to 2 hours late. If more than 2 hours, wait for next scheduled dose (don't double this dose).

What drug does:
Chemically related to marijuana, it probably regulates the vomiting control center in the brain.

Continued next column

 OVERDOSE

SYMPTOMS:
Mood changes; confusion and delusions; hallucinations; mental depression; nervousness; breathing difficulty; fast, slow or pounding heartbeat; fainting.
WHAT TO DO:
- **Dial 0 (operator) or 911 (emergency) for an ambulance or medical help. Then give first aid immediately.**
- **If patient is unconscious and not breathing, give mouth-to-mouth breathing. If there is no heartbeat, use cardiac massage and mouth-to-mouth breathing (CPR). Don't try to make patient vomit. If you can't get help quickly, take patient to nearest emergency facility.**
- **See emergency information on inside covers.**

Time lapse before drug works:
2 hours.

Don't take with:
Alcohol or any drug that depresses the central nervous system. (See Central Nervous System [CNS] Depressants in the Glossary.)

 POSSIBLE ADVERSE REACTIONS OR SIDE EFFECTS

SYMPTOMS	WHAT TO DO
Life-threatening:	
Mood changes; fainting; hallucinations; fast, slow or pounding heartbeat; confusion and delusions; mental depression; nervousness; breathing difficulty.	Seek emergency treatment.
Common:	
Dry mouth.	Continue. Call doctor when convenient.
Infrequent:	
Clumsiness, mental changes, drowsiness, headache, false sense of well-being.	Discontinue. Call doctor right away.
Rare:	
Blurred vision, dizziness on standing, appetite loss, muscle pain.	Discontinue. Call doctor right away.

WARNINGS & PRECAUTIONS

Don't take if:
- You are allergic to nabilone or marijuana.
- You have schizophrenic, manic or depressive states.

Before you start, consult your doctor:
- If you have abused drugs or are dependent on them, including alcohol.
- If you have had high blood pressure or heart disease.
- If you have had impaired liver function.

Over age 60:
Adverse reactions and side effects may be more frequent and severe than in younger persons. You may need smaller doses for shorter periods of time.

Pregnancy:
Studies inconclusive on harm to unborn child. Decide with your doctor whether drug benefits justify risk to unborn child.

Breast-feeding:
Drug passes into milk. Avoid drug or discontinue nursing until you finish medicine. Consult doctor for advice on maintaining milk supply.

Infants & children:
Not recommended for children 18 and younger. Use only under doctor's supervision.

Prolonged use:
- Avoid prolonged use. This medicine is intended to be used only during a cycle of cancer chemotherapy.
- Talk to your doctor about the need for follow-up medical examinations or laboratory studies to check blood pressure, heart function.

Skin & sunlight:
No problems expected.

Driving, piloting or hazardous work:
Don't drive or pilot aircraft until you learn how medicine affects you. Don't work around dangerous machinery. Don't climb ladders or work in high places. Danger increases if you drink alcohol or take medicine affecting alertness and reflexes.

Discontinuing:
No problems expected.

Others:
- Blood pressure should be measured regularly.
- Learn to count and recognize changes in your pulse.
- Get up from bed or chair slowly to avoid fainting.

POSSIBLE INTERACTION WITH OTHER DRUGS

GENERIC NAME OR DRUG CLASS	COMBINED EFFECT
Apomorphine	Decreases effect of apomorphine.
Central nervous system depressants, other*	Greater depression of the central nervous system.

POSSIBLE INTERACTION WITH OTHER SUBSTANCES

INTERACTS WITH	COMBINED EFFECT
Alcohol:	Dangerous depression of the central nervous system. Avoid.
Beverages:	None expected.
Cocaine:	Decreased nabilone effect. Avoid.
Foods:	None expected.
Marijuana:	None expected.
Tobacco:	None expected.

NAFARELIN

BRAND NAMES

Synarel

BASIC INFORMATION

Habit forming? No
Prescription needed? Yes
Available as generic? No
Drug class: Gonadotropin inhibitor

 USES

Treatment of endometriosis to relieve pain and reduce scattered implants of endometrial tissue.

 DOSAGE & USAGE INFORMATION

How to take:
Nasal spray—Follow instructions on package insert provided with your medicine.

When to take:
As directed by your doctor. Usually two times a day.

If you forget a dose:
Take as soon as you remember. Don't double this dose.

What drug does:
Reduces estrogen production from ovaries.

Time lapse before drug works:
May require 6 months for full effect.

Don't take with:
- Birth control pills.
- Nasal sprays to decongest the membranes in the nose.
- Any other medicine without consulting your doctor or pharmacist.

 OVERDOSE

SYMPTOMS:
None expected.
WHAT TO DO:
Overdose unlikely to threaten life. If person takes much larger amount than prescribed, call doctor, poison-control center or hospital emergency room for instructions.

 POSSIBLE ADVERSE REACTIONS OR SIDE EFFECTS

SYMPTOMS	WHAT TO DO
Life-threatening: None expected.	
Common: Hot flashes.	No action necessary.
Infrequent: Decreased sexual desire, vaginal dryness, headache, acne, swelling of hands and feet, reduction of breast size, weight gain, itchy scalp with flaking, muscle ache, nasal irritation.	Continue. Call doctor when convenient.
Rare: Insomnia, depression, weight loss.	Continue. Call doctor when convenient.

WARNINGS & PRECAUTIONS

Don't take if:
- You become pregnant.
- You have breast cancer.
- You are allergic to any of the ingredients in nafarelin.
- You have undiagnosed abnormal vaginal bleeding.

Before you start, consult your doctor:
- If you take birth control pills.
- If you have diabetes.
- If you have heart disease.
- If you have epilepsy.
- If you have kidney disease.
- If you have liver disease.
- If you have migraine headaches.
- If you need to use topical nasal decongestants.

Over age 60:
Adverse reactions and side effects may be more frequent and severe than in younger persons.

Pregnancy:
Risk to unborn child outweighs drug benefits. Don't use. Stop if you get pregnant.

Breast-feeding:
Unknown whether medicine filters into milk. Consult doctor.

Infants & children:
Not recommended.

Prolonged use:
- Full effect requires prolonged use. Don't discontinue without consulting doctor.
- Talk to your doctor about the need for follow-up medical examinations or laboratory studies to check liver function; mammogram.

Skin & sunlight:
No special problems expected.

Driving, piloting or hazardous work:
No special problems expected.

Discontinuing:
Don't discontinue without consulting doctor. Menstrual periods may be absent for 2 to 3 months after discontinuation.

Others:
- May alter blood sugar levels in diabetic persons.
- Interferes with accuracy of laboratory tests to study pituitary gonadotropic and gonadal functions.
- Experience with nafarelin has been limited to women 18 years of age and older.
- Bone density decreases during treatment phase, but recovers following treatment.

 ## POSSIBLE INTERACTION WITH OTHER DRUGS

GENERIC NAME OR DRUG CLASS	COMBINED EFFECT
Decongestant nasal sprays	Decreased absorption of nafarelin.

 ## POSSIBLE INTERACTION WITH OTHER SUBSTANCES

INTERACTS WITH	COMBINED EFFECT
Alcohol:	Excessive nervous system depression. Avoid.
Beverages: Caffeine drinks.	Rapid, irregular heartbeat. Avoid.
Cocaine:	May interfere with expected action of nafarelin. Avoid.
Foods:	None expected.
Marijuana:	May interfere with expected action of nafarelin. Avoid.
Tobacco:	Rapid, irregular heartbeat; increased leg cramps. Avoid.

NAFCILLIN

BRAND NAMES

Nafcil　　　　　**Unipen**
Nallpen

BASIC INFORMATION

Habit forming? No
Prescription needed? Yes
Available as generic? Yes
Drug class: Antibiotic (penicillin)

 USES

Treatment of bacterial infections that are susceptible to nafcillin.

 DOSAGE & USAGE INFORMATION

How to take:
* Tablets or capsules—Swallow with liquid on an empty stomach 1 hour before or 2 hours after eating.
* Liquid—Take with cold beverage. Liquid form is perishable and effective for only 7 days at room temperature. Effective for 14 days if stored in refrigerator. Don't freeze.

When to take:
Follow instructions on prescription label or side of package. Doses should be evenly spaced. For example, 4 times a day means every 6 hours.

If you forget a dose:
Take as soon as you remember. Continue regular schedule.

What drug does:
Destroys susceptible bacteria. Does not kill viruses.

Time lapse before drug works:
May be several days before medicine affects infection.

Don't take with:
Any other medicine without consulting your doctor or pharmacist.

 OVERDOSE

SYMPTOMS:
Severe diarrhea, nausea or vomiting.
WHAT TO DO:
Overdose unlikely to threaten life. If person takes much larger amount than prescribed, call doctor, poison-control center or hospital emergency room for instructions.

 POSSIBLE ADVERSE REACTIONS OR SIDE EFFECTS

SYMPTOMS	WHAT TO DO
Life-threatening:	
Hives, rash, intense itching, faintness soon after a dose (anaphylaxis).	Seek emergency treatment immediately.
Common:	
Dark or discolored tongue.	Continue. Tell doctor at next visit.
Infrequent:	
• Mild nausea, vomiting, diarrhea.	Continue. Call doctor when convenient.
• Bloody urine, face and ankle swelling.	Discontinue. Call doctor right away.
Rare:	
Unexplained bleeding or bruising, weakness, sore throat, fever, abdominal cramps, convulsions.	Discontinue. Call doctor right away.

WARNINGS & PRECAUTIONS

Don't take if:
You are allergic to nafcillin, cephalosporin antibiotics, other penicillins or penicillamine. Life-threatening reaction may occur.

Before you start, consult your doctor:
- If you are allergic to any substance or drug.
- If you take birth control pills.

Over age 60:
You may have skin reactions, particularly around genitals and anus.

Pregnancy:
Studies inconclusive on harm to unborn child. Animal studies show fetal abnormalities. Decide with your doctor whether drug benefits justify risk to unborn child.

Breast-feeding:
Drug passes into milk. Child may become sensitive to penicillins and have allergic reactions to penicillin drugs. Avoid nafcillin or discontinue nursing until you finish medicine. Consult doctor for advice on maintaining milk supply.

Infants & children:
No problems expected.

Prolonged use:
- You may become more susceptible to infections caused by germs not responsive to nafcillin.
- Talk to your doctor about the need for follow-up medical examinations or laboratory studies to check SGPT*, SGOT*.

Skin & sunlight:
No problems expected.

Driving, piloting or hazardous work:
Usually not dangerous. Most hazardous reactions likely to occur a few minutes after taking nafcillin.

Discontinuing:
Don't discontinue without doctor's advice until you complete prescribed dose, even though symptoms diminish or disappear.

Others:
- Absorption of this drug in oral form is unpredictable. Injections are more reliable.
- May interfere with the accuracy of some medical tests.
- Birth control pills may not be effective. Use additional birth-control methods.

POSSIBLE INTERACTION WITH OTHER DRUGS

GENERIC NAME OR DRUG CLASS	COMBINED EFFECT
Beta-adrenergic blockers*	Increased chance of anaphylaxis (see emergency information on inside front cover).
Birth control pills	Impaired contraceptive efficiency.
Chloramphenicol	Decreased effect of both drugs.
Erythromycins*	Decreased effect of both drugs.
Loperamide	Decreased nafcillin effect.
Paromomycin	Decreased effect of both drugs.
Probenecid	Increased effect of all penicillins.
Sodium benzoate & sodium phenylacetate	May reduce effect of sodium benzoate & sodium phenylacetate.
Tetracyclines*	Decreased effect of both drugs.
Troleandomycin	Decreased effect of both drugs.

POSSIBLE INTERACTION WITH OTHER SUBSTANCES

INTERACTS WITH	COMBINED EFFECT
Alcohol:	Occasional stomach irritation.
Beverages:	None expected.
Cocaine:	No proven problems.
Foods: Acidic fruits or juices, aged cheese, wines, syrups (if taken with).	Decreased antibiotic effect.
Marijuana:	No proven problems.
Tobacco:	None expected.

NALIDIXIC ACID

BRAND NAMES

NegGram

BASIC INFORMATION

Habit forming? No
Prescription needed? Yes
Available as generic? No
Drug class: Antimicrobial

 ## USES

Treatment for urinary tract infections.

 ## DOSAGE & USAGE INFORMATION

How to take:
• Tablet—Swallow with food or milk to lessen stomach irritation. If you can't swallow whole, crumble tablet and take with liquid or food.
• Liquid—Take with liquid or food.

When to take:
At the same times each day.

If you forget a dose:
Take as soon as you remember up to 2 hours late. If more than 2 hours, wait for next scheduled dose (don't double this dose).

What drug does:
Destroys bacteria susceptible to nalidixic acid.

Time lapse before drug works:
1 to 2 weeks.

Don't take with:
Any other medicine without consulting your doctor or pharmacist.

 ## OVERDOSE

SYMPTOMS:
Lethargy, stomach upset, behavioral changes, hyperglycemia, psychosis, convulsions and stupor.
WHAT TO DO:
• **Dial 0 (operator) or 911 (emergency) for an ambulance or medical help. Then give first aid immediately.**
• **If patient is unconscious and not breathing, give mouth-to-mouth breathing. If there is no heartbeat, use cardiac massage and mouth-to-mouth breathing (CPR). Don't try to make patient vomit. If you can't get help quickly, take patient to nearest emergency facility.**
• **See emergency information on inside covers.**

 ## POSSIBLE ADVERSE REACTIONS OR SIDE EFFECTS

SYMPTOMS	WHAT TO DO
Life-threatening:	
Hives, rash, intense itching, faintness soon after a dose (anaphylaxis).	Seek emergency treatment immediately.
Common:	
Rash; itchy skin; decreased, blurred or double vision; halos around lights or excess brightness; changes in color vision; nausea; vomiting; diarrhea.	Discontinue. Call doctor right away.
Infrequent:	
• Dizziness, drowsiness, sensitivity to sun, headache.	Continue. Call doctor when convenient.
• Dark urine, hallucinations, mood changes.	Discontinue. Call doctor right away.
Rare:	
Paleness, sore throat or fever, severe abdominal pain, pale stool, unusual bleeding or bruising, jaundice, fatigue, weakness, seizures, psychosis, joint pain, numbness or tingling in hands or feet.	Discontinue. Call doctor right away.

WARNINGS & PRECAUTIONS

Don't take if:
- You are allergic to nalidixic acid.
- You have a seizure disorder (epilepsy, convulsions).

Before you start, consult your doctor:
- If you plan to become pregnant within medication period.
- If you have or have had kidney or liver disease.
- If you have impaired circulation of the brain (hardened arteries).
- If you have Parkinson's disease.
- If you have diabetes (it may affect urine-sugar tests).

Over age 60:
Adverse reactions and side effects may be more frequent and severe than in younger persons.

Pregnancy:
Risk to unborn child outweighs drug benefits. Don't use, especially during first 3 months.

Breast-feeding:
Drug passes into milk. Avoid drug or discontinue nursing until you finish medicine. Consult doctor for advice on maintaining milk supply.

Infants & children:
Not recommended.

Prolonged use:
Talk to your doctor about the need for follow-up medical examinations or laboratory studies to check complete blood counts (white blood cell count, platelet count, red blood cell count, hemoglobin, hematocrit), liver function, kidney function.

Skin & sunlight:
May cause rash or intensify sunburn in areas exposed to sun or sunlamp.

Driving, piloting or hazardous work:
Avoid if you feel drowsy, dizzy or have vision problems. Otherwise, no problems expected.

Discontinuing:
Don't discontinue without consulting doctor. Dose may require gradual reduction if you have taken drug for a long time. Doses of other drugs may also require adjustment.

Others:
Periodic blood counts and liver- and kidney-function tests recommended.

POSSIBLE INTERACTION WITH OTHER DRUGS

GENERIC NAME OR DRUG CLASS	COMBINED EFFECT
Antacids*	Decreased absorption of nalidixic acid.
Anticoagulants, oral*	Increased anticoagulant effect.
Calcium supplements*	Decreased effect of nalidixic acid.
Nitrofurantoin	Decreased effect of nalidixic acid.
Probenecid	Decreased effect of nalidixic acid.
Vitamin C (in large doses)	Increased effect of nalidixic acid.

POSSIBLE INTERACTION WITH OTHER SUBSTANCES

INTERACTS WITH	COMBINED EFFECT
Alcohol:	Impaired alertness, judgment and coordination.
Beverages:	None expected.
Cocaine:	Impaired judgment and coordination.
Foods:	None expected.
Marijuana:	Impaired alertness, judgment and coordination.
Tobacco:	None expected.

NALTREXONE

BRAND NAMES

Trexan

BASIC INFORMATION

Habit forming? No
Prescription needed? Yes
Available as generic? No
Drug class: Narcotic antagonist

 USES

Treats detoxified former narcotic addicts. It helps maintain a drug-free state.

 DOSAGE & USAGE INFORMATION

How to take:
- *Don't take at all until detoxification has been accomplished.*
- Tablets—Swallow with liquid or food to lessen stomach irritation. If you can't swallow whole, crumble tablet and take with liquid or food.

When to take:
At the same time every day or every other day as directed.

If you forget a dose:
Follow detailed instructions from the one who prescribed for you.

What drug does:
Binds to opiod receptors in the central nervous system and prohibits the effects of narcotic drugs.

Time lapse before drug works:
1 hour.

Don't take with:
- Narcotics.
- Any other medicine without consulting your doctor or pharmacist.

 OVERDOSE

SYMPTOMS:
Seizures, coma.
WHAT TO DO:
- **Dial 0 (operator) or 911 (emergency) for an ambulance or medical help. Then give first aid immediately.**
- **See emergency information on inside covers.**

 POSSIBLE ADVERSE REACTIONS OR SIDE EFFECTS

SYMPTOMS	WHAT TO DO
Life-threatening:	
Hallucinations, very fast heartbeat, fainting, breathing difficulties.	Seek emergency treatment immediately.
Common:	
Skin rash, chills, constipation, appetite loss, irritability, insomnia, anxiety, headache, nausea, vomiting.	Continue. Call doctor when convenient.
Infrequent:	
• Nosebleeds, joint pain.	Discontinue. Call doctor right away.
• Abdominal pain, blurred vision, confusion, earache, fever, hallucinations, depression, diarrhea, common cold symptoms.	Continue. Call doctor when convenient.
Rare:	
• Pain, tenderness or color change in feet.	Discontinue. Call doctor right away.
• Ringing in ears, swollen glands, decreased sex drive.	Continue. Call doctor when convenient.

WARNINGS & PRECAUTIONS

Don't take if:
- You don't have close medical supervision.
- You are currently dependent on drugs.
- You have severe liver disease.

Before you start, consult your doctor:
If you have mild liver disease.

Over age 60:
Adverse reactions and side effects may be more frequent and severe than in younger persons. You may need smaller doses for shorter periods of time.

Pregnancy:
Risk to unborn child outweighs drug benefits. Don't use.

Breast-feeding:
Safety not established. Consult doctor.

Infants & children:
Not recommended.

Prolonged use:
- Not recommended.
- Talk to your doctor about the need for follow-up medical examinations or laboratory studies to check kidney function.

Skin & sunlight:
No problems expected.

Driving, piloting or hazardous work:
Don't drive or pilot aircraft until you learn how medicine affects you. Don't work around dangerous machinery. Don't climb ladders or work in high places. Danger increases if you drink alcohol or take medicine affecting alertness and reflexes.

Discontinuing:
Don't discontinue without consulting doctor. Dose may require gradual reduction if you have taken drug for a long time. Doses of other drugs may also require adjustment.

Others:
- Probably not effective in treating people addicted to substances other than opium or morphine derivatives.
- Must be given under close supervision by people experienced in using naltrexone to treat addicts.
- Attempting to use narcotics to overcome effects of naltrexone may lead to coma and death.
- Withdraw several days prior to expected surgery.

POSSIBLE INTERACTION WITH OTHER DRUGS

GENERIC NAME OR DRUG CLASS	COMBINED EFFECT
Narcotic medicines* (butorphenal, codeine, heroin, hydrocodone, hydromorphone, levorphanol, morphine, nalbuphine, opium, oxycodone, oxymorphone, paregoric, pentazocine, propoxyphene)	Precipitates withdrawal symptoms. May lead to arrest, coma and death.
Isoniazid	Increased risk of liver damage.

POSSIBLE INTERACTION WITH OTHER SUBSTANCES

INTERACTS WITH	COMBINED EFFECT
Alcohol:	Unpredictable effects. Avoid.
Beverages:	None expected.
Cocaine:	Unpredictable effects. Avoid.
Foods:	None expected.
Marijuana:	Unpredictable effects. Avoid.
Tobacco:	None expected.

NARCOTIC & ACETAMINOPHEN

BRAND AND GENERIC NAMES

See complete list of brand and generic names in the *Brand Name Directory,* page 922.

BASIC INFORMATION

Habit forming? Yes
Prescription needed? Yes
Available as generic? Yes
Drug class: Narcotic, analgesic, fever-reducer

USES

Relieves pain.

DOSAGE & USAGE INFORMATION

How to take:
- Tablet or capsule—Swallow with liquid. If you can't swallow whole, crumble tablet or open capsule and take with liquid or food.
- Drops or liquid—Dilute dose in beverage before swallowing.

When to take:
When needed. No more often than every 4 hours.

If you forget a dose:
Take as soon as you remember. Wait 4 hours for next dose.

What drug does:
- May affect hypothalamus—the part of the brain that helps regulate body heat and receives body's pain messages.
- Blocks pain messages to brain and spinal cord.
- Reduces sensitivity of brain's cough-control center.

Continued next column

OVERDOSE

SYMPTOMS:
Stomach upset; irritability; sweating, convulsions; deep sleep; slow breathing; slow pulse; flushed, warm skin; constricted pupils; coma.
WHAT TO DO:
- **Dial 0 (operator) or 911 (emergency) for an ambulance or medical help. Then give first aid immediately.**
- **If patient is unconscious and not breathing, give mouth-to-mouth breathing. If there is no heartbeat, use cardiac massage and mouth-to-mouth breathing (CPR). Don't try to make patient vomit. If you can't get help quickly, take patient to nearest emergency facility.**
- **See emergency information on inside covers.**

Time lapse before drug works:
15 to 30 minutes. May last 4 hours.

Don't take with:
- Other drugs with acetaminophen. Too much acetaminophen can damage liver and kidneys.
- Any other medicine without consulting your doctor or pharmacist.

POSSIBLE ADVERSE REACTIONS OR SIDE EFFECTS

SYMPTOMS	WHAT TO DO
Life-threatening:	
Irregular or slow heartbeat, difficult breathing, wheezing.	Discontinue. Seek emergency treatment.
Common:	
Dizziness, agitation, tiredness, dry mouth, headache.	Continue. Call doctor when convenient.
Infrequent:	
Abdominal pain, constipation, vomiting, confusion, pinpoint eye pupils, hallucinations, flushed face, face swelling, uncontrolled muscle movements, jaundice, nightmares, insomnia.	Discontinue. Call doctor right away.
Rare:	
• Itchy skin; rash; sore throat, fever, mouth sores; bruising and bleeding increased; painful or difficult urination; blood in urine; blurred vision.	Discontinue. Call doctor right away.
• Depression.	Continue. Call doctor when convenient.

WARNINGS & PRECAUTIONS

Don't take if:
- You are allergic to any narcotic or acetaminophen.
- Your symptoms don't improve after 2 days use. Call your doctor.

Before you start, consult your doctor:
- If you have bronchial asthma, kidney disease or liver damage.
- If you will have surgery within 2 months, including dental surgery, requiring general or spinal anesthesia.

Over age 60:
More likely to be drowsy, dizzy, unsteady or constipated. Don't exceed recommended dose. You can't eliminate drug as efficiently as younger persons. Use only if absolutely necessary.

Pregnancy:
Decide with your doctor whether drug benefits justify risk to unborn child. Abuse by pregnant woman will result in addicted newborn. Withdrawal of newborn can be life-threatening.

Breast-feeding:
Drug filters into milk. May harm child. Avoid.

Infants & children:
Not recommended.

Prolonged use:
- Causes psychological and physical dependence (addiction).
- May affect blood stream and cause anemia. Limit use to 5 days for children 12 and under, and 10 days for adults.

Skin & sunlight:
No problems expected.

Driving, piloting or hazardous work:
Don't drive or pilot aircraft until you learn how medicine affects you. Don't work around dangerous machinery. Don't climb ladders or work in high places. Danger increases if you drink alcohol or take medicine affecting alertness and reflexes, such as antihistamines, tranquilizers, sedatives, pain medicine, narcotics and mind-altering drugs.

Discontinuing:
Discontinue in 2 days if symptoms don't improve. Report to your doctor any symptoms that develop after discontinuing such as gooseflesh, irritability, insomnia, yawning, weakness, large eye pupils.

Others:
No problems expected.

POSSIBLE INTERACTION WITH OTHER DRUGS

GENERIC NAME OR DRUG CLASS	COMBINED EFFECT
Analgesics, other*	Increased analgesic effect.
Anticoagulants, other*	May increase anticoagulant effect. Prothrombin times should be monitored.
Anticholinergics*	Increased anticholinergic effect.
Antidepressants*	Increased sedative effect.
Antihistamines*	Increased sedative effect.
Carteolol	Increased narcotic effect. Dangerous sedation.
Mind-altering drugs*	Increased sedative effect.
Narcotics, other*	Increased narcotic effect.
Nitrates*	Excessive blood-pressure drop.
Phenobarbital and other barbiturates*	Quicker elimination and decreased effect of acetaminophen.
Phenothiazines*	Increased phenothiazine effect.
Sedatives*	Increased sedative effect.
Selegiline	Severe toxicity characterized by breathing difficulty, seizures, coma.
Sertraline	Increased depressive effects of both drugs.
Sleep inducers*	Increased sedative effect.
Sotalol	Increased narcotic effect. Dangerous sedation.
Terfenadine	Possible oversedation.
Tetracyclines*	May slow tetracycline absorption. Space doses 2 hours apart.
Tranquilizers*	Increased sedative effect.
Zidovudine	Increased toxicity of zidovudine.

POSSIBLE INTERACTION WITH OTHER SUBSTANCES

INTERACTS WITH	COMBINED EFFECT
Alcohol:	Increases alcohol's intoxicating effect. Long-term use may cause toxic effect in liver. Avoid.
Beverages:	None expected.
Cocaine:	Increased toxic effects of cocaine. Avoid.
Foods:	None expected.
Marijuana:	Impairs physical and mental performance. Avoid.
Tobacco:	None expected.

*See Glossary

NARCOTIC ANALGESICS

BRAND AND GENERIC NAMES

See complete list of brand and generic names in the *Brand Name Directory*, page 923.

BASIC INFORMATION

Habit forming? Yes
Prescription needed? Yes
Available as generic? Yes
Drug class: Narcotic

 USES

Relieves pain and diarrhea; suppresses cough.

 DOSAGE & USAGE INFORMATION

How to take:
- Tablet, capsule or extended-release tablet—Swallow with liquid. If you can't swallow whole, crumble tablet or open capsule and take with liquid or food.
- Drops or liquid—Dilute dose in beverage before swallowing.
- Transdermal—follow instructions on prescription.
- Nasal—Follow package instructions.

When to take:
When needed. No more often than every 4 hours.

If you forget a dose:
Take as soon as you remember. Wait 4 hours for next dose.

What drug does:
- Blocks pain messages to brain and spinal cord.
- Reduces sensitivity of brain's cough-control center.

Time lapse before drug works:
30 minutes.

Continued next column

 OVERDOSE

SYMPTOMS:
Deep sleep, slow breathing; slow pulse; respiratory arrest; flushed, warm skin; seizures; constricted pupils.
WHAT TO DO:
- **Dial 0 (operator) or 911 (emergency) for an ambulance or medical help. Then give first aid immediately.**
- **If patient is unconscious and not breathing, give mouth-to-mouth breathing. If there is no heartbeat, use cardiac massage and mouth-to-mouth breathing (CPR). Don't try to make patient vomit. If you can't get help quickly, take patient to nearest emergency facility.**
- **See emergency information on inside covers.**

Don't take with:
Any other medicine without consulting your doctor or pharmacist.

 POSSIBLE ADVERSE REACTIONS OR SIDE EFFECTS

SYMPTOMS	WHAT TO DO
Life-threatening:	
Hives, rash, intense itching, faintness soon after a dose (anaphylaxis); seizures; restlessness (severe); slow heartbeat; breathing difficulty.	Seek emergency treatment immediately.
Common:	
Dizziness, flushed face, difficult urination, unusual tiredness.	Continue. Call doctor when convenient.
Infrequent:	
• Severe constipation, abdominal pain, vomiting, nausea.	Discontinue. Call doctor right away.
• Dry mouth, headache, appetite loss, nightmares, decreased sex drive.	Continue. Call doctor when convenient.
Rare:	
• Hives, rash, itchy skin, face swelling, slow heartbeat, irregular breathing, hallucinations, jaundice, disorientation, fainting.	Discontinue. Call doctor right away.
• Depression, blurred vision, decreased mental performance, anxiety, insomnia, weakness and faintness when arising from bed or chair, euphoria, ears ringing.	Continue. Call doctor when convenient.

 WARNINGS & PRECAUTIONS

Don't take if:
- You are allergic to any narcotic.
- Diarrhea is due to toxic effect of drugs or poisons.

Before you start, consult your doctor:
- If you have impaired liver or kidney function.
- If you will have surgery within 2 months, including dental surgery, requiring general or spinal anesthesia.
- If you have asthma.

Over age 60:
More likely to be drowsy, dizzy, unsteady or constipated. Use only if absolutely necessary.

Pregnancy:
Decide with your doctor whether drug benefits justify risk to unborn child. Abuse by pregnant woman will result in addicted newborn. Withdrawal of newborn can be life-threatening.

Breast-feeding:
Drug filters into milk. May harm child. Avoid.

Infants & children:
Not recommended.

Prolonged use:
Causes psychological and physical dependence (addiction).

Skin & sunlight:
May cause rash or intensify sunburn in areas exposed to sun or sunlamp.

Driving, piloting or hazardous work:
Don't drive or pilot aircraft until you learn how medicine affects you. Don't work around dangerous machinery. Don't climb ladders or work in high places. Danger increases if you drink alcohol or take medicine affecting alertness and reflexes, such as antihistamines, tranquilizers, sedatives, pain medicine, narcotics and mind-altering drugs.

Discontinuing:
May be unnecessary to finish medicine. Follow doctor's instructions. Notify doctor of any withdrawal symptoms such as gooseflesh, irritability, insomnia, yawning, weakness, large eye pupils.

Others:
Some products contain tartrazine dye. Avoid, especially if you are allergic to aspirin.

 ## POSSIBLE INTERACTION WITH OTHER DRUGS

GENERIC NAME OR DRUG CLASS	COMBINED EFFECT
Analgesics, other*	Increased analgesic effect.
Anticoagulants, oral*	Possible increased anticoagulant effect.
Anticholinergics*	Increased anticholinergic effect.
Antidepressants*	Increased sedative effect.
Antihistamines*	Increased sedative effect.
Butorphanol	Possibly precipitates withdrawal with chronic narcotic use.
Carbamazepine	Increased carbamazepine effect with propoxyphene possible.

Carteolol	Increased narcotic effect. Dangerous sedation.
Cimetidine	Possible increased narcotic effect and toxicity.
Clozapine	Toxic effect on the central nervous system.
Ethinamate	Dangerous increased effects of ethinamate. Avoid combining.
Fluoxetine	Increased depressant effects of both drugs.
Guanfacine	May increase depressant effects of either drug.
Leucovorin	High alcohol content of leucovorin may cause adverse effects.
MAO inhibitors*	Serious toxicity (including death).
Methyprylon	Increased sedative effect, perhaps to dangerous level. Avoid.
Mind-altering drugs*	Increased sedative effect.
Molindone	Increased narcotic effect.
Nabilone	Greater depression of central nervous system.
Nalbuphine	Possibly precipitates withdrawal with chronic narcotic use.

Continued page 952

 ## POSSIBLE INTERACTION WITH OTHER SUBSTANCES

INTERACTS WITH	COMBINED EFFECT
Alcohol:	Increases alcohol's intoxicating effect. Avoid.
Beverages:	None expected.
Cocaine:	Increased cocaine toxic effects. Avoid.
Foods:	None expected.
Marijuana:	Impairs physical and mental performance. Avoid.
Tobacco:	None expected.

NARCOTIC & ASPIRIN

BRAND AND GENERIC NAMES

See complete list of brand and generic names in the *Brand Name Directory*, page 924.

BASIC INFORMATION

Habit forming? Yes
Prescription needed? Yes
Available as generic? Yes
Drug class: Narcotic, analgesic, anti-inflammatory (non-steroidal)

 USES

Reduces pain, fever, inflammation.

 DOSAGE & USAGE INFORMATION

How to take:
Tablet or capsule—Swallow with liquid. If you can't swallow whole, crumble tablet or open capsule and take with liquid or food.

When to take:
When needed. No more often than every 4 hours.

If you forget a dose:
Take as soon as you remember. Wait 4 hours for next dose.

What drug does:
- Affects hypothalamus, the part of the brain which regulates temperature by dilating small blood vessels in skin.
- Prevents clumping of platelets (small blood cells) so blood vessels remain open.

Continued next column

 OVERDOSE

SYMPTOMS:
Ringing in ears; nausea; vomiting; dizziness; fever; deep sleep; slow breathing; slow pulse; flushed, warm skin; constricted pupils; hallucinations; convulsions; coma.
WHAT TO DO:
- **Dial 0 (operator) or 911 (emergency) for an ambulance or medical help. Then give first aid immediately.**
- **If patient is unconscious and not breathing, give mouth-to-mouth breathing. If there is no heartbeat, use cardiac massage and mouth-to-mouth breathing (CPR). Don't try to make patient vomit. If you can't get help quickly, take patient to nearest emergency facility.**
- **See emergency information on inside covers.**

- Decreases prostaglandin effect.
- Suppresses body's pain messages.
- Reduces sensitivity of brain's cough-control center.

Time lapse before drug works:
30 minutes.

Don't take with:
- Tetracyclines. Space doses 1 hour apart.
- Any other medicine without consulting your doctor or pharmacist.

 POSSIBLE ADVERSE REACTIONS OR SIDE EFFECTS

SYMPTOMS	WHAT TO DO
Life-threatening:	
Hives, rash, intense itching, faintness soon after a dose (anaphylaxis); difficulty breathing.	Seek emergency treatment immediately.
Lump (caused by blood clot in vein) or pain over blood vessel; cold hands, feet; seizures; pin point pupils.	Discontinue. Seek emergency treatment.
Common:	
Headache (severe), slow heartbeat, excitement, vomiting of blood.	Discontinue. Call doctor right away.
Dizziness, red or flushed face, ringing in ears, unusual tiredness, frequent urination, heartburn, indigestion, fever, hallucinations, constipation.	Continue. Call doctor when convenient.
Infrequent:	
Abdominal pain or cramps, vomiting.	Discontinue. Call doctor right away.
Rare:	
Change in vision; black, bloody or tarry stool; blood in urine; jaundice; mental confusion; irregular breathing; face swelling.	Discontinue. Call doctor right away.
Depression, blurred vision.	Continue. Call doctor when convenient.

 WARNINGS & PRECAUTIONS

Don't take if:
- You are allergic to any narcotic or subject to any substance abuse.
- You have a peptic ulcer of stomach or duodenum or a bleeding disorder.

Before you start, consult your doctor:
- If you have impaired liver or kidney function, asthma or nasal polyps.
- If you have had stomach or duodenal ulcers, gout.
- If you will have surgery within 2 months, including dental surgery, requiring general or spinal anesthesia.

Over age 60:
- More likely to be drowsy, dizzy, unsteady or constipated. Use only if absolutely necessary.
- More likely to cause hidden bleeding in stomach or intestines. Watch for dark stools.

Pregnancy:
Risk to unborn child outweighs drug benefits. Don't use.

Breast-feeding:
Drug passes into milk and may harm child. Avoid drug or discontinue nursing until you finish medicine. Consult doctor for advice on maintaining milk supply.

Infants & children:
Not recommended.

Prolonged use:
- Causes psychological and physical dependence (addiction).
- Kidney damage. Periodic kidney-function test recommended.

Skin & sunlight:
May cause rash or intensify sunburn in areas exposed to sun or sunlamp.

Driving, piloting or hazardous work:
Don't drive or pilot aircraft until you learn how medicine affects you. Don't work around dangerous machinery. Don't climb ladders or work in high places. Danger increases if you drink alcohol or take medicine affecting alertness and reflexes, such as antihistamines, tranquilizers, sedatives, pain medicine, narcotics and mind-altering drugs.

Discontinuing:
May be unnecessary to finish medicine. Follow doctor's instructions. Notify doctor of any withdrawal symptoms such as gooseflesh, irritability, insomnia, yawning, weakness, large eye pupils.

Others:
- Aspirin can complicate surgery; illness; pregnancy, labor and delivery.
- Urine tests for blood sugar may be inaccurate.

POSSIBLE INTERACTION WITH OTHER DRUGS

GENERIC NAME OR DRUG CLASS	COMBINED EFFECT
Acebutolol	Decreased anti-hypertensive effect of acebutolol.
ACE inhibitors*: captopril, enalapril, lisinopril	Decreased effect of ACE inhibitors.
Allopurinol	Decreased allopurinol effect.
Antacids*	Decreased aspirin effect.
Anticoagulants*	Increased anti-coagulant effect. Abnormal bleeding.
Antidepressants*	Increased sedative effect.
Antidiabetics, oral*	Low blood sugar.
Aspirin, other	Likely aspirin toxicity.
Bumetanide	Possible aspirin toxicity.
Carteolol	Increased narcotic effect. Dangerous sedation.
Cortisone drugs*	Increased cortisone effect. Risk of ulcers and stomach bleeding.
Ethacrynic acid	Possible aspirin toxicity.

Continued page 953

POSSIBLE INTERACTION WITH OTHER SUBSTANCES

INTERACTS WITH	COMBINED EFFECT
Alcohol:	Possible stomach irritation and bleeding. Increases alcohol's intoxicating effect. Avoid.
Beverages:	None expected.
Cocaine:	Decreased cocaine toxic effects. Avoid.
Foods:	None expected.
Marijuana:	Impairs physical and mental performance. Avoid.
Tobacco:	None expected.

NATAMYCIN (Ophthalmic)

BRAND NAMES

Natacyn   Pimaricin

BASIC INFORMATION

Habit forming? No
Prescription needed? Yes
Available as generic? No
Drug class: Antifungal (ophthalmic).
Note: Limited availability. Must be ordered
  directly from manufacturer.

USES

Treats fungus infections of the eye.

DOSAGE & USAGE INFORMATION

How to use:
Eye drops
- Wash hands.
- Apply pressure to inside corner of eye with middle finger.
- Tilt head backward. Pull lower lid away from eye with index finger of the same hand.
- Drop eye drops into pouch and close eye. Don't blink.
- Continue pressure for 1 minute after placing medicine in eye.
- Keep eyes closed for 1 to 2 minutes.
- Don't touch applicator tip to any surface (including the eye). If you accidentally touch tip, clean with warm soap and water.
- Keep container tightly closed.
- Keep cool, but don't freeze.
- Wash hands immediately after using.

When to use:
As directed. Usually 1 drop in eye every 1 or 2 hours for 3 or 4 days, then every 3 to 4 hours.

If you forget a dose:
Use as soon as you remember.

What drug does:
Changes cell membrane of fungus causing loss of essential constituents of fungus cell.

Continued next column

OVERDOSE

SYMPTOMS:
None expected.
WHAT TO DO:
Not intended for internal use. If child accidentally swallows, call poison-control center.

Time lapse before drug works:
Starts to work immediately. May require 2 weeks or more to cure infection.

Don't use with:
Other eye drops without consulting your eye doctor.

POSSIBLE ADVERSE REACTIONS OR SIDE EFFECTS

SYMPTOMS	WHAT TO DO
Life-threatening: None expected.	
Common: None expected.	
Infrequent: Eye irritation not present before using natamycin.	Discontinue. Call doctor right away.
Rare: None expected.	

NATAMYCIN (Ophthalmic)

WARNINGS & PRECAUTIONS

Don't use if:
You are allergic to natamycin or any antifungal medicine.

Before you start, consult your doctor:
If you have allergies to any substance.

Over age 60:
No problems expected.

Pregnancy:
No problems expected, but check with doctor.

Breast-feeding:
No problems expected, but check with doctor.

Infants & children:
No problems expected.

Prolonged use:
May cause eye irritation.

Skin & sunlight:
No problems expected.

Driving, piloting or hazardous work:
No problems expected.

Discontinuing:
Don't discontinue without consulting your eye doctor.

Others:
- Keep cool, but don't freeze.
- Notify doctor if condition doesn't improve within 1 week.

POSSIBLE INTERACTION WITH OTHER DRUGS

GENERIC NAME OR DRUG CLASS	COMBINED EFFECT
Clinically significant interactions with oral or injected medicines unlikely.	

POSSIBLE INTERACTION WITH OTHER SUBSTANCES

INTERACTS WITH	COMBINED EFFECT
Alcohol:	None expected.
Beverages:	None expected.
Cocaine:	None expected.
Foods:	None expected.
Marijuana:	None expected.
Tobacco:	None expected.

NEOMYCIN (Oral)

BRAND NAMES

Mycifradin

BASIC INFORMATION

Habit forming? No
Prescription needed? Yes
Available as generic? Yes
Drug class: Antibiotic

 USES

- Clears intestinal tract of germs prior to surgery.
- Treats some causes of diarrhea.
- Lowers blood cholesterol.
- Lessens symptoms of hepatic coma.

 DOSAGE & USAGE INFORMATION

How to take:
Tablet—Swallow with liquid or food to lessen stomach irritation. If you can't swallow whole, crumble tablet and take with liquid or food.

When to take:
According to directions on prescription.

If you forget a dose:
Take as soon as you remember up to 2 hours late. If more than 2 hours, wait for next scheduled dose (don't double this dose).

What drug does:
Kills germs susceptible to neomycin.

Time lapse before drug works:
2 to 3 days.

Continued next column

 OVERDOSE

SYMPTOMS:
Loss of hearing, difficulty breathing, respiratory paralysis.
WHAT TO DO:
- **Dial 0 (operator) or 911 (emergency) for an ambulance or medical help. Then give first aid immediately.**
- **If patient is unconscious and not breathing, give mouth-to-mouth breathing. If there is no heartbeat, use cardiac massage and mouth-to-mouth breathing (CPR). Don't try to make patient vomit. If you can't get help quickly, take patient to nearest emergency facility.**
- **See emergency information on inside covers.**

Don't take with:
Any other medicine without consulting your doctor or pharmacist.

 POSSIBLE ADVERSE REACTIONS OR SIDE EFFECTS

SYMPTOMS	WHAT TO DO
Life-threatening: In case of overdose, see previous column.	
Common: Sore mouth or rectum, nausea, vomiting.	Continue. Call doctor when convenient.
Infrequent: None expected.	
Rare: Clumsiness, dizziness, rash, hearing loss, ringing or noises in ear, frothy stools, gaseousness, decreased frequency of urination, diarrhea.	Discontinue. Call doctor right away.

WARNINGS & PRECAUTIONS

Don't take if:
You are allergic to neomycin or any aminoglycoside. (See Interactions column.)

Before you start, consult your doctor:
- If you will have surgery within 2 months, including dental surgery, requiring general or spinal anesthesia.
- If you have hearing loss or loss of balance secondary to 8th cranial nerve disease.
- If you have intestinal obstruction.
- If you have myasthenia gravis, Parkinson's disease, kidney disease, ulcers in intestines.

Over age 60:
Adverse reactions and side effects may be more frequent and severe than in younger persons.

Pregnancy:
No proven harm to unborn child. Avoid if possible.

Breast-feeding:
Avoid if possible.

Infants & children:
Only under close medical supervision.

Prolonged use:
- Adverse effects more likely.
- Talk to your doctor about the need for follow-up medical examinations or laboratory studies to check hearing, kidney function.

Skin & sunlight:
No problems expected.

Driving, piloting or hazardous work:
No problems expected.

Discontinuing:
May be unnecessary to finish medicine. Follow doctor's instructions.

Others:
No problems expected.

POSSIBLE INTERACTION WITH OTHER DRUGS

GENERIC NAME OR DRUG CLASS	COMBINED EFFECT
Aminoglycosides*	Increased chance of toxic effect on hearing, kidneys, muscles.
Beta carotene	Decreased absorption of beta carotene.
Capreomycin	Increased chance of toxic effects on hearing, kidneys.
Cephalothin	Increased chance of toxic effect on kidneys.
Cisplatin	Increased chance of toxic effects on hearing, kidneys.
Ethacrynic acid	Increased chance of toxic effects on hearing, kidneys.
Furosemide	Increased chance of toxic effects on hearing, kidneys.
Mercaptomerin	Increased chance of toxic effects on hearing, kidneys.
Tiopronin	Increased risk of toxicity to kidneys.
Vancomycin	Increased chance of toxic effects on hearing, kidneys.

POSSIBLE INTERACTION WITH OTHER SUBSTANCES

INTERACTS WITH	COMBINED EFFECT
Alcohol:	Increased chance of toxicity. Avoid.
Beverages:	No problems expected.
Cocaine:	Increased chance of toxicity. Avoid.
Foods:	No problems expected.
Marijuana:	Increased chance of toxicity. Avoid.
Tobacco:	No problems expected.

*See Glossary

NEOMYCIN (Topical)

BRAND NAMES
Myciguent

BASIC INFORMATION

Habit forming? No
Prescription needed? No
Available as generic? Yes
Drug class: Antibacterial (topical)

 ## USES

Treats skin infections that may accompany
burns, superficial boils, insect bites or stings,
skin ulcers, minor surgical wounds.

 ## DOSAGE & USAGE INFORMATION

How to take:
- Cream, lotion, ointment—Bathe and dry area
before use. Apply small amount and rub
gently.
- May cover with gauze or bandage if desired.

When to take:
3 or 4 times daily, or as directed by doctor.

If you forget a dose:
Use as soon as you remember.

What drug does:
Kills susceptible bacteria by interfering with
bacterial DNA and RNA.

Time lapse before drug works:
Begins first day. May require treatment for a
week or longer to cure infection.

Don't take with:
Any other medicine without consulting your
doctor or pharmacist.

 ## OVERDOSE

SYMPTOMS:
None expected.
WHAT TO DO:
- Not for internal use. If child accidentally
swallows, call poison-control center.
- Dial 0 (operator) or 911 (emergency) for
an ambulance or medical help. Then give
first aid immediately.
- See emergency information on inside
covers.

 ## POSSIBLE ADVERSE REACTIONS OR SIDE EFFECTS

SYMPTOMS	WHAT TO DO
Life-threatening: None expected.	
Common: None expected.	
Infrequent: Itching, swollen, red skin.	Discontinue. Call doctor right away.
Rare: None expected.	

WARNINGS & PRECAUTIONS

Don't take if:
You are allergic to neomycin or any topical medicine.

Before you start, consult your doctor:
If any lesions on the skin are open sores.

Over age 60:
No problems expected.

Pregnancy:
No problems expected, but check with doctor.

Breast-feeding:
No problems expected, but check with doctor.

Infants & children:
No problems expected, but check with doctor.

Prolonged use:
No problems expected, but check with doctor.

Skin & sunlight:
No problems expected, but check with doctor.

Driving, piloting or hazardous work:
No problems expected, but check with doctor.

Discontinuing:
No problems expected, but check with doctor.

Others:
- Heat and moisture in bathroom medicine cabinet can cause breakdown of medicine. Store someplace else.
- Keep cool, but don't freeze.

POSSIBLE INTERACTION WITH OTHER DRUGS

GENERIC NAME OR DRUG CLASS	COMBINED EFFECT
Any other topical medication	Hypersensitivity reactions more likely to occur.

POSSIBLE INTERACTION WITH OTHER SUBSTANCES

INTERACTS WITH	COMBINED EFFECT
Alcohol:	None expected.
Beverages:	None expected.
Cocaine:	None expected.
Foods:	None expected.
Marijuana:	None expected.
Tobacco:	None expected.

NEOSTIGMINE

BRAND NAMES

Prostigmin

BASIC INFORMATION

Habit forming? No
Prescription needed? Yes
Available as generic? Yes
Drug class: Cholinergic, antimyasthenic

USES

- Diagnosis and treatment of myasthenia gravis.
- Treatment of urinary retention and abdominal distention.
- Antidote to adverse effects of muscle relaxants used in surgery.

DOSAGE & USAGE INFORMATION

How to take:
- Tablet—Swallow with liquid or food to lessen stomach irritation.
- Extended-release capsules and tablets—Swallow each dose whole with liquid; do not crush.

When to take:
As directed, usually 3 or 4 times a day.

If you forget a dose:
Take as soon as you remember up to 2 hours late. If more than 2 hours, wait for next scheduled dose (don't double this dose).

What drug does:
Inhibits the chemical activity of an enzyme (cholinesterase) so nerve impulses can cross the junction of nerves and muscles.

Continued in next column

OVERDOSE

SYMPTOMS:
Muscle weakness or paralysis, cramps, twitching or clumsiness; severe diarrhea, nausea, vomiting, stomach cramps or pain; breathing difficulty; confusion, irritability, nervousness, restlessness, fear; unusually slow heartbeat; seizures; blurred vision; extreme fatigue.
WHAT TO DO:
- **Dial 0 (operator) or 911 (emergency) for an ambulance or medical help. Then give first aid immediately.**
- **See emergency information on inside covers.**

Time lapse before drug works:
3 hours.

Don't take with:
Any other medicine without consulting your doctor or pharmacist.

POSSIBLE ADVERSE REACTIONS OR SIDE EFFECTS

SYMPTOMS	WHAT TO DO
Life-threatening:	
In case of overdose, see previous column.	
Common:	
• Mild diarrhea, nausea, vomiting, stomach cramps or pain.	Discontinue. Call doctor right away.
• Excess saliva, unusual sweating.	Continue. Call doctor when convenient.
Infrequent:	
• Confusion, irritability.	Discontinue. Seek emergency treatment.
• Constricted pupils, watery eyes, lung congestion, frequent urge to urinate.	Continue. Call doctor when convenient.
Rare:	
Bronchospasm, slow heartbeat, weakness.	Discontinue. Call doctor right away.

WARNINGS & PRECAUTIONS

Don't take if:
- You are allergic to any cholinergic or bromide.
- You take mecamylamine.

Before you start, consult your doctor:
- If you plan to become pregnant within medication period.
- If you have bronchial asthma.
- If you have heartbeat irregularities.
- If you have urinary obstruction or urinary-tract infection.

Over age 60:
Adverse reactions and side effects may be more frequent and severe than in younger persons.

Pregnancy:
No proven harm to unborn child. Avoid if possible. May increase contractions of the womb close to time of delivery.

Breast-feeding:
No problems expected, but consult doctor.

Infants & children:
Not recommended.

Prolonged use:
Medication may lose effectiveness. Discontinuing for a few days may restore effect.

Skin & sunlight:
No problems expected.

Driving, piloting or hazardous work:
Don't drive or pilot aircraft until you learn how medicine affects you. Don't work around dangerous machinery. Don't climb ladders or work in high places. Danger increases if you drink alcohol or take medicine affecting alertness and reflexes, such as antihistamines, tranquilizers, sedatives, pain medicine, narcotics and mind-altering drugs.

Discontinuing:
Don't discontinue without doctor's advice until you complete prescribed dose, even though symptoms diminish or disappear.

Others:
No problems expected.

POSSIBLE INTERACTION WITH OTHER DRUGS

GENERIC NAME OR DRUG CLASS	COMBINED EFFECT
Anesthetics, local or general*	Decreased neostigmine effect.
Antiarrhythmics*	Decreased neostigmine effect.
Anticholinergics*	Decreased neostigmine effect. May mask severe side effects.
Cholinergics, other*	Reduced intestinal-tract function. Possible brain and nervous-system toxicity.
Guanadrel	Decreased neostigmine effect.
Guanethridine	Decreased neostigmine effect.
Mecamylamine	Decreased neostigmine effect.
Nitrates*	Decreased neostigmine effect.
Procainamide	Decreased neostigmine effect.
Quinidine	Decreased neostigmine effect.
Tiremethaphan	Decreased neostigmine effect.

POSSIBLE INTERACTION WITH OTHER SUBSTANCES

INTERACTS WITH	COMBINED EFFECT
Alcohol:	No proven problems with small doses.
Beverages:	None expected.
Cocaine:	Decreased neostigmine effect. Avoid.
Foods:	None expected.
Marijuana:	No proven problems.
Tobacco:	No proven problems.

NIACIN (Vitamin B-3, Nicotinic Acid)

BRAND AND GENERIC NAMES

See complete list of brand and generic names in the *Brand Name Directory,* page 924.

There are numerous other multiple vitamin-mineral supplements available. Check labels.

BASIC INFORMATION

Habit forming? No
Prescription needed?
  Tablets: No
  Liquid, capsules: Yes
Available as generic? Yes
Drug class: Vitamin supplement, vasodilator, antihyperlipidemic

USES

- Replacement for niacin deficiency caused by inadequate diet.
- Treatment for vertigo (dizziness) and ringing in ears.
- Prevention of premenstrual headache.
- Reduction of blood levels of cholesterol and triglycerides.
- Treatment for pellagra.

DOSAGE & USAGE INFORMATION

How to take:
- Tablet, capsule or liquid—Swallow with liquid or food to lessen stomach irritation.
- Extended-release tablets or capsules— Swallow each dose whole.

When to take:
At the same times each day.

If you forget a dose:
Take as soon as you remember. Wait 4 hours for next dose.

Continued next column

OVERDOSE

SYMPTOMS:
Body flush, nausea, vomiting, abdominal cramps, diarrhea, weakness, lightheadedness, fainting, sweating.
WHAT TO DO:
Overdose unlikely to threaten life. If person takes much larger amount than prescribed, call doctor, poison-control center or hospital emergency room for instructions.

What drug does:
- Corrects niacin deficiency.
- Dilates blood vessels.
- In large doses, decreases cholesterol production.

Time lapse before drug works:
15 to 20 minutes.

Don't take with:
Any other medicine without consulting your doctor or pharmacist.

POSSIBLE ADVERSE REACTIONS OR SIDE EFFECTS

SYMPTOMS	WHAT TO DO
Life-threatening: None expected.	
Common: Dry skin.	Continue. Call doctor when convenient.
Infrequent: • Upper abdominal pain, diarrhea.	Discontinue. Call doctor right away.
• Headache, dizziness, faintness, temporary numbness and tingling in hands and feet.	Continue. Call doctor when convenient.
• "Hot" feeling, flush.	No action necessary.
Rare: Rash, itching, jaundice, double vision, weakness and faintness when arising from bed or chair.	Discontinue. Call doctor right away.

NIACIN (Vitamin B-3, Nicotinic Acid)

WARNINGS & PRECAUTIONS

Don't take if:
- You are allergic to niacin or any niacin-containing vitamin mixtures.
- You have impaired liver function.
- You have active peptic ulcer.

Before you start, consult your doctor:
- If you have sensitivity to tartrazine dye.
- If you have diabetes.
- If you have gout.
- If you have gallbladder or liver disease.

Over age 60:
Response to drug cannot be predicted. Dose must be individualized.

Pregnancy:
Risk to unborn child outweighs drug benefits. Don't use.

Breast-feeding:
Studies inconclusive. Consult doctor.

Infants & children:
- Use only under supervision.
- Keep vitamin-mineral supplements out of children's reach.

Prolonged use:
- May cause impaired liver function.
- Talk to your doctor about the need for follow-up medical examinations or laboratory studies to check liver function, blood sugar.

Skin & sunlight:
No problems expected.

Driving, piloting or hazardous work:
Avoid if you feel dizzy or faint. Otherwise, no problems expected.

Discontinuing:
May be unnecessary to finish medicine. Follow doctor's instructions.

Others:
- A balanced diet should provide all the niacin a healthy person needs and make supplements unnecessary. Best sources are meat, eggs and dairy products.
- Store in original container in cool, dry, dark place. Bathroom medicine chest too moist.
- Obesity reduces effectiveness.
- Some nicotinic acid products contain tartrazine dye. Read labels carefully if sensitive to tartrazine.

POSSIBLE INTERACTION WITH OTHER DRUGS

GENERIC NAME OR DRUG CLASS	COMBINED EFFECT
Antidiabetics*	Decreased anti-diabetic effect.
Beta-adrenergic blockers*	Excessively low blood pressure.
Guanethidine	Increased guanethidine effect.
Isoniazid	Decreased niacin effect.
Mecamylamine	Excessively low blood pressure.
Methyldopa	Excessively low blood pressure.
Pargyline	Excessively low blood pressure.
Probenecid	Decreased effect of probenecid.
Sulfinpyrazone	Decreased effect of sulfinpyrazone.

POSSIBLE INTERACTION WITH OTHER SUBSTANCES

INTERACTS WITH	COMBINED EFFECT
Alcohol:	Excessively low blood pressure. Use caution.
Beverages:	None expected.
Cocaine:	Increased flushing.
Foods:	None expected.
Marijuana:	None expected.
Tobacco:	Decreased niacin effect.

NICLOSAMIDE

BRAND NAMES

Niclocide

BASIC INFORMATION

Habit forming? No
Prescription needed? Yes
Available as generic? No
Drug class: Anthelmintic

 USES

Treats intestinal parasitic diseases including diphyllobothriasis, hymenolepiasis and taeniasis.

 DOSAGE & USAGE INFORMATION

How to take:
Chewable tablets—Chew completely or crush and mix with a small amount of liquid to make a paste.

When to take:
As a single dose after a light meal or as directed by doctor.

If you forget a dose:
Take as soon as you remember, then resume regular schedule.

What drug does:
Kills intestinal parasites.

Time lapse before drug works:
1 to 8 days.

Don't take with:
No special problems expected.

 OVERDOSE

SYMPTOMS:
None immediately.
WHAT TO DO:
- **Don't induce vomiting. Give a fast-acting laxative and an enema.**
- **Overdose unlikely to threaten life. If person takes much larger amount than prescribed, call doctor, poison-control center or hospital emergency room for instructions.**

 POSSIBLE ADVERSE REACTIONS OR SIDE EFFECTS

SYMPTOMS	WHAT TO DO
Life-threatening: None expected.	
Common: None expected.	
Infrequent: Stomach cramps, diarrhea, nausea.	Continue. Call doctor when convenient.
Rare: Rectal itching, dizziness, drowsiness, skin rash.	Continue. Call doctor when convenient.

WARNINGS & PRECAUTIONS

Don't take if:
You are allergic to niclosamide.

Before you start, consult your doctor:
If you have rectal bleeding, abdominal cramps or vomiting.

Over age 60:
Adverse reactions and side effects may be more frequent and severe than in younger persons.

Pregnancy:
No proven problems. Consult doctor.

Breast-feeding:
No problems expected, but consult doctor.

Infants & children:
Use only under close medical supervision.

Prolonged use:
Not intended for prolonged use.

Skin & sunlight:
No special problems expected.

Driving, piloting or hazardous work:
Don't drive or pilot aircraft until you learn how medicine affects you. Don't work around dangerous machinery. Don't climb ladders or work in high places. Danger increases if you drink alcohol or take medicine affecting alertness and reflexes, such as antihistamines, tranquilizers, sedatives, pain medicines, narcotics and mind-altering drugs.

Discontinuing:
Don't discontinue without medical advice.

Others:
Stool examinations by your doctor at 1-month and 3-month intervals following treatment may be necessary to determine the effectiveness of the medicine.

POSSIBLE INTERACTION WITH OTHER DRUGS

GENERIC NAME OR DRUG CLASS	COMBINED EFFECT
None expected.	

POSSIBLE INTERACTION WITH OTHER SUBSTANCES

INTERACTS WITH	COMBINED EFFECT
Alcohol:	Dizziness, drowsiness.
Beverages:	No proven problems.
Cocaine:	Dizziness, drowsiness.
Foods:	No proven problems.
Marijuana:	Dizziness, drowsiness.
Tobacco:	No proven problems.

NICOTINE (Skin Patch)

BRAND NAMES

Habitrol   PROSTEP
Nicoderm

BASIC INFORMATION

Habit Forming? Yes
Prescription needed? Yes
Available as generic? No
Drug class: Antismoking agent

 ## USES

As an aid to stop smoking. Used in conjunction with a comprehensive behavioral smoking cessation program.

 ## DOSAGE & USAGE INFORMATION

How to use:
Apply skin patch to clean, non-hairy site on the trunk or upper outer arm.

When to take:
Daily. Remove old patch and apply new patch to new location on the skin. Follow directions in the instruction packet that comes with the prescription.

If you forget a dose:
Remove old patch and apply new patch as soon as you remember. Return to regular schedule.

What drug does:
Delivers steady but gradually reduced supply of nicotine to the body for relief of smoking withdrawal symptoms. Reduces craving for cigarettes.

Time lapse before drug works:
2 to 4 hours.

Don't take with:
Any other medicine without consulting your doctor or pharmacist.

 ## OVERDOSE

SYMPTOMS:
None expected.
WHAT TO DO:
Overdose unlikely to threaten life. If person uses much larger amount than prescribed, call doctor, poison-control center or hospital emergency roon for instruction.

 ## POSSIBLE ADVERSE REACTIONS OR SIDE EFFECTS

SYMPTOMS	WHAT TO DO
Life-threatening: None expected.	
Common: Itching, redness, burning or skin rash at site of patch.	Continue. Call doctor when convenient.
Infrequent: Diarrhea, dizziness, indigestion, nervousness, strange dreams, muscle aches, constipation, sore throat, nausea, increased cough, pain, change in taste, excessive tiredness, change in menstruation, insomnia, headache.	Continue call doctor when convenient.
Rare: Mild chest pain, sinusitis, stomach pain, vomiting, dry mouth, numbness or tingling in hands or feet.	Continue. Call doctor when convenient.

NICOTINE (Skin Patch)

WARNINGS & PRECAUTIONS

Don't take if:
You are allergic to nicotine or any of the components in the skin patch.

Before you start, consult your doctor:
- If you are pregnant.
- If you have a skin disorder (such as eczema).
- If you are using other skin patch medication.
- If you have cardiovascular or peripheral vascular disease.
- If you have liver or kidney disease.
- If you have hyperthyroidism, insulin-dependent diabetes, pheochromocytoma, peptic ulcer disease or high blood pressure.

Over age 60:
Adverse reactions and side effects may be more frequent and severe than in younger persons.

Pregnancy:
Tobacco smoke and nicotine are harmful to the fetus. The specific effects of nicotine from the skin patch are unknown. Discuss the risks of both with your doctor.

Breast-feeding:
Drug passes into breast milk. Avoid drug or discontinue nursing until you finish medicine. Consult doctor for advice on maintaining milk supply.

Infants & children:
Not recommended.

Prolonged use:
Use for longer than 3 months not recommended.

Skin & sunlight:
No problems expected.

Driving, piloting or hazardous work:
No problems expected.

Discontinuing:
- Adverse reactions and side effects related to nicotine withdrawal may continue for some time.
- Entire course of treatment should take 8 to 12 weeks, depending on the size of the initial dose.

Others:
- Advise any doctor or dentist whom you consult that you take this medicine.
- May affect results of some medical tests.
- Keep both the used and unused skin patches out of the reach of children and pets. Dispose of old patches according to package instructions.
- For full benefit from this treatment, stop cigarette smoking as soon as you begin treatment.

POSSIBLE INTERACTION WITH OTHER DRUGS

GENERIC NAME OR DRUG CLASS	COMBINED EFFECT
Acetaminophen	Increased effect of acetaminophen.
Beta-adrenergic blockers*	Increased effect of beta blocker.
Caffeine-containing drugs	Increased effect of caffeine.
Imipramine	Increased effect of imipramine.
Insulin	May require insulin dosage adjustment.
Isoproterenol	Decreased effect of isoproterenol.
Labetalol	Increased effect of labetalol.
Oxazepam	Increased effect of oxazepam.
Pentazocine	Increased effect of pentazocine.
Phenylephrine	Decreased effect of phenylephrine.
Prazosin	Increased effect of prazosin.
Theophylline	Increased effect of theophylline.

POSSIBLE INTERACTION WITH OTHER SUBSTANCES

INTERACTS WITH	COMBINED EFFECT
Alcohol:	Increased cardiac irritability. Avoid.
Beverages: Caffeine drinks.	Increased cardiac irritability. Avoid.
Cocaine:	Increased cardiac irritability. Avoid.
Foods:	No proven problems.
Marijuana:	Increased toxic effects. Avoid.
Tobacco:	Increased adverse effects of nicotine. Avoid.

NICOTINE CHEWING GUM

BRAND NAMES

Nicorette

BASIC INFORMATION

Habit forming? Yes
Prescription needed? Yes
Available as generic? No
Drug class: Antismoking agent

 USES

Treats smoking addiction.

 DOSAGE & USAGE INFORMATION

How to take:
- Follow detailed instructions on patient instruction sheet provided with prescription.
- Chewing gum tablets—Chew gum pieces slowly for best effect.

When to take:
Follow detailed instructions on patient instruction sheet provided with prescription.

If you forget a dose:
Follow detailed instructions on patient instruction sheet provided with prescription.

What drug does:
Satisfies physical craving for nicotine in addicted persons and avoids peaks in blood nicotine level resulting from smoking.

Time lapse before drug works:
30 minutes.

Don't take with:
- Any other medicine without consulting your doctor or pharmacist.
- Coffee, soda or fruit juice within 15 minutes prior to chewing gum. They interfere with nicotine absorption.

 OVERDOSE

SYMPTOMS:
Vomiting, irregular heartbeat, mouth watering, abdominal pain, diarrhea, headache (severe), fainting, convulsions, coma.
WHAT TO DO:
- **Dial O (operator) or 911 (emergency) for an ambulance or medical help. Then give first aid immediately.**
- **See emergency information on inside cover.**

 POSSIBLE ADVERSE REACTIONS OR SIDE EFFECTS

SYMPTOMS	WHAT TO DO
Life-threatening:	
In case of overdose, see previous column.	
Frequent:	
Increased irritability causing heartbeat irregularity.	Continue. Call doctor when convenient.
Common:	
• Injury to loose teeth, jaw muscle ache.	Continue. Call doctor when convenient.
• Belching, mouth irritation or tingling, excessive salivation.	Continue. Tell doctor at next visit.
Infrequent:	
• Nausea and vomiting, abdominal pain.	Discontinue. Call doctor right away.
• Lightheadedness, headache, hiccups, constipation, coughing, dry mouth, appetite loss.	Continue. Call doctor when convenient.
Rare:	
Insomnia.	Continue. Tell doctor at next visit.

 WARNINGS & PRECAUTIONS

Don't take if:
- You are a non-smoker.
- You are pregnant or intend to become pregnant.
- You recently suffered a heart attack.

Before you start, consult your doctor:
- If you have coronary artery disease.
- If you have active temperomandibular joint disease.
- If you have severe angina.
- If you have peptic ulcer.

Over age 60:
Adverse reactions and side effects may be more frequent and severe than in younger persons.

Pregnancy:
Risk to unborn child outweighs drug benefits. Don't use.

Breast-feeding:
Drug passes into milk. Avoid drug or discontinue nursing until you finish medicine. Consult doctor for advice on maintaining milk supply.

Infants & children:
Don't use.

Prolonged use:
May cause addiction and greater likelihood of toxicity.

Skin & sunlight:
No problems expected.

Driving, piloting or hazardous work:
No problems expected.

Discontinuing:
May be unnecessary to finish medicine. Follow doctor's instructions.

Others:
- Children are very susceptible to toxic effects of nicotine; low doses can be fatal.
- Can cause tooth fillings to be pulled out.

POSSIBLE INTERACTION WITH OTHER DRUGS

GENERIC NAME OR DRUG CLASS	COMBINED EFFECT
Beta-adrenergic blockers*	Decreased blood pressure (slight).
Bronchodilators	Excessive absorption of bronchodilators.
Caffeine	Increased effect of caffeine.
Cortisone drugs*	Increased cortisone circulating in blood.
Furosemide	Increased effect of furosemide.

Glutethimide	Increased absorption of glutethimide.
Imipramine	Increased effect of imipramine.
Insulin	Excessive insulin absorption. Dosage adjustment required.
Pentazocine	Increased effect of pentazocine.
Phenacetin	Increased effect of phenacetin.
Propoxyphene	Decreased blood level of propoxyphene.
Propranolol	Excessive absorption of propranolol.
Theophylline	Increased effect of theophylline.

POSSIBLE INTERACTION WITH OTHER SUBSTANCES

INTERACTS WITH	COMBINED EFFECT
Alcohol:	Increased cardiac irritability. Avoid.
Beverages: Caffeine.	Increased cardiac irritability. Avoid any beverage with caffeine.
Cocaine:	Increased cardiac irritability. Avoid.
Foods:	No problems expected.
Marijuana:	Increased toxic effects. Avoid.
Tobacco:	Increased toxic effects. Avoid.

NIMODIPINE

BRAND NAMES

Nimotop

BASIC INFORMATION

Habit Forming? No
Prescription needed? Yes
Available as generic? No
Drug class: Calcium channel blocker

USES

Helps repair the damage caused by a ruptured blood vessel in the head (also called *ruptured aneurysm* or *subarachnoid hemorrhage*).

DOSAGE & USAGE INFORMATION

How to take:
Capsule—Swallow with liquid.

When to take:
Results are best if you begin taking within 96 hours after bleeding into the brain begins. Continue taking for 21 days or as directed by your physician.

If you forget a dose:
Take as soon as you remember up to 2 hours late. If more than 2 hours, wait for next scheduled dose (don't double this dose).

What drug does:
This is a calcium channel blocking drug that crosses easily from blood vessels into the brain, where it prevents spasms of the brain's arteries.

Continued next column

OVERDOSE

SYMPTOMS:
Unusally fast or unusually slow heartbeat, loss of consciousness, cardiac arrest.
WHAT TO DO:
- **Dial 0 (operator) or 911 (emergency) for an ambulance or medical help. Then give first aid immediately.**
- **If patient is unconscious and not breathing, give mouth-to-mouth breathing. If there is no heartbeat, use cardiac massage and mouth-to-mouth breathing (CPR). Don't try to make patient vomit. If you can't get help quickly, take patient to nearest emergency facility.**
- **See emergency information on inside covers.**

Time lapse before drug works:
1 to 2 hours.

Don't take with:
Any other medicine without consulting your doctor or pharmacist.

POSSIBLE ADVERSE REACTIONS OR SIDE EFFECTS

SYMPTOMS	WHAT TO DO
Life-threatening:	
In case of overdose. see previous column.	
Common:	
Tiredness, flushing, swelling of feet, ankles and abdomen.	Continue. Tell doctor at next visit.
Infrequent:	
● Unusually fast or unusually slow heartbeat, wheezing, cough, shortness of breath.	Discontinue. Call doctor right away.
● Dizziness; numbness or tingling in hands or feet; difficult urination.	Continue. Call doctor when convenient.
● Nausea, constipation.	Continue. Tell doctor at next visit.
Rare:	
● Transient blindness, increased angina.	Discontinue. Seek emergency treatment.
● Fainting, chest pain, fever, rash, jaundice, depression, psychosis.	Discontinue. Call doctor right away.
● Pain and swelling in joints, hair loss, vivid dreams.	Continue. Call doctor when convenient.
● Headache.	Continue. Tell doctor at next visit.

WARNINGS & PRECAUTIONS

Don't take if:
- You are allergic to any calcium channel blocking drug.
- You have very low blood pressure.

Before you start, consult your doctor:
- If you have kidney or liver disease.
- If you have high blood pressure.
- If you have heart disease other than coronary-artery disease.

Over age 60:
Adverse reactions and side effects may be more frequent and severe than in younger persons.

Pregnancy:
No proven harm to unborn child. Avoid if possible.

Breast-feeding:
Safety not established. Avoid if possible.

Infants & children:
Not recommended.

Prolonged use:
Talk to your doctor about the need for follow-up medical examinations or laboratory studies to check blood pressure, liver function, kidney function, ECG*.

Skin & sunlight:
Increased sensitivity to sunlight.

Driving, piloting or hazardous work:
Avoid if you feel dizzy. Otherwise, no problems expected.

Discontinuing:
Don't discontinue without doctor's advice until you complete prescribed dose, even though symptoms diminish or disappear.

Others:
- Learn to check your own pulse rate. If it drops to 50 beats per minute or lower, don't take nimodipine until you consult your doctor.
- Drug may lower blood-sugar level if daily dose is more than 60 mg.

 ## POSSIBLE INTERACTION WITH OTHER DRUGS

GENERIC NAME OR DRUG CLASS	COMBINED EFFECT
ACE inhibitors*: captopril, enalapril, lisinopril	Possible excessive potassium in blood. Dosages may need adjustment.
Antiarrhythmics*	Possible increased effect and toxicity of each drug.
Anticoagulants, oral*	Possible increased anticoagulant effect.
Anticonvulsants, hydantoin*	Increased anticonvulsant effect.
Antihypertensives*	Dangerous blood-pressure drop. Dosage may need adjustment.
Beta-adrenergic blockers*	Possible irregular heartbeat. May worsen congestive heart failure.
Betaxolol eye drops	May cause increased effect of nimodipine on heart function.
Calcium (large doses)	Possible decreased nimodipine effect.

Carbamazepine	May increase carbamazepine effect and toxicity.
Cimetidine	Possible increased nimodipine effect and toxicity.
Cyclosporine	Increased cyclosporine toxicity.
Disopyramide	May cause dangerously slow, fast or irregular heartbeat.
Diuretics*	Dangerous blood-pressure drop.
Levobutanol eye drops	May cause increased effect of nimodipine on heart function.
Lithium	Possible decreased lithium effect.
Nicardipine	Possible increased effect and toxicity of each drug.
Nitrates*	Reduced angina attacks.
Phenytoin	Possible decreased nimodipine effect.
Quinidine	Increased quinidine effect.
Rifampin	Decreased nimodipine effect.
Theophylline	May increase theophylline effect and toxicity.

Continued page 953

POSSIBLE INTERACTION WITH OTHER SUBSTANCES

INTERACTS WITH	COMBINED EFFECT
Alcohol:	Dangerously low blood pressure. Avoid.
Beverages:	None expected.
Cocaine:	Possible irregular heartbeat. Avoid.
Foods:	None expected.
Marijuana:	Possible irregular heartbeat. Avoid.
Tobacco:	Possible rapid heartbeat. Avoid.

*See Glossary

NITRATES

BRAND AND GENERIC NAMES

See complete list of brand and generic names in the *Brand Name Directory,* page 924.

BASIC INFORMATION

Habit forming? No
Prescription needed? Yes
Available as generic? Yes
Drug class: Antianginal (nitrate)

USES

- Reduces frequency and severity of angina attacks.
- Treats congestive heart failure.

DOSAGE & USAGE INFORMATION

How to take:
- Extended-release tablets or capsules—Swallow each dose whole with liquid.
- Chewable tablet—Chew tablet at earliest sign of angina, and hold in mouth for 2 minutes.
- Regular tablet or capsule—Swallow whole with liquid. Don't crush, chew or open.
- Buccal tablets (Nitrogard)—Allow to dissolve in side of mouth.
- Translingual spray (nitrolingual)—Spray under tongue according to instructions enclosed with prescription.
- Ointment—Apply as directed.
- Patches—Apply to skin according to package instructions.
- Sublingual tablets—Place under tongue every 3 to 5 minutes at earliest sign of angina. If you don't have complete relief with 3 or 4 tablets, call doctor.

Continued next column

OVERDOSE

SYMPTOMS:
Dizziness; blue fingernails and lips; feeling of pressure in head, fever, fainting; shortness of breath; weak, fast heartbeat; convulsions.
WHAT TO DO:
- **Dial 0 (operator) or 911 (emergency) for an ambulance or medical help. Then give first aid immediately.**
- **See emergency information on inside covers.**

When to take:
- Swallowed tablets—Take at the same times each day, 1 or 2 hours after meals.
- Sublingual tablets or spray—At onset of angina.
- Ointment—Follow prescription directions.
- Patches—According to physician's instructions.

If you forget a dose:
Take as soon as you remember up to 2 hours late. If more than 2 hours, wait for next scheduled dose (don't double this dose).

What drug does:
Relaxes blood vessels, increasing blood flow to heart muscle.

Time lapse before drug works:
- Sublingual tablets and spray—1 to 3 minutes.
- Other forms—15 to 30 minutes. Will not stop an attack, but may prevent attacks.

Don't take with:
Any other medicine without consulting your doctor or pharmacist.

POSSIBLE ADVERSE REACTIONS OR SIDE EFFECTS

SYMPTOMS	WHAT TO DO
Life-threatening:	
In case of overdose, see previous column.	
Common:	
Headache, flushed face and neck, dry mouth, nausea, vomiting, rapid heartbeat.	Continue. Tell doctor at next visit.
Infrequent:	
• Fainting.	Discontinue. Call doctor right away.
• Restlessness, blurred vision, dizziness.	Continue. Call doctor when convenient.
Rare:	
• Rash.	Discontinue. Call doctor right away.
• Severe irritation, peeling.	Continue. Call doctor when convenient.

WARNINGS & PRECAUTIONS

Don't take if:
You are allergic to nitrates, including nitroglycerin.

Before you start, consult your doctor:
- If you are taking non-prescription drugs.
- If you plan to become pregnant within medication period.
- If you have glaucoma.

- If you have reacted badly to any vasodilator drug.
- If you drink alcoholic beverages or smoke marijuana.

Over age 60:
Adverse reactions and side effects may be more frequent and severe than in younger persons.

Pregnancy:
No proven harm to unborn child. Avoid if possible.

Breast-feeding:
No problems expected. Consult your doctor.

Infants & children:
Not recommended.

Prolonged use:
- Drug may become less effective and require higher doses.
- Talk to your doctor about the need for follow-up medical examinations or laboratory studies to check blood pressure, heart rate.

Skin & sunlight:
No problems expected.

Driving, piloting or hazardous work:
Don't drive or pilot aircraft until you learn how medicine affects you. Don't work around dangerous machinery. Don't climb ladders or work in high places. Danger increases if you drink alcohol or take medicine affecting alertness and reflexes.

Discontinuing:
Except for sublingual tablets, don't discontinue without doctor's advice until you complete prescribed dose, even though symptoms diminish or disappear.

Others:
- If discomfort is not caused by angina, nitrate medication will not bring relief. Call doctor if discomfort persists.
- Periodic urine and laboratory blood studies of white cell counts recommended if you take nitrates.
- Keep sublingual tablets in original container. Always carry them with you, but keep from body heat if possible.
- Sublingual tablets produce a burning, stinging sensation when placed under the tongue. Replace supply if no burning or stinging is noted.

 POSSIBLE INTERACTION WITH OTHER DRUGS

GENERIC NAME OR DRUG CLASS	COMBINED EFFECT
Anticholinergics*	Increased internal eye pressure.
Antidepressants, tricyclic (TCA)*	Excessive blood pressure drop.
Antihypertensives*	Excessive blood pressure drop.
Beta-adrenergic blockers*	Excessive blood pressure drop.
Calcium channel blockers*	Decreased blood pressure.
Carteolol	Possible excessive blood pressure drop.
Cholinergics*	Decreased cholinergic effect.
Ephedrine	Decreased nitrate effect.
Guanfacine	Increased effects of both drugs.
Lisinopril	Possible excessive blood pressure drop.
Narcotics*	Excessive blood pressure drop.
Nicardipine	Reduced angina attacks.
Nimodipine	Reduced angina attacks.
Phenothiazines*	May decrease blood pressure.
Sotalol	Possible excessive blood pressure drop.
Sympathomimetics*	Possible reduced effects of both medicines.

 POSSIBLE INTERACTION WITH OTHER SUBSTANCES

INTERACTS WITH	COMBINED EFFECT
Alcohol:	Excessive blood pressure drop.
Beverages:	None expected.
Cocaine:	Reduced effectiveness of nitrates.
Foods:	None expected.
Marijuana:	Decreased nitrate effect.
Tobacco:	Decreased nitrate effect.

*See Glossary

NITROFURANTOIN

BRAND NAMES

Apo-Nitrofurantoin	Nephronex
Cyantin	Nifuran
Furadantin	Nitrex
Furalan	Nitrofan
Furaloid	Nitrofor
Furan	Nitrofuracot
Furanite	Novofuran
Furantoin	Ro-Antoin
Furatine	Sarodant
Furaton	Trantoin
Macrobid	Urotoin
Macrodantin	

BASIC INFORMATION

Habit forming? No
Prescription needed? Yes
Available as generic? Yes
Drug class: Antimicrobial

 USES

Treatment for urinary-tract infections.

 DOSAGE & USAGE INFORMATION

How to take:
- Tablet or capsule—Swallow with food or milk to lessen stomach irritation. If you can't swallow whole, crumble tablet or open capsule and take with liquid or food.
- Liquid—Shake well and take with food. Use a measuring spoon to ensure accuracy.

When to take:
At the same times each day.

If you forget a dose:
Take as soon as you remember up to 2 hours late. If more than 2 hours, wait for next scheduled dose (don't double this dose).

What drug does:
Prevents susceptible bacteria in the urinary tract from growing and multiplying.

Continued in next column

 OVERDOSE

SYMPTOMS:
Nausea, vomiting, abdominal pain, diarrhea.
WHAT TO DO:
Overdose unlikely to threaten life. If person takes much larger amount than prescribed, call doctor, poison-control center or hospital emergency room for instructions.

Time lapse before drug works:
1 to 2 weeks.

Don't take with:
Any other medicine without consulting your doctor or pharmacist.

 POSSIBLE ADVERSE REACTIONS OR SIDE EFFECTS

SYMPTOMS	WHAT TO DO
Life-threatening:	
Hives, rash, intense itching, faintness soon after a dose (anaphylaxis).	Seek emergency treatment immediately.
Common:	
• Diarrhea, appetite loss, nausea, vomiting, chest pain, cough, difficult breathing, chills or unexplained fever, abdominal pain.	Discontinue. Call doctor right away.
• Rusty colored or brown urine.	No action necessary.
Infrequent:	
• Rash, itchy skin, numbness, tingling or burning of face or mouth, fatigue, weakness.	Discontinue. Call doctor right away.
• Dizziness, headache, drowsiness, paleness (in children), discolored teeth (from liquid form).	Continue. Call doctor when convenient.
Rare:	
Jaundice.	Discontinue. Call doctor right away.

NITROFURANTOIN

WARNINGS & PRECAUTIONS

Don't take if:
- You are allergic to nitrofurantoin.
- You have impaired kidney function.
- You drink alcohol.

Before you start, consult your doctor:
- If you are prone to allergic reactions.
- If you are pregnant and within 2 weeks of delivery.
- If you have had kidney disease, lung disease, anemia, nerve damage, or G6PD deficiency (a metabolic deficiency).
- If you have diabetes. Drug may affect urine sugar tests.

Over age 60:
Adverse reactions and side effects may be more frequent and severe than in younger persons.

Pregnancy:
Risk to unborn child outweighs drug benefits, especially in last month of pregnancy. Don't use.

Breast-feeding:
Drug passes into milk. Avoid drug or discontinue nursing until you finish medicine. Consult doctor for advice on maintaining milk supply.

Infants & children:
Don't give to infants younger than 1 month. Use only under medical supervision for older children.

Prolonged use:
- Chest pain, cough, shortness of breath.
- Talk to your doctor about the need for follow-up medical examinations or laboratory studies to check liver function, lung function.

Skin & sunlight:
No problems expected.

Driving, piloting or hazardous work:
Avoid if you feel dizzy or drowsy. Otherwise, no problems expected.

Discontinuing:
Don't discontinue without consulting doctor. Dose may require gradual reduction if you have taken drug for a long time. Doses of other drugs may also require adjustment.

Others:
Periodic blood counts, liver-function tests, and chest X-rays recommended.

POSSIBLE INTERACTION WITH OTHER DRUGS

GENERIC NAME OR DRUG CLASS	COMBINED EFFECT
Dapsone	Increased risk of adverse effect on blood cells.
Didanosine	Increased risk of pancreatitis and peripheral neuropathy.
Isoniazid	Increased risk of liver damage.
Nalidixic acid	Decreased nitrofurantoin effect.
Neurotoxic medicines*	Increased risk of damage to nerve cells.
Phenobarbital	Decreased nitrofurantoin effect.
Probenecid	Increased nitrofurantoin effect.
Sulfinpyrazone	Possible nitrofurantoin toxicity.

POSSIBLE INTERACTION WITH OTHER SUBSTANCES

INTERACTS WITH	COMBINED EFFECT
Alcohol:	Possible disulfiram reaction.* Avoid.
Beverages:	None expected.
Cocaine:	No proven problems.
Foods:	None expected.
Marijuana:	None expected.
Tobacco:	None expected.

NORFLOXACIN

BRAND NAMES

Noroxin

BASIC INFORMATION

Habit forming? No
Prescription needed? Yes
Available as generic? No
Drug class: Antibacterial (antibiotic),
   fluoroquinolone

USES

- Treats infections of the kidney, ureter, bladder and urethra.
- Treats traveler's diarrhea, bacterial gastroenteritis.

DOSAGE & USAGE INFORMATION

How to take:
Tablet—On an empty stomach 1 hour before or 2 hours after meals. Take with lots of water.

When to take:
As directed. Usually every 12 hours on empty stomach.

If you forget a dose:
Take as soon as you remember up to 6 hours late. If more than 6 hours, wait for next scheduled dose (don't double this dose).

What drug does:
Interferes with nutrient necessary for growth and reproduction of bacteria. Will not kill viruses.

Time lapse before drug works:
2 hours to peak level in blood. May require 7 to 21 days of treatment to cure infections.

Don't take with:
- Food, antacids.
- Any other medicine without consulting your doctor or pharmacist.

OVERDOSE

SYMPTOMS:
Seizures
WHAT TO DO:
- **Dial 0 (operator) or 911 (emergency) for an ambulance or medical help. Then give first aid immediately.**
- **See emergency information on inside covers.**

POSSIBLE ADVERSE REACTIONS OR SIDE EFFECTS

SYMPTOMS	WHAT TO DO
Life-threatening:	
In case of overdose, see previous column.	
Common:	
Appetite loss.	Continue. Call doctor when convenient.
Infrequent:	
• Nausea, abdominal pains, insomnia, diarrhea, dizziness, fatigue, rash, crystals in urine.	Discontinue. Call doctor right away.
• Headache, depression, lightheadedness.	Continue. Call doctor when convenient.
Rare:	
• Seizures.	Discontinue. Seek emergency treatment.
• Joint pain, joint swelling, bloody urine, vision changes.	Discontinue. Call doctor right away.
• Dry mouth.	Continue. Call doctor when convenient.

WARNINGS & PRECAUTIONS

Don't take if:
You are allergic to any quinolone antibiotics.

Before you start, consult your doctor:
If you have chronic kidney disease with loss of kidney function.

Over age 60:
Adverse reactions and side effects may be more frequent and severe than in younger persons. Ask doctor about smaller doses.

Pregnancy:
Safety to unborn child unestablished. Avoid if possible.

Breast-feeding:
Drug passes into milk. Avoid drug or discontinue nursing until you finish medicine. Consult doctor for advice on maintaining milk supply.

Infants & children:
Not recommended if under 17 years old. Use only under close medical supervision.

Prolonged use:
No problems expected.

Skin & sunlight:
Eyes sensitive to sunlight.

Driving, piloting or hazardous work:
Avoid if you feel drowsy or dizzy.

Discontinuing:
No problems expected.

Others:
No problems expected.

POSSIBLE INTERACTION WITH OTHER DRUGS

GENERIC NAME OR DRUG CLASS	COMBINED EFFECT
Antacids*	Decreased absorption of norfloxacin.
Didanosine	Reduced norfloxacin effect.
Nitrofurantoin	Decreased norfloxacin effect.
Probenecid	Decreased effect of norfloxacin.
Theophylline	Increased effect and toxicity of theophylline.

POSSIBLE INTERACTION WITH OTHER SUBSTANCES

INTERACTS WITH	COMBINED EFFECT
Alcohol:	Decreased effect of norfloxacin.
Beverages:	None expected.
Cocaine:	Decreased effect of norfloxacin.
Foods:	None expected.
Marijuana:	Decreased effect of norfloxacin.
Tobacco:	May stimulate irritated gastrointestinal tract. Avoid.

NYLIDRIN

BRAND NAMES

Arlidin Forte   PMS Nylidrin

BASIC INFORMATION

Habit forming? No
Prescription needed? Yes
Available as generic? Yes
Drug class: Vasodilator

 ## USES

- May improve poor circulation in extremities.
- Reduces dizziness caused by poor circulation in inner ear.

 ## DOSAGE & USAGE INFORMATION

How to take:
Tablet—Swallow with liquid or food to lessen stomach irritation. If you can't swallow whole, crumble tablet and take with liquid or food.

When to take:
At the same times each day.

If you forget a dose:
Take as soon as you remember up to 2 hours late. If more than 2 hours, wait for next scheduled dose (don't double this dose).

What drug does:
Stimulates nerves that dilate blood vessels, increasing oxygen and nutrients.

Continued next column

 ## OVERDOSE

SYMPTOMS:
Blood-pressure drop; nausea, vomiting; rapid, irregular heartbeat, chest pain; blurred vision; metallic taste.
WHAT TO DO:
- **Dial 0 (operator) or 911 (emergency) for an ambulance or medical help. Then give first aid immediately.**
- **If patient is unconscious and not breathing, give mouth-to-mouth breathing. If there is no heartbeat, use cardiac massage and mouth-to-mouth breathing (CPR). Don't try to make patient vomit. If you can't get help quickly, take patient to nearest emergency facility.**
- **See emergency information on inside covers.**

Time lapse before drug works:
10 to 30 minutes.

Don't take with:
Any other medicine without consulting your doctor or pharmacist.

 ## POSSIBLE ADVERSE REACTIONS OR SIDE EFFECTS

SYMPTOMS	WHAT TO DO
Life-threatening:	
In case of overdose, see previous column.	
Common:	
• Chest pain.	Discontinue. Call doctor right away.
• Blurred vision, fever, decreased or difficult urination.	Continue. Call doctor when convenient.
Infrequent:	
• Rapid or irregular heartbeat.	Discontinue. Call doctor right away.
• Dizziness, weakness, tiredness.	Continue. Call doctor when convenient.
Rare:	
• Shakiness, chills.	Discontinue. Call doctor right away.
• Headache, nausea, vomiting, flushed face, nervousness.	Continue. Call doctor when convenient.

WARNINGS & PRECAUTIONS

Don't take if:
- You are allergic to any vasodilator drugs.
- You have had a heart attack or stroke within 4 weeks.
- You have an active peptic ulcer.

Before you start, consult your doctor:
- If you have had heart disease, heart-rhythm disorders (especially rapid heartbeat), a stroke or poor circulation to the brain.
- If you have glaucoma.
- If you have an overactive thyroid gland.
- If you plan to become pregnant within medication period.
- If you use tobacco.

Over age 60:
Adverse reactions and side effects may be more frequent and severe than in younger persons.

Pregnancy:
No proven harm to unborn child. Avoid if possible.

Breast-feeding:
No proven problems. Consult doctor.

Infants & children:
Not recommended.

Prolonged use:
No problems expected.

Skin & sunlight:
No problems expected.

Driving, piloting or hazardous work:
Don't drive or pilot aircraft until you learn how medicine affects you. Don't work around dangerous machinery. Don't climb ladders or work in high places. Danger increases if you drink alcohol or take medicine affecting alertness and reflexes, such as antihistamines, tranquilizers, sedatives, pain medicine, narcotics and mind-altering drugs.

Discontinuing:
Don't discontinue without consulting doctor. If your condition worsens, contact your doctor immediately. Dose may require gradual reduction if you have taken drug for a long time. Doses of other drugs may also require adjustment.

Others:
No problems expected.

POSSIBLE INTERACTION WITH OTHER DRUGS

GENERIC NAME OR DRUG CLASS	COMBINED EFFECT
Beta-adrenergic blockers*	Decreased effect of nylidrin.
Phenothiazines*	Increased blood level of phenothiazines.

POSSIBLE INTERACTION WITH OTHER SUBSTANCES

INTERACTS WITH	COMBINED EFFECT
Alcohol:	Possible increased stomach-acid secretion. Use with caution.
Beverages:	None expected.
Cocaine:	Increased adverse effects of nylidrin.
Foods:	None expected.
Marijuana:	None expected.
Tobacco:	Decreased nylidrin effect. Worsens circulation. Avoid.

NYSTATIN

BRAND NAMES

Dermacomb	Mykacet II
Myco II	Mytrex
Mycobiotic II	Nadostine
Mycogen II	Nilstat
Mycolog II	Nyaderm
Mycostatin	Nystaform
Myco-Triacet II	Nystex
Mykacet	Trisatin

BASIC INFORMATION

Habit forming? No
Prescription needed? Yes
Available as generic? Yes
Drug class: Antifungal

USES

Treatment of fungus infections of the mouth or vagina that are susceptible to nystatin.

DOSAGE & USAGE INFORMATION

How to take:
- Tablet—Swallow with liquid. If you can't swallow whole, crumble tablet and take with liquid or food.
- Ointment, cream or lotion—Use as directed by doctor and label.
- Liquid—Take as directed. Instruction varies by preparation.
- Lozenges—Take as directed on label.

When to take:
At the same time each day.

If you forget a dose:
Take as soon as you remember up to 2 hours late. If more than 2 hours, wait for next scheduled dose (don't double this dose).

Continued next column

OVERDOSE

SYMPTOMS:
Mild overdose may cause nausea, vomiting, diarrhea.
WHAT TO DO:
Overdose unlikely to threaten life. If person takes much larger amount than prescribed, call doctor, poison-control center or hospital emergency room for instructions.

What drug does:
Prevents growth and reproduction of fungus.

Time lapse before drug works:
Begins immediately. May require 3 weeks for maximum benefit, depending on location and severity of infection.

Don't take with:
Any other medicine without consulting your doctor or pharmacist.

POSSIBLE ADVERSE REACTIONS OR SIDE EFFECTS

SYMPTOMS	WHAT TO DO
Life-threatening: None expected.	
Common: (at high doses) Nausea, stomach pain, vomiting, diarrhea.	Discontinue. Call doctor right away.
Infrequent: Mild irritation, itch at application site.	Discontinue. Call doctor right away.
Rare: None expected.	

WARNINGS & PRECAUTIONS

Don't take if:
You are allergic to nystatin.

Before you start, consult your doctor:
If you plan to become pregnant within medication period.

Over age 60:
No problems expected.

Pregnancy:
No proven harm to unborn child. Avoid if possible.

Breast-feeding:
No proven problems. Consult doctor.

Infants & children:
No problems expected.

Prolonged use:
No problems expected.

Skin & sunlight:
No problems expected.

Driving, piloting or hazardous work:
No problems expected.

Discontinuing:
Don't discontinue without doctor's advice until you complete prescribed dose, even though symptoms diminish or disappear.

Others:
No problems expected.

POSSIBLE INTERACTION WITH OTHER DRUGS

GENERIC NAME OR DRUG CLASS	COMBINED EFFECT
None expected.	

POSSIBLE INTERACTION WITH OTHER SUBSTANCES

INTERACTS WITH	COMBINED EFFECT
Alcohol:	None expected.
Beverages:	None expected.
Cocaine:	None expected.
Foods:	None expected.
Marijuana:	None expected.
Tobacco:	None expected.

OFLOXACIN

BRAND NAMES

Floxin

BASIC INFORMATION

Habit forming? No
Prescription needed? Yes
Available as generic? No
Drug class: Antibacterial (antibiotic),
fluoroquinolone

 ## USES

- Treats infections of the kidney, ureter, bladder and urethra.
- Treats traveler's diarrhea, bacterial gastroenteritis.
- Treats gonorrhea and chlamydia infections.

 ## DOSAGE & USAGE INFORMATION

How to take:
Tablet—On an empty stomach 1 hour before or 2 hours after meals. Take with lots of water.

When to take:
As directed. Usually every 12 hours on empty stomach.

If you forget a dose:
Take as soon as you remember up to 6 hours late. If more than 6 hours, wait for next scheduled dose (don't double this dose).

What drug does:
Interferes with nutrient necessary for growth and reproduction of bacteria. Will not kill viruses.

Time lapse before drug works:
2 hours to peak level in blood. May require 7 to 21 days of treatment to cure infections.

Don't take with:
- Food, antacids.
- Any other medication without consulting your doctor or pharmacist.

 ## OVERDOSE

SYMPTOMS:
Seizures
WHAT TO DO:
- **Dial 0 (operator) or 911 (emergency) for an ambulance or medical help. Then give first aid immediately.**
- **See emergency information on inside covers.**

 ## POSSIBLE ADVERSE REACTIONS OR SIDE EFFECTS

SYMPTOMS	WHAT TO DO
Life-threatening:	
In case of overdose, see previous column.	
Common:	
Appetite loss.	Continue. Call doctor when convenient.
Infrequent:	
• Nausea, abdominal pains, insomnia, diarrhea, dizziness, fatigue, rash, crystals in urine.	Discontinue. Call doctor right away.
• Headache, depression, lightheadedness.	Continue. Call doctor when convenient.
Rare:	
• Seizures.	Discontinue. Seek emergency treatment.
• Joint pain, joint swelling, bloody urine, vision changes.	Discontinue. Call doctor right away.
• Dry mouth.	Continue. Call doctor when convenient.

WARNINGS & PRECAUTIONS

Don't take if:
You are allergic to any quinolone antibiotics.

Before you start, consult your doctor:
If you have chronic kidney disease with loss of kidney function.

Over age 60:
Adverse reactions and side effects may be more frequent and severe than in younger persons. Ask doctor about smaller doses.

Pregnancy:
Safety to unborn child unestablished. Avoid if possible.

Breast-feeding:
Drug passes into milk. Avoid drug or discontinue nursing until you finish medicine. Consult doctor for advice on maintaining milk supply.

Infants & children:
Not recommended if under 17 years old. Use only under close medical supervision.

Prolonged use:
No problems expected.

Skin & sunlight:
Eyes sensitive to sunlight.

Driving, piloting or hazardous work:
Avoid if you feel drowsy or dizzy.

Discontinuing:
No problems expected.

Others:
No problems expected.

POSSIBLE INTERACTION WITH OTHER DRUGS

GENERIC NAME OR DRUG CLASS	COMBINED EFFECT
Antacids*	Decreased absorption of ofloxacin.
Probenecid	Decreased effect of ofloxacin.

POSSIBLE INTERACTION WITH OTHER SUBSTANCES

INTERACTS WITH	COMBINED EFFECT
Alcohol:	Decreased effect of ofloxacin.
Beverages:	None expected.
Cocaine:	Decreased effect of ofloxacin.
Foods:	None expected.
Marijuana:	Decreased effect of ofloxacin.
Tobacco:	May stimulate irritated gastrointestinal tract. Avoid.

OLSALAZINE

BRAND NAMES

Dipentum

BASIC INFORMATION

Habit forming? No
Prescription needed? Yes
Available as generic? No
Drug class: Inflammatory bowel disease
  suppressant

 ## USES

To maintain remission of ulcerative colitis.
Generally prescribed when intolerance to
sulfasalazine exists.

 ## DOSAGE & USAGE
INFORMATION

How to take:
Capsule—Swallow with liquid or food to lessen
stomach irritation. If you can't swallow whole,
open capsule and take with liquid or food.

When to take:
Usually twice a day, or as directed on
prescription label.

If you forget a dose:
• Take as soon as possible.
• Skip if it is almost time for next dose.
• Don't double next dose.
• Notify your doctor if there are questions.

What drug does:
Inhibits prostaglandin production in the colon.

Time lapse before drug works:
1 hour.

Don't take with:
Any other medicine without consulting your
doctor or pharmacist.

 ## OVERDOSE

SYMPTOMS:
None expected.
WHAT TO DO:
**Overdose unlikely to threaten life. If person
takes much larger amount than prescribed,
call doctor, poison-control center or
hospital emergency room for instructions.**

 ## POSSIBLE
ADVERSE REACTIONS
OR SIDE EFFECTS

SYMPTOMS	WHAT TO DO
Life-threatening: Fever, sore throat, paleness, unusual bleeding (representing effect on blood, a rare complication).	Seek emergency treatment.
Common: Diarrhea, appetite loss, nausea, vomiting.	Continue. Call doctor when convenient.
Infrequent: Mood changes, sleeplessness, headache.	Continue. Call doctor when convenient.
Rare: Skin eruption (acne-like), muscle aches.	Continue. Call doctor when convenient.

WARNINGS & PRECAUTIONS

Don't take if:
- You are allergic to aspirin or any other salicylate.
- You are allergic to mesalamine.

Before you start, consult your doctor:
- If you have kidney disease.
- If you are taking any other prescription or non-prescription medicine.

Over age 60:
No special problems expected.

Pregnancy:
Risk to unborn child outweighs possible benefits. Don't use.

Breast-feeding:
Unknown effects.

Infants & children:
Effect not documented. Consult your family doctor or pediatrician.

Prolonged use:
Follow through with full prescribed course of treatment.

Skin & sunlight:
No special problems expected.

Driving, piloting or hazardous work:
Don't drive or pilot aircraft until you learn how medicine affects you. Don't work around dangerous machinery. Don't climb ladders or work in high places. Danger increases if you drink alcohol or take medicine affecting alertness and reflexes.

Discontinuing:
Don't discontinue without consulting doctor. Dose may require gradual reduction if you have taken drug for a long time. Doses of other drugs may also require adjustment.

Others:
Request your doctor to check blood counts and kidney function on a regular basis.

POSSIBLE INTERACTION WITH OTHER DRUGS

GENERIC NAME OR DRUG CLASS	COMBINED EFFECT
None expected since olsalazine is not appreciably absorbed from the gastrointestinal tract into the bloodstream.	

POSSIBLE INTERACTION WITH OTHER SUBSTANCES

INTERACTS WITH	COMBINED EFFECT
Alcohol:	Increased risk of gastrointestinal upset and/or bleeding.
Beverages: Highly spiced beverages.	Will irritate underlying condition that olsalazine treats.
Cocaine:	Avoid.
Foods: Highly spiced foods.	Will irritate underlying condition that olsalazine treats.
Marijuana:	Avoid.
Tobacco:	Will irritate underlying condition that olsalazine treats. Avoid.

OMEPRAZOLE

BRAND NAMES

Losec   Prilosec

BASIC INFORMATION

Habit forming? No
Prescription needed? Yes
Available as generic? No
Drug class: Antiulcer

USES

- Treats gastroesophageal reflux (splashing of stomach acid from the stomach up onto the lower end of the esophagus).
- Treats peptic ulcer in the stomach and duodenum.
- Treats any disorder associated with excess production of stomach acid.

DOSAGE & USAGE INFORMATION

How to take:
- Capsules—Swallow whole. Do not crush, chew or break open.
- If directed by your doctor, it is permissible and sometimes helpful to take with antacid medicine to relieve upper abdominal pain. Antacids may be used more than once daily if needed.

When to take:
Once daily, immediately before a meal (preferably breakfast), unless otherwise directed by your doctor.

If you forget a dose:
Take as soon as you remember up to 2 hours late. If more than 2 hours, wait for next scheduled dose (don't double this dose).

What drug does:
Prevents secretion of stomach acid no matter what its original cause.

Continued next column

OVERDOSE

SYMPTOMS:
Severe drowsiness, seizures, breathing difficulty, decreased body temperature.
WHAT TO DO:
- **Dial 0 (operator) or 911 (emergency) for an ambulance or medical help. Then give first aid immediately.**
- **See emergency information on inside covers.**

Time lapse before drug works:
30 minutes to 1 hour.

Don't take with:
- Tobacco, excess caffeine or spicy diet.
- Any other medicine without consulting your doctor or pharmacist.

POSSIBLE ADVERSE REACTIONS OR SIDE EFFECTS

SYMPTOMS	WHAT TO DO
Life-threatening: In case of overdose, see previous column.	
Common: Abdominal pain, itching skin.	Discontinue. Call doctor right away.
Infrequent: Muscle pain; dizziness, headache, drowsiness; chest pain, diarrhea, gaseousness.	Discontinue. Call doctor right away.
Rare: Weakness or unusual tiredness, sore throat, fever sores on mouth, unusual bleeding or bruising, cloudy urine, difficult or painful urination, painful nocturnal erections in males.	Discontinue. Call doctor right away.

OMEPRAZOLE

 ## WARNINGS & PRECAUTIONS

Don't take if:
You are allergic to omeprazole.

Before you start, consult your doctor:
- If you are allergic to any other medicines, foods, preservatives or dyes.
- If you have liver disease now or a history of liver disease in the past.

Over age 60:
No special problems expected.

Pregnancy:
Studies inconclusive on harm to unborn child. Animal studies show fetal abnormalities. Decide with your doctor whether drug benefits justify risk to unborn child.

Breast-feeding:
Safety not established. Best to avoid or discontinue nursing until you finish medicine. Consult doctor for advice on maintaining milk supply.

Infants & children:
Safety not established. Consult doctor.

Prolonged use:
May cause carcinoid tumors if taken for over 8 weeks.

Skin & sunlight:
No problems expected.

Driving, piloting or hazardous work:
Don't drive or pilot aircraft until you learn how medicine affects you. Don't work around dangerous machinery. Don't climb ladders or work in high places. Danger increases if you drink alcohol or take medicine affecting alertness and reflexes.

Discontinuing:
Don't discontinue without consulting doctor. Dose may require gradual reduction if you have taken drug for a long time. Doses of other drugs may also require adjustment.

Others:
- Treatment of ulcers usually requires 4 to 6 weeks, although symptoms may greatly improve in 1 or 2 weeks.
- May affect results of some medical tests.

 ## POSSIBLE INTERACTION WITH OTHER DRUGS

GENERIC NAME OR DRUG CLASS	COMBINED EFFECT
Anticoagulants* (warfarin, coumadin, indandione derivatives)	Increased anticoagulant effect. May require dosage adjustment.
Diazepam	Delayed excretion and therefore increased concentration of diazepam.
Phenytoin	Delayed excretion and therefore increased concentration of omeprazole.

 ## POSSIBLE INTERACTION WITH OTHER SUBSTANCES

INTERACTS WITH	COMBINED EFFECT
Alcohol:	Decreased omeprazole effect.
Beverages: Caffeine drinks.	Decreased omeprazole effect.
Cocaine:	None expected.
Foods: Spicy or highly seasoned.	Decreased omeprazole effect.
Marijuana:	None expected.
Tobacco:	Decreased omeprazole effect.

ORPHENADRINE

BRAND NAMES

Banflex	Myotrol
Blanex	Neocyten
Disipal	Noradex
Flexagin	Norflex
Flexain	O-Flex
Flexoject	Orflagen
Flexon	Orfro
K-Flex	Orphenate
Marflex	Tega-Flex
Myolin	

BASIC INFORMATION

Habit forming? Possibly
Prescription needed?
 U.S.: Yes
 Canada: No
Available as generic? Yes
Drug class: Muscle relaxant, anticholinergic, antihistamine, antiparkinsonism

USES

- Reduces muscle-strain discomfort.
- Relieves symptoms of Parkinson's disease.
- Adjunctive treatment to rest, analgesics and physical therapy for muscle spasms.

DOSAGE & USAGE INFORMATION

How to take:
Tablet or extended-release tablet—Swallow with liquid. If you can't swallow whole, crumble tablet and take with liquid or food.

When to take:
At the same times each day.

If you forget a dose:
Take as soon as you remember up to 6 hours late. If more than 6 hours, wait for next scheduled dose (don't double this dose).

Continued next column

OVERDOSE

SYMPTOMS:
Fainting, confusion, blurred vision, difficulty swallowing, difficulty breathing, decreased urination, widely dilated pupils, rapid heartbeat, rapid pulse, paralysis, convulsions, coma.
WHAT TO DO:
- **Dial 0 (operator) or 911 (emergency) for an ambulance or medical help. Then give first aid immediately.**
- **See emergency information on inside covers.**

What drug does:
Sedative and analgesic effects reduce spasm and pain in skeletal muscles.

Time lapse before drug works:
1 to 2 hours.

Don't take with:
Any other medicine without consulting your doctor or pharmacist.

POSSIBLE ADVERSE REACTIONS OR SIDE EFFECTS

SYMPTOMS	WHAT TO DO
Life-threatening:	
Extreme weakness; transient paralysis; temporary loss of vision; hives, rash, intense itching, faintness soon after a dose (anaphylaxis).	Seek emergency treatment immediately.
Common:	
None expected.	
Infrequent:	
• Weakness, headache, dizziness, agitation, drowsiness, tremor, confusion, rapid or pounding heartbeat, depression, hearing loss.	Discontinue. Call doctor right away.
• Dry mouth, nausea, vomiting, constipation, urinary hesitancy or retention, abdominal pain, muscle weakness.	Continue. Call doctor when convenient.
Rare:	
Rash, itchy skin, blurred vision, hallucinations.	Discontinue. Call doctor right away.

WARNINGS & PRECAUTIONS

Don't take if:
- You are allergic to orphenadrine.
- You are allergic to tartrazine dye.

Before you start, consult your doctor:
- If you have glaucoma.
- If you have myasthenia gravis.
- If you have difficulty emptying bladder.
- If you have had heart disease or heart-rhythm disturbance.
- If you have had a peptic ulcer.
- If you have prostate enlargement.

Over age 60:
Adverse reactions and side effects may be more frequent and severe than in younger persons.

Pregnancy:
Safety not established. Avoid if possible.

Breast-feeding:
No proven problems. Consult doctor.

Infants & children:
Not recommended for children younger than 12.

Prolonged use:
- Increased internal-eye pressure.
- Talk to your doctor about the need for follow-up medical examinations or laboratory studies to check complete blood counts (white blood cell count, platelet count, red blood cell count, hemoglobin, hematocrit), liver function, kidney function.

Skin & sunlight:
No problems expected.

Driving, piloting or hazardous work:
Don't drive or pilot aircraft until you learn how medicine affects you. Don't work around dangerous machinery. Don't climb ladders or work in high places. Danger increases if you drink alcohol or take medicine affecting alertness and reflexes, such as antihistamines, tranquilizers, sedatives, pain medicine, narcotics and mind-altering drugs.

Discontinuing:
May be unnecessary to finish medicine. Follow doctor's instructions.

Others:
No problems expected.

POSSIBLE INTERACTION WITH OTHER DRUGS

GENERIC NAME OR DRUG CLASS	COMBINED EFFECT
Anticholinergics*	Increased anticholinergic effect.
Antidepressants, tricyclic (TCA)*	Increased sedation.
Antihistamines*	Increased sedation.
Attapulgite	Decreased effect of orphenadrine.
Carteolol	Decreased antihistamine effect.
Chlorpromazine	Hypoglycemia (low blood sugar).
Contraceptives, oral*	Decreased contraceptive effect.
Griseofulvin	Decreased griseofulvin effect.
Levodopa	Increased effect of levodopa. (Improves effectiveness in treating Parkinson's disease.)
Nabilone	Greater depression of central nervous system.
Nitrates*	Increased internal-eye pressure.
Nizatidine	Increased nizatidine effect.
Phenylbutazone	Decreased phenylbutazone effect.
Potassium supplements*	Increased possibility of intestinal ulcers with oral potassium tablets.
Propoxyphene	Possible confusion, nervousness, tremors.
Sotalol	Increased antihistamine effect.

POSSIBLE INTERACTION WITH OTHER SUBSTANCES

INTERACTS WITH	COMBINED EFFECT
Alcohol:	Increased drowsiness. Avoid.
Beverages:	None expected.
Cocaine:	Decreased orphenadrine effect. Avoid.
Foods:	None expected.
Marijuana:	Increased drowsiness, mouth dryness, muscle weakness, fainting.
Tobacco:	None expected.

ORPHENADRINE, ASPIRIN & CAFFEINE

BRAND NAMES

Norgesic	N3 Gesic
Norgesic Forte	N3 Gesic Forte
Norphadrine	Orphenagesic
Norphadrine Forte	Orphenagesic Forte

BASIC INFORMATION

Habit forming? Yes
Prescription needed? Yes
Available as generic? No
**Drug class: Stimulant, vasoconstrictor,
    muscle relaxant, analgesic,
    anti-inflammatory (non-steroidal)**

USES

- Reduces muscle-strain discomfort.
- Reduces pain, fever, inflammation.
- Relieves swelling, stiffness, joint pain.
- Treatment for drowsiness and fatigue.

DOSAGE & USAGE INFORMATION

How to take:
Tablet—Swallow with liquid. If you can't swallow whole, crumble tablet and take with liquid or food.

When to take:
At the same times each day.

If you forget a dose:
Take as soon as you remember up to 2 hours late. If more than 2 hours, wait for next scheduled dose (don't double this dose).

What drug does:
- Sedative and analgesic effects reduce spasm and pain in skeletal muscles.
- Affects hypothalamus, the part of the brain which regulates temperature by dilating small blood vessels in skin.
- Prevents clumping of platelets (small blood cells) so blood vessels remain open.
- Decreases prostaglandin effect.

Continued next column

OVERDOSE

SYMPTOMS:
Fainting, confusion, widely dilated pupils, rapid pulse, ringing in ears, nausea, vomiting, dizziness, fever, deep and rapid breathing, excitement, rapid heartbeat, hallucinations, coma.
WHAT TO DO:
- **Dial 0 (operator) or 911 (emergency) for an ambulance or medical help. Then give first aid immediately.**
- **See emergency information on inside covers.**

- Suppresses body's pain messages.
- Constricts blood-vessel walls.
- Stimulates central nervous system.

Time lapse before drug works:
1 hour.

Don't take with:
- Tetracyclines. Space doses 1 hour apart.
- Non-prescription drugs without consulting doctor.
- Any other medicine without consulting your doctor or pharmacist.

POSSIBLE ADVERSE REACTIONS OR SIDE EFFECTS

SYMPTOMS	WHAT TO DO
Life-threatening:	
Hives, rash, intense itching, wheezing, faintness, soon after a dose (anaphylaxis), convulsions, fever.	Seek emergency treatment immediately.
Common:	
• Nausea, vomiting, abdominal cramps, nervousness, urgent urination, low blood sugar (hunger, anxiety, cold sweats, rapid pulse).	Discontinue. Call doctor right away.
• Ringing in ears, indigestion, heartburn, insomnia.	Continue. Call doctor when convenient.
Infrequent:	
• Weakness, headache, dizziness, drowsiness, agitation, tremor, confusion, irregular heartbeat, hearing loss, diarrhea, hallucinations.	Discontinue. Call doctor right away.
• Dry mouth, constipation.	Continue. Call doctor when convenient.
Rare:	
• Black or bloody vomit.	Discontinue. Seek emergency treatment.
• Change in vision; blurred vision; black, bloody or tarry stool; bloody urine; dilated pupils; uncontrolled movement of hands; sore throat; fever.	Discontinue. Call doctor right away.

WARNINGS & PRECAUTIONS

Don't take if:
- You need to restrict sodium in your diet. Buffered effervescent tablets and sodium salicylate are high in sodium.
- Aspirin has a strong vinegar-like odor, which means it has decomposed.

- You have a peptic ulcer of stomach or duodenum, a bleeding disorder, heart disease.
- You are allergic to any stimulant or orphenadrine.

Before you start, consult your doctor:
- If you have had stomach or duodenal ulcers, gout, heart disease or heart-rhythm disturbance, peptic ulcer.
- If you have asthma, nasal polyps, irregular heartbeat, hypoglycemia (low blood sugar), epilepsy, glaucoma, myasthenia gravis, difficulty emptying bladder, prostate enlargement.

Over age 60:
- More likely to cause hidden bleeding in stomach or intestines. Watch for dark stools.
- Adverse reactions and side effects may be more frequent and severe than in younger persons.

Pregnancy:
Risk to unborn child outweighs drug benefits. Don't use.

Breast-feeding:
Drug passes into milk. Avoid drug or discontinue nursing until you finish medicine. Consult doctor for advice on maintaining milk supply.

Infants & children:
- Overdose frequent and severe. Keep bottles out of children's reach.
- Consult doctor before giving to persons under age 18 who have fever and discomfort of viral illness, especially chicken pox and influenza. Probably increases risk of Reye's syndrome.
- Not recommended for children younger than 12.

Prolonged use:
- Kidney damage. Periodic kidney-function test recommended.
- Stomach ulcers more likely.
- Increased internal eye pressure.
- Talk to your doctor about the need for follow-up medical examinations or laboratory studies to check liver function, complete blood counts (white blood cell count, platelet count, red blood cell count, hemoglobin, hematocrit).

Skin & sunlight:
Aspirin combined with sunscreen may decrease sunburn.

Driving, piloting or hazardous work:
Don't drive or pilot aircraft until you learn how medicine affects you. Don't work around dangerous machinery. Don't climb ladders or work in high places. Danger increases if you drink alcohol or take medicine affecting alertness and reflexes, such as antihistamines, tranquilizers, sedatives, pain medicine, narcotics and mind-altering drugs.

Discontinuing:
- For chronic illness—Don't discontinue without doctor's advice until you complete prescribed dose, even though symptoms diminish or disappear.

- May be unnecessary to finish medicine if you take it for a short-term illness. Follow doctor's instructions.

Others:
- Aspirin can complicate surgery; illness; pregnancy, labor and delivery.
- For arthritis, don't change dose without consulting doctor.
- Urine tests for blood sugar may be inaccurate.
- May produce or aggravate fibrocystic breast disease in women.

 ## POSSIBLE INTERACTION WITH OTHER DRUGS

GENERIC NAME OR DRUG CLASS	COMBINED EFFECT
Acebutolol	Decreased antihypertensive effect of acebutolol.
Allopurinol	Decreased allopurinol effect.
Antacids*	Decreased aspirin effect.
Anticholinergics*	Increased anticholinergic effect.
Anticoagulants*	Increased anticoagulant effect. Abnormal bleeding.

Continued page 953

 ## POSSIBLE INTERACTION WITH OTHER SUBSTANCES

INTERACTS WITH	COMBINED EFFECT
Alcohol:	Possible stomach irritation and bleeding, increased drowsiness. Avoid.
Beverages: Caffeine drinks.	Increased caffeine effect.
Cocaine:	Decreased orphenadrine effect. Overstimulation. Avoid.
Foods:	No proven problems.
Marijuana:	Increased effect of drugs. May lead to dangerous, rapid heartbeat. Increased dry mouth. Avoid.
Tobacco:	Increased heartbeat. Avoid.

*See Glossary

OXACILLIN

BRAND NAMES

Bactocill   Prostaphlin

BASIC INFORMATION

Habit forming? No
Prescription needed? Yes
Available as generic? Yes
Drug class: Antibiotic (penicillin)

USES

Treatment of bacterial infections that are susceptible to oxacillin.

DOSAGE & USAGE INFORMATION

How to take:
- Capsules—Swallow with liquid on an empty stomach 1 hour before or 2 hours after eating.
- Liquid—Take with cold beverage. Liquid form is perishable and effective for only 7 days at room temperature. Effective for 14 days if stored in refrigerator. Don't freeze.

When to take:
Follow instructions on prescription label or side of package. Doses should be evenly spaced. For example, 4 times a day means every 6 hours.

If you forget a dose:
Take as soon as you remember. Continue regular schedule.

What drug does:
Destroys susceptible bacteria. Does not kill viruses.

Time lapse before drug works:
May be several days before medicine affects infection.

Don't take with:
Any other medicine without consulting your doctor or pharmacist.

OVERDOSE

SYMPTOMS:
Severe diarrhea, nausea or vomiting.
WHAT TO DO:
Overdose unlikely to threaten life. If person takes much larger amount than prescribed, call doctor, poison-control center or hospital emergency room for instructions.

POSSIBLE ADVERSE REACTIONS OR SIDE EFFECTS

SYMPTOMS	WHAT TO DO
Life-threatening:	
Hives, rash, intense itching, faintness soon after a dose (anaphylaxis).	Seek emergency treatment immediately.
Common:	
Dark or discolored tongue.	Continue. Tell doctor at next visit.
Infrequent:	
• Mild nausea, vomiting, diarrhea.	Continue. Call doctor when convenient.
• Bloody urine, face and ankle swelling.	Discontinue. Call doctor right away.
Rare:	
Unexplained bleeding or bruising, weakness, sore throat, fever, abdominal cramps, convulsions.	Discontinue. Call doctor right away.

WARNINGS & PRECAUTIONS

Don't take if:
You are allergic to oxacillin, cephalosporin antibiotics, or other penicillins. Life-threatening reaction may occur.

Before you start, consult your doctor:
- If you are allergic to any substance or drug.
- If you take birth control pills.

Over age 60:
You may have skin reactions, particularly around genitals and anus.

Pregnancy:
Studies inconclusive on harm to unborn child. Animal studies show fetal abnormalities. Decide with your doctor whether drug benefits justify risk to unborn child.

Breast-feeding:
Drug passes into milk. Child may become sensitive to penicillins and have allergic reactions to penicillin drugs. Avoid oxacillin or discontinue nursing until you finish medicine. Consult doctor for advice on maintaining milk supply.

Infants & children:
No problems expected.

Prolonged use:
- You may become more susceptible to infections caused by germs not responsive to oxacillin.
- Talk to your doctor about the need for follow-up medical examinations or laboratory studies to check SGPT*, SGOT*.

Skin & sunlight:
No problems expected.

Driving, piloting or hazardous work:
Usually not dangerous. Most hazardous reactions likely to occur a few minutes after taking oxacillin.

Discontinuing:
Don't discontinue without doctor's advice until you complete prescribed dose, even though symptoms diminish or disappear.

Others:
- May interfere with the accuracy of some medical tests.
- Birth control pills may not be effective. Use additional birth-control methods.

POSSIBLE INTERACTION WITH OTHER DRUGS

GENERIC NAME OR DRUG CLASS	COMBINED EFFECT
Beta-adrenergic blockers*	Increased chance of anaphylaxis (see emergency information on inside front cover).
Birth control pills	Impaired contraceptive efficiency.
Chloramphenicol	Decreased effect of both drugs.
Erythromycins*	Decreased effect of both drugs.
Loperamide	Decreased oxacillin effect.
Paromomycin	Decreased effect of both drugs.
Probenecid	Increased effect of all penicillins.
Sodium benzoate & sodium phenylacetate	May reduce effect of sodium benzoate & sodium phenylacetate.
Tetracyclines*	Decreased effect of both drugs.
Troleandomycin	Decreased effect of both drugs.

POSSIBLE INTERACTION WITH OTHER SUBSTANCES

INTERACTS WITH	COMBINED EFFECT
Alcohol:	Occasional stomach irritation.
Beverages:	None expected.
Cocaine:	No proven problems.
Foods: Acidic fruits or juices, aged cheese, wines, syrups (if taken with).	Decreased antibiotic effect.
Marijuana:	No proven problems.
Tobacco:	None expected.

OXTRIPHYLLINE & GUAIFENESIN

BRAND NAMES

Brondecon   Brondelate

BASIC INFORMATION

Habit forming? No
Prescription needed? Yes
Available as generic? No
Drug class: Bronchodilator (xanthine),
  cough/cold preparation

USES

- Treatment for bronchial asthma symptoms.
- Loosens mucus in respiratory passages from allergies and infections.

DOSAGE & USAGE INFORMATION

How to take:
Tablet or elixir—Swallow with liquid. If you can't swallow whole, crumble tablet and take with liquid or food.

When to take:
Most effective taken on empty stomach 1 hour before or 2 hours after eating. However, may take with food to lessen stomach upset.

If you forget a dose:
Take as soon as you remember up to 2 hours late. If more than 2 hours, wait for next scheduled dose (don't double this dose).

What drug does:
- Relaxes and expands bronchial tubes.
- Increases production of watery fluids to thin mucus so it can be coughed out or absorbed.

Time lapse before drug works:
15 to 30 minutes.

Don't take with:
- Any stimulant.
- Any other medicine without consulting your doctor or pharmacist.

OVERDOSE

SYMPTOMS:
Restlessness, irritability, confusion, delirium, convulsions, rapid pulse, nausea, vomiting, coma.
WHAT TO DO:
- **Dial 0 (operator) or 911 (emergency) for an ambulance or medical help. Then give first aid immediately.**
- **See emergency information on inside covers.**

POSSIBLE ADVERSE REACTIONS OR SIDE EFFECTS

SYMPTOMS	WHAT TO DO
Life-threatening:	
Difficult breathing, irregular or fast heartbeat.	Discontinue. Seek emergency treatment.
Common:	
Headache, irritability, nervousness, restlessness, insomnia, nausea, vomiting, abdominal pain, drowsiness.	Continue. Call doctor when convenient.
Infrequent:	
• Hives, rash, red or flushed face, diarrhea, heartburn, muscle twitching.	Discontinue. Call doctor right away.
• Dizziness, lightheadedness, appetite loss.	Continue. Call doctor when convenient.
Rare:	
None expected.	

WARNINGS & PRECAUTIONS

Don't take if:
- You are allergic to any cough or cold preparation containing guaifenesin or any bronchodilator.
- You have an active peptic ulcer.

Before you start, consult your doctor:
- If you have had impaired kidney or liver function.
- If you have gastritis, peptic ulcer, high blood pressure or heart disease.
- If you take medication for gout.

Over age 60:
Adverse reactions and side effects may be more frequent and severe than in younger persons. For drug to work, you must drink 8 to 10 glasses of fluid per day.

Pregnancy:
Risk to unborn child outweighs drug benefits. Don't use.

Breast-feeding:
Drug passes into milk. Avoid drug or discontinue nursing until you finish medicine. Consult doctor for advice on maintaining milk supply.

Infants & children:
Use only under medical supervision.

Prolonged use:
- Stomach irritation.
- Talk to your doctor about the need for follow-up medical examinations or laboratory studies to check serum oxtriphylline levels, lung function.

Skin & sunlight:
No problems expected.

Driving, piloting or hazardous work:
Avoid if lightheaded or dizzy. Otherwise, no problems expected.

Discontinuing:
May be unnecessary to finish medicine. Follow doctor's instructions.

Others:
No problems expected.

POSSIBLE INTERACTION WITH OTHER DRUGS

GENERIC NAME OR DRUG CLASS	COMBINED EFFECT
Allopurinol	Decreased allopurinol effect.
Anticoagulants*	Possible risk of bleeding.
Ephedrine	Increased effect of both drugs.
Epinephrine	Increased effect of both drugs.
Erythromycins*	Increased bronchodilator effect.
Furosemide	Increased furosemide effect.
Lincomycins*	Increased bronchodilator effect.
Lithium	Decreased lithium effect.
Probenecid	Decreased effect of both drugs.
Propranolol	Decreased bronchodilator effect.
Rauwolfia alkaloids*	Rapid heartbeat.
Sulfinpyrazone	Decreased sulfinpyrazone effect.
Troleandomycin	Increased bronchodilator effect.

POSSIBLE INTERACTION WITH OTHER SUBSTANCES

INTERACTS WITH	COMBINED EFFECT
Alcohol:	None expected.
Beverages: Caffeine drinks.	Nervousness and insomnia. You must drink 8 to 10 glasses of fluid per day for drug to work.
Cocaine:	Excess stimulation. Avoid.
Foods:	None expected.
Marijuana:	Slightly increased antiasthmatic effect of bronchodilator.
Tobacco:	Decreased bronchodilator effect and harmful for all conditions requiring bronchodilator treatment. Avoid.

OXYBUTYNIN

BRAND NAMES

Ditropan

BASIC INFORMATION

Habit forming? No
Prescription needed? Yes
Available as generic? Yes
Drug class: Antispasmodic (urinary tract)

USES

Reduces spasms of urinary bladder and urethra that cause symptoms of frequent urination, urgency, night-time urination and incontinence.

DOSAGE & USAGE INFORMATION

How to take:
Tablets or syrup—Swallow with water.

When to take:
At the same time every day. Do not take with food unless instructed to do so by doctor.

If you forget a dose:
Take as soon as you remember up to 2 hours late. If more than 2 hours, wait for next scheduled dose. Don't double this dose.

What drug does:
Blocks nerve impulses at parasympathetic nerve endings, preventing muscle contractions and gland secretions of organs involved.

Time lapse before drug works:
30 minutes to 1 hour.

Don't take with:
Any other medicine without consulting your doctor or pharmacist.

OVERDOSE

SYMPTOMS:
Unsteadiness, confusion, dizziness, severe drowsiness, fast heartbeat, fever, red face, hallucinations, difficult breathing.
WHAT TO DO:
Overdose unlikely to threaten life. If person takes much larger amount than prescribed, call doctor, poison-control center or hospital emergency room for instructions.

POSSIBLE ADVERSE REACTIONS OR SIDE EFFECTS

SYMPTOMS	WHAT TO DO
Life-threatening:	
In case of overdose, see previous column.	
Common:	
Constipation; decreased sweating; drowsiness; dryness of mouth, nose and throat.	Continue. Call doctor when convenient.
Infrequent:	
Difficult swallowing, decreased sexual ability, headache, difficult urination, sensitivity to light, nausea, vomiting, insomnia, tiredness.	Continue. Call doctor when convenient.
Rare:	
Skin rash, eye pain, blurred vision.	Discontinue. Call doctor right away.

WARNINGS & PRECAUTIONS

Don't take if:
- You are allergic to any anticholinergic.
- You have trouble with stomach bloating.
- You have difficulty emptying your bladder completely.
- You have narrow-angle glaucoma.
- You have severe ulcerative colitis.

Before you start, consult your doctor:
- If you have open-angle glaucoma.
- If you have angina or fast heartbeat.
- If you have chronic bronchitis or asthma.
- If you have hiatal hernia; liver, kidney or thyroid disease; enlarged prostate or myasthenia gravis.
- If you will have surgery within 2 months, including dental surgery, requiring general or spinal anesthesia.

Over age 60:
Adverse reactions and side effects may be more frequent and severe than in younger persons. You may require smaller doses for shorter periods of time.

Pregnancy:
No proven harm to unborn child, but avoid if possible.

Breast-feeding:
Decreases flow of breast milk.

Infants & children:
Not recommended for children under 5.

Prolonged use:
Side effects more likely.

Skin & sunlight:
No special problems expected.

Driving, piloting or hazardous work:
Don't drive or pilot aircraft until you learn how medicine affects you. Don't work around dangerous machinery. Don't climb ladders or work in high places. Danger increases if you drink alcohol or take medicine affecting alertness and reflexes.

Discontinuing:
May be unnecessary to finish medicine. Follow doctor's instructions.

Others:
Advise any doctor or dentist whom you consult that you take this medicine.

POSSIBLE INTERACTION WITH OTHER DRUGS

GENERIC NAME OR DRUG CLASS	COMBINED EFFECT
Anticholinergics*	Increased effect of oxybutynin.
Central nervous system (CNS) depressants*	Increased sedative effect.

POSSIBLE INTERACTION WITH OTHER SUBSTANCES

INTERACTS WITH	COMBINED EFFECT
Alcohol:	None expected.
Beverages:	None expected.
Cocaine:	Excessively rapid heartbeat. Avoid.
Foods:	None expected.
Marijuana:	Drowsiness and dry mouth.
Tobacco:	None expected.

PANCREATIN, PEPSIN, BILE SALTS, HYOSCYAMINE, ATROPINE, SCOPOLAMINE & PHENOBARBITAL

BRAND NAMES

Donnazyme

BASIC INFORMATION

Habit forming? Yes
Prescription needed? Yes
Available as generic? No
Drug class: Digestant, sedative,
  anticholinergic

 ## USES

- Replaces deficient digestive enzymes.
- Sometimes used to relieve indigestion.

 ## DOSAGE & USAGE INFORMATION

How to take:
Tablet—Swallow with liquid or food to lessen stomach irritation. If you can't swallow whole, crumble tablet and take with food or liquid.

When to take:
With or after meals.

If you forget a dose:
Skip it and resume schedule. Don't double-dose.

What drug does:
Blocks nerve impulses at parasympathetic nerve endings, preventing smooth muscle contraction and gland secretions.

Time lapse before drug works:
30 to 60 minutes.

Don't take with:
- Any medicine that will decrease mental alertness or reflexes, such as alcohol, other mind-altering drugs, cough/cold medicines,

Continued next column

 ## OVERDOSE

SYMPTOMS:
Hallucinations, excitement, breathing difficulty, irregular heartbeat (too fast or too slow), fainting, collapse, coma.
WHAT TO DO:
- **Dial 0 (operator) or 911 (emergency) for an ambulance or medical help. Then give first aid immediately.**
- **See emergency information on inside covers.**

antihistamines, allergy medicine, sedatives, tranquilizers (sleeping pills or "downers") barbiturates, seizure medicine, narcotics, other prescription medicine for pain, muscle relaxants, anesthetics.
- See Interaction column and consult doctor.

 ## POSSIBLE ADVERSE REACTIONS OR SIDE EFFECTS

SYMPTOMS	WHAT TO DO
Life-threatening:	
In case of overdose, see previous column.	
Common:	
• Constipation, decreased sweating, headache.	Discontinue. Call doctor right away.
• Drowsiness, dry mouth, frequent urination.	Continue. Call doctor when convenient.
Infrequent:	
• Blurred vision.	Discontinue. Call doctor right away.
• Diminished sex drive, swallowing difficulty, sensitivity to light, insomnia.	Continue. Call doctor when convenient.
Rare:	
• Jaundice; unusual bleeding or bruising; swollen feet and ankles; abdominal pain; sore throat, fever, mouth sores; rash; hives; vomiting; joint pain; eye pain; diarrhea; blood in urine.	Discontinue. Call doctor right away.
• Unusual tiredness.	Continue. Call doctor when convenient.

 ## WARNINGS & PRECAUTIONS

Don't take if:
- You are allergic to any of the drugs in this combination.
- You have trouble with stomach bloating, difficulty emptying your bladder completely, narrow-angle glaucoma, severe ulcerative colitis, porphyria.

Before you start, consult your doctor:
- If you have open-angle glaucoma, angina, chronic bronchitis or asthma, liver disease, hiatal hernia, enlarged prostate, myasthenia gravis, epilepsy, kidney or liver damage, anemia, chronic pain.

PANCREATIN, PEPSIN, BILE SALTS, HYOSCYAMINE, ATROPINE, SCOPOLAMINE & PHENOBARBITAL

- If you will have surgery within 2 months, including dental surgery, requiring general or spinal anesthesia.

Over age 60:
Adverse reactions and side effects may be more frequent and severe than in younger persons

Pregnancy:
Risk to unborn child outweighs drug benefits. Don't use.

Breast-feeding:
Drug passes into milk. Avoid drug or discontinue nursing until you finish medicine. Consult doctor for advice on maintaining milk supply.

Infants & children:
Use only under medical supervision.

Prolonged use:
- Chronic constipation, possible fecal impaction.
- May cause addiction, anemia, chronic intoxication.
- May lower body temperature, making exposure to cold temperatures hazardous.

Skin & sunlight:
May cause rash or intensify sunburn in areas exposed to sun or sunlamp.

Driving, piloting or hazardous work:
Don't drive or pilot aircraft until you learn how medicine affects you. Don't work around dangerous machinery. Don't climb ladders or work in high places. Danger increases if you drink alcohol or take medicine affecting alertness and reflexes, such as antihistamines, tranquilizers, sedatives, pain medicine, narcotics and mind-altering drugs.

Discontinuing:
- May be unnecessary to finish medicine. Follow doctor's instructions.
- If you develop withdrawal symptoms of hallucinations, agitation or sleeplessness after discontinuing, call doctor right away.

Others:
- Potential for abuse.
- Enzyme deficiencies probably better treated with identified separate substances rather than a mixture of components.

 POSSIBLE INTERACTION WITH OTHER DRUGS

GENERIC NAME OR DRUG CLASS	COMBINED EFFECT
Amantadine	Increased atropine effect.
Antacids*	Decreased absorption of scopolamine.
Anticholinergics, other*	Increased anticholinergic effect.
Anticoagulants, oral*	Decreased anticoagulant effect.
Antidepressants, tricyclic (TCA)*	Decreased antidepressant effect. Possible dangerous oversedation.
Antidiabetics, oral*	Increased phenobartital effect.
Antihistamines*	Increased atropine effect.
Aspirin	Decreased aspirin effect.
Attapulgite	Decreased anticholinergic effect.
Beta-adrenergic blockers*	Decreased effect of beta-adrenergic blocker.
Buclizine	Increased scopolamine effect.
Central nervous system (CNS) depressants*	Increased CNS depression.
Contraceptives, oral*	Decreased contraceptive effect.
Cortisone drugs*	Decreased cortisone effect.
Digitalis	Possible decreased absorption of digitalis.

Continued page 954

 POSSIBLE INTERACTION WITH OTHER SUBSTANCES

INTERACTS WITH	COMBINED EFFECT
Alcohol:	Possible fatal oversedation. Avoid.
Beverages:	None expected.
Cocaine:	Excessively rapid heartbeat. Avoid.
Foods:	None expected.
Marijuana:	Excessive sedation, drowsiness and dry mouth.
Tobacco:	May increase stomach acidity, decreasing the effectiveness of Donnazyme. Avoid.

PANCRELIPASE

BRAND NAMES

Cotazym	Lipancreatin
Cotazym E.C.S.	Pancoate
Cotazym-S	Pancrease
Cotazym-65B	Pancrease MT4
Creon	Pancrease MT10
Entolase	Pancrease MT16
Entolase-HP	Ultrase MT 12
Enzymase-16	Ultrase MT 20
Festal II	Ultrase MT 24
Ilozyme	Viokase
Ku-Zyme HP	Zymase

BASIC INFORMATION

Habit forming? No
Prescription needed? Yes
Available as generic? No
Drug class: Enzyme (pancreatic)

USES

- Replaces pancreatic enzyme deficiency caused by surgery or disease.
- Treats fatty stools (steatorrhea).

DOSAGE & USAGE INFORMATION

How to take:
- Tablets, capsules or delayed-release capsules—Swallow whole. Do not take with milk or milk products.
- Powder—Sprinkle on liquid or soft food.

When to take:
Before meals.

If you forget a dose:
Take as soon as you remember up to 2 hours late. If more than 2 hours, wait for next scheduled dose (don't double this dose).

What drug does:
Enhances digestion of proteins, carbohydrates and fats.

OVERDOSE

SYMPTOMS:
Shortness of breath, wheezing, diarrhea.
WHAT TO DO:
Overdose unlikely to threaten life. If person takes much larger amount than prescribed, call doctor, poison-control center or hospital emergency room for instructions.

Time lapse before drug works:
30 minutes.

Don't take with:
Any other medicine without consulting your doctor or pharmacist.

POSSIBLE ADVERSE REACTIONS OR SIDE EFFECTS

SYMPTOMS	WHAT TO DO
Life-threatening: None expected.	
Common: None expected.	
Infrequent: Diarrhea, asthma.	Discontinue. Call doctor right away.
Rare: • Rash, hives, blood in urine, swollen feet or legs, abdominal cramps.	Discontinue. Call doctor right away.
• Nausea, joint pain.	Continue. Call doctor when convenient.

WARNINGS & PRECAUTIONS

Don't take if:
You are allergic to pancreatin, pancrelipase, or pork.

Before you start, consult your doctor:
If you take any other medicines.

Over age 60:
Adverse reactions and side effects may be more frequent and severe than in younger persons.

Pregnancy:
Risk to unborn child outweighs drug benefits. Don't use.

Breast-feeding:
Drug passes into milk. Avoid drug or discontinue nursing until you finish medicine. Consult doctor for advice on maintaining milk supply.

Infants & children:
Under close medical supervision only.

Prolonged use:
No additional problems expected.

Skin & sunlight:
No problems expected.

Driving, piloting or hazardous work:
No problems expected.

Discontinuing:
Don't discontinue without consulting doctor. Dose may require gradual reduction if you have taken drug for a long time. Doses of other drugs may also require adjustment.

Others:
If you take powder form, avoid inhaling.

POSSIBLE INTERACTION WITH OTHER DRUGS

GENERIC NAME OR DRUG CLASS	COMBINED EFFECT
Calcium carbonate antacids*	Decreased effect of pancrelipase.
Magnesium hydroxide antacids*	Decreased effect of pancrelipase.

POSSIBLE INTERACTION WITH OTHER SUBSTANCES

INTERACTS WITH	COMBINED EFFECT
Alcohol:	Unknown.
Beverages: Milk.	Decreased effect of pancrelipase.
Cocaine:	Unknown.
Foods: Ice cream, milk products.	Decreased effect of pancrelipase.
Marijuana:	Decreased absorption of pancrelipase.
Tobacco:	Decreased absorption of pancrelipase.

PANTOTHENIC ACID (Vitamin B-5)

BRAND AND GENERIC NAMES

**CALCIUM
PANTOTHENATE**   Dexol T.D.

An ingredient in numerous multiple vitamin-mineral supplements. Check labels.

BASIC INFORMATION

**Habit forming? No
Prescription needed? No
Available as generic? Yes
Drug class: Vitamin supplement**

 USES

Prevents and treats vitamin B-5 deficiency.

 DOSAGE & USAGE INFORMATION

How to take:
Tablet—Swallow with liquid.

When to take:
At the same times each day.

If you forget a dose:
Take as soon as you remember, then resume regular schedule.

What drug does:
Acts as co-enzyme in carbohydrate, protein and fat metabolism.

Time lapse before drug works:
15 to 20 minutes.

Don't take with:
- Levodopa—Small amounts of pantothenic acid will nullify levodopa effect. Carbidopa-levodopa combination not affected by this interaction.
- Any other medicine without consulting your doctor or pharmacist.

 OVERDOSE

**SYMPTOMS:
None expected.
WHAT TO DO:
Overdose unlikely to threaten life.**

 **POSSIBLE
ADVERSE REACTIONS
OR SIDE EFFECTS**

SYMPTOMS	WHAT TO DO
Life-threatening: None expected.	
Common: Heartburn.	Discontinue. Seek emergency treatment.
Infrequent: Cramps.	Discontinue Call doctor right away.
Rare: Rash, hives, difficult breathing.	Discontinue. Seek emergency treatment.

PANTOTHENIC ACID (Vitamin B-5)

WARNINGS & PRECAUTIONS

Don't take if:
You are allergic to pantothenic acid.

Before you start, consult your doctor:
If you have hemophilia.

Over age 60:
No problems expected.

Pregnancy:
Don't exceed recommended dose.

Breast-feeding:
Don't exceed recommended dose.

Infants & children:
Don't exceed recommended dose.

Prolonged use:
Large doses for more than 1 month may cause toxicity.

Skin & sunlight:
No problems expected.

Driving, piloting or hazardous work:
No problems expected.

Discontinuing:
No problems expected.

Others:
Regular pantothenic acid supplements are recommended if you take chloramphenicol, cycloserine, ethionamide, hydralazine, immunosuppressants, isoniazid or penicillamine. These decrease pantothenic acid absorption and can cause anemia or tingling and numbness in hands and feet.

POSSIBLE INTERACTION WITH OTHER DRUGS

GENERIC NAME OR DRUG CLASS	COMBINED EFFECT
None expected.	

POSSIBLE INTERACTION WITH OTHER SUBSTANCES

INTERACTS WITH	COMBINED EFFECT
Alcohol:	None expected.
Beverages:	None expected.
Cocaine:	None expected.
Foods:	None expected.
Marijuana:	None expected.
Tobacco:	May decrease pantothenic acid absorption. Decreased pantothenic acid effect.

PAPAVERINE

BRAND NAMES

See complete list of brand names in the *Brand Name Directory*, page 924.

BASIC INFORMATION

Habit forming? No
Prescription needed? Yes
Available as generic? Yes
Drug class: Vasodilator

 USES

- May improve poor circulation in the extremities or brain.
- Injected into penis to produce erections.

 DOSAGE & USAGE INFORMATION

How to take:
- Tablet—Swallow with liquid or food to lessen stomach irritation. If you can't swallow whole, crumble tablet and take with liquid or food.
- Extended-release capsules—Swallow whole with liquid.
- Injections to penis—Follow doctor's instructions.

When to take:
At the same times each day.

If you forget a dose:
Take as soon as you remember up to 2 hours late. If more than 2 hours, wait for next scheduled dose (don't double this dose).

What drug does:
Relaxes and expands blood-vessel walls, allowing better distribution of oxygen and nutrients.

Time lapse before drug works:
30 to 60 minutes.

Don't take with:
- Non-prescription drugs without consulting doctor.
- Any other medicine without consulting your doctor or pharmacist.

 OVERDOSE

SYMPTOMS:
Weakness, fainting, flush, sweating, stupor, irregular heartbeat.
WHAT TO DO:
- **Dial 0 (operator) or 911 (emergency) for an ambulance or medical help. Then give first aid immediately.**
- **See emergency information on inside covers.**

 POSSIBLE ADVERSE REACTIONS OR SIDE EFFECTS

SYMPTOMS	WHAT TO DO
Life-threatening: None expected.	
Common:	
• Drowsiness, dizziness, headache, flushed face, stomach irritation, indigestion, nausea, mild constipation.	Continue. Call doctor when convenient.
• Dry mouth, throat.	Continue. Tell doctor at next visit.
Infrequent: Rash, itchy skin, blurred or double vision, weakness, fast heartbeat.	Discontinue. Call doctor right away.
Rare: Jaundice.	Discontinue. Call doctor right away.

WARNINGS & PRECAUTIONS

Don't take if:
You are allergic to papaverine.

Before you start, consult your doctor:
- If you plan to become pregnant within medication period.
- If you have had a heart attack, heart disease, angina or stroke.
- If you have Parkinson's disease.

Over age 60:
Adverse reactions and side effects may be more frequent and severe than in younger persons.

Pregnancy:
No proven harm to unborn child. Avoid if possible.

Breast-feeding:
Drug filters into milk. May harm child. Avoid.

Infants & children:
Not recommended.

Prolonged use:
No problems expected.

Skin & sunlight:
No problems expected.

Driving, piloting or hazardous work:
Don't drive or pilot aircraft until you learn how medicine affects you. Don't work around dangerous machinery. Don't climb ladders or work in high places. Danger increases if you drink alcohol or take medicine affecting alertness and reflexes, such as antihistamines, tranquilizers, sedatives, pain medicine, narcotics and mind-altering drugs.

Discontinuing:
May be unnecessary to finish medicine. If drug does not help in 1 to 2 weeks, consult doctor about discontinuing.

Others:
- Periodic liver-function tests recommended.
- Internal eye-pressure measurements recommended if you have glaucoma.

POSSIBLE INTERACTION WITH OTHER DRUGS

GENERIC NAME OR DRUG CLASS	COMBINED EFFECT
Levodopa	Decreased levodopa effect.
Narcotics*	Increased sedation.
Pain relievers*	Increased sedation.
Pergolide	Decreased pergolide effect.
Sedatives*	Increased sedation.
Sympathomimetics*	Reversal of the effect of papaverine.
Tranquilizers*	Increased sedation.

POSSIBLE INTERACTION WITH OTHER SUBSTANCES

INTERACTS WITH	COMBINED EFFECT
Alcohol:	None expected.
Beverages:	None expected.
Cocaine:	Decreased papaverine effect.
Foods:	None expected.
Marijuana:	None expected.
Tobacco:	Decrease in papaverine's dilation of blood vessels.

PARA-AMINOSALICYLIC ACID
(Aminosalicylate Sodium)

BRAND NAMES

Nemasol-Sodium   Tubasal
P.A.S.

BASIC INFORMATION

Habit forming? No
Prescription needed? Yes
Available as generic? No
Drug class: Antitubercular

 ## USES

Treatment for tuberculosis (TB).

 ## DOSAGE & USAGE INFORMATION

How to take:
- Tablet—Swallow with liquid or food to lessen stomach irritation.
- Powder—Dissolve dose in water. Stir well and drink all liquid.

When to take:
At the same times each day.

If you forget a dose:
Take as soon as you remember up to 2 hours late. If more than 2 hours, wait for next scheduled dose (don't double this dose).

What drug does:
- Prevents growth of TB germs.
- Makes TB germs more susceptible to other antituberculosis drugs.

Time lapse before drug works:
6 months.

Don't take with:
Any other medicine without consulting your doctor or pharmacist.

 ## OVERDOSE

SYMPTOMS:
Nausea, vomiting, diarrhea; rapid breathing; convulsions.
WHAT TO DO:
- **Dial 0 (operator) or 911 (emergency) for an ambulance or medical help. Then give first aid immediately.**
- **See emergency information on inside covers.**

 ## POSSIBLE ADVERSE REACTIONS OR SIDE EFFECTS

SYMPTOMS	WHAT TO DO
Life-threatening:	
In case of overdose, see previous column.	
Common:	
• Painful urination, chills, low back pain, nausea, vomiting.	Discontinue. Call doctor right away.
• Diarrhea or abdominal pain.	Continue. Call doctor when convenient.
Infrequent:	
• Confusion, blood in urine.	Discontinue. Call doctor right away.
• Headache; itchy, dry, puffy skin; rash; light sensitivity; sore throat; fever; swelling in front of neck; decreased sex drive in men; fatigue; weakness.	Continue. Call doctor when convenient.
• Menstrual irregularities, weight gain.	Continue. Tell doctor at next visit.
Rare:	
Jaundice.	Discontinue. Call doctor right away.

PARA-AMINOSALICYLIC ACID
(Aminosalicylate Sodium)

 WARNINGS & PRECAUTIONS

Don't take if:
- You are allergic to para-aminosalicylic acid, aspirin or other salicylates.
- Tablets have turned brownish or purplish.

Before you start, consult your doctor:
- If you have ulcers in stomach or duodenum.
- If you have liver or kidney disease.
- If you have epilepsy.
- If you have adrenal insufficiency.
- If you have heart disease or congestive heart failure.
- If you have cancer.
- If you have overactive thyroid.

Over age 60:
Adverse reactions and side effects may be more frequent and severe than in younger persons.

Pregnancy:
Risk to unborn child outweighs drug benefits. Don't use.

Breast-feeding:
No proven problems. Consult doctor.

Infants & children:
Use only under medical supervision.

Prolonged use:
- Enlarged thyroid gland and decreased function.
- Talk to your doctor about the need for follow-up medical examinations or laboratory studies to check liver function, kidney function.

Skin & sunlight:
Increased sensitivity to light.

Driving, piloting or hazardous work:
No problems expected.

Discontinuing:
No problems expected.

Others:
- Treatment may need to continue for several years or indefinitely.
- Periodic blood tests and liver- and kidney-function studies recommended.

 POSSIBLE INTERACTION WITH OTHER DRUGS

GENERIC NAME OR DRUG CLASS	COMBINED EFFECT
Aminobenzoic acid (PABA)	Decreased effect of para-aminosalicylic acid.
Anticoagulants, oral*	Increased anti-coagulant effect.
Anticonvulsants, hydantoin*	Increased anti-convulsant effect.
Aspirin	Stomach irritation.
Barbiturates*	Oversedation.
Folic acid	Decreased effect of folic acid.
Probenecid	Increased para-aminosalicylic acid effect. Possible toxicity.
Rifampin	Decreased rifampin effect.
Sulfa drugs*	Decreased effect of sulfa drugs.
Sulfinpyrazone	Increased para-aminosalicylic acid effect. Possible toxicity.
Tetracyclines*	Reduced absorption of para-aminosalicylic acid. Space doses 3 hours apart.

 POSSIBLE INTERACTION WITH OTHER SUBSTANCES

INTERACTS WITH	COMBINED EFFECT
Alcohol:	Possible liver disease.
Beverages:	None expected
Cocaine:	None expected.
Foods:	None expected.
Marijuana:	None expected.
Tobacco:	None expected, but tobacco smoking may slow recovery. Avoid.

*See Glossary

PARALDEHYDE

BRAND NAMES

Paral

BASIC INFORMATION

Habit forming? Yes
Prescription needed? Yes
Available as generic? Yes
Drug class: Anticonvulsant

USES

- Treats convulsions.
- Treats toxic symptoms caused by drugs that may produce convulsions.

DOSAGE & USAGE INFORMATION

How to take:
- Follow doctor's instructions.
- May be given orally, rectally or by injection into a muscle.

When to take:
Follow doctor's instructions.

If you forget a dose:
Take as soon as you remember up to 2 hours late. If more than 2 hours, wait for next scheduled dose (don't double this dose).

What drug does:
Depresses central nervous system.

Time lapse before drug works:
- Oral—30 minutes to 1 hour.
- Rectal—2 to 3 hours.

Don't take with:
Any other medicines (including over-the-counter drugs such as cough and cold medicines, laxatives, antacids, diet pills, caffeine, nose drops or vitamins) without consulting your doctor.

OVERDOSE

SYMPTOMS:
Decreased urination, breathing difficulty, confusion, slow heartbeat, weakness.
WHAT TO DO:
- **Dial 0 (operator) or 911 (emergency) for an ambulance or medical help. Then give first aid immediately.**
- **See emergency information on inside covers.**

POSSIBLE ADVERSE REACTIONS OR SIDE EFFECTS

SYMPTOMS	WHAT TO DO
Life-threatening:	
In case of overdose, see previous column.	
Common:	
• Skin rash, jaundice (yellow skin and eyes).	Discontinue. Call doctor right away.
• Drowsiness, nausea, halitosis.	Continue. Call doctor when convenient.
Infrequent:	
Clumsiness, dizziness, headache.	Continue. Call doctor when convenient.
Rare:	
Abdominal cramps.	Continue. Call doctor when convenient.

WARNINGS & PRECAUTIONS

Don't take if:
You know you are allergic to paraldehyde.

Before you start, consult your doctor:
- If you have chronic lung disease.
- If you have history of drug abuse.
- If you have liver disease.
- If you have peptic ulcer.
- If you have colitis.

Over age 60:
No special problems expected.

Pregnancy:
Risk to unborn child outweighs drug benefits. Don't use.

Breast-feeding:
Effect not documented. Consult your doctor.

Infants & children:
No special problems expected.

Prolonged use:
- May be habit forming.
- Talk to your doctor about the need for follow-up medical examinations or laboratory studies to check liver function.

Skin & sunlight:
No problems expected.

Driving, piloting or hazardous work:
Avoid if you feel confused, drowsy or dizzy.

Discontinuing:
May develop withdrawal symptoms, such as: convulsions, hallucinations, sweating, muscle cramps, nausea or vomiting, trembling. If you experience any of these, notify your doctor right away.

Others:
- Advise any doctor or dentist whom you consult that you take this medicine.
- May affect results in some medical tests.
- Strong odor of paraldehyde on breath lasts for 24 hours.

POSSIBLE INTERACTION WITH OTHER DRUGS

GENERIC NAME OR DRUG CLASS	COMBINED EFFECT
Central nervous system (CNS) depressants, other*	Possible oversedation. Avoid simultaneous use.
Clozapine	Toxic effect on the central nervous system.
Disulfiram	Increased paraldehyde effect. Avoid simultaneous use.
Sertraline	Increased depressive effects of both drugs.

POSSIBLE INTERACTION WITH OTHER SUBSTANCES

INTERACTS WITH	COMBINED EFFECT
Alcohol:	Dangerous sedation. Avoid.
Beverages:	No special problems expected.
Cocaine:	No special problems expected.
Foods:	No special problems expected.
Marijuana:	No special problems expected.
Tobacco:	No special problems expected.

PARAMETHASONE

BRAND NAMES

Haldrone

BASIC INFORMATION

Habit forming? No
Prescription needed? Yes
Available as generic? No
Drug class: Cortisone drug (adrenal corticosteroid)

USES

- Reduces inflammation caused by many different medical problems.
- Treatment for some allergic diseases, blood disorders, kidney diseases, asthma and emphysema.
- Replaces corticosteroid deficiencies.

DOSAGE & USAGE INFORMATION

How to take:
Tablet—Swallow with liquid or food to lessen stomach irritation. If you can't swallow whole, crumble tablet and take with liquid or food.

When to take:
At the same times each day. Take once-a-day or once-every-other-day doses in mornings.

If you forget a dose:
- Several-doses-per-day prescription—Take as soon as you remember up to 2 hours late. If more than 2 hours, wait for next scheduled dose (don't double this dose).
- Once-a-day dose or less—Wait for next dose. Double this dose.

What drug does:
Decreases inflammatory responses.

Time lapse before drug works:
2 to 4 days.

Don't take with:
Any other medicine without consulting your doctor or pharmacist.

OVERDOSE

SYMPTOMS:
Headache, convulsions, heart failure.
WHAT TO DO:
- **Dial 0 (operator) or 911 (emergency) for an ambulance or medical help. Then give first aid immediately.**
- **Additional emergency information on inside covers.**

POSSIBLE ADVERSE REACTIONS OR SIDE EFFECTS

SYMPTOMS	WHAT TO DO
Life-threatening:	
Rash, hives, intense itching, faintness soon after a dose (anaphylaxis).	Seek emergency treatment immediately.
Common:	
Acne, poor wound healing, indigestion, nausea, vomiting, thirst, constipation, gaseousness, unpleasant taste, diarrhea, headache, cough, dizziness, hoarseness, appetite gain or loss.	Continue. Call doctor when convenient.
Infrequent:	
• Black, bloody or tarry stool; various infections; swallowing difficulties.	Discontinue. Seek emergency treatment.
• Blurred vision, halos around lights, sore throat, fever, muscle cramps.	Discontinue. Call doctor right away.
• Mood change, fatigue, frequent urination, weight gain, round face, weakness, irregular menstrual periods, insomnia, restlessness, dry mouth, euphoria, nosebleeds.	Continue. Call doctor when convenient.
Rare:	
• Irregular heartbeat.	Discontinue. Seek emergency treatment.
• Rash, pancreatitis, numbness or tingling in hands or feet, thrombophlebitis, hallucinations, convulsions.	Discontinue. Call doctor right away.

WARNINGS & PRECAUTIONS

Don't take if:
- You are allergic to any cortisone drug.
- You have tuberculosis or fungus infection.
- You have herpes infection of eyes, lips or genitals.
- You have bone disease, thyroid disease, colitis, peptic ulcer, diabetes, myasthenia gravis, liver or kidney disease, diverticulitis, glaucoma, heart disease.

Before you start, consult your doctor:
- If you have had tuberculosis.
- If you have congestive heart failure, diabetes, peptic ulcer, glaucoma, underactive thyroid, high blood pressure, myasthenia gravis.
- If you have blood clots in legs or lungs.

Over age 60:
Adverse reactions and side effects may be more frequent and severe than in younger persons. Likely to aggravate edema, diabetes or ulcers. Likely to cause cataracts and osteoporosis (softening of the bones).

Pregnancy:
Risk to unborn child outweighs drug benefits. Don't use.

Breast-feeding:
Drug passes into milk. Avoid drug or discontinue nursing until you finish medicine. Consult doctor for advice on maintaining milk supply.

Infants & children:
Use only under medical supervision.

Prolonged use:
- Retards growth in children.
- Possible glaucoma, cataracts, diabetes, fragile bones and thin skin.
- Functional dependence.
- Talk to your doctor about the need for follow-up medical examinations or laboratory studies to check blood pressure, serum electrolytes, stools for blood.

Skin & sunlight:
No problems expected.

Driving, piloting or hazardous work:
No problems expected.

Discontinuing:
- Don't discontinue without doctor's advice until you complete prescribed dose, even though symptoms diminish or disappear.
- Drug affects your response to surgery, illness, injury or stress for 2 years after discontinuing. Tell anyone who takes medical care of you within 2 years about drug.

Others:
- Avoid immunizations if possible.
- Your resistance to infection is less while taking this medicine.
- Advise any doctor or dentist whom you consult that you take this medicine.
- Those who have inactive or "cured" tuberculosis may be subjected to a possible recurrence of active tuberculosis.
- Children who must take cortisone drugs may grow less well.

POSSIBLE INTERACTION WITH OTHER DRUGS

GENERIC NAME OR DRUG CLASS	COMBINED EFFECT
Amphotericin B	Potassium depletion.
Anticholinergics*	Possible glaucoma.
Anticoagulants, oral*	Decreased anti-coagulant effect.
Anticonvulsants, hydantoin*	Decreased para-methasone effect.
Antidiabetics, oral*	Decreased anti-diabetic effect.
Antihistamines*	Decreased para-methasone effect.
Aspirin	Increased para-methasone effect.
Attenuated virus vaccines*	Possible viral infection.
Barbiturates*	Decreased para-methasone effect. Oversedation.
Chloral hydrate	Decreased para-methasone effect.
Chlorthalidone	Potassium depletion.
Cholestyramine	Decreased para-methasone absorption.
Cholinergics*	Decreased cholinergic effect.
Colestipol	Decreased para-methasone absorption.
Contraceptives, oral*	Increased para-methasone effect.

Continued page 955

POSSIBLE INTERACTION WITH OTHER SUBSTANCES

INTERACTS WITH	COMBINED EFFECT
Alcohol:	Risk of stomach ulcers.
Beverages:	No proven problems.
Cocaine:	Overstimulation. Avoid.
Foods:	No proven problems.
Marijuana:	Decreased immunity.
Tobacco:	Increased para-methasone effect. Possible toxicity.

PAREGORIC

BRAND NAMES

Brown Mixture
Camphorated Opium
  Tincture
Laudanum
Opium Tincture

BASIC INFORMATION

Habit forming? Yes
Prescription needed? Yes
Available as generic? Yes
Drug class: Narcotic, antidiarrheal

USES

Reduces intestinal cramps and diarrhea.

DOSAGE & USAGE INFORMATION

How to take:
Drops or liquid—Dilute dose in beverage before swallowing.

When to take:
As needed for diarrhea, no more often than every 4 hours.

If you forget a dose:
Take as soon as you remember. Wait 4 hours for next dose.

What drug does:
Anesthetizes surface membranes of intestines and blocks nerve impulses.

Time lapse before drug works:
2 to 6 hours.

Don't take with:
Any other medicine without consulting your doctor or pharmacist.

OVERDOSE

SYMPTOMS:
Deep sleep; slow breathing; slow pulse; flushed, warm skin; constricted pupils.
WHAT TO DO:
- **Dial 0 (operator) or 911 (emergency) for an ambulance or medical help. Then give first aid immediately.**
- **If patient is unconscious and not breathing, give mouth-to-mouth breathing. If there is no heartbeat, use cardiac massage and mouth-to-mouth breathing (CPR). Don't try to make patient vomit. If you can't get help quickly, take patient to nearest emergency facility.**
- **See emergency information on inside covers.**

POSSIBLE ADVERSE REACTIONS OR SIDE EFFECTS

SYMPTOMS	WHAT TO DO
Life-threatening:	
In case of overdose, see previous column.	
Common:	
Dizziness, flushed face, unusual tiredness, difficult urination.	Continue. Call doctor when convenient.
Infrequent:	
Severe constipation, abdominal pain, vomiting.	Discontinue. Call doctor right away.
Rare:	
• Hives, rash, itchy skin, slow heartbeat, irregular breathing.	Discontinue. Call doctor right away.
• Depression.	Continue. Call doctor when convenient.

WARNINGS & PRECAUTIONS

Don't take if:
You are allergic to any narcotic.

Before you start, consult your doctor:
If you have impaired liver or kidney function.

Over age 60:
More likely to be drowsy, dizzy, unsteady or constipated.

Pregnancy:
No proven harm to unborn child. Avoid if possible.

Breast-feeding:
Drug filters into milk. May depress infant. Avoid.

Infants & children:
Use only under medical supervision.

Prolonged use:
Causes psychological and physical dependence.

Skin & sunlight:
No problems expected.

Driving, piloting or hazardous work:
Don't drive or pilot aircraft until you learn how medicine affects you. Don't work around dangerous machinery. Don't climb ladders or work in high places. Danger increases if you drink alcohol or take medicine affecting alertness and reflexes, such as antihistamines, tranquilizers, sedatives, pain medicine, narcotics and mind-altering drugs.

Discontinuing:
May be unnecessary to finish medicine. Follow doctor's instructions.

Others:
Great potential for abuse.

POSSIBLE INTERACTION WITH OTHER DRUGS

GENERIC NAME OR DRUG CLASS	COMBINED EFFECT
Analgesics*	Increased analgesic effect.
Antidepressants*	Increased sedation.
Antihistamines*	Increased sedation.
Carteolol	Increased narcotic effect. Dangerous sedation.
Central nervous system (CNS) depressants*	Increased central nerve system depression.
Clozapine	Toxic effect on the central nervous system.
Ethinamate	Dangerous increased effects of ethinamate. Avoid combining.
Fluoxetine	Increased depressant effects of both drugs.
Guanfacine	May increase depressant effects of either medicine.
Leucovorin	High alcohol content of leucovorin may cause adverse effects.
Methyprylon	May increase sedative effect to dangerous level. Avoid.
Mind-altering drugs*	Increased sedation.
Nabilone	Greater depression of central nervous system.
Narcotics, other*	Increased narcotic effect.
Phenothiazines*	Increased sedative effect of paregoric.
Sedatives*	Excessive sedation.
Sertraline	Increased depressive effects of both drugs.
Sleep inducers*	Increased effect of sleep inducers.
Sotalol	Increased narcotic effect. Dangerous sedation.
Tranquilizers*	Increased tranquilizer effect.

POSSIBLE INTERACTION WITH OTHER SUBSTANCES

INTERACTS WITH	COMBINED EFFECT
Alcohol:	Increases alcohol's intoxicating effect. Avoid.
Beverages:	None expected.
Cocaine:	None expected.
Foods:	None expected.
Marijuana:	Impairs physical and mental performance.
Tobacco:	None expected.

PEDICULISIDES (Topical)

BRAND AND GENERIC NAMES

A-200 Gel	Nix Creme Rinse
A-200 Shampoo	Ovide
Barc	PMS Lindane
Bio-Well	PERMETHRIN
Blue	Prioderm
Derbac	Pronto Lice Killing
Elimite Cream	Shampoo Kit
GBH	PYRETHRINS AND
G-well	PIPERONYL
Kwell	BUTOXIDE
Kwellada	Pyrinyl
Kwildane	R&C
Lice-Enz Foam and	RID
Comb Lice Killing	Scabene
Shampoo Kit	Thionex
Licetrol	TISIT
LINDANE	TISIT BLue
MALATHION	Triple X

BASIC INFORMATION

Habit forming? No
Prescription needed? Yes
Available as generic? Yes, some
Drug class: Pediculiside, scabicide

USES

- Treats scabies and lice infections of skin or scalp.
- Cream and lotion treats scabies.
- Shampoo treats lice infections.
- Carefully read patient instructions contained in package.

OVERDOSE

SYMPTOMS:
Rarely (toxic effects from too much absorbed through skin)—Vomiting, muscle cramps, dizziness, seizure, rapid heartbeat.
WHAT TO DO:
- **Not for internal use. If child accidentally swallows, call poison-control center.**
- **Dial 0 (operator) or 911 (emergency) for an ambulance or medical help. Then give first aid immediately.**
- **See emergency information on inside covers.**

DOSAGE & USAGE INFORMATION

How to use:
- Follow package directions.
- Wear plastic gloves when you apply.
- Bathe before applying.
- Use in well ventilated room.
- Use care not to apply more than directed.

When to use:
As directed on package.

If you forget a dose:
Use as soon as you remember.

What drug does:
Becomes absorbed into bodies of lice and scabies organisms, stimulates their central nervous system causing convulsions and death. Does not affect humans in this way.

Time lapse before drug works:
Cream or lotion requires 8 to 12 hours contact with skin.

Don't use with:
Other medicines for scabies or lice.

POSSIBLE ADVERSE REACTIONS OR SIDE EFFECTS

SYMPTOMS	WHAT TO DO
Life-threatening	
None expected.	
Common	
None expected.	
Infrequent	
None expected.	
Rare	
Skin irritation or rash.	Discontinue. Call doctor right away.

WARNINGS & PRECAUTIONS

Don't use if:
You are allergic to any medicine with lindane, pyrethrins or piperonyl butoxide.

Before you start, consult your doctor:
- If you are allergic to anything that touches your skin.
- If you are using any other medicines, creams, lotions or oils.

Over age 60:
Adverse reactions and side effects may be more frequent and severe than in younger persons. Ask doctor about smaller doses.

Pregnancy:
Avoid. May be absorbed through skin and harm baby.

Breast-feeding:
Drug filters into milk. May harm child. Avoid if possible.

Infants & children:
More likely to be toxic. Use only under close medical supervision.

Prolonged use:
Not recommended. Avoid.

Skin & sunlight:
No problems expected, but check with doctor.

Driving, piloting or hazardous work:
No problems expected, but check with doctor.

Discontinuing:
No problems expected, but check with doctor.

Others:
- Don't use on open sores or wounds.
- Put on freshly dry cleaned or washed clothing after treatment.
- After treatment, boil all bed sheets, covers and towels before using.
- Store items that can't be washed or cleaned in plastic bags for 2 weeks.
- Avoid inhaling or swallowing.
- Thoroughly clean house.
- Wash combs and hairbrushes in hot soapy water. Don't share with others.

POSSIBLE INTERACTION WITH OTHER DRUGS

GENERIC NAME OR DRUG CLASS	COMBINED EFFECT
Antimyasthenics*	Excessive absorption and chance of toxicity (with malathion only).
Cholinesterase inhibitors*	Excessive absorption and chance of toxicity (with malathion only).

POSSIBLE INTERACTION WITH OTHER SUBSTANCES

INTERACTS WITH	COMBINED EFFECT
Alcohol:	None expected.
Beverages:	None expected.
Cocaine:	None expected.
Foods:	None expected.
Marijuana:	None expected.
Tobacco:	None expected.

*See Glossary

PEMOLINE

BRAND NAMES

Cylert   Cylert Chewable

BASIC INFORMATION

Habit forming? Yes
Prescription needed? Yes
Available as generic? No
Drug class: Central nervous system
stimulant

USES

- Decreases overactivity and lengthens attention span in hyperactive children.
- Treatment of minimal brain dysfunction.

DOSAGE & USAGE INFORMATION

How to take:
- Tablet—Swallow with liquid or food to lessen stomach irritation. If you can't swallow whole, crumble tablet and take with liquid or food.
- Chewable tablets—Chew well before swallowing.

When to take:
At the same times each day.

If you forget a dose:
Take as soon as you remember up to 2 hours late. If more than 2 hours, wait for next scheduled dose (don't double this dose).

What drug does:
Stimulates brain to improve alertness, concentration and attention span. Calms the hyperactive child.

Continued next column

OVERDOSE

SYMPTOMS:
Rapid heartbeat, hallucinations, fever, confusion, convulsions, coma.
WHAT TO DO:
- **Dial 0 (operator) or 911 (emergency) for an ambulance or medical help. Then give first aid immediately.**
- **If patient is unconscious and not breathing, give mouth-to-mouth breathing. If there is no heartbeat, use cardiac massage and mouth-to-mouth breathing (CPR). Don't try to make patient vomit. If you can't get help quickly, take patient to nearest emergency facility.**
- **See emergency information on inside covers.**

Time lapse before drug works:
- 1 month or more for maximum effect on child.
- 30 minutes to stimulate adults.

Don't take with:
Any other medicine without consulting your doctor or pharmacist.

POSSIBLE ADVERSE REACTIONS OR SIDE EFFECTS

SYMPTOMS	WHAT TO DO
Life-threatening:	
In case of overdose, see previous column.	
Common:	
Insomnia.	Continue. Call doctor when convenient.
Infrequent:	
• Irritability, depression dizziness, headache, drowsiness, unusual movement of eyes, rapid heartbeat.	Discontinue. Call doctor right away.
• Rash, unusual movements of tongue, appetite loss, abdominal pain, nausea, weight loss.	Continue. Call doctor when convenient.
Rare:	
• Seizures.	Discontinue. Seek emergency treatment.
• Abnormal muscular movements, jaundice, hallucinations.	Discontinue. Call doctor right away.

WARNINGS & PRECAUTIONS

Don't take if:
You are allergic to pemoline.

Before you start, consult your doctor:
- If you have liver disease.
- If you have kidney disease.
- If patient younger than 6 years.
- If there is marked emotional instability.

Over age 60:
Adverse reactions and side effects may be more frequent and severe than in younger persons.

Pregnancy:
No proven harm to unborn child. Avoid if possible.

Breast-feeding:
No problems expected. Consult doctor.

Infants & children:
Use only under close medical supervision for children 6 or older.

Prolonged use:
- Rare possibility of physical growth retardation.
- Talk to your doctor about the need for follow-up medical examinations or laboratory studies to check liver function, growth charts.

Skin & sunlight:
No problems expected.

Driving, piloting or hazardous work:
Don't drive or pilot aircraft until you learn how medicine affects you. Don't work around dangerous machinery. Don't climb ladders or work in high places. Danger increases if you drink alcohol or take medicine affecting alertness and reflexes, such as antihistamines, tranquilizers, sedatives, pain medicine, narcotics and mind-altering drugs.

Discontinuing:
- Don't discontinue without consulting doctor. Dose may require gradual reduction if you have taken drug for a long time. Doses of other drugs may also require adjustment.
- If you notice any of the following symptoms after discontinuing, notify your doctor: Mental depression (severe), tiredness or weakness.

Others:
Dose must be carefully adjusted by doctor.

POSSIBLE INTERACTION WITH OTHER DRUGS

GENERIC NAME OR DRUG CLASS	COMBINED EFFECT
Loxapine	May increase toxic effects of both drugs.
Nabilone	Greater depression of central nervous system.

POSSIBLE INTERACTION WITH OTHER SUBSTANCES

INTERACTS WITH	COMBINED EFFECT
Alcohol:	More chance of depression. Avoid.
Beverages: Caffeine drinks.	May raise blood pressure. Avoid.
Cocaine:	Convulsions or excessive nervousness.
Foods:	No problems expected.
Marijuana:	Unknown.
Tobacco:	Unknown.

PENICILLAMINE

BRAND NAMES

Cuprimine
Depen

Distamine
Pendramine

BASIC INFORMATION

Habit forming? No
Prescription needed? Yes
Available as generic? No
Drug class: Chelating agent, antirheumatic,
antidote (heavy metal)

 USES

- Treatment for rheumatoid arthritis.
- Prevention of kidney stones.
- Treatment for heavy metal poisoning.

 DOSAGE & USAGE INFORMATION

How to take:
Tablets or capsules—With liquid on an empty
stomach 1 hour before or 2 hours after eating.

When to take:
At the same times each day.

If you forget a dose:
- 1 dose a day—Take as soon as you
remember up to 12 hours late. If more than
12 hours, wait for next scheduled dose (don't
double this dose).
- More than 1 dose a day—Take as soon as
you remember up to 2 hours late. If more
than 2 hours, wait for next scheduled dose
(don't double this dose).

What drug does:
- Combines with heavy metals so kidney can
excrete them.
- Combines with cysteine (amino acid found in
many foods) to prevent cysteine kidney
stones.
- May improve protective function of some
white-blood cells against rheumatoid arthritis.

Continued next column

 OVERDOSE

SYMPTOMS:
**Ulcers, sores, convulsions, coughing up
blood, coma.**
WHAT TO DO:
- **Dial 0 (operator) or 911 (emergency) for
an ambulance or medical help. Then give
first aid immediately.**
- **See emergency information on inside
covers.**

Time lapse before drug works:
2 to 3 months.

Don't take with:
Any other medicine without consulting your
doctor or pharmacist.

 POSSIBLE ADVERSE REACTIONS OR SIDE EFFECTS

SYMPTOMS	WHAT TO DO
Life-threatening:	
In case of overdose, see previous column.	
Common:	
Rash, itchy skin, swollen lymph glands, appetite loss, nausea, diarrhea, vomiting, decreased taste.	Discontinue. Call doctor right away.
Infrequent:	
Sore throat, fever, unusual bruising, swollen feet or legs, bloody or cloudy urine, weight gain, fatigue, weakness, joint pain.	Discontinue. Call doctor right away.
Rare:	
Double or blurred vision; pain; ringing in ears; ulcers, sores, white spots in mouth; difficult breathing; coughing up blood; jaundice; abdominal pain; skin blisters; peeling skin.	Discontinue. Call doctor right away.

PENICILLAMINE

WARNINGS & PRECAUTIONS

Don't take if:
- You are allergic to penicillamine.
- You have severe anemia.

Before you start, consult your doctor:
- If you have kidney disease.
- If you are allergic to any pencillin antibiotic.

Over age 60:
More likely to damage blood cells and kidneys.

Pregnancy:
Risk to unborn child outweighs drug benefits. Don't use.

Breast-feeding:
Safety not established. Consult doctor.

Infants & children:
Use only under medical supervision.

Prolonged use:
- May damage blood cells, kidney, liver.
- Talk to your doctor about the need for follow-up medical examinations or laboratory studies to check complete blood counts (white blood cell count, platelet count, red blood cell count, hemoglobin, hematocrit), kidney function, liver function.

Skin & sunlight:
No problems expected.

Driving, piloting or hazardous work:
No problems expected.

Discontinuing:
No problems expected.

Others:
Request laboratory studies on blood and urine every 2 weeks. Kidney- and liver-function studies recommended every 6 months.

POSSIBLE INTERACTION WITH OTHER DRUGS

GENERIC NAME OR DRUG CLASS	COMBINED EFFECT
Clozapine	Toxic effect on bone marrow.
Flecainide	Possible decreased blood cell production in bone marrow.
Gold compounds*	Damage to blood cells and kidney.
Immuno-suppressants*	Damage to blood cells and kidney.
Iron supplements*	Decreased effect of penicillamine. Wait 2 hours between doses.
Oxyphenbutazone	Damage to blood cells and kidney.
Phenylbutazone	Damage to blood cells and kidney.
Quinine	Damage to blood cells and kidney.
Tiopronin	Increased risk of toxicity to bone marrow and kidneys.
Tocainide	Possible decreased blood-cell production in bone marrow.
Zinc supplements	Increased need for zinc.

POSSIBLE INTERACTION WITH OTHER SUBSTANCES

INTERACTS WITH	COMBINED EFFECT
Alcohol:	Increased side effects of penicillamine.
Beverages:	None expected.
Cocaine:	Increased side effects of penicillamine.
Foods:	Possible decreased penicillamine effect by decreased absorption.
Marijuana:	Increased side effects of penicillamine.
Tobacco:	None expected.

*See Glossary

PENICILLIN G

BRAND AND GENERIC NAMES

Ayercillin
Bicillin
Bicillin L.A.
Crystapen
Crysticillin
Duracillin
Duracillin A.S.
Megacillin

Novopen-G
Pentids
Permapen
Pfizerpen
Pfizerpen-AS
PIPERACILLIN
Pipracil
Wycillin

BASIC INFORMATION

Habit forming? No
Prescription needed? Yes
Available as generic? Yes
Drug class: Antibiotic (penicillin)

 ## USES

Treatment of bacterial infections that are
susceptible to penicillin G.

 ## DOSAGE & USAGE INFORMATION

How to take:
- Tablet—Swallow with liquid on an empty
  stomach 1 hour before or 2 hours after
  eating.
- Liquid—Take with cold beverage. Liquid form
  is perishable and effective for only 7 days at
  room temperature. Effective for 14 days if
  stored in refrigerator. Don't freeze.

When to take:
Follow instructions on prescription label or side
of package. Doses should be evenly spaced.
For example, 4 times a day means every 6
hours.

If you forget a dose:
Take as soon as you remember. Continue
regular schedule.

What drug does:
Destroys susceptible bacteria. Does not kill
viruses.

Continued next column

 ## OVERDOSE

SYMPTOMS:
Severe diarrhea, nausea or vomiting.
WHAT TO DO:
**Overdose unlikely to threaten life. If person
takes much larger amount than prescribed,
call doctor, poison-control center or
hospital emergency room for instructions.**

Time lapse before drug works:
May be several days before medicine affects
infection.

Don't take with:
Any other medicine without consulting your
doctor or pharmacist.

 ## POSSIBLE ADVERSE REACTIONS OR SIDE EFFECTS

SYMPTOMS	WHAT TO DO
Life-threatening:	
Hives, rash, intense itching, faintness soon after a dose (anaphylaxis).	Seek emergency treatment immediately.
Common:	
Dark or discolored tongue.	Continue. Tell doctor at next visit.
Infrequent:	
• Mild nausea, vomiting, diarrhea.	Continue. Call doctor when convenient.
• Bloody urine, face and ankle swelling.	Discontinue. Call doctor right away.
Rare:	
Unexplained bleeding or bruising, weakness, sore throat, fever, abdominal cramps, convulsions.	Discontinue. Call doctor right away.

WARNINGS & PRECAUTIONS

Don't take if:
You are allergic to penicillin G, cephalosporin antibiotics, other penicillins. Life-threatening reaction may occur.

Before you start, consult your doctor:
- If you are allergic to any substance or drug.
- If you take birth control pills.

Over age 60:
You may have skin reactions, particularly around genitals and anus.

Pregnancy:
Studies inconclusive on harm to unborn child. Animal studies show fetal abnormalities. Decide with your doctor whether drug benefits justify risk to unborn child.

Breast-feeding:
Drug passes into milk. Child may become sensitive to penicillins and have allergic reactions to penicillin drugs. Avoid penicillin G or discontinue nursing until you finish medicine. Consult doctor for advice on maintaining milk supply.

Infants & children:
No problems expected.

Prolonged use:
- You may become more susceptible to infections caused by germs not responsive to penicillin G.
- Talk to your doctor about the need for follow-up medical examinations or laboratory studies to check SGPT*, SGOT*.

Skin & sunlight:
No problems expected.

Driving, piloting or hazardous work:
Usually not dangerous. Most hazardous reactions likely to occur a few minutes after taking penicillin G.

Discontinuing:
Don't discontinue without doctor's advice until you complete prescribed dose, even though symptoms diminish or disappear.

Others:
- Urine sugar test for diabetes may show false positive result.
- Birth control pills may not be effective. Use additional birth-control methods.

POSSIBLE INTERACTION WITH OTHER DRUGS

GENERIC NAME OR DRUG CLASS	COMBINED EFFECT
Beta-adrenergic blockers*	Increased chance of anaphylaxis (see emergency information on inside front cover).
Birth control pills	Impaired contraceptive efficiency.
Calcium supplements*	Decreased penicillin effect.
Chloramphenicol	Decreased effect of both drugs.
Cholestyramine	May decrease penicillin effect.
Colestipol	May decrease penicillin effect.
Erythromycins*	Decreased effect of both drugs.
Paromomycin	Decreased effect of both drugs.
Probenecid	Increased effect of all penicillins.
Sodium benzoate & sodium phenylacetate	May reduce effect of sodium benzoate & sodium phenylacetate.
Tetracyclines*	Decreased effect of both drugs.
Troleandomycin	Decreased effect of both drugs.

POSSIBLE INTERACTION WITH OTHER SUBSTANCES

INTERACTS WITH	COMBINED EFFECT
Alcohol:	Occasional stomach irritation.
Beverages:	None expected.
Cocaine:	No proven problems.
Foods: Acidic fruits or juices, aged cheese, wines, syrups (if taken with).	Decreased antibiotic effect.
Marijuana:	No proven problems.
Tobacco:	None expected.

*See Glossary

PENICILLIN V

BRAND NAMES

Apo-Pen-VK
Beepen-VK
Betapen-VK
Ledercillin VK
Nadopen-V
Novapen V
Novopen-VK
Pen Vee
Pen Vee K

Phenoxymethyl-
  penicillin
PVF
PVF K
Robicillin VK
V-Cillin K
VC-K
Veetids

BASIC INFORMATION

Habit forming? No
Prescription needed? Yes
Available as generic? Yes
Drug class: Antibiotic (penicillin)

 USES

- Treatment of bacterial infections that are susceptible to penicillin V.
- Prevention of streptococcal infections in susceptible persons such as those with heart valves damaged by rheumatic fever.

 DOSAGE & USAGE INFORMATION

How to take:
- Tablet—Swallow with liquid on an empty stomach 1 hour before meals or 2 hours after eating.
- Liquid—Take with cold beverage. Liquid form is perishable and effective for only 7 days at room temperature. Effective for 14 days if stored in refrigerator. Don't freeze.

When to take:
Follow instructions on prescription label or side of package. Doses should be evenly spaced. For example, 4 times a day means every 6 hours.

If you forget a dose:
Take as soon as you remember. Continue regular schedule.

Continued next column

 OVERDOSE

SYMPTOMS:
Severe diarrhea, nausea or vomiting.
WHAT TO DO:
Overdose unlikely to threaten life. If person takes much larger amount than prescribed, call doctor, poison-control center or hospital emergency room for instructions.

What drug does:
Destroys susceptible bacteria. Does not kill viruses.

Time lapse before drug works:
May be several days before penicillin V affects infection.

Don't take with:
Any other medicine without consulting your doctor or pharmacist.

 POSSIBLE ADVERSE REACTIONS OR SIDE EFFECTS

SYMPTOMS	WHAT TO DO
Life-threatening:	
Hives, rash, intense itching, faintness soon after a dose (anaphylaxis).	Seek emergency treatment immediately.
Common:	
Dark or discolored tongue.	Continue. Tell doctor at next visit.
Infrequent:	
• Mild nausea, vomiting, diarrhea.	Continue. Call doctor when convenient.
• Bloody urine, face and ankle swelling.	Discontinue. Call doctor right away.
Rare:	
Unexplained bleeding or bruising, weakness, sore throat, fever, abdominal cramps, convulsions.	Discontinue. Call doctor right away.

WARNINGS & PRECAUTIONS

Don't take if:
You are allergic to penicillin V, cephalosporin antibiotics, other penicillins or penicillamine. Life-threatening reaction may occur.

Before you start, consult your doctor:
- If you are allergic to any substance or drug.
- If you take birth control pills.

Over age 60:
You may have skin reactions, particularly around genitals and anus.

Pregnancy:
Studies inconclusive on danger to unborn child. Decide with your doctor whether drug benefits justify risk to unborn child.

Breast-feeding:
Drug passes into milk. Child may become sensitive to penicillin. Child more likely to have future allergic reactions to penicillin. Avoid penicillin V or discontinue nursing until you finish medicine. Consult doctor for advice on maintaining milk supply.

Infants & children:
No problems expected.

Prolonged use:
- You may become more susceptible to infections caused by germs not responsive to penicillin V.
- Talk to your doctor about the need for follow-up medical examinations or laboratory studies to check SGPT*, SGOT*.

Skin & sunlight:
No problems expected.

Driving, piloting or hazardous work:
Usually not dangerous. Most hazardous reactions likely to occur a few minutes after taking penicillin V.

Discontinuing:
Don't discontinue without doctor's advice until you have finished prescribed dose, even if symptoms diminish or disappear.

Others:
- May interfere with the accuracy of some medical tests.
- Birth control pills may not be effective. Use additional birth-control methods.

POSSIBLE INTERACTION WITH OTHER DRUGS

GENERIC NAME OR DRUG CLASS	COMBINED EFFECT
Beta-adrenergic blockers*	Increased chance of anaphylaxis (see emergency information on inside front cover).
Birth control pills	Impaired contraceptive efficiency.
Calcium supplements*	Decreased penicillin effect.
Chloramphenicol	Decreased effect of both drugs.
Cholestyramine	May decrease penicillin effect.
Colestipol	May decrease penicillin effect.
Erythromycins*	Decreased effect of both drugs.
Paromomycin	Decreased effect of both drugs.
Probenecid	Increased effect of all penicillins.
Sodium benzoate & sodium phenylacetate	May reduce effect of sodium benzoate & sodium phenylacetate.
Tetracyclines*	Decreased effect of both drugs.
Troleandomycin	Decreased effect of both drugs.

POSSIBLE INTERACTION WITH OTHER SUBSTANCES

INTERACTS WITH	COMBINED EFFECT
Alcohol:	Occasional stomach irritation.
Beverages:	None expected.
Cocaine:	No proven problems.
Foods: Acidic fruits or juices, aged cheese, wines, syrups (if taken with).	Decreased antibiotic effect.
Marijuana:	No proven problems.
Tobacco:	None expected.

PENTAMIDINE

BRAND NAMES

NebuPent   Pentacarinat
Pentam

BASIC INFORMATION

Habit forming? No
Prescription needed? Yes
Available as generic? No
Drug class: Antiprotozoal

USES

- Treats pneumocystis carinii, which is common in AIDS patients.
- Treats some tropical diseases such as leishmaniasis, African sleeping sickness and others.

DOSAGE & USAGE INFORMATION

How to take:
- Injection—Intramuscular or intravenous.
- Inhalation—Follow package instructions.

When to take:
According to doctor's instructions.

If you forget a dose:
Not likely to happen.

What drug does:
Interferes with RNA and DNA of infecting organisms.

Time lapse before drug works:
30 minutes to 1 hour.

Don't take with:
Any other medicines (including over-the-counter drugs such as cough and cold medicines, laxatives, antacids, diet pills, caffeine, nose drops or vitamins) without consulting your doctor.

OVERDOSE

SYMPTOMS:
None expected.
WHAT TO DO:
Overdose unlikely to threaten life. If person takes much larger amount than prescribed, call doctor, poison-control center or hospital emergency room for instructions.

POSSIBLE ADVERSE REACTIONS OR SIDE EFFECTS

SYMPTOMS	WHAT TO DO
Life-threatening:	
Unconsciousness, rapid pulse, cold sweats.	Seek emergency treatment immediately.
Common:	
• Flushed skin, fruit-like breath odor, increased thirst, increased urination, appetite loss, vision changes, chills, sweating, headache, nausea, nervousness.	Discontinue. Seek emergency treatment.
• Confusion, dizziness, fainting, hallucinations, skin rash, sore throat and fever.	Discontinue. Call doctor right away.
Infrequent:	
Hardness or pain at injection site.	Continue. Tell doctor at next visit.
Rare:	
Flushed face.	Continue. Tell doctor at next visit.

WARNINGS & PRECAUTIONS

Don't take if:
You know you are allergic to pentamidine.

Before you start, consult your doctor:
- If you have anemia or blood disorders.
- If you have heart disease, diabetes or kidney disease.

Over age 60:
Adverse reactions and side effects may be more frequent and severe than in younger persons. You may need smaller doses for shorter periods of time.

Pregnancy:
Unknown effects. Consult doctor.

Breast-feeding:
Unknown effects. Consult doctor.

Infants & children:
Unknown effects. Consult doctor.

Prolonged use:
Talk to your doctor about the need for follow-up medical examinations or laboratory studies to check blood sugar; blood pressure; kidney, liver and heart function; complete blood counts (white blood cell count, platelet count, red blood cell count, hemoglobin, hematocrit); ECG* and serum calcium.

Skin & sunlight:
No problems expected.

Driving, piloting or hazardous work:
Avoid if you feel confused, drowsy or dizzy.

Discontinuing:
No special problems expected.

Others:
- Advise any doctor or dentist whom you consult that you take this medicine.
- May affect results in some medical tests.
- Lie down during injections.
- Avoid exposure to people who have infectious diseases.

POSSIBLE INTERACTION WITH OTHER DRUGS

GENERIC NAME OR DRUG CLASS	COMBINED EFFECT
ACE inhibitors*	May increase bone marrow depression or make kidney damage more likely.
Antineoplastic (cancer-treating) drugs*	May increase bone marrow depression or make kidney damage more likely.
Clozapine	Toxic effect on bone marrow.
Tiopronin	Increased risk of toxicity to bone marrow and kidneys.

POSSIBLE INTERACTION WITH OTHER SUBSTANCES

INTERACTS WITH	COMBINED EFFECT
Alcohol:	Increased likelihood of adverse reactions. Avoid.
Beverages:	No special problems expected.
Cocaine:	Increased likelihood of adverse reactions. Avoid.
Foods:	No special problems expected.
Marijuana:	Increased likelihood of adverse reactions. Avoid.
Tobacco:	No special problems expected.

*See Glossary

PENTOXIFYLLINE

BRAND NAMES

Trental

BASIC INFORMATION

Habit forming? No
Prescription needed? Yes
Available as generic? No
Drug class: Hemorrheologic agent

USES

Reduces pain in legs caused by poor circulation.

DOSAGE & USAGE INFORMATION

How to take:
Extended-release tablets—Swallow whole with water and food.

When to take:
At mealtimes. Taking with food decreases the likelihood of irritating the stomach to cause nausea.

If you forget a dose:
Take as soon as you remember up to 3 hours late. If more than 3 hours, wait for next scheduled dose (don't double this dose).

What drug does:
- Reduces "stickiness" of red blood cells and improves flexibility of the red cells.
- Improves blood flow through blood vessels.

Time lapse before drug works:
1 hour. Several weeks for full effect on circulation.

Don't take with:
- Tobacco or medicines to treat hypertension.
- Any other medicine without consulting your doctor or pharmacist.

OVERDOSE

SYMPTOMS:
Drowsiness, flushed face, fainting, nervousness, convulsions, coma.
WHAT TO DO:
- **Dial 0 (operator) or 911 (emergency) for an ambulance or medical help. Then give first aid immediately.**
- **See emergency information on inside covers.**

POSSIBLE ADVERSE REACTIONS OR SIDE EFFECTS

SYMPTOMS	WHAT TO DO
Life-threatening: Chest pain, irregular heartbeat.	Discontinue. Seek emergency treatment.
Common: None expected.	
Infrequent: • Dizziness, headache, nausea, vomiting. low blood pressure, nose bleed, swollen feet and ankles, viral-like syndrome, nasal congestion, laryngitis, rash, itchy skin, blurred vision, abdominal pain.	Discontinue. Call doctor right away.
• Insomnia, nervousness, red eyes.	Continue. Call doctor when convenient.
Rare: None expected.	

WARNINGS & PRECAUTIONS

Don't take if:
You are allergic to pentoxifylline.

Before you start, consult your doctor:
- If you are allergic to caffeine, theophylline, theobromine, aminophyllin, dyphyllin, oxtriphylline, theobromine.
- If you have angina.

Over age 60:
Adverse reactions and side effects may be more frequent and severe than in younger persons. Ask doctor about smaller doses.

Pregnancy:
Safety to unborn child unestablished. Avoid if possible.

Breast-feeding:
Drug passes into milk. Avoid drug or discontinue nursing until you finish medicine. Consult doctor for advice on maintaining milk supply.

Infants & children:
Not recommended.

Prolonged use:
No problems expected.

Skin & sunlight:
No problems expected.

Driving, piloting or hazardous work:
Wait to see if drug causes drowsiness or dizziness. If none, no problems expected.

Discontinuing:
No problems expected.

Others:
Don't smoke.

 ## POSSIBLE INTERACTION WITH OTHER DRUGS

GENERIC NAME OR DRUG CLASS	COMBINED EFFECT
Anticoagulants, oral*	Possible decreased effect of anticoagulant.
Antihypertensives* (acebutolol, alseroxylen, amiloride, atenolol, butmetanide, captopril, chlorothiazide, chlorthalidone, clonidine, cyclothiazide, guanethidine, hydralazine, methyldopa, metoprolol, spironolactone, verapamil, nadolol, oxprenolol, pindolol, propranolol, timolol)	Possible increased effect of hypertensive medication.

 ## POSSIBLE INTERACTION WITH OTHER SUBSTANCES

INTERACTS WITH	COMBINED EFFECT
Alcohol:	Unknown. Best to avoid.
Beverages: Coffee, tea or other caffeine-containing beverages.	May decrease effectiveness of pentoxifylline.
Cocaine:	Reduced pentoxifylline effect.
Foods:	None expected.
Marijuana:	Decreased effect of pentoxifylline.
Tobacco:	Decreased effect of pentoxifylline.

PERGOLIDE

BRAND NAMES

Permax

BASIC INFORMATION

Habit forming? No
Prescription needed? Yes
Available as generic? No
Drug class: Antidyskinetic

 ## USES

Treats Parkinson's disease when used together with levodopa or carbidopa.

 ## DOSAGE & USAGE INFORMATION

How to take:
Tablets—Swallow with liquid. If you can't swallow whole, crumble tablet and take with liquid or food. Instructions to take on empty stomach mean 1 hour before or 2 hours after eating.

When to take:
Follow doctor's instructions. Usually 3 times a day.

If you forget a dose:
Take as soon as you remember up to 2 hours late. If more than 2 hours, wait for next scheduled dose (don't double this dose).

What drug does:
- Stimulates dopamine receptors in the central nervous system to make them more active.
- Lowers the required dosage of carbidopa and levodopa.

Time lapse before drug works:
Not documented.

Don't take with:
Any other medicines (including over-the-counter drugs such as cough and cold medicines, laxatives, antacids, diet pills, caffeine, nose drops or vitamins) without consulting your doctor or pharmacist.

 ## OVERDOSE

SYMPTOMS:
None expected.
WHAT TO DO:
Overdose unlikely to threaten life. If person takes much larger amount than prescribed, call doctor, poison-control center or hospital emergency room for instructions.

 ## POSSIBLE ADVERSE REACTIONS OR SIDE EFFECTS

SYMPTOMS	WHAT TO DO
Life-threatening:	
Seizures, chest pain, shortness of breath.	Seek emergency treatment immediately.
Common:	
• Confusion; hallucinations; painful urination; unusual movements of face, head, hands and tongue.	Discontinue. Seek emergency treatment.
• Abdominal pain, constipation, dizziness, nasal stuffiness.	Continue. Call doctor when convenient.
Infrequent:	
Chills, diarrhea, dry mouth, appetite loss, facial swelling, increased sex drive.	Continue. Call doctor when convenient.
Rare:	
Weakness, vision changes, fainting, increased sweating, nausea and vomiting.	Discontinue. Seek emergency treatment.

WARNINGS & PRECAUTIONS

Don't take if:
You are allergic to pergolide or any ergot preparation.

Before you start, consult your doctor:
• If you have heartbeat irregularities.
• If you have hallucinations.

Over age 60:
No special problems expected.

Pregnancy:
Risk to unborn child outweighs drug benefits. Don't use.

Breast-feeding:
Not recommended. Pergolide can prevent lactation.

Infants & children:
Effect not documented. Consult your pediatrician.

Prolonged use:
Request frequent blood pressure checks.

Skin & sunlight:
No problems expected.

Driving, piloting or hazardous work:
Don't drive or pilot aircraft until you learn how medicine affects you. Don't work around dangerous machinery. Don't climb ladders or work in high places. Danger increases if you drink alcohol or take medicine affecting alertness and reflexes.

Discontinuing:
No special problems expected.

Others:
• Advise any doctor or dentist whom you consult that you take this medicine.
• May affect results in some medical tests.

POSSIBLE INTERACTION WITH OTHER DRUGS

GENERIC NAME OR DRUG CLASS	COMBINED EFFECT
Chlorprothixene	Decreased pergolide effect.
Droperidol	Decreased pergolide effect.
Flupenthixol	Decreased pergolide effect.
Haloperidol	Decreased pergolide effect.
Loxapine	Decreased pergolide effect.
Methyldopa	Decreased pergolide effect.
Metoclopropamide	Decreased pergolide effect.
Molindone	Decreased pergolide effect.
Papaverine	Decreased pergolide effect.
Reserpine	Decreased pergolide effect.
Sertraline	Increased depressive effects of both drugs.
Thiothixene	Decreased pergolide effect.

POSSIBLE INTERACTION WITH OTHER SUBSTANCES

INTERACTS WITH	COMBINED EFFECT
Alcohol:	Increased likelihood of adverse reactions. Avoid.
Beverages:	No special problems expected.
Cocaine:	Increased likelihood of adverse reactions. Avoid.
Foods:	No special problems expected.
Marijuana:	Increased likelihood of adverse reactions. Avoid.
Tobacco:	No special problems expected.

PERPHENAZINE & AMITRIPTYLINE

BRAND NAMES

Elavil Plus
Etrafon
PMS Levazine

Proavil
Triamed
Triavil

BASIC INFORMATION

Habit forming? No
Prescription needed? Yes
Available as generic? Yes
Drug class: Tranquilizer (phenothiazine),
antidepressant

USES

- Decreases nausea, vomiting, hiccups.
- Gradually relieves, but doesn't cure, symptoms of depression, anxiety, agitation.
- Pain relief (sometimes).

DOSAGE & USAGE INFORMATION

How to take:
Tablet or liquid—Swallow with liquid.

When to take:
At the same time each day.

If you forget a dose:
Bedtime dose—If you forget your once-a-day bedtime dose, don't take it more than 3 hours late. If more than 3 hours, wait for next scheduled dose (don't double this dose).

What drug does:
- Suppresses brain's vomiting center.
- Suppresses brain centers that control abnormal emotions and behavior.
- Probably affects part of brain that controls messages between nerve cells.

Continued next column

OVERDOSE

SYMPTOMS:
Stupor, convulsions, hallucinations, coma.
WHAT TO DO:
- Dial 0 (operator) or 911 (emergency) for an ambulance or medical help. Then give first aid immediately.
- If patient is unconscious and not breathing, give mouth-to-mouth breathing. If there is no heartbeat, use cardiac massage and mouth-to-mouth breathing (CPR). Don't try to make patient vomit. If you can't get help quickly, take patient to nearest emergency facility.
- See emergency information on inside covers.

Time lapse before drug works:
- Nausea and vomiting—1 hour or less.
- Nervous and mental disorders—4-6 weeks.
- Begins in 1 to 2 weeks. May require 4 to 6 weeks for maximum benefit.

Don't take with:
- Antacid or medicine for diarrhea.
- Any other medicine without consulting your doctor or pharmacist.

POSSIBLE ADVERSE REACTIONS OR SIDE EFFECTS

SYMPTOMS	WHAT TO DO
Life-threatening: Seizures; irregular heartbeat; weak pulse; fainting; muscle spasms; uncontrolled muscle movements of tongue, face and other muscles (neuroleptic malignant syndrome*).	Discontinue. Seek emergency treatment.
Common: • Headache, nausea, vomiting, irregular heartbeat, drowsiness.	Discontinue. Call doctor right away.
• Insomnia, dry mouth, "sweet tooth," decreased sweating, runny nose, constipation.	Continue. Call doctor when convenient.
Infrequent: • Hallucinations, dizziness, tremor, blurred vision, eye pain, inflamed tongue, joint pain, back pain, hiccups.	Discontinue. Call doctor right away.
• Frequent urination, diminished sex drive, breast swelling, menstrual irregularities, nasal congestion.	Continue. Call doctor when convenient.
Rare: • Rash; itchy skin; jaundice; change in vision; sore throat, fever, mouth sores; abdominal pain.	Discontinue. Call doctor right away.
• Fatigue, weakness.	Continue. Call doctor when convenient.

WARNINGS & PRECAUTIONS

Don't take if:
- You are allergic to any phenothiazine, tricyclic antidepressant.
- You have a blood or bone-marrow disease, glaucoma, prostate trouble.
- You drink alcohol.
- You have had a heart attack within 6 weeks.
- You have taken MAO inhibitors within 2 weeks.
- Patient is younger than 12.

Before you start, consult your doctor:
- If you have asthma, emphysema or other lung disorder.
- If you have an enlarged prostate, heart disease, high blood pressure, stomach or intestinal problems, overactive thyroid, liver disease.
- If you take non-prescription ulcer medicine, asthma medicine or amphetamines.
- If you will have surgery within 2 months, including dental surgery, requiring general or spinal anesthesia.

Over age 60:
Adverse reactions and side effects may be more frequent and severe than in younger persons. More likely to develop involuntary movement of jaws, lips, tongue, chewing, difficult urination. Report this to your doctor immediately. Early treatment can help.

Pregnancy:
Risk to unborn child outweighs drug benefits. Don't use.

Breast-feeding:
Drug passes into milk. Avoid drug or discontinue nursing until you finish medicine. Consult doctor for advice on maintaining milk supply.

Infants & children:
Don't give to children younger than 12.

Prolonged use:
May lead to tardive dyskinesia (involuntary movement of jaws, lips, tongue, chewing).

Skin & sunlight:
May cause rash or intensify sunburn in areas exposed to sun or sunlamp. Skin may remain sensitive for 3 months after discontinuing.

Driving, piloting or hazardous work:
Don't drive or pilot aircraft until you learn how medicine affects you. Don't work around dangerous machinery. Don't climb ladders or work in high places. Danger increases if you drink alcohol or take medicine affecting alertness and reflexes, such as antihistamines, tranquilizers, sedatives, pain medicine, narcotics and mind-altering drugs.

Discontinuing:
- Nervous and mental disorders—Don't discontinue without doctor's advice until you complete prescribed dose, even though symptoms diminish or disappear.

- Dose may require gradual reduction if you have taken drug for a long time. Doses of other drugs may also require adjustment.

Others:
No problems expected.

POSSIBLE INTERACTION WITH OTHER DRUGS

GENERIC NAME OR DRUG CLASS	COMBINED EFFECT
Anticholinergics*	Increased anticholinergic effect, increased sedation.
Anticoagulants, oral*	Increased anticoagulant effect.
Antihistamines*	Increased antihistamine effect.
Appetite suppressants*	Decreased suppressant effect.
Barbiturates*	Decreased antidepressant effect. Increased sedation.
Cimetidine	Possible increased effect and toxicity of perphenazine and amitriptyline.
Clonidine	Possible decreased clonidine effect.
Dronabinol	Increased effect of both drugs.
Ethchlorvynol	Delirium.

Continued page 955

POSSIBLE INTERACTION WITH OTHER SUBSTANCES

INTERACTS WITH	COMBINED EFFECT
Alcohol: Beverages or medicines with alcohol.	Excessive intoxication. Avoid.
Beverages: Coffee.	Reduces effectiveness.
Cocaine:	Excessive intoxication. Avoid.
Foods:	None expected.
Marijuana:	Excessive drowsiness. Avoid.
Tobacco:	None expected.

*See Glossary

PHENAZOPYRIDINE

BRAND NAMES

Azo-Cheragan	Phenazodine
Azo-Gantanol	Pyrazodine
Azo-Gantrisin	Pyridiate
Azo-Standard	Pyridium
Azo-Sulfamethoxazole	Pyronium
Azo-Sulfisoxazole	Sul-Azo
Azo-Truxazole	Urodine
Baridium	Uro-Gantanol
Eridium	Urogesic
Geridium	Viridium
Phen-Azo	

BASIC INFORMATION

Habit forming? No
Prescription needed? Yes
Available as generic? Yes
Drug class: Analgesic (urinary)

USES

Relieves pain of lower urinary-tract irritation, as in cystitis, urethritis or prostatitis. Relieves symptoms only. Phenazopyridine alone does not cure infections.

DOSAGE & USAGE INFORMATION

How to take:
Tablet—Swallow with liquid or food to lessen stomach irritation.

When to take:
At the same times each day.

If you forget a dose:
Take as soon as you remember up to 2 hours late. If more than 2 hours, wait for next scheduled dose (don't double this dose).

What drug does:
Anesthetizes lower urinary tract. Relieves pain, burning, pressure and urgency to urinate.

Time lapse before drug works:
1 to 2 hours.

OVERDOSE

SYMPTOMS:
Shortness of breath, weakness.
WHAT TO DO:
Overdose unlikely to threaten life. If person takes much larger amount than prescribed, call doctor, poison-control center or hospital emergency room for instructions.

Don't take with:
Any other medicine without consulting your doctor or pharmacist.

POSSIBLE ADVERSE REACTIONS OR SIDE EFFECTS

SYMPTOMS	WHAT TO DO
Life-threatening:	
In case of overdose, see previous column.	
Common:	
Red-orange urine.	No action necessary.
Infrequent:	
Indigestion, fatigue, weakness, dizziness, abdominal pain.	Continue. Call doctor when convenient.
Rare:	
• Rash, jaundice, bluish skin color.	Discontinue. Call doctor right away.
• Headache.	Continue. Call doctor when convenient.

WARNINGS & PRECAUTIONS

Don't take if:
- You have hepatitis.
- You are allergic to any urinary analgesic.

Before you start, consult your doctor:
If you have kidney or liver disease.

Over age 60:
Adverse reactions and side effects may be more frequent and severe than in younger persons.

Pregnancy:
No proven harm to unborn child. Avoid if possible.

Breast-feeding:
No problems expected.

Infants & children:
Not recommended.

Prolonged use:
- Orange or yellow skin.
- Anemia. Occasional blood studies recommended.

Skin & sunlight:
No problems expected.

Driving, piloting or hazardous work:
No problems expected.

Discontinuing:
May be unnecessary to finish medicine. Follow doctor's instructions.

Others:
No problems expected.

POSSIBLE INTERACTION WITH OTHER DRUGS

GENERIC NAME OR DRUG CLASS	COMBINED EFFECT
None expected.	

POSSIBLE INTERACTION WITH OTHER SUBSTANCES

INTERACTS WITH	COMBINED EFFECT
Alcohol:	None expected.
Beverages:	None expected.
Cocaine:	None expected.
Foods:	None expected.
Marijuana:	None expected.
Tobacco:	None expected.

PHENOLPHTHALEIN

BRAND NAMES

Agoral	Ex-Lax Pills
Alophen	Feen-A-Mint Gum
Correctol	Medilax
Espotabs	Modane
Evac-U-Gen	Phenolax
Evac-U-Lax	Trilax
Ex-Lax	

BASIC INFORMATION

Habit forming? No
Prescription needed? No
Available as generic? No
Drug class: Laxative (stimulant)

 ## USES

Constipation relief.

 ## DOSAGE & USAGE INFORMATION

How to take:
- Tablet or wafer—Swallow with liquid. If you can't swallow whole, chew or crumble and take with liquid or food.
- Liquid—Drink 6 to 8 glasses of water each day, in addition to one taken with each dose.
- Chewable tablets—Chew thoroughly before swallowing.

When to take:
Usually at bedtime with a snack, unless directed otherwise.

If you forget a dose:
Take as soon as you remember.

What drug does:
Acts on smooth muscles of intestine wall to cause vigorous bowel movement.

Time lapse before drug works:
6 to 10 hours.

Continued next column

 ## OVERDOSE

SYMPTOMS:
Vomiting, electrolyte depletion.
WHAT TO DO:
- **Dial O (operator) or 911 (emergency) for an ambulance or medical help. Then give first aid immediately.**
- **See emergency information on inside cover.**

Don't take with:
- Don't take within 2 hours of taking another medicine. Laxative interferes with medicine absorption.
- Any other medicine without consulting your doctor or pharmacist.

 ## POSSIBLE ADVERSE REACTIONS OR SIDE EFFECTS

SYMPTOMS	WHAT TO DO
Life-threatening:	
In case of overdose, see previous column.	
Common:	
• Rectal irritation.	Continue. Call doctor when convenient.
• Pink to orange urine.	No action necessary.
Infrequent:	
• Dangerous potassium loss (thirst, weakness, heartbeat irregularity, paralysis, and diarrhea).	Discontinue. Call doctor right away.
• Belching, cramps, nausea.	Continue. Call doctor when convenient.
Rare:	
Irritability, confusion, headache, rash, difficult breathing, irregular heartbeat, muscle cramps, unusual tiredness or weakness, burning on urination.	Discontinue. Call doctor right away.

WARNINGS & PRECAUTIONS

Don't take if:
- You have symptoms of appendicitis, inflamed bowel or intestinal blockage.
- You are allergic to a stimulant laxative.
- You have missed a bowel movement for only 1 or 2 days.

Before you start, consult your doctor:
- If you have a colostomy or ileostomy.
- If you have congestive heart disease.
- If you have diabetes.
- If you have high blood pressure.
- If you have a laxative habit.
- If you have rectal bleeding.
- If you take other laxatives.

Over age 60:
Adverse reactions and side effects may be more frequent and severe than in younger persons.

Pregnancy:
Risk to mother and unborn child outweighs drug benefits. Don't use.

Breast-feeding:
Drug passes into milk. Avoid drug or discontinue nursing until you finish medicine. Consult doctor for advice on maintaining milk supply.

Infants & children:
Use only under medical supervision.

Prolonged use:
Don't take for more than 1 week unless under a doctor's supervision. May cause laxative dependence.

Skin & sunlight:
No problems expected.

Driving, piloting or hazardous work:
No problems expected.

Discontinuing:
May be unnecessary to finish medicine. Follow doctor's instructions.

Others:
Don't take to "flush out" your system or as a "tonic."

POSSIBLE INTERACTION WITH OTHER DRUGS

GENERIC NAME OR DRUG CLASS	COMBINED EFFECT
Antacids*	Tablet coating may dissolve too rapidly, irritating stomach or bowel.
Antihypertensives*	May cause dangerous low potassium level.
Digitalis	Increased digitalis toxicity due to decreased serum potassium level.
Diuretics*	May cause dangerous low potassium level.

POSSIBLE INTERACTION WITH OTHER SUBSTANCES

INTERACTS WITH	COMBINED EFFECT
Alcohol:	None expected.
Beverages: Milk.	Tablet coating may dissolve too rapidly, irritating stomach or bowel.
Cocaine:	None expected.
Foods:	None expected.
Marijuana:	None expected.
Tobacco:	None expected.

PHENOTHIAZINES

BRAND AND GENERIC NAMES

See complete list of brand and generic names in the *Brand Names Directory,* page 924.

BASIC INFORMATION

Habit forming? No
Prescription needed? Yes
Available as generic? Yes, for some.
Drug class: Tranquilizer, antiemetic (phenothiazine)

USES

- Stops nausea, vomiting, hiccups.
- Reduces anxiety, agitation.

DOSAGE & USAGE INFORMATION

How to take:
- Tablet or extended-release capsule—Swallow with liquid or food to lessen stomach irritation.
- Suppositories—Remove wrapper and moisten suppository with water. Gently insert into rectum, large end first.
- Drops or liquid—Dilute dose in beverage.

When to take:
- Nervous and mental disorders—Take at the same times each day.
- Nausea and vomiting—Take as needed, no more often than every 4 hours.

If you forget a dose:
- Nervous and mental disorders—Take up to 2 hours late. If more than 2 hours, wait for next scheduled dose (don't double this dose).
- Nausea and vomiting—Take as soon as you remember. Wait 4 hours for next dose.

What drug does:
- Suppresses brain's vomiting center.
- Suppresses brain centers that control abnormal emotions and behavior.

Time lapse before drug works:
- Nausea and vomiting—1 hour or less.
- Nervous and mental disorders—4 to 6 weeks.

Continued next column

OVERDOSE

SYMPTOMS:
Stupor, convulsions, coma.
WHAT TO DO:
- Dial 0 (operator) or 911 (emergency) for an ambulance or medical help. Then give first aid immediately.
- See emergency information on inside covers.

Don't take with:
- Antacid or medicine for diarrhea.
- Non-prescription drug for cough, cold or allergy.
- Any other medicine without consulting your doctor or pharmacist.

POSSIBLE ADVERSE REACTIONS OR SIDE EFFECTS

SYMPTOMS	WHAT TO DO
Life-threatening:	
Uncontrolled muscle movements of tongue, face and other muscles (neuroleptic malignant syndrome, rare).	Discontinue. Seek emergency treatment.
Common:	
• Muscle spasms of face and neck, unsteady gait.	Discontinue. Seek emergency treatment.
• Restlessness, tremor, drowsiness, blurred vision, lip smacking, worm-like movements of tongue.	Discontinue. Call doctor right away.
• Decreased sweating, dry mouth, stuffy nose, constipation.	Continue. Call doctor when convenient.
Infrequent:	
• Fainting.	Discontinue. Seek emergency treatment.
• Rash.	Discontinue. Call doctor right away.
• Difficult urination, decreased sex drive, swollen breasts, menstrual irregularities, dizziness.	Continue. Call doctor when convenient.
Rare:	
Vision changes, sore throat, fever, jaundice, abdominal pain, confusion, hot dry skin, prolonged penile erections.	Discontinue. Call doctor right away.

WARNINGS & PRECAUTIONS

Don't take if:
- You are allergic to any phenothiazine.
- You have a blood or bone-marrow disease.

Before you start, consult your doctor:
- If you will have surgery within 2 months, including dental surgery, requiring general or spinal anesthesia.
- If you have asthma, emphysema or other lung disorder; glaucoma; or prostate trouble.
- If you take non-prescription ulcer medicine, asthma medicine or amphetamines.

Over age 60:
Adverse reactions and side effects may be more frequent and severe than in younger persons. More likely to develop involuntary movement of jaws, lips, tongue, chewing. Report this to your doctor immediately. Early treatment can help.

Pregnancy:
Risk to unborn child outweighs drug benefits. Don't use.

Breast-feeding:
Drug passes into milk. Avoid drug or discontinue nursing until you finish medicine. Consult doctor for advice on maintaining milk supply.

Infants & children:
Don't give to children younger than 2.

Prolonged use:
- May lead to tardive dyskinesia (involuntary movement of jaws, lips, tongue, chewing).
- Talk to your doctor about the need for follow-up medical examinations or laboratory studies to check complete blood counts (white blood cell count, platelet count, red blood cell count, hemoglobin, hematocrit), blood pressure, liver function, eyes.

Skin & sunlight:
May cause rash or intensify sunburn in areas exposed to sun or sunlamp. Skin may remain sensitive for 3 months after discontinuing.

Driving, piloting or hazardous work:
Don't drive or pilot aircraft until you learn how medicine affects you. Don't work around dangerous machinery. Don't climb ladders or work in high places. Danger increases if you drink alcohol or take medicine affecting alertness and reflexes.

Discontinuing:
- Nervous and mental disorders—Don't discontinue without doctor's advice until you complete prescribed dose, even though symptoms diminish or disappear.
- Nausea and vomiting—May be unnecessary to finish medicine. Follow doctor's instructions.

Others:
- No problems expected.
- Advise any doctor or dentist whom you consult that you take this medicine.

POSSIBLE INTERACTION WITH OTHER DRUGS

GENERIC NAME OR DRUG CLASS	COMBINED EFFECT
Anticholinergics*	Increased anti-cholinergic effect.
Antidepressants, tricyclic (TCA)*	Increased phenothiazine effect.
Antihistamines*	Increased antihistamine effect.
Antihypertensives*	Severe low blood pressure.
Antithyroid agents*	Increased risk of blood disorders.
Appetite suppressants*	Decreased suppressant effect.
Bupropion	Increased risk of major seizures.
Calcium supplements*	Decreased phenothiazine effect.
Clozapine	Toxic effect on the central nervous system.
Dronabinol	Increased effects of both drugs. Avoid.
Guanethidine	Increased guanethidine effect.
Isoniazid	Increased risk of liver damage.
Levodopa	Decreased levodopa effect.
Lithium	Decreased lithium effect.
Mind-altering drugs*	Increased effect of mind-altering drugs.
Metrizamide	Increased seizures.
Metyrosine	Increased likelihood of toxic symptoms of each.
Molindone	Increased tranquilizer effect.
Nabilone	Greater depression of central nervous system.

Continued on page 955

POSSIBLE INTERACTION WITH OTHER SUBSTANCES

INTERACTS WITH	COMBINED EFFECT
Alcohol:	Dangerous over-sedation. Avoid
Beverages:	None expected.
Cocaine:	Decreased phenothiazine effect. Avoid.
Foods:	None expected.
Marijuana:	Drowsiness. May increase antinausea effect.
Tobacco:	None expected.

*See Glossary

PHENSUXIMIDE

BRAND NAMES

Milontin

BASIC INFORMATION

Habit forming? No
Prescription needed? Yes
Available as generic? No
Drug class: Anticonvulsant (succinimide)

USES

Controls seizures in treatment of epilepsy.

DOSAGE & USAGE INFORMATION

How to take:
Capsule—Swallow with liquid or food to lessen stomach irritation.

When to take:
Every day in regularly-spaced doses, according to prescription.

If you forget a dose:
Take as soon as you remember up to 2 hours late. If more than 2 hours, wait for next scheduled dose (don't double this dose).

What drug does:
Depresses nerve transmissions in part of brain that controls muscles.

Time lapse before drug works:
3 hours.

Don't take with:
Any other medicine without consulting your doctor or pharmacist.

OVERDOSE

SYMPTOMS:
Coma
WHAT TO DO:
- **Dial 0 (operator) or 911 (emergency) for an ambulance or medical help. Then give first aid immediately.**
- **If patient is unconscious and not breathing, give mouth-to-mouth breathing. If there is no heartbeat, use cardiac massage and mouth-to-mouth breathing (CPR). Don't try to make patient vomit. If you can't get help quickly, take patient to nearest emergency facility.**
- **See emergency information on inside covers.**

POSSIBLE ADVERSE REACTIONS OR SIDE EFFECTS

SYMPTOMS	WHAT TO DO
Life-threatening:	
In case of overdose, see previous column.	
Common:	
Nausea, vomiting, appetite loss, dizziness, drowsiness, hiccups, abdominal pain.	Continue. Call doctor when convenient.
Infrequent:	
Headache, irritability, mood change, tiredness.	Continue. Call doctor when convenient.
Rare:	
• Rash, sore throat, fever, unusual bleeding or bruising, depression, confusion, eye swelling, blood in urine, vaginal bleeding, gum swelling.	Discontinue. Call doctor right away.
• Swollen lymph glands.	Continue. Call doctor when convenient.

WARNINGS & PRECAUTIONS

Don't take if:
You are allergic to any succinimide anticonvulsant.

Before you start, consult your doctor:
- If you plan to become pregnant within medication period.
- If you take other anticonvulsants.
- If you have blood disease.
- If you have kidney or liver disease.

Over age 60:
Adverse reactions and side effects may be more frequent and severe than in younger persons.

Pregnancy:
Risk to unborn child outweighs drug benefits. Don't use.

Breast-feeding:
Drug passes into milk. Avoid drug or discontinue nursing.

Infants & children:
Use only under medical supervision.

Prolonged use:
Talk to your doctor about the need for follow-up medical examinations or laboratory studies to check complete blood counts (white blood cell count, platelet count, red blood cell count, hemoglobin, hematocrit), liver function, kidney function, urine.

Skin & sunlight:
No problems expected.

Driving, piloting or hazardous work:
Don't drive or pilot aircraft until you learn how medicine affects you. Don't work around dangerous machinery. Don't climb ladders or work in high places. Danger increases if you drink alcohol or take medicine affecting alertness and reflexes, such as antihistamines, tranquilizers, sedatives, pain medicine, narcotics and mind-altering drugs.

Discontinuing:
Don't discontinue without doctor's advice until you complete prescribed dose, even though symptoms diminish or disappear.

Others:
- Your response to medicine should be checked regularly by your doctor. Dose and schedule may have to be altered frequently to fit individual needs.
- Periodic blood-cell counts, kidney- and liver-function studies recommended.
- May discolor urine pink to red-brown. No action needed.

POSSIBLE INTERACTION WITH OTHER DRUGS

GENERIC NAME OR DRUG CLASS	COMBINED EFFECT
Anticonvulsants, other*	Increased effect of both drugs.
Antidepressants, tricyclic (TCA)*	May provoke seizures.
Antipsychotics*	May provoke seizures.
Haloperidol	Decreased haloperidol effect; changed seizure pattern.

POSSIBLE INTERACTION WITH OTHER SUBSTANCES

INTERACTS WITH	COMBINED EFFECT
Alcohol:	May provoke seizures.
Beverages:	None expected.
Cocaine:	May provoke seizures.
Foods:	None expected.
Marijuana:	May provoke seizures.
Tobacco:	None expected.

PHENYLEPHRINE

BRAND NAMES

See complete list of brand names in the *Brand Name Directory,* page 925.

BASIC INFORMATION

Habit forming? No
Prescription needed? No
Available as generic? Yes
Drug class: Sympathomimetic

 ## USES

Temporary relief of congestion of nose, sinuses and throat caused by allergies, colds or sinusitis.

 ## DOSAGE & USAGE INFORMATION

How to take:
According to package directions.

When to take:
As needed, no more often than every 4 hours.

If you forget a dose:
Take when you remember. Wait 4 hours for next dose. Never double a dose.

What drug does:
Contracts blood-vessel walls of nose, sinus and throat tissues, enlarging airways.

Time lapse before drug works:
5 to 30 minutes.

Don't take with:
- Non-prescription drugs for asthma, cough, cold, allergy, appetite suppressants, sleeping pills or drugs containing caffeine without consulting doctor.
- See Interaction column and consult doctor.

 ## OVERDOSE

SYMPTOMS:
Headache, heart palpitations, vomiting, blood-pressure rise, slow and forceful pulse.
WHAT TO DO:
- **Dial 0 (operator) or 911 (emergency) for an ambulance or medical help. Then give first aid immediately.**
- **See emergency information on inside covers.**

 ## POSSIBLE ADVERSE REACTIONS OR SIDE EFFECTS

SYMPTOMS	WHAT TO DO
Life-threatening:	
In case of overdose, see previous column.	
Common:	
• Fast or pounding heartbeat.	Discontinue. Call doctor right away.
• Headache or dizziness; shakiness; insomnia; burning, dryness, stinging inside nose; nervousness.	Continue. Call doctor when convenient.
Infrequent:	
Paleness.	Continue. Call doctor when convenient.
Rare:	
Unusual sweating.	Discontinue. Call doctor right away.

WARNINGS & PRECAUTIONS

Don't take if:
You are allergic to any sympathomimetic.

Before you start, consult your doctor:
- If you have high blood pressure.
- If you have heart disease.
- If you have diabetes.
- If you have overactive thyroid.
- If you have taken MAO inhibitors in past 2 weeks.

Over age 60:
Adverse reactions and side effects may be more frequent and severe than in younger persons.

Pregnancy:
Risk to unborn child outweighs drug benefits. Don't use.

Breast-feeding:
Drug passes into milk. Avoid drug or discontinue nursing until you finish medicine. Consult doctor for advice on maintaining milk supply.

Infants & children:
Use only under close supervision.

Prolonged use:
- Rebound* congestion and chemical irritation of nasal membranes.
- May cause functional dependence.
- Talk to your doctor about the need for follow-up medical examinations or laboratory studies to check blood pressure, ECG*.

Skin & sunlight:
No problems expected.

Driving, piloting or hazardous work:
No problems expected.

Discontinuing:
May be unnecessary to finish medicine. Follow doctor's instructions.

Others:
No problems expected.

POSSIBLE INTERACTION WITH OTHER DRUGS

GENERIC NAME OR DRUG CLASS	COMBINED EFFECT
Amphetamines*	Increased nervousness.
Antiasthmatics*	Nervous stimulation.
Antidepressants, tricyclic (TCA)*	Increased phenylephrine effect.
Antihypertensives*	Decreased antihypertensive effect.
Beta-adrenergic blockers*	Decreased effects of both drugs.
Digitalis	Decreased digitalis effect.
Furazolidine	Sudden, severe increase in blood pressure.
Guanadrel	Decreased effect of both drugs.
MAO inhibitors*	Dangerous blood-pressure rise.
Methyldopa	Possible increased blood pressure.
Nicotine	Decreased effect of phenylephrine.
Nitrates*	Possible decreased effects of both drugs.
Oxprenolol	Decreased effects of both drugs.
Phenothiazines*	Possible increased phenylephrine toxicity. Possible decreased phenylephrine effect.
Rauwolfia	Decreased rauwolfia effect.
Sedatives*	Decreased sedative effect.
Sympathomimetics, other*	Increased stimulant effect.
Tranquilizers*	Decreased tranquilizer effect.

POSSIBLE INTERACTION WITH OTHER SUBSTANCES

INTERACTS WITH	COMBINED EFFECT
Alcohol:	None expected.
Beverages: Caffeine drinks.	Excess brain stimulation.
Cocaine:	Excess brain stimulation.
Foods:	None expected.
Marijuana:	None expected.
Tobacco:	None expected.

PHENYLEPHRINE (Ophthalmic)

BRAND NAMES

Ak-Dilate
Ak-Nefrin
Dilatair
I-Phrine
Isopto Frin
Mydfrin

Neo-Synephrine
Ocugestrin
Ocu-Phrin
Prefrin Liquifilm
Relief

BASIC INFORMATION

Habit forming? No
Prescription needed? Yes, some strengths
Available as generic? No
Drug class: Mydriatic, decongestant

 ## USES

- High concentration drops—Dilates pupils.
- Low concentration drops (available without prescription)—Relieves minor eye irritations caused by colds, hay fever, dust, wind, swimming, sun, smog, hard contact lenses, eye strain, smoke.

 ## DOSAGE & USAGE INFORMATION

How to use:
Eye drops
- Wash hands.
- Apply pressure to inside corner of eye with middle finger.
- Continue pressure for 1 minute after placing medicine in eye.
- Tilt head backward. Pull lower lid away from eye with index finger of the same hand.
- Drop eye drops into pouch and close eye. Don't blink.
- Keep eyes closed for 1 to 2 minutes.
- Don't touch applicator tip to any surface (including the eye). If you accidentally touch tip, clean with warm soap and water.
- Keep container tightly closed.
- Keep cool, but don't freeze.
- Wash hands immediately after using.

Continued next column

 ## OVERDOSE

SYMPTOMS:
None expected.
WHAT TO DO:
Not intended for internal use. If child accidentally swallows, call poison-control center.

When to use:
As directed on label.

If you forget a dose:
Use as soon as you remember.

What drug does:
Acts on small blood vessels to make them constrict.

Time lapse before drug works:
15 to 90 minutes.

Don't use with:
- Other eye drops or ointment without consulting your eye doctor.
- Antidepressants, guanadrel, guanethidine, maprotiline, pargyline, any MAO inhibitor.

 ## POSSIBLE ADVERSE REACTIONS OR SIDE EFFECTS

SYMPTOMS	WHAT TO DO
Life-threatening None expected, unless you use much more than directed.	Discontinue. Call doctor right away.
Common None expected.	
Infrequent None expected, unless you use much more than directed. If too much is used—Burning or stinging eyes, headache, watery eyes, eye irritation not present before.	Continue. Call doctor when convenient.
Rare None expected, unless you use much more than directed. If too much gets absorbed—Paleness, dizziness, tremor, increased sweating, irregular or fast heartbeat.	Discontinue. Call doctor right away.

PHENYLEPHRINE (Ophthalmic)

WARNINGS & PRECAUTIONS

Don't use if:
- You are allergic to phenylephrine.
- You have glaucoma.

Before you start, consult your doctor:
- If you have heart disease with irregular heartbeat, high blood pressure, diabetes.
- If you take antidepressants, guanadrel, guanethidine, maprotiline, pargyline, any MAO inhibitor.

Over age 60:
Adverse reactions and side effects may be more frequent and severe than in younger persons. Ask doctor about smaller doses.

Pregnancy:
Safety to unborn child unestablished. Avoid if possible.

Breast-feeding:
Safety not established.

Infants & children:
Use only under close medical supervision.

Prolonged use:
Avoid if possible.

Skin & sunlight:
Sometimes causes increased sensitivity to sunlight.

Driving, piloting or hazardous work:
No problems expected.

Discontinuing:
No problems expected.

Others:
- Keep cool, but don't freeze.
- Consult doctor if condition doesn't improve in 3 to 4 days.

POSSIBLE INTERACTION WITH OTHER DRUGS

GENERIC NAME OR DRUG CLASS	COMBINED EFFECT
Clinically significant interactions with oral or injected medicines unlikely.	

POSSIBLE INTERACTION WITH OTHER SUBSTANCES

INTERACTS WITH	COMBINED EFFECT
Alcohol:	None expected.
Beverages:	None expected.
Cocaine:	None expected.
Foods:	None expected.
Marijuana:	None expected.
Tobacco:	None expected.

PHENYLPROPANOLAMINE

BRAND NAMES

See complete list of brand names in the *Brand Name Directory,* page 925.

BASIC INFORMATION

Habit forming? No
Prescription needed?
　High strength: Yes
　Low strength: No
Available as generic? Yes
Drug class: Sympathomimetic

USES

- Relieves bronchial asthma.
- Decreases congestion of breathing passages.
- Suppresses allergic reactions.
- Decreases appetite.

DOSAGE & USAGE INFORMATION

How to take:
- Tablet—Swallow with liquid. You may chew or crush tablet.
- Extended-release capsules—Swallow each dose whole.

When to take:
As needed, no more often than every 4 hours.

If you forget a dose:
Take up to 2 hours late. If more than 2 hours, wait for next dose (don't double this dose).

What drug does:
- Prevents cells from releasing allergy-causing chemicals (histamines).
- Relaxes muscles of bronchial tubes.
- Decreases blood-vessel size and blood flow, thus causing decongestion.

Time lapse before drug works:
30 to 60 minutes.

Continued next column

OVERDOSE

SYMPTOMS:
Severe anxiety, confusion, delirium, muscle tremors, rapid and irregular pulse.
WHAT TO DO:
- **Dial 0 (operator) or 911 (emergency) for an ambulance or medical help. Then give first aid immediately.**
- **See emergency information on inside covers.**

Don't take with:
- Non-prescription drugs for cough, cold, allergy or asthma without consulting doctor.
- See Interaction column and consult doctor.

POSSIBLE ADVERSE REACTIONS OR SIDE EFFECTS

SYMPTOMS	WHAT TO DO
Life-threatening:	
In case of overdose, see previous column.	
Common:	
• Rapid heartbeat.	Discontinue. Call doctor right away.
• Nervousness, headache, paleness.	Continue. Call doctor when convenient.
• Insomnia.	Continue. Tell doctor at next visit.
Infrequent:	
• Irregular heartbeat.	Discontinue. Call doctor right away.
• Dizziness, appetite loss, nausea, vomiting, difficult urination, nightmares, weakness.	Continue. Call doctor when convenient.
Rare:	
Tightness in chest.	Discontinue. Call doctor right away.

WARNINGS & PRECAUTIONS

Don't take if:
You are allergic to any sympathomimetic drug.

Before you start, consult your doctor:
- If you have high blood pressure, diabetes, overactive thyroid gland, difficulty urinating.
- If you have taken any MAO inhibitors in past 2 weeks.
- If you have taken digitalis preparations in the last 7 days.
- If you will have surgery within 2 months, including dental surgery, requiring general or spinal anesthesia.
- If you take any other over-the-counter medicine.

Over age 60:
More likely to develop high blood pressure, heart-rhythm disturbances, angina and to feel drug's stimulant effects.

Pregnancy:
No proven harm to unborn child. Avoid if possible.

Breast-feeding:
Safety not established. Consult doctor.

Infants & children:
Don't give to children under 6 years old.

Prolonged use:
- Excessive doses—Rare toxic psychosis.
- Men with enlarged prostate gland may have more urination difficulty.
- Talk to your doctor about the need for follow-up medical examinations or laboratory studies.

Skin & sunlight:
No known problems.

Driving, piloting or hazardous work:
No restrictions unless you feel dizzy.

Discontinuing:
May be unnecessary to finish medicine. Follow doctor's instructions.

Others:
No problems expected.

POSSIBLE INTERACTION WITH OTHER DRUGS

GENERIC NAME OR DRUG CLASS	COMBINED EFFECT
Anesthetics, general*	Increased phenyl-propanolamine effect.
Antidepressants, tricyclic (TCA)*	Increased effect of phenylpropanolamine. Excessive stimulation of heart and blood pressure.
Antihypertensives*	Decreased antihypertensive effect.
Beta-adrenergic blockers*	Decreased effects of both drugs.
Digitalis preparations*	Serious heart-rhythm disturbances.
Epinephrine	Increased epinephrine effect.
Ergot preparations*	Serious blood-pressure rise.

Guanethidine	Decreased effect of both drugs.
Guanadrel	Decreased effect of both drugs.
MAO inhibitors*	Increased phenyl-propanolamine effect. Dangerous blood-pressure rise.
Methyldopa	Possible increased blood pressure.
Nitrates*	Possible decreased effects of both drugs.
Phenothiazines*	Possible increased phenylpropanolamine toxicity. Possible decreased phenylpropanolamine effect.
Rauwolfia	Decreased rauwolfia effect.
Sympathomimetics*	Increased phenylpropanolamine effect.
Terazosin	Decreases effectiveness of terazosin.

POSSIBLE INTERACTION WITH OTHER SUBSTANCES

INTERACTS WITH	COMBINED EFFECT
Alcohol:	Increased sedation.
Beverages: Caffeine drinks.	Nervousness or insomnia.
Cocaine:	High risk of heartbeat irregularities and high blood pressure.
Foods:	None expected.
Marijuana:	Rapid heartbeat, possible heart-rhythm disturbance. Avoid.
Tobacco:	None expected.

PHENYTOIN

BRAND NAMES

Dilantin
Dilantin Infatabs
Dilantin Kapseals
Dilantin-125

Dilantin-30-Pediatric
Diphenylan
Diphenylhydantoin

BASIC INFORMATION

Habit forming? No
Prescription needed? Yes
Available as generic? Yes
Drug class: Anticonvulsant (hydantoin)

USES

- Prevents some forms of epileptic seizures.
- Stabilizes irregular heartbeat.

DOSAGE & USAGE INFORMATION

How to take:
- Capsule—Swallow with liquid.
- Chewable tablets—Chew carefully before swallowing.
- Suspension—Shake well before taking with liquid.

When to take:
At the same time each day.

If you forget a dose:
- If drug taken 1 time per day—Take as soon as you remember up to 12 hours late. If more than 12 hours, wait for next scheduled dose (don't double this dose).
- If taken several times per day—Take as soon as possible, then return to regular schedule.

What drug does:
Promotes sodium loss from nerve fibers. This lessens excitability and inhibits spread of nerve impulses.

Time lapse before drug works:
7 to 10 days continual use.

Don't take with:
Any other medicine without consulting your doctor or pharmacist.

OVERDOSE

SYMPTOMS:
Jerky eye movements; stagger; slurred speech; imbalance; drowsiness; blood-pressure drop; slow, shallow breathing; coma.
WHAT TO DO:
- **Dial 0 (operator) or 911 (emergency) for an ambulance or medical help. Then give first aid immediately.**
- **See emergency information on inside covers.**

POSSIBLE ADVERSE REACTIONS OR SIDE EFFECTS

SYMPTOMS	WHAT TO DO
Life-threatening: In case of overdose, see previous column.	
Common: Enlarged, tender, receding gums with increased likelihood of bleeding; nausea; vomiting; constipation; mild dizziness.	Continue. Call doctor when convenient.
Infrequent: • Hallucinations, confusion, slurred speech, stagger, rash, change in vision, agitation.	Discontinue. Call doctor right away.
• Headache, diarrhea, drowsiness, muscle twitching.	Continue. Call doctor when convenient.
• Increased body and facial hair, breast swelling, insomnia, decreased sex drive.	Continue. Tell doctor at next visit.
Rare: Sore throat, fever, abdominal pain, unusual bleeding or bruising, swollen lymph glands, jaundice.	Discontinue. Call doctor right away.

WARNINGS & PRECAUTIONS

Don't take if:
You are allergic to any hydantoin anticonvulsant.

Before you start, consult your doctor:
- If you have had impaired liver function or disease.
- If you will have surgery within 2 months, including dental surgery, requiring general or spinal anesthesia.

Over age 60:
Adverse reactions and side effects may be more frequent and severe than in younger persons.

Pregnancy:
Risk to unborn child outweighs drug benefits. Don't use.

Breast-feeding:
Drug passes into milk. Avoid drug or discontinue nursing until you finish medicine. Consult doctor for advice on maintaining milk supply.

Infants & children:
Use only under medical supervision.

Prolonged use:
- Weakened bones.
- Lymph gland enlargement.
- Possible liver damage.
- Numbness and tingling of hands and feet.
- Continual back-and-forth eye movements.
- Bleeding, swollen or tender gums.
- Talk to your doctor about the need for follow-up medical examinations or laboratory studies to check complete blood counts (white blood cell count, platelet count, red blood cell count, hemoglobin, hematocrit), liver function, EEG*.

Skin & sunlight:
May cause rash or intensify sunburn in areas exposed to sun or sunlamp.

Driving, piloting or hazardous work:
Don't drive or pilot aircraft until you learn how medicine affects you. Don't work around dangerous machinery. Don't climb ladders or work in high places. Danger increases if you drink alcohol or take medicine affecting alertness and reflexes.

Discontinuing:
Don't discontinue without consulting doctor. Dose may require gradual reduction if you have taken drug for a long time. Doses of other drugs may also require adjustment.

Others:
May cause learning disability.

POSSIBLE INTERACTION WITH OTHER DRUGS

GENERIC NAME OR DRUG CLASS	COMBINED EFFECT
Anticoagulants*	Increased effect of anticoagulant.
Antidepressants, tricyclic (TCA)*	Decreased phenytoin effect. Phenytoin dose requires adjustment.
Barbiturates*	Changed seizure pattern.
Carbamazepine	Possible increased phenytoin metabolism.
Carbonic anhydrase inhibitors*	Increased chance of bone disease.
Carteolol	Decreased carteolol effect.
Central nervous system (CNS) depressants*	Oversedation.
Chloramphenicol	Increased phenytoin effect.
Cimetidine	Increased phenytoin toxicity.

	COMBINED EFFECT
Contraceptives, oral*	Increased seizures. Menstrual irregularities.
Cortisone drugs*	Decreased cortisone effect.
Cyclosporine	May decrease cyclosporine effect.
Dextrothyroxine	Possible decreased dextrothyroxine effect.
Didanosine	Increased risk of peripheral neuropathy.
Digitalis preparations*	Decreased digitalis effect.
Disopyramide	Decreased disopyramide effect.
Disulfiram	Increased phenytoin effect.
Encainide	Increased effect of toxicity on heart muscle.
Estrogens*	Increased estrogen effect.
Fluconazole	Increased phenytoin effect.
Furosemide	Decreased furosemide effect.
Gold compounds*	Increased phenytoin blood levels. Phenytoin dose may require adjustment.
Griseofulvin	Increased griseofulvin effect.
Hypoglycemics, oral*	Possible decreased hypoglycemic effect.
Isoniazid	Increased phenytoin effect.

Continued page 956

POSSIBLE INTERACTION WITH OTHER SUBSTANCES

INTERACTS WITH	COMBINED EFFECT
Alcohol:	Possible decreased anticonvulsant effect. Use with caution.
Beverages:	None expected.
Cocaine:	Possible seizures.
Foods:	None expected.
Marijuana:	Drowsiness, unsteadiness, decreased anticonvulsant effect.
Tobacco:	None expected.

PILOCARPINE

BRAND NAMES

Adsorbocarpine
Akarpine
Almocarpine
I-Pilocarpine
Isopto Carpine
Minims Pilocarpine
Miocarpine
Ocu-Carpine

Ocusert Pilo
Pilocar
Pilokair
Pilopine HS
Piloptic
P.V. Carpine
P.V. Carpine
   Liquifilm

BASIC INFORMATION

Habit forming? No
Prescription needed?
   U.S.: Yes
   Canada: No
Available as generic? Yes
Drug class: Antiglaucoma

 ## USES

Treatment for glaucoma.

 ## DOSAGE & USAGE INFORMATION

How to take:
- Drops—Apply to eyes. Close eyes for 1 or 2 minutes to absorb medicine.
- Eye system—Follow label directions.
- Gel—Follow label directions.

When to use:
As directed on label.

Continued next column

 ## OVERDOSE

SYMPTOMS:
If swallowed—Nausea, vomiting, diarrhea, forceful urination, profuse sweating, rapid pulse, breathing difficulty, loss of consciousness.
WHAT TO DO:
- Dial 0 (operator) or 911 (emergency) for an ambulance or medical help. Then give first aid immediately.
- If patient is unconscious and not breathing, give mouth-to-mouth breathing. If there is no heartbeat, use cardiac massage and mouth-to-mouth breathing (CPR). Don't try to make patient vomit. If you can't get help quickly, take patient to nearest emergency facility.
- See emergency information on inside covers.

If you forget a dose:
Apply as soon as possible and return to prescribed schedule. Don't double dose.

What drug does:
Reduces internal-eye pressure.

Time lapse before drug works:
15 to 30 minutes.

Don't take with:
Any other medicine without consulting your doctor or pharmacist.

 ## POSSIBLE ADVERSE REACTIONS OR SIDE EFFECTS

SYMPTOMS	WHAT TO DO
Life-threatening:	
In case of overdose, see previous column.	
Common:	
Pain, blurred or altered vision.	Continue. Call doctor when convenient.
Infrequent:	
• Headache, eye irritation or twitching, nausea, vomiting, diarrhea, difficult breathing, muscle tremors.	Discontinue. Call doctor right away.
• Profuse sweating, unusual saliva flow.	Continue. Call doctor when convenient.
Rare:	
None expected.	

WARNINGS & PRECAUTIONS

Don't take if:
You are allergic to pilocarpine.

Before you start, consult your doctor:
- If you take sedatives, sleeping pills, tranquilizers, antidepressants, antihistamines, narcotics or mind-altering drugs.
- If you have asthma.
- If you have conjunctivitis (pink eye).

Over age 60:
Adverse reactions and side effects may be more frequent and severe than in younger persons.

Pregnancy:
No proven harm to unborn child. Avoid if possible.

Breast-feeding:
No proven problems. Consult doctor.

Infants & children:
Not recommended.

Prolonged use:
- You may develop tolerance for drug, making it ineffective.
- Talk to your doctor about the need for follow-up medical examinations to check eye pressure.

Skin & sunlight:
No problems expected.

Driving, piloting or hazardous work:
Don't drive or pilot aircraft until you learn how medicine affects you. Don't work around dangerous machinery. Don't climb ladders or work in high places. Danger increases if you drink alcohol or take medicine affecting alertness and reflexes, such as antihistamines, tranquilizers, sedatives, pain medicine, narcotics and mind-altering drugs.

Discontinuing:
Doctor may discontinue and substitute another drug to keep treatment effective.

Others:
- Can provoke asthma attack in susceptible individuals.
- Drops may impair vision for 2 to 3 hours.

POSSIBLE INTERACTION WITH OTHER DRUGS

GENERIC NAME OR DRUG CLASS	COMBINED EFFECT
Belladonna (ophthalmic)	Decreased pilocarpine effect.
Cyclopentolate	Decreased pilocarpine effect.

POSSIBLE INTERACTION WITH OTHER SUBSTANCES

INTERACTS WITH	COMBINED EFFECT
Alcohol:	May prolong alcohol's effect on brain.
Beverages:	None expected.
Cocaine:	Decreased pilocarpine effect. Avoid.
Foods:	None expected.
Marijuana (if prescribed):	Used once or twice weekly—May help lower internal eye pressure.
Tobacco:	None expected.

PODOPHYLLUM (Topical)

BRAND NAMES

Podofin

BASIC INFORMATION

Habit forming? No
Prescription needed? Yes
Available as generic? No
Drug class: Cytotoxic (topical)

USES

Treats venereal warts (*condylomata acuminata*).

DOSAGE & USAGE INFORMATION

How to use:
- Apply petroleum jelly on normal skin surrounding warts.
- With a glass applicator or cotton swab, carefully apply podophyllum to the warts.
- Wash hands immediately after application.
- Allow to remain on warts for 1 to 6 hours after application, then remove with soap and water.

When to use:
Follow doctor's instructions. Usually at 1-week intervals.

If you forget a dose:
Apply it as soon as you remember. Return to regular schedule.

What drug does:
Kills cells and erodes tissue.

Time lapse before drug works:
Up to 4 weeks.

Don't use with:
Any other medicines (including over-the-counter drugs such as cough and cold medicines, laxatives, antacids, diet pills, caffeine, nose drops or vitamins) without consulting your doctor.

OVERDOSE

SYMPTOMS:
The following symptoms occur when the body absorbs too much podophyllum: Seizures, painful urination, breathing difficulty, dizziness, heartbeat irregularity, hands and feet numb and tingling, abdominal pain, excitement, irritability.
WHAT TO DO:
- **Dial 0 (operator) or 911 (emergency) for an ambulance or medical help. Then give first aid immediately.**
- **See emergency information on inside covers.**

POSSIBLE ADVERSE REACTIONS OR SIDE EFFECTS

SYMPTOMS	WHAT TO DO
Life-threatening: In case of overdose, see previous column.	
Common: Burning, red skin.	Discontinue. Call doctor right away.
Infrequent: Skin rash, hallucinations, diarrhea, nausea and vomiting, unusual bleeding.	Discontinue. Call doctor right away.
Rare: In case of overdose, see previous column.	

PODOPHYLLUM (Topical)

WARNINGS & PRECAUTIONS

Don't use if:
Warts are crumbled and bleeding.

Before you start, consult your doctor:
If you have used podophyllum before.

Over age 60:
No special problems expected.

Pregnancy:
Risk to unborn child outweighs drug benefits.
Don't use.

Breast-feeding:
Drug passes into milk. Avoid drug or
discontinue nursing until you finish medicine.
Consult doctor for advice on maintaining milk
supply.

Infants & children:
No special problems expected.

Prolonged use:
Increased chance of adverse reactions.

Skin & sunlight:
No problems expected.

Driving, piloting or hazardous work:
Avoid if you feel confused, drowsy or dizzy.

Discontinuing:
No special problems expected.

Others:
- Advise any doctor or dentist whom you
  consult that you take this medicine.
- Keep away from eyes, nose and mouth.
- Don't use on moles or birthmarks.
- Don't use near heat or open flame.

POSSIBLE INTERACTION WITH OTHER DRUGS

GENERIC NAME OR DRUG CLASS	COMBINED EFFECT
None expected.	

POSSIBLE INTERACTION WITH OTHER SUBSTANCES

INTERACTS WITH	COMBINED EFFECT
Alcohol:	Increased chance of central nervous system stimulation. Avoid.
Beverages:	No special problems expected.
Cocaine:	Increased chance of central nervous system stimulation. Avoid.
Foods:	No special problems expected.
Marijuana:	Increased chance of central nervous system stimulation. Avoid.
Tobacco:	Podophyllum is flammable. Don't use while smoking.

POLOXAMER 188

BRAND NAMES

Alaxin   **Poloxalkol**

BASIC INFORMATION

Habit forming? No
Prescription needed? No
Available as generic? No
Drug class: Laxative (emollient)

 USES

Constipation relief.

 DOSAGE & USAGE INFORMATION

How to take:
Capsule—Swallow with liquid. Don't open capsules.

When to take:
At the same time each day, preferably bedtime.

If you forget a dose:
Take as soon as you remember. Wait 12 hours for next dose. Return to regular schedule.

What drug does:
Makes stool hold fluid so it is easier to pass.

Time lapse before drug works:
2 to 3 days of continual use.

Don't take with:
• Other medicines at same time. Wait 2 hours.
• Any other medicine without consulting your doctor or pharmacist.

 OVERDOSE

SYMPTOMS:
Appetite loss, nausea, vomiting, diarrhea.
WHAT TO DO:
Overdose unlikely to threaten life. If person takes much larger amount than prescribed, call doctor, poison-control center or hospital emergency room for instructions.

 POSSIBLE ADVERSE REACTIONS OR SIDE EFFECTS

SYMPTOMS	WHAT TO DO
Life-threatening: None expected.	
Common: None expected.	
Infrequent: Throat irritation (liquid only), intestinal and abdominal cramps.	Continue. Call doctor when convenient.
Rare: Rash.	Discontinue. Call doctor right away.

WARNINGS & PRECAUTIONS

Don't take if:
- You are allergic to any emollient laxative.
- You have abdominal pain and fever that might be appendicitis.

Before you start, consult your doctor:
- If you are taking other laxatives.
- To be sure constipation isn't a sign of a serious disorder.

Over age 60:
You must drink 6 to 8 glasses of fluid every 24 hours for drug to work.

Pregnancy:
No problems expected. Consult doctor.

Breast-feeding:
No problems expected.

Infants & children:
No problems expected.

Prolonged use:
Avoid. Overuse of laxatives may damage intestine lining.

Skin & sunlight:
No problems expected.

Driving, piloting or hazardous work:
No problems expected.

Discontinuing:
May be unnecessary to finish medicine. Follow doctor's instructions.

Others:
No problems expected.

POSSIBLE INTERACTION WITH OTHER DRUGS

GENERIC NAME OR DRUG CLASS	COMBINED EFFECT
Danthron	Possible liver damage.
Digitalis preparations*	Toxic absorption of digitalis.
Mineral oil	Increased mineral oil absorption into bloodstream. Avoid.
Phenolphthalein	Increased phenolphthalein absorption. Possible toxicity.

POSSIBLE INTERACTION WITH OTHER SUBSTANCES

INTERACTS WITH	COMBINED EFFECT
Alcohol:	None expected.
Beverages:	None expected.
Cocaine:	None expected.
Foods:	None expected.
Marijuana:	None expected.
Tobacco:	None expected.

POLYCARBOPHIL CALCIUM

BRAND NAMES

Equalactin   Mitrolan
FiberCon

BASIC INFORMATION

Habit forming? No
Prescription needed? No
Available as generic? No
Drug class: Laxative (bulk-forming),
   antidiarrheal

USES

- Relieves constipation and prevents straining for bowel movement.
- Stops diarrhea.

DOSAGE & USAGE INFORMATION

How to take:
- Tablets (laxative)—Swallow with 8 oz. cold liquid. Drink 6 to 8 glasses of water each day in addition to the one with each dose.
- Tablets (diarrhea)—Take without water at half-hour intervals.
- Chewable tablets—Chew well before swallowing.

When to take:
At the same times each day.

If you forget a dose:
Take as soon as you remember. Resume regular schedule.

What drug does:
Absorbs water, stimulating the bowel to form a soft, bulky stool and decreasing watery diarrhea.

Time lapse before drug works:
May require 2 or 3 days to begin, then works in 12 to 24 hours.

Don't take with:
- Any other medicine without consulting your doctor or pharmacist.
- Don't take within 2 hours of taking another medicine.

OVERDOSE

SYMPTOMS:
None expected.
WHAT TO DO:
Overdose unlikely to threaten life. If person takes much larger amount than prescribed, call doctor, poison-control center or hospital emergency room for instructions.

POSSIBLE ADVERSE REACTIONS OR SIDE EFFECTS

SYMPTOMS	WHAT TO DO
Life-threatening: None expected.	
Common: None expected.	
Infrequent: Swallowing difficulty, "lump in throat" sensation, nausea, vomiting, diarrhea.	Continue. Call doctor when convenient.
Rare: Itchy skin, rash, intestinal blockage, asthma.	Discontinue. Call doctor right away.

WARNINGS & PRECAUTIONS

Don't take if:
- You are allergic to any bulk-forming laxative.
- You have symptoms of appendicitis, inflamed bowel or intestinal blockage.
- You have missed a bowel movement for only 1 or 2 days.

Before you start, consult your doctor:
- If you have diabetes.
- If you have a laxative habit.
- If you have rectal bleeding.
- If you have difficulty swallowing.
- If you take other laxatives.

Over age 60:
Adverse reactions and side effects may be more frequent and severe than in younger persons.

Pregnancy:
Most bulk-forming laxatives contain sodium or sugars which may cause fluid retention. Avoid if possible.

Breast-feeding:
No problems expected.

Infants & children:
Use only under medical supervision.

Prolonged use:
Don't take for more than 1 week unless under a doctor's supervision. May cause laxative dependence.

Skin & sunlight:
No problems expected.

Driving, piloting or hazardous work:
No problems expected.

Discontinuing:
May be unnecessary to finish medicine. Follow doctor's instructions.

Others:
Don't take to "flush out" your system or as a "tonic."

POSSIBLE INTERACTION WITH OTHER DRUGS

GENERIC NAME OR DRUG CLASS	COMBINED EFFECT
Digitalis preparations*	Decreased digitalis effect.
Salicylates* (including aspirin)	Decreased salicylate effect.
Tetracyclines*	Decreased tetracycline effect.

POSSIBLE INTERACTION WITH OTHER SUBSTANCES

INTERACTS WITH	COMBINED EFFECT
Alcohol:	None expected.
Beverages:	None expected.
Cocaine:	None expected.
Foods:	None expected.
Marijuana:	None expected.
Tobacco:	None expected.

POTASSIUM IODIDE

BRAND NAMES

Pima
Thyro-Block

KI
SSKI

BASIC INFORMATION

Habit forming? No
Prescription needed? Yes
Available as generic? Yes
Drug class: Antihyperthyroid

 ## USES

- Treats overactive thyroid disease.
- Treats iodine deficiency.
- Formerly used to decrease thickness of bronchial secretions.

 ## DOSAGE & USAGE INFORMATION

How to take:
Take in full glass of water, fruit juice, milk or broth.

When to take:
- Take after meals and at bedtime with food or milk.
- Follow your doctor's instructions.

If you forget a dose:
Take as soon as you remember up to 2 hours late. If more than 2 hours, wait for next scheduled dose (don't double this dose).

What drug does:
Decreases release of thyroid hormone.

Time lapse before drug works:
Approximately 10 days.

Don't take with:
Any other medicines (including over-the-counter drugs such as cough and cold medicines, laxatives, antacids, diet pills, caffeine, nose drops or vitamins) without consulting your doctor.

 ## OVERDOSE

SYMPTOMS:
None expected.
WHAT TO DO:
Overdose unlikely to threaten life. If person takes much larger amount than prescribed, call doctor, poison-control center or hospital emergency room for instructions.

 ## POSSIBLE ADVERSE REACTIONS OR SIDE EFFECTS

SYMPTOMS	WHAT TO DO
Life-threatening: Black or tarry stools.	Discontinue. Seek emergency treatment.
Common: • Skin rash, swollen salivary glands.	Discontinue. Call doctor right away.
• Diarrhea, nausea, abdominal pain.	Continue. Call doctor when convenient.
Infrequent: Burning mouth, severe headache, increased salivation.	Discontinue. Call doctor right away.
Rare: Confusion, fever, heartbeat irregularities, feet and hands numb and tingling, swollen neck, unusual tiredness.	Discontinue. Call doctor right away.

WARNINGS & PRECAUTIONS

Don't take if:
You are intolerant of or allergic to potassium iodide.

Before you start, consult your doctor:
If you have kidney disease.

Over age 60:
No special problems expected.

Pregnancy:
Risk to unborn child outweighs drug benefits. Don't use.

Breast-feeding:
Drug passes into milk. Avoid drug or discontinue nursing until you finish medicine. Consult doctor for advice on maintaining milk supply.

Infants & children:
Avoid.

Prolonged use:
- Talk to your doctor about the need for follow-up medical examinations or laboratory studies to check serum potassium levels.
- If burning mouth, headache or salivation occur, discontinue and call doctor.

Skin & sunlight:
No problems expected.

Driving, piloting or hazardous work:
Avoid if you feel confused, drowsy or dizzy.

Discontinuing:
No special problems expected.

Others:
- Advise any doctor or dentist whom you consult that you take this medicine.
- Don't use if solution turns yellow.

POSSIBLE INTERACTION WITH OTHER DRUGS

GENERIC NAME OR DRUG CLASS	COMBINED EFFECT
ACE inhibitors*: captopril, enalapril, lisinopril	May raise potassium level in blood to toxic levels.
Antithyroid drugs*	Excessive effect of antithyroid drugs.
Lithium	Increased chance of producing a thyroid goiter.
Spironolactone	May raise potassium level in blood to toxic levels.
Triamterene	May raise potassium level in blood to toxic levels.

POSSIBLE INTERACTION WITH OTHER SUBSTANCES

INTERACTS WITH	COMBINED EFFECT
Alcohol:	No special problems expected.
Beverages:	No special problems expected.
Cocaine:	No special problems expected.
Foods: High in iodine.	Too much iodine in blood.
Marijuana:	No special problems expected.
Tobacco:	No special problems expected.

POTASSIUM PHOSPHATES

BRAND NAMES

K-Phos Original   Neutra-Phos K

BASIC INFORMATION

Habit forming? No
Prescription needed? Yes
Available as generic? No
Drug class: Electrolyte replenisher

USES

- Provides supplement of phosphorous for people with diseases which decrease phosphorous absorption from food.
- Treatment of hypercalcemia due to cancer.

DOSAGE & USAGE INFORMATION

How to take:
- Tablets—Dissolve tablets in 3/4 to 1 glass of water. Let tablets soak 2 to 5 minutes, then stir to completely dissolve.
- Oral solution—Follow directions on label.

When to take:
After meals or with food to prevent or lessen stomach irritation or loose stools.

If you forget a dose:
Take within 1 hour then return to original schedule. If later than 1 hour, skip dose. Don't double-dose.

What drug does:
- Provides supplemental phosphates.
- Makes uric acid.

Time lapse before drug works:
30-60 minutes.

Don't take with:
Any other medicine without consulting your doctor or pharmacist.

OVERDOSE

SYMPTOMS:
Irregular heartbeat, blood-pressure drop with weakness, coma, cardiac arrest.
WHAT TO DO:
- **Dial 0 (operator) or 911 (emergency) for an ambulance or medical help. Then give first aid immediately.**
- **See emergency information on inside covers.**

POSSIBLE ADVERSE REACTIONS OR SIDE EFFECTS

SYMPTOMS	WHAT TO DO
Life-threatening: Irregular heartbeat, shortness of breath, seizures.	Discontinue. Seek emergency treatment.
Common: Muscle cramps.	Discontinue. Call doctor right away.
Infrequent: Bone and joint pain, numbness or tingling in hands or feet, unusual tiredness, weakness, diarrhea, nausea, abdominal pain, vomiting, confusion, headache, dizziness.	Discontinue. Call doctor right away.
Rare: Foot and leg swelling.	Discontinue. Call doctor right away.

WARNINGS & PRECAUTIONS

Don't take if:
You have had allergic reaction to potassium, sodium or phosphates; severe kidney disease; severe burns.

Before you start, consult your doctor:
If you have heart problems, adrenal insufficiency, liver disease, high blood pressure, pregnancy, hypoparathyroidism, chronic kidney disease, osteomalacia, pancreatitis, rickets.

Over age 60:
Adverse reactions and side effects may be more frequent and severe than in younger persons. Ask doctor about smaller doses.

Pregnancy:
Risk to unborn child outweighs drug benefits. Don't use.

Breast-feeding:
No data available in humans.

Infants & children:
Use only under medical supervision.

Prolonged use:
Monitor ECG, serum calcium, phosphorous and potassium levels.

Skin & sunlight:
No problems expected.

Driving, piloting or hazardous work:
Avoid if medicine causes dizziness or confusion.

Discontinuing:
Don't discontinue without consulting doctor. Dose may require gradual reduction if you have taken drug for a long time. Doses of other drugs may also require adjustment.

Others:
Protect liquid medicine from freezing.

POSSIBLE INTERACTION WITH OTHER DRUGS

GENERIC NAME OR DRUG CLASS	COMBINED EFFECT
ACE inhibitors*: captopril, enalapril, lisinopril	Level of potassium in blood too high.
Antacids*	May decrease potassium absorption.
Calcium	Decreased potassium effect.
Cortisone drugs*	Increased fluid retention.
Digitalis preparations*	Level of potassium in blood too high.
Diuretics* (amiloride, spironolactone, triamterene)	Level of potassium in blood too high.
Male hormones*	Fluid retention.
Potassium supplements*	Level of potassium in blood too high.
Vitamin D (calcifidiol and calcitriol)	Level of phosphorous in blood too high.

POSSIBLE INTERACTION WITH OTHER SUBSTANCES

INTERACTS WITH	COMBINED EFFECT
Alcohol:	None expected.
Beverages: Salty drinks such as tomato juice, commercial thirst quenchers, salt substitutes.	Increased fluid retention.
Cocaine:	May cause irregular heartbeat.
Foods: Salty foods such as canned soups, potato chips, TV dinners, hot dogs, pickles.	Increased fluid retention.
Marijuana:	May cause irregular heartbeat.
Tobacco:	May aggravate irregular heartbeat.

*See Glossary

POTASSIUM & SODIUM PHOSPHATES

BRAND AND GENERIC NAMES

**DIBASIC POTASSIUM
& SODIUM
PHOSPHATES**
K-Phos M.F.
K-Phos Neutral
K-Phos 2

**MONOBASIC
POTASSIUM &
SODIUM
PHOSPHATES**
Neutra-Phos
Neutra-Phos-K
Uro-KP-Neutral

BASIC INFORMATION

Habit forming? No
Prescription needed? Yes
Available as generic? Yes
Drug class: Electrolyte replenisher

 USES

- Provides supplement of phosphorous for people with diseases which decrease phosphorous absorption from food.
- Treatment of hypercalcemia due to cancer.

 DOSAGE & USAGE INFORMATION

How to take:
- Tablets or capsules—Dissolve tablets or open capsules in 3/4 to 1 glass of water. Let tablets soak 2 to 5 minutes, then stir to completely dissolve.
- Oral solution—Take after meals with liquid to decrease stomach irritation.

When to take:
After meals or with food to prevent or lessen stomach irritation or loose stools.

If you forget a dose:
Take within 1 hour then return to original schedule. If later than 1 hour, skip dose. Don't double-dose.

Continued next column

 OVERDOSE

SYMPTOMS:
Irregular heartbeat, blood-pressure drop with weakness, coma, cardiac arrest.
WHAT TO DO:
- **Dial 0 (operator) or 911 (emergency) for an ambulance or medical help. Then give first aid immediately.**
- **See emergency information on inside covers.**

What drug does:
- Provides supplemental phosphates.
- Makes uric acid.

Time lapse before drug works:
30-60 minutes.

Don't take with:
Any other medicine without consulting your doctor or pharmacist.

 POSSIBLE ADVERSE REACTIONS OR SIDE EFFECTS

SYMPTOMS	WHAT TO DO
Life-threatening: Irregular heartbeat, difficult breathing, anxiety, weak legs, seizures.	Discontinue. Seek emergency treatment.
Common: None expected.	
Infrequent: Numbness or tingling in hands or feet, diarrhea, nausea, abdominal pain, vomiting, headache, dizziness, muscle cramps, swollen feet and ankles, thirst, weakness.	Discontinue. Call doctor right away.
Rare: Confusion.	Discontinue. Call doctor right away.

POTASSIUM & SODIUM PHOSPHATES

WARNINGS & PRECAUTIONS

Don't take if:
You have had allergic reaction to potassium, sodium or phosphates; severe kidney disease; severe burns.

Before you start, consult your doctor:
If you have heart problems, adrenal insufficiency, liver disease, high blood pressure, pregnancy, hypoparathyroidism, chronic kidney disease, osteomalacia, pancreatitis, rickets.

Over age 60:
Adverse reactions and side effects may be more frequent and severe than in younger persons. Ask doctor about smaller doses.

Pregnancy:
Risk to unborn child outweighs drug benefits. Don't use.

Breast-feeding:
No data available in humans.

Infants & children:
Use only under medical supervision.

Prolonged use:
Monitor ECG, serum calcium, phosphorous and potassium levels.

Skin & sunlight:
No problems expected.

Driving, piloting or hazardous work:
Avoid if medicine causes dizziness or confusion.

Discontinuing:
Don't discontinue without consulting doctor. Dose may require gradual reduction if you have taken drug for a long time. Doses of other drugs may also require adjustment.

Others:
Protect liquid medicine from freezing.

POSSIBLE INTERACTION WITH OTHER DRUGS

GENERIC NAME OR DRUG CLASS	COMBINED EFFECT
ACE inhibitors*: captopril, enalapril, lisinopril	Level of potassium in blood too high.
Antacids*	May decrease potassium absorption.
Calcium	Decreased potassium effect.
Cortisone drugs*	Increased fluid retention.
Digitalis preparations*	Level of potassium in blood too high.
Diuretics* (amiloride, spironolactone, triamterene)	Level of potassium in blood too high.
Male hormones*	Fluid retention.
Potassium supplements*	Level of potassium in blood too high.
Vitamin D (calcifidiol and calcitriol)	Level of phosphorous in blood too high.

POSSIBLE INTERACTION WITH OTHER SUBSTANCES

INTERACTS WITH	COMBINED EFFECT
Alcohol:	None expected.
Beverages: Salty drinks such as tomato juice, commercial thirst quenchers, salt substitutes.	Increased fluid retention.
Cocaine:	May cause irregular heartbeat.
Foods: Salty foods such as canned soups, potato chips, TV dinners, hot dogs, pickles.	Increased fluid retention.
Marijuana:	May cause irregular heartbeat.
Tobacco:	May aggravate irregular heartbeat.

POTASSIUM SUPPLEMENTS

BRAND AND GENERIC NAMES

See complete list of brand and generic names in the *Brand Name Directory*, page 926.

BASIC INFORMATION

Habit forming? No
Prescription needed? Yes
Available as generic? Yes
Drug class: Mineral supplement (potassium)

USES

- Treatment for potassium deficiency from diuretics, cortisone or digitalis medicines.
- Treatment for low potassium associated with some illnesses.

DOSAGE & USAGE INFORMATION

How to take:
- Tablet or capsule—Swallow with liquid or food to lessen stomach irritation. You may chew or crush tablet.
- Extended-release tablets or capsules—Swallow each dose whole with liquid.
- Effervescent tablets, granules, powder or liquid—Dilute dose in water.

When to take:
At the same time each day, preferably with food or immediately after meals.

If you forget a dose:
Take as soon as you remember. Don't double next dose.

What drug does:
Preserves or restores normal function of nerve cells, heart and skeletal-muscle cells, kidneys, and stomach-juice secretions.

Continued next column

OVERDOSE

SYMPTOMS:
Paralysis of arms and legs, irregular heartbeat, blood-pressure drop, convulsions, coma, cardiac arrest.
WHAT TO DO:
- **Dial 0 (operator) or 911 (emergency) for an ambulance or medical help. Then give first aid immediately.**
- **See emergency information on inside covers.**

Time lapse before drug works:
1 to 2 hours. Full benefit may require 12 to 24 hours.

Don't take with:
Any other medicine without consulting your doctor or pharmacist.

POSSIBLE ADVERSE REACTIONS OR SIDE EFFECTS

SYMPTOMS	WHAT TO DO
Life-threatening:	
In case of overdose, see previous column.	
Common:	
None expected.	
Infrequent:	
Diarrhea, nausea, vomiting, skin rash, abdominal pain.	Continue. Call doctor when convenient.
Rare:	
• Confusion; irregular heartbeat; difficult breathing; unusual fatigue; weakness; heaviness of legs; hemorrhage, perforation with enteric-coated tablets (rarely with wax matrix tablets); esophageal ulceration with tablets; bloody stools.	Discontinue. Call doctor right away.
• Numbness or tingling in hands or feet, anxiety.	Continue. Call doctor when convenient.

WARNINGS & PRECAUTIONS

Don't take if:
- You are allergic to any potassium supplement.
- You have acute or chronic kidney disease.

Before you start, consult your doctor:
- If you have Addison's disease or familial periodic paralysis.
- If you have heart disease.
- If you have intestinal blockage.
- If you have a stomach ulcer.
- If you use diuretics.
- If you use heart medicine.
- If you use laxatives or have chronic diarrhea.
- If you use salt substitutes or low-salt milk.

Over age 60:
Observe dose schedule strictly. Potassium balance is critical. Deviation above or below normal can have serious results.

Pregnancy:
No problems expected if you adhere strictly to prescribed dose.

POTASSIUM SUPPLEMENTS

Breast-feeding:
Studies inconclusive on harm to infant. Consult doctor.

Infants & children:
Use only under doctor's supervision.

Prolonged use:
- Slows absorption of vitamin B-12. May cause anemia.
- Request frequent lab tests to monitor potassium levels in blood, especially if you take digitalis preparations.

Skin & sunlight:
No problems expected.

Driving, piloting or hazardous work:
No problems expected.

Discontinuing:
Don't discontinue without consulting doctor. Dose may require gradual reduction if you have taken drug for a long time. Doses of other drugs may also require adjustment.

Others:
- Overdose or underdose serious. Frequent EKGs and laboratory blood studies to measure serum electrolytes and kidney function recommended.
- Prolonged diarrhea may call for increased dosage of potassium.
- Serious injury may necessitate temporary *decrease* in potassium.
- Some products contain tartrazine dye. Avoid, especially if you are allergic to aspirin.

POSSIBLE INTERACTION WITH OTHER DRUGS

GENERIC NAME OR DRUG CLASS	COMBINED EFFECT
ACE inhibitors*: captopril, enalapril, lisinopril	Possible increased potassium effect.
Amiloride	Dangerous rise in blood potassium.
Anticholinergics, other*	Increased possibility of intestinal ulcers, which sometimes occur with oral potassium tablets.
Atropine	Increased possibility of intestinal ulcers, which sometimes occur with oral potassium tablets.
Belladonna	Increased possibility of intestinal ulcers, which sometimes occur with oral potassium tablets.
Cortisone medicines*	Decreased effect of potassium.
Digitalis preparations*	Possible irregular heartbeat.
Diuretics, thiazide or loop*	Decreased potassium effect.
Laxatives*	Possible decreased potassium effect.
Non-steroidal anti-inflammatory drugs* (NSAIDs)	Increased risk of stomach irritation.
Spironolactone	Dangerous rise in blood potassium.
Triamterene	Dangerous rise in blood potassium.
Vitamin B-12	Extended-release tablets may decrease vitamin B-12 absorption and increase vitamin B-12 requirements.

POSSIBLE INTERACTION WITH OTHER SUBSTANCES

INTERACTS WITH	COMBINED EFFECT
Alcohol:	None expected.
Beverages: Salty drinks such as tomato juice, commercial thirst quenchers.	Increased fluid retention.
Cocaine:	May cause irregular heartbeat.
Foods: Salty foods.	Increased fluid retention.
Marijuana:	May cause irregular heartbeat.
Tobacco:	None expected.

PRAZOSIN

BRAND NAMES

Minipress

BASIC INFORMATION

Habit forming? No
Prescription needed? Yes
Available as generic? Yes
Drug class: Antihypertensive

 USES

- Treatment for high blood pressure.
- May improve congestive heart failure.
- Treatment for Raynaud's disease.

 DOSAGE & USAGE INFORMATION

How to take:
Tablet or capsule—Swallow with liquid. If you can't swallow whole, crumble tablet or open capsule and take with liquid or food.

When to take:
At the same times each day.

If you forget a dose:
Take as soon as you remember up to 2 hours late. If more than 2 hours, wait for next scheduled dose (don't double this dose).

What drug does:
Expands and relaxes blood-vessel walls to lower blood pressure.

Time lapse before drug works:
30 minutes.

Don't take with:
Any other medicine without consulting your doctor or pharmacist.

 OVERDOSE

SYMPTOMS:
Extreme weakness; loss of consciousness; cold, sweaty skin; weak, rapid pulse; coma.
WHAT TO DO:
- **Dial 0 (operator) or 911 (emergency) for an ambulance or medical help. Then give first aid immediately.**
- **If patient is unconscious and not breathing, give mouth-to-mouth breathing. If there is no heartbeat, use cardiac massage and mouth-to-mouth breathing (CPR). Don't try to make patient vomit. If you can't get help quickly, take patient to nearest emergency facility.**
- **See emergency information on inside covers.**

 POSSIBLE ADVERSE REACTIONS OR SIDE EFFECTS

SYMPTOMS	WHAT TO DO
Life-threatening:	
In case of overdose, see previous column.	
Common:	
● Rapid heartbeat.	Discontinue. Call doctor right away.
● Vivid dreams, drowsiness, dizziness.	Continue. Call doctor when convenient.
Infrequent:	
● Rash or itchy skin, blurred vision, shortness of breath, difficult breathing, chest pain.	Discontinue. Call doctor right away.
● Appetite loss, constipation or diarrhea, abdominal pain, nausea, vomiting, fluid retention, joint or muscle aches, weakness and faintness when arising from bed or chair.	Continue. Call doctor when convenient.
● Headache, irritability, depression, dry mouth, stuffy nose, increased urination.	Continue. Tell doctor at next visit.
Rare:	
Decreased sexual function, numbness or tingling in hands or feet.	Continue. Call doctor when convenient.

 WARNINGS & PRECAUTIONS

Don't take if:
- You are allergic to prazosin.
- You are depressed.
- You will have surgery within 2 months, including dental surgery, requiring general or spinal anesthesia.

Before you start, consult your doctor:
- If you experience lightheadedness or fainting with other antihypertensive drugs.
- If you are easily depressed.
- If you have impaired brain circulation or have had a stroke.
- If you have coronary heart disease (with or without angina).
- If you have kidney disease or impaired liver function.

Over age 60:
Begin with no more than 1 mg. per day for first 3 days. Increases should be gradual and supervised by your doctor. Don't stand while taking. Sudden changes in position may cause falls. Sit or lie down promptly if you feel dizzy. If you have impaired brain circulation or coronary heart disease, excessive lowering of blood pressure should be avoided. Report problems to your doctor immediately.

Pregnancy:
Studies inconclusive on harm to unborn child. Consult doctor.

Breast-feeding:
No proven problems. Consult doctor.

Infants & children:
Not recommended.

Prolonged use:
Talk to your doctor about the need for follow-up medical examinations or laboratory studies.

Skin & sunlight:
No problems expected.

Driving, piloting or hazardous work:
Don't drive or pilot aircraft until you learn how medicine affects you. Don't work around dangerous machinery. Don't climb ladders or work in high places.

Discontinuing:
Don't discontinue without doctor's advice until you complete prescribed dose, even though symptoms diminish or disappear.

Others:
First dose likely to cause fainting. Take it at night and get out of bed slowly next morning.

POSSIBLE INTERACTION WITH OTHER DRUGS

GENERIC NAME OR DRUG CLASS	COMBINED EFFECT
Amphetamines*	Decreased prazosin effect.
Antihypertensives, other*	Increased anti-hypertensive effect. Dosages may require adjustments.
Estrogen	Decreased effect of prazosin.
Guanfacine	Increased effect of both medicines.

Lisinopril	Increased antihypertensive effect. Dosage of each may require adjustment.
MAO inhibitors*	Blood pressure drop.
Nicardipine	Blood pressure drop. Dosages may require adjustment.
Nicotine	Increased prazosin effect.
Nifedipine	Weakness and faintness when arising from bed or chair.
Nimodipine	Dangerous blood pressure drop.
Nitrates*	Possible excessive blood pressure drop.
Non-steroidal anti-inflammatory drugs (NSAIDs)*	Decreased effect of prazosin.
Sotalol	Increased antihypertensive effect.
Sympathomimetics*	Decreased effect of prazosin.
Terazosin	Decreases effectiveness of terazosin.
Verapamil	Weakness and faintness when arising from bed or chair.

POSSIBLE INTERACTION WITH OTHER SUBSTANCES

INTERACTS WITH	COMBINED EFFECT
Alcohol:	Excessive blood pressure drop.
Beverages:	None expected.
Cocaine:	Increased risk of heart block and high blood pressure.
Foods:	None expected.
Marijuana:	Possible fainting. Avoid.
Tobacco:	Possible spasm of coronary arteries. Avoid.

PRAZOSIN & POLYTHIAZIDE

BRAND NAMES

Minizide

BASIC INFORMATION

Habit forming? No
Prescription needed? Yes
Available as generic? No
Drug class: Antihypertensive, diuretic (thiazide)

USES

- Controls, but doesn't cure, high blood pressure.
- Reduces fluid retention (edema) caused by conditions such as heart disorders and liver disease.
- Treatment for Raynaud's disease.

DOSAGE & USAGE INFORMATION

How to take:
Tablet or capsule—Swallow with 8 oz. of liquid. If you can't swallow whole, crumble tablet or open capsule and take with liquid or food. Don't exceed dose.

When to take:
At the same times each day.

If you forget a dose:
Take as soon as you remember up to 2 hours late. If more than 2 hours, wait for next scheduled dose (don't double this dose).

Continued next column

OVERDOSE

SYMPTOMS:
Extreme weakness; loss of consciousness; cold, sweaty skin; weak, rapid pulse; cramps; weakness; drowsiness; coma.
WHAT TO DO:
- **Dial 0 (operator) or 911 (emergency) for an ambulance or medical help. Then give first aid immediately.**
- **If patient is unconscious and not breathing, give mouth-to-mouth breathing. If there is no heartbeat, use cardiac massage and mouth-to-mouth breathing (CPR). Don't try to make patient vomit. If you can't get help quickly, take patient to nearest emergency facility.**
- **See emergency information on inside covers.**

What drug does:
- Expands and relaxes blood-vessel walls to lower blood pressure.
- Forces sodium and water excretion, reducing body fluid.
- Relaxes muscle cells of small arteries.
- Reduced body fluid and relaxed arteries lower blood pressure.

Time lapse before drug works:
4 to 6 hours. May require several weeks to lower blood pressure.

Don't take with:
- Non-prescription drugs without consulting doctor.
- See Interaction column and consult doctor.

POSSIBLE ADVERSE REACTIONS OR SIDE EFFECTS

SYMPTOMS	WHAT TO DO
Life-threatening:	
Irregular heartbeat, weak pulse, fast heartbeat, difficult breathing, chest pain.	Discontinue. Seek emergency treatment.
Common:	
Nightmares, vivid dreams, drowsiness, dizziness, dry mouth, stuffy nose.	Continue. Call doctor when convenient.
Infrequent:	
• Blurred vision, abdominal pain, nausea, vomiting, difficult breathing.	Discontinue. Call doctor right away.
• Mood change, headache, dry mouth, muscle pain, urgent urination, weakness, tiredness, weight gain or loss, runny nose, joint or muscle pain, agitation, depression, rash, appetite loss, weakness and faintness when arising from bed or chair, constipation.	Continue. Call doctor when convenient.
Rare:	
• Sore throat, fever, mouth sores; jaundice.	Discontinue. Call doctor right away.
• Diminished sex drive, numbness or tingling in hands or feet.	Continue. Call doctor when convenient.

WARNINGS & PRECAUTIONS

Don't take if:
- You are allergic to any thiazide diuretic drug or prazosin.
- You are depressed.
- You will have surgery within 2 months, including dental surgery, requiring general or spinal anesthesia.

Before you start, consult your doctor:
- If you are allergic to any sulfa drug.
- If you have gout, impaired brain circulation or have had a stroke, coronary heart disease (with or without angina), kidney disease or impaired liver function.
- If you experience lightheadedness or fainting with other antihypertensive drugs.
- If you are easily depressed.

Over age 60:
- Adverse reactions and side effects may be more frequent and severe than in younger persons, especially dizziness and excessive potassium loss.
- Don't stand while taking. Sudden changes in position may cause falls. Sit or lie down promptly if you feel dizzy. If you have impaired brain circulation or coronary heart disease, excessive lowering of blood pressure should be avoided. Report problems to your doctor immediately.

Pregnancy:
Risk to unborn child outweighs drug benefits. Don't use.

Breast-feeding:
Drug passes into milk. Avoid drug or discontinue nursing until you finish medicine. Consult doctor for advice on maintaining milk supply.

Infants & children:
Not recommended.

Prolonged use:
- You may need medicine to treat high blood pressure for the rest of your life.
- Talk to your doctor about the need for follow-up medical examinations or laboratory studies.

Skin & sunlight:
May cause rash or intensify sunburn in areas exposed to sun or sunlamp.

Driving, piloting or hazardous work:
Don't drive or pilot aircraft until you learn how medicine affects you. Don't work around dangerous machinery. Don't climb ladders or work in high places. Danger increases if you drink alcohol or take medicine affecting alertness and reflexes, such as antihistamines, tranquilizers, sedatives, pain medicine, narcotics and mind-altering drugs.

Discontinuing:
Don't discontinue without consulting doctor.

Others:
- First dose likely to cause fainting. Take it at night and get out of bed slowly next morning.
- Hot weather and fever may cause dehydration and drop in blood pressure. Dose may require temporary adjustment. Weigh daily and report any unexpected weight decreases to your doctor.
- May cause rise in uric acid, leading to gout.
- May cause blood-sugar rise in diabetics.

POSSIBLE INTERACTION WITH OTHER DRUGS

GENERIC NAME OR DRUG CLASS	COMBINED EFFECT
Acebutolol	Increased antihypertensive effect. Dosages may require adjustments.
ACE inhibitors*: captopril, enalapril lisinopril	Decreased blood pressure.
Allopurinol	Decreased allopurinol effect.
Amphetamines*	Decreased prazosin effect.
Amphotericin B	Increased potassium.
Antidepressants, tricyclic (TCA)*	Dangerous drop in blood pressure. Avoid combination unless under medical supervision.

Continued page 956

POSSIBLE INTERACTION WITH OTHER SUBSTANCES

INTERACTS WITH	COMBINED EFFECT
Alcohol:	Dangerous blood pressure drop. Avoid.
Beverages:	None expected.
Cocaine:	Increased risk of heart block and high blood pressure.
Foods: Licorice.	Excessive potassium loss that causes dangerous heart rhythms.
Marijuana:	Possible fainting, increased blood pressure. Avoid.
Tobacco:	Possible spasm of coronary arteries. Avoid.

*See Glossary

PREDNISOLONE

BRAND NAMES

See complete list of brand names in the *Brand Name Directory*, page 927.

BASIC INFORMATION

Habit forming? No
Prescription needed? Yes
Available as generic? Yes
Drug class: Cortisone drug (adrenal corticosteroid)

USES

- Reduces inflammation caused by many different medical problems.
- Treatment for some allergic diseases, blood disorders, kidney diseases, asthma and emphysema.
- Replaces corticosteroid deficiencies.

DOSAGE & USAGE INFORMATION

How to take:
Tablet or liquid—Swallow with liquid or food to lessen stomach irritation. If you can't swallow whole, crumble tablet and take with liquid or food.

When to take:
At the same times each day. Take once-a-day or once-every-other-day doses in mornings.

If you forget a dose:
- Several-doses-per-day prescription—Take as soon as you remember up to 2 hours late. If more than 2 hours, wait for next scheduled dose (don't double this dose).
- Once-a-day dose or less—Wait for next dose. Double this dose.

What drug does:
Decreases inflammatory responses.

Time lapse before drug works:
2 to 4 days.

Don't take with:
Any other medicine without consulting your doctor or pharmacist.

OVERDOSE

SYMPTOMS:
Headache, convulsions, heart failure.
WHAT TO DO:
- **Dial 0 (operator) or 911 (emergency) for an ambulance or medical help. Then give first aid immediately.**
- **See emergency information on inside covers.**

POSSIBLE ADVERSE REACTIONS OR SIDE EFFECTS

SYMPTOMS	WHAT TO DO
Life-threatening:	
Hives, rash, intense itching, faintness soon after a dose (anaphylaxis).	Seek emergency treatment immediately.
Common:	
Acne, poor wound healing, thirst, indigestion, nausea, vomiting, constipation, gaseousness, unpleasant taste, diarrhea, headache, cough, dizziness, hoarseness, appetite gain or loss.	Continue. Call doctor when convenient.
Infrequent:	
• Black, bloody or tarry stool; various infections; swallowing difficulties.	Discontinue. Seek emergency treatment.
• Blurred vision, halos around lights, sore throat, fever, muscle cramps, swollen legs or feet.	Discontinue. Call doctor right away.
• Mood change, fatigue, insomnia, weakness, restlessness, frequent urination, weight gain, round face, irregular menstrual periods, dry mouth, euphoria, nosebleeds.	Continue. Call doctor when convenient.
Rare:	
• Irregular heartbeat.	Discontinue. Seek emergency treatment.
• Rash, numbness or tingling of hands or feet, pancreatitis, hallucinations, thrombophlebitis, convulsions.	Discontinue. Call doctor right away.

WARNINGS & PRECAUTIONS

Don't take if:
- You are allergic to any cortisone drug.
- You have tuberculosis or fungus infection.
- You have herpes infection of eyes, lips or genitals.
- You have bone disease, thyroid disease, colitis, peptic ulcer, diabetes, myasthenia gravis, liver or kidney disease, diverticulitis, glaucoma, heart disease.

Before you start, consult your doctor:
- If you have had tuberculosis.
- If you have congestive heart failure, diabetes, peptic ulcer, glaucoma, underactive thyroid, high blood pressure, myasthenia gravis, blood clots in legs or lungs.

Over age 60:
Adverse reactions and side effects may be more frequent and severe than in younger persons. Likely to aggravate edema, diabetes or ulcers. Likely to cause cataracts and osteoporosis (softening of the bones).

Pregnancy:
Risk to unborn child outweighs drug benefits. Don't use.

Breast-feeding:
Drug passes into milk. Avoid drug or discontinue nursing until you finish medicine. Consult doctor for advice on maintaining milk supply.

Infants & children:
Use only under medical supervision.

Prolonged use:
- Retards growth in children.
- Possible glaucoma, cataracts, diabetes, fragile bones and thin skin.
- Functional dependence.
- Talk to your doctor about the need for follow-up medical examinations or laboratory studies to check blood pressure, serum electrolytes, stools for blood.

Skin & sunlight:
No problems expected.

Driving, piloting or hazardous work:
No problems expected.

Discontinuing:
- Don't discontinue without doctor's advice until you complete prescribed dose, even though symptoms diminish or disappear.
- Drug affects your response to surgery, illness, injury or stress for 2 years after discontinuing. Tell anyone who takes medical care of you within 2 years about drug.

Others:
- Avoid immunizations if possible.
- Your resistance to infection is less while taking this medicine.
- Advise any doctor or dentist whom you consult that you take this medicine.
- Those who have inactive or "cured" tuberculosis may be subjected to a possible recurrence of active tuberculosis.
- Children who must take cortisone drugs may grow less well.

POSSIBLE INTERACTION WITH OTHER DRUGS

GENERIC NAME OR DRUG CLASS	COMBINED EFFECT
Amphotericin B	Potassium depletion.
Anticholinergics*	Possible glaucoma.
Anticoagulants, oral*	Decreased anticoagulant effect.
Anticonvulsants, hydantoin*	Decreased prednisolone effect.
Antidiabetics, oral*	Decreased antidiabetic effect.
Antihistamines*	Decreased prednisolone effect.
Aspirin	Increased prednisolone effect.
Attenuated virus vaccines*	Possible viral infection.
Barbiturates*	Decreased prednisolone effect. Oversedation.
Beta-adrenergic blockers*	Decreased prednisolone effect.
Chloral hydrate	Decreased prednisolone effect.
Chlorthalidone	Potassium depletion.
Cholestyramine	Decreased prednisolone absorption effect.
Cholinergics*	Decreased cholinergic effect.
Colestipol	Decreased prednisolone absorption effect.
Contraceptives, oral*	Increased prednisolone effect.

Continued page 957

POSSIBLE INTERACTION WITH OTHER SUBSTANCES

INTERACTS WITH	COMBINED EFFECT
Alcohol:	Risk of stomach ulcers.
Beverages:	No proven problems.
Cocaine:	Overstimulation. Avoid.
Foods:	No proven problems.
Marijuana:	Decreased immunity.
Tobacco:	Increased prednisolone effect. Possible toxicity.

*See Glossary

PREDNISONE

BRAND NAMES

Apo-Prednisone	Prednicen-M
Deltasone	Prednisone Intensol
Liquid-Pred	Sterapred
Meticorten	Winpred
Orasone	

BASIC INFORMATION

Habit forming? No
Prescription needed? Yes
Available as generic? Yes
Drug class: Cortisone drug (adrenal corticosteroid)

 USES

- Reduces inflammation caused by many different medical problems.
- Treatment for some allergic diseases, blood disorders, kidney diseases, asthma and emphysema.
- Replaces corticosteroid deficiencies.

 DOSAGE & USAGE INFORMATION

How to take:
Tablet or liquid—Swallow with liquid or food to lessen stomach irritation. If you can't swallow whole, crumble tablet.

When to take:
At the same times each day. Take once-a-day or once-every-other-day doses in mornings.

If you forget a dose:
- Several-doses-per-day prescription—Take as soon as you remember up to 2 hours late. If more than 2 hours, wait for next scheduled dose (don't double this dose).
- Once-a-day dose or less—Wait for next dose. Double this dose.

What drug does:
Decreases inflammatory responses.

Time lapse before drug works:
2 to 4 days.

Continued next column

 OVERDOSE

SYMPTOMS:
Headache, convulsions, heart failure.
WHAT TO DO:
- **Dial 0 (operator) or 911 (emergency) for an ambulance or medical help. Then give first aid immediately.**
- **See emergency information on inside covers.**

Don't take with:
Any other medicine without consulting your doctor or pharmacist.

 POSSIBLE ADVERSE REACTIONS OR SIDE EFFECTS

SYMPTOMS	WHAT TO DO
Life-threatening:	
Hives, rash, intense itching, faintness soon after a dose (anaphylaxis).	Seek emergency treatment immediately.
Common:	
Acne, poor wound healing, thirst, indigestion, nausea, vomiting, constipation, gaseousness, unpleasant taste, diarrhea, headache, cough, dizziness, hoarseness, appetite gain or loss.	Continue. Call doctor when convenient.
Infrequent:	
• Black, bloody or tarry stool; various infections; swallowing difficulties.	Discontinue. Seek emergency treatment.
• Blurred vision, halos around lights, sore throat, fever, muscle cramps, swollen legs or feet.	Discontinue. Call doctor right away.
• Mood change, fatigue, insomnia, weakness, restlessness, frequent urination, weight gain, round face, irregular menstrual periods, dry mouth, euphoria, nosebleeds.	Continue. Call doctor when convenient.
Rare:	
• Irregular heartbeat.	Discontinue. Seek emergency treatment.
• Skin rash, fever, joint pain, acute psychosis, hair loss, pancreatitis, numbness or tingling in hands or feet, convulsions, thrombophlebitis, hallucinations.	Discontinue. Call doctor right away.

 WARNINGS & PRECAUTIONS

Don't take if:
- You are allergic to any cortisone drug.
- You have tuberculosis or fungus infection.
- You have herpes infection of eyes, lips or genitals.

- You have bone disease, thyroid disease, colitis, peptic ulcer, diabetes, myasthenia gravis, liver or kidney disease, diverticulitis, glaucoma, heart disease.

Before you start, consult your doctor:
- If you have had tuberculosis.
- If you have congestive heart failure.
- If you have diabetes.
- If you have peptic ulcer.
- If you have glaucoma.
- If you have underactive thyroid.
- If you have high blood pressure.
- If you have myasthenia gravis.
- If you have blood clots in legs or lungs.

Over age 60:
Adverse reactions and side effects may be more frequent and severe than in younger persons. Likely to aggravate edema, diabetes or ulcers. Likely to cause cataracts and osteoporosis (softening of the bones).

Pregnancy:
Risk to unborn child outweighs drug benefits. Don't use.

Breast-feeding:
Drug passes into milk. Avoid drug or discontinue nursing until you finish medicine. Consult doctor for advice on maintaining milk supply.

Infants & children:
Use only under medical supervision.

Prolonged use:
- Retards growth in children.
- Possible glaucoma, cataracts, diabetes, fragile bones and thin skin.
- Functional dependence.
- Talk to your doctor about the need for follow-up medical examinations or laboratory studies to check blood pressure, serum electrolytes, stools for blood.

Skin & sunlight:
No problems expected.

Driving, piloting or hazardous work:
No problems expected.

Discontinuing:
- Don't discontinue without doctor's advice until you complete prescribed dose, even though symptoms diminish or disappear.
- Drug affects your response to surgery, illness, injury or stress for 2 years after discontinuing. Tell anyone who takes medical care of you within 2 years about drug.

Others:
- Avoid immunizations if possible.
- Your resistance to infection is less while taking this medicine.
- Advise any doctor or dentist whom you consult that you take this medicine.

- Those who have inactive or "cured" tuberculosis may be subjected to a possible recurrence of active tuberculosis.
- Children who must take cortisone drugs may grow less well.

 ## POSSIBLE INTERACTION WITH OTHER DRUGS

GENERIC NAME OR DRUG CLASS	COMBINED EFFECT
Amphotericin B	Potassium depletion.
Anticholinergics*	Possible glaucoma.
Anticoagulants, oral*	Decreased anti-coagulant effect.
Anticonvulsants, hydantoin*	Decreased prednisone effect.
Antidiabetics, oral*	Decreased anti-diabetic effect.
Antihistamines*	Decreased prednisone effect.
Aspirin	Increased prednisone effect.
Attenuated virus vaccines*	Possible viral infection.
Barbiturates*	Decreased prednisone effect. Oversedation.
Chloral hydrate	Decreased prednisone effect.
Chlorthalidone	Potassium depletion.
Cholestyramine	Decreased prednisone absorption.
Cholinergics*	Decreased cholinergic effect.
Colestipol	Decreased prednisone absorption.

Continued page 957

 ## POSSIBLE INTERACTION WITH OTHER SUBSTANCES

INTERACTS WITH	COMBINED EFFECT
Alcohol:	Risk of stomach ulcers.
Beverages:	No proven problems.
Cocaine:	Overstimulation. Avoid.
Foods:	No proven problems.
Marijuana:	Decreased immunity.
Tobacco:	Increased prednisone effect. Possible toxicity.

*See Glossary

PRIMAQUINE

GENERIC NAMES

PRIMAQUINE

BASIC INFORMATION

Habit forming? No
Prescription needed? Yes
Available as generic? Yes
Drug class: Antiprotozoal (antimalarial)

USES

- Treats some forms of malaria.
- Prevents relapses of some forms of malaria.
- Treats pneumocystis carinii pneumonia (used in combination with clindamycin).

DOSAGE & USAGE INFORMATION

How to take:
Tablets—Take with meals or antacids to minimize stomach irritation.

When to take:
At the same time each day, according to instructions on prescription label.

If you forget a dose:
Take as soon as you remember up to 2 hours late. If more than 2 hours, wait for next scheduled dose. Don't double this dose.

What drug does:
Alters the properties of DNA in malaria organisms to prevent them from multiplying.

Time lapse before drug works:
2 to 3 hours.

Don't take with:
Any other medicine without consulting your doctor or pharmacist.

OVERDOSE

SYMPTOMS:
None expected.
WHAT TO DO:
Overdose unlikely to threaten life. If person takes much larger amount than prescribed, call doctor, poison-control center or hospital emergency room for instructions.

POSSIBLE ADVERSE REACTIONS OR SIDE EFFECTS

SYMPTOMS	WHAT TO DO
Life-threatening: None expected.	
Common: None expected.	
Infrequent: Dark urine; back, leg or stomach pain; appetite loss; pale skin; fever.	Discontinue. Call doctor right away.
Rare: Blue fingernails, lips and skin; dizziness; difficult breathing; extraordinary tiredness; sore throat; fever.	Discontinue. Call doctor right away.

WARNINGS & PRECAUTIONS

Don't take if:
- You have G6PD deficiency.
- You are hypersensitive to primaquine.

Before you start, consult your doctor:
If you are Black, Oriental, Asian or of Mediterranean origin.

Over age 60:
No special problems expected.

Pregnancy:
No proven harm to unborn child, but avoid if possible.

Breast-feeding:
Drug passes into milk. Avoid drug or discontinue nursing until you finish medicine. Consult doctor for advice on maintaining milk supply.

Infants & children:
No special problems expected.

Prolonged use:
No special problems expected.

Skin & sunlight:
No special problems expected.

Driving, piloting or hazardous work:
No special problems expected.

Discontinuing:
No special problems expected.

Others:
- If you are Black, Asian, Oriental or of Mediterranean origin, insist on a test for G6PD deficiency before taking this medicine.
- Advise any doctor or dentist whom you consult that you take this medicine.

POSSIBLE INTERACTION WITH OTHER DRUGS

GENERIC NAME OR DRUG CLASS	COMBINED EFFECT
Hemolytics*, other	Increased risk of serious side effects affecting the blood.
Quinacrine	Increased toxic effects of primaquine.

POSSIBLE INTERACTION WITH OTHER SUBSTANCES

INTERACTS WITH	COMBINED EFFECT
Alcohol:	Possible liver toxicity. Avoid.
Beverages:	None expected.
Cocaine:	None expected.
Foods:	None expected.
Marijuana:	None expected.
Tobacco:	None expected.

PRIMIDONE

BRAND NAMES

Apo-Primidone   Mysoline
Myidone   Sertan

BASIC INFORMATION

Habit forming? No
Prescription needed? Yes
Available as generic? Yes
Drug class: Anticonvulsant

USES

Prevents some forms of epileptic seizures.

DOSAGE & USAGE INFORMATION

How to take:
- Tablet—Swallow with liquid. If you can't swallow whole, crumble tablet and take with liquid or food.
- Liquid—If desired, dilute dose in beverage before swallowing.

When to take:
Daily in regularly spaced doses, according to doctor's prescription.

If you forget a dose:
Take as soon as you remember up to 2 hours late. If more than 2 hours, wait for next scheduled dose (don't double this dose).

What drug does:
Probably inhibits repetitious spread of impulses along nerve pathways.

Continued next column

OVERDOSE

SYMPTOMS:
Slow, shallow breathing; weak, rapid pulse; confusion, deep sleep, coma.
WHAT TO DO:
- **Dial 0 (operator) or 911 (emergency) for an ambulance or medical help. Then give first aid immediately.**
- **If patient is unconscious and not breathing, give mouth-to-mouth breathing. If there is no heartbeat, use cardiac massage and mouth-to-mouth breathing (CPR). Don't try to make patient vomit. If you can't get help quickly, take patient to nearest emergency facility.**
- **See emergency information on inside covers.**

Time lapse before drug works:
2 to 3 weeks.

Don't take with:
Any other medicine without consulting your doctor or pharmacist.

POSSIBLE ADVERSE REACTIONS OR SIDE EFFECTS

SYMPTOMS	WHAT TO DO
Life-threatening:	
In case of overdose, see previous column.	
Common:	
• Difficult breathing.	Discontinue. Call doctor right away.
• Confusion, change in vision.	Continue. Call doctor when convenient.
• Clumsiness, dizziness, drowsiness.	Continue. Tell doctor at next visit.
Infrequent:	
• Unusual excitement, particularly in children; nausea; vomiting.	Discontinue. Call doctor right away.
• Headache, fatigue, weakness.	Continue. Call doctor when convenient.
Rare:	
• Rash or hives, appetite loss, acute psychosis, hair loss, fever, joint pain.	Discontinue. Call doctor right away.
• Swollen eyelids or legs.	Continue. Call doctor when convenient.
• Decreased sexual ability.	Continue. Tell doctor at next visit.

WARNINGS & PRECAUTIONS

Don't take if:
- You are allergic to any barbiturate.
- You have had porphyria.

Before you start, consult your doctor:
- If you have had liver, kidney or lung disease or asthma.
- If you have lupus.

Over age 60:
Adverse reactions and side effects may be more frequent and severe than in younger persons.

Pregnancy:
Studies inconclusive on harm to unborn child. Animal studies show fetal abnormalities. Decide with your doctor whether drug benefits justify risk to unborn child.

Breast-feeding:
Drug filters into milk. May harm child. Avoid.

Infants & children:
Use only under medical supervision.

Prolonged use:
- Enlarged lymph and thyroid glands.
- Anemia.
- Rickets in children and osteomalacia (insufficient calcium to bones) in adults.
- Talk to your doctor about the need for follow-up medical examinations or laboratory studies to check complete blood counts (white blood cell count, platelet count, red blood cell count, hemoglobin, hematocrit), liver function, kidney function.

Skin & sunlight:
None expected.

Driving, piloting or hazardous work:
Don't drive or pilot aircraft until you learn how medicine affects you. Don't work around dangerous machinery. Don't climb ladders or work in high places. Danger increases if you drink alcohol or take medicine affecting alertness and reflexes.

Discontinuing:
Don't discontinue abruptly or without doctor's advice until you complete prescribed dose, even though symptoms diminish or disappear.

Others:
- Tell doctor if you become ill or injured and must interrupt dose schedule.
- Periodic laboratory blood tests of drug level recommended.

 POSSIBLE INTERACTION WITH OTHER DRUGS

GENERIC NAME OR DRUG CLASS	COMBINED EFFECT
Anticoagulants, oral*	Decreased primidone effect.
Anticonvulsants, other*	Changed seizure pattern.
Antidepressants*	Increased antidepressant effect.
Antidiabetics*	Increased effect of primidone sedation.
Antihistamines*	Increased effect of primidone sedation.
Aspirin	Decreased aspirin effect.
Carbamazepine	Unpredictable increase or decrease of primidone effect.
Carbonic anhydrase inhibitors*	Possible decreased primidone effect.

Central nervous system (CNS) depressants*	Increased CNS depressant effects.
Contraceptives, oral*	Decreased contraceptive effect.
Cortisone drugs*	Decreased cortisone effect.
Cyclosporine	Decreased effect of cyclosporine.
Digitalis preparations*	Decreased digitalis effect.
Disulfiram	Possible increased primidone effect.
Estrogens*	Decreased estrogen effect.
Griseofulvin	Possible decreased griseofulvin effect.
Isoniazid	Decreased primidone effect.
Leucovorin (large dose)	May counteract anticonvulsant effect of primidone.
Loxapine	Decreased anticonvulsant effect of primidone.
MAO inhibitors*	Increased effect of primidone sedation.
Metronidazole	Possible decreased metronidazole effect.
Mind-altering drugs*	Increased effect of mind-altering drugs.

Continued page 958

 POSSIBLE INTERACTION WITH OTHER SUBSTANCES

INTERACTS WITH	COMBINED EFFECT
Alcohol:	Dangerous sedative effect. Avoid.
Beverages:	None expected.
Cocaine:	Decreased primidone effect.
Foods:	Possible need for more vitamin D.
Marijuana:	Decreased anticonvulsant effect of primidone. Drowsiness, unsteadiness.
Tobacco:	None expected.

PROBENECID

BRAND NAMES

Benacen
Benemid
Benuryl

Parbenem
Polycillin-PRB
Probalan

BASIC INFORMATION

Habit forming? No
Prescription needed? Yes
Available as generic? Yes
Drug class: Antigout

 ## USES

* Treatment for chronic gout.
* Increases blood levels of penicillins and cephalosporins.

 ## DOSAGE & USAGE INFORMATION

How to take:
Tablet—Swallow with liquid or food to lessen stomach irritation. If you can't swallow whole, crumble tablet and take with liquid or food.

When to take:
At the same time each day.

If you forget a dose:
Take as soon as you remember up to 12 hours late. If more than 12 hours, wait for next scheduled dose (don't double this dose).

What drug does:
* Forces kidneys to excrete uric acid.
* Reduces amount of penicillin excreted in urine.

Time lapse before drug works:
May require several months of regular use to prevent acute gout.

Don't take with:
* Non-prescription drugs containing aspirin or caffeine.
* Any other medicine without consulting your doctor or pharmacist.

 ## OVERDOSE

SYMPTOMS:
Breathing difficulty, severe nervous agitation, vomiting, seizures, convulsions, delirium, coma.
WHAT TO DO:
* **Dial 0 (operator) or 911 (emergency) for an ambulance or medical help. Then give first aid immediately.**
* **See emergency information on inside covers.**

 ## POSSIBLE ADVERSE REACTIONS OR SIDE EFFECTS

SYMPTOMS	WHAT TO DO
Life-threatening:	
In case of overdose, see previous column.	
Common:	
Headache, appetite loss, nausea, vomiting.	Continue. Call doctor when convenient.
Infrequent:	
• Blood in urine, low back pain. worsening gout.	Discontinue. Call doctor right away.
• Dizziness, flushed face, itchy skin.	Continue. Call doctor when convenient.
• Painful or frequent urination, sore gums.	Continue. Tell doctor at next visit.
Rare:	
Sore throat, fever and chills; difficult breathing; unusual bleeding or bruising; red, painful joint; jaundice; foot, leg or face swelling.	Discontinue. Call doctor right away.

 ## WARNINGS & PRECAUTIONS

Don't take if:
* You are allergic to any uricosuric.
* You have acute gout.
* Patient is younger than 2.

Before you start, consult your doctor:
* If you have had kidney stones or kidney disease.
* If you have a peptic ulcer.
* If you have bone-marrow or blood-cell disease.

Over age 60:
Adverse reactions and side effects may be more frequent and severe than in younger persons.

Pregnancy:
Studies inconclusive on harm to unborn child. Animal studies show fetal abnormalities. Decide with your doctor whether drug benefits justify risk to unborn child.

Breast-feeding:
No proven problems.

Infants & children:
Not recommended.

Prolonged use:
- Possible kidney damage.
- Talk to your doctor about the need for follow-up medical examinations or laboratory studies to check serum uric acid, urine uric acid.

Skin & sunlight:
No problems expected.

Driving, piloting or hazardous work:
Avoid if you feel dizzy. Otherwise, no problems expected.

Discontinuing:
Don't discontinue without consulting doctor. Dose may require gradual reduction if you have taken drug for a long time. Doses of other drugs may also require adjustment.

Others:
If signs of gout attack develop while taking medicine, consult doctor.

POSSIBLE INTERACTION WITH OTHER DRUGS

GENERIC NAME OR DRUG CLASS	COMBINED EFFECT
Allopurinol	Increased effect of each drug.
Anticoagulants, oral*	Increased anti-coagulant effect.
Aspirin	Decreased probenecid effect.
Bismuth subsalicylate	Decreased effect of probenecid.
Cefixime	Increased cefixime effect.
Cephalosporins*	Increased cephalosporin effect.
Ciprofloxacin	May cause kidney dysfunction.
Dapsone	Increased dapsone effect. Increased toxicity.
Diclofenac	Increased diclofenac effect.
Diuretics, thiazide*	Decreased probenecid effect.
Hypoglycemics, oral*	Increased hypo-glycemic effect.
Indomethacin	Increased adverse effects of indomethacin.
Methotrexate	Increased methotrexate toxicity.
Nitrofurantoin	Incresed effect of nitrofurantoin.
Non-steroidal anti-inflammatory drugs* (NSAIDs)	Increased toxic risk.
Para-aminosalicylic acid	Increased effect of para-aminosalicylic acid.
Penicillins*	Enhanced penicillin effect.
Pyrazinamide	Decreased probenecid effect.
Salicylates*	Decreased probenecid effect.
Sodium benzoate & sodium phenylacetate	May reduce effect of sodium benzoate & sodium phenylacetate.
Sulfa drugs*	Slows elimination. May cause harmful accumulation of sulfa.
Thioguanine	More likelihood of toxicity of both drugs.
Zidovudine	Increased zidovudine toxicity risk.

POSSIBLE INTERACTION WITH OTHER SUBSTANCES

INTERACTS WITH	COMBINED EFFECT
Alcohol:	Decreased probenecid effect.
Beverages: Caffeine drinks.	Loss of probenecid effectiveness.
Cocaine:	None expected.
Foods:	None expected.
Marijuana:	Daily use— Decreased probenecid effect.
Tobacco:	None expected.

PROBENECID & COLCHICINE

BRAND NAMES

Colabid
Col Benemid
Col-Probencid
Proben-C

BASIC INFORMATION

Habit forming? No
Prescription needed? Yes
Available as generic? Yes
Drug class: Antigout

USES

- Increases blood levels of penicillins and cephalosporins.
- Relieves joint pain, inflammation, swelling from gout.
- Also used for familial Mediterranean fever, dermatitis herpetiformis.

DOSAGE & USAGE INFORMATION

How to take:
Tablet—Swallow with liquid or food to lessen stomach irritation. If you can't swallow whole, crumble tablet and take with liquid or food.

When to take:
At the same time each day.

If you forget a dose:
Take as soon as you remember up to 12 hours late. If more than 12 hours, wait for next scheduled dose (don't double this dose).

What drug does:
- Forces kidneys to excrete uric acid.
- Reduces amount of penicillin excreted in urine.
- Decreases acidity of joint tissues and prevents deposits of uric-acid crystals.

Continued next column

OVERDOSE

SYMPTOMS:
Breathing difficulty, severe nervous agitation, convulsions, bloody urine, diarrhea, vomiting, muscle weakness, fever, stupor, seizures, delirium, coma.
WHAT TO DO:
- **Dial 0 (operator) or 911 (emergency) for an ambulance or medical help. Then give first aid immediately.**
- **See emergency information on inside covers.**

Time lapse before drug works:
12 to 48 hours.

Don't take with:
- Non-prescription drugs containing aspirin or caffeine.
- Any other medicine without consulting your doctor or pharmacist.

POSSIBLE ADVERSE REACTIONS OR SIDE EFFECTS

SYMPTOMS	WHAT TO DO
Life-threatening: Blood in urine; convulsions; severe muscle weakness; difficult breathing; burning feeling of stomach, throat or skin; worsening gout.	Discontinue. Seek emergency treatment.
Common: Diarrhea, headache, abdominal pain.	Discontinue. Call doctor right away.
Infrequent: • Back pain; painful, difficult urination.	Discontinue. Call doctor right away.
• Dizziness, red or flushed face, urgent urination, sore gums, hair loss.	Continue. Call doctor when convenient.
Rare: Sudden decrease in urine output; nausea; vomiting; mood change; fever; chills; diarrhea; jaundice; numbness or tingling in hands or feet; rash; sore throat, fever, mouth sores; swollen face, feet and ankles; unexplained bleeding or bruising; weight gain or loss; low white or red blood cells.	Discontinue. Call doctor right away.

WARNINGS & PRECAUTIONS

Don't take if:
You are allergic to any uricosuric or colchicine.

Before you start, consult your doctor:
- If you have had kidney stones, kidney disease, heart or liver disease, peptic ulcers or ulcerative colitis.
- If you have bone-marrow or blood-cell disease.
- If you will have surgery within 2 months, including dental surgery, requiring general or spinal anesthesia.

PROBENECID & COLCHICINE

Over age 60:
Adverse reactions and side effects may be more frequent and severe than in younger persons. Colchicine has a narrow margin of safety for people in this age group.

Pregnancy:
Risk to unborn child outweighs drug benefits. Don't use.

Breast-feeding:
No problems expected, but consult doctor.

Infants & children:
Not recommended.

Prolonged use:
- Possible kidney damage.
- Permanent hair loss.
- Anemia. Request blood counts.
- Numbness or tingling in hands and feet.
- Talk to your doctor about the need for follow-up medical examinations or laboratory studies to check serum uric acid, urine uric acid.

Skin & sunlight:
No problems expected.

Driving, piloting or hazardous work:
Don't drive or pilot aircraft until you learn how medicine affects you. Don't work around dangerous machinery. Don't climb ladders or work in high places. Danger increases if you drink alcohol or take medicine affecting alertness and reflexes, such as antihistamines, tranquilizers, sedatives, pain medicine, narcotics and mind-altering drugs.

Discontinuing:
- May be unnecessary to finish medicine. Follow doctor's instructions.
- Stop taking if severe digestive upsets occur before symptoms are relieved.

Others:
- If signs of gout attack develop while taking medicine, consult doctor.
- Limit each course of treatment to 8 mg. Don't exceed 3 mg. per 24 hours.
- Decreased sperm count in males.

POSSIBLE INTERACTION WITH OTHER DRUGS

GENERIC NAME OR DRUG CLASS	COMBINED EFFECT
Acetohexamide	Increased acetohexamide effect.
Allopurinol	Increased effect of each drug.
Anticoagulants*	Irregular effect on anti-coagulation, sometimes increased, sometimes decreased. Follow prothrombin times.
Antidepressants*	Oversedation.
Antihistamines*	Oversedation.
Antihypertensives*	Decreased antihypertensive effect.
Appetite suppressants*	Increased suppressant effect.
Bismuth subsalicylate	Decreased effect of probenecid.
Cefixime	Increased cefixime effect.
Cephalosporins*	Increased cephalosporin effect.
Dapsone	Increased dapsone effect. Increased toxicity.
Diclofenac	Increased diclofenac effect.
Diuretics, thiazide*	Decreased probenecid effect.
Indomethacin	Increased adverse effects of indomethacin.
Methotrexate	Increased methotrexate effect.
Mind-altering drugs*	Oversedation.
Narcotics*	Oversedation.
Nitrofurantoin	Increased nitrofurantoin effect.
Non-steroidal anti-inflammatory drugs* (NSAIDs)	Increased toxic risk.

Continued page 958

POSSIBLE INTERACTION WITH OTHER SUBSTANCES

INTERACTS WITH	COMBINED EFFECT
Alcohol:	Decreased probenecid effect.
Beverages: Caffeine drinks.	Loss of probenecid effectiveness.
Herbal teas.	Increased colchicine effect. Avoid.
Cocaine:	Overstimulation. Avoid.
Foods:	No proven problems.
Marijuana:	Decreased colchicine and probenecid effect.
Tobacco:	No proven problems.

*See Glossary

PROBUCOL

BRAND NAMES

Lorelco

BASIC INFORMATION

Habit forming? No
Prescription needed? Yes
Available as generic? No
Drug class: Antihyperlipidemic

USES

Lowers cholesterol level in blood in persons with type IIa hyperlipoproteinemia.

DOSAGE & USAGE INFORMATION

How to take:
Tablet—Swallow with liquid. If you can't swallow whole, crumble tablet and take with liquid or food.

When to take:
With morning and evening meals.

If you forget a dose:
Take as soon as you remember up to 2 hours late. If more than 2 hours, wait for next scheduled dose (don't double this dose).

What drug does:
Reduces serum cholesterol without reducing liver cholesterol.

Time lapse before drug works:
3 to 4 months.

Don't take with:
Other medicines or vitamins. Separate by 1 to 2 hours.

OVERDOSE

SYMPTOMS:
None reported.
WHAT TO DO:
Overdose unlikely to threaten life. If person takes much larger amount than prescribed, call doctor, poison-control center or hospital emergency room for instructions.

POSSIBLE ADVERSE REACTIONS OR SIDE EFFECTS

SYMPTOMS	WHAT TO DO
Life-threatening: None expected.	
Common: Bloating, diarrhea, nausea, vomiting, abdominal pain, flatus.	Continue. Call doctor when convenient.
Infrequent:	
• Dizziness, headache.	Discontinue. Call doctor right away.
• Numbness or tingling in feet, toes, fingers, face.	Continue. Call doctor when convenient.
Rare:	
• Swelling of hands, face, feet, mouth.	Discontinue. Seek emergency treatment.
• Rash.	Discontinue. Call doctor right away.

WARNINGS & PRECAUTIONS

Don't take if:
You are allergic to probucol.

Before you start, consult your doctor:
- If you have liver disease such as cirrhosis.
- If you have heartbeat irregularity.
- If you have congestive heart failure that is not under control.
- If you have gallstones.

Over age 60:
Adverse reactions and side effects may be more frequent and severe than in younger persons.

Pregnancy:
No proven problems. Avoid if possible. Continue using birth-control methods for 6 months after discontinuing medicine.

Breast-feeding:
Not recommended. Animal studies show drug passes into milk. Studies not available for human beings.

Infants & children:
Not recommended. Safety and dosage have not been established.

Prolonged use:
Request serum cholesterol and serum triglyceride laboratory studies every 2 to 4 months.

Skin & sunlight:
No problems expected.

Driving, piloting or hazardous work:
If medicine does not cause dizziness, no problems expected.

Discontinuing:
Don't discontinue without consulting doctor. Dose may require gradual reduction if you have taken drug for a long time. Doses of other drugs may also require adjustment.

Others:
Medicine works best in conjunction with low-fat, low-cholesterol diet and an active, regular exercise program.

POSSIBLE INTERACTION WITH OTHER DRUGS

GENERIC NAME OR DRUG CLASS	COMBINED EFFECT
Chenodiol	Decreased chenodiol effect.
Clofibrate	Combination no more effective than one drug only, so don't take both.

POSSIBLE INTERACTION WITH OTHER SUBSTANCES

INTERACTS WITH	COMBINED EFFECT
Alcohol:	May aggravate liver problems. Avoid.
Beverages:	None expected.
Cocaine:	None expected.
Foods:	None expected.
Marijuana:	None expected.
Tobacco:	None expected.

PROCAINAMIDE

BRAND NAMES

Procan SR   Pronestyl
Promine   Pronestyl SR

BASIC INFORMATION

Habit forming? No
Prescription needed? Yes
Available as generic? Yes
Drug class: Antiarrhythmic

 USES

Stabilizes irregular heartbeat.

 DOSAGE & USAGE INFORMATION

How to take:
- Tablet or capsule—Swallow with liquid.
- Extended-release tablets—Swallow each dose whole. Do not crush them.

When to take:
Best taken on empty stomach, 1 hour before or 2 hours after meals. If necessary, may be taken with food or milk to lessen stomach upset.

If you forget a dose:
Take as soon as you remember up to 2 hours late. If more than 2 hours, wait for next scheduled dose (don't double this dose).

What drug does:
Slows activity of pacemaker (rhythm-control center of heart) and delays transmission of electrical impulses.

Time lapse before drug works:
30 to 60 minutes.

Don't take with:
Any other medicine without consulting your doctor or pharmacist.

 OVERDOSE

SYMPTOMS:
Fast and irregular heartbeat, confusion, stupor, decreased blood pressure, fainting, cardiac arrest.
WHAT TO DO:
- **Dial 0 (operator) or 911 (emergency) for an ambulance or medical help. Then give first aid immediately.**
- **See emergency information on inside covers.**

 POSSIBLE ADVERSE REACTIONS OR SIDE EFFECTS

SYMPTOMS	WHAT TO DO
Life-threatening: Hives, rash, intense itching, faintness soon after dose (anaphylaxis); convulsions.	Seek emergency treatment immediately.
Common: Diarrhea, appetite loss, nausea, vomiting, bitter taste.	Continue. Call doctor when convenient.
Infrequent: • Joint pain, painful breathing.	Discontinue. Call doctor right away.
• Dizziness.	Continue. Call doctor when convenient.
Rare: • Hallucinations, depression, confusion, psychosis, itchy skin, rash, sore throat, fever, jaundice, unusual bleeding or bruising.	Discontinue. Call doctor right away.
• Headache, fatigue.	Continue. Call doctor when convenient.

 WARNINGS & PRECAUTIONS

Don't take if:
- You are allergic to procainamide.
- You have myasthenia gravis.

Before you start, consult your doctor:
- If you are allergic to local anesthetics that end in "caine."
- If you have had liver or kidney disease or impaired kidney function.
- If you have had lupus.
- If you take digitalis preparations.
- If you will have surgery within 2 months, including dental surgery, requiring general or spinal anesthesia.

Over age 60:
Adverse reactions and side effects may be more frequent and severe than in younger persons.

Pregnancy:
No proven harm to unborn child. Avoid if possible.

Breast-feeding:
No proven problems. Consult doctor.

Infants & children:
Not recommended.

Prolonged use:
- May cause lupus-like illness.
- Talk to your doctor about the need for follow-up medical examinations or laboratory studies to check ANA titers*, blood pressure, complete blood counts (white blood cell count, platelet count, red blood cell count, hemoglobin, hematocrit).

Skin & sunlight:
No problems expected.

Driving, piloting or hazardous work:
Use caution if you feel dizzy or weak. Otherwise, no problems expected.

Discontinuing:
Don't discontinue without doctor's advice until you complete prescribed dose, even though symptoms diminish or disappear.

Others:
Some products contain tartrazine dye. Avoid, especially if you are allergic to aspirin.

POSSIBLE INTERACTION WITH OTHER DRUGS

GENERIC NAME OR DRUG CLASS	COMBINED EFFECT
Acetazolamide	Increased procainamide effect.
Ambenonium	Decreased ambenonium effect.
Aminoglycosides*	Possible severe muscle weakness, impaired breathing.
Antiarrhythmics, other*	Increased likelihood of adverse reactions with either drug. Possible increased effect of both drugs.
Antihypertensives*	Increased antihypertensive effect.
Antimyasthenics*	Decreased antimyasthenic effect.
Anticholinergics*	Increased anticholinergic effect.

Cimetidine	Increased procainamide effect.
Dapsone	Increased risk of adverse effect on blood cells.
Encainide	Increased effect of toxicity on heart muscle.
Guanfacine	Increased effect of both medicines.
Kanamycin	Possible severe muscle weakness, impaired breathing.
Neomycin	Possible severe muscle weakness, impaired breathing.
Nicardipine	Possible increased effect and toxicity of each drug.
Nizatidine	Increased effect and toxicity of procainamide.
Pimozide	Increased risk of heartbeat irregularities.
Propafenone	Increased effect of both drugs and increased risk of toxicity.

POSSIBLE INTERACTION WITH OTHER SUBSTANCES

INTERACTS WITH	COMBINED EFFECT
Alcohol:	None expected.
Beverages: Caffeine drinks, iced drinks.	Irregular heartbeat.
Cocaine:	Decreased procainamide effect.
Foods:	None expected.
Marijuana:	None expected.
Tobacco:	Decreased procainamide effect.

PROCARBAZINE

BRAND NAMES

Matulane   Natulan

BASIC INFORMATION

Habit forming? No
Prescription needed? Yes
Available as generic? No
Drug class: Antineoplastic

USES

Treatment for some kinds of cancer.

DOSAGE & USAGE INFORMATION

How to take:
Capsule—Swallow with liquid after light meal. Don't drink fluids with meals. Drink extra fluids between meals. Avoid sweet or fatty foods.

When to take:
At the same time each day.

If you forget a dose:
Take as soon as you remember. Don't double dose ever.

What drug does:
Inhibits abnormal cell reproduction. Procarbazine is an alkylating agent and an MAO inhibitor.

Time lapse before drug works:
Up to 6 weeks for full effect.

Don't take with:
Any other medicine without consulting your doctor or pharmacist.

OVERDOSE

SYMPTOMS:
Restlessness, agitation, fever, convulsions, bleeding.
WHAT TO DO:
- **Dial 0 (operator) or 911 (emergency) for an ambulance or medical help. Then give first aid immediately.**
- **If patient is unconscious and not breathing, give mouth-to-mouth breathing. If there is no heartbeat, use cardiac massage and mouth-to-mouth breathing (CPR). Don't try to make patient vomit. If you can't get help quickly, take patient to nearest emergency facility.**
- **See emergency information on inside covers.**

POSSIBLE ADVERSE REACTIONS OR SIDE EFFECTS

SYMPTOMS	WHAT TO DO
Life-threatening:	
In case of overdose, see previous column.	
Common:	
• Nausea, vomiting, decreased urination, numbness or tingling in hands or feet, hair loss, rapid or pounding heartbeat, shortness of breath.	Discontinue. Call doctor right away.
• Fatigue, weakness, confusion.	Continue. Call doctor when convenient.
• Dizziness when changing position, dry mouth, inflamed tongue, constipation, difficult urination.	Continue. Tell doctor at next visit.
Infrequent:	
• Fainting.	Discontinue. Seek emergency treatment.
• Severe headache; abnormal bleeding or bruising; muscle, joint or chest pain, enlarged eye pupils; black tarry stools; bloody urine.	Discontinue. Call doctor right away.
• Hallucinations, insomnia, nightmares, diarrhea, swollen feet or legs, nervousness, eyes sensitive to light, cough or hoarseness, mouth sores, depression.	Continue. Call doctor when convenient.
• Diminished sex drive.	Continue. Tell doctor at next visit.
Rare:	
Rash, stiff neck, jaundice, fever, sore throat, vomiting blood, wheezing.	Discontinue. Call doctor right away.

WARNINGS & PRECAUTIONS

Don't take if:
- You are allergic to any MAO inhibitor.
- You have heart disease, congestive heart failure, heart-rhythm irregularities or high blood pressure.
- You have liver or kidney disease.

Before you start, consult your doctor:
- If you are alcoholic.
- If you have asthma.
- If you have had a stroke.

- If you have diabetes or epilepsy.
- If you have overactive thyroid.
- If you have schizophrenia.
- If you have Parkinson's disease.
- If you have adrenal-gland tumor.
- If you will have surgery within 2 months, including dental surgery, requiring general or spinal anesthesia.

Over age 60:
Not recommended.

Pregnancy:
Avoid if possible.

Breast-feeding:
Safety not established. Consult doctor.

Infants & children:
Not recommended.

Prolonged use:
- May be toxic to liver.
- Talk to your doctor about the need for follow-up medical examinations or laboratory studies to check complete blood counts (white blood cell count, platelet count, red blood cell count, hemoglobin, hematocrit), bone marrow, kidney function.

Skin & sunlight:
May cause rash or intensify sunburn in areas exposed to sun or sunlamp.

Driving, piloting or hazardous work:
Don't drive or pilot aircraft until you learn how medicine affects you. Don't work around dangerous machinery. Don't climb ladders or work in high places. Danger increases if you drink alcohol or take medicine affecting alertness and reflexes.

Discontinuing:
- Don't discontinue without doctor's advice until you complete prescribed dose, even though symptoms diminish or disappear.
- Follow precautions regarding foods, drinks and other medicines for 2 weeks after discontinuing.

Others:
- May affect blood-sugar levels in patients with diabetes.
- Fever may indicate that MAO inhibitor dose requires adjustment.

POSSIBLE INTERACTION WITH OTHER DRUGS

GENERIC NAME OR DRUG CLASS	COMBINED EFFECT
Amphetamines*	Blood pressure rise to life-threatening level.
Anticonvulsants*	Changed seizure pattern.
Antidepressants, tricyclic (TCA)*	Blood pressure rise to life-threatening level.

Antidiabetics, oral and insulin*	Excessively low blood sugar.
Antihistamines*	Increased sedation.
Barbiturates*	Increased sedation.
Bone marrow depressants*	Increased toxicity to bone marrow.
Buspirone	Elevated blood pressure.
Caffeine	Irregular heartbeat or high blood pressure.
Carbamazepine	Fever, seizures. Avoid.
Central nervous system (CNS) depressants*	Increased CNS depression.
Clozapine	Toxic effect on bone marrow and central nervous system.
Cyclobenzaprine	Fever, seizures. Avoid.
Dextromethorphan	Fever, hypertension.
Diuretics*	Excessively low blood pressure.
Doxapam	Increased blood pressure.
Ethinamate	Dangerous increased effects of ethinamate. Avoid combining.
Fluoxetine	Increased depressant effects of both drugs.

Continued on page 958

POSSIBLE INTERACTION WITH OTHER SUBSTANCES

INTERACTS WITH	COMBINED EFFECT
Alcohol:	Increased sedation to dangerous level. Disulfiram-like reaction.
Beverages: Caffeine drinks.	Irregular heartbeat or high blood pressure.
Drinks containing tyramine*	Blood pressure rise to life-threatening level.
Cocaine:	Overstimulation. Possibly fatal.
Foods: Foods containing tyramine*	Blood pressure rise to life-threatening level.
Marijuana:	Overstimulation. Avoid.
Tobacco:	No proven problems.

*See Glossary

PROGESTINS

BRAND AND GENERIC NAMES

See complete list of brand and generic names in the *Brand Names Directory,* page 927.

BASIC INFORMATION

Habit forming? No
Prescription needed? Yes
Available as generic? Yes, for some.
Drug class: Female sex hormone (progestin)

USES

- Treatment for menstrual or uterine disorders caused by progestin imbalance.
- Contraceptive (when combined with estrogens in birth control pills).
- Treatment for cancer of breast and uterus.
- Treatment for toxic sleep apnea.
- Female hormone imbalance.

DOSAGE & USAGE INFORMATION

How to take:
- Tablet—Swallow with liquid or food to lessen stomach irritation. You may crumble tablet.
- Injection—Under doctor's supervision.

When to take:
At the same time each day.

If you forget a dose:
- Menstrual disorders—Take up to 2 hours late. If more than 2 hours, wait for next dose (don't double this dose).
- Contraceptive—Consult your doctor. You may need to use another birth-control method until next period.

What drug does:
- Creates a uterine lining similar to pregnancy that prevents bleeding.
- Suppresses a pituitary gland hormone responsible for ovulation.
- Stimulates cervical mucus, which stops sperm penetration and prevents pregnancy.

Continued next column

OVERDOSE

SYMPTOMS:
Nausea, vomiting, fluid retention, breast discomfort or enlargement, vaginal bleeding.
WHAT TO DO:
Overdose unlikely to threaten life. If person takes much larger amount than prescribed, call doctor, poison-control center or hospital emergency room for instructions.

Time lapse before drug works:
- Menstrual disorders—24 to 48 hours.
- Contraception—3 weeks.
- Cancer—May require 2 to 3 months regular use for maximum benefit.

Don't take with:
Any other medicine without consulting your doctor or pharmacist.

POSSIBLE ADVERSE REACTIONS OR SIDE EFFECTS

SYMPTOMS	WHAT TO DO
Life-threatening: Blood clot in leg, brain or lung; hives, rash, intense itching, faintness soon after a dose (anaphylaxis).	Seek emergency treatment immediately.
Common: Appetite or weight changes, swollen feet or ankles, unusual tiredness or weakness, menstrual cycle changes.	Continue. Tell doctor at next visit.
Infrequent: • Prolonged vaginal bleeding, pain in calf.	Discontinue. Call doctor right away.
• Depression.	Continue. Call doctor when convenient.
• Acne, increased facial or body hair, nausea, tender breasts, headache, enlarged clitoris.	Continue. Tell doctor at next visit.
Rare: • Rash, stomach or side pain, jaundice, fever, vision changes.	Discontinue. Call doctor right away.
• Amenorrhea, hair loss, insomnia, brown skin spots, voice change.	Continue. Call doctor when convenient.

WARNINGS & PRECAUTIONS

Don't take if:
- You are allergic to any progestin hormone.
- You may be pregnant.
- You have liver or gallbladder disease.
- You have had thrombophlebitis, embolism or stroke.
- You have unexplained vaginal bleeding.
- You have had breast or uterine cancer.

Before you start, consult your doctor:
- If you have heart or kidney disease.
- If you have diabetes.
- If you have a seizure disorder.
- If you suffer migraines.
- If you are easily depressed.

Over age 60:
No special problems expected.

Pregnancy:
May harm child. Discontinue at first sign of pregnancy.

Breast-feeding:
Drug passes into milk. Avoid drug or discontinue nursing until you finish medicine. Consult doctor for advice on maintaining milk supply.

Infants & children:
Use only for female children under medical supervision.

Prolonged use:
No problems expected.

Skin & sunlight:
No problems expected.

Driving, piloting or hazardous work:
No problems expected.

Discontinuing:
Consult doctor. This medicine stays in the body and causes fetal abnormalities. Wait at least 3 months before becoming pregnant.

Others:
- Patients with diabetes must be monitored closely.
- Symptoms of blood clot in leg, brain or lung are: chest, groin, leg pain; sudden, severe headache; loss of coordination; vision change; shortness of breath; slurred speech.
- May affect results in some medical tests.
- Advise any doctor or dentist whom you consult that you take this medicine.

POSSIBLE INTERACTION WITH OTHER DRUGS

GENERIC NAME OR DRUG CLASS	COMBINED EFFECT
Bromocriptine	Decreased bromocriptine effect.
Hypoglycemics, oral*	Decreased effect of oral hypoglycemics.
Insulin	Decreased effect of insulin.
Phenobarbital	Decreased progestin effect.
Phenothiazines*	Increased phenothiazine effect.
Phenylbutazone	Decreased progestin effect.
Rifampin	Decreased contraceptive effect.

POSSIBLE INTERACTION WITH OTHER SUBSTANCES

INTERACTS WITH	COMBINED EFFECT
Alcohol:	None expected.
Beverages:	None expected.
Cocaine:	Decreased progestin effect.
Foods: Salt.	Fluid retention.
Marijuana:	Possible menstrual irregularities or bleeding between periods.
Tobacco: All forms.	Possible blood clots in lung, brain, legs. Avoid.

PROPAFENONE

BRAND NAMES

Rhythmol

BASIC INFORMATION

Habit forming? No
Prescription needed? Yes
Available as generic? No
Drug class: Antiarrhythmic

 USES

Treats severe heartbeat irregularities (life-threatening ventricular rhythm disturbances).

 DOSAGE & USAGE INFORMATION

How to take:
Tablet—Swallow with liquid or food to lessen stomach irritation. If you can't swallow whole, crumble tablet and take with liquid or food.

When to take:
At the same time each day, according to instructions on prescription label.

If you forget a dose:
Take as soon as you remember up to 2 hours late. If more than 2 hours, wait for next scheduled dose. Don't double this dose.

What drug does:
Slows electrical activity in the heart to decrease the excitability of the heart muscle.

Time lapse before drug works:
3-1/2 hours to 1 week for full effect. Begins working almost immediately.

Don't take with:
Any other medicine (including non-prescription drugs such as cough and cold medicines, nose drops, vitamins, laxatives, antacids, diet pills, or caffeine) without consulting your doctor or pharmacist.

 OVERDOSE

SYMPTOMS:
Very rapid heart rate that is also irregular.
WHAT TO DO:
Overdose unlikely to threaten life. If person takes much larger amount than prescribed, call doctor, poison-control center or hospital emergency room for instructions.

 POSSIBLE ADVERSE REACTIONS OR SIDE EFFECTS

SYMPTOMS	WHAT TO DO
Life-threatening:	
Severe chest pain, severe shortness of breath.	Seek emergency treatment.
Common:	
• Faster or more irregular heartbeat.	Discontinue. Call doctor right away.
• Taste change, dizziness.	Continue. Call doctor when convenient.
Infrequent:	
• Blurred vision, skin rash.	Discontinue. Call doctor right away.
• Constipation, diarrhea.	Continue. Call doctor when convenient.
• Dry mouth, nausea.	Continue. Tell doctor at next visit.
Rare:	
Fever, chills, trembling, joint pain, slow heartbeat.	Discontinue. Call doctor right away.

WARNINGS & PRECAUTIONS

Don't take if:
You are allergic to propafenone.

Before you start, consult your doctor:
- If you have asthma or bronchospasm.
- If you have congestive heart failure.
- If you have liver disease or kidney disease.
- If you have a recent history of heart attack.
- If you have a pacemaker.

Over age 60:
More likely to have decreased kidney function and require dosage modification.

Pregnancy:
No proven harm to unborn child, but avoid if possible.

Breast-feeding:
No proven problems.

Infants & children:
Safety and efficacy not established.

Prolonged use:
Don't discontinue without consulting doctor. Dose may require gradual reduction if you have taken drug for a long time. Dosages of other drugs may also require adjustment.

Skin & sunlight:
No special problems expected.

Driving, piloting or hazardous work:
Don't drive or pilot aircraft until you learn how medicine affects you. Don't work around dangerous machinery. Don't climb ladders or work in high places. Danger increases if you drink alcohol or take medicine affecting alertness and reflexes.

Discontinuing:
Don't discontinue without consulting doctor. Dose may require gradual reduction if you have taken drug for a long time. Doses of other drugs may also require adjustment.

Others:
- Advise any doctor or dentist whom you consult that you take this medicine, especially if you are to be anesthetized.
- Report changes in symptoms to your doctor and return for periodic visits to check progress.
- Carry or wear a medical I.D. card or bracelet.

POSSIBLE INTERACTION WITH OTHER DRUGS

GENERIC NAME OR DRUG CLASS	COMBINED EFFECT
Anesthetics, local (e.g., prior to dental procedures)	May increase risk of side effects.
Anticoagulants*	May require anticoagulant dosage adjustment.
Beta-adrenergic blockers*	Increased beta blocker effect.
Digitalis preparations*	Increased digitalis absorption. May require decreased dosage of digitalis preparation.

POSSIBLE INTERACTION WITH OTHER SUBSTANCES

INTERACTS WITH	COMBINED EFFECT
Alcohol:	Unpredictable effect on heartbeat. Avoid.
Beverages: Caffeine drinks.	Increased heartbeat irregularity. Avoid.
Cocaine:	Increased heartbeat irregularity. Avoid.
Foods:	None expected.
Marijuana:	Increased heartbeat irregularity. Avoid.
Tobacco:	Increased heartbeat irregularity. Avoid.

PROPANTHELINE

BRAND NAMES

Pro-Banthine   Propanthel

BASIC INFORMATION

Habit forming? No
Prescription needed?
  High strength: Yes
  Low strength: No
Available as generic? Yes
Drug class: Antispasmodic, anticholinergic

USES

- Reduces spasms of digestive system, bladder and urethra.
- Treats peptic ulcers.

DOSAGE & USAGE INFORMATION

How to take:
Tablet—Swallow with liquid or food to lessen stomach irritation.

When to take:
30 minutes before meals (unless directed otherwise by doctor).

If you forget a dose:
Take as soon as you remember up to 2 hours late. If more than 2 hours, wait for next scheduled dose (don't double this dose).

What drug does:
Blocks nerve impulses at parasympathetic nerve endings, preventing muscle contractions and gland secretions of organs involved.

Time lapse before drug works:
15 to 30 minutes.

Don't take with:
Any other medicine without consulting your doctor or pharmacist.

OVERDOSE

SYMPTOMS:
Dilated pupils, blurred vision, rapid pulse and breathing, dizziness, fever, hallucinations, confusion, slurred speech, agitation, flushed face, convulsions, coma.
WHAT TO DO:
- **Dial 0 (operator) or 911 (emergency) for an ambulance or medical help. Then give first aid immediately.**
- **See emergency information on inside covers.**

POSSIBLE ADVERSE REACTIONS OR SIDE EFFECTS

SYMPTOMS	WHAT TO DO
Life-threatening:	
Hives, rash, intense itching, faintness soon after a dose (anaphylaxis).	Seek emergency treatment immediately.
Common:	
• Confusion, delirium, rapid heartbeat.	Discontinue. Call doctor right away.
• Nausea, vomiting, decreased sweating.	Continue. Call doctor when convenient.
• Constipation, loss of taste.	Continue. Tell doctor at next visit.
• Dry ears, nose, throat, mouth.	No action necessary.
Infrequent:	
• Headache, difficult urination, nasal congestion, altered taste, impotence.	Continue. Call doctor when convenient.
• Lightheadedness.	Discontinue. Call doctor right away.
Rare:	
Rash or hives, eye pain, blurred vision.	Discontinue. Call doctor right away.

WARNINGS & PRECAUTIONS

Don't take if:
- You are allergic to any anticholinergic.
- You have trouble with stomach bloating.
- You have difficulty emptying your bladder completely.
- You have narrow-angle glaucoma.
- You have severe ulcerative colitis.

Before you start, consult your doctor:
- If you have open-angle glaucoma.
- If you have angina.
- If you have chronic bronchitis or asthma.
- If you have hiatal hernia.
- If you have liver, kidney or thyroid disease.
- If you have enlarged prostate.
- If you have myasthenia gravis.
- If you have peptic ulcer.
- If you will have surgery within 2 months, including dental surgery, requiring general or spinal anesthesia.

Over age 60:
Adverse reactions and side effects may be more frequent and severe than in younger persons.

Pregnancy:
Studies inconclusive on harm to unborn child. Decide with your doctor whether drug benefits justify risk to unborn child.

Breast-feeding:
Drug passes into milk and decreases milk flow. Avoid drug or discontinue nursing until you finish medicine. Consult doctor for advice on maintaining milk supply.

Infants & children:
Use only under medical supervision.

Prolonged use:
Chronic constipation, possible fecal impaction. Consult doctor immediately.

Skin & sunlight:
No problems expected.

Driving, piloting or hazardous work:
Use disqualifies you for piloting aircraft. Otherwise, no problems expected.

Discontinuing:
May be unnecessary to finish medicine. Follow doctor's instructions.

Others:
Advise any doctor or dentist whom you consult that you take this medicine.

POSSIBLE INTERACTION WITH OTHER DRUGS

GENERIC NAME OR DRUG CLASS	COMBINED EFFECT
Amantadine	Increased propantheline effect.
Antacids*	Decreased propantheline effect.
Anticholinergics, other*	Increased propantheline effect.
Antidepressants, tricyclic (TCA)*	Increased propantheline effect. Increased sedation.
Antidiarrhea preparations*	Reduced propantheline effect.
Antihistamines*	Increased propantheline effect.
Attapulgite	Decreased propantheline effect.
Buclizine	Increased propantheline effect.
Cortisone drugs*	Increased internal eye pressure.
Digitalis	Possible decreased absorption of digitalis.
Haloperidol	Increased internal eye pressure.
Ketoconazole	Decreased ketoconazole effect.
MAO inhibitors*	Increased propantheline effect.
Meperidine	Increased propantheline effect.
Methylphenidate	Increased propantheline effect.
Molindone	Increased anti-cholinergic effect.
Nitrates*	Increased internal eye pressure.
Nizatidine	Increased nizatidine effect.
Orphenadrine	Increased propantheline effect.
Phenothiazines*	Increased propantheline effect.
Pilocarpine	Loss of pilocarpine effect in glaucoma treatment.
Potassium supplements*	Increased possibility of intestinal ulcers with oral potassium tablets.
Quinidine	Increased propantheline effect.
Sedatives* or central nervous system (CNS) depressants*	Increased sedative effect of both drugs.
Terfenadine	Possible increased propantheline effect.
Vitamin C	Decreased propantheline effect. Avoid large doses of vitamin C.

POSSIBLE INTERACTION WITH OTHER SUBSTANCES

INTERACTS WITH	COMBINED EFFECT
Alcohol:	None expected.
Beverages:	None expected.
Cocaine:	Excessively rapid heartbeat. Avoid.
Foods:	None expected.
Marijuana:	Drowsiness and dry mouth.
Tobacco:	None expected.

*See Glossary

PROTECTANT (Ophthalmic)

BRAND AND GENERIC NAMES

Gonak
Goniosol
HYDROXYPROPYL
   CELLULOSE
HYDROXYPROPYL
   METHYL-CELLULOSE
Isopto Alkaline
Isopto Plain
Isopto Tears

Just Tears
Lacril (ophthalmic)
Lacrisert
Moisture Drops
Tearisol
Tears Naturale
Tears Renewed
Ultra Tears

BASIC INFORMATION

Habit forming? No
Prescription needed? Yes
Available as generic? No
Drug class: Protectant (ophthalmic),
   artificial tears

USES

- Relieves eye dryness and irritation caused by inadequate flow of tears.
- Moistens contact lenses and artificial eyes.

DOSAGE & USAGE INFORMATION

How to use:
Eye drops
- Wash hands.
- Apply pressure to inside corner of eye with middle finger.
- Continue pressure for 1 minute after placing medicine in eye.
- Tilt head backward. Pull lower lid away from eye with index finger of the same hand.
- Drop eye drops into pouch and close eye. Don't blink.
- Keep eyes closed for 1 to 2 minutes.
- Don't touch applicator tip to any surface (including the eye). If you accidentally touch tip, clean with warm soap and water.
- Keep container tightly closed.
- Keep cool, but don't freeze.
- Wash hands immediately after using.

Continued next column

OVERDOSE

SYMPTOMS:
None expected.
WHAT TO DO:
Not intended for internal use. If child accidentally swallows, call poison-control center.

When to use:
As directed. Usually every 3 or 4 hours.

If you forget a dose:
Use as soon as you remember.

What drug does:
- Stabilizes and thickens tear film.
- Lubricates and protects eye.

Time lapse before drug works:
2 to 10 minutes.

Don't use with:
Other eye drops without consulting your doctor.

POSSIBLE ADVERSE REACTIONS OR SIDE EFFECTS

SYMPTOMS	WHAT TO DO
Life-threatening None expected.	
Common None expected.	
Infrequent Eye irritation not present before using artificial tears.	Discontinue. Call doctor right away.
Rare None expected.	

PROTECTANT (Ophthalmic)

 ## WARNINGS & PRECAUTIONS

Don't use if:
You are allergic to any artificial tears.

Before you start, consult your doctor:
If you use any other eye drops.

Over age 60:
No problems expected.

Pregnancy:
No problems expected, but check with doctor.

Breast-feeding:
No problems expected, but check with doctor.

Infants & children:
Don't use.

Prolonged use:
Don't use for more than 3 or 4 days.

Skin & sunlight:
No problems expected.

Driving, piloting or hazardous work:
No problems expected.

Discontinuing:
May not need all the medicine in container. If symptoms disappear, stop using.

Others:
- Keep cool, but don't freeze.
- Check with your doctor if eye irritation continues or becomes worse.

 ## POSSIBLE INTERACTION WITH OTHER DRUGS

GENERIC NAME OR DRUG CLASS	COMBINED EFFECT
Clinically significant interactions with oral or injected medicines unlikely.	

 ## POSSIBLE INTERACTION WITH OTHER SUBSTANCES

INTERACTS WITH	COMBINED EFFECT
Alcohol:	None expected.
Beverages:	None expected.
Cocaine:	None expected.
Foods:	None expected.
Marijuana:	None expected.
Tobacco:	None expected.

PSEUDOEPHEDRINE

BRAND NAMES

See complete list of brand names in the *Brand Name Directory*, page 927.

BASIC INFORMATION

Habit forming? No
Prescription needed?
  U.S.: High strength—Yes
       Low strength—No
  Canada: No
Available as generic? Yes
Drug class: Sympathomimetic

 ## USES

Reduces congestion of nose, sinuses and throat from allergies and infections.

 ## DOSAGE & USAGE INFORMATION

How to take:
- Tablet—Swallow with liquid. You may chew or crush tablet.
- Extended-release capsules—Swallow each dose whole.
- Syrup—Take as directed on label.
- Drops—Place directly on tongue and swallow.

When to take:
- At the same times each day.
- To prevent insomnia, take last dose of day a few hours before bedtime.

If you forget a dose:
Take up to 2 hours late. If more than 2 hours, wait for next dose (don't double this dose).

What drug does:
Decreases blood volume in nasal tissues, shrinking tissues and enlarging airways.

Continued next column

 ## OVERDOSE

SYMPTOMS:
Nervousness, restlessness, headache, rapid or irregular heartbeat, sweating, nausea, vomiting, anxiety, confusion, delirium, muscle tremors, convulsions, hallucinations.
WHAT TO DO:
- **Dial 0 (operator) or 911 (emergency) for an ambulance or medical help. Then give first aid immediately.**
- **See emergency information on inside covers.**

Time lapse before drug works:
15 to 20 minutes.

Don't take with:
- Non-prescription drugs with caffeine without consulting doctor.
- Any other medicine without consulting your doctor or pharmacist.

 ## POSSIBLE ADVERSE REACTIONS OR SIDE EFFECTS

SYMPTOMS	WHAT TO DO
Life-threatening:	
In case of overdose, see previous column.	
Common:	
Agitation, insomnia.	Continue. Tell doctor at next visit.
Infrequent:	
• Nausea or vomiting, irregular or slow heartbeat, difficult breathing, unusually fast or pounding heartbeat, painful or difficult urination, increased sweating, trembling.	Discontinue. Call doctor right away.
• Dizziness, headache, shakiness, weakness.	Continue. Call doctor when convenient.
• Paleness.	Continue. Tell doctor at next visit.
Rare:	
Hallucinations, seizures.	Discontinue. Seek emergency treatment.

WARNINGS & PRECAUTIONS

Don't take if:
You are allergic to any sympathomimetic drug.

Before you start, consult your doctor:
- If you have overactive thyroid or diabetes.
- If you have taken any MAO inhibitors in past 2 weeks.
- If you take digitalis preparations or have high blood pressure or heart disease.
- If you will have surgery within 2 months, including dental surgery, requiring general or spinal anesthesia.
- If you have urination difficulty.

Over age 60:
Adverse reactions and side effects may be more frequent and severe than in younger persons.

Pregnancy:
No proven harm to unborn child. Avoid if possible.

Breast-feeding:
Drug passes into milk. Avoid drug or discontinue nursing until you finish medicine. Consult doctor for advice on maintaining milk supply.

Infants & children:
Keep dose low or avoid.

Prolonged use:
No proven problems.

Skin & sunlight:
No problems expected.

Driving, piloting or hazardous work:
Avoid if you feel dizzy. Otherwise, no problems expected..

Discontinuing:
May be unnecessary to finish medicine. Follow doctor's instructions.

Others:
No problems expected.

POSSIBLE INTERACTION WITH OTHER DRUGS

GENERIC NAME OR DRUG CLASS	COMBINED EFFECT
Antihypertensives*	Decreased antihypertensive effect.
Beta-adrenergic blockers*	Decreased effect of both drugs.
Calcium supplements*	Increased pseudoephedrine effect.
Digitalis preparations*	Irregular heartbeat.
Epinephrine	Increased epinephrine effect. Excessive heart stimulation and blood-pressure increase.
Ergot preparations*	Serious blood-pressure rise.
Guanadrel	Decreased effect of both drugs.
Guanethidine	Decreased effect of both drugs.
MAO inhibitors*	Increased pseudoephedrine effect.
Methyldopa	Possible increased blood pressure.
Nitrates*	Possible decreased effects of both drugs.
Phenothiazines*	Possible increased pseudoephedrine toxicity. Possible decreased pseudoephedrine effect.
Rauwolfia	Decreased rauwolfia effect.
Sympathomimetics*	Increased pseudoephedrine effect.
Terazosin	Decreases effectiveness of terazosin.

POSSIBLE INTERACTION WITH OTHER SUBSTANCES

INTERACTS WITH	COMBINED EFFECT
Alcohol:	None expected.
Beverages: Caffeine drinks.	Nervousness or insomnia.
Cocaine:	High risk of heartbeat irregularities and high blood pressure.
Foods:	None expected.
Marijuana:	Rapid heartbeat.
Tobacco:	None expected.

PSORALENS

BRAND AND GENERIC NAMES

8-Mop
METHOXSALEN
Methoxsalen Lotion
 (Topical)
Oxsoralen

Oxsoralen-Ultra
Oxsoralen (Topical)
TRIOXSALEN
Trisoralen
UltraMOP

BASIC INFORMATION

Habit forming? No
Prescription needed? Yes
Available as generic? No
Drug class: Repigmenting agent (psoralen)

 ## USES

- Repigmenting skin affected with vitiligo (absence of skin pigment).
- Treatment for psoriasis, when other treatments haven't helped.
- Treatment for mycosis fungoides.

 ## DOSAGE & USAGE INFORMATION

How to take or apply:
- Tablet or capsule—Swallow with liquid or food to lessen stomach irritation.
- Topical—As directed by doctor.

When to take or apply:
2 to 4 hours before exposure to sunlight or sunlamp.

If you forget a dose:
Take as soon as you remember. Delay sun exposure for at least 2 hours after taking.

What drug does:
Helps pigment cells when used in conjunction with ultraviolet light.

Time lapse before drug works:
- For vitiligo, 6 to 9 months.
- For psoriasis, 10 weeks or longer.
- For tanning, 3 to 4 days.

Don't take with:
Any other medicine which causes skin sensitivity to sun. Ask pharmacist.

 ## OVERDOSE

SYMPTOMS:
Blistering skin, swelling feet and legs.
WHAT TO DO:
Overdose unlikely to threaten life. If person takes much larger amount than prescribed, call doctor, poison-control center or hospital emergency room for instructions.

 ## POSSIBLE ADVERSE REACTIONS OR SIDE EFFECTS

SYMPTOMS	WHAT TO DO
Life-threatening:	
None expected.	
Common:	
● Increased skin sensitivity to sun.	Always protect from overexposure.
● Increased eye sensitivity to sunlight.	Always protect with wrap-around sunglasses.
● Nausea.	Continue. Call doctor when convenient.
Infrequent:	
● Skin red and sore.	Discontinue. Call doctor right away.
● Dizziness, headache, depression, leg cramps, insomnia.	Continue. Call doctor when convenient.
Rare:	
Hepatitis with jaundice, blistering and peeling.	Discontinue. Call doctor right away.

 ## WARNINGS & PRECAUTIONS

Don't take if:
- You are allergic to any other psoralen.
- You are unwilling or unable to remain under close medical supervision.

Before you start, consult your doctor:
- If you have heart or liver disease.
- If you have allergy to sunlight.
- If you have cataracts.
- If you have albinism.
- If you have lupus erythematosis, porphyria, chronic infection, skin cancer or peptic ulcer.
- If you will have surgery within 2 months, including dental surgery, requiring general or spinal anesthesia.

Over age 60:
Adverse reactions and side effects may be more frequent and severe than in younger persons.

Pregnancy:
Risk to unborn child outweighs drug benefits. Don't use.

Breast-feeding:
Drug passes into milk. Avoid drug or discontinue nursing until you finish medicine. Consult doctor for advice on maintaining milk supply.

Infants & children:
Not recommended.

Prolonged use:
- Increased chance of toxic effects.
- Talk to your doctor about the need for follow-up medical examinations or laboratory studies to check ANA titers*, complete blood counts (white blood cell count, platelet count, red blood cell count, hemoglobin, hematocrit), liver function, kidney function, eyes.

Skin & sunlight:
Too much can burn skin. Cover skin for 24 hours before and 8 hours following treatments.

Driving, piloting or hazardous work:
No problems expected. Protect eyes and skin from bright light.

Discontinuing:
Skin may remain sensitive for some time after treatment stops. Use extra protection from sun.

Others:
- Use sunblock on lips.
- Don't use just to make skin tan.
- Don't use hard gelatin capsules interchangeably with soft gelatin capsules.

POSSIBLE INTERACTION WITH OTHER DRUGS

GENERIC NAME OR DRUG CLASS	COMBINED EFFECT
Any medicine causing sensitization to sunlight, such as acetohexamide, amitriptyline, anthralin, barbiturates, bendroflumethiazide, carbamazepine, chlordiazepoxide, chloroquine, chlorothiazide, chloropromazine, chloropropamide, chlortetracycline, chlorthalidone, clindamycin, coal tar derivatives, cyproheptadine, demeclocycline, desipramine, diethylstilbrestrol, diphenhydramine, doxepin, doxycycline, estrogen, fluphenazine, gold preparations, glyburide, griseofulvin, hydrochlorothiazide,	Greatly increased likelihood of extreme sensitivity to sunlight.

hydroflumethiazide, imipramine, lincomycin, mesoridazine, methacycline, nalidixic acid, nortriptyline, oral contraceptives, oxyphenbutazone, oxytetracycline, perphenazine, phenobarbital, phenylbutazone, phenytoin, prochlorperazine, promazine, promethazine, protriptyline, pyrazinamide, sulfonamides, tetracycline, thioridazine, thiazide diuretics, tolazamide, tolbutamide, tranylcypromine, triamterene, trifluoperazine, trimeprazine, trimipramine, triprolidine

POSSIBLE INTERACTION WITH OTHER SUBSTANCES

INTERACTS WITH	COMBINED EFFECT
Alcohol:	May increase chance of liver toxicity.
Beverages: Lime drinks.	Avoid—toxic.
Cocaine:	Increased chance of toxicity. Avoid.
Foods: Those containing furocoumarin (limes, parsley, figs, parsnips, carrots, celery, mustard).	May cause toxic effects to psoralens.
Marijuana:	Increased chance of toxicity. Avoid.
Tobacco:	May cause uneven absorption of medicine. Avoid.

*See Glossary

PSYLLIUM

BRAND NAMES

See complete list of brand names in the *Brand Name Directory*, page 929.

BASIC INFORMATION

Habit forming? No
Prescription needed? No
Available as generic? No
Drug class: Laxative (bulk-forming)

 USES

Relieves constipation and prevents straining for bowel movement.

 DOSAGE & USAGE INFORMATION

How to take:
- Powder or granules—Dilute dose in 8 oz. cold water or fruit juice.
- Wafers or chewable pieces—Chew and swallow with liquid.

When to take:
At the same time each day, preferably morning.

If you forget a dose:
Take as soon as you remember. Resume regular schedule.

What drug does:
Absorbs water, stimulating the bowel to form a soft, bulky stool.

Time lapse before drug works:
May require 2 or 3 days to begin, then works in 12 to 24 hours.

Don't take with:
- Any other medicine without consulting your doctor or pharmacist.
- Don't take within 2 hours of taking another medicine.

 OVERDOSE

SYMPTOMS:
None expected.
WHAT TO DO:
Overdose unlikely to threaten life. If person takes much larger amount than prescribed, call doctor, poison-control center or hospital emergency room for instructions.

 POSSIBLE ADVERSE REACTIONS OR SIDE EFFECTS

SYMPTOMS	WHAT TO DO
Life-threatening None expected.	
Common: None expected.	
Infrequent: Swallowing difficulty, "lump in throat" sensation.	Continue. Call doctor when convenient.
Rare: Rash, itchy skin, asthma.	Discontinue. Call doctor right away.

WARNINGS & PRECAUTIONS

Don't take if:
- You are allergic to any bulk-forming laxative.
- You have symptoms of appendicitis, inflamed bowel or intestinal blockage.
- You have missed a bowel movement for only 1 or 2 days.

Before you start, consult your doctor:
- If you have diabetes.
- If you have kidney disease.
- If you have a laxative habit.
- If you have rectal bleeding.
- If you have difficulty swallowing.
- If you take other laxatives.

Over age 60:
Adverse reactions and side effects may be more frequent and severe than in younger persons.

Pregnancy:
Most bulk-forming laxatives contain sodium or sugars which may cause fluid retention. Avoid if possible.

Breast-feeding:
No problems expected.

Infants & children:
Use only under medical supervision.

Prolonged use:
Don't take for more than 1 week unless under a doctor's supervision. May cause laxative dependence.

Skin & sunlight:
No problems expected.

Driving, piloting or hazardous work:
No problems expected.

Discontinuing:
May be unnecessary to finish medicine. Follow doctor's instructions.

Others:
Don't take to "flush out" your system, or as a "tonic."

POSSIBLE INTERACTION WITH OTHER DRUGS

GENERIC NAME OR DRUG CLASS	COMBINED EFFECT
Digitalis preparations*	Decreased digitalis effect.
Salicylates* (including aspirin)	Decreased salicylate effect.

POSSIBLE INTERACTION WITH OTHER SUBSTANCES

INTERACTS WITH	COMBINED EFFECT
Alcohol:	None expected.
Beverages:	None expected.
Cocaine:	None expected.
Foods:	None expected.
Marijuana:	None expected.
Tobacco:	None expected.

---

*See Glossary

PYRANTEL

BRAND NAMES

Antiminth
Aut
Cobantril
Combantrin

Lombriareu
Reese's Pinworm
  Medicine
Trilombrin

BASIC INFORMATION

Habit forming? No
Prescription needed? Yes
Available as generic? Yes
Drug class: Anthelmintic

 ## USES

Treats intestinal parasitic disease caused by *Ascaris lumbricoides* (common roundworm), *Enterobiasis vermicularis* (pinworms), hookworm infections and other intestinal parasites.

 ## DOSAGE & USAGE INFORMATION

How to take:
- Tablets—Swallow with liquid. If you can't swallow whole, crumble tablet and take with liquid or food. Instructions to take on empty stomach mean 1 hour before or 2 hours after eating.
- Oral suspension—Swallow with liquid or food to lessen stomach irritation.

When to take:
Usually as a single dose following a light meal. Some parasites may require 3 days of treatment.

If you forget a dose:
Take as soon as you remember, then resume regular schedule.

What drug does:
Forces intestinal parasites to loosen their grip on the membrane lining the intestine so that the body can expel them in the stool.

Continued next column

 ## OVERDOSE

SYMPTOMS:
None expected.
WHAT TO DO:
Overdose unlikely to threaten life. If person takes much larger amount than prescribed, call doctor, poison-control center or hospital emergency room for instructions.

Time lapse before drug works:
1 to 3 days.

Don't take with:
Other drugs without talking to your doctor or pharmacist.

 ## POSSIBLE ADVERSE REACTIONS OR SIDE EFFECTS

SYMPTOMS	WHAT TO DO
Life-threatening: None expected.	
Common: None expected.	
Infrequent: Dizziness, drowsiness, headache, insomnia, abdominal cramps, diarrhea, nausea.	Discontinue. Call doctor right away.
Rare: Skin rash.	Discontinue. Call doctor right away.

PYRANTEL

WARNINGS & PRECAUTIONS

Don't take if:
You are allergic to pyrantel.

Before you start, consult your doctor:
If you have colitis, stomach ulcer, diverticulitis.

Over age 60:
No special problems expected.

Pregnancy:
No proven problems. Consult doctor.

Breast-feeding:
No problems expected, but consult doctor.

Infants & children:
Use only under close medical supervision.

Prolonged use:
Not intended for prolonged use.

Skin & sunlight:
No special problems expected.

Driving, piloting or hazardous work:
Don't drive or pilot aircraft until you learn how medicine affects you. Don't work around dangerous machinery. Don't climb ladders or work in high places. Danger increases if you drink alcohol or take medicines affecting alertness and reflexes, such as antihistamines, tranquilizers, sedatives, pain medicines, narcotics and mind-altering drugs.

Discontinuing:
Don't discontinue without doctor's advice until you complete prescribed dose even though symptoms diminish or disappear.

Others:
- Patients with some intestinal parasites may be anemic and need iron supplements for treatment. Consult doctor.
- For pinworms, all members of the household should be treated simultaneously.
- Treatment may need to be repeated several weeks later.

POSSIBLE INTERACTION WITH OTHER DRUGS

GENERIC NAME OR DRUG CLASS	COMBINED EFFECT
None expected	

POSSIBLE INTERACTION WITH OTHER SUBSTANCES

INTERACTS WITH	COMBINED EFFECT
Alcohol:	Dizziness, drowsiness.
Beverages:	No proven problems.
Cocaine:	Dizziness, drowsiness.
Foods:	No proven problems.
Marijuana:	Dizziness, drowsiness.
Tobacco:	No proven problems.

PYRIDOSTIGMINE

BRAND NAMES

Mestinon   Regonol
Mestinon Timespans

BASIC INFORMATION

Habit forming? No
Prescription needed? Yes
Available as generic? No
Drug class: Cholinergic, antimyasthenics

USES

- Diagnosis and treatment of myasthenia gravis.
- Treatment of urinary retention and abdominal distention.
- Antidote to adverse effects of muscle relaxants used in surgery.

DOSAGE & USAGE INFORMATION

How to take:
- Tablet or syrup—Swallow with liquid or food to lessen stomach irritation.
- Extended-release tablets—Swallow each dose whole. If you take regular tablets, you may chew or crush them.

When to take:
As directed, usually 3 or 4 times a day.

If you forget a dose:
Take as soon as you remember up to 2 hours late. If more than 2 hours, wait for next scheduled dose (don't double this dose).

What drug does:
Inhibits the chemical activity of an enzyme (cholinesterase) so nerve impulses can cross the junction of nerves and muscles.

Continued next column

OVERDOSE

SYMPTOMS:
Muscle weakness or paralysis, cramps, twitching or clumsiness; severe diarrhea, nausea, vomiting, stomach cramps or pain; breathing difficulty; confusion, irritability, nervousness, restlessness, fear; unusually slow heartbeat; seizures; blurred vision; extreme fatigue.
WHAT TO DO:
- **Dial 0 (operator) or 911 (emergency) for an ambulance or medical help. Then give first aid immediately.**
- **See emergency information on inside covers.**

Time lapse before drug works:
3 hours.

Don't take with:
Any other medicine without consulting your doctor or pharmacist.

POSSIBLE ADVERSE REACTIONS OR SIDE EFFECTS

SYMPTOMS	WHAT TO DO
Life-threatening:	
In case of overdose, see previous column.	
Common:	
• Mild diarrhea, nausea, vomiting, stomach cramps or pain.	Discontinue. Call doctor right away.
• Excess saliva, unusual sweating.	Continue. Call doctor when convenient.
Infrequent:	
• Confusion, irritability.	Discontinue. Seek emergency treatment.
• Constricted pupils, watery eyes, lung congestion, frequent urge to urinate.	Continue. Call doctor when convenient.
Rare:	
Bronchospasm, slow heartbeat, weakness.	Discontinue. Call doctor right away.

WARNINGS & PRECAUTIONS

Don't take if:
- You are allergic to any cholinergic or bromide.
- You take mecamylamine.

Before you start, consult your doctor:
- If you plan to become pregnant within medication period.
- If you have bronchial asthma.
- If you have heartbeat irregularities.
- If you have urinary obstruction or urinary-tract infection.

Over age 60:
Adverse reactions and side effects may be more frequent and severe than in younger persons.

Pregnancy:
No proven harm to unborn child. Avoid if possible. May increase contractions of the womb close to time of delivery.

Breast-feeding:
No problems expected, but consult doctor.

Infants & children:
Not recommended.

Prolonged use:
Medication may lose effectiveness. Discontinuing for a few days may restore effect.

Skin & sunlight:
No problems expected.

Driving, piloting or hazardous work:
Don't drive or pilot aircraft until you learn how medicine affects you. Don't work around dangerous machinery. Don't climb ladders or work in high places. Danger increases if you drink alcohol or take medicine affecting alertness and reflexes, such as antihistamines, tranquilizers, sedatives, pain medicine, narcotics and mind-altering drugs.

Discontinuing:
Don't discontinue without doctor's advice until you complete prescribed dose, even though symptoms diminish or disappear.

Others:
No problems expected.

POSSIBLE INTERACTION WITH OTHER DRUGS

GENERIC NAME OR DRUG CLASS	COMBINED EFFECT
Anesthetics, local or general*	Decreased pyridostigmine effect.
Antiarrhythmics*	Decreased pyridostigmine effect.
Anticholinergics*	Decreased pyridostigmine effect. May mask severe side effects.
Cholinergics, other*	Reduced intestinal-tract function. Possible brain and nervous-system toxicity.
Guanadrel	Decreased pyridostigmine effect.
Guanethidine	Decreased pyridostigmine effect.
Mecamylamine	Decreased pyridostigmine effect.
Nitrates*	Decreased pyridostigmine effect.
Procainamide	Decreased pyridostigmine effect.
Quinidine	Decreased pyridostigmine effect.

POSSIBLE INTERACTION WITH OTHER SUBSTANCES

INTERACTS WITH	COMBINED EFFECT
Alcohol:	No proven problems with small doses.
Beverages:	None expected.
Cocaine:	Decreased pyridostigmine effect. Avoid.
Foods:	None expected.
Marijuana:	No proven problems.
Tobacco:	No proven problems.

PYRIDOXINE (Vitamin B-6)

BRAND NAMES

Beesix   Rodex
Hexa-Betalin   Tex Six T.R.
Pyroxine

BASIC INFORMATION

Habit forming? No
Prescription needed?
  High strength: Yes
  Low strength: No
Available as generic? Yes
Drug class: Vitamin supplement

 USES

- Prevention and treatment of pyridoxine deficiency.
- Treatment of some forms of anemia.
- Treatment of INH (isonicotinic acid hydrozide), cycloserine poisoning.

 DOSAGE & USAGE INFORMATION

How to take:
- Tablets—Swallow with liquid.
- Extended-release capsules—Swallow each dose whole with liquid.

When to take:
At the same times each day.

If you forget a dose:
Take as soon as you remember, then resume regular schedule.

What drug does:
Acts as co-enzyme in carbohydrate, protein and fat metabolism.

Time lapse before drug works:
15 to 20 minutes.

Don't take with:
- Levodopa—Small amounts of pyridoxine will nullify levodopa effect. Carbidopa-levodopa combination not affected by this interaction.
- Any other medicine without consulting your doctor or pharmacist.

 OVERDOSE

SYMPTOMS:
None expected.
WHAT TO DO:
Overdose unlikely to threaten life.

 POSSIBLE ADVERSE REACTIONS OR SIDE EFFECTS

SYMPTOMS	WHAT TO DO
Life-threatening: None expected.	
Common: None expected.	
Infrequent: Nausea, headache.	Discontinue. Call doctor right away.
Rare: Numbness or tingling in hands or feet (large doses).	Discontinue. Call doctor right away.

WARNINGS & PRECAUTIONS

Don't take if:
You are allergic to pyridoxine.

Before you start, consult your doctor:
If you are pregnant or breast-feeding.

Over age 60:
No problems expected.

Pregnancy:
Don't exceed recommended dose.

Breast-feeding:
Don't exceed recommended dose.

Infants & children:
Don't exceed recommended dose.

Prolonged use:
Large doses for more than 1 month may cause toxicity.

Skin & sunlight:
No problems expected.

Driving, piloting or hazardous work:
No problems expected.

Discontinuing:
No problems expected.

Others:
Regular pyridoxine supplements recommended if you take chloramphenicol, cycloserine, ethionamide, hydralazine, immunosuppressants, isoniazid or penicillamine. These decrease pyridoxine absorption and can cause anemia or tingling and numbness in hands and feet.

POSSIBLE INTERACTION WITH OTHER DRUGS

GENERIC NAME OR DRUG CLASS	COMBINED EFFECT
Contraceptives, oral*	Decreased pyridoxine effect.
Cycloserine	Decreased pyridoxine effect.
Ethionamide	Decreased pyridoxine effect.
Hydralazine	Decreased pyridoxine effect.
Hypnotics, barbiturates*	Decreased hypnotic effect.
Immuno-suppressants*	Decreased pyridoxine effect.
Isoniazid	Decreased pyridoxine effect.
Levodopa	Decreased levodopa effect.
Penicillamine	Decreased pyridoxine effect.
Phenobarbital	Possible decreased phenobarbital effect.
Phenytoin	Decreased phenytoin effect.

POSSIBLE INTERACTION WITH OTHER SUBSTANCES

INTERACTS WITH	COMBINED EFFECT
Alcohol:	None expected.
Beverages:	None expected.
Cocaine:	None expected.
Foods:	None expected.
Marijuana:	None expected.
Tobacco:	May decrease pyridoxine absorption. Decreased pyridoxine effect.

PYRVINIUM

BRAND NAMES

Vanquin   Viprynium

BASIC INFORMATION

Habit forming? No
Prescription needed? Yes
Available as generic? No
Drug class: Anthelmintic

 ## USES

Treatment for pinworm infestation.

 ## DOSAGE & USAGE INFORMATION

How to take:
Tablet—Swallow whole with food or liquid. Don't crush or chew tablet.

When to take:
According to label instructions. Usually a single dose, which may be repeated in 2 or 3 weeks.

If you forget a dose:
Take when remembered.

What drug does:
Interferes with a metabolic process in the infecting parasite and kills it.

Time lapse before drug works:
12 hours.

Don't take with:
- Non-prescription drugs for pinworms.
- Any other medicine without consulting your doctor or pharmacist.

 ## OVERDOSE

SYMPTOMS:
Increased severity of adverse reactions and side effects.
WHAT TO DO:
Overdose unlikely to threaten life. If person takes much larger amount than prescribed, call doctor, poison-control center or hospital emergency room for instructions.

 ## POSSIBLE ADVERSE REACTIONS OR SIDE EFFECTS

SYMPTOMS	WHAT TO DO
Life-threatening: None expected.	
Common: Urine turns red.	No action necessary. This always happens.
Infrequent: None expected.	
Rare: • Rash.	Discontinue. Call doctor right away.
• Dizziness, stomach cramps, nausea, vomiting.	Continue. Call doctor when convenient.

WARNINGS & PRECAUTIONS

Don't take if:
You are allergic to any anthelmintic drug.

Before you start, consult your doctor:
• If you have kidney or liver disease.
• If you have a bowel disease or inflammation.

Over age 60:
Adverse reactions and side effects may be more frequent and severe than in younger persons.

Pregnancy:
No proven harm to unborn child. Avoid if possible.

Breast-feeding:
No problems expected, but consult doctor.

Infants & children:
No problems expected.

Prolonged use:
Not recommended.

Skin & sunlight:
May cause rash or intensify sunburn in areas exposed to sun or sunlamp.

Driving, piloting or hazardous work:
Avoid if you feel dizzy. Otherwise, no problems expected.

Discontinuing:
Don't discontinue without doctor's advice until you complete prescribed dose, even though symptoms diminish or disappear.

Others:
• This medicine is a dye that permanently stains most materials. Teeth will be stained a few days. Stool and vomit may be red.
• Pinworm infestations are highly contagious. All family members should be treated at the same time.

POSSIBLE INTERACTION WITH OTHER DRUGS

GENERIC NAME OR DRUG CLASS	COMBINED EFFECT
None expected.	

POSSIBLE INTERACTION WITH OTHER SUBSTANCES

INTERACTS WITH	COMBINED EFFECT
Alcohol:	None expected.
Beverages:	None expected.
Cocaine:	None expected.
Foods:	None expected.
Marijuana:	None expected.
Tobacco:	None expected.

QUINACRINE

BRAND NAMES

Atabrine

BASIC INFORMATION

Habit forming? No
Prescription needed? Yes
Available as generic? Yes
Drug class: Antiprotozoal

 ## USES

Treats disease caused by the intestinal parasite *Giardia lamblia*.

 ## DOSAGE & USAGE INFORMATION

How to take:
Tablets—Swallow with full glass of water, tea or fruit juice. If you can't swallow whole, crumble tablet and mix with jam or chocolate syrup.

When to take:
After meals.

If you forget a dose:
Take as soon as you remember up to 2 hours late. If more than 2 hours, wait for next scheduled dose (don't double this dose).

What drug does:
Destroys *Gardia lamblia* parasites in the gastrointestinal system.

Continued next column

 ## OVERDOSE

SYMPTOMS:
Severe abdominal cramps, convulsions, severe diarrhea, fainting, irregular heartbeat, restlessness.
WHAT TO DO:
- **Dial 0 (operator) or 911 (emergency) for an ambulance or medical help. Then give first aid immediately.**
- **If patient is unconscious and not breathing, give mouth-to-mouth breathing. If there is no heartbeat, use cardiac massage and mouth-to-mouth breathing (CPR). Don't try to make patient vomit. If you can't get help quickly, take patient to nearest emergency facility.**
- **See emergency information on inside covers.**

Time lapse before drug works:
1 day.

Don't take with:
Any other medicine without consulting your doctor or pharmacist.

 ## POSSIBLE ADVERSE REACTIONS OR SIDE EFFECTS

SYMPTOMS	WHAT TO DO
Life-threatening:	
In case of overdose, see previous column.	
Common:	
● Dizziness, nausea, headache.	Discontinue. Call doctor right away.
● Yellow eyes, skin, urine (due to dye-like characteristics of quinacrine).	Report to doctor, but no action necessary.
Infrequent:	
● Mild abdominal cramps; mild diarrhea; appetite loss; skin rash, itching or peeling.	Discontinue. Call doctor right away.
● Mood changes.	Continue. Call doctor when convenient.
Rare:	
Hallucinations, nightmares.	Discontinue. Call doctor right away.

WARNINGS & PRECAUTIONS

Don't take if:
You are allergic to quinacrine.

Before you start, consult your doctor:
- If you have porphyria.
- If you have had psoriasis.
- If you have a history of severe mental disorders.
- If you are on a low-salt, low-sugar or other special diet.

Over age 60:
No special problems.

Pregnancy:
Studies inconclusive on harm to unborn child. Decide with your doctor whether drug benefits justify risk to unborn child. Treatment best begun after child has been delivered.

Breast-feeding:
No problems documented.

Infants & children:
Children tolerate quinacrine poorly. Quinacrine may cause vomiting due to bitter taste. Try crushing tablets in jam, honey or chocolate syrup.

Prolonged use:
- Can cause eye problems, liver disease, aplastic anemia. Don't use for more than 5 days.
- Talk to your doctor about the need for follow-up medical examinations or laboratory studies to check stools for giardiasis.

Skin & sunlight:
No problems expected.

Driving, piloting or hazardous work:
Don't drive or pilot aircraft until you learn how medicine affects you. Don't work around dangerous machinery. Don't climb ladders or work in high places. Danger increases if you drink alcohol or take medicine affecting alertness and reflexes, such as antihistamines, tranquilizers, sedatives, pain medicine, narcotics and mind-altering drugs.

Discontinuing:
Don't discontinue before 5 days without consulting doctor.

Others:
Request 3 stool exams several days apart.

 POSSIBLE INTERACTION WITH OTHER DRUGS

GENERIC NAME OR DRUG CLASS	COMBINED EFFECT
Primaquine	Decreased effect of primaquine.

 POSSIBLE INTERACTION WITH OTHER SUBSTANCES

INTERACTS WITH	COMBINED EFFECT
Alcohol:	Increased adverse effects of both. Avoid.
Beverages:	Increased adverse effects of both. Avoid.
Cocaine:	Increased adverse effects of both. Avoid.
Foods:	Increased adverse effects of both. Avoid.
Marijuana:	Increased adverse effects of both. Avoid.
Tobacco:	Increased adverse effects of both. Avoid.

QUINIDINE

BRAND NAMES

Apo-Quinidine	Quinaglute Dura-Tabs
Cardioquin	Quinalan
Cin-Quin	Quinate
Duraquin	Quinidex Extentabs
Novoquinidin	Quinora

BASIC INFORMATION

Habit forming? No
Prescription needed?
 U.S.: Yes
 Canada: No
Available as generic? Yes
Drug class: Antiarrhythmic

USES

Corrects heart rhythm disorders.

DOSAGE & USAGE INFORMATION

How to take:
- Tablet or capsule—Swallow with liquid or food to lessen stomach irritation.
- Extended-release tablets—Swallow each dose whole. Don't crush them.

When to take:
At the same times each day.

If you forget a dose:
Take as soon as you remember up to 2 hours late. If more than 2 hours, wait for next scheduled dose (don't double this dose).

What drug does:
Delays nerve impulses to the heart to regulate heartbeat.

Continued next column

OVERDOSE

SYMPTOMS:
Confusion, severe blood-pressure drop, lethargy, breathing difficulty, fainting, seizures, coma.
WHAT TO DO:
- **Dial 0 (operator) or 911 (emergency) for an ambulance or medical help. Then give first aid immediately.**
- **If patient is unconscious and not breathing, give mouth-to-mouth breathing. If there is no heartbeat, use cardiac massage and mouth-to-mouth breathing (CPR). Don't try to make patient vomit. If you can't get help quickly, take patient to nearest emergency facility.**
- **See emergency information on inside covers.**

Time lapse before drug works:
2 to 4 hours.

Don't take with:
Any other medicine without consulting your doctor or pharmacist.

POSSIBLE ADVERSE REACTIONS OR SIDE EFFECTS

SYMPTOMS	WHAT TO DO
Life-threatening: Hives, rash, intense itching, faintness soon after a dose (anaphylaxis); wheezing.	Seek emergency treatment immediately.
Common: Bitter taste, diarrhea, nausea, vomiting, appetite loss, abdominal pain.	Discontinue. Call doctor right away.
Infrequent: • Dizziness, lightheadedness, fainting, headache, confusion, rash, change in vision, difficult breathing, rapid heartbeat.	Discontinue. Call doctor right away.
• Ringing in ears.	Continue. Call doctor when convenient.
Rare: • Unusual bleeding or bruising, difficulty or pain on swallowing, fever, joint pain, jaundice, hepatitis.	Discontinue. Call doctor right away.
• Weakness.	Continue. Call doctor when convenient.

WARNINGS & PRECAUTIONS

Don't take if:
- You are allergic to quinidine.
- You have an active infection.

Before you start, consult your doctor:
About any drug you take, including non-prescription drugs.

Over age 60:
Adverse reactions and side effects may be more frequent and severe than in younger persons.

Pregnancy:
Risk to unborn child outweighs drug benefits. Don't use.

Breast-feeding:
Drug filters into milk. May harm child. Avoid.

QUINIDINE

Infants & children:
No problems expected.

Prolonged use:
Talk to your doctor about the need for follow-up medical examinations or laboratory studies to check complete blood counts (white blood cell count, platelet count, red blood cell count, hemoglobin, hematocrit), liver function, kidney function, serum potassium levels, ECG*.

Skin & sunlight:
No problems expected.

Driving, piloting or hazardous work:
Don't drive or pilot aircraft until you learn how medicine affects you. Don't work around dangerous machinery. Don't climb ladders or work in high places. Danger increases if you drink alcohol or take medicine affecting alertness and reflexes, such as antihistamines, tranquilizers, sedatives, pain medicine, narcotics and mind-altering drugs.

Discontinuing:
Don't discontinue without doctor's advice until you complete prescribed dose, even though symptoms diminish or disappear.

Others:
No problems expected.

 POSSIBLE INTERACTION WITH OTHER DRUGS

GENERIC NAME OR DRUG CLASS	COMBINED EFFECT
Alkalizers, urinary	Slows quinidine elimination, increases effect and toxicity.
Antiarrhythmics*	May increase or decrease effect or toxicity of quinidine.
Anticholinergics*	Increased anticholinergic effect.
Anticoagulants, oral*	Possible increased anticoagulant effect.
Antihypertensives*	Increased antihypertensive effect.
Beta-adrenergic blockers*	May slow heartbeat excessively.
Cholinergics*	Decreased cholinergic effect.
Cimetidine	Increased quinidine effect.
Dapsone	Increased risk of adverse effect on blood cells.
Digitalis preparations*	May slow heartbeat excessively. Dose adjustments may be needed.
Encainide	Increased effect of toxicity on heart muscle.
Flecainide	Possible irregular heartbeat.
Guanfacine	Increased effect of both medicines.
Nicardipine	Possible increased effect and toxicity of each drug.
Nifedipine	Possible decreased quinidine effect.
Nimodipine	Increased quinidine effect.
Phenobarbital	Decreased quinidine effect.
Phenothiazines*	Possible increased quinidine effect.
Phenytoin	Decreased quinidine effect.
Pimozide	Increased risk of heartbeat irregularities.
Propafenone	Increased effect of both drugs and increased risk of toxicity.
Rauwolfia alkaloids*	Possibly disturbs heart rhythms.
Tocainide	Increased possibility of adverse reactions from either drug.
Rifampin	Decreased quinidine effect.
Verapamil	Hypotension.

 POSSIBLE INTERACTION WITH OTHER SUBSTANCES

INTERACTS WITH	COMBINED EFFECT
Alcohol:	None expected.
Beverages: Caffeine drinks.	Causes rapid heartbeat. Use sparingly.
Cocaine:	Irregular heartbeat. Avoid.
Foods:	None expected.
Marijuana:	Can cause fainting.
Tobacco:	Irregular heartbeat. Avoid.

*See Glossary

QUININE

BRAND NAMES

NovoQuinine	Quiphile
Quinamm	Q-Vel
Quindan	Strema

BASIC INFORMATION

Habit forming? No
Prescription needed?
  High strength: Yes
  Low strength: No
Available as generic? Yes
Drug class: Antiprotozoal

USES

- Treatment or prevention of malaria.
- Relief of muscle cramps.

DOSAGE & USAGE INFORMATION

How to take:
Tablet or capsule—Swallow with liquid or food to lessen stomach irritation.

When to take:
- Prevention—At the same time each day, usually at bedtime.
- Treatment—At the same times each day in evenly spaced doses.

If you forget a dose:
- Prevention—Take as soon as you remember up to 12 hours late. If more than 12 hours, wait for next scheduled dose (don't double this dose).
- Treatment—Take as soon as you remember up to 2 hours late. If more than 2 hours, wait for next scheduled dose (don't double this dose).

Continued next column

OVERDOSE

SYMPTOMS:
Severe impairment of vision and hearing; severe nausea, vomiting, diarrhea; shallow breathing, fast heartbeat; apprehension, confusion, delirium.
WHAT TO DO:
Dial 0 (operator) or 911 (emergency) for an ambulance or medical help. Then give first aid immediately.

What drug does:
- Reduces contractions of skeletal muscles.
- Increases blood flow.
- Interferes with genes in malaria micro-organisms.

Time lapse before drug works:
May require several days or weeks for maximum effect.

Don't take with:
Any other medicine without consulting your doctor or pharmacist.

POSSIBLE ADVERSE REACTIONS OR SIDE EFFECTS

SYMPTOMS	WHAT TO DO
Life-threatening: In case of overdose, see previous column.	
Common:	
Blurred vision or change in vision, eyes sensitive to light.	Discontinue. Call doctor right away.
Dizziness, headache, abdominal discomfort, mild nausea, vomiting, diarrhea.	Continue. Call doctor when convenient.
Ringing or buzzing in ears, impaired hearing.	Continue. Tell doctor at next visit.
Infrequent:	
Rash, hives, itchy skin, difficult breathing.	Discontinue. Call doctor right away.
Rare:	
Sore throat, fever, unusual bleeding or bruising, unusual tiredness or weakness, angina.	Discontinue. Call doctor right away.

WARNINGS & PRECAUTIONS

Don't take if:
You are allergic to quinine or quinidine.

Before you start, consult your doctor:
- If you plan to become pregnant within medication period.
- If you have asthma.
- If you have eye disease, hearing problems or ringing in the ears.
- If you have heart disease.
- If you have myasthenia gravis.

Over age 60:
Adverse reactions and side effects may be more frequent and severe than in younger persons.

Pregnancy:
Risk to unborn child outweighs drug benefits. Don't use.

Breast-feeding:
Drug filters into milk. May harm child. Avoid.

Infants & children:
Use only under medical supervision.

Prolonged use:
May develop headache, blurred vision, nausea, temporary hearing loss, but seldom need to discontinue because of these symptoms.

Skin & sunlight:
Increased sensitivity to sunlight.

Driving, piloting or hazardous work:
Avoid if you feel dizzy or have blurred vision. Otherwise, no problems expected.

Discontinuing:
Don't discontinue without doctor's advice until you complete prescribed dose, even though symptoms diminish or disappear.

Others:
Don't confuse with quinidine, a medicine for heart-rhythm problems.

POSSIBLE INTERACTION WITH OTHER DRUGS

GENERIC NAME OR DRUG CLASS	COMBINED EFFECT
Antacids* (with aluminum hydroxide)	Decreased quinine effect.
Anticoagulants, oral*	Increased anti-coagulant effect.
Dapsone	Increased risk of adverse effect on blood cells.
Digitalis	Possible increased digitalis effect.
Digoxin	Possible increased digoxin effect.
Mefloquine	Increased risk of heartbeat irregularities.
Quinidine	Possible toxic effects of quinine.
Sodium bicarbonate	Possible toxic effects of quinine.

POSSIBLE INTERACTION WITH OTHER SUBSTANCES

INTERACTS WITH	COMBINED EFFECT
Alcohol:	No proven problems.
Beverages:	None expected.
Cocaine:	No proven problems.
Foods:	None expected.
Marijuana:	No proven problems.
Tobacco:	None expected.

RADIO-PHARMACEUTICALS

BRAND NAMES

See complete list of brand names in the
Brand Name Directory, page 929.

BASIC INFORMATION

Habit forming? No
Prescription needed? Yes
Available as generic? Yes
Drug class: Radio-pharmaceuticals

USES

To help establish an accurate diagnosis for
many medical problems, such as pernicious
anemia, malabsorption, iron metabolism, cancer,
abscess, infection, cerebrospinal fluid flow,
blood volume, kidney diseases, lung diseases,
pancreas diseases, red blood cell disorders,
spleen diseases, thyroid diseases, thyroid
cancer, brain diseases or tumor, bladder
diseases, eye tumors, liver diseases, heart
diseases, bone diseases, bone marrow
diseases.

DOSAGE & USAGE INFORMATION

How to take:
- As directed by nuclear medicine specialist.
  Most are given intravenously by the doctor,
  some are taken by mouth.
- Drink lots of liquids and urinate often after test
  to decrease possible radiation effect on the
  kidneys and urinary bladder.

When to take:
According to individual instructions.

If you forget a dose:
Take as soon as you remember.

What drug does:
Very small quantities of radioactive substances
concentrate in various organs of the body and
become measurable. Pictures or readings of the
organ or system under study become possible.

Time lapse before drug works:
Varies between products.

Don't take with:
Any other medicine without consulting doctor.

OVERDOSE

SYMPTOMS:
None expected.
WHAT TO DO:
None expected.

POSSIBLE ADVERSE REACTIONS OR SIDE EFFECTS

SYMPTOMS	WHAT TO DO
Life-threatening:	
Hives, rash, intense itching, faintness soon after a dose (anaphylaxis).	Seek emergency treatment immediately.
Common:	
Appetite loss.	Call doctor when convenient.
Infrequent:	
Drowsiness; fast heartbeat; swollen feet, ankles, hands or throat; abdominal pain; rash; hives; nausea; vomiting, headache; red or flushed face; fever; fainting.	Call doctor right away.
Rare:	
Constipation, coughing, sneezing, runny nose, wheezing.	Call doctor right away.

WARNINGS & PRECAUTIONS

Don't take if:
You are allergic to the prescribed drug.

Before you start, consult your doctor:
- If you have had allergic reactions to human serum albumin.
- If you are allergic to anything.

Over age 60:
Adverse reactions and side effects may be more frequent and severe than in younger persons. Ask doctor about smaller doses.

Pregnancy:
Avoid during pregnancy if possible.

Breast-feeding:
Drug passes into milk. Avoid drug or discontinue nursing until you finish medicine. Consult doctor for advice on maintaining milk supply.

Infants & children:
No problems expected.

Prolonged use:
Not intended for prolonged use.

Skin & sunlight:
No problems expected.

Driving, piloting or hazardous work:
No problems expected.

Discontinuing:
No problems expected.

Others:
Some of these agents may accumulate in the urinary bladder. To decrease chance of excessive radiation, drink 8 oz. of fluid every 1 hour for 10 to 12 hours following the test, unless otherwise specified by your doctor.

POSSIBLE INTERACTION WITH OTHER DRUGS

GENERIC NAME OR DRUG CLASS	COMBINED EFFECT
None expected.	

POSSIBLE INTERACTION WITH OTHER SUBSTANCES

INTERACTS WITH	COMBINED EFFECT
Alcohol:	None expected.
Beverages:	None expected.
Cocaine:	None expected.
Foods:	None expected.
Marijuana:	None expected.
Tobacco:	None expected.

RAUWOLFIA ALKALOIDS

BRAND AND GENERIC NAMES

See complete list of brand and generic names in the *Brand Name Directory*, page 929.

BASIC INFORMATION

Habit forming? No
Prescription needed? Yes
Available as generic? Yes
Drug class: Antihypertensive, tranquilizer (rauwolfia alkaloid)

 ## USES

- Treatment for high blood pressure.
- Tranquilizer for mental and emotional disturbances.

 ## DOSAGE & USAGE INFORMATION

How to take:
Tablet or timed-release capsule—Swallow with liquid or food to lessen stomach irritation. If you can't swallow whole, crumble tablet or open capsule and take with liquid or food.

When to take:
At the same times each day.

If you forget a dose:
Take as soon as you remember up to 2 hours late. If more than 2 hours, wait for next scheduled dose (don't double this dose).

What drug does:
- Interferes with nerve impulses and relaxes blood-vessel muscles, reducing blood pressure.
- Suppresses brain centers that control emotions.

Time lapse before drug works:
3 weeks continual use required to determine effectiveness.

Don't take with:
Any other medicine without consulting your doctor or pharmacist.

 ## OVERDOSE

SYMPTOMS:
Drowsiness; slow, weak pulse; slow, shallow breathing; diarrhea; coma; flush; low body temperature; pinpoint pupils.
WHAT TO DO:
- Dial 0 (operator) or 911 (emergency) for an ambulance or medical help. Then give first aid immediately.
- See emergency information on inside covers.

 ## POSSIBLE ADVERSE REACTIONS OR SIDE EFFECTS

SYMPTOMS	WHAT TO DO
Life-threatening:	
In case of overdose, see previous column.	
Common:	
• Depression, dizziness.	Continue. Call doctor when convenient.
• Headache, faintness, drowsiness, lethargy, red eyes, stuffy nose, impotence, diminished sex drive, diarrhea, dry mouth.	Continue. Tell doctor at next visit.
Infrequent:	
• Black stool; bloody vomit; chest pain; shortness of breath; irregular or slow heartbeat; stiffness in muscles, bones, joints.	Discontinue. Call doctor right away.
• Trembling hands, foot and leg swelling.	Continue. Call doctor when convenient.
Rare:	
• Rash or itchy skin, sore throat, fever, abdominal pain, nausea, vomiting, unusual bleeding or bruising, jaundice.	Discontinue. Call doctor right away.
• Painful urination, nightmares.	Continue. Call doctor when convenient.

 ## WARNINGS & PRECAUTIONS

Don't take if:
- You are allergic to any rauwolfia alkaloid.
- You are depressed.
- You have active peptic ulcer.
- You have ulcerative colitis.

Before you start, consult your doctor:
- If you have been depressed.
- If you have had peptic ulcer, ulcerative colitis or gallstones.
- If you have epilepsy.
- If you will have surgery within 2 months, including dental surgery, requiring general or spinal anesthesia.

Over age 60:
Adverse reactions and side effects may be more frequent and severe than in younger persons.

Pregnancy:
Studies inconclusive on harm to unborn child. Animal studies show fetal abnormalities. Decide with your doctor whether drug benefits justify risk to unborn child.

Breast-feeding:
Drug passes into milk. Avoid drug or discontinue nursing until you finish medicine. Consult doctor for advice on maintaining milk supply.

Infants & children:
Not recommended.

Prolonged use:
- Causes cancer in laboratory animals. Consult your doctor if you have family or personal history of cancer.
- Talk to your doctor about the need for follow-up medical examinations or laboratory studies.

Skin & sunlight:
No problems expected.

Driving, piloting or hazardous work:
Avoid if you feel drowsy, dizzy or faint. Otherwise, no problems expected.

Discontinuing:
Don't discontinue without consulting doctor. Dose may require gradual reduction if you have taken drug for a long time. Doses of other drugs may also require adjustment.

Others:
Consult your doctor if you do isometric exercises. These raise blood pressure. Drug may intensify blood-pressure rise.

POSSIBLE INTERACTION WITH OTHER DRUGS

GENERIC NAME OR DRUG CLASS	COMBINED EFFECT
Anticoagulants, oral*	Unpredictable increased or decreased effect of anticoagulant.
Anticonvulsants*	Serious change in seizure pattern.
Antidepressants*	Increased antidepressant effect.
Antihistamines*	Increased antihistamine effect.
Antihypertensives, other*	Increased effect of rauwolfia.
Aspirin	Decreased aspirin effect.
Beta-adrenergic blockers*	Increased effect of rauwolfia alkaloids. Excessive sedation.
Carteolol	Increased antihypertensive effect.
Clozapine	Toxic effect on the central nervous system.

Digitalis preparations*	Possible irregular heartbeat.
Dronabinol	Increased effects of both drugs. Avoid.
Ethinamate	Dangerous increased effects of ethinamate. Avoid combining.
Fluoxetine	Increased depressant effects of both drugs.
Guanfacine	May increase depressant effects of either medicine.
Leucovorin	High alcohol content of leucovorin may cause adverse effects.
Levodopa	Decreased levodopa effect.
Lisinopril	Increased antihypertensive effect. Dosage of each may require adjustment.
Loxapine	May increase toxic effects of both drugs.
MAO inhibitors*	Severe depression.
Methyprylon	May increase sedative effect to dangerous level. Avoid.

Continued on page 959

POSSIBLE INTERACTION WITH OTHER SUBSTANCES

INTERACTS WITH	COMBINED EFFECT
Alcohol:	Increased intoxication. Use with extreme caution.
Beverages: Carbonated drinks.	Decreased rauwolfia alkaloids effect.
Cocaine:	Increased risk of heart block and high blood pressure.
Foods: Spicy foods.	Possible digestive upset.
Marijuana:	Occasional use—Mild drowsiness. Daily use—Moderate drowsiness, low blood pressure, depression.
Tobacco:	No problems expected.

*See Glossary

RAUWOLFIA & THIAZIDE DIURETICS

BRAND AND GENERIC NAMES

See complete list of brand and generic names in the *Brand Name Directory*, page 929.

BASIC INFORMATION

Habit forming? No
Prescription needed? Yes
Available as generic? Yes
Drug class: Antihypertensive, diuretic, tranquilizer

USES

- Controls, but doesn't cure, high blood pressure.
- Reduces fluid retention (edema).

DOSAGE & USAGE INFORMATION

How to take:
Tablet—Swallow with liquid. If you can't swallow whole, crumble tablet and take with liquid or food.

When to take:
At the same time each day.

If you forget a dose:
Take as soon as you remember up to 2 hours late. If more than 2 hours, wait for next scheduled dose (don't double this dose).

What drug does:
- Forces sodium and water excretion, reducing body fluid.
- Reduced body fluid and relaxed arteries lower blood pressure.
- Interferes with nerve impulses and relaxes blood-vessel muscles, reducing blood pressure.
- Suppresses brain centers that control emotion.

Continued next column

OVERDOSE

SYMPTOMS:
Cramps; weakness; drowsiness; pinpoint pupils; slow, weak pulse; slow, shallow breathing; diarrhea; flush; low body temperature; coma.
WHAT TO DO:
- **Dial 0 (operator) or 911 (emergency) for an ambulance or medical help. Then give first aid immediately.**
- **See emergency information on inside covers.**

Time lapse before drug works:
3 weeks continual use required to determine effectiveness.

Don't take with:
Any other prescription or non-prescription drugs without consulting your doctor or pharmacist.

POSSIBLE ADVERSE REACTIONS OR SIDE EFFECTS

SYMPTOMS	WHAT TO DO
Life-threatening: Irregular heartbeat, weak pulse, hives, black stool, bloody vomit.	Discontinue. Seek emergency treatment.
Common: Lethargy, drowsiness, tremor, depression, red eyes, runny nose, diarrhea, dry mouth.	Continue. Call doctor when convenient.
Infrequent: • Blurred vision, abdominal pain, nausea, vomiting, irregular heartbeat, joint pain.	Discontinue. Call doctor right away.
• Dizziness, mood change, headache, dry mouth, weakness, tiredness, weight gain or loss, foot and leg swelling.	Continue. Call doctor when convenient.
Rare: • Sore throat, fever, mouth sores; jaundice; unexplained bleeding or bruising.	Discontinue. Call doctor right away.
• Rash, painful or difficult urination, tremor, impotence, nightmares.	Continue. Call doctor when convenient.

WARNINGS & PRECAUTIONS

Don't take if:
- You are allergic to any thiazide diuretic drug or any rauwolfia alkaloid.
- You are depressed.
- You have active peptic ulcer or ulcerative colitis.

Before you start, consult your doctor:
- If you are allergic to any sulfa drug.
- If you have gout, liver, pancreas or kidney disorder, epilepsy.
- If you have had peptic ulcer, ulcerative colitis or gallstones.
- If you have been depressed.

- If you will have surgery within 2 months, including dental surgery, requiring general or spinal anesthesia.

Over age 60:
Adverse reactions and side effects may be more frequent and severe than in younger persons, especially dizziness and excessive potassium loss.

Pregnancy:
Risk to unborn child outweighs drug benefits. Don't use.

Breast-feeding:
Drug passes into milk. Avoid drug or discontinue nursing until you finish medicine. Consult doctor for advice on maintaining milk supply.

Infants & children:
Not recommended.

Prolonged use:
- You may need medicine to treat high blood pressure for the rest of your life.
- Causes cancer in laboratory animals. Consult your doctor if you have family or personal history of cancer.
- Talk to your doctor about the need for follow-up medical examinations or laboratory studies to check blood pressure.

Skin & sunlight:
May cause rash or intensify sunburn in areas exposed to sun or sunlamp.

Driving, piloting or hazardous work:
Don't drive or pilot aircraft until you learn how medicine affects you. Don't work around dangerous machinery. Don't climb ladders or work in high places. Danger increases if you drink alcohol or take medicine affecting alertness and reflexes, such as antihistamines, tranquilizers, sedatives, pain medicine, narcotics and mind-altering drugs.

Discontinuing:
Don't discontinue without consulting doctor. Dose may require gradual reduction if you have taken drug for a long time. Doses of other drugs may also require adjustment.

Others:
- Hot weather and fever may cause dehydration and drop in blood pressure. Dose may require temporary adjustment. Weigh daily and report any unexpected weight decreases to your doctor.
- May cause rise in uric acid, leading to gout.
- May cause blood-sugar rise in diabetics.
- Consult your doctor if you do isometric exercises. These raise blood pressure. Drug may intensify blood-pressure rise.

POSSIBLE INTERACTION WITH OTHER DRUGS

GENERIC NAME OR DRUG CLASS	COMBINED EFFECT
Anticoagulants, oral*	Unpredictable increased or decreased effect of anticoagulant.
Anticonvulsants*	Serious change in seizure pattern.
Antidepressants, tricyclic (TCA)*	Dangerous drop in blood pressure. Avoid combination unless under medical supervision.
Antihistamines*	Increased antihistamine effect.
Antihypertensives*	Increased effect of rauwolfia.
Aspirin	Decreased aspirin effect.
Barbiturates*	Increased hydro-chlorothiazide effect.
Beta-adrenergic blockers*	Increased effect of rauwolfia alkaloids. Excessive sedation.

Continued page 959

POSSIBLE INTERACTION WITH OTHER SUBSTANCES

INTERACTS WITH	COMBINED EFFECT
Alcohol:	Increased intoxication. Dangerous blood pressure drop. Avoid.
Beverages: Carbonated drinks.	Decreased rauwolfia effect.
Cocaine:	Increased risk of heart block and high blood pressure.
Foods: Spicy foods.	Possible digestive upset.
Licorice.	Excessive potassium loss that causes dangerous heart rhythms.
Marijuana:	Occasional use—Mild drowsiness. Daily use—Moderate drowsiness, low blood pressure, depression.
Tobacco:	No proven problems.

RESERPINE & HYDRALAZINE

BRAND NAMES

Serpasil-Apresoline

BASIC INFORMATION

Habit forming? No
Prescription needed? Yes
Available as generic? No
Drug class: Antihypertensive, tranquilizer
(rauwolfia alkaloid)

 ## USES

Treatment for high blood pressure and
congestive heart failure.

 ## DOSAGE & USAGE INFORMATION

How to take:
Tablet—Swallow with liquid or food to lessen
stomach irritation. If you can't swallow whole,
crumble tablet and take with liquid or food.

When to take:
At the same times each day.

If you forget a dose:
Take as soon as you remember up to 2 hours
late. If more than 2 hours, wait for next
scheduled dose (don't double this dose).

What drug does:
- Interferes with nerve impulses and relaxes blood-
vessel muscles, reducing blood pressure.
- Suppresses brain centers that control emotions.

Continued next column

 ## OVERDOSE

SYMPTOMS:
**Drowsiness, slow, shallow breathing; pinpoint
pupils; diarrhea; flush; low body temperature;
rapid, weak heartbeat; fainting; extreme
weakness; cold, sweaty skin; coma.**
WHAT TO DO:
- **Dial 0 (operator) or 911 (emergency) for
an ambulance or medical help. Then give
first aid immediately.**
- **If patient is unconscious and not
breathing, give mouth-to-mouth
breathing. If there is no heartbeat, use
cardiac massage and mouth-to-mouth
breathing (CPR). Don't try to make patient
vomit. If you can't get help quickly, take
patient to nearest emergency facility.**
- **See emergency information on inside
covers.**

Time lapse before drug works:
Regular use for several weeks may be
necessary to determine drug's effectiveness.

Don't take with:
- Non-prescription drugs containing alcohol
without consulting doctor.
- Any other medicine without consulting your
doctor or pharmacist.

 ## POSSIBLE ADVERSE REACTIONS OR SIDE EFFECTS

SYMPTOMS	WHAT TO DO
Life-threatening:	
Fainting, black stool, black vomit, chest pain, rapid or irregular heartbeat.	Discontinue. Seek emergency treatment.
Common:	
• Nausea, vomiting.	Discontinue. Call doctor right away.
• Headache, diarrhea, drowsiness, runny nose, appetite loss, dry mouth.	Continue. Call doctor when convenient.
Infrequent:	
• Rash, hives, chest pain, joint pain.	Discontinue. Call doctor right away.
• Confusion; dizziness; red or flushed face; irritated, red, watery eyes; constipation; joint stiffness; weakness, depression, foot and leg swelling.	Continue. Call doctor when convenient.
Rare:	
• Unexplained bleeding or bruising, sore throat, swollen lymph glands, abdominal pain, jaundice, weakness and faintness when arising from bed or chair.	Discontinue. Call doctor right away.
• Numbness, tingling, burning feeling in feet and hands; nasal congestion; impotence; nightmares.	Continue. Call doctor when convenient.

 ## WARNINGS & PRECAUTIONS

Don't take if:
- If you are allergic to any rauwolfia alkaloid,
hydralazine or tartrazine dye.
- You are depressed.
- You have active peptic ulcer, ulcerative colitis,
or history of coronary-artery disease or
rheumatic heart disease.

Before you start, consult your doctor:
- If you have been depressed.
- If you have had peptic ulcer, ulcerative colitis, gallstones, lupus, a stroke, kidney disease or impaired kidney function.
- If you have epilepsy.
- If you will have surgery within 2 months, including dental surgery, requiring general or spinal anesthesia.

Over age 60:
Adverse reactions and side effects may be more frequent and severe than in younger persons.

Pregnancy:
Risk to unborn child outweighs drug benefits. Don't use.

Breast-feeding:
Drug passes into milk. Avoid drug or discontinue nursing until you finish medicine. Consult doctor for advice on maintaining milk supply.

Infants & children:
Not recommended.

Prolonged use:
- Causes cancer in laboratory animals. Consult your doctor if you have family or personal history of cancer.
- May cause lupus (a connective tissue illness with arthritis, anemia and kidney malfunction).
- Possible psychosis.
- May cause numbness, tingling in hands or feet.
- Talk to your doctor about the need for follow-up medical examinations or laboratory studies.

Skin & sunlight:
No problems expected.

Driving, piloting or hazardous work:
Don't drive or pilot aircraft until you learn how medicine affects you. Don't work around dangerous machinery. Don't climb ladders or work in high places. Danger increases if you drink alcohol or take medicine affecting alertness and reflexes, such as antihistamines, tranquilizers, sedatives, pain medicine, narcotics and mind-altering drugs.

Discontinuing:
Don't discontinue without consulting doctor. Dose may require gradual reduction if you have taken drug for a long time. Doses of other drugs may also require adjustment.

Others:
- Consult your doctor if you do isometric exercises. These raise blood pressure. Drug may intensify blood-pressure rise.
- Vitamin B-6 diet supplement may be advisable. Consult doctor.
- Some products contain tartrazine dye. Avoid, especially if you are allergic to aspirin.

POSSIBLE INTERACTION WITH OTHER DRUGS

GENERIC NAME OR DRUG CLASS	COMBINED EFFECT
Amphetamines*	Decreased hydralazine effect.
Anticoagulants, oral*	Unpredictable increased or decreased effect of anticoagulant.
Anticonvulsants*	Serious change in seizure pattern.
Antidepressants*	Increased antidepressant effect.
Antihistamines*	Increased antihistamine effect.
Antihypertensives, other*	Increased antihypertensive effect.
Aspirin	Decreased aspirin effect.
Beta-adrenergic blockers*	Increased effect of rauwolfia alkaloids. Excessive sedation.
Carteolol	Increased antihypertensive effect.
Diazoxide	Increased antihypertensive effect.

Continued page 960

POSSIBLE INTERACTION WITH OTHER SUBSTANCES

INTERACTS WITH	COMBINED EFFECT
Alcohol:	Increased intoxication. Avoid.
Beverages: Carbonated drinks.	Decreased rauwolfia alkaloids effect.
Cocaine:	Dangerous blood pressure rise. Avoid.
Foods: Spicy foods.	Possible digestive upset.
Marijuana:	Occasional use—Mild drowsiness. Daily use—Moderate drowsiness, low blood pressure, depression.
Tobacco:	Possible angina attacks.

*See Glossary

RESERPINE, HYDRALAZINE & HYDROCHLOROTHIAZIDE

BRAND NAMES

Cam-Ap-Es	Ser-Ap-Es
Cherapas	Serpazide
Ser-A-Gen	Tri-Hydroserpine
Seralazide	Unipres

BASIC INFORMATION

Habit forming? No
Prescription needed? Yes
Available as generic? Yes
Drug class: Antihypertensive

USES

- Treatment for high blood pressure and congestive heart failure.
- Reduces fluid retention (edema).

DOSAGE & USAGE INFORMATION

How to take:
Tablet—Swallow with liquid. If you can't swallow whole, crumble tablet and take with liquid or food.

When to take:
At the same times each day.

If you forget a dose:
Take as soon as you remember up to 2 hours late. If more than 2 hours, wait for next scheduled dose (don't double this dose).

What drug does:
- Interferes with nerve impulses and relaxes blood-vessel muscles, reducing blood pressure.
- Suppresses brain centers that control emotions.
- Forces sodium and water excretion, reducing body fluid. Reduced body fluid and relaxed arteries lower blood pressure.

Continued next column

OVERDOSE

SYMPTOMS:
Drowsiness; slow, shallow breathing; pinpoint pupils; diarrhea; flush; low body temperature; rapid, weak heartbeat; fainting; extreme weakness; cold, sweaty skin; cramps, coma.
WHAT TO DO:
- **Dial 0 (operator) or 911 (emergency) for an ambulance or medical help. Then give first aid immediately.**
- **See emergency information on inside covers.**

Time lapse before drug works:
Regular use for several weeks may be necessary to determine drug's effectiveness.

Don't take with:
- Non-prescription drugs containing alcohol without consulting doctor.
- Any other medicine without consulting your doctor or pharmacist.

POSSIBLE ADVERSE REACTIONS OR SIDE EFFECTS

SYMPTOMS	WHAT TO DO
Life-threatening:	
Rapid or irregular heartbeat, weak pulse, fainting, black stool, black or bloody vomit, chest pain.	Discontinue. Seek emergency treatment.
Common:	
• Nausea, vomiting.	Discontinue. Call doctor right away.
• Headache, diarrhea, drowsiness, runny nose, appetite loss.	Continue. Call doctor when convenient.
Infrequent:	
• Blurred vision, chest pain, abdominal pain, rash, hives, joint pain.	Discontinue. Call doctor right away.
• Dizziness; mood change; headache; dry mouth; weakness; tiredness; weight gain or loss; eyes red, watery, irritated; confusion; constipation; red or flushed face; joint stiffness; depression; anxiety; foot and leg swelling.	Continue. Call doctor when convenient.
Rare:	
• Jaundice; unexplained bleeding or bruising; sore throat, fever, mouth sores; weakness and faintness when arising from bed or chair.	Discontinue. Call doctor right away.
• Numbness, tingling, burning feeling in feet and hands; nasal congestion; impotence; nightmares.	Continue. Call doctor when convenient.

WARNINGS & PRECAUTIONS

Don't take if:
- You are allergic to any rauwolfia alkaloid, hydralazine, any thiazide diuretic drug, or tartrazine dye.

RESERPINE, HYDRALAZINE & HYDROCHLOROTHIAZIDE

- You are depressed.
- You have active peptic ulcer, ulcerative colitis, history of coronary-artery disease or rheumatic heart disease.

Before you start, consult your doctor:
- If you have been depressed.
- If you have had peptic ulcer, ulcerative colitis, gallstones, kidney disease or impaired kidney function, lupus or a stroke.
- If you have epilepsy, gout, liver, pancreas or kidney disorder.
- If you feel pain in chest, neck or arms on physical exertion.
- If you are allergic to any sulfa drug.
- If you will have surgery within 2 months, including dental surgery, requiring general or spinal anesthesia.

Over age 60:
Adverse reactions and side effects may be more frequent and severe than in younger persons, especially dizziness and excessive potassium loss.

Pregnancy:
Risk to unborn child outweighs drug benefits. Don't use.

Breast-feeding:
Drug passes into milk. Avoid drug or discontinue nursing until you finish medicine.

Infants & children:
Not recommended.

Prolonged use:
- Causes cancer in laboratory animals. Consult your doctor if you have family or personal history of cancer.
- Possible psychosis.
- May cause lupus; numbness, tingling in hands or feet.
- Talk to your doctor about the need for follow-up medical examinations or laboratory studies.

Skin & sunlight:
May cause rash or intensify sunburn in areas exposed to sun or sunlamp.

Driving, piloting or hazardous work:
Don't drive or pilot aircraft until you learn how medicine affects you. Don't work around dangerous machinery. Don't climb ladders or work in high places. Danger increases if you drink alcohol or take medicine affecting alertness and reflexes.

Discontinuing:
Don't discontinue without consulting doctor. Dose may require gradual reduction if you have taken drug for a long time. Doses of other drugs may also require adjustment.

Others:
- Consult your doctor if you do isometric exercises. These raise blood pressure. Drug may intensify blood-pressure rise.

- Vitamin B-6 supplement may be advisable. Consult doctor.
- Hot weather and fever may cause dehydration and drop in blood pressure. Dose may require temporary adjustment. Weigh daily and report any unexpected weight decreases to your doctor.
- May cause rise in uric acid, leading to gout.
- May cause blood-sugar rise in diabetics.
- Some products contain tartrazine dye. Avoid, especially if you are allergic to aspirin.

 POSSIBLE INTERACTION WITH OTHER DRUGS

GENERIC NAME OR DRUG CLASS	COMBINED EFFECT
Acebutolol	Possible increased effects of drugs.
Allopurinol	Decreased allopurinol effect.
Amphetamines*	Decreased hydralazine effect.
Anticoagulants, oral*	Unpredictable increased or decreased effect of anticoagulant.

Continued page 960

 POSSIBLE INTERACTION WITH OTHER SUBSTANCES

INTERACTS WITH	COMBINED EFFECT
Alcohol:	Increased intoxication. Avoid.
Beverages: Carbonated drinks.	Decreased rauwolfia alkaloids effect.
Cocaine:	Dangerous blood pressure rise. Avoid.
Foods: Spicy foods.	Possible digestive upset.
Licorice.	Excessive potassium loss that causes dangerous heart rhythms.
Marijuana:	Weakness on standing. May increase blood pressure. Occasional use—Mild drowsiness. Daily use—Moderate drowsiness, low blood pressure, depression.
Tobacco:	Possible angina attacks.

*See Glossary

RIBAVIRIN

BRAND NAMES

Tribavirin   Virazole
Virazid

BASIC INFORMATION

Habit forming? No
Prescription needed? Yes
Available as generic? No
Drug class: Antiviral

USES

- Treats severe viral pneumonia.
- Treats influenza A and B with some success.
- It does *not* treat other viruses such as the common cold.

DOSAGE & USAGE INFORMATION

How to take:
By inhalation of a fine mist through mouth. Requires a special sprayer attached to oxygen mask, face mask for infants or hood.

When to take:
As ordered by your doctor.

If you forget a dose:
Use as soon as you remember.

What drug does:
Kills virus or prevents its growth.

Time lapse before drug works:
Begins working in 1 hour. May require treatment for 12 to 18 hours per day for 3 to 7 days.

Don't take with:
Any other medicine without consulting your doctor or pharmacist.

OVERDOSE

SYMPTOMS:
None expected.
WHAT TO DO:
Overdose unlikely to threaten life. If person takes much larger amount than prescribed, call doctor, poison-control center or hospital emergency room for instructions.

POSSIBLE ADVERSE REACTIONS OR SIDE EFFECTS

SYMPTOMS	WHAT TO DO
Life-threatening: None expected.	
Common: None expected.	
Infrequent: Blurred vision; dizziness; fainting; eye irritation; eyes more sensitive to light; red, swollen or itchy eyes.	Discontinue. Call doctor right away.
Rare: Difficult breathing.	Discontinue. Call doctor right away.

WARNINGS & PRECAUTIONS

Don't take if:
You are allergic to ribavirin.

Before you start, consult your doctor:
If you are now on low-salt, low-sugar or any special diet.

Over age 60:
Adverse reactions and side effects may be more frequent and severe than in younger persons. Ask doctor about smaller doses.

Pregnancy:
Risk to unborn child outweighs drug benefits. Don't use.

Breast-feeding:
Drug passes into milk. Avoid drug or discontinue nursing until you finish medicine. Consult doctor for advice on maintaining milk supply.

Infants & children:
Use only under close medical supervision.

Prolonged use:
No problems expected.

Skin & sunlight:
Increased sensitivity to light.

Driving, piloting or hazardous work:
Don't drive or pilot aircraft until you learn how medicine affects you. Don't work around dangerous machinery. Don't climb ladders or work in high places. Danger increases if you drink alcohol or take medicine affecting alertness and reflexes, such as antihistamines, tranquilizers, sedatives, pain medicine, narcotics and mind-altering drugs.

Discontinuing:
Don't discontinue without consulting doctor. Dose may require gradual reduction if you have taken drug for a long time. Doses of other drugs may also require adjustment.

Others:
Ribavirin is indicated for use in treatment of severe viral pneumonia caused by repiratory syncytial virus (RSV) in hospitalized infants and young children.

POSSIBLE INTERACTION WITH OTHER DRUGS

GENERIC NAME OR DRUG CLASS	COMBINED EFFECT
Zidovudine	Decreased effect of ribavirin and zidovudine.

POSSIBLE INTERACTION WITH OTHER SUBSTANCES

INTERACTS WITH	COMBINED EFFECT
Alcohol:	None expected.
Beverages:	None expected.
Cocaine:	None expected.
Foods:	None expected.
Marijuana:	None expected.
Tobacco:	None expected.

RIBOFLAVIN (Vitamin B-2)

BRAND NAMES

Many multivitamin preparations. Check labels.

BASIC INFORMATION

Habit forming? No
Prescription needed? No
Available as generic? Yes
Drug class: Vitamin supplement

 ## USES

- Dietary supplement to ensure normal growth and health.
- Dietary supplement to treat symptoms caused by deficiency of B-2: sores in mouth, eyes sensitive to light, itching and peeling skin.

 ## DOSAGE & USAGE INFORMATION

How to take:
Tablet—Swallow with liquid or food to lessen stomach irritation. If you can't swallow whole, crumble tablet and take with liquid or food.

When to take:
At the same times each day.

If you forget a dose:
Take as soon as you remember. Resume regular schedule. Don't double dose.

What drug does:
Promotes normal growth and health.

Time lapse before drug works:
Requires continual intake.

Don't take with:
Any other medicine without consulting your doctor or pharmacist.

 ## OVERDOSE

SYMPTOMS:
Dark urine, nausea, vomiting.
WHAT TO DO:
Overdose unlikely to threaten life. If person takes much larger amount than prescribed, call doctor, poison-control center or hospital emergency room for instructions.

 ## POSSIBLE ADVERSE REACTIONS OR SIDE EFFECTS

SYMPTOMS	WHAT TO DO
Life-threatening: None expected.	
Common: Urine yellow in color.	No action necessary.
Infrequent: None expected.	
Rare: None expected.	

RIBOFLAVIN (Vitamin B-2)

 WARNINGS & PRECAUTIONS

Don't take if:
- You are allergic to any B vitamin.
- You have chronic kidney failure.

Before you start, consult your doctor:
If you are pregnant or plan pregnancy.

Over age 60:
No problems expected.

Pregnancy:
Recommended. Consult doctor.

Breast-feeding:
Recommended. Consult doctor.

Infants & children:
Consult doctor.

Prolonged use:
No problems expected.

Skin & sunlight:
No problems expected.

Driving, piloting or hazardous work:
No problems expected.

Discontinuing:
No problems expected.

Others:
A balanced diet should provide all the vitamin B-2 a healthy person needs and make supplements unnecessary during periods of good health. Best sources are milk, meats and green leafy vegetables.

 POSSIBLE INTERACTION WITH OTHER DRUGS

GENERIC NAME OR DRUG CLASS	COMBINED EFFECT
Anticholinergics*	Possible increased riboflavin absorption.
Antidepressants, tricyclic (TCA)*	Decreased riboflavin effect.
Phenothiazines*	Decreased riboflavin effect.
Probenecid	Decreased riboflavin effect.

 POSSIBLE INTERACTION WITH OTHER SUBSTANCES

INTERACTS WITH	COMBINED EFFECT
Alcohol:	Prevents uptake and absorption of vitamin B-2.
Beverages:	No problems expected.
Cocaine:	No problems expected.
Foods:	No problems expected.
Marijuana:	No problems expected.
Tobacco:	Prevents absorption of vitamin B-2 and other vitamins and nutrients.

RIFAMPIN

BRAND NAMES

Rifadin

Rifamate

Rifampicin

Rimactane

Rofact

BASIC INFORMATION

Habit forming? No
Prescription needed? Yes
Available as generic? No
Drug class: Antibiotic (rifamycin)

USES

Treatment for tuberculosis and other infections. Requires daily use for 1 to 2 years.

DOSAGE & USAGE INFORMATION

How to take:
Capsule—Swallow with liquid. If you can't swallow whole, open capsule and take with liquid or small amount of food. For child, mix with small amount of applesauce or jelly.

When to take:
1 hour before or 2 hours after a meal.

If you forget a dose:
Take as soon as you remember up to 2 hours late. If more than 2 hours, wait for next scheduled dose (don't double this dose).

What drug does:
Prevents multiplication of tuberculosis germs.

Continued next column

OVERDOSE

SYMPTOMS:
Slow, shallow breathing; weak, rapid pulse; cold, sweaty skin; coma.
WHAT TO DO:
- **Dial 0 (operator) or 911 (emergency) for an ambulance or medical help. Then give first aid immediately.**
- **If patient is unconscious and not breathing, give mouth-to-mouth breathing. If there is no heartbeat, use cardiac massage and mouth-to-mouth breathing (CPR). Don't try to make patient vomit. If you can't get help quickly, take patient to nearest emergency facility.**
- **See emergency information on inside covers.**

Time lapse before drug works:
Usually 2 weeks. May require 1 to 2 years without missed doses for maximum benefit.

Don't take with:
Any other medicine without consulting your doctor or pharmacist.

POSSIBLE ADVERSE REACTIONS OR SIDE EFFECTS

SYMPTOMS	WHAT TO DO
Life-threatening:	
In case of overdose, see previous column.	
Common:	
Diarrhea; reddish urine, stool, saliva, sweat and tears.	Continue. Call doctor when convenient.
Infrequent:	
• Rash; flushed, itchy skin of face and scalp; blurred vision; difficult breathing; nausea, vomiting; abdominal cramps.	Discontinue. Call doctor right away.
• Dizziness, unsteady gait, confusion, muscle or bone pain, heartburn, flatulence, chills.	Continue. Call doctor when convenient.
• Headache, fever.	Continue. Tell doctor at next visit.
Rare:	
• Sore throat, mouth or tongue; jaundice.	Discontinue. Call doctor right away.
• Appetite loss, less urination.	Continue. Call doctor when convenient.

WARNINGS & PRECAUTIONS

Don't take if:
- You are allergic to rifampin.
- You wear soft contact lenses.

Before you start, consult your doctor:
If you are alcoholic or have liver disease.

Over age 60:
Adverse reactions and side effects may be more frequent and severe than in younger persons.

Pregnancy:
Studies inconclusive on harm to unborn child. Animal studies show fetal abnormalities. Decide with your doctor whether drug benefits justify risk to unborn child.

Breast-feeding:
No proven problems. Consult doctor.

Infants & children:
Use only under medical supervision.

Prolonged use:
- You may become more susceptible to infections caused by germs not responsive to rifampin.
- Talk to your doctor about the need for follow-up medical examinations or laboratory studies to check liver function.

Skin & sunlight:
No problems expected.

Driving, piloting or hazardous work:
Don't drive or pilot aircraft until you learn how medicine affects you. Don't work around dangerous machinery. Don't climb ladders or work in high places. Danger increases if you drink alcohol or take medicine affecting alertness and reflexes, such as antihistamines, tranquilizers, sedatives, pain medicine, narcotics and mind-altering drugs.

Discontinuing:
Don't discontinue without doctor's advice until you complete prescribed dose, even though symptoms diminish or disappear.

Others:
Reddish tears may discolor soft contact lenses.

 POSSIBLE INTERACTION WITH OTHER DRUGS

GENERIC NAME OR DRUG CLASS	COMBINED EFFECT
Anticoagulants, oral*	Decreased anti-coagulant effect.
Barbiturates*	Decreased barbiturate effect.
Chloramphenicol	Decreased effect of both drugs.
Clozapine	Toxic effect on bone marrow.
Contraceptives, oral*	Decreased contra-ceptive effect.
Cortisone drugs*	Decreased effect of cortisone drugs.
Cyclosporine	Decreased effect of both drugs.
Dapsone	Decreased dapsone effect.
Digitoxin	Decreased digitoxin effect.
Disopyramide	Decreased disopyramide effect.
Estrogens* (including contraceptive pills)	Decreased effect of both drugs.
Flecainide	Possible decreased blood-cell production in bone marrow.
Isoniazid	Possible toxicity to liver.
Ketoconazole	Increased risk of liver toxicity.
Methadone	Decreased methadone effect.
Nicardipine	Decreased nicardipine effect.
Nimodipine	Decreased nimodipine effect.
Para-aminosalicylic acid	Decreased rifampin effect.
Probenecid	Possible toxicity to liver.
Quinidine	Decreased effect of both drugs.
Tiopronin	Increased risk of toxicity to bone marrow and kidneys.
Tocainide	Possible decreased blood-cell production in bone marrow.
Tolbutamide and other oral antidiabetics*	Decreased tolbutamide effect.
Trimethoprim	Decreased trimethoprim effect.

 POSSIBLE INTERACTION WITH OTHER SUBSTANCES

INTERACTS WITH	COMBINED EFFECT
Alcohol:	Possible toxicity to liver.
Beverages:	None expected.
Cocaine:	No proven problems.
Foods:	None expected.
Marijuana:	No proven problems.
Tobacco:	None expected.

*See Glossary

RITODRINE

BRAND NAMES

Yutopar

BASIC INFORMATION

Habit forming? No
Prescription needed? Yes
Available as generic? Yes
Drug class: Labor inhibitor, beta-adrenergic stimulator

USES

Halts premature labor in pregnancies of 20 or more weeks.

DOSAGE & USAGE INFORMATION

How to take:
Tablet—Swallow with liquid or food to lessen stomach irritation. If you can't swallow whole, crumble tablet and take with liquid or food.

When to take:
Every 4 to 6 hours until term.

If you forget a dose:
Take as soon as you remember up to 2 hours late. If more than 2 hours, wait for next scheduled dose (don't double this dose).

What drug does:
Inhibits contractions of uterus (womb).

Time lapse before drug works:
30 to 60 minutes (oral form). Faster intravenously.

Don't take with:
Any other medicine without consulting your doctor or pharmacist.

OVERDOSE

SYMPTOMS:
Rapid, irregular heartbeat to 120 or more; shortness of breath.
WHAT TO DO:
- **Dial 0 (operator) or 911 (emergency) for an ambulance or medical help. Then give first aid immediately.**
- **If patient is unconscious and not breathing, give mouth-to-mouth breathing. If there is no heartbeat, use cardiac massage and mouth-to-mouth breathing (CPR). Don't try to make patient vomit. If you can't get help quickly, take patient to nearest emergency facility.**
- **See emergency information on inside covers.**

POSSIBLE ADVERSE REACTIONS OR SIDE EFFECTS

SYMPTOMS	WHAT TO DO
Life-threatening:	
Hives, rash, intense itching, faintness soon after a dose (anaphylaxis).	See emergency treatment immediately.
Common:	
Irregular heartbeat, fast heartbeat.	Discontinue. Call doctor right away.
Infrequent:	
• Shortness of breath.	Discontinue. Call doctor right away.
• Nervousness, trembling, headache, nausea, vomiting.	Continue. Call doctor when convenient.
Rare:	
Rash, angina, jaundice.	Discontinue. Call doctor right away.

WARNINGS & PRECAUTIONS

Don't take if:
- You have heart disease.
- You have eclampsia.
- You have lung congestion.
- You have infection in the uterus.
- You have an overactive thyroid.
- You have a bleeding disorder.

Before you start, consult your doctor:
- If you have asthma.
- If you have diabetes.
- If you have high blood pressure.
- If you have pre-eclampsia.

Over age 60:
Not used.

Pregnancy:
Ritodrine crosses placenta, but animal studies show that it causes no effects on fetuses. Benefits versus risks must be assessed by you and your doctor.

Breast-feeding:
Not applicable.

Infants & children:
Not used.

Prolonged use:
Talk to your doctor about the need for follow-up medical examinations or laboratory studies to check blood sugar, ECG*, fluid and electrolytes.

Skin & sunlight:
No problems expected.

Driving, piloting or hazardous work:
Don't drive or pilot aircraft until you learn how medicine affects you. Don't work around dangerous machinery. Don't climb ladders or work in high places. Danger increases if you drink alcohol or take medicine affecting alertness and reflexes, such as antihistamines, tranquilizers, sedatives, pain medicine, narcotics and mind-altering drugs.

Discontinuing:
Don't discontinue without consulting doctor. Dose may require gradual reduction if you have taken drug for a long time. Doses of other drugs may also require adjustment.

Others:
No problems expected.

POSSIBLE INTERACTION WITH OTHER DRUGS

GENERIC NAME OR DRUG CLASS	COMBINED EFFECT
Adrenal corticosteroids*	Increased chance of fluid in lungs of mother. Avoid.
Anesthetics, general*	Possible cardiac arrhythmias or hypotension.
Beta-adrenergic blockers*	Decreased effect of ritodrine.
Diazoxide	Possible cardiac arrhythmias or hypotension.
Magnesium sulfate	Possible cardiac arrhythmias or hypotension.
Meperidine	Possible cardiac arrhythmias or hypotension.
Sympathomimetics*	Increased side effects of both.

POSSIBLE INTERACTION WITH OTHER SUBSTANCES

INTERACTS WITH	COMBINED EFFECT
Alcohol:	Increased adverse effects. Avoid.
Beverages:	No problems expected.
Cocaine:	Injury to fetus. Avoid.
Foods:	No problems expected.
Marijuana:	Injury to fetus. Avoid.
Tobacco:	Injury to fetus. Avoid.

SALICYLATES

BRAND AND GENERIC NAMES

See complete list of brand and generic names in the *Brand Name Directory*, page 929.

BASIC INFORMATION

Habit forming? No
Prescription needed? For some
Available as generic? Yes
Drug class: Analgesic, anti-inflammatory (non-steroidal)

USES

- Reduces pain, fever, inflammation.
- Relieves swelling, stiffness, joint pain of arthritis or rheumatism.
- Decreases risk of myocardial infarction in unstable angina (aspirin only).

DOSAGE & USAGE INFORMATION

How to take:
- Tablet or capsule—Swallow with liquid.
- Extended-release tablets—Swallow each dose whole.
- Suppositories—Remove wrapper and moisten suppository with water. Gently insert into rectum, large end first.

When to take:
Pain, fever, inflammation—As needed, no more often than every 4 hours.

If you forget a dose:
- Pain, fever—Take as soon as you remember. Wait 4 hours for next dose.
- Arthritis—Take as soon as you remember up to 2 hours late. Return to regular schedule.

What drug does:
- Affects hypothalamus, the part of the brain that regulates temperature by dilating small blood vessels in skin.
- Prevents clumping of platelets (small blood cells) so blood vessels remain open.

Continued next column

OVERDOSE

SYMPTOMS:
Ringing in ears; nausea; vomiting; dizziness; fever; deep, rapid breathing; hallucinations; convulsions; coma.
WHAT TO DO:
- **Dial 0 (operator) or 911 (emergency) for an ambulance or medical help. Then give first aid immediately.**
- **See emergency information on inside covers.**

- Decreases prostaglandin effect.
- Suppresses body's pain messages.

Time lapse before drug works:
30 minutes for pain, fever, arthritis.

Don't take with:
- Tetracyclines. Space doses 1 hour apart.
- Any other medicine without consulting your doctor or pharmacist.

POSSIBLE ADVERSE REACTIONS OR SIDE EFFECTS

SYMPTOMS	WHAT TO DO
Life-threatening:	
Hives, rash, intense itching, faintness soon after a dose (anaphylaxis); black or bloody vomit; blood in urine.	Seek emergency treatment immediately.
Common:	
• Nausea, vomiting, abdominal pain.	Discontinue. Seek emergency treatment.
• Heartburn, indigestion.	Continue. Call doctor when convenient.
• Ringing in ears.	Continue. Tell doctor at next visit.
Infrequent:	
None expected.	
Rare:	
• Black stools, unexplained fever.	Discontinue. Seek emergency treatment.
• Rash, hives, itchy skin, diminished vision, shortness of breath, wheezing, jaundice.	Discontinue. Call doctor right away.
• Drowsiness, headache.	Continue. Call doctor when convenient.

WARNINGS & PRECAUTIONS

Don't take if:
- You need to restrict sodium in your diet. Buffered effervescent tablets and sodium salicylate are high in sodium.
- Salicylates have a strong vinegar-like odor, which means it has decomposed.
- You have a peptic ulcer of stomach or duodenum.
- You have a bleeding disorder.

Before you start, consult your doctor:
- If you have had stomach or duodenal ulcers.
- If you have had gout.
- If you have asthma or nasal polyps.

Over age 60:
More likely to cause hidden bleeding in stomach or intestines. Watch for dark stools.

Pregnancy:
Risk to unborn child outweighs drug benefits.
Don't use.

Breast-feeding:
Drug passes into milk. Avoid drug or discontinue nursing until you finish medicine. Consult doctor for advice on maintaining milk supply.

Infants & children:
- Overdose frequent and severe. Keep bottles out of children's reach.
- Consult doctor before giving to persons under age 18 who have fever and discomfort of viral illness, especially chicken pox and influenza. Probably increases risk of Reye's syndrome.

Prolonged use:
- Kidney damage. Periodic kidney-function test recommended.
- Talk to your doctor about the need for follow-up medical examinations or laboratory studies to check liver function.

Skin & sunlight:
Aspirin combined with sunscreen may decrease sunburn.

Driving, piloting or hazardous work:
No restrictions unless you feel drowsy.

Discontinuing:
For chronic illness—Don't discontinue without doctor's advice until you complete prescribed dose, even though symptoms diminish or disappear.

Others:
- Salicylates can complicate surgery, pregnancy, labor and delivery, and illness.
- For arthritis—Don't change dose without consulting doctor.
- Urine tests for blood sugar may be inaccurate.

 ## POSSIBLE INTERACTION WITH OTHER DRUGS

GENERIC NAME OR DRUG CLASS	COMBINED EFFECT
ACE inhibitors*: captopril, enalapril, lisinopril	Decreased ACE inhibitor effect.
Acetaminophen	Increased risk of kidney damage (high, prolonged dose of each).
Allopurinol	Decreased allopurinol effect.
Antacids*	Decreased salicylate effect.
Anticoagulants*	Increased anticoagulant effect. Abnormal bleeding.

Antidiabetics, oral*	Low blood sugar.
Aspirin, other	Likely salicylate toxicity.
Beta-adrenergic blockers*	Decreased antihypertensive effect.
Bismuth subsalicylate	Increased risk of salicylate toxicity.
Bumetanide	Decreased diuretic effect.
Calcium supplements*	Increased salicylate effect.
Carteolol	Decreased antihypertensive effect of carteolol.
Cortisone drugs*	Increased cortisone effect. Risk of ulcers and stomach bleeding.
Ethacrynic acid	Decreased diuretic effect.
Furosemide	Possible salicylate toxicity.
Gold compounds*	Increased likelihood of kidney damage.
Indomethacin	Risk of stomach bleeding and ulcers.
Insulin	Decreased blood sugar.
Methotrexate	Increased methotrexate effect and toxicity.
Non-steroidal anti-inflammatory drugs (NSAIDs)*	Risk of stomach bleeding and ulcers.
Para-aminosalicylic acid	Possible salicylate toxicity.

Continued page 961

 ## POSSIBLE INTERACTION WITH OTHER SUBSTANCES

INTERACTS WITH	COMBINED EFFECT
Alcohol:	Possible stomach irritation and bleeding. Avoid.
Beverages:	None expected.
Cocaine:	None expected.
Foods:	None expected.
Marijuana:	Possible increased pain relief, but marijuana may slow body's recovery. Avoid.
Tobacco:	None expected.

SCOPOLAMINE (Hyoscine)

BRAND NAMES

See complete list of brand names in the *Brand Name Directory,* page 929.

BASIC INFORMATION

Habit forming? No
Prescription needed?
  High strength: Yes
  Low strength: No
Available as generic? Yes
Drug class: Antispasmodic, anticholinergic

USES

- Reduces spasms of digestive system, bladder and urethra.
- Relieves painful menstruation.
- Prevents motion sickness.

DOSAGE & USAGE INFORMATION

How to take:
- Capsules—Swallow with liquid or food to lessen stomach irritation.
- Drops—Dilute dose in beverage.
- Skin discs—Clean application site. Change application sites with each dose.

When to take:
- Motion sickness—Apply disc 30 minutes before departure.
- Other uses—Take 30 minutes before meals (unless directed otherwise by doctor).

If you forget a dose:
Take up to 2 hours late. If more than 2 hours, wait for next dose (don't double this dose).

What drug does:
Blocks nerve impulses at parasympathetic nerve endings, preventing muscle contractions and gland secretions of organs involved.

Continued next column

OVERDOSE

SYMPTOMS:
Dilated pupils, blurred vision, rapid pulse and breathing, dizziness, fever, hallucinations, confusion, slurred speech, agitation, flushed face, convulsions, coma.
WHAT TO DO:
- **Dial 0 (operator) or 911 (emergency) for an ambulance or medical help. Then give first aid immediately.**
- **See emergency information on inside covers.**

Time lapse before drug works:
15 to 30 minutes.

Don't take with:
Any other medicine without consulting your doctor or pharmacist.

POSSIBLE ADVERSE REACTIONS OR SIDE EFFECTS

SYMPTOMS	WHAT TO DO
Life-threatening:	
Hives, rash, intense itching, faintness soon after a dose (anaphylaxis).	Seek emergency treatment immediately.
Common:	
Confusion, delirium, rapid heartbeat.	Discontinue. Call doctor right away.
Nausea, vomiting, decreased sweating.	Continue. Call doctor when convenient.
Constipation, loss of taste.	Continue. Tell doctor at next visit.
Dryness in ears, nose, throat, mouth.	No action necessary.
Infrequent:	
Headache, difficult urination, nasal congestion, altered taste.	Continue. Call doctor when convenient.
Lightheadedness.	Discontinue. Call doctor right away.
Rare:	
Rash or hives, eye pain, blurred vision.	Discontinue. Call doctor right away.

WARNINGS & PRECAUTIONS

Don't take if:
- You are allergic to any anticholinergic.
- You have trouble with stomach bloating.
- You have difficulty emptying your bladder completely.
- You have narrow-angle glaucoma.
- You have severe ulcerative colitis.

Before you start, consult your doctor:
- If you have open-angle glaucoma, angina, chronic bronchitis or asthma, hiatal hernia, liver disease, enlarged prostate, myasthenia gravis, peptic ulcer, kidney or thyroid disease.
- If you will have surgery within 2 months, including dental surgery, requiring general or spinal anesthesia.

Over age 60:
Adverse reactions and side effects may be more frequent and severe than in younger persons.

Pregnancy:
Studies inconclusive on harm to unborn child. Animal studies show fetal abnormalities. Decide with your doctor whether drug benefits justify risk to unborn child.

Breast-feeding:
Drug passes into milk and decreases milk flow. Avoid drug or discontinue nursing until you finish medicine. Consult doctor for advice on maintaining milk supply.

Infants & children:
Use only under medical supervision.

Prolonged use:
Chronic constipation, possible fecal impaction. Consult doctor immediately.

Skin & sunlight:
No problems expected.

Driving, piloting or hazardous work:
Use disqualifies you for piloting aircraft. Otherwise, no problems expected.

Discontinuing:
May be unnecessary to finish medicine. Follow doctor's instructions.

Others:
Advise any doctor or dentist whom you consult that you take this medicine.

POSSIBLE INTERACTION WITH OTHER DRUGS

GENERIC NAME OR DRUG CLASS	COMBINED EFFECT
Amantadine	Increased scopolamine effect.
Antacids*	Decreased scopolamine effect.
Anticholinergics, other*	Increased scopolamine effect.
Antidepressants, tricyclic (TCA)*	Increased scopolamine effect. Increased sedation.
Antidiarrheals*	Decreased scopolamine effect.
Antihistamines*	Increased scopolamine effect.
Attapulgite	Decreased scopolamine effect.
Buclizine	Increased scopolamine effect.
Clozapine	Toxic effect on the central nervous system.
Cortisone drugs*	Increased internal eye pressure.
Digitalis	Possible decreased absorption of scopolamine.
Encainide	Increased effect of toxicity on heart muscle.

Ethinamate	Dangerous increased effects of ethinamate. Avoid combining.
Fluoxetine	Increased depressant effects of both drugs.
Guanfacine	May increase depressant effects of either medicine.
Haloperidol	Increased internal eye pressure.
Ketoconazole	Decreased ketoconazole effect.
Leucovorin	High alcohol content of leucovorin may cause adverse effects.
MAO inhibitors*	Increased scopolamine effect.
Meperidine	Increased scopolamine effect.
Methylphenidate	Increased scopolamine effect.
Methyprylon	May increase sedative effect to dangerous level. Avoid.
Molindone	Increased anticholinergic effect.
Nabilone	Greater depression of central nervous system.
Nitrates*	Increased internal eye pressure.
Nizatidine	Increased nizatidine effect.
Orphenadrine	Increased scopolamine effect.
Phenothiazines*	Increased scopolamine effect.

Continued page 961

POSSIBLE INTERACTION WITH OTHER SUBSTANCES

INTERACTS WITH	COMBINED EFFECT
Alcohol:	None expected.
Beverages:	None expected.
Cocaine:	Excessively rapid heartbeat. Avoid.
Foods:	None expected.
Marijuana:	Drowsiness, dry mouth.
Tobacco:	None expected.

*See Glossary

SELEGILINE

BRAND NAMES

Eldepryl   **Movergan**
Jumex   **Procythol**
Jumexal

BASIC INFORMATION

All the information in this chart applies only when selegiline is given with other drugs that treat Parkinson's disease.

Habit forming? No
Prescription needed? Yes
Available as generic? No
Drug class: Antidyskinetic

USES

- Treats Parkinson's disease (*paralysis agitans*) when given with levodopa or the combination of levodopa and carbidopa.
- Treats mental depression when taken alone.

DOSAGE & USAGE INFORMATION

How to take:
Tablets—Swallow with liquid. If you can't swallow whole, crumble tablet and take with liquid or food. Instructions to take on empty stomach mean 1 hour before or 2 hours after eating.

When to take:
Usually taken at breakfast and lunch to minimize nausea or insomnia. Don't take after mid-afternoon.

Continued in next column

OVERDOSE

SYMPTOMS:
Mouth-opening difficulty; neck and heel muscle spasm; sweating; irregular, fast heartbeat; reflexes hyperactive; cold or clammy skin; chest pain; agitation; fainting; seizures; coma. Symptoms can develop 12 to 48 hours after ingestion.
WHAT TO DO:
- **Dial 0 (operator) or 911 (emergency) for an ambulance or medical help. Then give first aid immediately.**
- **If patient is unconsciousness and not breathing, give mouth-to-mouth breathing. If there is no heartbeat, use cardiac massage and mouth-to-mouth breathing (CPR). Don't try to make patient vomit. If you can't get help quickly, take patient to nearest emergency facility.**
- **See emergency information on inside covers.**

If you forget a dose:
Take as soon as you remember up to 2 hours late. If more than 2 hours, wait for next scheduled dose (don't double this dose).

What drug does:
Inhibits action of monoamine oxidase Type B (MAO B), a major chemical enzyme in the brain. Doses higher than recommended can cause high blood pressure.

Time lapse before drug works:
2 hours.

Don't take with:
- Any foods containing tyramine, such as cheese; wine; beer; non-alcoholic beer; liqueurs; yeast extracts; bean pods; pickled or smoked fish, meat, chicken, turkey or other poultry; fermented sausage (summer sausage, salami, pepperoni); bologna; overripe fruit; caffeine.
- Any other medicines (including over-the-counter drugs such as cough and cold medicines, laxatives, antacids, diet pills, nose drops or vitamins) without consulting your doctor.
- Study Interaction column.

POSSIBLE ADVERSE REACTIONS OR SIDE EFFECTS

SYMPTOMS	WHAT TO DO
Life-threatening:	
• In case of overdose, see previous column.	
• Severe chest pain, enlarged pupils, heartbeat irregularities, severe nausea and vomiting, stiff neck.	Seek emergency treatment.
Common:	
• Mood changes, unusual or uncontrolled body movements, hallucinations, head-ache, lip smacking, difficult urination.	Discontinue. Call doctor right away.
• Abdominal pain, dizziness, dry mouth, insomnia, mild nausea.	Continue. Call doctor when convenient.
Infrequent:	
• Chest pain, heartbeat irregularities, wheez-ing, swollen feet, speech difficulty, bloody or black stools.	Discontinue. Seek emergency treatment.

- Constipation; anxiety; tiredness; eyelid spasm; unpleasant taste; blurred vision; leg pain; ears ringing; chills; skin rash; lips or mouth burning; drowsiness; frequent, decreased urination.

Continue. Call doctor when convenient.

Rare:
Weight loss, heartburn, jaw clenching or teeth gnashing, impaired memory, uncontrolled body movements.

Continue. Call doctor when convenient.

WARNINGS & PRECAUTIONS

Don't take if:
You are allergic to selegiline.

Before you start, consult your doctor:
If you have a past medical history of peptic ulcer.

Over age 60:
Adverse reactions and side effects may be more frequent and severe than in younger persons. You may need smaller doses for shorter periods of time.

Pregnancy:
No proven harm to unborn child, but avoid if possible.

Breast-feeding:
No proven harm, but avoid if possible.

Infants & children:
Not recommended.

Prolonged use:
Talk to your doctor about the need for follow-up medical examinations or laboratory studies to check complete blood counts (white blood cell count, platelet count, red blood cell count, hemoglobin, hematocrit), stomach x-rays.

Skin & sunlight:
Increased sensitivity to ultraviolet rays from sun or sunlamps. Avoid overexposure.

Driving, piloting or hazardous work:
Don't drive or pilot aircraft until you learn how medicine affects you. Don't work around dangerous machinery. Don't climb ladders or work in high places. Danger increases if you drink alcohol or take medicine affecting alertness and reflexes.

Discontinuing:
No special problems expected.

Others:
- Avoid sudden rises from lying-down or sitting positions.
- Advise any doctor or dentist whom you consult that you take this medicine.
- May affect results in some medical tests.

POSSIBLE INTERACTION WITH OTHER DRUGS

GENERIC NAME OR DRUG CLASS	COMBINED EFFECT
Caffeine (high doses)	Can cause same symptoms as tyramine-containing foods.* (See "Don't take with" information block on previous page.)
Levodopa	Increased risk of adverse reactions.
Meperdine	Possibly severe drop in blood pressure. Avoid.
Narcotics*	Severe toxic reaction leading to seizures, coma, and/or death.
Sertraline	Increased depressive effects of both drugs.

POSSIBLE INTERACTION WITH OTHER SUBSTANCES

INTERACTS WITH	COMBINED EFFECT
Alcohol:	Can cause severe toxicity. Avoid.
Beverages: Drinks containing large quantities of caffeine.	Can cause severe toxicity. Avoid.
Cocaine:	High blood pressure, rapid heartbeat. Avoid.
Foods: Tyramine-containing*. (See "Don't take with" information block on previous page.)	Severe toxicity, perhaps leading to death. *Carefully avoid.*
Marijuana:	Rapid heart rate. Avoid.
Tobacco:	Rapid heart rate. Avoid.

SENNA

BRAND NAMES

Black-Draught
  Lax Senna
Fletcher's Castoria
Senexon

Senokot
Senolax
X-Prep Liquid

BASIC INFORMATION

Habit forming? No
Prescription needed? No
Available as generic? No
Drug class: Laxative (stimulant)

 USES

Constipation relief.

 DOSAGE & USAGE INFORMATION

How to take:
- Tablet—Swallow with liquid. If you can't swallow whole, chew or crumble tablet and take with liquid or food.
- Liquid, granules—Drink 6 to 8 glasses of water each day, in addition to one taken with each dose.
- Suppositories—Remove wrapper and moisten suppository with water. Gently insert larger end into rectum. Push well into rectum with finger.

When to take:
Usually at bedtime with a snack, unless directed otherwise.

If you forget a dose:
Take as soon as you remember.

What drug does:
Acts on smooth muscles of intestine wall to cause vigorous bowel movement.

Time lapse before drug works:
6 to 10 hours.

Continued next column

 OVERDOSE

SYMPTOMS:
Vomiting, electrolyte depletion.
WHAT TO DO:
Overdose unlikely to threaten life. If person takes much larger amount than prescribed, call doctor, poison-control center or hospital emergency room for instructions.

Don't take with:
- See Interaction column and consult doctor.
- Don't take within 2 hours of taking another medicine. Laxative interferes with medicine absorption.

 POSSIBLE ADVERSE REACTIONS OR SIDE EFFECTS

SYMPTOMS	WHAT TO DO
Life-threatening: None expected.	
Common:	
• Rectal irritation.	Continue. Call doctor when convenient.
• Yellow-brown or red-violet urine.	No action necessary.
Infrequent:	
• Dangerous potassium loss (thirst, weakness, heartbeat irregularity, paralysis, nausea and diarrhea).	Discontinue. Call doctor right away.
• Belching, cramps, nausea.	Continue. Call doctor when convenient.
Rare:	
• Irritability, headache, confusion, rash, difficult breathing, irregular heartbeat, muscle cramps, unusual tiredness or weakness.	Discontinue. Call doctor right away.
• Burning on urination.	Continue. Call doctor when convenient.

WARNINGS & PRECAUTIONS

Don't take if:
- You have symptoms of appendicitis, inflamed bowel or intestinal blockage.
- You are allergic to a stimulant laxative.
- You have missed a bowel movement for only 1 or 2 days.

Before you start, consult your doctor:
- If you have a colostomy or ileostomy.
- If you have congestive heart disease.
- If you have diabetes.
- If you have high blood pressure.
- If you have a laxative habit.
- If you have rectal bleeding.
- If you take other laxatives.

Over age 60:
Adverse reactions and side effects may be more frequent and severe than in younger persons.

Pregnancy:
Risk to mother and unborn child outweighs drug benefits. Don't use.

Breast-feeding:
Drug passes into milk. Avoid drug or discontinue nursing until you finish medicine. Consult doctor for advice on maintaining milk supply.

Infants & children:
Use only under medical supervision.

Prolonged use:
Don't take for more than 1 week unless under a doctor's supervision. May cause laxative dependence.

Skin & sunlight:
No problems expected.

Driving, piloting or hazardous work:
No problems expected.

Discontinuing:
May be unnecessary to finish medicine. Follow doctor's instructions.

Others:
- Don't take to "flush out" your system or as a "tonic."
- May cause urine to get discolored. No action necessary.

POSSIBLE INTERACTION WITH OTHER DRUGS

GENERIC NAME OR DRUG CLASS	COMBINED EFFECT
Antihypertensives*	May cause dangerous low potassium level.
Digitalis	Increased digitalis toxicity.
Diuretics*	May cause dangerous low potassium level.

POSSIBLE INTERACTION WITH OTHER SUBSTANCES

INTERACTS WITH	COMBINED EFFECT
Alcohol:	None expected.
Beverages:	None expected.
Cocaine:	None expected.
Foods:	None expected.
Marijuana:	None expected.
Tobacco:	None expected.

**See Glossary

SENNOSIDES A & B

BRAND NAMES

Glysennid   **Gentle Nature**
Nytilax

BASIC INFORMATION

Habit forming? No
Prescription needed? No
Available as generic? No
Drug class: Laxative (stimulant)

USES

Constipation relief.

DOSAGE & USAGE INFORMATION

How to take:
- Tablet—Swallow with liquid. If you can't swallow whole, chew or crumble tablet and take with liquid or food.
- Liquid, granules—Drink 6 to 8 glasses of water each day, in addition to one taken with each dose.

When to take:
Usually at bedtime with a snack, unless directed otherwise.

If you forget a dose:
Take as soon as you remember.

What drug does:
Acts on smooth muscles of intestine wall to cause vigorous bowel movement.

Time lapse before drug works:
6 to 10 hours.

Don't take with:
- Any other medicine without consulting your doctor or pharmacist.
- Don't take within 2 hours of taking another medicine. Laxative interferes with medicine absorption.

OVERDOSE

SYMPTOMS:
Vomiting, electrolyte depletion.
WHAT TO DO:
Overdose unlikely to threaten life. If person takes much larger amount than prescribed, call doctor, poison-control center or hospital emergency room for instructions.

POSSIBLE ADVERSE REACTIONS OR SIDE EFFECTS

SYMPTOMS	WHAT TO DO
Life-threatening:	
None expected.	
Common:	
• Rectal irritation.	Continue. Call doctor when convenient.
• Yellow-brown or red-violet urine.	No action necessary.
Infrequent:	
• Dangerous potassium loss (thirst, weakness, heartbeat irregularity, paralysis, nausea and diarrhea).	Discontinue. Call doctor right away.
• Belching, cramps, nausea.	Continue. Call doctor when convenient.
Rare:	
• Irritability, headache, confusion, rash, difficult breathing, irregular heartbeat, muscle cramps, unusual tiredness or weakness.	Discontinue. Call doctor right away.
• Burning on urination.	Continue. Call doctor when convenient.

WARNINGS & PRECAUTIONS

Don't take if:
- You have symptoms of appendicitis, inflamed bowel or intestinal blockage.
- You are allergic to a stimulant laxative.
- You have missed a bowel movement for only 1 or 2 days.

Before you start, consult your doctor:
- If you have a colostomy or ileostomy.
- If you have congestive heart disease.
- If you have diabetes.
- If you have high blood pressure.
- If you have a laxative habit.
- If you have rectal bleeding.
- If you take other laxatives.

Over age 60:
Adverse reactions and side effects may be more frequent and severe than in younger persons.

Pregnancy:
Risk to mother and unborn child outweighs drug benefits. Don't use.

Breast-feeding:
Drug passes into milk. Avoid drug or discontinue nursing until you finish medicine. Consult doctor for advice on maintaining milk supply.

Infants & children:
Use only under medical supervision.

Prolonged use:
Don't take for more than 1 week unless under a doctor's supervision. May cause laxative dependence.

Skin & sunlight:
No problems expected.

Driving, piloting or hazardous work:
No problems expected.

Discontinuing:
May be unnecessary to finish medicine. Follow doctor's instructions.

Others:
- Don't take to "flush out" your system or as a "tonic."
- May cause urine to get discolored. No action necessary.

POSSIBLE INTERACTION WITH OTHER DRUGS

GENERIC NAME OR DRUG CLASS	COMBINED EFFECT
Antihypertensives*	May cause dangerous low potassium level.
Digitalis	Increased digitalis toxicity.
Diuretics*	May cause dangerous low potassium level.

POSSIBLE INTERACTION WITH OTHER SUBSTANCES

INTERACTS WITH	COMBINED EFFECT
Alcohol:	None expected.
Beverages:	None expected.
Cocaine:	None expected.
Foods:	None expected.
Marijuana:	None expected.
Tobacco:	None expected.

SERTRALINE

BRAND NAMES

Zoloft

BASIC INFORMATION

Habit forming? No
Prescription needed? Yes
Available as generic? No
Drug class: Antidepressant

 ## USES

Treats mental depression.

 ## DOSAGE & USAGE INFORMATION

How to take:
Tablets—Swallow with liquid. If you can't
swallow whole, crumble tablet and take with
liquid or food.

When to take:
Once daily, either in the morning or in the
evening.

If you forget a dose:
Take as soon as you remember up to 2 hours
late. If more than 2 hours, wait for next
scheduled dose (don't double this dose).

What drug does:
Inhibits uptake of serotonin in the central
nervous system, preventing depression.

Time lapse before drug works:
1 to 4 weeks.

Don't take with:
- Any monoamine oxidase (MAO) inhibitor* (or
  within 14 days of discontinuing an MAO
  inhibitor). To do so may cause serious or
  even fatal reactions.
- Any other non-prescription drugs without
  consulting your doctor.

 ## OVERDOSE

SYMPTOMS:
Seizures, agitation, violent vomiting.
WHAT TO DO:
- **Dial 0 (operator) or 911 (emergency) for
  an ambulance or medical help. Then give
  first aid immediately.**
- **See emergency information on inside
  covers.**

 ## POSSIBLE ADVERSE REACTIONS OR SIDE EFFECTS

SYMPTOMS	WHAT TO DO
Life-threatening: In case of overdose, see previous column.	
Common: Weight loss, dry mouth, sweating, headache, insomnia.	Continue. Call doctor when convenient.
Infrequent: • Nausea, diarrhea, tremor, fatigue.	Continue. Call doctor when convenient.
• Palpitations, dizziness.	Discontinue. Call doctor right away.
Rare: Mania, chest pain, skin rash.	Discontinue. Call doctor right away.

WARNINGS & PRECAUTIONS

Don't take if:
- You have epilepsy.
- You have an allergy to sertraline.

Before you start, consult your doctor:
If you have severe liver or kidney disease.

Over age 60:
Adverse reactions may be more frequent and severe than in younger persons. You may need smaller doses for shorter periods of time.

Pregnancy:
No proven problems. Don't take unless essential.

Breast-feeding:
Unknown effects.

Infants & children:
Not recommended.

Prolonged use:
No special problems expected.

Skin & sunlight:
No special problems expected.

Driving, piloting or hazardous work:
Don't drive or pilot aircraft until you learn how the medicine affects you. Don't work around dangerous machinery. Don't climb ladders or work in high places.

Discontinuing:
Don't discontinue without consulting doctor. Dose may require gradual reduction if you have taken drug for a long time. Doses of other drugs may also require adjustment.

Others:
- Advise any doctor or dentist whom you consult that you take this medicine.
- May affect results of some medical tests.

POSSIBLE INTERACTION WITH OTHER DRUGS

GENERIC NAME OR DRUG CLASS	COMBINED EFFECT
Central nervous system (CNS) depressants*	Increases depressive effects of both drugs.

POSSIBLE INTERACTION WITH OTHER SUBSTANCES

INTERACTS WITH	COMBINED EFFECT
Alcohol:	May increase depression.
Beverages:	No proven problems.
Cocaine:	Decreased effect of sertraline.
Foods:	No proven problems.
Marijuana:	Decreased effect of sertraline.
Tobacco:	No proven problems.

*See Glossary

SIMETHICONE

BRAND NAMES

DI-Gel
Extra Stength Gas-X
Gas-X
Gelusil
Mygel
Mylanta
Mylicon
Mylicon-80
Mylicon-125

Ovol
Ovol-40
Ovol-80
Phazyme
Phazyme 95
Phazyme 125
Riopan Plus
Silain

BASIC INFORMATION

Habit forming? No
Prescription needed? No
Available as generic? Yes, for some
Drug class: Antiflatulent

USES

- Treatment for retention of abdominal gas.
- Used prior to x-ray of abdomen to reduce gas shadows.

DOSAGE & USAGE INFORMATION

How to take:
- Tablet or capsule—Swallow with liquid.
- Liquid—Dissolve in water. Drink complete dose.
- Chewable tablets—Chew completely. Don't swallow whole.

When to take:
After meals and at bedtime.

If you forget a dose:
Take when remembered if needed.

What drug does:
Reduces surface tension of gas bubbles in stomach.

Time lapse before drug works:
10 minutes.

Don't take with:
Any other medicine without consulting your doctor or pharmacist.

OVERDOSE

SYMPTOMS:
None expected.
WHAT TO DO:
Overdose unlikely to threaten life.

POSSIBLE ADVERSE REACTIONS OR SIDE EFFECTS

SYMPTOMS	WHAT TO DO
Life-threatening: None expected.	
Common: None expected.	
Infrequent: None expected.	
Rare: None expected.	

WARNINGS & PRECAUTIONS

Don't take if:
You are allergic to simethicone.

Before you start, consult your doctor:
No problems expected.

Over age 60:
No problems expected.

Pregnancy:
No proven harm to unborn child. Avoid if possible.

Breast-feeding:
No problems expected.

Infants & children:
Not recommended.

Prolonged use:
No problems expected.

Skin & sunlight:
No problems expected.

Driving, piloting or hazardous work:
No problems expected.

Discontinuing:
May be unnecessary to finish medicine. Discontinue when symptoms disappear.

Others:
No problems expected.

POSSIBLE INTERACTION WITH OTHER DRUGS

GENERIC NAME OR DRUG CLASS	COMBINED EFFECT
None expected.	

POSSIBLE INTERACTION WITH OTHER SUBSTANCES

INTERACTS WITH	COMBINED EFFECT
Alcohol:	None expected.
Beverages:	None expected.
Cocaine:	None expected.
Foods:	None expected.
Marijuana:	None expected.
Tobacco:	None expected.

*See Glossary

SODIUM BENZOATE AND SODIUM PHENYLACETATE

BRAND NAMES

Ucephan

BASIC INFORMATION

Habit forming? No
Prescription needed? Yes
Available as generic? No
Drug class: Antihyperammonemia

USES

Treats and prevents the condition (including coma) caused by too much ammonia in the blood.

DOSAGE & USAGE INFORMATION

How to take:
Oral solution—Dilute in milk or baby formula. Be careful not to splash it on skin or clothing since odor may linger.

When to take:
Take with meals and as directed by your doctor or nurse.

If you forget a dose:
Take as soon as you remember up to 2 hours late. If more than 2 hours, wait for next scheduled dose (don't double this dose).

What drug does:
Prevents the body from producing excessive ammonia caused by the breakdown of protein.

Time lapse before drug works:
Within 1 hour.

Don't take with:
- Penicillin, probenecid, valproic acid. Avoid high-protein foods while drug is needed.
- Any other medicine without consulting your doctor or pharmacist.

OVERDOSE

SYMPTOMS:
Fainting, coma, excessive drowsiness, shortness of breath, vomiting.
WHAT TO DO:
- **Dial 0 (operator) or 911 (emergency) for an ambulance or medical help. Then give first aid immediately.**
- **See emergency information on inside covers.**

POSSIBLE ADVERSE REACTIONS OR SIDE EFFECTS

SYMPTOMS	WHAT TO DO
Life-threatening: In case of overdose, see previous column	
Common; Nausea, vomiting.	Call doctor right away.
Infrequent: None expected with normal doses unless there is other underlying disease.	
Rare: None expected with normal doses unless there is other underlying disease.	

SODIUM BENZOATE AND SODIUM PHENYLACETATE

WARNINGS & PRECAUTIONS

Don't take if:
You are allergic to sodium benzoate and sodium phenylacetate.

Before you start, consult your doctor:
- If you have edema from any medical problem, such as kidney disease, toxemia of pregnancy, congestive heart failure.
- If you have peptic ulcer disease.

Over age 60:
May require dosage adjustment if kidney function is impaired due to normal aging.

Pregnancy:
Safety not established. Consult doctor.

Breast-feeding:
Safety not established. Best to avoid or discontinue nursing until you finish medicine. Consult doctor for advice on maintaining milk supply.

Infants & children:
Infants with low birth weight are particularly vulnerable to toxic effects. Use only under close supervision of a medical professional.

Prolonged use:
No special problems expected.

Skin & sunlight:
No special problems expected.

Driving, piloting or hazardous work:
Don't drive or pilot aircraft until you learn how medicine affects you. Don't work around dangerous machinery. Don't climb ladders or work in high places. Danger increases if you drink alcohol or take medicine affecting alertness and reflexes.

Discontinuing:
No special problems expected.

Others:
- Sometimes used at the same times as amino acid supplements.
- May affect results of some medical tests.
- Laboratory studies needed on a frequent basis to determine serum ammonia concentrations.

POSSIBLE INTERACTION WITH OTHER DRUGS

GENERIC NAME OR DRUG CLASS	COMBINED EFFECT
Penicillins*	May reduce the effects of sodium benzoate and sodium phenylacetate.
Probenecid	May reduce the effects of sodium benzoate and sodium phenylacetate.
Valproic acid	May reduce the effects of sodium benzoate and sodium phenylacetate.

POSSIBLE INTERACTION WITH OTHER SUBSTANCES

INTERACTS WITH	COMBINED EFFECT
Alcohol:	Avoid. May worsen the condition being treated.
Beverages:	None expected.
Cocaine:	None expected.
Foods: Foods high in protein.	Avoid. May worsen the condition being treated.
Marijuana:	None expected.
Tobacco:	None expected.

SODIUM BICARBONATE

BRAND NAMES

Arm & Hammer Pure
  Baking Soda
Bell/ans

Citrocarbonate
Soda Mint

BASIC INFORMATION

Habit forming? No
Prescription needed? No
Available as generic? Yes
Drug class: Alkalizer, antacid

 USES

- Treats metobolic acidosis.
- Alkalinizes urine to reduce uric acid kidney stones.
- Treats hyperacidity of the stomach that is present with indigestion, gastroesophageal reflux and peptic ulcer disease.

 DOSAGE & USAGE INFORMATION

How to take:
- Tablets—Swallow with liquid. If you can't swallow whole, crumble tablet and take with liquid or food.
- Powder—Mix in a glass of water and drink.
- Effervescent sodium bicarbonate—Mix in a glass of cold water and drink.

When to take:
- For hyperacidity—1 to 3 hours after meals.
- For kidney stones—According to prescription instructions.

If you forget a dose:
Take as soon as you remember up to 2 hours late. If more than 2 hours, wait for next scheduled dose (don't double this dose).

What drug does:
- Buffers acid in the stomach.
- Increases excretion of bicarbonate in the urine to help dissolve uric acid stones.

Continued next column

 OVERDOSE

SYMPTOMS:
Excessive swelling of feet and lower legs.
WHAT TO DO:
Overdose unlikely to threaten life. If person takes much larger amount than prescribed, call doctor, poison-control center or hospital emergency room for instructions.

Time lapse before drug works:
Works immediately, but the duration of effect is short.

Don't take with:
- Non-prescription drugs without consulting doctor.
- See Interaction column and consult doctor.

 POSSIBLE ADVERSE REACTIONS OR SIDE EFFECTS

SYMPTOMS	WHAT TO DO
Life-threatening: None expected.	
Common: None expected.	
Infrequent: • Stomach cramps that continue.	Discontinue. Call doctor right away.
• Nausea, headache, appetite loss (with long-term use).	Continue. Call doctor when convenient.
Rare: Muscle pain or twitching, nervousness, breathing difficulty, mild swelling of feet or lower legs (with large doses).	Discontinue. Call doctor right away.

WARNINGS & PRECAUTIONS

Don't take if:
You are allergic to sodium bicarbonate.

Before you start, consult your doctor:
If you have heart disease, kidney disease or toxemia of pregnancy.

Over age 60:
Adverse reactions and side effects may be more frequent and severe than in younger persons.

Pregnancy:
May cause weight gain and swelling of feet and ankles. Avoid if you have high blood pressure.

Breast-feeding:
No problems expected, but consult doctor.

Infants & children:
Not recommended. Safety and dosage have not been established.

Prolonged use:
Don't use for longer than prescribed or recommended. May cause sodium overload.

Skin & sunlight:
No special problems expected.

Driving, piloting or hazardous work:
No special problems expected.

Discontinuing:
May be unnecessary to finish medicine. Follow doctor's instructions.

Others:
- Heat and moisture in bathroom medicine cabinet can cause breakdown of medicine. Store someplace else.
- May interfere with the accuracy of some medical tests (especially acidosis and urinalysis tests).

POSSIBLE INTERACTION WITH OTHER DRUGS

GENERIC NAME OR DRUG CLASS	COMBINED EFFECT
Adrenocorticoids	Sodium overload.
Cortisone	Sodium overload.
Ketoconazole	Decreased absorption of ketoconazole.
Mecamylamine	Reduced mecamylamine effect.
Tetracyclines*	Greatly reduced absorption of tetracyclines.
Any other medicine	Decreased absorption of other medicine if taken within 1 to 2 hours of taking sodium bicarbonate.

POSSIBLE INTERACTION WITH OTHER SUBSTANCES

INTERACTS WITH	COMBINED EFFECT
Alcohol:	Decreased effectiveness of sodium bicarbonate.
Beverages:	None expected.
Cocaine:	None expected.
Foods:	None expected.
Marijuana:	None expected.
Tobacco:	Decreased effectiveness of sodium bicarbonate.

SODIUM FLUORIDE

BRAND NAMES

Denta-Fl
Flo-Tab
Fluor-A-Day
Fluorident
Fluoritab
Fluorodex
Flura
Karidium
Luride

Luride-SF
Nafeen
Pediaflor
Pedi-Dent
Solu-Flur
Stay-Flo
Studaflor
Thera-Flur

Numerous other multiple vitamin-mineral supplements. Check labels.

BASIC INFORMATION

Habit forming? No
Prescription needed? Yes
Available as generic? No
Drug class: Mineral supplement (fluoride)

 ## USES

- Reduces tooth cavities.
- Treatment for osteoporosis.

 ## DOSAGE & USAGE INFORMATION

How to take:
- Tablet—Swallow with liquid or crumble tablet and take with liquid (*not* milk) or food.
- Liquid—Measure with dropper and take directly or with liquid.
- Chewable tablets—Chew slowly and thoroughly before swallowing.

When to take:
Usually at bedtime after teeth are thoroughly brushed.

Continued next column

 ## OVERDOSE

SYMPTOMS:
Stomach cramps or pain, nausea, faintness, vomiting (possibly bloody), diarrhea, black stools, shallow breathing, muscle spasms, seizures, arrhythmias.
WHAT TO DO:
- Dial 0 (operator) or 911 (emergency) for an ambulance or medical help. Then give first aid immediately.
- See emergency information on inside covers.

If you forget a dose:
Take as soon as you remember. Don't double a forgotten dose. Return to schedule.

What drug does:
Provides supplemental fluoride to combat tooth decay.

Time lapse before drug works:
8 weeks to provide maximum effect.

Don't take with:
- Any other medicine simultaneously.
- See Interaction column.

 ## POSSIBLE ADVERSE REACTIONS OR SIDE EFFECTS

SYMPTOMS	WHAT TO DO
Life-threatening:	
In case of overdose, see previous column.	
Common:	
Constipation, appetite loss.	Continue. Call doctor when convenient.
Infrequent:	
• Rash.	Discontinue. Call doctor right away.
• Tooth discoloration.	Continue. Call doctor when convenient.
Rare:	
• Severe upsets (digestive) only with overdose.	Discontinue. Seek emergency treatment.
• Sores in mouth and lips, bone aching, stiffness.	Discontinue. Call doctor right away.

WARNINGS & PRECAUTIONS

Don't take if:
- Your water supply contains 0.7 parts fluoride per million. Too much fluoride stains teeth permanently.
- You are allergic to any fluoride-containing product.
- You have underactive thyroid.

Before you start, consult your doctor:
Not necessary.

Over age 60:
No problems expected.

Pregnancy:
No problems expected.

Breast-feeding:
No problems expected.

Infants & children:
No problems expected except accidental overdose. Keep vitamin-mineral supplements out of children's reach.

Prolonged use:
Excess may cause discolored teeth and decreased calcium in blood.

Skin & sunlight:
No problems expected.

Driving, piloting or hazardous work:
No problems expected.

Discontinuing:
No problems expected.

Others:
- Store in original plastic container. Fluoride decomposes glass.
- Some products contain tartrazine dye. Avoid, especially if you are allergic to aspirin.

POSSIBLE INTERACTION WITH OTHER DRUGS

GENERIC NAME OR DRUG CLASS	COMBINED EFFECT
Calcium supplements*	Decreased effect of calcium and fluoride.

POSSIBLE INTERACTION WITH OTHER SUBSTANCES

INTERACTS WITH	COMBINED EFFECT
Alcohol:	None expected.
Beverages: Milk.	Prevents absorption of fluoride. Space dose 2 hours before or after milk.
Cocaine:	None expected.
Foods:	None expected.
Marijuana:	None expected.
Tobacco:	None expected.

SODIUM PHOSPHATE

BRAND NAMES

Fleet Enema   Sal Hepatica
Fleet Phospho-Soda

BASIC INFORMATION

Habit forming? No
Prescription needed? No
Available as generic? Yes
Drug class: Laxative (hyperosmotic)

USES

Constipation relief.

DOSAGE & USAGE INFORMATION

How to take:
Liquid, effervescent tablet or powder—Dilute
dose in beverage before swallowing.

When to take:
Usually once a day, preferably in the morning.

If you forget a dose:
Take as soon as you remember up to 8 hours
before bedtime. If later, wait for next scheduled
dose (don't double this dose). Don't take at
bedtime.

What drug does:
Draws water into bowel from other body tissues.
Causes distention through fluid accumulation,
which promotes soft stool and accelerates bowel
motion.

Time lapse before drug works:
30 minutes to 3 hours.

Don't take with:
Any other medicine without consulting your
doctor or pharmacist.

OVERDOSE

SYMPTOMS:
**Fluid depletion, weakness, vomiting,
fainting.**
WHAT TO DO:
**Overdose unlikely to threaten life. If person
takes much larger amount than prescribed,
call doctor, poison-control center or
hospital emergency room for instructions.**

POSSIBLE ADVERSE REACTIONS OR SIDE EFFECTS

SYMPTOMS	WHAT TO DO
Life-threatening: In case of overdose, see previous column.	
Common: Weakness.	Continue. Call doctor when convenient.
Infrequent: • Irregular heartbeat.	Discontinue. Call doctor right away.
• Increased thirst, gaseousness, cramps, diarrhea, nausea.	Continue. Tell doctor at next visit.
Rare: Dizziness, confusion, tiredness or weakness.	Continue. Call doctor when convenient.

SODIUM PHOSPHATE

WARNINGS & PRECAUTIONS

Don't take if:
- You are allergic to any hyperosmotic laxative.
- You have symptoms of appendicitis, inflamed bowel or intestinal blockage.
- You have missed a bowel movement for only 1 or 2 days.

Before you start, consult your doctor:
- If you have congestive heart disease.
- If you have diabetes.
- If you have high blood pressure.
- If you have a colostomy or ileostomy.
- If you have kidney disease.
- If you have a laxative habit.
- If you have rectal bleeding.
- If you take another laxative.

Over age 60:
Adverse reactions and side effects may be more frequent and severe than in younger persons.

Pregnancy:
Salt content may cause fluid retention and swelling. Avoid if possible.

Breast-feeding:
No problems expected.

Infants & children:
Use only under medical supervision.

Prolonged use:
Don't take for more than 1 week unless under a doctor's supervision. May cause laxative dependence.

Skin & sunlight:
No problems expected.

Driving, piloting or hazardous work:
No problems expected.

Discontinuing:
May be unnecessary to finish medicine. Follow doctor's instructions.

Others:
- Don't take to "flush out" your system or as a "tonic."
- Don't take within 2 hours of taking another medicine.

POSSIBLE INTERACTION WITH OTHER DRUGS

GENERIC NAME OR DRUG CLASS	COMBINED EFFECT
Chlordiazepoxide	Decreased chlordiazepoxide effect.
Chlorpromazine	Decreased chlorpromazine effect.
Dicumarol	Decreased dicumarol effect.
Digoxin	Decreased digoxin effect.
Diuretics, potassium-sparing*	Excessive potassium loss.
Isoniazid	Decreased isoniazid effect.
Mexiletine	May decrease effectiveness of mexiletine.
Potassium supplements*	Reduced potassium supplements effect.
Tetracyclines*	Possible intestinal blockage.

POSSIBLE INTERACTION WITH OTHER SUBSTANCES

INTERACTS WITH	COMBINED EFFECT
Alcohol:	None expected.
Beverages:	None expected.
Cocaine:	None expected.
Foods:	None expected.
Marijuana:	None expected.
Tobacco:	None expected.

SPIRONOLACTONE

BRAND NAMES

Aldactone   Sincomen
Novospiroton

BASIC INFORMATION

Habit forming? No
Prescription needed? Yes
Available as generic? Yes
Drug class: Antihypertensive, diuretic

USES

- Reduces high blood pressure.
- Prevents fluid retention.

DOSAGE & USAGE INFORMATION

How to take:
Tablet—Swallow with liquid or food to lessen stomach irritation. If you can't swallow whole, crumble tablet and take with liquid or food.

When to take:
- 1 dose a day—Take after breakfast.
- More than 1 dose a day—Take last dose no later than 6 p.m.

If you forget a dose:
- 1 dose a day—Take as soon as you remember up to 12 hours late. If more than 12 hours, wait for next scheduled dose (don't double this dose).
- More than 1 dose a day—Take as soon as you remember. Wait 6 hours for next dose.

What drug does:
- Increases sodium and water excretion through increased urine production, decreasing body fluid and blood pressure.
- Retains potassium.

Time lapse before drug works:
3 to 5 days.

Continued next column

OVERDOSE

SYMPTOMS:
Thirst, drowsiness, confusion, fatigue, weakness, nausea, vomiting, irregular heartbeat, excessive blood-pressure drop.
WHAT TO DO:
- **Dial 0 (operator) or 911 (emergency) for an ambulance or medical help. Then give first aid immediately.**
- **See emergency information on inside covers.**

Don't take with:
Any other medicine without consulting your doctor or pharmacist.

POSSIBLE ADVERSE REACTIONS OR SIDE EFFECTS

SYMPTOMS	WHAT TO DO
Life-threatening:	
In case of overdose, see previous column.	
Common:	
Drowsiness or headache, thirst, nausea, vomiting, diarrhea, abdominal cramping, muscle cramps.	Continue. Call doctor when convenient.
Infrequent:	
• Confusion, irregular heartbeat, shortness of breath, constipation, breast tenderness, unusual sweating.	Discontinue. Call doctor right away.
• Numbness, tingling in hands or feet; menstrual irregularities; change in sex drive; dizziness; energy loss.	Continue. Call doctor when convenient.
Rare:	
• Rash or itchy skin, fever.	Discontinue. Call doctor right away.
• Deep voice in women, excess hair growth, voice change, enlarged clitoris in women.	Continue. Tell doctor at next visit.

WARNINGS & PRECAUTIONS

Don't take if:
- You are allergic to spironolactone.
- You have impaired kidney function.
- Your serum potassium level is high.

Before you start, consult your doctor:
- If you have had kidney or liver disease.
- If you will have surgery within 2 months, including dental surgery, requiring general or spinal anesthesia.

Over age 60:
- Limit use to 2 to 3 weeks if possible.
- Adverse reactions and side effects may be more frequent and severe than in younger persons.
- Heat or fever can reduce blood pressure. May require dose adjustment.
- Overdose and extended use may cause blood clots.

Pregnancy:
No proven harm to unborn child. Avoid if possible.

Breast-feeding:
No proven problems. Consult doctor.

Infants & children:
Use only under medical supervision.

Prolonged use:
- Potassium retention with irregular heartbeat, unusual weakness and confusion.
- Talk to your doctor about the need for follow-up medical examinations or laboratory studies to check blood pressure, kidney function, ECG* and serum electrolytes.

Skin & sunlight:
Increased sensitivity to sunlight.

Driving, piloting or hazardous work:
Avoid if you feel drowsy. Otherwise, no problems expected.

Discontinuing:
Consult doctor about adjusting doses of other drugs.

Others:
No problems expected.

POSSIBLE INTERACTION WITH OTHER DRUGS

GENERIC NAME OR DRUG CLASS	COMBINED EFFECT
ACE inhibitors*: captopril, enalapril, lisinopril	Possible excessive potassium in blood.
Amiloride	Dangerous potassium retention.
Anticoagulants, oral*	Possible decreased anticoagulant effect.
Antihypertensives, other*	Increased antihypertensive effect.
Aspirin	Decreased spironolactone effect.
Carteolol	Increased antihypertensive effect.
Cyclosporine	Possible excessive potassium in blood.
Digitalis preparations*	Decreased digitalis effect.
Diuretics, other*	Increased effect of both drugs. Beneficial if needed and dose is correct.
Laxatives*	Reduced potassium levels.
Lithium	Likely lithium toxicity.
Nicardipine	Blood pressure drop. Dosages may require adjustment.
Nimodipine	Dangerous blood pressure drop.
Nitrates*	Excessive blood pressure drop.
Potassium iodide	May raise potassium level in blood to toxic levels.
Potassium supplements*	Dangerous potassium retention, causing possible heartbeat irregularity.
Salicylates*	May decrease spironolactone effect.
Sodium bicarbonate	Reduces high potassium levels.
Sotalol	Increased antihypertensive effect.
Terazosin	Decreases effectiveness of terazosin.
Triamterene	Dangerous potassium retention.

POSSIBLE INTERACTION WITH OTHER SUBSTANCES

INTERACTS WITH	COMBINED EFFECT
Alcohol:	None expected.
Beverages: Low-salt milk.	Possible potassium toxicity.
Cocaine:	Increased risk of heart block and high blood pressure.
Foods: Salt.	Don't restrict unless directed by doctor.
Salt substitutes.	Possible potassium toxicity.
Marijuana:	Increased thirst, fainting.
Tobacco:	None expected.

SPIRONOLACTONE & HYDROCHLOROTHIAZIDE

BRAND NAMES

Aldactazide   Spirozide
Novospirozine

BASIC INFORMATION

Habit forming? Yes
Prescription needed? Yes
Available as generic? Yes
Drug class: Antihypertensive, diuretic
(thiazide)

USES

- Controls, but doesn't cure, high blood pressure.
- Reduces fluid retention (edema).

DOSAGE & USAGE INFORMATION

How to take:
Tablet—Swallow with liquid. If you can't swallow whole, crumble tablet and take with liquid or food.

When to take:
- 1 dose a day—Take after breakfast.
- More than 1 dose a day—Take last dose no later than 6 p.m.

If you forget a dose:
- 1 dose a day—Take as soon as you remember up to 12 hours late. If more than 12 hours, wait for next scheduled dose (don't double this dose).
- More than 1 dose a day—Take as soon as you remember. Wait 6 hours for next dose.

What drug does:
- Increases sodium and water excretion through increased urine production.
- Retains potassium.
- Relaxes muscle cells of small arteries.
- Reduced body fluid and relaxed arteries lower blood pressure.

Continued next column

OVERDOSE

SYMPTOMS:
Thirst, drowsiness, confusion, fatigue, weakness, nausea, vomiting, cramps, irregular heartbeat, weak pulse, excessive blood-pressure drop, coma.
WHAT TO DO:
- **Dial 0 (operator) or 911 (emergency) for an ambulance or medical help. Then give first aid immediately.**
- **See emergency information on inside covers.**

Time lapse before drug works:
4 to 6 hours. May require several weeks to lower blood pressure.

Don't take with:
Any other medicine without consulting your doctor or pharmacist.

POSSIBLE ADVERSE REACTIONS OR SIDE EFFECTS

SYMPTOMS	WHAT TO DO
Life-threatening: Irregular heartbeat, weak pulse, shortness of breath.	Discontinue. Seek emergency treatment.
Common: Drowsiness, headache, thirst, abdominal cramping, muscle cramps.	Continue. Call doctor when convenient.
Infrequent: • Blurred vision, abdominal pain, nausea, vomiting, constipation, breast tenderness.	Discontinue. Call doctor right away.
• Dizziness, mood change, headache, dry mouth, menstrual irregularities, diminished sex drive, increased sweating, weakness, tiredness, weight gain or loss, confusion, numbness or tingling in hands or feet, diarrhea.	Continue. Call doctor when convenient.
Rare: • Sore throat, fever, rash, jaundice.	Discontinue. Call doctor right away.
• Excess growth of hair, deep voice in in women, enlarged clitoris in women.	Continue. Call doctor when convenient.

WARNINGS & PRECAUTIONS

Don't take if:
You are allergic to any thiazide diuretic drug.

Before you start, consult your doctor:
- If you are allergic to any sulfa drug.
- If you have gout, liver, pancreas or kidney disorder.
- If you have had kidney or liver disease.
- If you will have surgery within 2 months, including dental surgery, requiring general or spinal anesthesia.

SPIRONOLACTONE & HYDROCHLOROTHIAZIDE

Over age 60:
- Adverse reactions and side effects may be more frequent and severe than in younger persons, especially dizziness and excessive potassium loss.
- Limit use to 2 to 3 weeks if possible.
- Heat or fever can reduce blood pressure. May require dose adjustment.
- Overdose and extended use may cause blood clots.

Pregnancy:
Risk to unborn child outweighs drug benefits. Don't use.

Breast-feeding:
Drug passes into milk. Avoid drug or discontinue nursing until you finish medicine.

Infants & children:
Use only under medical supervision.

Prolonged use:
- You may need medicine to treat high blood pressure for the rest of your life.
- Potassium retention with irregular heartbeat, unusual weakness and confusion.
- Talk to your doctor about the need for follow-up medical examinations or laboratory studies to check blood pressure, kidney function, ECG* and serum electrolytes.

Skin & sunlight:
May cause rash or intensify sunburn in areas exposed to sun or sunlamp.

Driving, piloting or hazardous work:
Don't drive or pilot aircraft until you learn how medicine affects you. Don't work around dangerous machinery. Don't climb ladders or work in high places. Danger increases if you drink alcohol or take medicine affecting alertness and reflexes.

Discontinuing:
- Don't discontinue without medical advice.
- Consult doctor about adjusting doses of other drugs.

Others:
- Hot weather and fever may cause dehydration and drop in blood pressure. Dose may require temporary adjustment. Weigh daily and report any unexpected weight decreases to your doctor.
- May cause rise in uric acid, leading to gout.
- May cause blood-sugar rise in diabetics.

 POSSIBLE INTERACTION WITH OTHER DRUGS

GENERIC NAME OR DRUG CLASS	COMBINED EFFECT
ACE inhibitors*: captopril, enalapril, lisinopril	Possible excessive potassium in blood.
Allopurinol	Decreased allopurinol effect.
Anticoagulants, oral*	Decreased anticoagulant effect.
Antidepressants, tricyclic (TCA)*	Dangerous drop in blood pressure. Avoid combination unless under medical supervision.
Antidiabetics, oral*	Increased blood sugar.
Antihypertensives, other*	Increased antihypertensive effect.
Aspirin	Decreased spironolactone effect.
Barbiturates*	Increased hydrochlorothiazide effect.
Carteolol	Increased antihypertensive effect.
Cholestyramine	Decreased hydrochlorothiazide effect.
Cortisone drugs*	Excessive potassium loss that causes dangerous heart rhythms.
Cyclosporine	Possible excessive potassium in blood.

Continued page 961

 POSSIBLE INTERACTION WITH OTHER SUBSTANCES

INTERACTS WITH	COMBINED EFFECT
Alcohol:	Dangerous blood-pressure drop.
Beverages: Low-salt milk.	Possible potassium toxicity.
Cocaine:	Decreased spironolactone effect.
Foods: Salt.	Don't restrict unless directed by doctor.
Salt substitutes.	Possible potassium toxicity.
Marijuana:	May increase blood pressure. Increased thirst, fainting.
Tobacco:	None expected.

*See Glossary

SUCRALFATE

BRAND NAMES

Carafate   Sulcrate

BASIC INFORMATION

Habit forming? No
Prescription needed? Yes
Available as generic? No
Drug class: Antiulcer

 ## USES

Treatment of duodenal ulcer.

 ## DOSAGE & USAGE INFORMATION

How to take:
Tablet—Take as directed on an empty stomach.

When to take:
1 hour before meals and at bedtime. Allow 2 hours to elapse before taking other prescription medicines.

If you forget a dose:
Take as soon as you remember up to 2 hours late. If more than 2 hours, wait for next scheduled dose (don't double this dose).

What drug does:
Covers ulcer site and protects from acid, enzymes and bile salts.

Time lapse before drug works:
Begins in 30 minutes. May require several days to relieve pain.

Don't take with:
Any other medicine without consulting your doctor or pharmacist.

 ## OVERDOSE

SYMPTOMS:
None expected.
WHAT TO DO:
Overdose unlikely to threaten life. If person takes much larger amount than prescribed, call doctor, poison-control center or hospital emergency room for instructions.

 ## POSSIBLE ADVERSE REACTIONS OR SIDE EFFECTS

SYMPTOMS	WHAT TO DO
Life-threatening: None expected.	
Common: Constipation.	Continue. Call doctor when convenient.
Infrequent: ● Diarrhea.	Discontinue. Call doctor right away.
● Dizziness, sleepiness, rash, itchy skin, abdominal pain, indigestion, vomiting, nausea, dry mouth.	Continue. Call doctor when convenient.
Rare: Back pain.	Continue. Call doctor when convenient.

SUCRALFATE

WARNINGS & PRECAUTIONS

Don't take if:
You are allergic to sucralfate.

Before you start, consult your doctor:
If you will have surgery within 2 months, including dental surgery, requiring general or spinal anesthesia.

Over age 60:
Adverse reactions and side effects may be more frequent and severe than in younger persons.

Pregnancy:
No proven harm to unborn child. Avoid if possible.

Breast-feeding:
Unknown effects.

Infants & children:
Safety not established.

Prolonged use:
Request blood counts if medicine needed longer than 8 weeks.

Skin & sunlight:
No problems expected.

Driving, piloting or hazardous work:
Don't drive or pilot aircraft until you learn how medicine affects you. Don't work around dangerous machinery. Don't climb ladders or work in high places. Danger increases if you drink alcohol or take medicine affecting alertness and reflexes, such as antihistamines, tranquilizers, sedatives, pain medicine, narcotics and mind-altering drugs.

Discontinuing:
Don't discontinue without consulting doctor. Dose may require gradual reduction if you have taken drug for a long time. Doses of other drugs may also require adjustment.

Others:
No problems expected.

POSSIBLE INTERACTION WITH OTHER DRUGS

GENERIC NAME OR DRUG CLASS	COMBINED EFFECT
Cimetidine	Possible decreased absorption of cimetidine if taken simultaneously.
Phenytoin	Possible decreased absorption of phenytoin if taken simultaneously.
Tetracyclines*	Possible decreased absorption of tetracycline if taken simultaneously.
Vitamins A, D, E, K	Decreased vitamin absorption.

POSSIBLE INTERACTION WITH OTHER SUBSTANCES

INTERACTS WITH	COMBINED EFFECT
Alcohol:	Irritates ulcer. Avoid.
Beverages: Caffeine.	Irritates ulcer. Avoid.
Cocaine:	May make ulcer worse. Avoid.
Foods:	No problems expected.
Marijuana:	May make ulcer worse. Avoid.
Tobacco:	May make ulcer worse. Avoid.

SULFACYTINE

BRAND NAMES

Renoquid

BASIC INFORMATION

Habit forming? No
Prescription needed? Yes
Available as generic? No
Drug class: Sulfa (sulfonamide)

 USES

Treatment for urinary tract infections responsive to this drug.

 DOSAGE & USAGE INFORMATION

How to take:
Tablet—Swallow with liquid. Instructions to take on empty stomach mean 1 hour before or 2 hours after eating.

When to take:
At the same times each day, evenly spaced.

If you forget a dose:
Take as soon as you remember up to 2 hours late. If more than 2 hours, wait for next scheduled dose (don't double this dose).

What drug does:
Interferes with a nutrient (folic acid) necessary for growth and reproduction of bacteria. Will not attack viruses.

Time lapse before drug works:
2 to 5 days to affect infection.

Don't take with:
Any other medicine without consulting your doctor or pharmacist.

 OVERDOSE

SYMPTOMS:
Less urine, bloody urine, coma.
WHAT TO DO:
- **Dial 0 (operator) or 911 (emergency) for an ambulance or medical help. Then give first aid immediately.**
- **See emergency information on inside covers.**

 POSSIBLE ADVERSE REACTIONS OR SIDE EFFECTS

SYMPTOMS	WHAT TO DO
Life-threatening:	
In case of overdose, see previous column.	
Common:	
• Itchy skin, rash.	Discontinue. Call doctor right away.
• Headache, vomiting, nausea, diarrhea, appetite loss, skin sensitive to sun.	Continue. Call doctor when convenient.
Infrequent:	
• Red, peeling or blistering skin; sore throat; fever; swallowing difficulty; unusual bruising; aching joints or muscles; jaundice.	Discontinue. Call doctor right away.
• Dizziness, tiredness, weakness.	Continue. Call doctor when convenient.
Rare:	
Painful urination, low back pain, numbness or tingling in hands or feet, bloody urine, neck swelling.	Discontinue. Call doctor right away.

 WARNINGS & PRECAUTIONS

Don't take if:
You are allergic to any sulfa drug.

Before you start, consult your doctor:
- If you are allergic to carbonic anhydrase inhibitors, oral antidiabetics, thiazide or loop diuretics.
- If you are allergic by nature.
- If you have liver or kidney disease.
- If you have porphyria.
- If you have developed anemia from use of any drug.

Over age 60:
Adverse reactions and side effects may be more frequent and severe than in younger persons.

Pregnancy:
Risk to unborn child outweighs drug benefits. Don't use.

Breast-feeding:
Drug passes into milk. Avoid drug or discontinue nursing until you finish medicine. Consult doctor for advice on maintaining milk supply.

Infants & children:
Don't give to infants younger than 1 month.

Prolonged use:
- May enlarge thyroid gland.
- You may become more susceptible to infections caused by germs not responsive to this drug.
- Request frequent blood counts, liver- and kidney-function studies.

Skin & sunlight:
May cause rash or intensify sunburn in areas exposed to sun or sunlamp.

Driving, piloting or hazardous work:
Avoid if you feel dizzy. Otherwise, no problems expected.

Discontinuing:
Don't discontinue without doctor's advice until you complete prescribed dose, even though symptoms diminish or disappear.

Others:
- Drink 2 quarts of liquid each day to prevent adverse reactions.
- If you require surgery, tell anesthetist you take sulfa. Pentothal anesthesia should not be used.

POSSIBLE INTERACTION WITH OTHER DRUGS

GENERIC NAME OR DRUG CLASS	COMBINED EFFECT
Aminobenzoates	Possible decreased sulfa effect.
Anticoagulants, oral*	Increased anti-coagulant effect.
Anticonvulsants, hydantoin* and antidiabetic drugs*	Toxic effect on brain.
Aspirin	Increased sulfa effect.
Calcium supplements*	Decreased sulfa effect.

Clozapine	Toxic effect on the central nervous system.
Hepatotoxic agents*	Increased liver toxicity.
Isoniazid	Possible anemia.
Mecamylamine	Decreased antibiotic effect.
Methenamine	Possible kidney blockage.
Methotrexate	Increased methotrexate effect.
Oxyphenbutazone	Increased sulfa effect.
Para-aminosalicylic acid	Decreased sulfa effect.
Penicillins*	Decreased penicillin effect.
Phenylbutazone	Increased sulfa effect.
Probenecid	Increased sulfa effect.
Sulfinpyrazone	Increased sulfa effect.
Sulfonureas*	May increase hypo-glycemic action.
Tiopronin	Increased risk of toxicity to kidneys.
Trimethoprim	Increased sulfa effect.
Zidovudine	Increased risk of toxic effects of zidovudine.

POSSIBLE INTERACTION WITH OTHER SUBSTANCES

INTERACTS WITH	COMBINED EFFECT
Alcohol:	Increased alcohol effect.
Beverages: Less than 2 quarts of fluid daily.	Kidney damage.
Cocaine:	None expected.
Foods:	None expected.
Marijuana:	None expected.
Tobacco:	None expected.

*See Glossary

SULFADOXINE AND PYRIMETHAMINE

BRAND NAMES

Fansidar

BASIC INFORMATION

Habit forming? No
Prescription needed? Yes
Available as generic? No
Drug class: Antiprotozoal

USES

- Treats malaria (*plasmodium faciparum*).
- Helps prevent malaria when traveling to areas where it exists.
- Also used to prevent isosporiasis in patients with acquired immunodeficiency disease.

DOSAGE & USAGE INFORMATION

How to take:
Tablets—Swallow with liquid. If you can't swallow whole, crumble tablet and take with liquid or food. Instructions to take on empty stomach mean 1 hour before or 2 hours after eating.

When to take:
Follow doctor's instructions.

If you forget a dose:
Take as soon as you remember. If close to time for next dose, skip this one and wait for next scheduled dose. Don't double dose.

What drug does:
The sulfa component kills bacteria; the pyrimethamine works to kill malaria organisms in red blood cells or human tisue.

Time lapse before drug works:
2 to 6 hours.

Continued next column

OVERDOSE

SYMPTOMS:
Appetite loss, sore throat and fever, seizure, coma.
WHAT TO DO:
- **Dial 0 (operator) or 911 (emergency) for an ambulance or medical help. Then give first aid immediately.**
- **See emergency information on inside front covers.**

Don't take with:
- Any other medicines (including over-the-counter drugs such as cough and cold medicines, laxatives, antacids, diet pills, caffeine, nose drops or vitamins) without consulting your doctor.
- Mefloquine.

POSSIBLE ADVERSE REACTIONS OR SIDE EFFECTS

SYMPTOMS	WHAT TO DO
Life-threatening:	
In case of overdose, see previous column.	
Common:	
Loss or change of taste; diarrhea; skin rash; pale skin; sore throat; sore, red tongue; mouth ulcers; fever; excessive bleeding; tiredness, light sensitivity.	Discontinue. Call doctor right away.
Infrequent:	
Aching joints, fever, skin blisters or peeling, jaundice (yellow skin and eyes).	Discontinue. Call doctor right away.
Rare:	
Bloody urine, burning on urination, back pain, swollen neck.	Discontinue. Call doctor right away.

SULFADOXINE AND PYRIMETHAMINE

 ## WARNINGS & PRECAUTIONS

Don't take if:
You know you are allergic to sulfa drugs, furosemide, thiazide diuretics, carbonase anhydrase inhibitors.

Before you start, consult your doctor:
- If you have AIDS.
- If you have anemia, seizures, G6PD deficiency, liver disease, porphyria, kidney disease.
- If you can't tolerate sulfa drugs.

Over age 60:
Adverse reactions and side effects may be more frequent and severe than in younger persons. You may need smaller doses for shorter periods of time.

Pregnancy:
Use birth control so you won't get pregnant while in an endemic malaria area. Fansidar should not be taken during pregnancy if it can possibly be avoided.

Breast-feeding:
Drug passes into milk. Avoid drug or discontinue nursing until you finish medicine. Consult doctor for advice on maintaining milk supply.

Infants & children:
Don't use in infants under 2 months old.

Prolonged use:
Talk to your doctor about the need for follow-up medical examinations or laboratory studies to check complete blood counts (white blood cell count, platelet count, red blood cell count, hemoglobin, hematocrit) and urinalyses.

Skin & sunlight:
Increased sensitivity to sunlight.

Driving, piloting or hazardous work:
Avoid if you feel confused, drowsy or dizzy.

Discontinuing:
Don't discontinue for 4 to 6 weeks after you leave endemic malaria areas.

Others:
- Advise any doctor or dentist whom you consult that you take this medicine.
- May affect results in some medical tests.
- Sleep under mosquito netting while in endemic areas. Wear long-sleeved shirts and long pants.
- Report to your doctor if you develop any symptoms of illness while you take Fansidar—even if the symptoms seem minor.

 ## POSSIBLE INTERACTION WITH OTHER DRUGS

GENERIC NAME OR DRUG CLASS	COMBINED EFFECT
Anticoagulants*	Increased risk of toxicity.
Anticonvulsants*	Increased risk of toxicity.
Antidiabetics*	Increased risk of toxicity.
Bone marrow depressants*	Increased risk of bleeding or other toxic symptoms.
Clozapine	Toxic effect on the central nervous system.
Contraceptives, oral*	Reduced reliability of the pill.
Hepatotoxic medicines*	Increased risk of liver toxicity.
Methenamine	Increased risk of kidney toxicity.
Methotrexate	Increased risk of toxicity.
Zidovudine	Increased risk of liver toxicity.

 ## POSSIBLE INTERACTION WITH OTHER SUBSTANCES

INTERACTS WITH	COMBINED EFFECT
Alcohol:	Nausea and vomiting. Avoid.
Beverages:	No special problems expected.
Cocaine:	Increased likelihood of adverse reactions or seizures. Avoid.
Foods:	No special problems expected.
Marijuana:	Increased likelihood of adverse reactions. Avoid.
Tobacco:	No special problems expected.

SULFAMETHOXAZOLE

BRAND NAMES

See complete list of brand names in the *Brand Names Directory*, page 929.

BASIC INFORMATION

Habit forming? No
Prescription needed? Yes
Available as generic? Yes
Drug class: Sulfa (sulfonamide)

 ## USES

Treatment for urinary tract infections responsive to this drug.

 ## DOSAGE & USAGE INFORMATION

How to take:
- Tablet—Swallow with liquid. Instructions to take on empty stomach mean 1 hour before or 2 hours after eating.
- Liquid—Shake carefully before measuring.

When to take:
At the same times each day, evenly spaced.

If you forget a dose:
Take as soon as you remember up to 2 hours late. If more than 2 hours, wait for next scheduled dose (don't double this dose).

What drug does:
Interferes with a nutrient (folic acid) necessary for growth and reproduction of bacteria. Will not attack viruses.

Time lapse before drug works:
2 to 5 days to affect infection.

Don't take with:
Any other medicine without consulting your doctor or pharmacist.

 ## OVERDOSE

SYMPTOMS:
Less urine, bloody urine, coma.
WHAT TO DO:
- **Dial 0 (operator) or 911 (emergency) for an ambulance or medical help. Then give first aid immediately.**
- **See emergency information on inside covers.**

 ## POSSIBLE ADVERSE REACTIONS OR SIDE EFFECTS

SYMPTOMS	WHAT TO DO
Life-threatening:	
In case of overdose, see previous column.	
Common:	
• Itchy skin, rash.	Discontinue. Call doctor right away.
• Headache, nausea, vomiting, diarrhea, appetite loss, skin sensitive to sun.	Continue. Call doctor when convenient.
Infrequent:	
• Red, peeling or blistering skin; sore throat; fever; swallowing difficulty; unusual bruising; aching joints or muscles; jaundice.	Discontinue. Call doctor right away.
• Dizziness, weakness, tiredness.	Continue. Call doctor when convenient.
Rare:	
Painful urination; low back pain; numbness, tingling, burning feeling in feet and hands, bloody urine, neck swelling.	Discontinue. Call doctor right away.

 ## WARNINGS & PRECAUTIONS

Don't take if:
You are allergic to any sulfa drug.

Before you start, consult your doctor:
- If you are allergic to carbonic anhydrase inhibitors, oral antidiabetics or thiazide or loop diuretics.
- If you are allergic by nature.
- If you have liver or kidney disease.
- If you have porphyria.
- If you have developed anemia from use of any drug.

SULFAMETHOXAZOLE

Over age 60:
Adverse reactions and side effects may be more frequent and severe than in younger persons.

Pregnancy:
Risk to unborn child outweighs drug benefits. Don't use.

Breast-feeding:
Drug passes into milk. Avoid drug or discontinue nursing until you finish medicine. Consult doctor for advice on maintaining milk supply.

Infants & children:
Don't give to infants younger than 1 month.

Prolonged use:
- May enlarge thyroid gland.
- You may become more susceptible to infections caused by germs not responsive to this drug.
- Request frequent blood counts, liver- and kidney-function studies.

Skin & sunlight:
May cause rash or intensify sunburn in areas exposed to sun or sunlamp.

Driving, piloting or hazardous work:
Avoid if you feel dizzy. Otherwise, no problems expected.

Discontinuing:
Don't discontinue without doctor's advice until you complete prescribed dose, even though symptoms diminish or disappear.

Others:
- Drink 2 quarts of liquid each day to prevent adverse reactions.
- If you require surgery, tell anesthetist you take sulfa. Pentothal anesthesia should not be used.

 ## POSSIBLE INTERACTION WITH OTHER DRUGS

GENERIC NAME OR DRUG CLASS	COMBINED EFFECT
Aminobenzoates	Possible decreased sulfa effect.
Anticoagulants, oral*	Increased anticoagulant effect.
Anticonvulsants, hydantoin* and antidiabetic drugs*	Toxic effect on brain.
Aspirin	Increased sulfa effect.
Calcium supplements*	Decreased sulfa effect.
Clozapine	Toxic effect on the central nervous system.
Hepatotoxic agents*	Increased liver toxicity.
Isoniazid	Possible anemia.
Mecamylamine	Decreased antibiotic effect.
Methenamine	Possible kidney blockage.
Methotrexate	Increased methotrexate effect.
Oxyphenbutazone	Increased sulfa effect.
Para-aminosalicylic acid	Decreased sulfa effect.
Penicillins*	Decreased penicillin effect.
Phenylbutazone	Increased sulfa effect.
Probenecid	Increased sulfa effect.
Sulfinpyrazone	Increased sulfa effect.
Sulfonureas*	May increase hypoglycemic action.
Trimethoprim	Increased sulfa effect.
Zidovudine	Increased risk of toxic effects of zidovudine.

 ## POSSIBLE INTERACTION WITH OTHER SUBSTANCES

INTERACTS WITH	COMBINED EFFECT
Alcohol:	Increased alcohol effect.
Beverages: Less than 2 quarts of fluid daily.	Kidney damage.
Cocaine:	None expected.
Foods:	None expected.
Marijuana:	None expected.
Tobacco:	None expected.

*See Glossary

SULFASALAZINE

BRAND NAMES

Azaline
Azulfidine
Azulfidine En-Tabs
PMS Sulfasalazine
PMS Sulfasalazine
  EC

Salazopyrin
Salazosulfapyridine
Salicylazosulfa-
  pyridine
S.A.S.
S.A.S. Enteric

BASIC INFORMATION

Habit forming? No
Prescription needed? Yes
Available as generic? Yes
Drug class: Sulfa (sulfonamide)

 ## USES

Treatment for ulceration and bleeding during active phase of ulcerative colitis.

 ## DOSAGE & USAGE INFORMATION

How to take:
- Tablet—Swallow with liquid. Instructions to take on empty stomach mean 1 hour before or 2 hours after eating.
- Liquid—Shake carefully before measuring.

When to take:
At the same times each day, evenly spaced.

If you forget a dose:
Take as soon as you remember up to 2 hours late. If more than 2 hours, wait for next scheduled dose (don't double this dose).

What drug does:
Anti-inflammatory action reduces tissue destruction in colon.

Time lapse before drug works:
2 to 5 days.

Don't take with:
Any other medicine without consulting your doctor or pharmacist.

 ## OVERDOSE

SYMPTOMS:
Less urine, bloody urine, coma.
WHAT TO DO:
- **Dial 0 (operator) or 911 (emergency) for an ambulance or medical help. Then give first aid immediately.**
- **See emergency information on inside covers.**

 ## POSSIBLE ADVERSE REACTIONS OR SIDE EFFECTS

SYMPTOMS	WHAT TO DO
Life-threatening:	
In case of overdose, see previous column.	
Common:	
• Itchy skin, rash.	Discontinue. Call doctor right away.
• Headache, nausea, vomiting, diarrhea, appetite loss, skin sensitive to sun.	Continue. Call doctor when convenient.
• Orange urine.	Continue. Tell doctor at next visit.
Infrequent:	
• Red, peeling or blistering skin; sore throat; fever; swallowing difficulty; unusual bruising; aching joints or muscles; jaundice.	Discontinue. Call doctor right away.
• Dizziness, tiredness, weakness, impotence.	Continue. Call doctor when convenient.
Rare:	
Painful urination; low back pain; numbness, tingling, burning feeling in feet and hands, bloody urine, neck swelling.	Discontinue. Call doctor right away.

 ## WARNINGS & PRECAUTIONS

Don't take if:
You are allergic to any sulfa drug.

Before you start, consult your doctor:
- If you are allergic to carbonic anhydrase inhibitors, oral antidiabetics or thiazide or loop diuretics.
- If you are allergic by nature.
- If you have liver or kidney disease.
- If you have porphyria.
- If you have developed anemia from use of any drug.

Over age 60:
Adverse reactions and side effects may be more frequent and severe than in younger persons.

Pregnancy:
Risk to unborn child outweighs drug benefits. Don't use.

Breast-feeding:
Drug passes into milk. Avoid drug or discontinue nursing until you finish medicine. Consult doctor for advice on maintaining milk supply.

Infants & children:
Don't give to infants younger than 1 month.

Prolonged use:
- May enlarge thyroid gland.
- You may become more susceptible to infections caused by germs not responsive to this drug.
- Request frequent blood counts, liver- and kidney-function studies.

Skin & sunlight:
May cause rash or intensify sunburn in areas exposed to sun or sunlamp.

Driving, piloting or hazardous work:
Avoid if you feel dizzy. Otherwise, no problems expected.

Discontinuing:
Don't discontinue without doctor's advice until you complete prescribed dose, even though symptoms diminish or disappear.

Others:
- Drink 2 quarts of liquid each day to prevent adverse reactions.
- If you require surgery, tell anesthetist you take sulfa. Pentothal anesthesia should not be used.

 ## POSSIBLE INTERACTION WITH OTHER DRUGS

GENERIC NAME OR DRUG CLASS	COMBINED EFFECT
Aminobenzoates	Possible decreased sulfa effect.
Antibiotics*	Decreased sulfa effect.
Anticoagulants, oral*	Increased anticoagulant effect.
Anticonvulsants, hydantoin* and antidiabetic drugs*	Toxic effect on brain.
Aspirin	Increased sulfa effect.
Calcium supplements*	Decreased sulfa effect.

Clozapine	Toxic effect on the central nervous system.
Digoxin	Decreased digoxin effect.
Hepatotoxic agents*	Increased liver toxicity.
Iron supplements*	Decreased sulfa effect.
Isoniazid	Possible anemia.
Mecamylamine	Decreased antibiotic effect.
Methenamine	Possible kidney blockage.
Methotrexate	Increased methotrexate effect.
Oxyphenbutazone	Increased sulfa effect.
Para-aminosalicylic acid	Decreased sulfa effect.
Penicillins*	Decreased penicillin effect.
Phenylbutazone	Increased sulfa effect.
Probenecid	Increased sulfa effect.
Sulfinpyrazone	Increased sulfa effect.
Sulfonureas*	May increase hypo-glycemic action.
Trimethoprim	Increased sulfa effect.
Vitamin C	Possible kidney damage. Avoid large doses of vitamin C.
Zidovudine	Increased risk of toxic effects of zidovudine.

 ## POSSIBLE INTERACTION WITH OTHER SUBSTANCES

INTERACTS WITH	COMBINED EFFECT
Alcohol:	Increased alcohol effect.
Beverages: Less than 2 quarts of fluid daily.	Kidney damage.
Cocaine:	None expected.
Foods:	None expected.
Marijuana:	None expected.
Tobacco:	None expected.

SULFINPYRAZONE

BRAND NAMES

Antazone
Anturan
Anturane
Apo-Sulfinpyrazone
Novopyrazone

BASIC INFORMATION

Habit forming? No
Prescription needed? Yes
Available as generic? Yes
Drug class: Antigout

USES

- Treatment for chronic gout.
- Reduces severity of recurrent heart attack. (This use is experimental and not yet approved by F.D.A.)

DOSAGE & USAGE INFORMATION

How to take:
Tablet or capsule—Swallow with liquid or food to lessen stomach irritation. If you can't swallow whole, crumble tablet or open capsule and take with liquid or food.

When to take:
At the same times each day.

If you forget a dose:
Take as soon as you remember up to 2 hours late. If more than 2 hours, wait for next scheduled dose (don't double this dose).

Continued next column

OVERDOSE

SYMPTOMS:
Breathing difficulty, vomiting, imbalance, seizures, convulsions, coma.
WHAT TO DO:
- **Dial 0 (operator) or 911 (emergency) for an ambulance or medical help. Then give first aid immediately.**
- **If patient is unconscious and not breathing, give mouth-to-mouth breathing. If there is no heartbeat, use cardiac massage and mouth-to-mouth breathing (CPR). Don't try to make patient vomit. If you can't get help quickly, take patient to nearest emergency facility.**
- **See emergency information on inside covers.**

What drug does:
Reduces uric-acid level in blood and tissues by increasing amount of uric acid secreted in urine by kidneys.

Time lapse before drug works:
May require 6 months to prevent gout attacks.

Don't take with:
Any other medicine without consulting your doctor or pharmacist.

POSSIBLE ADVERSE REACTIONS OR SIDE EFFECTS

SYMPTOMS	WHAT TO DO
Life-threatening: In case of overdose, see previous column.	
Common: None expected.	
Infrequent:	
• Painful or difficult urination, worsening gout.	Discontinue. Call doctor right away.
• Rash, nausea, vomiting, abdominal pain, low back pain.	Continue. Call doctor when convenient.
Rare:	
• Black, bloody or tarry stools.	Discontinue. Seek emergency treatment.
• Sore throat; fever; unusual bleeding or bruising; red, painful joints; blood in urine; fatigue or weakness.	Discontinue. Call doctor right away.

WARNINGS & PRECAUTIONS

Don't take if:
- You are allergic to any uricosuric.
- You have acute gout.
- You have active ulcers (stomach or duodenal), enteritis or ulcerative colitis.
- You have blood-cell disorders.
- You are allergic to oxyphenbutazone or phenylbutazone.

Before you start, consult your doctor:
If you have kidney or blood disease.

Over age 60:
Adverse reactions and side effects may be more frequent and severe than in younger persons. You require lower dose because of decreased kidney function.

Pregnancy:
Studies inconclusive on harm to unborn child. Animal studies show fetal abnormalities. Decide with your doctor whether drug benefits justify risk to unborn child.

Breast-feeding:
No proven problems. Consult doctor.

Infants & children:
Not recommended.

Prolonged use:
- Possible kidney damage.
- Talk to your doctor about the need for follow-up medical examinations or laboratory studies to check complete blood counts (white blood cell count, platelet count, red blood cell count, hemoglobin, hematocrit), kidney function, serum uric acid and urine uric acid.

Skin & sunlight:
No problems expected.

Driving, piloting or hazardous work:
No problems expected.

Discontinuing:
Don't discontinue without consulting doctor. Dose may require gradual reduction if you have taken drug for a long time. Doses of other drugs may also require adjustment.

Others:
- Drink 10 to 12 glasses of water each day you take this medicine.
- Periodic blood and urine laboratory tests recommended.

POSSIBLE INTERACTION WITH OTHER DRUGS

GENERIC NAME OR DRUG CLASS	COMBINED EFFECT
Allopurinol	Increased effect of each drug.
Anticoagulants, oral*	Increased anti-coagulant effect.
Antidiabetics, oral*	Increased antidiabetic effect.
Aspirin	Bleeding tendency. Decreased sulfin-pyrazone effect.
Bismuth subsalicylate	Decreased effect of sulfinpyrazone.

Cephalexin	Increased effect of cephalexin.
Cephradine	Increased effect of cephradine.
Cholestyramine	Decreased sulfin-pyrazone effect.
Contraceptives, oral*	Increased bleeding between menstrual periods.
Diuretics*	Decreased sulfin-pyrazone effect.
Penicillins*	Increased penicillin effect.
Salicylates*	Bleeding tendency. Decreased sulfin-pyrazone effect.
Sulfa drugs*	Increased effect of sulfa drugs.
Thioguanine	May need increased dosage of sulfinpyrazone.

POSSIBLE INTERACTION WITH OTHER SUBSTANCES

INTERACTS WITH	COMBINED EFFECT
Alcohol:	Decreased sulfin-pyrazone effect.
Beverages: Caffeine drinks.	Decreased sulfin-pyrazone effect.
Cocaine:	None expected.
Foods:	None expected.
Marijuana:	Occasional use—None expected. Daily use—May increase blood level of uric acid.
Tobacco:	None expected.

*See Glossary

SULFISOXAZOLE

BRAND NAMES

See complete list of brand names in the *Brand Name Directory,* page 930.

BASIC INFORMATION

Habit forming? No
Prescription needed? Yes
Available as generic? Yes
Drug class: Sulfa (sulfonamide)

 ## USES

Treatment for urinary tract infections responsive to this drug.

 ## DOSAGE & USAGE INFORMATION

How to take:
- Tablet—Swallow with liquid. Instructions to take on empty stomach mean 1 hour before or 2 hours after eating.
- Liquid—Shake carefully before measuring.

When to take:
At the same times each day, evenly spaced.

If you forget a dose:
Take as soon as you remember up to 2 hours late. If more than 2 hours, wait for next scheduled dose (don't double this dose).

What drug does:
Interferes with a nutrient (folic acid) necessary for growth and reproduction of bacteria. Will not attack viruses.

Time lapse before drug works:
2 to 5 days to affect infection.

Don't take with:
Any other medicine without consulting your doctor or pharmacist.

 ## OVERDOSE

SYMPTOMS:
Less urine, bloody urine, coma.
WHAT TO DO:
- **Dial 0 (operator) or 911 (emergency) for an ambulance or medical help. Then give first aid immediately.**
- **See emergency information on inside covers.**

 ## POSSIBLE ADVERSE REACTIONS OR SIDE EFFECTS

SYMPTOMS	WHAT TO DO
Life-threatening:	
In case of overdose, see previous column.	
Common:	
● Itchy skin, rash.	Discontinue. Call doctor right away.
● Headache, nausea, vomiting, diarrhea, appetite loss, skin sensitive to sun.	Continue. Call doctor when convenient.
Infrequent:	
● Red, peeling or blistering skin; sore throat; fever; swallowing difficulty; unusual bruising; aching joints or muscles; jaundice.	Discontinue. Call doctor right away.
● Dizziness, tiredness, weakness.	Continue. Call doctor when convenient.
Rare:	
Painful urination; low back pain; numbness, tingling, burning feeling in feet and hands, bloody urine, neck swelling.	Discontinue. Call doctor right away.

 ## WARNINGS & PRECAUTIONS

Don't take if:
You are allergic to any sulfa drug.

Before you start, consult your doctor:
- If you are allergic to carbonic anhydrase inhibitors, oral antidiabetics or thiazide or loop diuretics.
- If you are allergic by nature.
- If you have liver or kidney disease.
- If you have porphyria.
- If you have developed anemia from use of any drug.

Over age 60:
Adverse reactions and side effects may be more frequent and severe than in younger persons.

Pregnancy:
Risk to unborn child outweighs drug benefits. Don't use.

Breast-feeding:
Drug passes into milk. Avoid drug or discontinue nursing until you finish medicine. Consult doctor for advice on maintaining milk supply.

Infants & children:
Don't give to infants younger than 1 month.

Prolonged use:
- May enlarge thyroid gland.
- You may become more susceptible to infections caused by germs not responsive to this drug.
- Request frequent blood counts, liver- and kidney-function studies.

Skin & sunlight:
May cause rash or intensify sunburn in areas exposed to sun or sunlamp.

Driving, piloting or hazardous work:
Avoid if you feel dizzy. Otherwise, no problems expected.

Discontinuing:
Don't discontinue without doctor's advice until you complete prescribed dose, even though symptoms diminish or disappear.

Others:
- Drink 2 quarts of liquid each day to prevent adverse reactions.
- If you require surgery, tell anesthetist you take sulfa.

 POSSIBLE INTERACTION WITH OTHER DRUGS

GENERIC NAME OR DRUG CLASS	COMBINED EFFECT
Aminobenzoates	Possible decreased sulfisoxazole effect.
Anticoagulants, oral*	Increased anticoagulant effect.
Anticonvulsants, hydantoin* and antidiabetic drugs*	Toxic effect on brain.
Aspirin	Increased sulfa effect.
Calcium supplements*	Decreased sulfa effect.
Clozapine	Toxic effect on the central nervous system.
Flecainide	Possible decreased blood-cell production in bone marrow.

Hepatotoxic agents*	Increased liver toxicity.
Isoniazid	Possible anemia.
Mecamylamine	Decreased antibiotic effect.
Methenamine	Possible kidney blockage.
Methotrexate	Increased possibility of toxic side effects from methotrexate.
Oxyphenbutazone	Increased sulfa effect.
Para-aminosalicylic acid	Decreased sulfa effect.
Penicillins*	Decreased penicillin effect.
Phenylbutazone	Increased sulfa effect.
Probenecid	Increased sulfa effect.
Sulfinpyrazone	Increased sulfa effect.
Sulfonureas*	May increase hypoglycemic action.
Tocainide	Possible decreased blood-cell production in bone marrow.
Trimethoprim	Increased sulfa effect.
Zidovudine	Increased risk of toxic effect of zidovudine.

 POSSIBLE INTERACTION WITH OTHER SUBSTANCES

INTERACTS WITH	COMBINED EFFECT
Alcohol:	Increased alcohol effect.
Beverages: Less than 2 quarts of fluid daily.	Kidney damage.
Cocaine:	None expected.
Foods:	None expected.
Marijuana:	None expected.
Tobacco:	None expected.

SULFONAMIDES & PHENAZOPYRIDINE

BRAND AND GENERIC NAMES

Azo Gantanol
Azo Gantrisin
Azo-Sulfamethoxazole
Azo-Sulfisoxazole
Sulfafurazole &
  Phenazopyridine

SULFAMETHOXA-
  ZOLE & PHENAZO-
  PYRIDINE
SULFISOXAZOLE &
  PHENAZO-
  PYRIDINE
Uro-Gantanol

BASIC INFORMATION

Habit forming? No
Prescription needed? Yes
Available as generic? Yes
Drug class: Analgesic (urinary), sulfonamide

USES

- Treatment for infections responsive to this drug.
- Relieves pain of lower urinary-tract irritation, as in cystitis, urethritis or prostatitis.

DOSAGE & USAGE INFORMATION

How to take:
Tablet—Swallow with liquid. Instructions to take on empty stomach mean 1 hour before or 2 hours after eating.

When to take:
At the same times each day, after meals.

If you forget a dose:
Take as soon as you remember up to 2 hours late. If more than 2 hours, wait for next scheduled dose (don't double this dose).

What drug does:
- Interferes with a nutrient (folic acid) necessary for growth and reproduction of bacteria. Will not attack viruses.
- Anesthetizes lower urinary tract. Relieves pain, burning, pressure and urgency to urinate.

Continued next column

OVERDOSE

SYMPTOMS:
Less urine, bloody urine, shortness of breath, weakness, coma.
WHAT TO DO:
- **Dial 0 (operator) or 911 (emergency) for an ambulance or medical help. Then give first aid immediately.**
- **See emergency information on inside covers.**

Time lapse before drug works:
2 to 5 days to affect infection.

Don't take with:
Any other medicine without consulting your doctor or pharmacist.

POSSIBLE ADVERSE REACTIONS OR SIDE EFFECTS

SYMPTOMS	WHAT TO DO
Life-threatening:	
In case of overdose, see previous column.	
Common:	
• Rash, itchy skin.	Discontinue. Call doctor right away.
• Dizziness, diarrhea, headache, appetite loss, nausea, vomiting, skin sensitive to sun.	Continue. Call doctor when convenient.
Infrequent:	
• Joint pain; swallowing difficulty; pale skin; blistering; peeling of skin; sore throat, fever, mouth sores; unexplained bleeding or bruising; jaundice.	Discontinue. Call doctor right away.
• Abdominal pain, indigestion, weakness, tiredness.	Continue. Call doctor when convenient.
Rare:	
Back pain; neck swelling; numbness, tingling, burning feeling in feet and hands; bloody urine; painful urination.	Discontinue. Call doctor right away.

WARNINGS & PRECAUTIONS

Don't take if:
- You are allergic to any sulfa drug or urinary analgesic.
- You have hepatitis.

Before you start, consult your doctor:
- If you are allergic to carbonic anhydrase inhibitors, oral antidiabetics or thiazide or loop diuretics.
- If you are allergic by nature.
- If you have liver or kidney disease, porphyria.
- If you have developed anemia from use of any drug.
- If you have G6PD deficiency.

SULFONAMIDES & PHENAZOPYRIDINE

Over age 60:
Adverse reactions and side effects may be more frequent and severe than in younger persons.

Pregnancy:
Risk to unborn child outweighs drug benefits. Don't use.

Breast-feeding:
Drug passes into milk. Avoid drug or discontinue nursing until you finish medicine. Consult doctor for advice on maintaining milk supply.

Infants & children:
Don't give to infants younger than 1 month.

Prolonged use:
- May enlarge thyroid gland.
- You may become more susceptible to infections caused by germs not responsive to this drug.
- Request frequent blood counts, liver- and kidney-function studies.
- Orange or yellow skin.
- Anemia. Occasional blood studies recommended.

Skin & sunlight:
May cause rash or intensify sunburn in areas exposed to sun or sunlamp.

Driving, piloting or hazardous work:
Avoid if you feel dizzy. Otherwise, no problems expected.

Discontinuing:
Don't discontinue without doctor's advice until you complete prescribed dose, even though symptoms diminish or disappear.

Others:
- Drink 2 quarts of liquid each day to prevent adverse reactions.
- If you require surgery, tell anesthetist you take sulfa.
- Will probably cause urine to be reddish orange. Requires no action.
- May stain fabrics.

POSSIBLE INTERACTION WITH OTHER DRUGS

GENERIC NAME OR DRUG CLASS	COMBINED EFFECT
Aminobenzoates	Possible decreased sulfa effect.
Anticoagulants, oral*	Increased anticoagulant effect.
Anticonvulsants, hydantoin* and antidiabetic drugs	Toxic effect on brain.
Aspirin	Increased sulfa effect.
Clozapine	Toxic effect on the central nervous system.
Didanosine	Increased risk of pancreatitis.
Hepatotoxic agents*	Increased liver toxicity.
Isoniazid	Possible anemia.
Mecamylamine	Decreased antibiotic effect.
Methenamine	Possible kidney blockage.
Methotrexate	Increased methotrexate effect.
Oxyphenbutazone	Increased sulfa effect.
Para-aminosalicylic acid	Decreased sulfa effect.
Penicillins*	Decreased penicillin effect.
Phenylbutazone	Increased sulfa effect.
Probenecid	Increased sulfa effect.
Sulfinpyrazone	Increased sulfa effect.
Sulfonureas*	May increase hypoglycemic action.
Trimethoprim	Increased sulfa effect.
Zidovudine	Increased risk of toxic effects of zidovudine.

POSSIBLE INTERACTION WITH OTHER SUBSTANCES

INTERACTS WITH	COMBINED EFFECT
Alcohol:	Increased alcohol effect.
Beverages: Less than 2 quarts of fluid daily.	Kidney damage.
Cocaine:	None expected.
Foods:	None expected.
Marijuana:	None expected.
Tobacco:	None expected.

TAMOXIFEN

BRAND NAMES

Nolvadex   Tamofen
Nolvadex-D   Tamone
Novo-Tamoxifen

BASIC INFORMATION

Habit forming? No
Prescription needed? Yes
Available as generic? No
Drug class: Antineoplastic

 USES

Treats advanced breast cancer.

 DOSAGE & USAGE INFORMATION

How to take:
* Tablets—Swallow with liquid. If you can't swallow whole, crumble tablet and take with liquid or food. Instructions to take on empty stomach mean 1 hour before or 2 hours after eating.
* Enteric-coated tablets—Swallow whole.

When to take:
Follow doctor's instructions.

If you forget a dose:
Skip the missed dose and return to regular schedule. Don't double dose.

What drug does:
Blocks uptake of estradiol and inhibits growth of cancer cells.

Time lapse before drug works:
* 4 to 10 weeks.
* With bone metastases—several months.

Don't take with:
Any other medicines (including over-the-counter drugs such as cough and cold medicines, laxatives, antacids, diet pills, caffeine, nose drops or vitamins) without consulting your doctor.

 OVERDOSE

SYMPTOMS:
None expected.
WHAT TO DO:
Overdose unlikely to threaten life. If person takes much larger amount than prescribed, call doctor, poison-control center or hospital emergency room for instructions.

 POSSIBLE ADVERSE REACTIONS OR SIDE EFFECTS

SYMPTOMS	WHAT TO DO
Life-threatening: Leg pain, shortness of breath.	Seek emergency treatment immediately.
Common: Hot flashes, nausea and vomiting, weight gain.	Continue. Call doctor when convenient.
Infrequent: Headache, dry skin, menstrual irregularities, vaginal itching.	Continue. Call doctor when convenient.
Rare: Blurred vision, confusion, sleepiness.	Discontinue. Call doctor right away.

WARNINGS & PRECAUTIONS

Don't take if:
You are allergic to tamoxifen.

Before you start, consult your doctor:
- If you have cataracts.
- If you have blood disorders.

Over age 60:
Adverse reactions and side effects may be more frequent and severe than in younger persons. You may need smaller doses for shorter periods of time.

Pregnancy:
Risk to unborn child outweighs drug benefits. Don't use.

Breast-feeding:
Effect not documented. Consult your doctor.

Infants & children:
Not intended for use in children.

Prolonged use:
Talk to your doctor about the need for follow-up medical examinations or laboratory studies to check complete blood counts (white blood cell count, platelet count, red blood cell count, hemoglobin, hematocrit) and serum calcium.

Skin & sunlight:
No problems expected.

Driving, piloting or hazardous work:
Avoid if you feel confused, drowsy or dizzy.

Discontinuing:
No special problems expected.

Others:
- Advise any doctor or dentist whom you consult that you take this medicine.
- May affect results in some medical tests.

POSSIBLE INTERACTION WITH OTHER DRUGS

GENERIC NAME OR DRUG CLASS	COMBINED EFFECT
Antacids*	Decreased tamoxifen effect.
Estrogens*	Decreased tamoxifen effect.
Famotidine	Decreased tamoxifen effect.
H$_2$ antagonist antihistamines*	Decreased tamoxifen effect.
Ranitidine	Decreased tamoxifen effect.

POSSIBLE INTERACTION WITH OTHER SUBSTANCES

INTERACTS WITH	COMBINED EFFECT
Alcohol:	No special problems expected.
Beverages:	No special problems expected.
Cocaine:	No special problems expected.
Foods:	No special problems expected.
Marijuana:	No special problems expected.
Tobacco:	No special problems expected.

*See Glossary

TERAZOSIN

BRAND NAMES

Hytrin

BASIC INFORMATION

Habit forming? No
Prescription needed? Yes
Available as generic? No
Drug class: Antihypertensive

USES

Treats high blood pressure.

DOSAGE & USAGE INFORMATION

How to take:
Tablet—Swallow with liquid or food to lessen stomach irritation. If you can't swallow whole, crumble tablet and take with liquid or food.

When to take:
Once a day (usually) at bedtime.

If you forget a dose:
Take as soon as you remember. Don't ever double the dose.

What drug does:
Relaxes smooth muscle in arteries, reducing blood pressure. Terazosin doesn't cure hypertension, but controls it. Persons with hypertension may need lifelong treatment.

Time lapse before drug works:
15 minutes.

Continued next column

OVERDOSE

SYMPTOMS:
Difficult breathing, vomiting, fainting, slow heartbeat, coma, diminished reflexes.
WHAT TO DO:
- **Dial 0 (operator) or 911 (emergency) for an ambulance or medical help. Then give first aid immediately.**
- **If patient is unconscious and not breathing, give mouth-to-mouth breathing. If there is no heartbeat, use cardiac massage and mouth-to-mouth breathing (CPR). Don't try to make patient vomit. If you can't get help quickly, take patient to nearest emergency facility.**
- **See emergency information on inside covers.**

Don't take with:
Any other drug (especially over-the-counter medicines containing alcohol) without consulting your doctor.

POSSIBLE ADVERSE REACTIONS OR SIDE EFFECTS

SYMPTOMS	WHAT TO DO
Life-threatening: In case of overdose, see previous column.	
Common: Headache, dizziness, tiredness or weakness.	Continue. Call doctor right away.
Infrequent: • Chest pain; lightheadedness on arising from bed or chair (more likely to occur with first dose); increased or rapid heartbeat, fainting, nausea and vomiting.	Discontinue. Call doctor right away.
• Fluid retention and weight gain.	Continue. Call doctor when convenient.
Rare: Back pain, joint pain, blurred vision, stuffy nose, drowsiness.	Continue. Call doctor when convenient.

WARNINGS & PRECAUTIONS

Don't take if:
- You are allergic to any alpha-adrenergic blocker.
- You are under age 12.

Before you start, consult your doctor:
- If you will have surgery within 2 months, including dental surgery, requiring general or spinal anesthesia.
- If you have heart disease or chronic kidney disease.
- If you have a peripheral circulation disorder (intermittent claudication, Buerger's disease).
- If you have history of depression.

Over age 60:
More sensitivity to drug causing weakness, fainting episodes, low temperature.

Pregnancy:
Studies inconclusive on harm to unborn child.
Decide with your doctor whether drug benefits
justify risk to unborn child.

Breast-feeding:
No proven problems.

Infants & children:
Not recommended for children. Adequate
studies not complete.

Prolonged use:
Talk to your doctor about the need for follow-up
medical examinations or laboratory studies.

Skin & sunlight:
No problems expected.

Driving, piloting or hazardous work:
Don't drive or pilot aircraft until you learn how
medicine affects you. Don't work around
dangerous machinery. Don't climb ladders or
work in high places. Danger increases if you
drink alcohol or take medicine affecting
alertness and reflexes, such as antihistamines,
tranquilizers, sedatives, pain medicine, narcotics
and mind-altering drugs.

Discontinuing:
- Don't discontinue without consulting doctor.
  Dose may require gradual reduction if you
  have taken drug for a long time. Doses of
  other drugs may also require adjustment.
- Stopping abruptly may cause rebound high
  blood pressure, anxiety, chest pain, insomnia,
  headache, nausea, irregular heartbeat,
  flushed face, sweating.

Others:
- Avoid becoming overheated.
- Check blood pressure frequently.

POSSIBLE INTERACTION WITH OTHER DRUGS

GENERIC NAME OR DRUG CLASS	COMBINED EFFECT
Diclofenac	Decreases effectiveness of terazosin. Causes sodium and fluid retention.
Diuretics, loop*	Decreased effectiveness of terazosin.
Estrogens*	Decreases effectiveness of terazosin.

Lisinopril	Increased antihypertensive effect. Dosage of each may require adjustment.
Nicardipine	Blood pressure drop. Dosages may require adjustment.
Nimodipine	Dangerous blood pressure drop.
Non-steroidal anti-inflammatory drugs (NSAIDs)*	Decreases effectiveness of terazosin. Causes sodium and fluid retention.
Other medicines to treat high blood pressure (antihypertensives*)	Decreases effectiveness of terazosin.
Sympathomimetics*	Decreases effectiveness of terazosin.

POSSIBLE INTERACTION WITH OTHER SUBSTANCES

INTERACTS WITH	COMBINED EFFECT
Alcohol:	Increased sensitivity to sedative effect of alcohol and very low blood pressure. Avoid.
Beverages: Caffeine drinks.	Decreased terazosin effect.
Cocaine:	Blood pressure rise. Avoid.
Foods:	No problems expected.
Marijuana:	Weakness on standing.
Tobacco:	No problems expected.

TERFENADINE

BRAND NAMES

Seldane   Seldane D

BASIC INFORMATION

Habit forming? No
Prescription needed? Yes
Available as generic? No
Drug class: Antihistamine, H₁ receptor antagonist

USES

Reduces allergic symptoms such as hay fever, hives, rash or itching. Less likely to cause drowsiness than most other antihistamines.

DOSAGE & USAGE INFORMATION

How to take:
Tablet—Swallow with water or food to lessen stomach irritation.

When to take:
Follow prescription instructions.

If you forget a dose:
Take as soon as you remember up to 2 hours late. If more than 2 hours, wait for next scheduled dose (don't double this dose).

What drug does:
Blocks effects of histamine, a chemical produced by the body as a result of contact with an allergen.

Time lapse before drug works:
1 to 2 hours; maximum effect at 3 to 4 hours.

Don't take with:
Any other medicine without consulting your doctor or pharmacist.

OVERDOSE

SYMPTOMS:
Headache, nausea, confusion, heartbeat rhythm disturbance.
WHAT TO DO:
- **Dial 0 (operator) or 911 (emergency) for an ambulance or medical help. Then give first aid immediately.**
- **See emergency information on inside covers.**

POSSIBLE ADVERSE REACTIONS OR SIDE EFFECTS

SYMPTOMS	WHAT TO DO
Life-threatening:	
In case of overdose, see previous column.	
Common:	
None expected.	
Infrequent:	
• Nausea, vomiting sore throat, itching.	Discontinue. Call doctor right away.
• Fatigue, headache, dizziness, weakness.	Continue. Call doctor when convenient.
Rare:	
• Swollen lips. difficult breathing	Discontinue. Seek emergency treatment.
• Irregular heartbeat, nightmares, frequent urination, wheezing.	Discontinue. Call doctor right away.
• Thinning hair.	Continue. Call doctor when convenient.

WARNINGS & PRECAUTIONS

Don't take if:
You are allergic to terfenadine.

Before you start, consult your doctor:
- If you have liver disease.
- If you are allergic to other antihistamines.
- If you have an enlarged prostrate or glaucoma.
- If you are under age 12.
- If you are allergic to any substance or any medicine.
- If you are pregnant or expect to become pregnant.
- If you have asthma.
- If you will have surgery within 2 months, including dental surgery, requiring general or spinal anesthesia.
- If you plan to have skin tests for allergies.

Over age 60:
Don't exceed recommended dose. Take only on advise of your doctor.

Pregnancy:
No proven harm to unborn child. Avoid if possible.

Breast-feeding:
Drug may pass into milk although this has not been proven. Consult doctor for advice on using while breast feeding.

Infants & children:
Safety and effectiveness in children under age 12 have not been established.

Prolonged use:
Take only on advice of your doctor.

Skin & sunlight:
No problems expected.

Driving, piloting or hazardous work:
Don't drive or pilot aircraft until you learn how medicine affects you. Sedation and dizziness are less likely to occur with terfenadine than with other antihistamines.

Discontinuing:
No problems expected.

Others:
No problems expected.

POSSIBLE INTERACTION WITH OTHER DRUGS

GENERIC NAME OR DRUG CLASS	COMBINED EFFECT
Carteolol	Decreased antihistamine effect.
Ketoconazole	Life-threatening heartbeat irregularity. Avoid.
Nabilone	Greater depression of central nervous system.
Sotalol	Increased antihistamine effect.

POSSIBLE INTERACTION WITH OTHER SUBSTANCES

INTERACTS WITH	COMBINED EFFECT
Alcohol:	Possible oversedation.
Beverages:	None expected.
Cocaine:	Decreased terfenadine effect.
Foods:	None expected.
Marijuana:	None expected.
Tobacco:	None expected.

TERPIN HYDRATE

BRAND AND GENERIC NAMES

Chexit
CODEINE AND
   TERPIN HYDRATE
DEXTROMETHOR-
   PHAN HYDROBRO-
   MIDE AND TERPIN
   HYDRATE
Prunicodeine
Terphan
Terpin-Dex

Terpin Hydrate and
   Codeine Syrup
Terpin Hydrate
   Elixir
Tricodene #1
Tricodene NN
   Cough and Cold
   Medication
Tussagesic

BASIC INFORMATION

Habit forming? Yes
Prescription needed? No
Available as generic? Yes
Drug class: Expectorant

USES

Decreases cough due to simple bronchial irritation.

DOSAGE & USAGE INFORMATION

How to take:
Follow each dose with 8 oz. water or food to decrease gastric distress. Works better in combination with a cool-air vaporizer.

When to take:
3 to 4 times each day, spaced at least 4 hours apart.

If you forget a dose:
Take as soon as you remember. Wait 4 hours for next dose.

What drug does:
Loosens mucus in bronchial tubes to make mucus easier to cough up.

Time lapse before drug works:
10 to 15 minutes.

Don't take with:
Any other medicine without consulting your doctor or pharmacist.

OVERDOSE

SYMPTOMS:
Nausea, drowsiness.
WHAT TO DO:
Overdose unlikely to threaten life. If person takes much larger amount than prescribed, call doctor, poison-control center or hospital emergency room for instructions.

POSSIBLE ADVERSE REACTIONS OR SIDE EFFECTS

SYMPTOMS	WHAT TO DO
Life-threatening: None expected.	
Common: None expected.	
Infrequent: Nausea, vomiting, abdominal pain.	Continue. Call doctor when convenient.
Rare: Symptoms of alcohol intoxication, especially in children.	Discontinue. Call doctor right away.

WARNINGS & PRECAUTIONS

Don't take if:
- You are allergic to terpin hydrate.
- You are a recovering or active alcoholic.

Before you start, consult your doctor:
If you plan to become pregnant within medication period.

Over age 60:
No problems expected.

Pregnancy:
Risk to unborn child outweighs drug benefits. Don't use.

Breast-feeding:
Drug filters into milk. May harm child. Avoid.

Infants & children:
Use only under medical supervision.

Prolonged use:
Habit forming.

Skin & sunlight:
No problems expected.

Driving, piloting or hazardous work:
Don't drive or pilot aircraft until you learn how medicine affects you. Don't work around dangerous machinery. Don't climb ladders or work in high places. Danger increases if you drink alcohol or take medicine affecting alertness and reflexes, such as antihistamines, tranquilizers, sedatives, pain medicine, narcotics and mind-altering drugs.

Discontinuing:
May be unnecessary to finish medicine. Follow doctor's instructions.

Others:
- Exceeding recommended doses may cause intoxication; drug is 42.5% alcohol.
- Frequently combined with codeine, which increases hazards.

POSSIBLE INTERACTION WITH OTHER DRUGS

GENERIC NAME OR DRUG CLASS	COMBINED EFFECT
Antidepressants*	Increased sedation.
Antihistamines*	Increased sedation
Central nervous system (CNS) depressants*	Increased sedative effect of both.
Disulfiram	Possible disulfiram reaction*.
Muscle relaxants*	Increased sedation.
Narcotics*	Increased sedation.
Sedatives*	Increased sedation.
Sleep inducers*	Increased sedation.
Tranquilizers*	Increased sedation.

POSSIBLE INTERACTION WITH OTHER SUBSTANCES

INTERACTS WITH	COMBINED EFFECT
Alcohol:	Contains alcohol. Increased sedative effect of both drugs. Avoid.
Beverages:	None expected.
Cocaine:	Unpredictable effect on nervous system. Avoid.
Foods:	None expected.
Marijuana:	Unpredictable effect on nervous system. Avoid.
Tobacco:	None expected.

*See Glossary

TESTOLACTONE

BRAND NAMES

Teslac

BASIC INFORMATION

Habit forming? No
Prescription needed? Yes
Available as generic? No
Drug class: Antineoplastic

 USES

Treats advanced breast cancer.

 DOSAGE & USAGE INFORMATION

How to take:
Tablets—Swallow with liquid. If you can't swallow whole, crumble tablet and take with liquid or food. Instructions to take on empty stomach mean 1 hour before or 2 hours after eating.

When to take:
Follow doctor's instructions.

If you forget a dose:
Take as soon as you remember up to 2 hours late. If more than 2 hours, wait for next scheduled dose (don't double this dose).

What drug does:
Inhibits growth of cancer cells.

Time lapse before drug works:
6 to 12 weeks.

Don't take with:
Any other medicines (including over-the-counter drugs such as cough and cold medicines, laxatives, antacids, diet pills, caffeine, nose drops or vitamins) without consulting your doctor.

 OVERDOSE

SYMPTOMS:
None expected.
WHAT TO DO:
Overdose unlikely to threaten life. If person takes much larger amount than prescribed, call doctor, poison-control center or hospital emergency room for instructions.

 POSSIBLE ADVERSE REACTIONS OR SIDE EFFECTS

SYMPTOMS	WHAT TO DO
Life-threatening: None expected.	
Common: Appetite loss.	Continue. Call doctor when convenient.
Infrequent: Diarrhea; swollen feet and legs; numb and tingling fingers, toes, face.	Continue. Call doctor when convenient.
Rare: Red tongue.	Continue. Call doctor when convenient.

TESTOLACTONE

WARNINGS & PRECAUTIONS

Don't take if:
You are allergic to testosterone.

Before you start, consult your doctor:
- If you have heart disease.
- If you have kidney disease.

Over age 60:
Adverse reactions and side effects may be more frequent and severe than in younger persons. You may need smaller doses for shorter periods of time.

Pregnancy:
Risk to unborn child outweighs drug benefits. Don't use.

Breast-feeding:
Effect not documented. Consult your doctor.

Infants & children:
Not recommended.

Prolonged use:
Talk to your doctor about the need for follow-up medical examinations or laboratory studies to check serum calcium levels.

Skin & sunlight:
No problems expected.

Driving, piloting or hazardous work:
No problems expected.

Discontinuing:
No special problems expected.

Others:
- Advise any doctor or dentist whom you consult that you take this medicine.
- May affect results in some medical tests.

POSSIBLE INTERACTION WITH OTHER DRUGS

GENERIC NAME OR DRUG CLASS	COMBINED EFFECT
Anticoagulants*	Increased anticoagulant effect.

POSSIBLE INTERACTION WITH OTHER SUBSTANCES

INTERACTS WITH	COMBINED EFFECT
Alcohol:	No special problems expected.
Beverages:	No special problems expected.
Cocaine:	No special problems expected.
Foods:	No special problems expected.
Marijuana:	No special problems expected.
Tobacco:	No special problems expected.

TESTOSTERONE & ESTRADIOL

BRAND AND GENERIC NAMES

See complete list of brand and generic names in the *Brand Name Directory*, page 930.

BASIC INFORMATION

Habit forming? No
Prescription needed? Yes
Available as generic? Yes
Drug class: Androgens-estrogens

USES

- Prevents breast fullness in new mothers after childbirth.
- Relieves menopause symptoms such as unnecessary sweating, hot flashes, chills, faintness and dizziness.

DOSAGE & USAGE INFORMATION

How to take:
Given by injection, deeply intramuscular.

When to take:
When directed.

If you forget a dose:
Check with your doctor.

What drug does:
- Restores normal estrogen level in tissues.
- Stimulates cells that produce male sex characteristics.
- Replaces hormone deficiencies.
- Stimulates red-blood-cell production.
- Suppresses production of estrogen.

Time lapse before drug works:
10 to 20 days.

Don't take with:
Any other medicine without consulting your doctor or pharmacist.

OVERDOSE

SYMPTOMS:
Headache (severe), coordination loss, vision changes, chest pain, shortness of breath (sudden), speech slurring.
WHAT TO DO:
Overdose unlikely to threaten life. If person takes much larger amount than prescribed, call doctor, poison-control center or hospital emergency room for instructions.

POSSIBLE ADVERSE REACTIONS OR SIDE EFFECTS

SYMPTOMS	WHAT TO DO
Life-threatening:	
• In case of overdose, see previous column.	
• Hives, black stool, black or bloody vomit, intense itching, weakness, loss of consciousness.	Discontinue. Seek emergency treatment.
Common:	
• Red or flushed face; rash; swollen, tender breasts.	Discontinue. Call doctor right away.
• Depression, irritability, dizziness, confusion, acne or oily skin (females), enlarged clitoris, deepened voice, appetite loss, increased sex drive, unnatural hair growth, headache, constipation.	Continue. Call doctor when convenient.
Infrequent:	
• Nausea, vomiting, diarrhea, unusual vaginal bleeding or discharge, uncontrolled muscle movements.	Discontinue. Call doctor right away.
• Swollen feet and ankles, migraine headache.	Continue. Call doctor when convenient.
Rare:	
• Jaundice, abdominal pain.	Discontinue. Call doctor right away.
• Brown blotches on skin; hair loss; sore throat, fever, mouth sores.	Continue. Call doctor when convenient.

WARNINGS & PRECAUTIONS

Don't take if:
- You are allergic to any male hormone or any estrogen-containing drugs.
- You have impaired liver function.
- You have had blood clots, stroke or heart attack.
- You have unexplained vaginal bleeding.

Before you start, consult your doctor:
- If you might be pregnant or plan to become pregnant within 3 months.
- If you have heart disease, arteriosclerosis, diabetes, liver disease, high blood pressure, asthma, congestive heart failure, kidney disease or gallstones.
- If you have high level of blood calcium.

- If you have had migraine headaches, epilepsy or porphyria.
- If you have had cancer of breast or reproductive organs, fibrocystic breast disease, fibroid tumors of the uterus or endometriosis.

Over age 60:
- May stimulate sexual activity.
- Can make high blood pressure or heart disease worse.
- Controversial. You and your doctor must decide if drug risks outweigh benefits.

Pregnancy:
Risk to unborn child outweighs drug benefits. Don't use.

Breast-feeding:
Drug passes into milk. Avoid drug or discontinue nursing until you finish medicine. Consult doctor for advice on maintaining milk supply.

Infants & children:
Not recommended.

Prolonged use:
- Increased growth of fibroid tumors of uterus.
- Possible kidney stones.
- Unnatural hair growth and deep voice in women.
- Talk to your doctor about the need for follow-up medical examinations or laboratory studies to check pap smear, liver function, mammogram, complete blood counts (white blood cell count, platelet count, red blood cell count, hemoglobin, hematocrit).
- Possible breast lumps, jaundice, sore throat, fever. If any of these occur, call your doctor.

Skin & sunlight:
May cause rash or intensify sunburn in areas exposed to sun or sunlamp.

Driving, piloting or hazardous work:
No problems expected.

Discontinuing:
You may need to discontinue estrogens periodically. Consult your doctor.

Others:
- In rare instances, may cause blood clot in lung, brain or leg. Symptoms are *sudden* severe headache, coordination loss, vision change, chest pain, breathing difficulty, slurred speech, pain in legs or groin. Seek emergency treatment immediately.
- Will not increase strength in athletes.
- Carefully read the paper delivered with your prescription called "Information for the Patient."
- Don't smoke.

POSSIBLE INTERACTION WITH OTHER DRUGS

GENERIC NAME OR DRUG CLASS	COMBINED EFFECT
Anticoagulants, oral*	Increased effect of of anticoagulant.
Anticonvulsants, hydantoin*	Increased seizures.
Antidiabetics, oral*	Unpredictable increase or decrease in blood sugar.
Antifibrinolytic agents*	Increased possibility of blood clotting.
Carbamazepine	Increased seizures.
Chlorzoxazone	Decreased androgen effect.
Cholestyramine	Decreased cholestyramine effect.
Clofibrate	Decreased clofibrate effect.
Colestipol	Decreased colestipol effect.
Insulin	Unpredictable increase or decrease in blood sugar.
Nicotinic acid	Decreased nicotinic acid.

Continued on page 962

POSSIBLE INTERACTION WITH OTHER SUBSTANCES

INTERACTS WITH	COMBINED EFFECT
Alcohol:	None expected.
Beverages:	None expected.
Cocaine:	No proven problems.
Foods: Salt.	Excessive fluid retention (edema). Decrease salt intake while taking male hormones.
Marijuana:	Decreased blood levels of androgens. Possible menstrual irregularities and bleeding between periods.
Tobacco:	Increased risk of blood clots leading to stroke or heart attack.

---

*See Glossary

TETRACYCLINES

BRAND AND GENERIC NAMES

See complete list of brand and generic names in the *Brand Name Directory*, page 930.

BASIC INFORMATION

Habit forming? No
Prescription needed? Yes
Available as generic? Yes
Drug class: Antibiotic (tetracycline)

 ## USES

- Treatment for infections susceptible to any tetracycline. Will not cure virus infections such as colds or flu.
- Treatment for acne.

 ## DOSAGE & USAGE INFORMATION

How to take:
- Tablet or capsule—Take on empty stomach 1 hour before or 2 hours after eating. If you can't swallow whole, crumble tablet or open capsule and take with liquid or food.
- Liquid—Shake well. Take with measuring spoon.

When to take:
At the same times each day, evenly spaced.

If you forget a dose:
Take as soon as you remember up to 2 hours late. If more than 2 hours, wait for next scheduled dose (don't double this dose).

What drug does:
Prevents germ growth and reproduction.

Time lapse before drug works:
- Infections—May require 5 days to affect infection.
- Acne—May require 4 weeks to affect acne.

Don't take with:
Any other medicine without consulting your doctor or pharmacist.

 ## OVERDOSE

SYMPTOMS:
Severe nausea, vomiting, diarrhea.
WHAT TO DO:
Overdose unlikely to threaten life. If person takes much larger amount than prescribed, call doctor, poison-control center or hospital emergency room for instructions.

 ## POSSIBLE ADVERSE REACTIONS OR SIDE EFFECTS

SYMPTOMS	WHAT TO DO
Life-threatening:	
Hives, rash, intense itching faintness soon after a dose (anaphylaxis).	Seek emergency treatment immediately.
Common:	
• Sore mouth or tongue, nausea, vomiting, diarrhea.	Discontinue. Seek emergency treatment.
• Itching around rectum and genitals.	Discontinue. Call doctor right away.
• Vaginal discharge due to yeast, abdominal discomfort.	Continue. Call doctor when convenient.
• Dark tongue.	Continue. Tell doctor at next visit.
Infrequent:	
• Headache, rash.	Discontinue. Call doctor right away.
• Excessive thirst, increased urination, dizziness (minocycline).	Continue. Call doctor when convenient.
Rare:	
Blurred vision, jaundice.	Discontinue. Call doctor right away.

 ## WARNINGS & PRECAUTIONS

Don't take if:
You are allergic to any tetracycline antibiotic.

Before you start, consult your doctor:
- If you have kidney or liver disease.
- If you have lupus.
- If you have myasthenia gravis.

Over age 60:
Dosage usually less than in younger adults. More likely to cause itching around rectum. Ask your doctor how to prevent it.

Pregnancy:
Risk to unborn child outweighs drug benefits. Don't use.

Breast-feeding:
Drug passes into milk. Avoid drug or discontinue nursing until you finish medicine. Consult doctor for advice on maintaining milk supply.

Infants & children:
May cause permanent teeth malformation or discoloration in children less than 8 years old. Don't use.

Prolonged use:
- You may become more susceptible to infections caused by germs not responsive to tetracycline.
- May cause rare problems in liver, kidney or bone marrow. Periodic laboratory blood studies, liver- and kidney-function tests recommended if you use drug a long time.

Skin & sunlight:
May cause rash or intensify sunburn in areas exposed to sun or sunlamp.

Driving, piloting or hazardous work:
No problems expected.

Discontinuing:
Don't discontinue without doctor's advice until you complete prescribed dose, even though symptoms diminish or disappear.

Others:
Avoid using outdated drug.

 POSSIBLE INTERACTION WITH OTHER DRUGS

GENERIC NAME OR DRUG CLASS	COMBINED EFFECT
Antacids*	Decreased tetracycline effect.
Anticoagulants, oral*	Increased anticoagulant effect.
Bismuth subsalicylate	Decreased absorption of tetracycline.
Calcium supplements*	Decreased tetracycline effect.
Cefixime	Decreased antibiotic effect of cefixime.
Cholestyramine or colestipol	Decreased tetracycline effect.
Contraceptives, oral*	Decreased contraceptive effect.
Desmopressin	Possible decreased desmopressin effect.
Digitalis preparations*	Increased digitalis effect.
Etretinate	Increased chance of adverse reactions of etretinate.
Lithium	Increased lithium effect.

Mineral supplements* (iron, calcium, magnesium, zinc)	Decreased tetracycline absorption. Separate doses by 1 to 2 hours.
Penicillins*	Decreased penicillin effect.
Sodium bicarbonate	Greatly reduced absorption of tetracycline.
Tiopronin	Increased risk of toxicity to kidneys (except doxycycline and minocycline).
Zinc supplements	Decreased absorption of tetracycline if taken within 2 hours of each other.

 POSSIBLE INTERACTION WITH OTHER SUBSTANCES

INTERACTS WITH	COMBINED EFFECT
Alcohol:	Possible liver damage. Avoid.
Beverages: Milk.	Decreased tetracycline absorption. Take dose 2 hours after or 1 hour before drinking.
Cocaine:	No proven problems.
Foods: Dairy products.	Decreased tetracycline absorption. Take dose 2 hours after or 1 hour before eating.
Marijuana:	No interactions expected, but marijuana may slow body's recovery. Avoid.
Tobacco:	None expected.

*See Glossary

THEOPHYLLINE, EPHEDRINE & BARBITURATES

BRAND NAMES

Azma Aid
Phedral-C.T.
Primatene "P"
  Formula
Tedral
Tedral SA

Tedrigen
T.E.P.
Theodrine
Theodrine Pediatric
Theofed
Theofedral

BASIC INFORMATION

Habit forming? Yes
Prescription needed? Some yes, others no
Available as generic? Some yes, others no
Drug class: Bronchodilator, barbiturate, sympathomimetic, sedative

USES

- Treatment for bronchial asthma symptoms.
- Decreases congestion of breathing passages.
- Suppresses allergic reactions.
- Reduces anxiety or nervous tension (low dose).

DOSAGE & USAGE INFORMATION

How to take:
- Tablet or elixir—Swallow with liquid.
- Extended-release tablets—Swallow each dose whole. If you take regular tablets, you may chew or crush them.

When to take:
Most effective taken on empty stomach 1 hour before or 2 hours after eating. However, may take with food to lessen stomach upset.

Continued next column

OVERDOSE

SYMPTOMS:
Restlessness, irritability, anxiety, confusion, hallucinations, vomiting blood, delirium, muscle tremors, convulsions, rapid and irregular pulse, coma.
WHAT TO DO:
- **Dial 0 (operator) or 911 (emergency) for an ambulance or medical help. Then give first aid immediately.**
- **See emergency information on inside covers.**

If you forget a dose:
Take as soon as you remember up to 2 hours late. If more than 2 hours, wait for next scheduled dose (don't double this dose).

What drug does:
- Relaxes and expands bronchial tubes.
- Prevents cells from releasing allergy-causing chemicals (histamines).
- Decreases blood-vessel size and blood flow, thus causing decongestion.
- May partially block nerve impulses at nerve-cell connections.

Time lapse before drug works:
15 to 30 minutes.

Don't take with:
- Non-prescription drugs with ephedrine, pseudoephedrine or epinephrine.
- Non-prescription drugs for cough, cold, allergy or asthma without consulting doctor.
- Any other medicine without consulting your doctor or pharmacist.

POSSIBLE ADVERSE REACTIONS OR SIDE EFFECTS

SYMPTOMS	WHAT TO DO
Life-threatening:	
Difficult breathing, uncontrollable rapid heart rate, loss of consciousness.	Discontinue. Seek emergency treatment.
Common:	
● Headache, irritability, nervousness, restlessness, insomnia, nausea, vomiting, abdominal pain, irregular heartbeat, "hangover" effect.	Discontinue. Call doctor right away.
● Dizziness, light-headedness, paleness, heartburn.	Continue. Call doctor when convenient.
Infrequent:	
● Rash; hives; red or flushed face; appetite loss; diarrhea; cough; confusion; slurred speech; eyelid, face, lip swelling; joint pain.	Discontinue. Call doctor right away.
● Frequent urination.	Continue. Call doctor when convenient.
Rare:	
Agitation; sore throat, fever, mouth sores; jaundice.	Discontinue. Call doctor right away.

THEOPHYLLINE, EPHEDRINE & BARBITURATES

WARNINGS & PRECAUTIONS

Don't take if:
- You are allergic to any bronchodilator or barbiturate.
- You are allergic to ephedrine or any sympathomimetic drug.
- You have an active peptic ulcer or porphyria.

Before you start, consult your doctor:
- If you have gastritis, peptic ulcer, high blood pressure or heart disease, diabetes, overactive thyroid gland, difficulty urinating, epilepsy, kidney or liver damage, asthma, anemia, chronic pain, taken any MAO inhibitor in past 2 weeks, taken digitalis preparations in the last 7 days.
- If you have had impaired kidney or liver function.
- If you take medication for gout.
- If you will have surgery within 2 months, including dental surgery, requiring general or spinal anesthesia.

Over age 60:
- Adverse reactions and side effects may be more frequent and severe than in younger persons. Use small doses.
- More likely to develop high blood pressure, heart-rhythm disturbances, angina and to feel drug's stimulant effects.

Pregnancy:
Risk to unborn child outweighs drug benefits. Don't use.

Breast-feeding:
Drug passes into milk. Avoid drug or discontinue nursing until you finish medicine.

Infants & children:
Use only under medical supervision.

Prolonged use:
- Stomach irritation.
- Excessive doses—Rare toxic psychosis.
- Men with enlarged prostate gland may have more urination difficulty.
- May cause addiction, anemia, chronic intoxication.
- May lower body temperature, making exposure to cold temperatures hazardous.

Skin & sunlight:
May cause rash or intensify sunburn in areas exposed to sun or sunlamp.

Driving, piloting or hazardous work:
Don't drive or pilot aircraft until you learn how medicine affects you. Don't work around dangerous machinery. Don't climb ladders or work in high places. Danger increases if you drink alcohol or take medicine affecting alertness and reflexes.

Discontinuing:
- May be unnecessary to finish medicine. Follow doctor's instructions.
- If you develop withdrawal symptoms of hallucinations, agitation or sleeplessness after discontinuing, call doctor right away.

Others:
Potential for abuse.

POSSIBLE INTERACTION WITH OTHER DRUGS

GENERIC NAME OR DRUG CLASS	COMBINED EFFECT
Allopurinol	Decreased allopurinol effect.
Anticoagulants, oral*	Decreased anticoagulant effect.
Anticonvulsants*	Changed seizure patterns.
Antidepressants, tricyclic (TCA)*	Decreased antidepressant effect. Possible dangerous oversedation.
Antidiabetics, oral*	Increased phenobarbital effect.

Continued page 962

POSSIBLE INTERACTION WITH OTHER SUBSTANCES

INTERACTS WITH	COMBINED EFFECT
Alcohol:	Possible fatal oversedation. Avoid.
Beverages: Caffeine drinks.	Nervousness or insomnia.
Cocaine:	High risk of heartbeat irregularities and high blood pressure.
Foods:	None expected.
Marijuana:	Rapid heartbeat, possible heart-rhythm disturbance.
Tobacco:	Decreased bronchodilator effect.

THEOPHYLLINE, EPHEDRINE, GUAIFENESIN & BARBITURATES

BRAND NAMES

Bronkolixir
Bronkotabs
Guaiaphed

Mudrane GG
Quibron Plus

BASIC INFORMATION

Habit forming? Yes (barbiturates)
Prescription needed? Yes
Available as generic? Yes
Drug class: Bronchodilator (xanthine),
  cough/cold preparation, sympatho-
  mimetic, sedative

USES

- Treatment for symptoms of bronchial asthma, emphysema, chronic bronchitis.
- Relieves wheezing, coughing and shortness of breath.

DOSAGE & USAGE INFORMATION

How to take:
Tablet, capsule or elixir—Swallow with liquid.

When to take:
Most effective taken on empty stomach 1 hour before or 2 hours after eating. However, may take with food to lessen stomach upset.

If you forget a dose:
Take as soon as you remember up to 2 hours late. If more than 2 hours, wait for next scheduled dose (don't double this dose).

Continued next column

OVERDOSE

SYMPTOMS:
Restlessness, irritability, confusion, hallucinations, muscle tremors, severe anxiety, rapid and irregular pulse, mild weakness, nausea, vomiting blood, delirium, coma.
WHAT TO DO:
- **Overdose unlikely to threaten life. Depending on severity of symptoms and amount taken, call doctor, poison-control center or hospital emergency room for instructions.**
- **Dial 0 (operator) or 911 (emergency) for an ambulance or medical help. Then give first aid immediately.**
- **See emergency information on inside covers.**

What drug does:
- Relaxes and expands bronchial tubes.
- Prevents cells from releasing allergy-causing chemicals (histamines).
- Relaxes muscles of bronchial tubes.
- Decreases blood-vessel size and blood flow, thus causing decongestion.
- Increases production of watery fluids to thin mucus so it can be coughed out or absorbed.
- May partially block nerve impulses at nerve-cell connections.

Time lapse before drug works:
30 to 60 minutes.

Don't take with:
- Non-prescription drugs with ephedrine, pseudoephedrine or epinephrine.
- Non-prescription drugs for cough, cold, allergy or asthma without consulting doctor.
- See Interaction column and consult doctor.

POSSIBLE ADVERSE REACTIONS OR SIDE EFFECTS

SYMPTOMS	WHAT TO DO
Life-threatening:	
Difficult breathing, uncontrollable rapid heart rate, loss of consciousness.	Discontinue. Seek emergency treatment.
Common:	
• Headache, irritability, nervousness, restlessness, insomnia, nausea, vomiting, abdominal pain, irregular heartbeat.	Discontinue. Call doctor right away.
• Dizziness, lightheadedness, paleness, heartburn.	Continue. Call doctor when convenient.
Infrequent:	
• Skin rash or hives, red or flushed face, appetite loss, diarrhea, abdominal pain.	Discontinue. Call doctor right away.
• Frequent urination.	Continue. Call doctor when convenient.
Rare:	
None expected.	

THEOPHYLLINE, EPHEDRINE, GUAIFENESIN & BARBITURATES

WARNINGS & PRECAUTIONS

Don't take if:
- You are allergic to any bronchodilator, ephedrine, any sympathomimetic drug, cough or cold preparation containing guaifenesin.
- You have an active peptic ulcer.

Before you start, consult your doctor:
- If you have had impaired kidney or liver function.
- If you have gastritis, peptic ulcer, high blood pressure, heart disease, diabetes, overactive thyroid gland, difficulty urinating, epilepsy, anemia, chronic pain, taken any MAO inhibitor in past 2 weeks, taken digitalis preparations in the last 7 days.
- If you take medication for gout.
- If you will have surgery within 2 months, including dental surgery, requiring general or spinal anesthesia.

Over age 60:
- Adverse reactions and side effects may be more frequent and severe than in younger persons. Use small doses. For drug to work, you must drink 8 to 10 glasses of fluid per day.
- More likely to develop high blood pressure, heart-rhythm disturbances, angina and to feel drug's stimulant effects.

Pregnancy:
Risk to unborn child outweighs drug benefits. Don't use.

Breast-feeding:
Drug passes into milk. Avoid drug or discontinue nursing until you finish medicine. Consult doctor for advice on maintaining milk supply.

Infants & children:
Use only under medical supervision.

Prolonged use:
- Stomach irritation.
- Excessive doses—Rare toxic psychosis.
- Men with enlarged prostate gland may have more urination difficulty.
- May cause addiction, anemia, chronic intoxication.
- May lower body temperature, making exposure to cold temperature hazardous.

Skin & sunlight:
May cause rash or intensify sunburn in areas exposed to sun or sunlamp.

Driving, piloting or hazardous work:
Don't drive or pilot aircraft until you learn how medicine affects you. Don't work around dangerous machinery. Don't climb ladders or work in high places. Danger increases if you drink alcohol or take medicine affecting alertness and reflexes, such as antihistamines, tranquilizers, sedatives, pain medicine, narcotics and mind-altering drugs.

Discontinuing:
- May be unnecessary to finish medicine. Follow doctor's instructions.
- If you develop withdrawal symptoms of hallucinations, agitation or sleeplessness after discontinuing, call doctor right away.

Others:
Great potential for abuse.

POSSIBLE INTERACTION WITH OTHER DRUGS

GENERIC NAME OR DRUG CLASS	COMBINED EFFECT
Allopurinol	Decreased allopurinol effect.
Anticonvulsants*	Changed seizure patterns.

Continued page 963

POSSIBLE INTERACTION WITH OTHER SUBSTANCES

INTERACTS WITH	COMBINED EFFECT
Alcohol:	Possible fatal oversedation. Avoid.
Beverages:	You must drink 8 to 10 glasses of fluid per day for drug to work.
Caffeine drinks.	Nervousness and insomnia.
Cocaine:	High risk of heartbeat irregularities and high blood pressure.
Foods:	None expected.
Marijuana:	Excessive sedation, rapid heartbeat, possible heart-rhythm disturbance. Avoid.
Tobacco:	Decreased bronchodilator effect. Smoking is damaging to all problems this medicine treats. Avoid.

THEOPHYLLINE, EPHEDRINE & HYDROXYZINE

BRAND NAMES

Brophed
Hydrophed
Hydrophed D.F.
Marax

Marax D.F.
T.E.H. Compound
Theozine

BASIC INFORMATION

Habit forming? No
Prescription needed? Yes
Available as generic? Yes
Drug class: Bronchodilator (xanthine), sympathomimetic, antihistamine

USES

- Treatment for symptoms of bronchial asthma, emphysema, chronic bronchitis.
- Relieves wheezing, coughing and shortness of breath.

DOSAGE & USAGE INFORMATION

How to take:
Tablet, capsule or syrup—Swallow with liquid.

When to take:
Most effective taken on empty stomach 1 hour before or 2 hours after eating. However, may take with food to lessen stomach upset.

If you forget a dose:
Take as soon as you remember up to 2 hours late. If more than 2 hours, wait for next scheduled dose (don't double this dose).

Continued next column

OVERDOSE

SYMPTOMS:
Restlessness, irritability, confusion, hallucinations, severe anxiety, muscle tremors, rapid and irregular pulse, agitation, purposeless movements, vomiting blood, delirium, convulsions, coma.
WHAT TO DO:
- **Dial 0 (operator) or 911 (emergency) for an ambulance or medical help. Then give first aid immediately.**
- **See emergency information on inside covers.**

What drug does:
- Relaxes and expands bronchial tubes.
- Prevents cells from releasing allergy-causing chemicals (histamines).
- Relaxes muscles of bronchial tubes.
- Decreases blood-vessel size and blood flow, thus causing decongestion.
- May reduce activity in areas of the brain that influence emotional stability.

Time lapse before drug works:
15 to 60 minutes.

Don't take with:
- Non-prescription drugs with ephedrine, pseudoephedrine or epinephrine.
- Non-prescription drugs for cough, cold, allergy or asthma without consulting doctor.
- See Interaction column and consult doctor.

POSSIBLE ADVERSE REACTIONS OR SIDE EFFECTS

SYMPTOMS	WHAT TO DO
Life-threatening:	
Difficult breathing, uncontrollable rapid heart rate, loss of consciousness.	Discontinue. Seek emergency treatment.
Common:	
• Headache, irritability, nervousness, restlessness, insomnia, nausea, vomiting, abdominal pain, irregular heartbeat.	Discontinue. Call doctor right away.
• Dizziness, lightheadedness, paleness, heartburn.	Continue. Call doctor when convenient.
Infrequent:	
• Skin rash or hives, red or flushed face, appetite loss, diarrhea, abdominal pain.	Discontinue. Call doctor right away.
• Frequent urination.	Continue. Call doctor when convenient.
Rare:	
Tremor.	Discontinue. Call doctor right away.

THEOPHYLLINE, EPHEDRINE & HYDROXYZINE

WARNINGS & PRECAUTIONS

Don't take if:
- You are allergic to any bronchodilator, ephedrine, any sympathomimetic drug, or antihistamine.
- You have an active peptic ulcer.

Before you start, consult your doctor:
- If you have had impaired kidney or liver function.
- If you have gastritis, peptic ulcer, high blood pressure, heart disease, diabetes, overactive thyroid gland, difficulty urinating, epilepsy, taken any MAO inhibitor in past 2 weeks, taken digitalis preparations in the last 7 days.
- If you take medication for gout.
- If you will have surgery within 2 months, including dental surgery, requiring general or spinal anesthesia.

Over age 60:
- Adverse reactions and side effects may be more frequent and severe than in younger persons.
- More likely to develop increased urination difficulty, high blood pressure, heart-rhythm disturbances, angina and to feel drug's stimulant effects.

Pregnancy:
Risk to unborn child outweighs drug benefits. Don't use.

Breast-feeding:
Drug passes into milk. Avoid drug or discontinue nursing until you finish medicine. Consult doctor for advice on maintaining milk supply.

Infants & children:
Use only under medical supervision.

Prolonged use:
- Stomach irritation.
- Excessive doses—Rare toxic psychosis.
- Men with enlarged prostate gland may have more urination difficulty.
- Tolerance develops and reduces effectiveness.

Skin & sunlight:
No problems expected.

Driving, piloting or hazardous work:
Don't drive or pilot aircraft until you learn how medicine affects you. Don't work around dangerous machinery. Don't climb ladders or work in high places. Danger increases if you drink alcohol or take medicine affecting alertness and reflexes, such as antihistamines, tranquilizers, sedatives, pain medicine, narcotics and mind-altering drugs.

Discontinuing:
Don't discontinue without consulting doctor. Dose may require gradual reduction if you have taken drug for a long time. Doses of other drugs may also require adjustment.

Others:
No problems expected.

POSSIBLE INTERACTION WITH OTHER DRUGS

GENERIC NAME OR DRUG CLASS	COMBINED EFFECT
Allopurinol	Decreased allopurinol effect.
Antidepressants, tricyclic (TCA) *	Increased effect of ephedrine. Excess stimulation of heart and blood pressure.
Antihistamines *	Increased hydroxyzine effect.
Antihypertensives *	Decreased antihypertensive effect.
Beta-adrenergic blockers *	Decreased effect of drugs.
Carteolol	Decreased antihistamine effect.

Continued page 964

POSSIBLE INTERACTION WITH OTHER SUBSTANCES

INTERACTS WITH	COMBINED EFFECT
Alcohol:	Increased sedation and intoxication. Avoid.
Beverages: Caffeine drinks.	Nervousness and insomnia.
Cocaine:	High risk of heartbeat irregularities and high blood pressure.
Foods:	None expected.
Marijuana:	Slightly increased anti-asthmatic effect of bronchodilator. Rapid heartbeat, possible heart-rhythm disturbance.
Tobacco:	Decreased bronchodilator effect. Smoking is damaging to all problems this medicine treats. Avoid.

*See Glossary

THEOPHYLLINE & GUAIFENESIN

BRAND NAMES

Asbron G
Asbron G Inlay
  Tablets
Bronchial
Elixophyllin-GG
Glyceryl T
Lanophyllin-GG
Mudrane GG2

Q-B
Quiagen
Quibron
Slo-Phyllin GG
Syncophylate-GG
Theocolate
Theolair-Plus
Theolate

BASIC INFORMATION

Habit forming? No
Prescription needed? Yes
Available as generic? Yes
Drug class: Bronchodilator, expectorant

 ## USES

- Treatment for bronchial asthma symptoms.
- Loosens mucus in respiratory passages.
- Relieves coughing, wheezing, shortness of breath.

 ## DOSAGE & USAGE INFORMATION

How to take:
Tablet, capsule, elixir or syrup—Swallow with liquid.

When to take:
Most effective taken on empty stomach 1 hour before or 2 hours after eating. However, may take with food to lessen stomach upset.

If you forget a dose:
Take as soon as you remember up to 2 hours late. If more than 2 hours, wait for next scheduled dose (don't double this dose).

Continued next column

 ## OVERDOSE

SYMPTOMS:
Restlessness, irritability, confusion, hallucinations, drowsiness, mild weakness, nausea, vomiting blood, delirium, convulsions, rapid pulse, coma.
WHAT TO DO:
- **Dial 0 (operator) or 911 (emergency) for an ambulance or medical help. Then give first aid immediately.**
- **See emergency information on inside covers.**

What drug does:
- Relaxes and expands bronchial tubes.
- Increases production of watery fluids to thin mucus so it can be coughed out or absorbed.

Time lapse before drug works:
15 to 30 minutes.

Don't take with:
Any other medicine without consulting your doctor or pharmacist.

 ## POSSIBLE ADVERSE REACTIONS OR SIDE EFFECTS

SYMPTOMS	WHAT TO DO
Life-threatening:	
Difficult breathing, uncontrollable heart rate, loss of consciousness.	Discontinue. Seek emergency treatment.
Common:	
• Headache, irritability, nervousness, restlessness, insomnia, drowsiness, nausea, vomiting.	Discontinue. Call doctor right away.
• Dizziness, lightheadedness, diarrhea, abdominal pain, heartburn.	Continue. Call doctor when convenient.
Infrequent:	
Skin rash or hives, red or flushed face, appetite loss, diarrhea.	Discontinue. Call doctor right away.
Rare:	
None expected.	

 ## WARNINGS & PRECAUTIONS

Don't take if:
- You are allergic to any bronchodilator or cough or cold preparation containing guaifenesin.
- You have an active peptic ulcer.

Before you start, consult your doctor:
- If you have had impaired kidney or liver function.
- If you have gastritis, peptic ulcer, high blood pressure or heart disease.
- If you take medication for gout.

THEOPHYLLINE & GUAIFENESIN

Over age 60:
Adverse reactions and side effects may be more frequent and severe than in younger persons. For drug to work, you must drink 8 to 10 glasses of fluid per day.

Pregnancy:
Risk to unborn child outweighs drug benefits. Don't use.

Breast-feeding:
Drug passes into milk. Avoid drug or discontinue nursing until you finish medicine. Consult doctor for advice on maintaining milk supply.

Infants & children:
Use only under medical supervision.

Prolonged use:
Stomach irritation.

Skin & sunlight:
No problems expected.

Driving, piloting or hazardous work:
Avoid if lightheaded, drowsy or dizzy. Otherwise, no problems expected.

Discontinuing:
May be unnecessary to finish medicine. Follow doctor's instructions.

Others:
No problems expected.

 POSSIBLE INTERACTION WITH OTHER DRUGS

GENERIC NAME OR DRUG CLASS	COMBINED EFFECT
Allopurinol	Decreased allopurinol effect.
Anticoagulants*	Possible risk of bleeding.
Ciprofloxacin	Increased possibility of central nervous system poisoning, such as nausea, vomiting, restlessness, palpitations.
Clarithromycin	Increased concentration of theophylline.
Ephedrine	Increased effect of both drugs.
Epinephrine	Increased effect of both drugs.
Erythromycins*	Increased bronchodilator effect.
Finasteride	Decreased theophylline effect.
Furosemide	Increased furosemide effect.
Lincomycins*	Increased bronchodilator effect.
Lithium	Decreased lithium effect.
Moricizine	Decreased bronchodilator effect.
Nicotine	Increased bronchodilator effect.
Probenecid	Decreased effect of both drugs.
Propranolol	Decreased bronchodilator effect.
Rauwolfia alkaloids*	Rapid heartbeat.
Sulfinpyrazone	Decreased sulfinpyrazone effect.
Ticlopidine	Increased theophylline effect.
Troleandomycin	Increased bronchodilator effect.

 POSSIBLE INTERACTION WITH OTHER SUBSTANCES

INTERACTS WITH	COMBINED EFFECT
Alcohol:	No proven problems.
Beverages:	You must drink 8 to 10 glasses of fluid per day for drug to work.
Caffeine drinks.	Nervousness and insomnia.
Cocaine:	Excess stimulation. Avoid.
Foods:	None expected.
Marijuana:	Slightly increased antiasthmatic effect of bronchodilator.
Tobacco:	Decreased bronchodilator effect. Cigarette smoking makes worse all problems that this medicine treats. Avoid.

THIABENDAZOLE

BRAND NAMES

Foldan
Mintezol
Mintezol (Topical)
Minzolum
Triasox

BASIC INFORMATION

Habit forming? No
Prescription needed? Yes
Available as generic? No
Drug class: Anthelmintic

USES

Treatment of parasite infestations.

DOSAGE & USAGE INFORMATION

How to take or apply:
- Tablet—Swallow with liquid or food to lessen stomach irritation.
- Topical suspension—Apply to end of each tunnel or burrow made by worm.
- Chewable tablets—Chew thoroughly before swallowing.

When to take or apply:
- Tablet—According to instructions on prescription, after meals.
- Topical—2 to 4 times daily up to 14 days.

If you forget a dose:
Take as soon as you remember up to 2 hours late. If more than 2 hours, wait for next scheduled dose (don't double this dose).

What drug does:
Kills larvae and adult worms.

Continued next column

OVERDOSE

SYMPTOMS:
Aching, fever, blistered skin, seizures.
WHAT TO DO:
- **Dial 0 (operator) or 911 (emergency) for an ambulance or medical help. Then give first aid immediately.**
- **If patient is unconscious and not breathing, give mouth-to-mouth breathing. If there is no heartbeat, use cardiac massage and mouth-to-mouth breathing (CPR). Don't try to make patient vomit. If you can't get help quickly, take patient to nearest emergency facility.**
- **See emergency information on inside covers.**

Time lapse before drug works:
Varies according to degree of infestation.

Don't take with:
Any other medicine without consulting your doctor or pharmacist.

POSSIBLE ADVERSE REACTIONS OR SIDE EFFECTS

SYMPTOMS	WHAT TO DO
Life-threatening:	
In case of overdose, see previous column.	
Common:	
Nausea, vomiting, abdominal pain.	Discontinue. Call doctor right away.
Dizziness, headache, drowsiness, appetite loss, bedwetting.	Continue. Call doctor when convenient.
Asparagus-like odor of urine.	Continue. Tell doctor at next visit.
Infrequent:	
Redness, blistering with fever, rash with itchy skin, aching joints and muscles, chills and fever.	Discontinue. Call doctor right away.
Ringing or buzzing in ears, numbness or tingling in hands and feet, swollen lymph nodes, diarrhea.	Continue. Call doctor when convenient.
Rare:	
Blurred or yellow vision, seizures.	Discontinue. Call doctor right away.

WARNINGS & PRECAUTIONS

Don't take if:
You are allergic to thiabendazole.

Before you start, consult your doctor:
• If you have kidney disease.
• If you have liver disease.

Over age 60:
Adverse reactions and side effects may be more frequent and severe than in younger persons.

Pregnancy:
Risk to unborn child outweighs drug benefits. Don't use.

Breast-feeding:
Unknown effect. Consult doctor.

Infants & children:
Use only under medical supervision.

Prolonged use:
Request follow-up sputum and stool exams 2 to 3 weeks following treatment.

Skin & sunlight:
No problems expected.

Driving, piloting or hazardous work:
Don't drive or pilot aircraft until you learn how medicine affects you. Don't work around dangerous machinery. Don't climb ladders or work in high places. Danger increases if you drink alcohol or take medicine affecting alertness and reflexes, such as antihistamines, tranquilizers, sedatives, pain medicine, narcotics and mind-altering drugs.

Discontinuing:
May be unnecessary to finish medicine. Follow doctor's instructions.

Others:
• To prevent reinfection: Deworm household pets regularly. Cover sand boxes. Cook all pork until well done.
• Patients who take thiabendazole may excrete urine that smells like asparagus.

POSSIBLE INTERACTION WITH OTHER DRUGS

GENERIC NAME OR DRUG CLASS	COMBINED EFFECT
Theophylline	Increased theophylline effect.

POSSIBLE INTERACTION WITH OTHER SUBSTANCES

INTERACTS WITH	COMBINED EFFECT
Alcohol:	Decreased thiabendazole effect.
Beverages:	No problems expected.
Cocaine:	Decreased thiabendazole effect.
Foods:	Take with foods to decrease nausea.
Marijuana:	Decreased thiabendazole effect.
Tobacco:	May decrease absorption of medicine.

THIAMINE (Vitamin B-1)

BRAND NAMES

Betalin S	Bewon
Betaxin	Biamine

Numerous other multiple vitamin-mineral supplements. Check labels.

BASIC INFORMATION

Habit forming? No
Prescription needed? No
Available as generic? Yes
Drug class: Vitamin supplement

 ## USES

- Dietary supplement to promote normal growth, development and health.
- Treatment for beri-beri (a thiamine-deficiency disease).
- Dietary supplement for alcoholism, cirrhosis, overactive thyroid, infection, breast-feeding, absorption diseases, pregnancy, prolonged diarrhea, burns.

 ## DOSAGE & USAGE INFORMATION

How to take:
Tablet or liquid—Swallow with beverage or food to lessen stomach irritation.

When to take:
At the same time each day.

If you forget a dose:
Take when remembered. Return to regular schedule.

What drug does:
- Promotes normal growth and development.
- Combines with an enzyme to metabolize carbohydrates.

Time lapse before drug works:
15 minutes.

Don't take with:
Any other medicine without consulting your doctor or pharmacist.

 ## OVERDOSE

SYMPTOMS:
Increased severity of adverse reactions and side effects.
WHAT TO DO:
Overdose unlikely to threaten life. If person takes much larger amount than prescribed, call doctor, poison-control center or hospital emergency room for instructions.

 ## POSSIBLE ADVERSE REACTIONS OR SIDE EFFECTS

SYMPTOMS	WHAT TO DO
Life-threatening:	
Hives, rash, intense itching, faintness soon after a dose (anaphylaxis) (injection only).	Seek emergency treatment immediately.
Common:	
None expected.	
Infrequent:	
None expected.	
Rare:	
• Wheezing.	Discontinue. Seek emergency treatment.
• Rash or itchy skin.	Discontinue. Call doctor right away.

WARNINGS & PRECAUTIONS

Don't take if:
You are allergic to any B vitamin.

Before you start, consult your doctor:
If you have liver or kidney disease.

Over age 60:
No problems expected.

Pregnancy:
No problems expected.

Breast-feeding:
No problems expected.

Infants & children:
No problems expected.

Prolonged use:
No problems expected.

Skin & sunlight:
No problems expected.

Driving, piloting or hazardous work:
No problems expected.

Discontinuing:
No problems expected.

Others:
A balanced diet should provide enough thiamine for healthy people to make supplement unnecessary. Best dietary sources of thiamine are whole-grain cereals and meats.

POSSIBLE INTERACTION WITH OTHER DRUGS

GENERIC NAME OR DRUG CLASS	COMBINED EFFECT
Barbiturates*	Decreased thiamine effect.

POSSIBLE INTERACTION WITH OTHER SUBSTANCES

INTERACTS WITH	COMBINED EFFECT
Alcohol:	None expected.
Beverages: Carbonates, citrates (additives listed on many beverage labels).	Decreased thiamine effect.
Cocaine:	None expected.
Foods: Carbonates, citrates (additives listed on many food labels).	Decreased thiamine effect.
Marijuana:	None expected.
Tobacco:	None expected.

THIOGUANINE

BRAND NAMES

Lanvis

BASIC INFORMATION

Habit forming? No
Prescription needed? Yes
Available as generic? Yes
Drug class: Antineoplastic

 USES

Treats some forms of leukemia.

 DOSAGE & USAGE INFORMATION

How to take:
Tablets—Swallow with liquid. If you can't swallow whole, crumble tablet and take with liquid or food. Instructions to take on empty stomach mean 1 hour before or 2 hours after eating.

When to take:
According to doctor's instructions.

If you forget a dose:
Skip the missed dose and return to regular schedule. Don't double dose.

What drug does:
Interferes with growth of cancer cells.

Time lapse before drug works:
Varies greatly among patients.

Don't take with:
Any other medicines (including over-the-counter drugs such as cough and cold medicines, laxatives, antacids, diet pills, caffeine, nose drops or vitamins) without consulting your doctor.

 OVERDOSE

SYMPTOMS:
None expected.
WHAT TO DO:
Overdose unlikely to threaten life. If person takes much larger amount than prescribed, call doctor, poison-control center or hospital emergency room for instructions.

 POSSIBLE ADVERSE REACTIONS OR SIDE EFFECTS

SYMPTOMS	WHAT TO DO
Life-threatening: Black, tarry stools.	Discontinue. Seek emergency treatment.
Common:	
• Appetite loss, diarrhea, skin rash.	Continue. Call doctor when convenient.
• Nausea.	No action necessary.
Infrequent: Bloody urine; hoarseness or cough; fever or chills; lower back or side pain; painful or difficult urination; red spots on skin; unusual bleeding or bruising; joint pain; swollen feet and legs; unsteady gait.	Discontinue. Call doctor right away.
Rare: Mouth and lip sores; jaundice (yellow skin and eyes).	Discontinue. Call doctor right away.

WARNINGS & PRECAUTIONS

Don't take if:
- You are allergic to thioguanine.
- You have chicken pox or shingles.

Before you start, consult your doctor:
- If you have gout.
- If you have an infection.
- If you have kidney or liver disease.
- If you have had radiation or cancer chemotherapy within 6 weeks.

Over age 60:
Adverse reactions and side effects may be more frequent and severe than in younger persons. You may need smaller doses for shorter periods of time.

Pregnancy:
- Risk to unborn child outweighs drug benefits. Don't use.
- Don't use birth control pills for contraception.

Breast-feeding:
Drug may pass into milk. Avoid drug or discontinue nursing until you finish medicine. Consult doctor for advice on maintaining milk supply.

Infants & children:
No special problems expected.

Prolonged use:
- Increased likelihood of side effects.
- Talk to your doctor about the need for follow-up medical examinations or laboratory studies to check kidney and liver function, serum uric acid, and complete blood counts (white blood cell count, platelet count, red blood cell count, hemoglobin, hematocrit).

Skin & sunlight:
No problems expected.

Driving, piloting or hazardous work:
No problems expected.

Discontinuing:
Report to your doctor any of these symptoms that occur after discontinuing: black, tarry stools; bloody urine; hoarseness or cough; fever or chills; lower back or side pain; painful or difficult urination; red spots on skin; unusual bleeding or bruising.

Others:
- Advise any doctor or dentist whom you consult that you take this medicine.
- May affect results in some medical tests.
- Don't use birth control pills for contraception.

POSSIBLE INTERACTION WITH OTHER DRUGS

GENERIC NAME OR DRUG CLASS	COMBINED EFFECT
Antithyroid agents*	More likelihood of toxicity of both drugs.
Azathioprine	More likelihood of toxicity of both drugs.
Chloramphenicol	More likelihood of toxicity of both drugs.
Clozapine	Toxic effect on bone marrow.
Colchicine	May need increased dosage of colchicine.
Flucytosine	More likelihood of toxicity of both drugs.
Interferon	More likelihood of toxicity of both drugs.
Levamisole	Increased risk of bone marrow depression.
Plicamycin	More likelihood of toxicity of both drugs.
Probenecid	More likelihood of toxicity of both drugs.
Sulfinpyrazone	May need increased dosage of sulfinpyrazone.
Tiopronin	Increased risk of toxicity to bone marrow.
Zidovudine	More likelihood of toxicity of both drugs.

POSSIBLE INTERACTION WITH OTHER SUBSTANCES

INTERACTS WITH	COMBINED EFFECT
Alcohol:	Increased side effects.
Beverages:	No special problems expected.
Cocaine:	Increased side effects.
Foods:	No special problems expected.
Marijuana:	No special problems expected.
Tobacco:	No special problems expected.

THIOTHIXENE

BRAND NAMES

Navane

BASIC INFORMATION

Habit forming? No
Prescription needed? Yes
Available as generic? No
Drug class: Tranquilizer (thioxanthine),
antiemetic

 ## USES

- Reduces anxiety, agitation, psychosis.
- Stops vomiting, hiccups.

 ## DOSAGE & USAGE INFORMATION

How to take:
- Capsule—Swallow with liquid. If you can't swallow whole, open capsule and take with liquid or food.
- Syrup—Dilute dose in beverage before swallowing.

When to take:
At the same time each day.

If you forget a dose:
Take as soon as you remember up to 2 hours late. If more than 2 hours, wait for next scheduled dose (don't double this dose).

What drug does:
Corrects imbalance of nerve impulses.

Time lapse before drug works:
3 weeks.

Continued next column

 ## OVERDOSE

SYMPTOMS:
Drowsiness, dizziness, weakness, muscle rigidity, twitching, tremors, confusion, dry mouth, blurred vision, rapid pulse, shallow breathing, low blood pressure, convulsions, coma.
WHAT TO DO:
- **Dial 0 (operator) or 911 (emergency) for an ambulance or medical help. Then give first aid immediately.**
- **If patient is unconscious and not breathing, give mouth-to-mouth breathing. If there is no heartbeat, use cardiac massage and mouth-to-mouth breathing (CPR). Don't try to make patient vomit. If you can't get help quickly, take patient to nearest emergency facility.**
- **See emergency information on inside covers.**

Don't take with:
Any other medicine without consulting your doctor or pharmacist.

 ## POSSIBLE ADVERSE REACTIONS OR SIDE EFFECTS

SYMPTOMS	WHAT TO DO
Life-threatening:	
Uncontrolled muscle movements of tongue, face and other muscles (neuroleptic malignant syndrome, rare).	Discontinue. Seek emergency treatment.
Common:	
• Fainting, jerky and involuntary movements, blurred vision, restlessness, rapid heartbeat.	Discontinue. Call doctor right away.
• Dizziness, drowsiness, constipation, muscle spasms, shuffling walk, decreased sweating, increased appetite, weight gain, sensitivity to light.	Continue. Call doctor when convenient.
• Dry mouth, nasal congestion.	Continue. Tell doctor at next visit.
Infrequent:	
• Rash, abdominal pain.	Discontinue. Call doctor right away.
• Less sexual ability, difficult urination.	Continue. Call doctor when convenient.
• Menstrual irregularities, swollen breasts, milk secretion by breasts.	Continue. Tell doctor at next visit.
Rare:	
Sore throat, fever, jaundice, lip smacking, cheek puffing, chewing movements of mouth, heatstroke, bleeding or bruising.	Discontinue. Call doctor right away.

 ## WARNINGS & PRECAUTIONS

Don't take if:
- You are allergic to any thioxanthine or phenothiazine tranquilizer.
- You have serious blood disorder.
- You have Parkinson's disease.
- Patient is younger than 12.

Before you start, consult your doctor:
- If you have had liver or kidney disease.
- If you have epilepsy, glaucoma, prostate trouble.
- If you have high blood pressure or heart disease (especially angina).

- If you use alcohol daily.
- If you will have surgery within 2 months, including dental surgery, requiring general or spinal anesthesia.

Over age 60:
Adverse reactions and side effects may be more frequent and severe than in younger persons.

Pregnancy:
No proven harm to unborn child. Avoid if possible.

Breast-feeding:
Studies inconclusive. Consult your doctor.

Infants & children:
Not recommended.

Prolonged use:
- Pigment deposits in lens and retina of eye.
- Involuntary movements of jaws, lips, tongue (tardive dyskinesia).
- Talk to your doctor about the need for follow-up medical examinations or laboratory studies to check complete blood counts (white blood cell count, platelet count, red blood cell count, hemoglobin, hematocrit), liver function, eyes.

Skin & sunlight:
May cause rash or intensify sunburn in areas exposed to sun or sunlamp.

Driving, piloting or hazardous work:
Don't drive or pilot aircraft until you learn how medicine affects you. Don't work around dangerous machinery. Don't climb ladders or work in high places. Danger increases if you drink alcohol or take medicine affecting alertness and reflexes.

Discontinuing:
Don't discontinue without consulting doctor. Dose may require gradual reduction if you have taken drug for a long time. Doses of other drugs may also require adjustment.

Others:
Hot temperatures increase chance of heat stroke.

 ## POSSIBLE INTERACTION WITH OTHER DRUGS

GENERIC NAME OR DRUG CLASS	COMBINED EFFECT
Anticholinergics*	Increased anticholinergic effect.
Anticonvulsants*	Change in seizure pattern.
Antidepressants, tricyclic (TCA)*	Increased thiothixene effect. Excessive sedation.
Antihistamines*	Increased thiothixene effect. Excessive sedation.

Antihypertensives*	Excessively low blood pressure.
Barbiturates*	Increased thiothixene effect. Excessive sedation.
Bethanechol	Decreased bethanechol effect.
Bupropion	Increased risk of major seizures.
Dronabinol	Increased effects of both drugs. Avoid.
Guanethidine	Decreased guanethidine effect.
Levodopa	Decreased levodopa effect.
MAO inhibitors*	Excessive sedation.
Mind-altering drugs*	Increased thiothixene effect. Excessive sedation.
Narcotics*	Increased thiothixene effect. Excessive sedation.
Pergolide	Decreased pergolide effect.
Procarbazine	Increased sedation.
Sedatives*	Increased thiothixene effect. Excessive sedation.
Sertraline	Increased depressive effects of both drugs.
Sleep inducers*	Increased thiothixene effect. Excessive sedation.
Tranquilizers*	Increased thiothixene effect. Excessive sedation.

 ## POSSIBLE INTERACTION WITH OTHER SUBSTANCES

INTERACTS WITH	COMBINED EFFECT
Alcohol:	Excessive brain depression. Avoid.
Beverages:	None expected.
Cocaine:	Decreased thiothixene effect. Avoid.
Foods:	None expected.
Marijuana:	Daily use—Fainting likely, possible psychosis.
Tobacco:	None expected.

*See Glossary

THYROID HORMONES

BRAND NAMES

Cytomel
Eltroxin
Euthroid
Levothyroxine
Levothroid
Levoxine
LIOTRIX

LIOTHYRONINE
Proloid
Synthroid
THYROGLOBULIN
THYROID
Thyrolar
THYROXINE

BASIC INFORMATION

Habit forming? No
Prescription needed? Yes
Available as generic? No
Drug class: Thyroid hormone

 USES

Replacement for thyroid hormone deficiency.

 DOSAGE & USAGE INFORMATION

How to take:
Tablet—Swallow with liquid.

When to take:
At the same time each day before a meal or on awakening.

If you forget a dose:
Take as soon as you remember up to 12 hours late. If more than 12 hours, wait for next scheduled dose (don't double this dose).

What drug does:
Increases cell metabolism rate.

Time lapse before drug works:
48 hours.

Don't take with:
Any other medicine without consulting your doctor or pharmacist.

 OVERDOSE

SYMPTOMS:
"Hot" feeling, heart palpitations, nervousness, sweating, hand tremors, insomnia, rapid and irregular pulse, headache, irritability, diarrhea, weight loss, muscle cramps, angina, congestive heart failure possible.
WHAT TO DO:
Overdose unlikely to threaten life. If person takes much larger amount than prescribed, call doctor, poison-control center or hospital emergency room for instructions.

 POSSIBLE ADVERSE REACTIONS OR SIDE EFFECTS

SYMPTOMS	WHAT TO DO
Life-threatening:	
In case of overdose, see previous column.	
Common:	
• Tremor, headache, irritability, insomnia.	Discontinue. Call doctor right away.
• Appetite change, diarrhea, leg cramps, menstrual irregularities, fever, heat sensitivity, unusual sweating, weight loss, nervousness.	Continue. Call doctor when convenient.
Infrequent:	
Hives, rash, vomiting, chest pain, rapid and irregular heartbeat, shortness of breath.	Discontinue. Call doctor right away.
Rare:	
None expected.	

WARNINGS & PRECAUTIONS

Don't take if:
- You have had a heart attack within 6 weeks.
- You have no thyroid deficiency, but want to use this to lose weight.

Before you start, consult your doctor:
- If you have heart disease or high blood pressure.
- If you have diabetes.
- If you have Addison's disease, have had adrenal gland deficiency or use epinephrine, ephedrine or isoproterenol for asthma.

Over age 60:
More sensitive to thyroid hormone. May need smaller doses.

Pregnancy:
Considered safe if for thyroid deficiency only.

Breast-feeding:
Present in milk. Considered safe if dose is correct.

Infants & children:
Use only under medical supervision.

Prolonged use:
- No problems expected if dose is correct.
- Talk to your doctor about the need for follow-up medical examinations or laboratory studies to check thyroid, heart.

Skin & sunlight:
No problems expected.

Driving, piloting or hazardous work:
No problems expected.

Discontinuing:
Don't discontinue without consulting doctor. Dose may require gradual reduction if you have taken drug for a long time. Doses of other drugs may also require adjustment.

Others:
- Digestive upsets, tremors, cramps, nervousness, insomnia or diarrhea may indicate need for dose adjustment.
- Different brands can cause different results. Do not change brands without consulting doctor.

POSSIBLE INTERACTION WITH OTHER DRUGS

GENERIC NAME OR DRUG CLASS	COMBINED EFFECT
Amphetamines*	Increased amphetamine effect.
Anticoagulants, oral*	Increased anticoagulant effect.
Antidepressants, tricyclic (TCAs)*	Increased antidepressant effect. Irregular heartbeat.
Antidiabetics*	Antidiabetic may require adjustment.
Aspirin (large doses, continuous use)	Increased effect of thyroid hormone.
Barbiturates*	Decreased barbiturate effect.
Beta-adrenergic blockers*	Possible decreased effect of beta blockers.
Cholestyramine	Decreased effect of thyroid hormone.
Colestipol	Decreased effect of thyroid hormone.
Contraceptives, oral*	Decreased effect of thyroid hormone.
Cortisone drugs*	Requires dose adjustment to prevent cortisone deficiency.
Digitalis preparations*	Decreased digitalis effect.
Ephedrine	Increased ephedrine effect.
Epinephrine	Increased epinephrine effect.
Estrogens*	Decreased effect of thyroid hormone.
Methylphenidate	Increased methylphenidate effect.
Phenytoin	Possible decreased effect of thyroid hormone.
Sympathomimetics*	Increased risk of rapid or irregular heartbeat.

POSSIBLE INTERACTION WITH OTHER SUBSTANCES

INTERACTS WITH	COMBINED EFFECT
Alcohol:	None expected.
Beverages:	None expected.
Cocaine:	Excess stimulation. Avoid.
Foods: Soybeans.	Heavy consumption interferes with thyroid function.
Marijuana:	None expected.
Tobacco:	None expected.

TICARCILLIN

BRAND NAMES

Ticar

BASIC INFORMATION

Habit forming? No
Prescription needed? Yes
Available as generic? No
Drug class: Antibiotic (penicillin)

 ## USES

Treatment of bacterial infections that are
susceptible to ticarcillin.

 ## DOSAGE & USAGE INFORMATION

How to take:
By injection only.

When to take:
Follow doctor's instructions.

If you forget a dose:
Consult doctor.

What drug does:
Destroys susceptible bacteria. Does not kill
viruses.

Time lapse before drug works:
May be several days before medicine affects
infection.

Don't take with:
Any other medicine without consulting your
doctor or pharmacist.

 ## OVERDOSE

SYMPTOMS:
**Severe diarrhea, nausea, edema or
vomiting.**
WHAT TO DO:
**Overdose unlikely to threaten life. If person
takes much larger amount than prescribed,
call doctor, poison-control center or
hospital emergency room for instructions.**

 ## POSSIBLE ADVERSE REACTIONS OR SIDE EFFECTS

SYMPTOMS	WHAT TO DO
Life-threatening: Hives, rash, intense itching, faintness soon after a dose (anaphylaxis).	Seek emergency treatment immediately.
Common: Dark or discolored tongue.	Continue. Tell doctor at next visit.
Infrequent: • Mild nausea, vomiting, diarrhea.	Continue. Call doctor when convenient.
• Bloody urine, face or ankle swelling.	Discontinue. Call doctor right away.
Rare: Unexplained bleeding or bruising, weakness, hoarseness, heartbeat irregularities, sore throat, fever, abdominal cramps, convulsions.	Discontinue. Call doctor right away.

WARNINGS & PRECAUTIONS

Don't take if:
You are allergic to ticarcillin, cephalosporin antibiotics, or other penicillins. Life-threatening reaction may occur.

Before you start, consult your doctor:
• If you are allergic to any substance or drug.
• If you take birth control pills.

Over age 60:
You may have skin reactions, particularly around genitals and anus.

Pregnancy:
Studies inconclusive on harm to unborn child. Animal studies show fetal abnormalities. Decide with your doctor whether drug benefits justify risk to unborn child.

Breast-feeding:
Drug passes into milk. Child may become sensitive to penicillins and have allergic reactions to penicillin drugs. Avoid ticarcillin or discontinue nursing until you finish medicine. Consult doctor for advice on maintaining milk supply.

Infants & children:
No problems expected.

Prolonged use:
• You may become more susceptible to infections caused by germs not responsive to ticarcillin.
• Talk to your doctor about the need for follow-up medical examinations or laboratory studies to check SGPT*, SGOT*.

Skin & sunlight:
No problems expected.

Driving, piloting or hazardous work:
Usually not dangerous. Most hazardous reactions likely to occur a few minutes after taking ticarcillin.

Discontinuing:
Don't discontinue without doctor's advice until you complete prescribed dose, even though symptoms diminish or disappear.

Others:
• May interfere with the accuracy of some medical tests.
• Birth control pills may not be effective. Use additional birth-control methods.

POSSIBLE INTERACTION WITH OTHER DRUGS

GENERIC NAME OR DRUG CLASS	COMBINED EFFECT
Beta-adrenergic blockers*	Increased chance of anaphylaxis (see emergency information on inside front cover).
Birth control pills	Impaired contraceptive efficiency.
Chloramphenicol	Decreased effect of both drugs.
Erythromycins*	Decreased effect of both drugs.
Loperamide	Decreased ticarcillin effect.
Paromomycin	Decreased effect of both drugs.
Probenecid	Increased effect of all penicillins.
Tetracyclines*	Decreased effect of both drugs.
Troleandomycin	Decreased effect of both drugs.

POSSIBLE INTERACTION WITH OTHER SUBSTANCES

INTERACTS WITH	COMBINED EFFECT
Alcohol:	Occasional stomach irritation.
Beverages:	None expected.
Cocaine:	No proven problems.
Foods: Acidic fruits or juices, aged cheese, wines, syrups (if taken with).	Decreased antibiotic effect.
Marijuana:	No proven problems.
Tobacco:	None expected.

TICLOPIDINE

BRAND NAMES

Ticlid

BASIC INFORMATION

Habit forming? No
Prescription needed? Yes
Available as generic? No
Drug class: Platelet aggregation inhibitor

 USES

Decreases the risk of stroke in patients who
have warning signs of stroke or who have had
strokes caused by blood clots.

 DOSAGE & USAGE INFORMATION

How to take:
Tablets—Swallow with liquid. If you can't
swallow whole, crumble tablet and take with
liquid or food.

When to take:
Twice a day with food or as directed.

If you forget a dose:
Take as soon as you remember up to 2 hours
late. If more than 2 hours, wait for next
scheduled dose (don't double this dose).

What drug does:
Inhibits the clumping of platelets and thereby
prevents blood clotting.

Time lapse before drug works:
2 hours.

Don't take with:
Any other drugs (particularly aspirin) without
consulting doctor or pharmacist.

 OVERDOSE

SYMPTOMS:
Bloody vomit or excessive bleeding from
gums, nose or rectum.
WHAT TO DO:
Dial 0 (operator) or 911 (emergency) for an
ambulance or medical help. Then give first
aid immediately.

 POSSIBLE ADVERSE REACTIONS OR SIDE EFFECTS

SYMPTOMS	WHAT TO DO
Life-threatening:	
None expected.	
Common:	
• Diarrhea, elevated level of cholesterol in blood.	Continue. Call doctor when convenient.
• Nausea, skin rash, abdominal pain.	Discontinue. Call doctor right away.
Infrequent:	
• Unusual bleeding or bruising.	Discontinue. Seek emergency treatment.
• Headache.	Continue. Call doctor when convenient.
Rare:	
• Sore throat, mouth ulcers, fever, chills.	Discontinue. Seek emergency treatment.
• Dizziness, loss of appetite, gaseousness.	Continue. Call doctor when convenient.

WARNINGS & PRECAUTIONS

Don't take if:
- You are allergic to ticlopidine.
- You have reduced white blood cells (neutropenia).

Before you start, consult your doctor:
- If you have liver disease, kidney disease, peptic ulcers or diverticulitis.
- If you have any bleeding disorder.

Over age 60:
No special problems expected.

Pregnancy:
Use during pregnancy only if clearly needed. Consult doctor.

Breast-feeding:
Safety not established. Consult doctor.

Infants & children:
Not recommended. Safety has not been established.

Prolonged use:
No special problems expected.

Skin & sunlight:
No special problems expected.

Driving, piloting or hazardous work:
Don't drive or pilot aircraft until you learn how the medicine affects you. Don't work around dangerous machinery. Don't climb ladders or work in high places.

Discontinuing:
No special problems expected.

Others:
- Advise any doctor or dentist whom you consult that you take this medicine. This is particularly important if any surgery is scheduled.
- May affect results of some medical tests.
- Report any unusual bleeding to your doctor.

 POSSIBLE INTERACTION WITH OTHER DRUGS

GENERIC NAME OR DRUG CLASS	COMBINED EFFECT
Antacids*	Decreased ticlopidine effect.
Aspirin	Increased effects of both drugs.
Cimetidine	Increased ticlopidine effect.
Digoxin	Slightly decreased digoxin effect.
Theophylline	Increased theophylline effect.

 POSSIBLE INTERACTION WITH OTHER SUBSTANCES

INTERACTS WITH	COMBINED EFFECT
Alcohol:	Increased likelihood of bleeding. Avoid.
Beverages:	No proven problems.
Cocaine:	No proven problems.
Foods:	Best to take with foods to prevent stomach upset.
Marijuana:	No proven problems.
Tobacco:	No proven problems.

TIOPRONIN

BRAND NAMES

Capen
Captimer
Epatiol
Mucolysin
Sutilan

Thiola
Thiosol
Tioglis
Vincol

BASIC INFORMATION

Habit forming? No
Prescription needed? Yes
Available as generic? No
Drug class: Antiurolithic

 ## USES

Prevents the formation of kidney stones when
there is too much cystine in the urine.

 ## DOSAGE & USAGE INFORMATION

How to take:
Tablets—Swallow with liquid. If you can't
swallow whole, crumble tablet and take with
liquid or food. Instructions to take on empty
stomach mean 1 hour before or 2 hours after
eating.

When to take:
3 times daily (once approximately every 8 hours).

If you forget a dose:
Take as soon as you remember up to 2 hours
late. If more than 2 hours, wait for next
scheduled dose (don't double this dose).

What drug does:
Removes high levels of cystine from the body.

Time lapse before drug works:
Works immediately.

Don't take with:
- Medicines that are known to cause kidney
  damage or depress bone marrow.
- Any other medicine without consulting your
  doctor or pharmacist.

 ## OVERDOSE

SYMPTOMS:
**None expected. If massive overdose is
suspected, follow instructions below.**
WHAT TO DO:
- **Dial 0 (operator) or 911 (emergency) for
  an ambulance or medical help. Then give
  first aid immediately.**
- **See emergency information on inside
  covers.**

 ## POSSIBLE ADVERSE REACTIONS OR SIDE EFFECTS

SYMPTOMS	WHAT TO DO
Life-threatening:	
In case of overdose, see previous column	
Common:	
• Skin rash, itching skin, mouth sores, mouth ulcers.	Discontinue. Call doctor right away.
• Abdominal pain, gaseousness, diarrhea, nausea or vomiting.	Continue. Call doctor when convenient.
Infrequent:	
• Cloudy urine, chills, breathing difficulty, joint pain.	Discontinue. Call doctor right away.
• Impaired smell or taste.	Continue. Call doctor when convenient.
Rare:	
None expected.	

WARNINGS & PRECAUTIONS

Don't take if:
You are allergic to tiopronin or penicillamine.

Before you start, consult your doctor:
If you have had any of the following in the past:
- Agranulocytosis*
- Aplastic anemia*
- Thrombocytopenia*
- Impaired kidney function

Over age 60:
May require dosage adjustment if kidney function is impaired due to normal aging.

Pregnancy:
No studies reported, but similar drugs cause harmful effects on the unborn child. Best to avoid during pregnancy.

Breast-feeding:
Drug passes into milk. Avoid or discontinue nursing until you finish medicine. Consult doctor for advice on maintaining milk supply.

Infants & children:
Safety not established. Consult doctor.

Prolonged use:
No special problems expected.

Skin & sunlight:
No special problems expected.

Driving, piloting or hazardous work:
Don't drive or pilot aircraft until you learn how medicine affects you. Don't work around dangerous machinery. Don't climb ladders or work in high places. Danger increases if you drink alcohol or take medicine affecting alertness and reflexes.

Discontinuing:
No special problems expected.

Others:
- Advise any doctor or dentist whom you consult that you take this medicine.
- May affect results of some medical tests.

POSSIBLE INTERACTION WITH OTHER DRUGS

GENERIC NAME OR DRUG CLASS	COMBINED EFFECT
Bone marrow depressants*	May increase possibility of toxic effects of tiopronin.
Medications toxic to kidneys (nephrotoxins)*	May increase possibility of toxic effects of tiopronin.

POSSIBLE INTERACTION WITH OTHER SUBSTANCES

INTERACTS WITH	COMBINED EFFECT
Alcohol:	None expected.
Beverages: Water	Enhances effects of tiopronin. Drink 8 to 10 glasses daily.
Cocaine:	None expected.
Foods:	None expected.
Marijuana:	None expected.
Tobacco:	None expected.

TOCAINIDE

BRAND NAMES

Tonocard

BASIC INFORMATION

Habit forming? No
Prescription needed? Yes
Available as generic? No
Drug class: Antiarrhythmic

 ## USES

Stabilizes irregular heartbeat, particularly irregular contractions of the ventricles of the heart or a too rapid heart rate.

 ## DOSAGE & USAGE INFORMATION

How to take:
Tablet—Swallow with food, water or milk. Dosage may need to be changed according to individual response.

When to take:
Take at regular times each day. For example, instructions to take 3 times a day means every 8 hours.

If you forget a dose:
Take as soon as you remember up to 4 hours late. If more than 4 hours, wait for next scheduled dose (don't double this dose).

What drug does:
Decreases excitability of cells of heart muscle.

Time lapse before drug works:
30 minutes to 2 hours.

Don't take with:
- Any other medicine without consulting your doctor or pharmacist.
- Wear identification information that states that you take this medicine so during an emergency a physician will know to avoid additional medicines that might be harmful or dangerous.

 ## OVERDOSE

SYMPTOMS:
Convulsions, depressed breathing, cardiac arrest.
WHAT TO DO:
- **Dial 0 (operator) or 911 (emergency) for an ambulance or medical help. Then give first aid immediately.**
- **See emergency information on inside covers.**

 ## POSSIBLE ADVERSE REACTIONS OR SIDE EFFECTS

SYMPTOMS	WHAT TO DO
Life-threatening:	
In case of overdose, see previous column.	
Common:	
• Nausea, vomiting, lightheadedness, dizziness.	Discontinue. Call doctor right away.
• Appetite loss.	Continue. Call doctor when convenient.
Infrequent:	
• Trembling, headache.	Discontinue. Call doctor right away.
• Numbness or tingling in hands or feet.	Continue. Call doctor when convenient.
Rare:	
• Sore throat, unexplained bleeding or bruising, fever, chills, blurred vision, may accelerate heart rate or worsen irregular heartbeat, cough, difficult breathing, wheezing, double vision, disorientation, shakiness, seizures, blisters.	Discontinue. Call doctor right away.
• Rash, swollen feet and ankles, unusual sweating.	Continue. Call doctor when convenient.

 ## WARNINGS & PRECAUTIONS

Don't take if:
- You are allergic to tocainide or anesthetics whose names end in "caine."
- You have myasthenia gravis.

Before you start, consult your doctor:
- If you have congestive heart failure.
- If you are pregnant or plan to become pregnant.
- If you take anticancer drugs, trimethoprim, pyrimethamine, primaquine, phenylbutazone, penicillamine or oxyphenbutazone. These may affect blood-cell production in bone marrow.
- If you take any other heart medicine such as digitalis, flucystosine, colchicine, chloramphenicol, beta-adrenergic blockers or azathioprine. These can worsen heartbeat irregularity.

- If you will have surgery within 2 months, including dental surgery, requiring general, local or spinal anesthesia.
- If you have liver or kidney disease.

Over age 60:
Adverse reactions and side effects may be more frequent and severe than in younger persons.

Pregnancy:
No proven harm to unborn child. Nevertheless, avoid if possible.

Breast-feeding:
Avoid if possible.

Infants & children:
Not recommended. Safety and dosage have not been established.

Prolonged use:
Request periodic lab studies on blood, liver function, potassium levels, X-ray, ECG*.

Skin & sunlight:
No problems expected.

Driving, piloting or hazardous work:
Use caution if medicine causes you to feel dizzy or weak. Otherwise, no problems expected.

Discontinuing:
Don't discontinue without consulting doctor, even though symptoms diminish or disappear.

Others:
No problems expected.

POSSIBLE INTERACTION WITH OTHER DRUGS

GENERIC NAME OR DRUG CLASS	COMBINED EFFECT
Antiarrhythmics, others*	Increased possibility of adverse reactions from either drug.
Beta-adrenergic blockers*	Irregular heartbeat. May worsen congestive heart failure.
Bone marrow depressants* such as anticancer drugs, azathioprine, chloramphenicol, colchicine, flucytosine, oxyphenbutazone, penicillamine, phenylbutazone, primaquine, pyrimethamine, trimethoprim	Decreased production of blood cells in bone marrow.
Cimetidine	May increase tocainide effect and toxicity.
Clozapine	Toxic effect on bone marrow.
Encainide	Increased effect of toxicity on heart muscle.
Guanfacine	Increased effect of both medicines.
Nicardipine	Increased effect and toxicity of each drug.
Nimodipine	Increased likelihood of adverse effect from either drug.
Propafenone	Increased effect of both drugs and increased risk of toxicity.
Tiopronin	Increased risk of toxicity to bone marrow.

POSSIBLE INTERACTION WITH OTHER SUBSTANCES

INTERACTS WITH	COMBINED EFFECT
Alcohol:	Possible irregular heartbeat. Avoid.
Beverages: Caffeine drinks, iced drinks.	Possible irregular heartbeat.
Cocaine:	Possible light-headedness, dizziness, quivering, convulsions.
Foods:	None expected.
Marijuana:	None expected.
Tobacco:	Possible irregular heartbeat.

TRAZODONE

BRAND NAMES

Desyrel   Trialodine
Trazon

BASIC INFORMATION

Habit forming? No
Prescription needed? Yes
Available as generic? Yes
Drug class: Antidepressant (non-tricyclic)

USES

- Treats mental depression.
- Treats anxiety.

DOSAGE & USAGE INFORMATION

How to take:
Tablet—Swallow with liquid or food to lessen stomach irritation. If you can't swallow whole, crumble tablet and take with liquid or food.

When to take:
According to prescription directions. Bedtime dose usually higher than other doses.

If you forget a dose:
Take as soon as you remember up to 2 hours late. If more than 2 hours, wait for next scheduled dose (don't double this dose).

What drug does:
Inhibits serotonin uptake in brain cells.

Time lapse before drug works:
2 to 4 weeks for full effect.

Don't take with:
Any other medicine without consulting your doctor or pharmacist.

OVERDOSE

SYMPTOMS:
Fainting, irregular heartbeat, respiratory arrest, chest pain, seizures, coma.
WHAT TO DO:
- **Dial 0 (operator) or 911 (emergency) for an ambulance or medical help. Then give first aid immediately.**
- **If patient is unconscious and not breathing, give mouth-to-mouth breathing. If there is no heartbeat, use cardiac massage and mouth-to-mouth breathing (CPR). Don't try to make patient vomit. If you can't get help quickly, take patient to nearest emergency facility.**
- **See emergency information on inside covers.**

POSSIBLE ADVERSE REACTIONS OR SIDE EFFECTS

SYMPTOMS	WHAT TO DO
Life-threatening:	
In case of overdose, see previous column.	
Common:	
Drowsiness.	Continue. Call doctor when convenient.
Infrequent:	
• Prolonged penile erections.	Seek emergency treatment immediately.
• Tremor, fainting, incoordination, blood pressue rise or drop, rapid heartbeat, shortness of breath.	Discontinue. Call doctor right away.
• Disorientation, confusion, fatigue, dizziness on standing, headache, nervousness, rash, itchy skin, blurred vision, ringing in ears, dry mouth, bad taste, diarrhea, nausea, vomiting, constipation, aching, menstrual changes, diminished sex drive, nightmares, vivid dreams.	Continue. Call doctor when convenient.
Rare:	
Unusual excitement	Discontinue. Call doctor right away.

WARNINGS & PRECAUTIONS

Don't take if:
- You are allergic to trazodone.
- You are thinking about suicide.

Before you start, consult your doctor:
- If you have heart rhythm problem.
- If you have any heart disease.
- If you will have surgery within 2 months, including dental surgery, requiring general or spinal anesthesia.

Over age 60:
Adverse reactions and side effects may be more frequent and severe than in younger persons.

Pregnancy:
Risk to unborn child outweighs drug benefits. Don't use.

Breast-feeding:
Drug passes into milk. Avoid drug or discontinue nursing until you finish medicine. Consult doctor for advice on maintaining milk supply.

Infants & children:
Not recommended.

Prolonged use:
Occasional blood counts, especially if you have fever and sore throat.

Skin & sunlight:
No problems expected.

Driving, piloting or hazardous work:
Don't drive or pilot aircraft until you learn how medicine affects you. Don't work around dangerous machinery. Don't climb ladders or work in high places. Danger increases if you drink alcohol or take medicine affecting alertness and reflexes, such as antihistamines, tranquilizers, sedatives, pain medicine, narcotics and mind-altering drugs.

Discontinuing:
Don't discontinue without consulting doctor. Dose may require gradual reduction if you have taken drug for a long time. Doses of other drugs may also require adjustment.

Others:
Electroshock therapy should be avoided.

POSSIBLE INTERACTION WITH OTHER DRUGS

GENERIC NAME OR DRUG CLASS	COMBINED EFFECT
Antidepressants, other*	Excess drowsiness.
Antihistamines*	Excess drowsiness.
Antihypertensives*	Possible too low blood pressure. Avoid.
Barbiturates*	Too low blood pressure. Avoid.
Central nervous system (CNS) depressants*	Increased sedation.

Clozapine	Toxic effect on the central nervous system.
Digitalis preparations*	Possible increased digitalis level in blood.
Guanfacine	Increased effect of both medicines.
MAO inhibitors*	May add to toxic effect of each.
Nabilone	Greater depression of central nervous system.
Narcotics*	Excess drowsiness.
Phenytoin	Possible increased phenytoin level in blood.
Sedatives*	Excess drowsiness.
Sertraline	Increased depressive effects of both drugs.
Tranquilizers*	Excess drowsiness.

POSSIBLE INTERACTION WITH OTHER SUBSTANCES

INTERACTS WITH	COMBINED EFFECT
Alcohol:	Excess sedation. Avoid.
Beverages: Caffeine.	May add to heartbeat irregularity. Avoid.
Cocaine:	May add to heartbeat irregularity. Avoid.
Foods:	No problems expected.
Marijuana:	May add to heartbeat irregularity. Avoid.
Tobacco:	May add to heartbeat irregularity. Avoid.

TRETINOIN (Topical)

BRAND NAMES

Retin-A Cream
Retin-A Cream
  Regimen Kit
Retin-A Gel
Retin-A Gel
  Regimen Kit
Retin-A Solution
Retinoic Acid

Stieva-A Cream
Stieva-A Cream
  Forte
Stieva-A Gel
Stieva-A Solution
Vitamin A Acid
  Cream
Vitamin A Acid Gel

BASIC INFORMATION

Habit forming? No
Prescription needed? Yes
Available as generic? Yes
Drug class: Anti-acne (topical)

USES

Treatment for acne, psoriasis, ichthyosis, keratosis, folliculitis, flat warts.

DOSAGE & USAGE INFORMATION

How to use:
Wash skin with non-medicated soap, pat dry, wait 20 minutes before applying.
- Cream or gel—Apply to affected areas with fingertips and rub in gently.
- Solution—Apply to affected areas with gauze pad or cotton swab. Avoid getting too wet so medicine doesn't drip into eyes, mouth, lips or inside nose.
- Follow manufacturer's directions on container.

When to use:
At the same time each day.

If you forget an application:
Use as soon as you remember.

What drug does:
Increases skin-cell turnover so skin layer peels off more easily.

Continued next column

OVERDOSE

SYMPTOMS:
None expected.
WHAT TO DO:
If person swallows drug, call doctor, poison-control center or hospital emergency room for instructions.

Time lapse before drug works:
2 to 3 weeks. May require 6 weeks for maximum improvement.

Don't use with:
- Benzoyl peroxide. Apply 12 hours apart.
- Any other medicine without consulting your doctor or pharmacist.

POSSIBLE ADVERSE REACTIONS OR SIDE EFFECTS

SYMPTOMS	WHAT TO DO
Life-threatening: None expected.	
Common:	
• Pigment change in treated area, warmth or stinging, peeling.	Continue. Tell doctor at next visit.
• Sensitivity to wind or cold.	No action necessary.
Infrequent: Blistering, crusting, severe burning, swelling.	Discontinue. Call doctor right away.
Rare: None expected.	

WARNINGS & PRECAUTIONS

Don't take if:
- You are allergic to tretinoin.
- You are sunburned, windburned or have an open skin wound.

Before you start, consult your doctor:
If you have eczema.

Over age 60:
Not recommended.

Pregnancy:
No proven harm to unborn child. Avoid if possible.

Breast-feeding:
No problems expected.

Infants & children:
Not recommended.

Prolonged use:
No problems expected.

Skin & sunlight:
- May cause rash or intensify sunburn in areas exposed to sun or sunlamp.
- In some animal studies, tretinoin caused skin tumors to develop faster when treated area was exposed to ultraviolet light (sunlight or sunlamp). No proven similar effects in humans.

Driving, piloting or hazardous work:
No problems expected.

Discontinuing:
Don't discontinue without doctor's advice until you complete prescribed dose, even though symptoms diminish or disappear.

Others:
Acne may get worse before improvement starts in 2 or 3 weeks. Don't wash face more than 2 or 3 times daily.

POSSIBLE INTERACTION WITH OTHER DRUGS

GENERIC NAME OR DRUG CLASS	COMBINED EFFECT
Antiacne topical preparations, other*	Severe skin irritation.
Cosmetics (medicated)	Severe skin irritation.
Etretinate	Increased chance of toxicity of each drug.
Skin preparations with alcohol	Severe skin irritation.
Soaps or cleansers (abrasive)	Severe skin irritation.

POSSIBLE INTERACTION WITH OTHER SUBSTANCES

INTERACTS WITH	COMBINED EFFECT
Alcohol:	None expected.
Beverages:	None expected.
Cocaine:	None expected.
Foods:	None expected.
Marijuana:	None expected.
Tobacco:	None expected.

TRIAMCINOLONE

BRAND NAMES

See complete list of brand names in the *Brand Name Directory*, page 930.

BASIC INFORMATION

Habit forming? No
Prescription needed? Yes
Available as generic? Yes
Drug class: Cortisone drug (adrenal corticosteroid)

USES

- Reduces inflammation caused by many different medical problems.
- Treatment for some allergic diseases, blood disorders, kidney diseases, asthma and emphysema.
- Replaces corticosteroid deficiencies.

DOSAGE & USAGE INFORMATION

How to take:
- Tablet or syrup—Swallow with liquid or food to lessen stomach irritation. If you can't swallow whole, crumble tablet.
- Aerosol—Follow package instructions.

When to take:
At the same times each day. Take once-a-day or once-every-other-day doses in mornings.

If you forget a dose:
- Several-doses-per-day prescription—Take as soon as you remember up to 2 hours late. If more than 2 hours, wait for next scheduled dose (don't double this dose).
- Once-a-day dose or less—Wait for next dose. Double this dose.

What drug does:
Decreases inflammatory responses.

Time lapse before drug works:
2 to 4 days.

Don't take with:
Any other medicine without consulting your doctor or pharmacist.

OVERDOSE

SYMPTOMS:
Headache, convulsions, heart failure.
WHAT TO DO:
- **Dial 0 (operator) or 911 (emergency) for an ambulance or medical help. Then give first aid immediately.**
- **See emergency information on inside covers.**

POSSIBLE ADVERSE REACTIONS OR SIDE EFFECTS

SYMPTOMS	WHAT TO DO
Life-threatening:	
Hives, rash, intense itching, faintness soon after a dose (anaphylaxis).	Seek emergency treatment immediately.
Common:	
Acne, thirst, indigestion, nausea, vomiting, poor wound healing, decreased growth in children, constipation, gaseousness, unpleasant taste, diarrhea, headache, cough, dizziness, hoarseness, appetite gain or loss.	Continue. Call doctor when convenient.
Infrequent:	
• Black, bloody or tarry stool; various infections; swallowing difficulties.	Discontinue. Seek emergency treatment.
• Blurred vision, halos around lights, muscle cramps, swollen legs and feet, sore throat, fever.	Discontinue. Call doctor right away.
• Mood change, fatigue, weakness, insomnia, restlessness, frequent urination, weight gain, round face, menstrual irregularities, dry mouth, euphoria, nosebleeds.	Continue. Call doctor when convenient.
Rare:	
• Irregular heartbeat.	Discontinue. Seek emergency treatment.
• Rash, pancreatitis, numbness or tingling in hands or feet, thrombophlebitis, hallucinations, convulsions.	Discontinue. Call doctor right away.

WARNINGS & PRECAUTIONS

Don't take if:
- You are allergic to any cortisone drug.
- You have tuberculosis or fungus infection.
- You have herpes infection of eyes, lips or genitals.
- You have bone disease, thyroid disease, colitis, peptic ulcer, diabetes, myasthenia gravis, liver or kidney disease, diverticulitis, glaucoma, heart disease.

Before you start, consult your doctor:
- If you have had tuberculosis.
- If you have congestive heart failure, diabetes, peptic ulcer, glaucoma, underactive thyroid, high blood pressure, myasthenia gravis, blood clots in legs or lungs.

Over age 60:
Adverse reactions and side effects may be more frequent and severe than in younger persons. Likely to aggravate edema, diabetes or ulcers. Likely to cause cataracts and osteoporosis (softening of the bones).

Pregnancy:
Risk to unborn child outweighs drug benefits. Don't use.

Breast-feeding:
Drug passes into milk. Avoid drug or discontinue nursing until you finish medicine. Consult doctor for advice on maintaining milk supply.

Infants & children:
Use only under medical supervision.

Prolonged use:
- Retards growth in children.
- Possible glaucoma, cataracts, diabetes, fragile bones and thin skin.
- Functional dependence.
- Talk to your doctor about the need for follow-up medical examinations or laboratory studies to check blood pressure, serum electrolytes, stools for blood.

Skin & sunlight:
No problems expected.

Driving, piloting or hazardous work:
No problems expected.

Discontinuing:
- Don't discontinue without doctor's advice until you complete prescribed dose, even though symptoms diminish or disappear.
- Drug affects your response to surgery, illness, injury or stress for 2 years after discontinuing. Tell anyone who takes medical care of you within 2 years about drug.

Others:
- Avoid immunizations if possible.
- Your resistance to infection is less while taking this medicine.
- Advise any doctor or dentist whom you consult that you take this medicine.

POSSIBLE INTERACTION WITH OTHER DRUGS

GENERIC NAME OR DRUG CLASS	COMBINED EFFECT
Amphotericin B	Potassium depletion.
Anticholinergics*	Possible glaucoma.
Anticoagulants, oral*	Decreased anticoagulant effect.
Anticonvulsants, hydantoin*	Decreased triamcinolone effect.
Antidiabetics, oral*	Decreased antidiabetic effect.
Antihistamines*	Decreased triamcinolone effect.
Aspirin	Increased triamcinolone effect.
Attenuated virus vaccines*	Possible viral infection.
Barbiturates*	Decreased triamcinolone effect. Oversedation.
Chloral hydrate	Decreased triamcinolone effect.
Chlorthalidone	Potassium depletion.
Cholestyramine	Decreased triamcinolone absorption.
Cholinergics*	Decreased cholinergic effect.
Colestipol	Decreased triamcinolone absorption.
Contraceptives, oral*	Increased triamcinolone effect.
Digitalis preparations*	Dangerous potassium depletion. Possible digitalis toxicity.
Diuretics, thiazide*	Potassium depletion.
Ephedrine	Decreased triamcinolone effect.
Estrogens*	Increased triamcinolone effect.
Ethacrynic acid	Potassium depletion.

Continued page 965

POSSIBLE INTERACTION WITH OTHER SUBSTANCES

INTERACTS WITH	COMBINED EFFECT
Alcohol:	Risk of stomach ulcers.
Beverages:	No proven problems.
Cocaine:	Overstimulation. Avoid.
Foods:	No proven problems.
Marijuana:	Decreased immunity.
Tobacco:	Increased triamcinolone effect. Possible toxicity.

*See Glossary

TRIAMTERENE

BRAND NAMES

Dyrenium

BASIC INFORMATION

Habit forming? No
Prescription needed? Yes
Available as generic? No
Drug class: Antihypertensive, diuretic

USES

- Reduces fluid retention (edema).
- Reduces potassium loss.

DOSAGE & USAGE INFORMATION

How to take:
Capsule—Swallow with liquid or food to lessen stomach irritation. If you can't swallow whole, open capsule and take with liquid or food.

When to take:
- 1 dose per day—Take after breakfast.
- More than 1 dose per day—Take last dose no later than 6 p.m.

If you forget a dose:
Take as soon as you remember up to 6 hours late. If more than 6 hours, wait for next scheduled dose (don't double this dose).

What drug does:
Increases urine production to eliminate sodium and water from body while conserving potassium.

Continued next column

OVERDOSE

SYMPTOMS:
Lethargy, nausea, vomiting, hypotension, irregular heartbeat, coma.
WHAT TO DO:
- **Dial 0 (operator) or 911 (emergency) for an ambulance or medical help. Then give first aid immediately.**
- **If patient is unconscious and not breathing, give mouth-to-mouth breathing. If there is no heartbeat, use cardiac massage and mouth-to-mouth breathing (CPR). Don't try to make patient vomit. If you can't get help quickly, take patient to nearest emergency facility.**
- **See emergency information on inside covers.**

Time lapse before drug works:
2 hours. May require 2 to 3 days for maximum benefit.

Don't take with:
Any other medicine without consulting your doctor or pharmacist.

POSSIBLE ADVERSE REACTIONS OR SIDE EFFECTS

SYMPTOMS	WHAT TO DO
Life-threatening:	
Hives, rash, intense itching, faintness soon after a dose (anaphylaxis).	Seek emergency treatment immediately.
Common:	
Constipation, decreased interest in sex.	Continue. Call doctor when convenient.
Infrequent:	
• Drowsiness, thirst, dry mouth, confusion, irregular heartbeat, shortness of breath, kidney stones, unusual tiredness, weakness, fever and chills, cracked mouth corners, black stools, dry mouth.	Discontinue. Call doctor right away.
• Diarrhea.	Continue. Call doctor when convenient.
• Anxiety.	Continue. Tell doctor at next visit.
Rare:	
• Rash, sore throat, red or inflamed tongue, unusual bleeding or bruising.	Discontinue. Call doctor right away.
• Headache.	Continue. Tell doctor at next visit.

WARNINGS & PRECAUTIONS

Don't take if:
- You are allergic to triamterene.
- You have had severe liver or kidney disease.

Before you start, consult your doctor:
- If you have gout, diabetes, kidney stones.
- If you will have surgery within 2 months, including dental surgery, requiring general or spinal anesthesia.

Over age 60:
- Warm weather or fever can decrease blood pressure. Dose may require adjustment.
- Extended use can increase blood clots.

Pregnancy:
No proven harm to unborn child. Avoid if possible.

Breast-feeding:
Safety not established. Consult doctor.

Infants & children:
Used infrequently. Use only under medical supervision.

Prolonged use:
- Potassium retention which may lead to heart-rhythm problems.
- Talk to your doctor about the need for follow-up medical examinations or laboratory studies to check blood pressure, kidney function, ECG* and serum electrolytes.

Skin & sunlight:
May cause rash or intensify sunburn in areas exposed to sun or sunlamp.

Driving, piloting or hazardous work:
Avoid if you feel drowsy or confused. Otherwise, no problems expected.

Discontinuing:
Don't discontinue without consulting doctor. Dose may require gradual reduction if you have taken drug for a long time. Doses of other drugs may also require adjustment.

Others:
No problems expected.

POSSIBLE INTERACTION WITH OTHER DRUGS

GENERIC NAME OR DRUG CLASS	COMBINED EFFECT
ACE inhibitors*: captopril, enalapril, lisinopril	Possible excessive potassium in blood.
Amiloride	Dangerous retention of potassium.
Amiodarone	Increased risk of heartbeat irregularity due to low potassium.
Antihypertensives, other*	Increased effect of other antihypertensives.
Calcium supplements*	Increased calcium in blood.
Carteolol	Increased antihypertensive effect.

	COMBINED EFFECT
Cyclosporine	Possible excessive potassium in blood.
Digitalis preparations*	Possible decreased digitalis effect.
Indomethacin	Possible acute renal failure.
Lithium	Increased lithium effect.
Nicardipine	Blood pressure drop. Dosages may require adjustment.
Nimodipine	Dangerous blood pressure drop.
Nitrates*	Excessive blood pressure drop.
Potassium supplements*	Possible excessive potassium retention.
Potassium iodide	May raise potassium level in blood to toxic levels.
Sotalol	Increased antihypertensive effect.
Spironolactone	Dangerous retention of potassium.
Terazosin	Decreases effectiveness of terazosin.

POSSIBLE INTERACTION WITH OTHER SUBSTANCES

INTERACTS WITH	COMBINED EFFECT
Alcohol:	None expected.
Beverages:	None expected.
Cocaine:	Increased risk of heart block and high blood pressure.
Foods: Salt.	Don't restrict unless directed by doctor.
Marijuana:	Daily use—Fainting likely.
Tobacco:	None expected.

TRIAMTERENE & HYDROCHLOROTHIAZIDE

BRAND NAMES

Apo-Triazide   Maxzide
Dyazide   Novotriamzide

BASIC INFORMATION

Habit forming? No
Prescription needed? Yes
Available as generic? Yes
Drug class: Diuretic

USES

- Reduces fluid retention (edema).
- Reduces potassium loss.
- Controls, but doesn't cure, high blood pressure.

DOSAGE & USAGE INFORMATION

How to take:
Tablet or capsule—Swallow with liquid. If you can't swallow whole, crumble tablet or open capsule and take with liquid or food.

When to take:
- 1 dose per day—Take after breakfast.
- More than 1 dose per day—Take last dose no later than 6 p.m.

If you forget a dose:
Take as soon as you remember up to 6 hours late. If more than 6 hours, wait for next scheduled dose (don't double this dose).

What drug does:
- Increases urine production to eliminate sodium and water from body while conserving potassium.
- Forces sodium and water excretion, reducing body fluid.
- Relaxes muscle cells of small arteries.
- Reduced body fluid and relaxed arteries lower blood pressure.

Continued next column

OVERDOSE

SYMPTOMS:
Lethargy, irregular heartbeat, cramps, nausea, vomiting, hypotension, weakness, drowsiness, weak pulse, coma.
WHAT TO DO:
- **Dial 0 (operator) or 911 (emergency) for an ambulance or medical help. Then give first aid immediately.**
- **See emergency information on inside covers.**

Time lapse before drug works:
4 to 6 hours. May require several weeks to lower blood pressure.

Don't take with:
Any prescription or non-prescription drugs without consulting your doctor.

POSSIBLE ADVERSE REACTIONS OR SIDE EFFECTS

SYMPTOMS	WHAT TO DO
Life-threatening: Irregular heartbeat, weak pulse, shortness of breath; hives, rash, intense itching, faintness soon after a dose (anaphylaxis).	Discontinue. Seek emergency treatment.
Common: • Mood change, muscle cramps.	Discontinue. Call doctor right away.
• Numbness or tingling in hands or feet, constipation, decreased interest in sex.	Continue. Call doctor when convenient.
Infrequent: • Blurred vision, abdominal pain, nausea, vomiting, kidney stones, fever and chills, red tongue, cracked mouth corners, black stools, dry mouth.	Discontinue. Call doctor right away.
• Dizziness, mood change, headache, weakness, tiredness, weight gain or loss.	Continue. Call doctor when convenient.
Rare: Sore throat, mouth sores, jaundice, rash, joint or muscle pain, hives, unexplained bleeding or bruising.	Discontinue. Call doctor right away.

WARNINGS & PRECAUTIONS

Don't take if:
- If you are allergic to triamterene or any thiazide diuretic drug.
- If you have had severe liver or kidney disease.

Before you start, consult your doctor:
- If you have gout, diabetes, liver, pancreas or kidney disorder.
- You are allergic to any sulfa drug.
- If you will have surgery within 2 months, including dental surgery, requiring general or spinal anesthesia.

TRIAMTERENE & HYDROCHLOROTHIAZIDE

Over age 60:
- Adverse reactions and side effects may be more frequent and severe than in younger persons, especially dizziness and excessive potassium loss.
- Warm weather or fever can decrease blood pressure. Dose may require adjustment.
- Extended use can increase blood clots.

Pregnancy:
Risk to unborn child outweighs drug benefits. Don't use.

Breast-feeding:
Drug passes into milk. Avoid drug or discontinue nursing until you finish medicine. Consult doctor for advice on maintaining milk supply.

Infants & children:
Used infrequently. Use only under medical supervision.

Prolonged use:
- Potassium retention which may lead to heart-rhythm problems.
- Talk to your doctor about the need for follow-up medical examinations or laboratory studies to check blood pressure, kidney function, ECG* and serum electrolytes.

Skin & sunlight:
May cause rash or intensify sunburn in areas exposed to sun or sunlamp.

Driving, piloting or hazardous work:
Don't drive or pilot aircraft until you learn how medicine affects you. Don't work around dangerous machinery. Don't climb ladders or work in high places. Danger increases if you drink alcohol or take medicine affecting alertness and reflexes, such as antihistamines, tranquilizers, sedatives, pain medicine, narcotics and mind-altering drugs.

Discontinuing:
Don't discontinue without consulting doctor. Dose may require gradual reduction if you have taken drug for a long time. Doses of other drugs may also require adjustment.

Others:
- Hot weather and fever may cause dehydration and drop in blood pressure. Dose may require temporary adjustment. Weigh daily and report any unexpected weight decreases to your doctor.
- May cause rise in uric acid, leading to gout.
- May cause blood-sugar rise in diabetics.

 POSSIBLE INTERACTION WITH OTHER DRUGS

GENERIC NAME OR DRUG CLASS	COMBINED EFFECT
ACE inhibitors*: captopril, enalapril, lisinopril	Decreased blood pressure.
Allopurinol	Decreased allopurinol effect.
Amiloride	Dangerous retention of potassium.
Amphotericin B	Increased potassium.
Antidepressants*	Dangerous drop in blood pressure. Avoid combination unless under medical supervision.
Antihypertensives*	Increased hypertensive effect.
Barbiturates*	Increased hydro-chlorothiazide effect.
Beta-adrenergic blockers*	Increased antihypertensive effect. Dosages of both drugs may require adjustment.
Cholestyramine	Decreased hydro-chlorothiazide effect.
Cortisone drugs*	Excessive potassium loss that causes dangerous heart rhythms.
Digitalis preparations*	Excessive potassium loss that causes dangerous heart rhythms.
Diuretics, thiazide*	Increased effect of other thiazide diuretics.
Indapamide	Increased diuretic effect.

Continued page 965

 POSSIBLE INTERACTION WITH OTHER SUBSTANCES

INTERACTS WITH	COMBINED EFFECT
Alcohol:	Dangerous blood pressure drop.
Beverages:	None expected.
Cocaine:	Decreased triamterene effect.
Foods: Salt.	Don't restrict unless directed by doctor.
Marijuana:	Daily use—Fainting likely.
Tobacco:	Decreases drug's effectiveness.

*See Glossary

TRIAZOLAM

BRAND NAMES

Apo-Triazo   Novotriolam
Halcion

BASIC INFORMATION

Habit forming? Yes
Prescription needed? Yes
Available as generic? Yes
Drug class: Sedative (hypnotic)

USES

- Treatment for insomnia.
- Prevention or treatment of transient insomnia associated with sudden sleep schedule changes such as travel across several time zones.

DOSAGE & USAGE INFORMATION

How to take:
Tablet—Swallow with liquid If you can't swallow whole, crumble tablet and take with liquid or food.

When to take:
At the same time each day, according to instructions on prescription label.

If you forget a dose:
Take as soon as you remember up to 2 hours late. If more than 2 hours, wait for next scheduled dose (don't double this dose).

What drug does:
Affects limbic system of brain, the part that controls emotions.

Time lapse before drug works:
2 hours. May take 6 weeks for full benefit.

Continued next column

OVERDOSE

SYMPTOMS:
Drowsiness, weakness, tremor, stupor, coma.
WHAT TO DO:
- **Dial 0 (operator) or 911 (emergency) for an ambulance or medical help. Then give first aid immediately.**
- **If patient is unconscious and not breathing, give mouth-to-mouth breathing. If there is no heartbeat, use cardiac massage and mouth-to-mouth breathing (CPR). Don't try to make patient vomit. If you can't get help quickly, take patient to nearest emergency facility.**
- **See emergency information on inside covers.**

Don't take with:
Any prescription or non-prescription drugs without consulting your doctor.

POSSIBLE ADVERSE REACTIONS OR SIDE EFFECTS

SYMPTOMS	WHAT TO DO
Life-threatening:	
In case of overdose, see previous column.	
Common:	
Clumsiness, drowsiness, dizziness.	Continue. Call doctor when convenient.
Infrequent:	
• Amnesia, hallucinations, confusion, depression, irritability, rash, itch, vision changes, sore throat, fever, chills, dry mouth.	Discontinue. Call doctor right away.
• Constipation or diarrhea, nausea, vomiting, difficult urination, vivid dreams, behavior changes, abdominal pain, headache.	Continue. Call doctor when convenient.
Rare:	
• Slow heartbeat, breathing difficulty.	Discontinue. Seek emergency treatment.
• Mouth, throat ulcers; jaundice.	Discontinue. Call doctor right away.
• Decreased sex drive.	Continue. Call doctor when convenient.

WARNINGS & PRECAUTIONS

Don't take if:
- You are allergic to any benzodiazepine.
- You have myasthenia gravis.
- You are an active or recovering alcoholic.
- Patient is younger than 6 months.

Before you start, consult your doctor:
- If you have liver, kidney or lung disease.
- If you have diabetes, epilepsy or porphyria.
- If you have glaucoma.

Over age 60:
Adverse reactions and side effects may be more frequent and severe than in younger persons. You may need smaller doses for shorter periods of time. You may develop agitation, rage or a "hangover" effect.

Pregnancy:
Risk to unborn child outweighs drug benefits. Don't use.

Breast-feeding:
Drug passes into milk. Avoid drug or discontinue nursing until you finish medicine. Consult doctor for advice on maintaining milk supply.

Infants & children:
Use only under medical supervision for children older than 6 months.

Prolonged use:
May impair liver function.

Skin & sunlight:
No problems expected.

Driving, piloting or hazardous work:
Don't drive or pilot aircraft until you learn how medicine affects you. Don't work around dangerous machinery. Don't climb ladders or work in high places. Danger increases if you drink alcohol or take medicine affecting alertness and reflexes.

Discontinuing:
Don't discontinue without consulting doctor. Dose may require gradual reduction if you have taken drug for a long time. Doses of other drugs may also require adjustment.

Others:
- Hot weather, heavy exercise and profuse sweat may reduce excretion and cause overdose.
- Blood sugar may rise in diabetics, requiring insulin adjustment.
- Don't use for insomnia more than 4-7 days.
- Advise any doctor or dentist whom you consult that you take this medicine.
- Triazolam has a very short duration of action in the body.

POSSIBLE INTERACTION WITH OTHER DRUGS

GENERIC NAME OR DRUG CLASS	COMBINED EFFECT
Anticonvulsants*	Change in seizure frequency or severity.
Antidepressants*	Increased sedative effect of both drugs.
Antihistamines*	Increased sedative effect of both drugs.
Antihypertensives*	Excessively low blood pressure.
Cimetadine	Increased triazolam effect.
Clozapine	Toxic effect on the central nervous system.
Contraceptives, oral*	Increased triazolam effect.
Disulfiram	Increased triazolam effect.
Dronabinol	Increased effects of both drugs. Avoid.
Erythromycins*	Increased triazolam effect.
Isoniazid	Increased triazolam effect.
Ketoconazole	Increased triazolam effect.
Levodopa	Possible decreased levodopa effect.
MAO inhibitors*	Convulsions, deep sedation, rage.
Molindone	Increased tranquilizer effect.
Nabilone	Greater depression of central nervous system.
Narcotics*	Increased sedative effect of both drugs.
Nicotine	Increased triazolam effect.
Nizatidine	Increased effect and toxicity of triazolam.
Omeprazole	Delayed excretion of triazolam causing increased amount of triazolam in blood.
Probenecid	Increased triazolam effect.
Sedatives*	Increased sedative effect of both drugs.
Sleep inducers*	Increased sedative effect of both drugs.
Tranquilizers*	Increased sedative effect of both drugs.
Zidovudine	Increased toxicity of zidovudine.

POSSIBLE INTERACTION WITH OTHER SUBSTANCES

INTERACTS WITH	COMBINED EFFECT
Alcohol:	Heavy sedation. Avoid.
Beverages:	None expected.
Cocaine:	Decreased triazolam effect.
Foods:	None expected.
Marijuana:	Heavy sedation. Avoid.
Tobacco:	Decreased triazolam effect.

*See Glossary

TRICYCLIC ANTIDEPRESSANTS

BRAND AND GENERIC NAMES

See complete list of brand and generic names in the *Brand Name Directory,* page 930.

BASIC INFORMATION

Habit forming? No
Prescription needed? Yes
Available as generic? Yes
Drug class: Antidepressant (tricyclic)

 ## USES

- Gradually relieves, but doesn't cure, symptoms of depression.
- Imipramine is also used to decrease bedwetting.
- Pain relief (sometimes).
- Clomipramine is used to treat obsessive-compulsive disorder.
- Protriptyline may be used to treat attention-deficit disorder.

 ## DOSAGE & USAGE INFORMATION

How to take:
Tablet, capsule or syrup—Swallow with liquid.

When to take:
At the same time each day, usually at bedtime.

If you forget a dose:
Bedtime dose—If you forget your once-a-day bedtime dose, don't take it more than 3 hours late. If more than 3 hours, wait for next scheduled dose. Don't double this dose.

Continued next column

 ## OVERDOSE

SYMPTOMS:
Hallucinations, drowsiness, enlarged pupils, respiratory failure, fever, cardiac arrhythmias, convulsions, coma.
WHAT TO DO:
- **Dial 0 (operator) or 911 (emergency) for an ambulance or medical help. Then give first aid immediately.**
- **If patient is unconscious and not breathing, give mouth-to-mouth breathing. If there is no heartbeat, use cardiac massage and mouth-to-mouth breathing (CPR). Don't try to make patient vomit. If you can't get help quickly, take patient to nearest emergency facility.**
- **See emergency information on inside covers.**

What drug does:
Probably affects part of brain that controls messages between nerve cells.

Time lapse before drug works:
Begins in 1 to 2 weeks. May require 4 to 6 weeks for maximum benefit.

Don't take with:
Any prescription or non-prescription drugs without consulting your doctor.

 ## POSSIBLE ADVERSE REACTIONS OR SIDE EFFECTS

SYMPTOMS	WHAT TO DO
Life-threatening:	
In case of overdose, see previous column.	
Common:	
• Tremor.	Discontinue. Call doctor right away.
• Headache, dry mouth or unpleasant taste, constipation or diarrhea, nausea, indigestion, fatigue, weakness, drowsiness, nervousness, anxiety, excessive sweating	Continue. Call doctor when convenient.
• Insomnia, "sweet tooth."	Continue. Tell doctor at next visit.
Infrequent:	
• Convulsions.	Discontinue. Seek emergency treatment.
• Hallucinations, shakiness, dizziness, fainting, blurred vision, eye pain, vomiting, irregular heartbeat or slow pulse, inflamed tongue, abdominal pain, jaundice, hair loss, rash, fever, chills, joint pain, palpitations, hiccups, visual changes.	Discontinue. Call doctor right away.
• Difficult or frequent urination; decreased sex drive; muscle aches; abnormal dreams; nasal congestion; weakness and faintness when arising from bed or chair; back pain.	Continue. Call doctor when convenient.
Rare:	
Itchy skin; sore throat; involuntary movements of jaw, lips and tongue; nightmares; confusion; swollen breasts; swollen testicles.	Discontinue. Call doctor right away.

WARNINGS & PRECAUTIONS

Don't take if:
- You are allergic to any tricyclic antidepressant.
- You drink alcohol.
- You have had a heart attack within 6 weeks.
- You have glaucoma.
- You have taken MAO inhibitors within 2 weeks.
- Patient is younger than 12.

Before you start, consult your doctor:
- If you will have surgery within 2 months, including dental surgery, requiring general or spinal anesthesia.
- If you have an enlarged prostate.
- If you have heart disease or high blood pressure.
- If you have stomach or intestinal problems.
- If you have an overactive thyroid.
- If you have asthma.
- If you have liver disease.

Over age 60:
More likely to develop urination difficulty and side effects such as seizures, hallucinations, shaking, dizziness, fainting, headache, insomnia.

Pregnancy:
Studies inconclusive on harm to unborn child. Animal studies show fetal abnormalities. Decide with your doctor whether drug benefits justify risk to unborn child.

Breast-feeding:
Drug passes into milk. Avoid drug or discontinue nursing until you finish medicine. Consult doctor about maintaining milk supply.

Infants & children:
Don't give to children younger than 12 except under medical supervision.

Prolonged use:
Talk to your doctor about the need for follow-up medical examinations or laboratory studies to check complete blood counts (white blood cell count, platelet count, red blood cell count, hemoglobin, hematocrit), blood pressure, eyes, teeth.

Skin & sunlight:
May cause rash or intensify sunburn in areas exposed to sun or sunlamp.

Driving, piloting or hazardous work:
Don't drive or pilot aircraft until you learn how medicine affects you. Don't work around dangerous machinery. Don't climb ladders or work in high places. Danger increases if you drink alcohol or take medicine affecting alertness and reflexes.

Discontinuing:
- Don't discontinue without consulting doctor. Dose may require gradual reduction if you have taken drug for a long time. Doses of other drugs may also require adjustment.

- Withdrawal symptoms such as convulsions, muscle cramps, nightmares, insomnia, abdominal pain. Call your physician right away if any of these occur.

Others:
No problems expected.

POSSIBLE INTERACTION WITH OTHER DRUGS

GENERIC NAME OR DRUG CLASS	COMBINED EFFECT
Anticoagulants, oral*	Possible increased anticoagulant effect.
Anticholinergics*	Increased anticholinergic effect.
Antihistamines*	Increased antihistamine effect.
Barbiturates*	Decreased antidepressant effect. Increased sedation.
Benzodiazepines*	Increased sedation.
Bupropion	Increased risk of major seizures.
Central nervous system (CNS) depressants*	Excessive sedation.

Continued page 966

POSSIBLE INTERACTION WITH OTHER SUBSTANCES

INTERACTS WITH	COMBINED EFFECT
Alcohol: Beverages or medicines with alcohol.	Excessive intoxication. Avoid.
Beverages:	None expected.
Cocaine:	Increased risk of heartbeat irregularity.
Foods: Breads, crackers, cookies, cheeses, peanut butter, corn, lentils, cranberries, plums, prunes, peanuts, Brazil nuts, walnuts, pastas, bacon, meat, fowl, eggs, fish (if taken with).	Decreased effectiveness of the antidepressant.
Marijuana:	Excessive drowsiness. Avoid.
Tobacco:	Possible decreased tricyclic antidepressant effect.

TRILOSTANE

BRAND NAMES

Modrastane

BASIC INFORMATION

Habit forming? No
Prescription needed? Yes
Available as generic? No
Drug class: Antiadrenal

 ## USES

Temporary treatment of Cushing's syndrome until surgery on adrenals or radiation to pituitary gland can be performed.

 ## DOSAGE & USAGE INFORMATION

How to take:
Capsules—Swallow with liquid. If you can't swallow whole, open capsule and take with liquid or food. Instructions to take on empty stomach mean 1 hour before or 2 hours after eating.

When to take:
Follow doctor's instructions.

If you forget a dose:
Take as soon as you remember up to 2 hours late. If more than 2 hours, wait for next scheduled dose (don't double this dose).

What drug does:
Decreases function of the adrenal cortex.

Time lapse before drug works:
8 hours.

Don't take with:
Any other medicines (including over-the-counter drugs such as cough and cold medicines, laxatives, antacids, diet pills, caffeine, nose drops or vitamins) without consulting your doctor.

 ## OVERDOSE

SYMPTOMS:
None expected.
WHAT TO DO:
Overdose unlikely to threaten life. If person takes much larger amount than prescribed, call doctor, poison-control center or hospital emergency room for instructions.

 ## POSSIBLE ADVERSE REACTIONS OR SIDE EFFECTS

SYMPTOMS	WHAT TO DO
Life-threatening: None expected.	
Common: Diarrhea, abdominal pain.	Discontinue. Call doctor right away.
Infrequent: Muscle ache, bloating, watery eyes, nausea, increased salivation, flushing, burning mouth or nose.	Continue. Call doctor when convenient.
Rare: Darkening skin, tiredness, appetite loss, depression, skin rash, vomiting.	Continue. Call doctor when convenient.

WARNINGS & PRECAUTIONS

Don't take if:
You know you are allergic to trilostane.

Before you start, consult your doctor:
- If you have an infection.
- If you will have surgery while taking.
- If you have a head injury.
- If you have kidney disease.

Over age 60:
Adverse reactions and side effects may be more frequent and severe than in younger persons. You may need smaller doses for shorter periods of time.

Pregnancy:
Risk to unborn child outweighs drug benefits. Don't use.

Breast-feeding:
Safety not established. Consult doctor.

Infants & children:
Effect not documented. Consult your pediatrician.

Prolonged use:
- Not intended for prolonged use.
- Talk to your doctor about the need for follow-up medical examinations or laboratory studies to check serum electrolytes and urinary 17 - hydroxycorticosteroid.

Skin & sunlight:
No problems expected.

Driving, piloting or hazardous work:
Avoid if you feel confused, drowsy or dizzy.

Discontinuing:
No special problems expected.

Others:
- Advise any doctor or dentist whom you consult that you take this medicine.
- May affect results in some medical tests.

POSSIBLE INTERACTION WITH OTHER DRUGS

GENERIC NAME OR DRUG CLASS	COMBINED EFFECT
Aminoglutethimide	Too much decrease in adrenal function.
Mitotane	Too much decrease in adrenal function.

POSSIBLE INTERACTION WITH OTHER SUBSTANCES

INTERACTS WITH	COMBINED EFFECT
Alcohol:	No special problems expected.
Beverages:	No special problems expected.
Cocaine:	No special problems expected.
Foods:	No special problems expected.
Marijuana:	No special problems expected.
Tobacco:	No special problems expected.

*See Glossary

TRIMEPRAZINE

BRAND NAMES

Panectyl   Temaril

BASIC INFORMATION

Habit forming? No
Prescription needed? Yes
Available as generic? Yes
Drug class: Tranquilizer (phenothiazine),
antihistamine

USES

Relieves itching of hives, skin allergies,
chickenpox.

DOSAGE & USAGE INFORMATION

How to take:
* Tablet or syrup—Swallow with liquid or food
to lessen stomach irritation.
* Extended-release capsules—Swallow each
dose whole. If you take regular tablets, you
may chew or crush them.

When to take:
At the same times each day.

If you forget a dose:
Take as soon as you remember up to 2 hours
late. If more than 2 hours, wait for next
scheduled dose (don't double this dose).

What drug does:
Blocks histamine action in skin.

Time lapse before drug works:
1 to 2 hours.

Don't take with:
* Antacid or medicine for diarrhea.
* Non-prescription drug for cough, cold or
allergy.
* Any other medicine without consulting your
doctor or pharmacist.

OVERDOSE

SYMPTOMS:
**Fast heartbeat, flushed face, shortness of
breath, clumsiness, drowsiness, muscle
spasms, jerking movements of head and
face.**
WHAT TO DO:
* **Dial 0 (operator) or 911 (emergency) for
an ambulance or medical help. Then give
first aid immediately.**
* **See emergency information on inside
covers.**

POSSIBLE ADVERSE REACTIONS OR SIDE EFFECTS

SYMPTOMS	WHAT TO DO
Life-threatening:	
In case of overdose, see previous column.	
Common:	
• Restlessness, tremor, drowsiness, tiredness, weakness.	Discontinue. Call doctor right away.
• Decreased sweating, dry mouth, nasal congestion, constipation.	Continue. Call doctor when convenient.
Infrequent:	
• Fainting.	Discontinue. Seek emergency treatment.
• Rash, muscle spasms of face and neck, unsteady gait.	Discontinue. Call doctor right away.
• Difficult urination, less interest in sex, swollen breasts, menstrual irregularities, dizziness, nausea, vomiting.	Continue. Call doctor when convenient.
Rare:	
Change in vision, sore throat, fever, jaundice, confusion, nightmares, unusual excitement.	Discontinue. Call doctor right away.

WARNINGS & PRECAUTIONS

Don't take if:
* You are allergic to any phenothiazine.
* You have a blood or bone-marrow disease.

Before you start, consult your doctor:
* If you will have surgery within 2 months,
including dental surgery, requiring general or
spinal anesthesia.
* If you have asthma, emphysema or other
lung disorder.
* If you take non-prescription ulcer medicine,
asthma medicine or amphetamines.

Over age 60:
Adverse reactions and side effects may be more
frequent and severe than in younger persons.
More likely to develop tardive dyskinesia
(involuntary movement of jaws, lips, tongue,
chewing). Report this to your doctor
immediately. Early treatment can help.

Pregnancy:
Risk to unborn child outweighs drug benefits.
Don't use.

Breast-feeding:
Drug passes into milk. Avoid drug or discontinue nursing until you finish medicine. Consult doctor for advice on maintaining milk supply.

Infants & children:
Don't give to children younger than 2.

Prolonged use:
- May lead to tardive dyskinesia (involuntary movement of jaws, lips, tongue, chewing).
- Talk to your doctor about the need for follow-up medical examinations or laboratory studies to check complete blood counts (white blood cell count, platelet count, red blood cell count, hemoglobin, hematocrit), liver function, eyes.

Skin & sunlight:
May cause rash or intensify sunburn in areas exposed to sun or sunlamp. Skin may remain sensitive for 3 months after discontinuing.

Driving, piloting or hazardous work:
Don't drive or pilot aircraft until you learn how medicine affects you. Don't work around dangerous machinery. Don't climb ladders or work in high places. Danger increases if you drink alcohol or take medicine affecting alertness and reflexes.

Discontinuing:
May be unnecessary to finish medicine. Follow doctor's instructions.

Others:
No problems expected.

 ## POSSIBLE INTERACTION WITH OTHER DRUGS

GENERIC NAME OR DRUG CLASS	COMBINED EFFECT
Antacids*	Decreased trimeprazine effect.
Anticholinergics*	Increased anticholinergic effect.
Anticonvulsants, hydantoin*	Increased anticonvulsant effect.
Antidepressants, tricyclic (TCA)*	Increased trimeprazine effect.
Antihistamines, other*	Increased antihistamine effect.
Antithyroid drugs*	Increased risk of bone marrow depression.
Appetite suppressants*	Decreased suppressant effect.
Barbiturates*	Oversedation.
Carteolol	Decreased antihistamine effect.

Central nervous system (CNS) depressants*	Dangerous degree of sedation.
Clozapine	Toxic effect on the central nervous system.
Dronabinol	Increased effects of both drugs. Avoid.
Epinephrine	Epinephrine effect decreased.
Ethinamate	Dangerous increased effects of ethinamate. Avoid combining.
Extrapyramidal reaction-causing medicines*	Increases frequency and severity of extrapyramidal reactions.
Fluoxetine	Increased depressant effects of both drugs.
Guanfacine	May increase depressant effects of either medicine.
Guanethidine	Decreased guanethidine effect.
Leucovorin	High alcohol content of leucovorin may cause adverse effects.
Levodopa	Decreased levodopa effect.
MAO inhibitors*	Increased trimeprazine effect.
Metyrosine	Increased likelihood of toxic symptoms of each.
Methyprylon	May increase sedative effect to dangerous level. Avoid.

Continued on page 966

 ## POSSIBLE INTERACTION WITH OTHER SUBSTANCES

INTERACTS WITH	COMBINED EFFECT
Alcohol:	Dangerous oversedation.
Beverages:	None expected.
Cocaine:	Decreased effect of trimeprazine. Avoid.
Foods:	None expected.
Marijuana:	Drowsiness.
Tobacco:	None expected.

*See Glossary

TRIMETHOBENZAMIDE

BRAND NAMES

Tebamide
Tegamide
Ticon

Tigan
Tiject-20

BASIC INFORMATION

Habit forming? No
Prescription needed? Yes
Available as generic? Yes
Drug class: Antiemetic

 ## USES

Reduces nausea and vomiting.

 ## DOSAGE & USAGE INFORMATION

How to take:
- Capsule—Swallow with liquid. If you can't swallow whole, open capsule and take with liquid or food.
- Suppositories—Remove wrapper and moisten suppository with water. Gently insert larger end into rectum. Push well into rectum with finger.

When to take:
When needed, no more often than label directs.

If you forget a dose:
Take when you remember. Wait as long as label directs for next dose.

What drug does:
Possibly blocks nerve impulses to brain's vomiting centers.

Time lapse before drug works:
20 to 40 minutes.

Continued next column

 ## OVERDOSE

SYMPTOMS:
Confusion, convulsions, coma.
WHAT TO DO:
- **Dial 0 (operator) or 911 (emergency) for an ambulance or medical help. Then give first aid immediately.**
- **If patient is unconscious and not breathing, give mouth-to-mouth breathing. If there is no heartbeat, use cardiac massage and mouth-to-mouth breathing (CPR). Don't try to make patient vomit. If you can't get help quickly, take patient to nearest emergency facility.**
- **See emergency information on inside covers.**

Don't take with:
Any other prescription or non-prescription drugs without consulting doctor.

 ## POSSIBLE ADVERSE REACTIONS OR SIDE EFFECTS

SYMPTOMS	WHAT TO DO
Life-threatening: In case of overdose, see previous column.	
Common: None expected.	
Infrequent:	
• Rash, blurred vision, low blood pressure.	Discontinue. Call doctor right away.
• Dizziness, headache, drowsiness, diarrhea, muscle cramps, unusual tiredness.	Continue. Call doctor when convenient.
Rare:	
• Convulsions.	Discontinue. Seek emergency treatment.
• Seizures, tremor, depression, sore throat, fever, repeated vomiting, back pain, jaundice, Parkinson symptoms, neck spasms.	Discontinue. Call doctor right away.

 ## WARNINGS & PRECAUTIONS

Don't take if:
- You are allergic to trimethobenzamide.
- You are allergic to local anesthetics and have suppository form.

Before you start, consult your doctor:
If you have reacted badly to antihistamines.

Over age 60:
More susceptible to low blood pressure and sedative effects of this drug.

Pregnancy:
No proven harm to unborn child. Avoid if possible.

Breast-feeding:
No proven problems. Avoid if possible.

Infants & children:
- Injectable form not recommended.
- Avoid during viral infections. Drug may contribute to Reye's syndrome.

Prolonged use:
- Damages blood-cell production of bone marrow.
- Causes Parkinson-like symptoms of tremors, rigidity.

Skin & sunlight:
Possible sun sensitivity. Use caution.

Driving, piloting or hazardous work:
- Use disqualifies you for piloting aircraft.
- Don't drive until you learn how medicine affects you. Don't work around dangerous machinery. Don't climb ladders or work in high places. Danger increases if you drink alcohol or take medicine affecting alertness and reflexes, such as antihistamines, tranquilizers, sedatives, pain medicine, narcotics and mind-altering drugs.

Discontinuing:
May be unnecessary to finish medicine. Follow doctor's instructions.

Others:
No problems expected.

POSSIBLE INTERACTION WITH OTHER DRUGS

GENERIC NAME OR DRUG CLASS	COMBINED EFFECT
Antidepressants*	Increased sedative effect.
Antihistamines*	Increased sedative effect.
Barbiturates*	Increased effect of both drugs.
Belladonna	Increased effect of both drugs.
Cholinergics*	Increased effect of both drugs.
Clozapine	Toxic effect on the central nervous system.
Ethinamate	Dangerous increased effects of ethinamate. Avoid combining.
Fluoxetine	Increased depressant effects of both drugs.
Guanfacine	May increase depressant effects of either medicine.
Leucovorin	High alcohol content of leucovorin may cause adverse effects.
Methyprylon	May increase sedative effect to dangerous level. Avoid.
Mind-altering drugs*	Increased effect of mind-altering drug.
Nabilone	Greater depression of central nervous system.
Narcotics*	Increased sedative effect.
Phenothiazines*	Increased effect of both drugs.
Sedatives*	Increased sedative effect.
Sertraline	Increased depressive effects of both drugs.
Sleep inducers*	Increased effect of sleep inducer.
Tranquilizers*	Increased sedative effect.

POSSIBLE INTERACTION WITH OTHER SUBSTANCES

INTERACTS WITH	COMBINED EFFECT
Alcohol:	Oversedation. Avoid.
Beverages:	None expected.
Cocaine:	None expected.
Foods:	None expected.
Marijuana:	Increased antinausea effect.
Tobacco:	None expected.

TRIMETHOPRIM

BRAND NAMES

Apo-Sulfatrim	Sulfamethoprim
Bactrim	Sulfaprim
Bethaprim	Sulfatrim
Cheragan with TMP	Sulfoxaprim
Cotrim	Sulmeprim
Novotrimel	Triazole
Proloprim	Trimeth-Sulfa
Protrin	Trimpex
Roubac	Trisulfam
Septra	Uroplus
SMZ-TMP	

BASIC INFORMATION

Habit forming? No
Prescription needed? Yes
Available as generic? Yes
Drug class: Antimicrobial

USES

- Treatment for urinary-tract infections susceptible to trimethoprim.
- Helps prevent recurrent urinary-tract infections if taken once a day.

DOSAGE & USAGE INFORMATION

How to take:
Tablet—Swallow with liquid or food to lessen stomach irritation.

When to take:
Space doses evenly in 24 hours to keep constant amount in urine.

If you forget a dose:
Take as soon as possible. Wait 5 to 6 hours before next dose. Then return to regular schedule.

What drug does:
Stops harmful bacterial germs from multiplying. Will not kill viruses.

Continued in next column

OVERDOSE

SYMPTOMS:
Nausea, vomiting, diarrhea.
WHAT TO DO:
Overdose unlikely to threaten life. If person takes much larger amount than prescribed, call doctor, poison-control center or hospital emergency room for instructions.

Time lapse before drug works:
2 to 5 days.

Don't take with:
Any other medicine without consulting your doctor or pharmacist.

POSSIBLE ADVERSE REACTIONS OR SIDE EFFECTS

SYMPTOMS	WHAT TO DO
Life-threatening:	
None expected.	
Common:	
● Rash, itchy skin.	Discontinue. Seek emergency treatment.
● Unusual taste.	Continue. Call doctor when convenient.
Infrequent:	
● Diarrhea, nausea, vomiting, abdominal pain.	Discontinue. Call doctor right away.
● Headache, appetite loss, sore mouth or tongue.	Continue. Call doctor when convenient.
Rare:	
● Blue fingernails, lips and skin; difficult breathing.	Discontinue. Seek emergency treatment.
● Sore throat, fever, anemia, jaundice, unusual bleeding or bruising.	Discontinue. Call doctor right away.

876

WARNINGS & PRECAUTIONS

Don't take if:
- You are allergic to trimethoprim or any sulfa drug.
- You are anemic due to folic acid deficiency.

Before you start, consult your doctor:
If you have had liver or kidney disease.

Over age 60:
- Reduced liver and kidney function may require reduced dose.
- More likely to have severe anal and genital itch.
- Increased susceptibility to anemia.

Pregnancy:
Studies inconclusive on harm to unborn child. Animal studies show fetal abnormalities. Decide with your doctor whether drug benefits justify risk to unborn child.

Breast-feeding:
No proven harm to unborn child. Avoid if possible.

Infants & children:
Use under medical supervision only.

Prolonged use:
- Anemia.
- Talk to your doctor about the need for follow-up medical examinations or laboratory studies to check complete blood counts (white blood cell count, platelet count, red blood cell count, hemoglobin, hematocrit).

Skin & sunlight:
May cause rash or intensify sunburn in areas exposed to sun or sunlamp.

Driving, piloting or hazardous work:
No problems expected.

Discontinuing:
Don't discontinue without doctor's advice until you complete prescribed dose, even though symptoms diminish or disappear.

Others:
No problems expected.

POSSIBLE INTERACTION WITH OTHER DRUGS

GENERIC NAME OR DRUG CLASS	COMBINED EFFECT
Bone marrow depressants*	Increased possibility of bone marrow supression.
Clozapine	Toxic effect on bone marrow.
Tiopronin	Increased risk of toxicity to bone marrow.

POSSIBLE INTERACTION WITH OTHER SUBSTANCES

INTERACTS WITH	COMBINED EFFECT
Alcohol:	Increased alcohol effect with Bactrim or Septra.
Beverages:	None expected.
Cocaine:	No proven problems.
Foods:	None expected.
Marijuana:	None expected.
Tobacco:	None expected.

URSODIOL

BRAND NAMES

Actigall

BASIC INFORMATION

Habit forming? No
Prescription needed? Yes
Available as generic? No
Drug class: Anticholethitic

 ## USES

Dissolves cholesterol gallstones in selected patients who either can't tolerate surgery or don't require surgery for other reasons. Not used when surgery is clearly indicated.

 ## DOSAGE & USAGE INFORMATION

How to take:
Tablets—Swallow with liquid or food to lessen stomach irritation. If you can't swallow whole, crumble tablet and take with liquid or food.

When to take:
With meals, 2 or 3 times a day according to your doctor's instructions.

If you forget a dose:
Take as soon as you remember up to 2 hours late. If more than 2 hours, wait for next scheduled time. Don't double this dose.

What drug does:
Decreases secretion of cholesterol into bile by suppressing production and secretion of cholesterol by the liver. Ursodiol will not help gallstone problems unless the gallstones are made of cholesterol. It works best when the stones are small.

Time lapse before drug works:
Unpredictable. Varies among patients.

Don't take with:
Any other medicine without consulting your doctor or pharmacist.

 ## OVERDOSE

SYMPTOMS: Severe diarrhea.
WHAT TO DO:
Overdose not expected to threaten life. If person takes much larger amount than prescribed, call doctor, poison-control center or hospital emergency room for instructions.

 ## POSSIBLE ADVERSE REACTIONS OR SIDE EFFECTS

SYMPTOMS	WHAT TO DO
Life-threatening: None expected.	
Common: None expected.	
Infrequent: None expected.	
Rare: Diarrhea.	Continue. Call doctor when convenient.

WARNINGS & PRECAUTIONS

Don't take if:
You can't tolerate other bile acids.

Before you start, consult your doctor:
- If you have complications of gallstones, such as infection or obstruction of the bile ducts.
- If you have had pancreatitis.
- If you have had chronically impaired liver function.
- If you take any other medicines for any reason.

Over age 60:
No special problems expected.

Pregnancy:
Studies have not been performed to determine effects on unborn child. Decide with your doctor whether drug benefits justify risk to unborn child.

Breast-feeding:
Unknown, but no documented problems.

Infants & children:
Not recommended. Adequate studies have not been performed.

Prolonged use:
- No special problems expected.
- Talk to your doctor about the need for follow-up medical examinations or laboratory studies to check kidney function.

Skin & sunlight:
No problems expected.

Driving, piloting or hazardous work:
Don't pilot aircraft until you learn how medicine affects you. Don't work around dangerous machinery. Don't climb ladders or work in high places. Danger increases if you drink alcohol or take medicine affecting alertness and reflexes, such as antihistamines, tranquilizers, sedatives, pain medicine, narcotics and mind-altering drugs.

Discontinuing:
Don't discontinue without consulting doctor.

Others:
Plan regular visits to your doctor while you take ursodiol. Have ultrasound and liver-function studies done at appropriate intervals. Liver damage is unlikely, but theoretically could happen.

POSSIBLE INTERACTION WITH OTHER DRUGS

GENERIC NAME OR DRUG CLASS	COMBINED EFFECT
Antacids* (aluminum-containing)	Decreased absorption of ursodiol.
Cholestyramine	Decreased absorption of ursodiol.
Clofibrate	Decreased effect of ursodiol.
Colestipol	Decreased absorption of ursodiol.
Estrogens*	Decreased effect of ursodiol.
Progesterone	Decreased effect of ursodiol.

POSSIBLE INTERACTION WITH OTHER SUBSTANCES

INTERACTS WITH	COMBINED EFFECT
Alcohol:	None expected, unless you have impaired liver function from alcohol abuse.
Beverages:	None expected.
Cocaine:	None expected.
Foods:	None expected.
Marijuana:	None expected.
Tobacco:	None reported. However, tobacco may possibly impair intestinal absorption from the intestinal tract. Better to avoid.

*See Glossary

VALPROIC ACID (Dipropylacetic Acid)

BRAND NAMES

Dalpro	Depakene
Depa	Myproic Acid

BASIC INFORMATION

Habit forming? No
Prescription needed? Yes
Available as generic? Yes
Drug class: Anticonvulsant

 USES

Controls petit mal (absence) seizures in treatment of epilepsy.

 DOSAGE & USAGE INFORMATION

How to take:
Capsule or syrup—Swallow with liquid or food to lessen stomach irritation.

When to take:
Once a day.

If you forget a dose:
Take as soon as you remember. Don't ever double dose.

What drug does:
Increases concentration of gamma aminobutyric acid, which inhibits nerve transmission in parts of brain.

Time lapse before drug works:
1 to 4 hours.

Don't take with:
Any other medicine without consulting your doctor or pharmacist.

 OVERDOSE

SYMPTOMS:
Coma
WHAT TO DO:
- Dial 0 (operator) or 911 (emergency) for an ambulance or medical help. Then give first aid immediately.
- If patient is unconscious and not breathing, give mouth-to-mouth breathing. If there is no heartbeat, use cardiac massage and mouth-to-mouth breathing (CPR). Don't try to make patient vomit. If you can't get help quickly, take patient to nearest emergency facility.
- See emergency information on inside covers.

 POSSIBLE ADVERSE REACTIONS OR SIDE EFFECTS

SYMPTOMS	WHAT TO DO
Life-threatening:	
In case of overdose, see previous column.	
Common:	
Menstrual irregularities. nausea, vomiting, abdominal cramps, diarrhea, tremor, weight gain.	Continue. Call doctor when convenient.
Infrequent:	
• Rash, blood spots under skin, hair loss, bleeding (heart and lungs), easy bruising.	Discontinue. Call doctor right away.
• Sleepiness, weakness, easily upset emotionally, depression, psychic changes, headache, incoordination, appetite change, constipation.	Continue. Call doctor when convenient.
Rare:	
• Double vision, unusual movements of eyes (nystagmus), swelling of feet, ankles and abdomen; jaundice; increased bleeding tendency.	Discontinue. Call doctor right away.
• Anemia (paleness, fatigue).	Continue. Call doctor when convenient.

 WARNINGS & PRECAUTIONS

Don't take if:
You are allergic to valproic acid.

Before you start, consult your doctor:
- If you have blood, kidney or liver disease.
- If you will have surgery within 2 months, including dental surgery, requiring general or spinal anesthesia.

Over age 60:
Adverse reactions and side effects may be more frequent and severe than in younger persons.

Pregnancy:
Risk to unborn child exists. Avoid if possible.

Breast-feeding:
Unknown effect.

VALPROIC ACID (Dipropylacetic Acid)

Infants & children:
Under close medical supervision only.

Prolonged use:
Request periodic blood tests, liver- and kidney-function tests.

Skin & sunlight:
No problems expected.

Driving, piloting or hazardous work:
Don't drive or pilot aircraft until you learn how medicine affects you. Don't work around dangerous machinery. Don't climb ladders or work in high places. Danger increases if you drink alcohol or take medicine affecting alertness and reflexes, such as antihistamines, tranquilizers, sedatives, pain medicine, narcotics and mind-altering drugs.

Discontinuing:
Don't discontinue without consulting doctor. Dose may require gradual reduction if you have taken drug for a long time. Doses of other drugs may also require adjustment.

Others:
No problems expected.

 ## POSSIBLE INTERACTION WITH OTHER DRUGS

GENERIC NAME OR DRUG CLASS	COMBINED EFFECT
Anticoagulants*	Increased chance of bleeding.
Aspirin	Increased chance of bleeding.
Central nervous system (CNS) depressants*	Increased sedative effect.
Clonazepam	May prolong seizure.
Clozapine	Toxic effect on bone marrow.
Didanosine	Increased risk of pancreatitis.
Dipyridamole	Increased chance of bleeding.
Flecainide	Possible decreased blood cell production in bone marrow.
Isoniazid	Increased risk of liver damage.
Levocarnitine	Decreased levocarnitine. Patients taking valproic acid may need to take the supplement levocarnitine.

MAO inhibitors*	Increased sedative effect.
Nabilone	Greater depression of central nervous system.
Phenobarbital	Increases chance of toxicity.
Phenytoin	Unpredictable. Dose may require adjustment.
Primidone	Increased chance of toxicity.
Sertraline	Increased depressive effects of both drugs.
Sodium benzoate & sodium phenylacetate	May reduce effect of sodium benzoate & sodium phenylacetate.
Sulfinpyrazone	Increased chance of bleeding.
Tiopronin	Increased risk of toxicity to bone marrow.
Tocainide	Possible decreased blood cell production in bone marrow.

 ## POSSIBLE INTERACTION WITH OTHER SUBSTANCES

INTERACTS WITH	COMBINED EFFECT
Alcohol:	Deep sedation. Avoid.
Beverages:	No problems expected.
Cocaine:	Increased brain sensitivity. Avoid.
Foods:	No problems expected.
Marijuana:	Increased brain sensitivity. Avoid.
Tobacco:	Decreased valproic acid effect.

VANCOMYCIN

BRAND NAMES

Vancocin

BASIC INFORMATION

Habit forming? No
Prescription needed? Yes
Available as generic? No
Drug class: Antibiotic

USES

- Treats colitis when caused by *clostridium* infections.
- Treats some forms of severe diarrhea.

DOSAGE & USAGE INFORMATION

How to take:
- Capsules—Swallow with liquid. If you can't swallow whole, open capsule and take with liquid or food. Instructions to take on empty stomach mean 1 hour before or 2 hours after eating.
- Oral solution—Use the calibrated measuring device. Swallow with other liquid to prevent nausea.
- There is also an injectable form. This information applies to the oral form only.

When to take:
According to doctor's instructions. Usually every 6 hours.

If you forget a dose:
Take as soon as you remember up to 2 hours late. If more than 2 hours, wait for next scheduled dose (don't double this dose).

What drug does:
Kills bacterial cells.

Time lapse before drug works:
None. Works right away. This medicine is not absorbed to a great extent through the intestinal tract.

Continued in next column

OVERDOSE

SYMPTOMS:
None expected.
WHAT TO DO:
Overdose unlikely to threaten life. If person takes much larger amount than prescribed, call doctor, poison-control center or hospital emergency room for instructions.

Don't take with:
Any other medicines (including over-the-counter drugs such as cough and cold medicines, laxatives, antacids, diet pills, caffeine, nose drops or vitamins) without consulting your doctor.

POSSIBLE ADVERSE REACTIONS OR SIDE EFFECTS

SYMPTOMS	WHAT TO DO
Life-threatening: None expected.	
Common: Bitter taste.	Continue. Tell doctor at next visit.
Infrequent: Nausea or vomiting.	Continue. Tell doctor at next visit.
Rare: Hearing loss, ears ringing or buzzing.	Discontinue. Call doctor right away.

WARNINGS & PRECAUTIONS

Don't take if:
You are allergic to vancomycin.

Before you start, consult your doctor:
- If you have hearing problems.
- If you have severe kidney disease.
- If you have intestinal obstruction.

Over age 60:
Adverse reactions and side effects may be more frequent and severe than in younger persons. You may need smaller doses for shorter periods of time.

Pregnancy:
Safety not established. Consult doctor.

Breast-feeding:
No special problems expected.

Infants & children:
No special problems expected.

Prolonged use:
Talk to your doctor about the need for follow-up medical examinations or laboratory studies to check hearing acuity, kidney function, vancomycin serum concentration and urinalyses.

Skin & sunlight:
No problems expected.

Driving, piloting or hazardous work:
No problems expected.

Discontinuing:
No special problems expected.

Others:
- Advise any doctor or dentist whom you consult that you take this medicine.
- May affect results in some medical tests.

POSSIBLE INTERACTION WITH OTHER DRUGS

GENERIC NAME OR DRUG CLASS	COMBINED EFFECT
Aminoglycosides*	Increased chance of hearing loss or kidney damage.
Amphotericin B by injection	Increased chance of hearing loss or kidney damage.
Bacitracin by injection	Increased chance of hearing loss or kidney damage.
Bumetanide by injection	Increased chance of hearing loss or kidney damage.
Capreomycin	Increased chance of hearing loss or kidney damage.
Cholestyramine	Increased chance of hearing loss or kidney damage. Decreased therapeutic effect of vancomycin.
Cisplatin	Increased chance of hearing loss or kidney damage.
Colestipol	Increased chance of hearing loss or kidney damage. Decreased therapeutic effect of vancomycin.
Cyclosporine	Increased chance of hearing loss or kidney damage.
Ethacrynic acid by injection	Increased chance of hearing loss or kidney damage.
Furosemide by injection	Increased chance of hearing loss or kidney damage.
Paromomycin	Increased chance of hearing loss or kidney damage.
Polymyxins*	Increased chance of hearing loss or kidney damage.
Streptozocin	Increased chance of hearing loss or kidney damage.
Tiopronin	Increased risk of toxicity to kidneys.

POSSIBLE INTERACTION WITH OTHER SUBSTANCES

INTERACTS WITH	COMBINED EFFECT
Alcohol:	No special problems expected.
Beverages:	No special problems expected.
Cocaine:	No special problems expected.
Foods:	No special problems expected.
Marijuana:	No special problems expected.
Tobacco:	No special problems expected.

VITAMIN A

BRAND NAMES

Acon
Afaxin
Alphalin

Aquasol A
Dispatabs
Sust-A

Numerous multiple vitamin-mineral supplements. Check labels.

BASIC INFORMATION

Habit forming? No
Prescription needed? No
Available as generic? Yes
Drug class: Vitamin supplement

 USES

- Dietary supplement to ensure normal growth and health, especially eyes and skin.
- Beta carotene form (Solatene) decreases severity of sun exposure in patients with porphyria.

 DOSAGE & USAGE INFORMATION

How to take:
- Drops or capsule—Swallow with liquid. If you can't swallow whole, open capsule and take with liquid or food.
- Oral solution—Swallow with liquid.

When to take:
At the same time each day.

If you forget a dose:
Take as soon as you remember. Resume regular schedule.

What drug does:
- Prevents night blindness.
- Promotes normal growth and health.

Continued in next column

 OVERDOSE

SYMPTOMS:
Increased adverse reactions and side effects. Jaundice (rare, but may occur with large doses), malaise, vomiting, irritability, bleeding gums, seizures, double vision, peeling skin.
WHAT TO DO:
If person takes much larger amount than prescribed, call doctor, poison-control center or hospital emergency room for instructions.

Time lapse before drug works:
Requires continual intake.

Don't take with:
Any other medicine without consulting your doctor or pharmacist.

 POSSIBLE ADVERSE REACTIONS OR SIDE EFFECTS

SYMPTOMS	WHAT TO DO
Life-threatening:	
In case of overdose, see previous column.	
Common:	
None expected.	
Infrequent:	
Confusion; dizziness; drowsiness; headache; irritability; dry, cracked lips; peeling skin; hair loss; sensitvity to light.	Continue. Call doctor when convenient.
Rare:	
• Bulging soft spot on baby's head, double vision, bone or joint pain, abdominal pain, frequent urination.	Discontinue. Call doctor right away.
• Diarrhea, appetite loss, nausea, vomiting.	Continue. Call doctor when convenient.

WARNINGS & PRECAUTIONS

Don't take if:
You have chronic kidney failure.

Before you start, consult your doctor:
If you have any kidney disorder.

Over age 60:
No problems expected.

Pregnancy:
Don't take more than 6,000 units daily.

Breast-feeding:
No problems expected.

Infants & children:
- Avoid large doses.
- Keep vitamin-mineral supplements out of children's reach.

Prolonged use:
No problems expected.

Skin & sunlight:
Increased sensitivity to light.

Driving, piloting or hazardous work:
No problems expected.

Discontinuing:
Don't discontinue without doctor's advice until you complete prescribed dose, even though symptoms diminish or disappear.

Others:
- Don't exceed dose. Too much over a long time may be harmful.
- A balanced diet should provide all the vitamin A a healthy person needs and prevent need for supplements. Best sources are liver, yellow-orange fruits and vegetables, dark-green, leafy vegetables, milk, butter and margarine.

POSSIBLE INTERACTION WITH OTHER DRUGS

GENERIC NAME OR DRUG CLASS	COMBINED EFFECT
Anticoagulants*	Increased anticoagulant effect with large doses (over 10,000 I.U.) of vitamin A.
Calcium supplements*	Decreased vitamin effect.
Cholestyramine	Decreased vitamin A absorption.
Colestipol	Decreased vitamin absorption.
Contraceptives, oral*	Increased vitamin A levels.
Isotretinoin	Increased toxic effect of each.
Mineral oil (long-term)	Decreased vitamin A absorption.
Neomycin	Decreased vitamin absorption.
Vitamin A derivatives, other	Increased toxicity risk.
Vitamin E (excess dose)	Vitamin A depletion.

POSSIBLE INTERACTION WITH OTHER SUBSTANCES

INTERACTS WITH	COMBINED EFFECT
Alcohol:	None expected.
Beverages:	None expected.
Cocaine:	None expected.
Foods:	None expected.
Marijuana:	None expected.
Tobacco:	None expected.

VITAMIN B-12 (Cyanocobalamin)

BRAND AND GENERIC NAMES

See complete list of brand and generic names in the *Brand Name Directory*, page 930.

BASIC INFORMATION

Habit forming? No
Prescription needed? No
Available as generic? Yes
Drug class: Vitamin supplement

USES

- Dietary supplement for normal growth, development and health.
- Treatment for nerve damage.
- Treatment for pernicious anemia.
- Treatment and prevention of vitamin B-12 deficiencies in people who have had stomach or intestines surgically removed.
- Prevention of vitamin B-12 deficiency in strict vegetarians and persons with absorption diseases.

DOSAGE & USAGE INFORMATION

How to take:
- Tablets—Swallow with liquid.
- Injection—Follow doctor's directions.

When to take:
- Oral—At the same time each day.
- Injection—Follow doctor's directions.

If you forget a dose:
Take when remembered. Don't double next dose. Resume regular schedule.

What drug does:
Acts as enzyme to promote normal fat and carbohydrate metabolism and protein synthesis.

Time lapse before drug works:
15 minutes.

Don't take with:
Any other medicine without consulting your doctor or pharmacist.

OVERDOSE

SYMPTOMS:
Increased adverse reactions and side effects.
WHAT TO DO:
Overdose unlikely to threaten life. If person takes much larger amount than prescribed, call doctor, poison-control center or hospital emergency room for instructions.

POSSIBLE ADVERSE REACTIONS OR SIDE EFFECTS

SYMPTOMS	WHAT TO DO
Life-threatening:	
Hives, rash, intense itching, faintness soon after a dose (anaphylaxis).	Seek emergency treatment immediately.
Common:	
None expected.	
Infrequent:	
None expected.	
Rare:	
• Itchy skin, wheezing.	Discontinue. Call doctor right away.
• Diarrhea.	Continue. Call doctor when convenient.

VITAMIN B-12 (Cyanocobalamin)

WARNINGS & PRECAUTIONS

Don't take if:
You have Leber's disease (optic nerve atrophy).

Before you start, consult your doctor:
- If you have gout.
- If you have heart disease.

Over age 60:
Don't take more than 100 mg. per day unless prescribed by your doctor.

Pregnancy:
No problems expected.

Breast-feeding:
No problems expected.

Infants & children:
No problems expected.

Prolonged use:
No problems expected.

Skin & sunlight:
No problems expected.

Driving, piloting or hazardous work:
No problems expected.

Discontinuing:
Don't discontinue without doctor's advice until you complete prescribed dose, even though symptoms diminish or disappear.

Others:
- A balanced diet should provide all the vitamin B-12 a healthy person needs and make supplements unnecessary. Best sources are meat, fish, egg yolk and cheese.
- Tablets should be used only for diet supplements. All other uses of vitamin B-12 require injections.
- Don't take large doses of vitamin C (1,000 mg. or more per day) unless prescribed by your doctor.

POSSIBLE INTERACTION WITH OTHER DRUGS

GENERIC NAME OR DRUG CLASS	COMBINED EFFECT
Anticonvulsants*	Decreased absorption of vitamin B-12.
Chloramphenicol	Decreased vitamin B-12 effect.
Cholestyramine	Decreased absorption of vitamin B-12.
Cimetidine	Decreased absorption of vitamin B-12.
Colchicine	Decreased absorption of vitamin B-12.
Famotidine	Decreased absorption of vitamin B-12.
H2 antagonists*	Decreased absorption of vitamin B-12.
Neomycin	Decreased absorption of vitamin B-12.
Para-aminosalicylic acid	Decreased effects of para-aminosalicyclic acid.
Potassium (extended-release forms)	Decreased absorption of vitamin B-12.
Ranitidine	Decreased absorption of vitamin B-12.
Vitamin C (ascorbic acid)	Destroys vitamin B-12 if taken at same time. Take 2 hours apart.

POSSIBLE INTERACTION WITH OTHER SUBSTANCES

INTERACTS WITH	COMBINED EFFECT
Alcohol:	Decreased absorption of vitamin B-12.
Beverages:	None expected.
Cocaine:	None expected.
Foods:	None expected.
Marijuana:	None expected.
Tobacco:	None expected.

VITAMIN C (Ascorbic Acid)

BRAND NAMES
See complete list of brand names in the Brand Name Directory, page 930.

BASIC INFORMATION

Habit forming? No
Prescription needed? No
Available as generic? Yes
Drug class: Vitamin supplement

 ## USES

- Prevention and treatment of scurvy and other vitamin-C deficiencies.
- Treatment of anemia.
- Maintenance of acid urine.

 ## DOSAGE & USAGE INFORMATION

How to take:
- Tablets, capsules, liquid—Swallow with 8 oz. water.
- Extended-release tablets—Swallow whole.
- Drops—Squirt directly into mouth or mix with liquid or food.
- Chewable tablets—Chew well before swallowing.

When to take:
1, 2 or 3 times per day, as prescribed on label.

If you forget a dose:
Take as soon as you remember. Return to regular schedule.

What drug does:
- May help form collagen.
- Increases iron absorption from intestine.
- Contributes to hemoglobin and red-blood-cell production in bone marrow.

Time lapse before drug works:
1 week.

Don't take with:
Any other medicine without consulting your doctor or pharmacist.

 ## OVERDOSE

SYMPTOMS:
Diarrhea, vomiting, dizziness.
WHAT TO DO:
Overdose unlikely to threaten life. If person takes much larger amount than prescribed, call doctor, poison-control center or hospital emergency room for instructions.

 ## POSSIBLE ADVERSE REACTIONS OR SIDE EFFECTS

SYMPTOMS	WHAT TO DO
Life-threatening: None expected.	
Common: None expected.	
Infrequent: • Mild diarrhea, nausea, vomiting.	Discontinue. Call doctor right away.
• Flushed face.	Continue. Call doctor when convenient.
Rare: • Kidney stones with high doses, anemia, abdominal pain.	Discontinue. Call doctor right away.
• Headache.	Continue. Tell doctor at next visit.

WARNINGS & PRECAUTIONS

Don't take if:
You are allergic to vitamin C.

Before you start, consult your doctor:
- If you have sickle-cell or other anemia.
- If you have had kidney stones.
- If you have gout.

Over age 60:
Don't take more than 100 mg. per day unless prescribed by your doctor.

Pregnancy:
No proven harm to unborn child. Avoid large doses.

Breast-feeding:
Avoid large doses.

Infants & children:
- Avoid large doses.
- Keep vitamin-mineral supplements out of children's reach.

Prolonged use:
Large doses for longer than 2 months may cause kidney stones.

Skin & sunlight:
No problems expected.

Driving, piloting or hazardous work:
No problems expected.

Discontinuing:
No problems expected.

Others:
- Store in cool, dry place.
- May cause inaccurate tests for sugar in urine or blood in stool.
- May cause crisis in patients with sickle-cell anemia.
- A balanced diet should provide all the vitamin C a healthy person needs and make supplements unnecessary. Best sources are citrus, strawberries, cantaloupe and raw peppers.
- Don't take large doses of vitamin C (1,000 mg. or more per day) unless prescribed by your doctor.
- Some products contain tartrazine dye. Avoid, if allergic (especially aspirin hypersensitivity).

POSSIBLE INTERACTION WITH OTHER DRUGS

GENERIC NAME OR DRUG CLASS	COMBINED EFFECT
Amphetamines*	Possible decreased amphetamine effect.
Anticholinergics*	Possible decreased anticholinergic effect.
Anticoagulants, oral*	Possible decreased anticoagulant effect.
Antidepressants, tricyclic (TCA)*	Possible decreased antidepressant effect.
Aspirin	Decreased vitamin C effect and salicylate excretion.
Barbiturates*	Decreased vitamin C effect. Increased barbiturate effect.
Cellulose sodium phosphate	Decreased vitamin C effect.
Contraceptives, oral*	Decreased vitamin C effect.
Estrogens*	Increased likelihood of adverse effects from estrogen with 1 gm or more of vitamin C per day.
Iron supplements*	Increased iron absorption.
Mexiletine	Possible decreased effectiveness of mexiletine.
Quinidine	Possible decreased quinidine effect.
Salicylates*	Decreased vitamin C effect and salicylate excretion. May lead to salicylate toxicity.
Tranquilizers* (phenothiazine)	May decrease phenothiazine effect if no vitamin C deficiency exists.

POSSIBLE INTERACTION WITH OTHER SUBSTANCES

INTERACTS WITH	COMBINED EFFECT
Alcohol:	None expected.
Beverages:	None expected.
Cocaine:	None expected.
Foods:	None expected.
Marijuana:	None expected.
Tobacco:	Increased requirement for vitamin C.

*See Glossary

VITAMIN D

BRAND AND GENERIC NAMES

Calciferol
CALCIFEDIOL
Calcijex
CALCITRIOL
Calderol
Deltalin
DHT
DHT Intensol

DIHYDROTA-
  CHYSTEROL
Drisdol
ERGOCALCIFEROL
Hytakerol
Ostoforte
Radiostol
Radiostol Forte
Rocaltrol

Numerous other multiple vitamin-mineral supplements. Check labels.

BASIC INFORMATION

Habit forming? No
Prescription needed?
  Low strength: No
  High strength: Yes
Available as generic? Yes
Drug class: Vitamin supplement

USES

- Dietary supplement.
- Prevention of rickets (bone disease).
- Treatment for hypocalcemia (low blood calcium) in kidney disease.
- Treatment for postoperative muscle contractions.
- Daily supplement for people who must use sunscreen daily.

DOSAGE & USAGE INFORMATION

How to take:
- Tablet, capsule or liquid—Swallow with liquid.
- Drops—Dilute dose in beverage.
- Injection—Take under doctor's supervision.

Continued next column

OVERDOSE

SYMPTOMS:
Severe stomach pain, nausea, vomiting, weight loss; bone and muscle pain; increased urination, cloudy urine; mood or mental changes (possible psychosis); high blood pressure, irregular heartbeat; eye irritation or light sensitivity; itchy skin.
WHAT TO DO:
Overdose unlikely to threaten life. If person takes much larger amount than prescribed, call doctor, poison-control center or hospital emergency room for instructions.

When to take:
As directed, usually once a day at the same time each day.

If you forget a dose:
Take up to 12 hours late. If more than 12 hours, wait for next dose (don't double this dose).

What drug does:
- Maintains growth and health.
- Prevents rickets.
- Essential so body can use calcium and phosphate.

Time lapse before drug works:
2 hours. May require 2 to 3 weeks of continual use for maximum effect.

Don't take with:
Non-prescription drugs or drugs in Interaction column without consulting doctor.

POSSIBLE ADVERSE REACTIONS OR SIDE EFFECTS

SYMPTOMS	WHAT TO DO
Life-threatening:	
In case of overdose, see previous column.	
Common:	
None expected.	
Infrequent:	
Headache, metallic taste in mouth, thirst, dry mouth, constipation, appetite loss, nausea, vomiting, weakness, cloudy urine, sensitivity to light.	Continue. Call doctor when convenient.
Rare:	
• Increased urination, pink eye, psychosis, severe abdominal pain, fever.	Discontinue. Call doctor right away.
• Muscle pain, bone pain, diarrhea.	Continue. Tell doctor when convenient.

WARNINGS & PRECAUTIONS

Don't take if:
You are allergic to medicine containing vitamin D.

Before you start, consult your doctor:
- If you plan to become pregnant while taking vitamin D.
- If you have epilepsy.
- If you have heart or blood-vessel disease.
- If you have kidney disease.

Over age 60:
Adverse reactions and side effects may be more frequent and severe than in younger persons.

Pregnancy:
Risk to unborn child outweighs drug benefits. Don't use.

Breast-feeding:
No problems expected, but consult doctor.

Infants & children:
- Avoid large doses.
- Keep vitamins out of children's reach.

Prolonged use:
- No problems expected.
- Talk to your doctor about the need for follow-up medical examinations or laboratory studies to check kidney function, liver function, serum calcium.

Skin & sunlight:
Increased sensitivity to light.

Driving, piloting or hazardous work:
No problems expected.

Discontinuing:
Don't discontinue without doctor's advice until you complete prescribed dose, even though symptoms diminish or disappear.

Others:
- Don't exceed dose. Too much over a long time may be harmful.
- A balanced diet should provide all the vitamin D a healthy person needs and make supplements unnecessary. Best sources are fish and vitamin-D fortified milk and bread.
- Some products contain tartrazine dye. Avoid, if allergic (especially aspirin hypersensitivity).
- Sunscreen prevents the body from manufacturing vitamin D from sunshine. Take supplementary vitamin D if you use sunscreen daily. Ask doctor for dosage.

POSSIBLE INTERACTION WITH OTHER DRUGS

GENERIC NAME OR DRUG CLASS	COMBINED EFFECT
Antacids* (magnesium-containing)	Possible excess magnesium.
Anticonvulsants, hydantoin*	Decreased vitamin D effect.
Calcium (high doses)	Excess calcium in blood.
Calcium channel blockers*	Possible decreased effect of calcium-channel blockers.
Calcium supplements*	Excessive absorption of vitamin D.
Cholestyramine	Decreased vitamin D effect.
Colestipol	Decreased vitamin D absorption.
Cortisone	Decreased vitamin D effect.
Digitalis preparations*	Heartbeat irregularities.
Diuretics, thiazide*	Possible increased calcium.
Mineral oil	Decreased vitamin D effect.
Neomycin	Decreased vitamin D absorption.
Nicardipine	Decreased nicardipine effect.
Phenobarbital	Decreased vitamin D effect.
Phosphorous preparations*	Accumulation of excess phosphorous.
Rifampin	Possible decreased vitamin D effect.
Vitamin D, other	Possible toxicity.

POSSIBLE INTERACTION WITH OTHER SUBSTANCES

INTERACTS WITH	COMBINED EFFECT
Alcohol:	None expected.
Beverages:	None expected.
Cocaine:	None expected.
Foods:	None expected.
Marijuana:	None expected.
Tobacco:	None expected.

*See Glossary

VITAMIN E

BRAND NAMES

Aquasol E   Epsilan-M
Chew-E   Pheryl-E
Eprolin   Viterra E
Numerous other multiple vitamin-mineral supplements. Check labels.

BASIC INFORMATION

Habit forming? No
Prescription needed? No
Available as generic? Yes
Drug class: Vitamin supplement

USES

- Dietary supplement to promote normal growth, development and health.
- Treatment and prevention of vitamin-E deficiency, especially in premature or low birth-weight infants.
- Treatment for fibrocystic disease of the breast.
- Treatment for circulatory problems to the lower extremities.
- Treatment for sickle-cell anemia.
- Treatment for lung toxicity from air pollution.

DOSAGE & USAGE INFORMATION

How to take:
- Tablet or capsule—Swallow with liquid or food to lessen stomach irritation.
- Drops—Dilute dose in beverage before swallowing or squirt directly into mouth.
- Injection—Take under doctor's supervision.

When to take:
At the same times each day.

If you forget a dose:
Take when you remember. Don't double next dose.

What drug does:
- Promotes normal growth and development.
- Prevents oxidation in body.

Continued next column

OVERDOSE

SYMPTOMS:
Nausea, vomiting, fatigue.
WHAT TO DO:
Overdose unlikely to threaten life. If person takes much larger amount than prescribed, call doctor, poison-control center or hospital emergency room for instructions.

Time lapse before drug works:
Not determined.

Don't take with:
Any other medicine without consulting your doctor or pharmacist.

POSSIBLE ADVERSE REACTIONS OR SIDE EFFECTS

SYMPTOMS	WHAT TO DO
Life-threatening: None expected.	
Common: Breast enlargement, dizziness, headache.	Continue. Call doctor when convenient.
Infrequent: Nausea, abdominal pain, muscle aches, pain in lower legs, fever, tiredness, weakness.	Continue. Call doctor when convenient.
Rare: Blurred vision, diarrhea.	Discontinue. Call doctor right away.

WARNINGS & PRECAUTIONS

Don't take if:
You are allergic to vitamin E.

Before you start, consult your doctor:
- If you have had blood clots in leg veins (thrombophlebitis).
- If you have liver disease.

Over age 60:
No problems expected. Avoid excessive doses.

Pregnancy:
No problems expected with normal daily requirements. Don't exceed prescribed dose.

Breast-feeding:
No problems expected.

Infants & children:
Use only under medical supervision.

Prolonged use:
Toxic accumulation of vitamin E. Don't exceed recommended dose.

Skin & sunlight:
No problems expected.

Driving, piloting or hazardous work:
No problems expected.

Discontinuing:
No problems expected.

Others:
A balanced diet should provide all the vitamin E a healthy person needs and make supplements unnecessary. Best sources are vegetable oils, whole-grain cereals, liver.

POSSIBLE INTERACTION WITH OTHER DRUGS

GENERIC NAME OR DRUG CLASS	COMBINED EFFECT
Anticoagulants, oral*	Increased anticoagulant effect.
Cholestyramine	Decreased vitamin E absorption.
Colestipol	Decreased vitamin E absorption.
Iron supplements*	Possible decreased effect of iron supplement in patients with iron-deficiency anemia. Decreased vitamin E effect in healthy persons.
Mineral oil	Decreased vitamin E effect.
Neomycin	Decreased vitamin E absorption.
Vitamin A	Recommended dose of vitamin E— Increased benefit and decreased toxicity of vitamin A. Excess dose of vitamin E— Vitamin A depletion.

POSSIBLE INTERACTION WITH OTHER SUBSTANCES

INTERACTS WITH	COMBINED EFFECT
Alcohol:	None expected.
Beverages:	None expected.
Cocaine:	None expected.
Foods:	None expected.
Marijuana:	None expected.
Tobacco:	None expected.

VITAMIN K

BRAND AND GENERIC NAMES

AquaMEPHYTON
Konakion
Menadione
MENADIOL

Mephyton
PHYTONADIONE
Synkayvite

BASIC INFORMATION

Habit forming? No
Prescription needed? No
Available as generic? No
Drug class: Vitamin supplement

 USES

- Dietary supplement.
- Treatment for bleeding disorders and malabsorption diseases due to vitamin K deficiency.
- Treatment for hemorrhagic disease of the newborn.
- Treatment for bleeding due to overdose of oral anticoagulants.

 DOSAGE & USAGE INFORMATION

How to take:
- Usually given by injection in hospital or doctor's office.
- Tablet—Swallow with liquid. If you can't swallow whole, crumble tablet and take with liquid or food.

When to take:
At the same time each day.

If you forget a dose:
Take as soon as you remember up to 12 hours late. If more than 12 hours, wait for next scheduled dose (don't double this dose).

What drug does:
- Promotes growth, development and good health.
- Supplies a necessary ingredient for blood clotting.

Continued next column

 OVERDOSE

SYMPTOMS:
Nausea, vomiting.
WHAT TO DO:
Overdose unlikely to threaten life. If person takes much larger amount than prescribed, call doctor, poison-control center or hospital emergency room for instructions.

Time lapse before drug works:
15 to 30 minutes to support blood clotting.

Don't take with:
Any other medicine without consulting your doctor or pharmacist.

 POSSIBLE ADVERSE REACTIONS OR SIDE EFFECTS

SYMPTOMS	WHAT TO DO
Life-threatening: None expected.	
Common: None expected.	
Infrequent: Unusual taste, face flushing.	Continue. Call doctor when convenient.
Rare: Rash, hives.	Discontinue. Call doctor right away.

WARNINGS & PRECAUTIONS

Don't take if:
- You are allergic to vitamin K.
- You have G6PD deficiency.
- You have liver disease.

Before you start, consult your doctor:
If you are pregnant.

Over age 60:
No problems expected.

Pregnancy:
Don't exceed dose.

Breast-feeding:
No problems expected.

Infants & children:
Phytonadione is the preferred form for hemorrhagic disease of the newborn.

Prolonged use:
Talk to your doctor about the need for follow-up medical examinations or laboratory studies to check prothrombin time.

Skin & sunlight:
No problems expected.

Driving, piloting or hazardous work:
No problems expected.

Discontinuing:
No problems expected.

Others:
- Tell all doctors and dentists you consult that you take this medicine.
- Don't exceed dose. Too much over a long time may be harmful.
- A balanced diet should provide all the vitamin K a healthy person needs and make supplements unnecessary. Best sources are green, leafy vegetables, meat or dairy products.

POSSIBLE INTERACTION WITH OTHER DRUGS

GENERIC NAME OR DRUG CLASS	COMBINED EFFECT
Anticoagulants, oral*	Decreased anti-coagulant effect.
Cholestyramine	Decreased vitamin K effect.
Colestipol	Decreased vitamin K absorption.
Dapsone	Increased risk of adverse effect on blood cells.
Mineral oil (long-term)	Vitamin K deficiency.
Neomycin	Decreased vitamin K absorption.
Sulfa drugs*	Vitamin K deficiency.

POSSIBLE INTERACTION WITH OTHER SUBSTANCES

INTERACTS WITH	COMBINED EFFECT
Alcohol:	None expected.
Beverages:	None expected.
Cocaine:	None expected.
Foods:	None expected.
Marijuana:	None expected.
Tobacco:	None expected.

VITAMINS & FLUORIDE

BRAND AND GENERIC NAMES

Adeflor
Cari-Tab
Mulvidren-F
Poly-Vi-Flor
Tri-Vi-Flor
Vi-Daylin/F
Vi-Penta F

MULTIPLE VITAMINS & FLUORIDE
VITAMINS A, D & C & FLUORIDE

BASIC INFORMATION

Habit forming? No
Prescription needed? Yes
Available as generic? No
Drug class: Vitamins, minerals

USES

- Reduces incidence of tooth cavities (fluoride). Children who need supplements should take until age 16.
- Prevents deficiencies of vitamin included in formula (some contain multiple vitamins whose content varies among products, others contain only vitamins A, D and C).

DOSAGE & USAGE INFORMATION

How to take:
- Chewable tablets—Chew or crush before swallowing.
- Oral liquid—Measure with specially marked dropper. May mix with food, fruit juice, cereal.

When to take:
- Bedtime or with or just after meals.
- If at bedtime, brush teeth first.

If you forget a dose:
Take as soon as you remember up to 2 hours late. If more than 2 hours, wait for next scheduled dose (don't double this dose).

Continued next column

OVERDOSE

SYMPTOMS:
Minor overdose—Black, brown or white spots on teeth.
Massive overdose—Shallow breathing, black or tarry stools, bloody vomit.
WHAT TO DO:
- **Dial 0 (operator) or 911 (emergency) for an ambulance or medical help. Then give first aid immediately.**
- **See emergency information on inside covers.**

What drug does:
Provides supplemental fluoride to combat tooth decay.

Time lapse before drug works:
8 weeks to provide maximum benefit.

Don't take with:
- Other medicine simultaneously.
- Any other medicine without consulting your doctor or pharmacist.

POSSIBLE ADVERSE REACTIONS OR SIDE EFFECTS

SYMPTOMS	WHAT TO DO
Life-threatening:	
Fainting, bloody vomit, bloody or black stool, breathing difficulty.	Discontinue. Seek emergency treatment.
Common:	
White, black or brown spots on teeth; nausea; vomiting.	Discontinue. Call doctor right away.
Infrequent:	
• Drowsiness; abdominal pain; increased salivation; watery eyes; weight loss; sore throat, fever, mouth sores; constipation; bone pain; rash; muscle stiffness; weakness; tremor; agitation.	Discontinue. Call doctor right away.
• Diarrhea.	Continue. Call doctor when convenient.
Rare:	
None expected.	

VITAMINS & FLUORIDE

WARNINGS & PRECAUTIONS

Don't take if:
- Your water supply contains 0.7 parts fluoride per million. Too much fluoride stains teeth permanently.
- You are allergic to any fluoride-containing product.
- You have underactive thyroid.

Before you start, consult your doctor or dentist:
For proper dosage.

Over age 60:
No problems expected.

Pregnancy:
No problems expected.

Breast-feeding:
No problems expected.

Infants & children:
No problems expected in children over 3 years of age except accidental overdose. Keep vitamin-mineral supplements out of children's reach.

Prolonged use:
Excess may cause discolored teeth and decreased calcium in blood.

Skin & sunlight:
No problems expected.

Driving, piloting or hazardous work:
No problems expected.

Discontinuing:
No problems expected.

Others:
- Store in original plastic container. Fluoride decomposes glass.
- Check with dentist once or twice a year to keep cavities at a minimum. Topical applications of fluoride may also be helpful.
- Fluoride probably not necessary if water contains about 1 part per million of fluoride or more. Check with health department.
- Don't freeze.
- Don't keep outdated medicine.

POSSIBLE INTERACTION WITH OTHER DRUGS

GENERIC NAME OR DRUG CLASS	COMBINED EFFECT
Iron supplements*	Decreased effect of any vitamin E if present in multivitamin product.
Vitamin A	May lead to vitamin A toxicity if vitamin A is in combination.
Vitamin D	May lead to vitamin D toxicity if vitamin D is in combination.

POSSIBLE INTERACTION WITH OTHER SUBSTANCES

INTERACTS WITH	COMBINED EFFECT
Alcohol:	None expected.
Beverages: Milk.	Prevents absorption of fluoride. Space dose 2 hours before or after milk.
Cocaine:	None expected.
Foods:	None expected.
Marijuana:	None expected.
Tobacco:	None expected.

XYLOMETAZOLINE & OXYMETAZOLINE (Nasal)

BRAND NAMES

See complete list of brand names in the *Brand Name Directory,* page 930.

BASIC INFORMATION

Habit forming? No
Prescription needed? No
Available as generic? Yes
Drug class: Sympathomimetic

 ## USES

Relieves congestion of nose, sinuses and throat from allergies and infections.

 ## DOSAGE & USAGE INFORMATION

How to take:
Nasal solution, nasal spray—Use as directed on label. Avoid contamination. Don't use same container for more than 1 person.

When to take:
When needed, no more often than every 4 hours.

If you forget a dose:
Take as soon as you remember. Wait 4 hours for next dose.

What drug does:
Constricts walls of small arteries in nose, sinuses and eustachian tubes.

Time lapse before drug works:
5 to 30 minutes.

Continued next column

 ## OVERDOSE

SYMPTOMS:
Headache, sweating, anxiety, agitation, rapid and irregular heartbeat.
WHAT TO DO:
* **Dial 0 (operator) or 911 (emergency) for an ambulance or medical help. Then give first aid immediately.**
* **If patient is unconscious and not breathing, give mouth-to-mouth breathing. If there is no heartbeat, use cardiac massage and mouth-to-mouth breathing (CPR). If you can't get help quickly, take patient to nearest emergency facility.**
* **See emergency information on inside covers.**

Don't take with:
* Non-prescription drugs for allergy, cough or cold without consulting doctor.
* Any other medicine without consulting your doctor or pharmacist.

 ## POSSIBLE ADVERSE REACTIONS OR SIDE EFFECTS

SYMPTOMS	WHAT TO DO
Life-threatening:	
In case of overdose, see previous column.	
Common:	
Runny, stuffy, burning, dry or stinging nose; sneezing; fast, irregular or pounding heartbeat.	Continue. Call doctor when convenient.
Infrequent:	
Headache or lightheadedness, insomnia, nervousness.	Continue. Call doctor when convenient.
Rare:	
None expected.	

WARNINGS & PRECAUTIONS

Don't take if:
You are allergic to any sympathomimetic nasal spray.

Before you start, consult your doctor:
- If you have heart disease or high blood pressure.
- If you have diabetes.
- If you have overactive thyroid.
- If you have taken MAO inhibitors in past 2 weeks.

Over age 60:
Adverse reactions and side effects may be more frequent and severe than in younger persons.

Pregnancy:
No proven harm to unborn child. Avoid if possible.

Breast-feeding:
No proven problems. Consult doctor.

Infants & children:
Don't give to children younger than 2.

Prolonged use:
Drug may lose effectiveness, cause increased congestion (rebound effect*) and irritate nasal membranes.

Skin & sunlight:
No problems expected.

Driving, piloting or hazardous work:
No problems expected.

Discontinuing:
May be unnecessary to finish medicine. Follow doctor's instructions.

Others:
No problems expected.

POSSIBLE INTERACTION WITH OTHER DRUGS

GENERIC NAME OR DRUG CLASS	COMBINED EFFECT
Antidepressants, tricyclic (TCA)*	Increased xylometazoline effect.
Beta-adrenergic blockers*	Decreased effects of both drugs.
Guanadrel	Decreased effect of both drugs.
MAO inhibitors*	Dangerous blood-pressure rise.
Methyldopa	Possible increased blood pressure.
Minoxidil	Decreased minoxidil effect.
Nitrates*	Possible decreased effects of both drugs.
Phenothiazines*	Possible increased xylometazoline toxicity. Possible decreased xylometazoline effect.
Rauwolfia	Decreased rauwolfia effect.
Sympathomimetics*	Increased effect of both drugs, especially harmful side effects.
Terazosin	Decreases effectiveness of terazosin.

POSSIBLE INTERACTION WITH OTHER SUBSTANCES

INTERACTS WITH	COMBINED EFFECT
Alcohol:	None expected.
Beverages: Caffeine drinks.	Nervousness or insomnia.
Cocaine:	High risk of heartbeat irregularities and high blood pressure.
Foods:	None expected.
Marijuana:	Overstimulation. Avoid.
Tobacco:	None expected.

ZIDOVUDINE (AZT, Azidothymidine)

BRAND NAMES

Apo-Zidovudine   Retrovir

BASIC INFORMATION

Habit forming? No
Prescription needed? Yes
Available as generic? No
Drug class: Antiviral

USES

Treatment of selected adult patients infected with HIV (human immunodeficiency virus), AIDS (acquired immune deficiency syndrome) and advanced ARC (AIDS-related complex). Does not cure the infection.

DOSAGE & USAGE INFORMATION

How to take:
- Capsule—Swallow with liquid.
- Syrup—Take with liquid.

When to take:
Every 4 hours around the clock unless instructed otherwise.

If you forget a dose:
Take as soon as you remember.

What drug does:
Inhibits reproduction of some viruses, including HIV virus (the virus that causes AIDS).

Time lapse before drug works:
May require several weeks of treatment for full effect. Absorption is rapid.

Don't take with:
- High-fat meals.
- Any other medicine without consulting your doctor or pharmacist.

OVERDOSE

SYMPTOMS:
Unusual bleeding or bruising, severe nausea and vomiting, seizures, unsteady gait.
WHAT TO DO:
- **Dial 0 (operator) or 911 (emergency) for an ambulance or medical help. Then give first aid immediately.**
- **See emergency information on inside covers.**

POSSIBLE ADVERSE REACTIONS OR SIDE EFFECTS

SYMPTOMS	WHAT TO DO
Life-threatening:	
Lip or tongue swelling.	Discontinue. Seek emergency treatment.
Common:	
• Pale skin (anemia), chills, diarrhea.	Discontinue. Call doctor right away.
• Severe headache, nausea, insomnia, diarrhea.	Continue. Call doctor when convenient.
Infrequent:	
Sweating, fever, appetite loss, abdominal pain, vomiting, aching muscles, dizziness, numbness in hands and feet, shortness of breath, skin rash, strange taste, nervousness, itching, mouth sores, discolored nails.	Continue. Call doctor when convenient.
Rare:	
Constipation, confusion, fainting, unexplained bleeding.	Discontinue. Call doctor right away.

WARNINGS & PRECAUTIONS

Don't take if:
You are allergic to any component of this capsule.

Before you start, consult your doctor:
- If you know you have a low white-blood-cell count or severe anemia.
- If you have severe kidney or liver disease.

Over age 60:
Elimination may be slower.

Pregnancy:
Should not be used in pregnancy except when zidovudine is clearly indicated.

Breast-feeding:
Not recommended for HIV-positive mothers.

Infants & children:
Not recommended.

ZIDOVUDINE (AZT, Azidothymidine)

Prolonged use:
Talk to your doctor about the need for follow-up medical examinations or laboratory studies to check complete blood counts (white blood cell count, platelet count, red blood cell count, hemoglobin, hematocrit).

Skin & sunlight:
No problems expected.

Driving, piloting, or hazardous work:
Don't drive or pilot aircraft until you learn how medicine affects you. Don't work around dangerous machinery. Don't climb ladders or work in high places. Danger increases if you drink alcohol or take medicine affecting alertness and reflexes, such as antihistamines, tranquilizers, sedatives, pain medicine, narcotics and mind-altering drugs.

Discontinuing:
Don't discontinue without consulting your doctor. Dose may require gradual reduction if you have taken drug for a long time. Doses of other drugs may also require adjustment.

Others:
- Zidovudine does *not cure* HIV virus infections. Transfusions or dose modification may be necessary if toxicity develops.
- Have blood counts followed closely during treatment to detect anemia or lowered white-blood-cell count.
- Zidovudine does not reduce risk of transmitting disease to others.
- Healing after dental procedures may be delayed.
- X-ray treatments may worsen anemia.
- Patients with AIDS or ARC may continue to develop complications, including opportunistic infections such as pneumocistis carnii pneumonia.

 POSSIBLE INTERACTION WITH OTHER DRUGS

GENERIC NAME OR DRUG CLASS	COMBINED EFFECT
Acetaminophen	May increase toxic effects of zidovudine. Avoid.
Acyclovir	Lethargy, convulsions.
Aspirin	May increase toxic effects of zidovudine.
Benzodiazepines	May increase toxic effects of zidovudine. Avoid.
Bone marrow depressants*	Increased bone marrow toxicity.
Cimetidine	May increase toxic effects of zidovudine. Avoid.
Clarithromycin	Decreased zidovudine effect.
Clozapine	Toxic effect on bone marrow.
Ganciclovir	Increased toxicity of both drugs. Use combination with caution only when essential.
Indomethacin	May increase toxic effects of zidovudine.
Levamisole	Increased risk of bone marrow depression.
Morphine	May increase toxic effects of zidovudine. Avoid.
Probenecid	May increase toxic effects of zidovudine.
Ribavirin	Decreased zidovudine effect.
Sulfadoxine and pyrimethamine	Increased risk of liver toxicity.
Sulfa drugs*	May increase toxic effects of zidovudine. Avoid.
Thioguanine	More likelihood of toxicity of both drugs.
Tiopronin	Increased risk of toxicity to bone marrow.

 POSSIBLE INTERACTION WITH OTHER SUBSTANCES

INTERACTS WITH	COMBINED EFFECT
Alcohol:	Unknown. Best to avoid.
Beverages:	None expected.
Cocaine:	Unknown. Best to avoid.
Foods:	None expected.
Marijuana:	Unknown. Best to avoid.
Tobacco:	None expected.

ZINC SUPPLEMENTS

BRAND NAMES

Egozinc
Orazinc
Verazinc
ZINC CHLORIDE
ZINC GLUCONATE

ZINC SULFATE
Zinc-220
Zincate
Zinkaps-220

Numerous multiple vitamin supplements.
Check label.

BASIC INFORMATION

Habit forming? No
Prescription needed? No
Available as generic? No
Drug class: Nutritional supplement (mineral)

 USES

- Treats zinc deficiency that may lead to growth retardation, appetite loss, changes in taste or smell, skin eruptions, slow wound healing, decreased immune function, diarrhea or impaired night vision.
- In absence of a deficiency, is used to treat burns, eating disorders, liver disorders, prematurity in infants, intestinal diseases, parasitism, kidney disorders, skin disorders and stress.
- May be useful as a supplement for those who are breast-feeding or pregnant (under a doctor's supervision).

 DOSAGE & USAGE INFORMATION

How to take:
Tablet or capsule—Swallow with liquid. If you can't swallow whole, crumble tablet or open capsule and take with liquid or food.

When to take:
At the same time each day, according to a doctor's instructions or the package label.

Continued next column

 OVERDOSE

SYMPTOMS:
Dizziness, yellow eyes and skin, shortness of breath, chest pain, vomiting.
WHAT TO DO:
- **Have patient drink lots of water.**
- **Dial 0 (operator) or 911 (emergency) for an ambulance or medical help. Then give first aid immediately.**

If you forget a dose:
Take as soon as you remember up to 2 hours late. If more than 2 hours, wait for next scheduled dose (don't double this dose).

What drug does:
Required by the body for the utilization of many enzymes, nucleic acids and proteins and for cell growth.

Time lapse before drug works:
2 hours.

Don't take with:
See Interaction column and consult doctor.

 POSSIBLE ADVERSE REACTIONS OR SIDE EFFECTS

SYMPTOMS	WHAT TO DO
Life-threatening:	
In case of overdose, see previous column.	
Common:	
None expected.	
Infrequent:	
None expected.	
Rare:	
• Indigestion, heartburn, nausea and vomiting (only with large doses).	Continue. Call doctor when convenient.
• Fever, chills, sore throat, ulcers in throat or mouth, unusual tiredness or weakness (only with large doses).	Discontinue. Call doctor right away.

WARNINGS & PRECAUTIONS

Don't take if:
You have an upper respiratory infection (zinc makes this worse).

Before you start, consult your doctor:
If you are pregnant or breast-feeding.

Over age 60:
No special problems expected. Nutritional supplements may be helpful if the diet is restricted in any way.

Pregnancy:
Adequate zinc intake is important. Consult a doctor.

Breast-feeding:
Adequate zinc intake important. Consult a doctor.

Infants & children:
Normal daily requirements vary with age. Consult a doctor.

Prolonged use:
No special problems expected.

Skin & sunlight:
No special problems expected.

Driving, piloting or hazardous work:
No special problems expected.

Discontinuing:
No special problems expected.

Others:
The best natural sources of zinc are red meats, oysters, herring, peas and beans.

 ## POSSIBLE INTERACTION WITH OTHER DRUGS

GENERIC NAME OR DRUG CLASS	COMBINED EFFECT
Copper supplements	Inhibited absorption of copper.
Diuretics, thiazide*	Increased need for zinc.
Folic acid	Increased need for zinc.
Iron supplements*	Increased need for zinc
Penicillamine	Increased need for zinc.
Tetracyclines*	Decreased absorption of tetracycline if taken within 2 hours of each other.

 ## POSSIBLE INTERACTION WITH OTHER SUBSTANCES

INTERACTS WITH	COMBINED EFFECT
Alcohol:	May increase need for zinc.
Beverages:	No proven problems.
Cocaine:	No proven problems.
Foods: High-fiber.	May decrease zinc absorption.
Marijuana:	No proven problems.
Tobacco:	May increase need for zinc.

Brand and Generic Name Directory

The following drugs are alphabetized by generic name or drug class, shown in large capital letters. The brand and generic names that follow each title in this list are the complete list referred to on the drug charts. Generic names are in all capital letters on the lists.

ACETAMINOPHEN
Abenol
Acephen
Aceta
Acetaminophen Uniserts
Actamin
Actamin Extra
Actimol
Alba-Temp 300
Allerest No-Drowsiness
Amaphen
Aminofen
Aminofen Max
Anacin-3
Anatuss
Anatuss with Codeine
Anoquan
Anuphen
Apacet
Apacet Extra Strength
Apacet Oral Solution
APAP
Apo-Acetaminophen
Aspirin-Free Excedrin Caplets
Atasol
Atasol Forte
Bancap
Banesin
Benadryl Allergy/Sinus Headache
    Caplets
Beta-Phed
Bromo-Seltzer
Bucet
Butace
Campain
Chexit
Children's Anacin 3
Children's Genapap
Children's Panadol
Children's Ty-Tab
Children's Tylenol
Co-Apap
Co-Tylenol
Coldrine
Colrex Compound
Comtrex
Comtrex Daytime Caplets
Comtrex Multi-Symptom Cold
    Reliever
Comtrex Multi-Symptom Hot Flu
    Relief
Comtrex Multi-Symptom Non-
    Drowsy Caplets
Comtrex Nighttime
Conacetol
Conar-A
Congespirin
Congespirin for Children Cold
    Tablets
Congespirin for Children Liquid
    Cold Medicine
Contac Jr. Children's Cold
    Medicine
Contac Maximum Strength Sinus
    Caplets

Contac Severe Cold Formula
Contac Severe Cold Formula
    Night Strength
CoTylenol Cold Medication
Covangesic
Dapa
Datril Extra Strength
DayCare
DayQuil Liquicaps
DayQuil Non-Drowsy Cold/Flu
Dilotab
Dolanex
Dolmar
Dorcol Children's Fever and Pain
    Reducer
Drinophen
Dristan
Dristan Cold
Dristan Cold and Flu
Dristan Maximum Strength
    Caplets
Drixoral Plus
Drixoral Sinus
Duadacin
Effervescent Tylenol Cold
Endolor
Esgic
Excedrin
Exdol
Exdol Strong
Ezol
Febridyne
Femcet
Fendol
Feverall Sprinkle Caps
Fevernol Children's Strength
Fevernol Junior Strength
Fioricet
Genapap
Genapap Extra Strength
Genebs
Genebs Extra Strength
Genex
Halenol
Halenol Extra Strength
Hycomine Compound
Improved Sino-Tuss
Infants' Anacin-3
Infants Genapap
Isopap
Kolephrin/DM
Korigesic
Liquiprin Children's Elixir
Liquiprin Infants' Drops
Meda Cap
Meda Tab
Medi-Flu
Medi-Flu Caplets
Medigesic
Midrin
Myapap Elixir
Naldegesic
Neo Citran Sinus Medicine
Neopap
NyQuil Liquicaps

NyQuil Nighttime Colds Medicine
Nytime Cold Medicine Liquid
Omnicol
Oraphen-PD
Ornex No Drowsiness Caplets
Pacaps
Panadol
Panadol Junior Strength
Panex
Panex 500
Paracetamol
Parafon Forte
Pedric
Pertussin PM
PhenAPAP No. 2
Phenaphen
Phrenilin
Presalin
Remcol-C
Repan
Rhinocaps
Robigesic
Robitussin Night Relief
Robitussin Night Relief Colds
    Formula Liquid
Rogesic
Rounox
Saleto-CF
Saleto D
Sedapap-10
Semcet
Sinarest
Sinarest No-Drowsiness
Sine-Aid
Sine-Aid Maximum Strength
Sine-Aid Maximum Strength
    Caplets
Sine-Off Maximum Strength
    Allergy
Sine-Off Maximum Strength-No
    Drowsiness
Singlet
Sinubid
Sinulin
Sinus Excedrin No Drowsiness
Sinus Excedrin No Drowsiness
    Caplets
Sinutab
Sinutab II Maximum Strength
Sinutab Maximum Strength
    without Drowsiness
Sinutab Maximum Strength
    without Drowsiness Caplets
Sinutab No Drowsiness
Sinutab No Drowsiness Extra
    Strength
St. Joseph Aspirin Free
St. Joseph Cold Tablets for
    Children
Sudafed Severe Cold Formula
Sudafed Sinus Maximum
    Strength
Sudafed Sinus Maximum
    Strength Caplets
Summit

Super-Anahist
Suppap
Tapanol
Tapanol Extra Strength
Tapar
Tempra
Tempra Double Strength
Tencet
Tenol
TheraFlu/Flu & Cold
TheraFlu/Flu, Cold & Cough
TheraFlu Nighttime Maximum
  Strength
Triad
Triaminicin
Triaminicin w/Codeine
Triaprin
Tussagesic
Two-Dyne
Ty-Cold Cold Formula
Ty Pap
Ty-Tab Extra Strength
Ty-Tab
Tylenol
Tylenol Allergy Sinus Gelcaps
Tylenol Cold and Flu
Tylenol Cold Medication
Tylenol Cold Medication,
  Non-Drowsy
Tylenol Cold Night Time
Tylenol Cough
Tylenol Extra Strength
Tylenol Junior Strength
Tylenol Sinus Maximum Strength
Tylenol Sinus Maximum Strength
  Caplets
Tylenol Sinus Medication
Tylenol Sinus Medication Extra
  Strength
Valadol
Valadol Liquid
Valorin
Valorin Extra
Vicks Formula 44M Multi-
  symptom Cough Mixture

ACETAMINOPHEN & SALICYLATES

ACETAMINOPHEN & ASPIRIN
ACETAMINOPHEN &
  SALICYLAMIDE
ACETAMINOPHEN & SODIUM
  SALICYLATE
ACETAMINOPHEN, ASPIRIN &
  SALICYLAMIDE
Arthralgin
Buffets II
Duoprin
Duradyne
Excedrin
Gelpirin
Gemnisyn
Goody's Extra Strength Tablets
Goody's Headache Powders
Presalin
Rid-A-Pain Compound
S-A-C
Salatin
Saleto
Salocol
Salphenyl
Supac

Tenol Plus
Tri-Pain
Trigesic
Vanquish

ADRENOCORTICOIDS (Topical)

9-1-1
Aclovate
Acticort-100
Adcortyl
Aeroseb-Dex
Aeroseb-HC
Ala-Cort
Ala-Scalp HP
ALCLOMETASONE (Topical)
Allercort
Alphaderm
Alphatrex
AMCINONIDE (Topical)
Anusol 2.5%, PD
Aristocort
Aristocort A
Aristocort C
Aristocort D
Aristocort R
Bactine
Barriere-HC
Beben
BECLOMETHASONE (Topical)
Beta-Val
Betacort Scalp Lotion
Betaderm
Betaderm Scalp Lotion
Betamethacot
BETAMETHASONE (Topical)
Betatrex
Betnovate
Bio-Syn
CaldeCORT Anti-Itch
CaldeCORT-Light
Carmol-HC
Celestoderm-V
Cetacort
CLOBETASOL (Topical)
CLOBETASONE (Topical)
CLOCORTOLONE (Topical)
Cloderm
Cordran
Cordran SP
Cort-Dome
Cortacet
Cortaid
Cortate
Cortef
Cortef Feminine Itch
Corticaine
Corticreme
Cortifair
CORTISOL
Cortoderm
Cortril
Cultivate
Cyclocort
Decaderm
Decadron
Decaspray
Delacort
Dermabet
Dermacort
DermiCort
Dermovate

Dermovate Scalp Application
Dermtex HC
DESONIDE (Topical)
DesOwen
DESOXIMETASONE (Topical)
DEXAMETHASONE (Topical)
DIFLORASONE (Topical)
DIFLUCORTOLONE (Topical)
Diprosone
Drenison
Ectosone
Ectosone Scalp Lotion
Efcortelan
Elcom
Elocon
Emo-Cort
Epifoam
Eumovate
Florene E
Florone
Fludonid
Fludroxycortide
FLUMETHASONE (Topical)
Fluocet
Fluocin
FLUOCINOLONE (Topical)
FLUOCINONIDE (Topical)
Fluoderm
Fluolar
Fluonide
FLURANDRENOLIDE (Topical)
Flutex
FLUTICASONE
Foille Cort
Gly-Cort
Gynecort
Gynecort 10
H2 Cort
Halciderm
HALCINONIDE (Topical)
HALOBETASOL
Halog
Halog E
HI-Cor
Hyderm
Hydro-Tex
HYDROCORTISONE (Dental)
HYDROCORTISONE (Rectal)
HYDROCORTISONE (Topical)
Hytone
Kenac
Kenalog
Kenalog-H
Keronel
Lacticare-HC
Lanacort
Lanacort 10
Lemoderm
Licon
Lidemol
Lidex
Lidex-E
Locacorten
Locoid
Lotrisone
Lyderm
Maxiflor
Maxivate
Medrol
Metaderm
METHYLPREDNISOLONE (Topical)
Metosyn
Metosyn FAPG

905

MOMETASONE (Topical)
My Cort
Nerisone
Novobetamet
Novohydrocort
Nutracort
Pentacort
Pharma-Cort
Prevex B
Prevex HC
Propaderm
Psorcon
Rederm
Rhulicort
Sential
S-T Cort
Sarna HC
Synacort
Synalar
Synamol
Synandone
Synemol
Temovate
Texacort-Scalp Solution
Topicort
Topsyn
Triaderm
TRIAMCINOLONE (Dental)
TRIAMCINOLONE (Topical)
Trianide
Trymex
Ultravate
Unicort
Uticort
Valisone
Valisone Scalp Lotion
Valnac
Vioform-Hydrocortisone
Westcort
Some of these brands are
    available as oral medicine.
    Look under specific generic
    name for each brand.

ANDROGENS
Anabolin
Anabolin LA 100
Anadrol
Anapolon 50
Anavar
Andro 100
Andro-Cyp 100
Andro-LA 200
Android
Android-F
Android-T
Androlone
Andronaq-50
Andronaq-LA
Andronate
Andropository 100
Andryl 200
Deca-Durabolin
Delatest
Delatestryl
Dep Andro
Depo-Testosterone
Depotest
Durabolin
Duratest
Durathate 200
ETHYLESTRENOL

Everone
FLUOXYMESTERONE
Halotestin
Histerone
Hybolin Decanoate
Hybolin-Improved
Kabolin
Malogen
Malogex
Maxibolin
Metandren
METHYLTESTOSTERONE
Nancrobolic L.A.
Nandrobolic
NANDROLONE
Neo-Durabolic
Ora-Testryl
Oreton
OXANDROLONE
OXYMETHOLONE
STANOZOLOL
T-Cypionate
Testa-C
Testamone 100
Testaqua
Testex
Testoject-50
Testoject-LA
Testone L.A.
TESTOSTERONE
Testred
Testred-Cypionate 200
Testrin P.A.
Virilon
Virolon IM
Winstrol

ANESTHETICS (Topical)
Americaine
Aminobenzoate
Bactine
BENZOCAINE
BENZOCAINE & MENTHOL
Benzocal
BUTACAINE
BUTAMBEN
Butesin Picrate
Butyl Aminobenzoate
CAPSAICIN
Cinchocaine
CYCLOMETHYCAINE
DIBUCAINE
DIPERODON
DYCLONINE
EMLA
Ethyl Aminobenzoate
LIDOCAINE
LIDOCAINE AND PRILOCAINE
Lignocaine
Mercurochrome II
Nupercainal Cream
Nupercainal Ointment
Pontocaine Cream
Pontocaine Ointment
PRAMOXINE
Prax
TETRACAINE
TETRACAINE & MENTHOL
Tronothane
Unguentine
Unguentine Plus
Unguentine Spray

Xylocaine
Zostrix
Zostrix-HP

ANGIOTENSIN-CONVERTING ENZYME (ACE) INHIBITORS
Accupril
Altace
Apo-Capto
BENAZEPRIL
Capoten
CAPTOPRIL
ENALAPRIL
FOSINOPRIL
LISINOPRIL
Lotensin
Monopril
Prinivil
QUINAPRIL
RAMIPRIL
Syn-Captopril
Vasotec
Zestril

ANGIOTENSIN-CONVERTING ENZYME (ACE) INHIBITORS & HYDROCHLORO-THIAZIDE
Capozide
CAPTOPRIL & HYDROCHLOROTHIAZIDE
ENALAPRIL & HYDROCHLOROTHIAZIDE
LISINOPRIL & HYDROCHLOROTHIAZIDE
Prinzide
Vaseretic
Zestoretic

ANTACIDS
Advanced Formula Di-Gel
Alamag
Algenic Alka
Algenic Alka Improved
Algicon
Alka-Mints
Alkets
Alma-Mag Improved
Alma-Mag #4 Improved
Almacone
Almacone II
ALternaGEL
Alu-Cap
Alu-Tab
Aludrox
Alumid
Alumid Plus
Alumid Plus II
ALUMINA AND MAGNESIA
ALUMINA AND MAGNESIUM CARBONATE
ALUMINA AND MAGNESIUM TRISILICATE
ALUMINA, MAGNESIA, AND CALCIUM CARBONATE
ALUMINA, MAGNESIA, AND SIMETHICONE

ALUMINA, MAGNESIUM
    CARBONATE, AND CALCIUM
    CARBONATE
ALUMINA, MAGNESIUM
    TRISILICATE, AND SODIUM
    BICARBONATE
ALUMINUM CARBONATE, BASIC
ALUMINUM HYDROXIDE
Amitone
Amphojel
Amphojel Plus
Amphojel Plus
Amphojel 500
AntaGel
AntaGel-II
Antiflux
Basaljel
Bisodol
Calcilac
Calcitrel
CALCIUM AND MAGNESIUM
    CARBONATES
CALCIUM AND MAGNESIUM
    CARBONATES AND
    MAGNESIUM OXIDE
CALCIUM CARBONATE
CALCIUM CARBONATE AND
    MAGNESIA
CALCIUM CARBONATE AND
    SIMETHICONE
CALCIUM CARBONATE,
    MAGNESIA, AND
    SIMETHICONE
Calglycine
Camalox
Chooz
Creamalin
Delcid
Di-Gel
DialumeDicarbosil
DIHYDROXYALUMINUM
    AMINOACETATE
DIHYDROXYALUMINUM
    AMINOACETATE, MAGNESIA,
    AND ALUMINA
DIHYDROXYALUMINUM SODIUM
    CARBONATE
Diovol Ex
Diovol Plus
Duracid
Equilet
Escot
Gas-Is-gon
Gaviscon
Gaviscon Extra Strength Relief
    Formula
Gaviscon-2
Gelamal
Gelusil
Gelusil Extra-Strength
Gelusil-M
Gelusil-II
Genalac
Glycate
Gustalac
Kudrox Double Strength
Liquimint
Losotron Plus
Lowsium
Lowsium Plus
Maalox
Maalox No. 1
Maalox No. 2

Maalox Plus
Maalox Plus, Extra Strength
Maalox TC
Maalox Whip, Extra Strength
Mag-Ox 400
MAGALDRATE
MAGALDRATE AND
    SIMETHICONE
Magmalin
Magnagel
Magnatril
MAGNESIUM CARBONATE AND
    SODIUM BICARBONATE
MAGNESIUM HYDROXIDE
MAGNESIUM OXIDE
MAGNESIUM TRISILICATE,
    ALUMINA, AND MAGNESIUM
    CARBONATE
MAGNESIUM TRISILICATE,
    ALUMINA, AND MAGNESIA
Mallamint
Maox
Mi-Acid
Mintox
Mygel
Mygel II
Mylanta
Mylanta-2 Extra Strength
Mylanta-2 PlainMylanta-II
Nephrox
Neutralca-S
Newtrogel II
Noralac
Pama No. 1
Par-Mag
Parviscon
Phillips' Milk of Magnesia
Riopan
Riopan Extra Strength
Riopan Plus
Riopan Plus 2
Riopan Plus Extra Strength
Robalate
Rolaids
Rolaids Calcium Rich
Rolaids Sodium Free
Rulox
Rulox No. 1
Rulox No. 2
Silain-Gel
Simaal Gel
Simaal 2 Gel
SIMETHICONE, ALUMINA,
    CALCIUM CARBONATE, AND
    MAGNESIA
SIMETHICONE, ALUMINA,
    MAGNESIUM CARBONATE,
    AND MAGNESIA
Spastosed
Tempo
Titracid
Titralac
Titralac Plus
Tralmag
Triconsil
Tums
Tums E-X
Tums Liquid Extra Strength
Tums Liquid Extra Strength
    w/Simethicone
Univol
Uro-Mag
WinGel

ANTI-ACNE (Topical)

Acne-Aid Gel
Acno
Acnomel-Acne Cream
Acnomel Cake
Acnotex
Anti-acne
Antinea
Aveeno Acne Bar
Aveeno Cleansing Bar
Bensulfoid Cream
Buf-Puf
Buf-Puf Acne Cleansing Bar with
    Vitamin E
Buf-Puf Medicated Maximum
    Strength Pads
Buf-Puf Medicated Regular
    Strength Pads
Calicylic
Clear Away
Clear by Design Medicated
    Cleansing Pads
Clearasil Adult Care Medicated
Clearasil Adult Care Medicated
    Blemish Stick
Clearasil Clearstick Maximum
    Strength Topical Solution
Clearasil Clearstick Regular
    Strength Topical Solution
Clearasil Double Textured Pads
    Maximum Strength
Clearasil Double Textured Pads
    Regular Strength
Clearasil Medicated Deep
    Cleanser Topical Solution
Compound W Gel
Compound W Liquid
Cuplex Gel
Cuticura Ointment
Derma & Soft Creme
Diasporal Cream
Duofilm
Duoplant
Duoplant Topical Solution
Fostex CM
Fostex Medicated Cleansing Bar
Fostex Medicated Cleansing
Fostex Regular Strength
    Medicated Cleansing Cream
Fostex Medicated Cleansing
    Liquid
Fostex Regular Strength
    Medicated Cleansing Bar
Fostex Regular Strength
    Medicated Cleansing Cream
Fostex Regular Strength
    Medicated Cover-Up
Fostril Cream
Fostril Lotion
Freezone
Gordofilm
Hydrosalic
Ionax Astringent Skin Cleanser
    Topical Solution
Ionil Plus Shampoo
Ionil Shampoo
Keralyt
Keratex Gel
Lactisol
Liquimat
Listerex Golden Scrub
Listerex Golden Scrub Lotion

Listerex Herbal Scrub Lotion
Mediplast
Meted Maximum Strength Anti-
Dandruff Shampoo with
Conditioners
Night Cast R
Night Cast Regular Formula
Mask-Lotion
Night Cast Special Formula
Mask-Lotion
Noxzema Anti-Acne Gel
Noxzema Anti-Acne Pads
Maximum Strength
Noxzema Anti-Acne Pads
Regular Strength
Occlusal Topical Solution
Occlusal-HP Topical Solution
Off-Ezy
Off-Ezy Topical Solution Corn &
Callus Removal Kit
Off-Ezy Topical Solution Wart
Removal Kit
Oxy Clean
Oxy Clean Maximum Strength
Oxy Clean Medicated Cleanser
Oxy Clean Medicated Pads
Maximum Strength
Oxy Clean Medicated Pads
Sensitive Skin
Oxy Clean Medicated Soap
Oxy Clean Regular Strength
Oxy Clean Regular Strength
Medicated Cleanser Topical
Solution
Oxy Clean Regular Strength
Medicated Pads
Oxy Clean Sensitive Skin
Cleanser Topical Solution
Oxy Clean Sensitive Skin Pads
Oxy Night Watch Maximum
Strength Lotion
Oxy Night Watch Night Time
Acne Medication Extra
Strength Lotion
Oxy Night Watch Night Time
Acne Medication Regular
Strength Lotion
Oxy Night Watch Sensitive Skin
Lotion
Oxy Sensitive Skin Vanishing
Formula Lotion
P&S
Paplex
Paplex Ultra
Pernox Lemon Medicated Scrub
Cleanser
Pernox Lotion Lathering
Abradant Scrub Cleanser
Pernox Lotion Lathering Scrub
Cleanser
Pernox Regular Medicated Scrub
Cleanser
Postacne
Propa pH Medicated Acne Cream
Maximum Strength
Propa pH Medicated Cleansing
Pads Maximum Strength
Propa pH Medicated Cleansing
Pads Sensitive Skin
Propa pH Perfectly Clear Skin
Cleanser Topical Solution Oily
Skin
Propa pH Perfectly Clear Skin

Cleanser Topical Solution
Sensitive Skin Formula
R.A.
RESORCINOL
RESORCINOL & SULFUR
Rezamid Lotion
Salac
Salacid
Sal-Acid Plaster
Salactic Film Topical Solution
Sal-Clens Plus Shampoo
Sal-Clens Shampoo
SALICYLIC ACID
SALICYLIC ACID & SULFUR
Saligel
Salonil
Sal-Plant Gel Topical Solution
Sastid
Sastid (AL) Scrub
Sastid Plain
Sastid Plain Shampoo and Acne
Wash
Sastid Soap
Sebasorb Liquid
Sebex
Sebulex Antiseborrheic
Treatment and Conditioning
Shampoo
Sebulex Antiseborrheic
Treatment Shampoo
Sebulex Conditioning Shampoo
Sebulex Cream Medicated
Shampoo
Sebulex Medcicated Dandruff
Shampoo with Conditioners
Sebulex Medicated Shampoo
Sebulex Regular Medicated
Dandruff Shampoo
Sebulex Shampoo
Stri-Dex
Stri-Dex Dual Textured Pads
Maximum Strength
Stri-Dex Dual Textured Pads
Regular Strength
Stri-Dex Dual Textured Pads
Sensitive Skin
Stri-Dex Maximum Strength Pads
Stri-Dex Regular Strength Pads
Stri-Dex Super Scrub Pads
Sulfo-Lac
Sulforcin
SULFUR (Topical)
Sulsal Soap
Tersac Cleansing Gel
Therac Lotion
Trans-Ver-Sal
Vanseb
Verukan Topical Solution
Verukan-HP Topical Solution
Viranol
Wart-Off Topical Solution
Xseb

ANTIBACTERIALS
(Ophthalmic)

Achromycin
Ak-Chlor Ophthalmic Ointment
Ak-Sulf
Alcomicin
Aureomycin
Bleph-10
Cetamide

Chibroxin
Chloracol Ophthalmic Solution
CHLORAMPHENICOL (Ophthalmic)
Chlorofair Ophthalmic Ointment
Chlorofair Ophthalmic Solution
Chloromycetin Ophthalmic
Ointment
Chloromycetin Ophthalmic
Solution
Chloroptic Ophthalmic Solution
Chloroptic S.O.P.
CHLORTETRACYCLINE
Cortisporin-Ophthalmic
Econochlor Ophthalmic Ointment
Econochlor Ophthalmic Solution
ERYTHROMYCIN (Ophthalmic)
Fenicol Ophthalmic Ointment
Gantrisin
Garamycin
Genoptic
Gentacidin
Gentafair
Gentak
GENTAMICIN
Gentrasul
I-Chlor Ophthalmic Solution
I-Sulfacet
Ilotycin
Isopto Cetamide
Isopto Fenicol
Mycitracin
NEOMYCIN
NEOMYCIN, POLYMIXIN B &
BACITRACIN
NEOMYCIN, POLYMIXIN B &
CORTISOL
NEOMYCIN, POLYMIXIN B &
GRAMICIDIN
NEOMYCIN, POLYMIXIN B &
HYDROCORTISONE
Neosporin
Neotricin
Ocu-Chlor Ophthalmic Ointment
Ocu-Chlor Ophthalmic Solution
Ocu-Mycin
Ocu-Sul-10
Ocu-Sul-15
Ocu-Sul-30
Ocusulf-10
Ophthacet
Ophthochlor Ophthalmic
Solution
Ophtho-Chloram Ophthalmic
Solution
Pentamycetin Ophthalmic
Ointment
Pentamycetin Ophthalmic
Solution
Sodium Sulamyd
Sopamycetin Ophthalmic
Ointment
Sopamycetin Ophthalmic
Solution
Spectro-Chlor Ophthalmic
Ointment
Spectro-Chlor Ophthalmic
Solution
Spectro-Genta
Spectro-Sulf
Steri-Units Sulfacetamide
SULFACETAMIDE (Ophthalmic)
Sulfair
Sulfair 10

Sulfair 15
Sulfair Forte
Sulfamide
SULFONAMIDES (Ophthalmic)
Sulten-10
TETRACYCLINE (Ophthalmic)

ANTIBACTERIALS (Topical)

BACITRACIN
Bactine First Aid Antibiotic
Bactroban
CHLORAMPHENICOL (Topical)
Chloromycetin
Cleocin T
CLINDAMYCIN
Flamazine
Folile
G-Myticin
Garamycin
Gentamar
GENTAMICIN
MUPIROCIN
Myciguent
Mycitracin
NEOMYCIN
NEOMYCIN & POLYMYXIN B
NEOMYCIN, POLYMYXIN B & BACITRACIN
Neo-Polycin
Neosporin
Topisporan

ANTIBACTERIALS, ANTIFUNGALS (Topical)

CICLIPIROX
Ciloxam
CLIOQUINOL
CLIOQUINOL & Exelderm
HYDROCORTISONE
Dermacomb
Flint SSD
IODOCHLORHYDROXYQUIN
IODOCHLORHYDROXYQUIN & HYDROCORTISONE
Loprox
Lotrisone
Mycobiotic
Mycogen
Mytrex
Racet
Silvadene
SILVER SULFADIAZINE
Sildimac
Thermazene
Tristatin
Vioform
Vioform-Hydrocortisone

ANTIDIABETIC AGENTS

ACETOHEXAMIDE
Alpha-Glibenclamide
Apo-Chlorpropamide
Apo-Tolbutamide
CHLORPROPAMIDE
DiaBeta
Diabinese
Dimelor
Euglucon
GLIPIZIDE
Glucamide

Glucotrol
GLYBURIDE
Micronase
Mobenol
Novobutamide
Novopropamide
Oramide
Orinase
Storzolamide
Tolamide
TOLAZAMIDE
TOLBUTAMIDE
Tolinase

ANTIDYSKINETICS

Akineton
Aparkane
Apo-Benztropine
Apo-Trihex
Artane
Artane Sequels
Bensylate
BENZTROPINE
BIPERIDEN
CARBIDOPA AND LEVODOPA
Cogentin
ETHOPROPAZINE
Kemadrin
Novohexidyl
Parsidol
Parsitan
PIMOZIDE Orap
PMS Benztropine
PMS Procyclidine
Procyclid
PROCYCLIDINE
Trihexane
Trihexy
TRIHEXYPHENIDYL

ANTIFUNGALS (Topical)

Aftate for Athlete's Foot Aerosol Spray Liquid
Aftate for Athlete's Foot Aerosol Spray Powder
Aftate for Athlete's Foot Gel
Aftate for Athlete's Foot Sprinkle Powder
Aftate for Jock Itch Aerosol Spray Powder
Aftate for Jock Itch Gel
Aftate for Jock Itch Sprinkle Powder
AMPHOTERACIN B
Caldesene Medicated Powder
Canesten Cream
Canesten Solution
CICLOPIROX
Ciloxam
CLOTRIMAZOLE
Cruex Aerosol Powder
Cruex Antifungal Cream
Cruex Antifungal Powder
Cruex Antifungal Spray Powder
Cruex Cream
Cruex Powder
Decylenes
Decylenes Powder
Desenex Aerosol Powder
Desenex Antifungal Cream
Desenex Antifungal Liquid
Desenex Antifungal Ointment

Desenex Antifungal Penetrating Foam
Desenex Antifungal Powder
Desenex Antifungal Spray Powder
Desenex Ointment
Desenex Powder
Desenex Solution
ECONAZOLE
Ecostatin
Exelderm
Flamazine
Fungizone
Genaspore Cream
Gordochom Solution
KETOCONAZOLE (Topical)
Lotriderm
Lotrimin Cream
Lotrimin Lotion
Lotrimin Ointment
Lotrisone
Micatin
MICONAZOLE
Monistat-Derm
Mycelex
Mycelex Troches
Myclo Cream
Myclo Solution
Miclo Spray
Mycostatin
Nadostine
NAFTIFINE
Naftin
Nilstat
Nizoral Shampoo
NP-27 Cream
NP-27 Powder
NP-27 Solution
NP-27 Spray Powder
Nyaderm
NYSTATIN
Nystex
Pitrex Cream
Spectazole
SULCONAZOLE
Tinactin Aerosol Liquid
Tinactin Aerosol Powder
Tinactin Antifungal Deodorant Powder Aerosol
Tinactin Cream
Tinactin Jock Itch Aerosol Powder
Tinactin Jock Itch Cream
Tinactin Jock Itch Spray Powder
Tinactin Plus Powder
Tinactin Powder
Tinactin Solution
Ting Antifungal Cream
Ting Antifungal Powder
Ting Antifungal Spray Liquid
Ting Antifungal Spray Powder
TOLNAFTATE
UNDECYLENIC ACID
Zeasorb-AF Powder

ANTIFUNGALS (Vaginal)

BUTOCONAZOLE
Canesten Cream
Canesten Lotion
Cicloprox
Ciloxam
CLOTRIMAZOLE
ECONAZOLE

Ecostatin
FemCare
Femstat
Genapax
Gentian Violet
Gyne-Lotrimin
Gyno-Trosyd
Lotrimin Cream
MICONAZOLE
Monistat
Monistat 3
Monistat 7
Mycelex-G
Myclo
Mycostatin
Nadostine
Nilstat
Nyaderm
NYSTATIN
Terazol 3
Terazol 7
TERCONAZOLE
TIOCONAZOLE

ANTIHISTAMINES

Actacin
Actagen-C Cough
Actidil
Actifed
Actifed 12-Hour
Actifed DM
Actifed w/Codeine Cough
Alamine
Alamine-C Liquid
Alersule
Alka-Seltzer Plus Maximum
    Strength Sinus Allergy
Aller-Chlor
Alleract
Allerest
Allerest 12 Hour
Allerest 12 Hour Caplets
Allerdryl
Allerfrin
Allerfrin w/Codeine
Allergy Formula Sinutab
Allergy Relief Medicine
AllerMax
Allerphed
Allert
Amaril D
Amaril D Spantab
Ambay Cough
Ambenyl Cough
Ambophen Expectorant
Anamine
Anamine HD
Anamine TD
Anatuss
Anatuss w/Codeine
Apo-Dimenhydrinate
Aprodrine
A.R.M. Maximum Strength
    Caplets
ASTEMIZOLE
Atrofed
Atrohist Sprinkle
AZATADINE
Bayaminicol
Baydec DM Drops
Bayhistine DH
BC Cold Powder

Beldin Cough
Belix
Ben-Allergin-50
Bena-D
Bena-D 50
Benadryl
Benadryl Allergy/Sinus Headache
    Caplets
Benadryl Complete Allergy
Benadryl Decongestant
Benahist 10
Benahist 50
Benaphen
Benoject-10
Benoject-50
Benylin Cold
Benylin Cough
Benylin Decongestant
Benylin w/Codeine
Benylin-DM
Biphetane DC Cough
Brexin
Brexin-L.A.
Bromanate DC Cough
Bromatap
Bromatapp
Brombay
Bromfed
Bromfed-AT
Bromfed-DM
Bromfed-PD
BROMODIPHENHYDRAMINE
Bromophen T.D.
Bromphen
Bromphen DC
BROMPHENIRAMINE
Brompheril
Bronkotuss Expectorant
Brotane DX Cough
Bydramine Cough
Caldomine-DH Forte
Caldomine-DH Pediatric
Calm X
Calmylin w/Codeine
CARBINOXAMINE
Carbinoxamine Compound
Carbiset
Carbodec DM Drops
Carbodec TR
Cardec-S
Cenafed Plus
Cerose-DM
Cheracol Plus
Cheracol Sinus
Children's Nyquil Nighttime Cold
    Medicine
Chexit
Chlo-Amine
Chlor-100
Chlorafed
Chlorafed H.S. Timecelles
Chlorafed Timecelles
Chlorate
Chlorgest-HD
Chlor-Niramine
Chlorphed
CHLORPHENIRAMINE
Chlor-Pro
Chlor-Pro 10
Chlor-Rest
Chlorspan-12

Chlortab-4
Chlortab-8
Chlor-Trimeton
Chlor-Trimeton Decongestant
Chlor-Trimeton Repetabs
Chlor-Tripolon
Chlor-Tripolon Decongestant
Citra Forte
Claritin
CLEMASTINE FUMARATE
Clistin
CoActifed
CoActifed Expectorant
Co-Apap
Codehist DH
Codimal-A
Codimal DH
Codimal DM
Codimal-LA Half
Codimal PH
Colrex Compound
Colrex Cough
Coltab Children's
Comhist
Comhist LA
Compoz
Comtrex Multi-Symptom Cold
    Reliever
Comtrex Multi-Symptom Hot Flu
    Relief
Comtrex Nighttime
Condrin LA
Conjec-B
Contact 12-Hour
Contac Severe Cold Formula
Contac Severe Cold Formula
    Night Strength
Cophene No. 2
Cophene-B
Cophene-S
Cophene-X
Cophene-XP
Co-Pyronil 2
Corcidin w/Codeine
Coristex-DH
Coristine-DH
Corsym
CoTylenol Cold Medication
Cremacoat 4 Throat Coating
    Cough Medicine
CYPROHEPTADINE
Dallergy Jr.
Dallergy-D
Decohist
Deconamine
Deconamine SR
Decongestabs
Dehist
Demazin
Demazin Repetabs
Dexaphen SA
DEXBROMPHENIRAMINE
Dexchlor
DEXCHLORPHENIRAMINE
Dexbrompheniramine
Dexophed
Diahist
Diamine T.D.
Dihistine
Dihistine DH
Dihydrex
Dimaphen S.A.
DIMENHYDRINATE

Dimentabs
Dimetane
Dimetane-DC Cough
Dimetane Decongestant
Dimetane-DX Cough
Dimetane Expectorant
Dimetane Expectorant-C
Dimetane Expectorant-DC
Dimetane Extentabs
Dimetane-Ten
Dimetapp
Dimetapp-DM
Dimetapp Extentabs
Dimetapp Maximum Strength
    Liquigels
Dimetapp Oral Infant Drops
Dimetapp w/Codeine
Dinate
Diphen Cough
Diphenacen-10
Diphenacen-50
Diphenadryl
DIPHENHYDRAMINE
DIPHENYLPYRALINE
Disobrom
Disophrol
Disophrol Chronotabs
Dommanate
Donatussin
Donatussin Drops
Dondril
Dorcol Children's Cold Formula
Dormarex 2
Dormin
DOXYLAMINE
Dramamine
Dramamine Chewable
Dramamine Liquid
Dramanate
Dramilin
Dramocen
Dramoject
Dristan Cold
Dristan Cold and Flu
Drixoral
Drixoral Plus
Drixtab
Drize
Duralex
Dura-Tap PD
Dura-Vent/A
Dymenate
Effervescent Tylenol Cold
Efficol Cough Whip (Cough
    Suppressant/Decongestant/
    Antihistamine)
Efricon Expectorant Liquid
Endafed
Endal HD
Endal-HD Plus
Father John's Medicine Plus
Fedahist
Fedahist Decongestant
Fedahist Gyrocaps
Fedahist Timecaps
Fenylhist
Fynex
Genac
Genallerate
Genamin
Genatap
Gencold
Gentab LA

Gravol
Gravol L/A
Guistrey Fortis
Hismanal
Hispril
Histabid Duracaps
Histadyl E.C.
Histafed C
Histaject Modified
Histalet
Histalet DM
Histalet Forte
Histamic
Histatab Plus
Histatan
Histatuss Pediatric
Hista-Vadrin
Histor-D
Hycomine
Hycomine Compound
Hycomine-S Pediatric
Hydramine
Hydramine Cough
Hydrate
Hydril
Hyrexin-50
Improved Sino-Tuss
Insomnal
Isoclor Timesules
Kierist
Kolephrin/DM
Kolephrin NN Liquid
Kophane
Kophane Cough and Cold
    Formula
Kronofed-A
Kronofed-A Jr.
Lanatuss Expectorant
LORATADINE
Mallergan-VC w/Codeine
Marmine
Medatussin Plus
Meda Syrup Forte
Medi-Flu
Medi-Flu Caplets
Midahist DH
Motion-Aid
Myfed
Myfedrine Plus
Myhistine DH
Myidil
Myminic
Myphetane DC Cough
Myphetapp
Naldecon
Naldecon Pediatric
Naldelate
Naldelate Pediatric Syrup
Nalgest
Napril
Nasahist
Nasahist B
Nauseatol
ND Clear T.D.
ND Stat Revised
Nervine Night-time Sleep-Aid
New-Decongest Pediatric Syrup
Nolahist
Nolamine
Noradryl
Norafed
Noraminic
Nordryl

Nordryl Cough
Normatane
Normatane DC
Novafed A
Novahistex
Novahistex C
Novahistex DH
Novahistex DH Expectorant
Novahistex DM
Novahistine
Novahistine DH
Novahistine DH Expectorant
Novahistine DH Liquid
Novodimenate
Novopheniram
NyQuil Liquicaps
NyQuil Nighttime Colds Medicine
Nytime Cold Medicine Liquid
Nytol w/DPH
Omni-Tuss
Omnicol
Optimine
Oragest S.R.
Oraminic II
Oraminic Spancaps
Ornade
Ornade A.F.
Ornade Expectorant
Ornade Spansules
Ornade-DM 10
Ornade-DM 15
Ornade-DM 30
Orthoxicol Cough
Panadyl
Par Decon
PBZ
PBZ-SR
PediaCare Allergy
Pediacare Children's Cold Relief
    Night Rest Cough-Cold
    Formula
PediaCare Children's Cough-Cold
    Formula
Pediacare Cold Formula
Pediacof Cough
Pelamine
Penntuss
Periactin
Pertussin PM
Pfeiffer's Allergy
Phanadex
Phenameth VC w/Codeine
Phenergan VC
Phenergan VC w/Codeine
Phenergan w/Codeine
Phenergan w/Dextromethorphan
Phenergan-D
Phenetron
Phenetron Lanacaps
PHENINDAMINE
PHENIRAMINE
Phentox Compound
PHENYLTOLOXAMINE
Pherazine VC
Pherazine VC w/Codeine
PMS-Dimenhydrinate
Poladex T.D.
Polaramine
Polaramine Expectorant
Polaramine Repetabs
Polargen
Poly-Histine-CS
Poly-Histine-D

Poly-Histine-D Ped
Prometh VC Plain
Poly-Histine-DM
Prometh VC w/Codeine
PROMETHAZINE
Promethazine and Codeine
Promethazine VC
Prominicol Cough
Prominicol Cough
Promist HD Liquid
Pseudo-Car DM
Pseudo-Chlor
Pseudodine C Cough
Pseudo-gest Plus
P-V-Tussin
Pyribenzamine
PYRILAMINE
Pyrilamine Maleate Tablets
Quelidrine Cough
Reidamine
Remcol-C
Rentamine
Resaid S.R.
Resporal TR
Rhinolar-EX
Rhinosyn-DM
Rinade B.I.D.
Robitussin A-C
Robitussin Night Relief
Robitussin Night Relief Colds
    Formula Liquid
Robitussin w/Codeine
Rondec
Rondec Drops
Rondec-DM
Rondec-DM Drops
Rondec-TR
R-Tannate
Ru-Tuss
Ru-Tuss II
Ru-Tuss w/Hydrocodone Liquid
Ryna
Ryna-C Liquid
Rynatan
Rynatuss
Rynatuss Pediatric
Seldane-D
Silphen
Sinucon Pediatric Drops
Sinusol-B
Sleep-Eze 3
Snaplets Multi
Snaplets-D
Sominex Liquid
Statuss Expectorant
Statuss Green
Sudafed Plus
Tamine S.R.
Tavist
Tavist-1
Tavist-D
T-Dry
T-Dry Junior
Telachlor
Teldrin
TheraFlu/Flu & Cold
TheraFlu/Flu, Cold & Cough
TheraFlu Nighttime Maximum
    Strength
T-Koff
Travamine

Triacin C Cough
Triaminic
Triaminic Allergy
Triaminic Chewables
Triaminic Cold
Triaminic Expectorant
Triaminic Expectorant DH
Triaminic Nite Light
Triaminic Oral Infant Drops
Triaminic TR
Triaminic-12
Triaminic-DM Expectorant
Triaminicin w/Codeine
Triaminicol DM
Triaminicol Multi-Symptom Relief
Tricodene Forte
Tricodene NN
Trifed
Trifed-C Cough
Trimedine Liquid
Trinalin Repetabs
Trind
Trind DM Liquid
Tri-Nefrin Extra Strength
Trinex
Triofed
Triotann
Tripalgin Cold
Trip-Tone
TRIPELENNAMINE
Tri-Phen-Chlor
Tri-Phen-Chlor T.D.
Triphenyl
Triphenyl T.D.
Tripodrine
Triposed
TRIPROLIDINE
Tritann Pediatric
Trymegen
Tusquelin
Tuss-Ornade Spansules
Tussafed
Tussagesic
Tussaminic DH Forte
Tussaminic DH Pediatric
Tussanil DH
Tussanil Plain
Tussar DM
Tussar SF
Tussar-2
Tussionex
Tussirex w/Codeine Liquid
Tusstat
Twilite
Ty-Cold Cold Formula
Tylenol Allergy Sinus Gelcaps
Tylenol Cold and Flu
Tylenol Cold Medication
Tylenol Cold Night Time
Unisom Nighttime Sleep Aid
Valdrene
Vanex-HD
Vasominic T.D.
Veltane
Veltap
Vicks Formula 44 Cough Mixture
Viro-Med
Wehamine
Wehdryl

ANTI-INFLAMMATORY DRUGS, NON-STEROIDAL (NSAIDs)

Aches-N-Pain
Advil
Advil Caplets
Alka-Butazolidin
Alka-Phenylbutazone
Alkabutazone
Airheumat
Amersol
Anaprox
Anaprox DS
Ansaid
Apo-Diclo
Apo-Ibuprofen
Apo-Indomethacin
Apo-Keto
Apo-Keto-E
Apo-Naproxen
Apo-Piroxicam
Apsifen
Apsifen-F
Brufen
Butacote
Butazone
Children's Advil
Clinoril
CoAdvil
DICLOFENAC
DIFLUNISAL
Dolgesic
Dolobid
ETODOLAC
Excedrin-IB Caplets
Excedrin-IB Tablets
Feldene
FENOPROFEN
Fenopron
FLOCTAFENINE
FLURBIPROFEN
Froben
Genpril
Haltran
Ibren
Ibumed
Ibuprin
Ibupro-600
IBUPROFEN
Ibutex
Idarac
Ifen
Imbrilon
Indameth
Indocid
Indocid SR
Indocin
Indocin SR
Indolar SR
INDOMETHACIN
Intrabutazone
KETOPROFEN
Lidifen
Lodine
Meclofen
MECLOFENAMATE
Meclomen
Medipren
MEFENAMIC ACID
Midol 200

Motrin
Motrin-IB
Motrin-IB Caplets
NABUMETONE
Nalfon
Nalfon 200
Naprosyn
NAPROXEN
Naxen
Novo-Sundac
Novobutazone
Novomethacin
Novonaprox
Novopirocam
Novoprofen
Nu-Indo
Nu-Pirox
Nuprin
Nuprin Caplets
Orudis
Orudis-E
Pamprin-IB
Paxofen
PediaProfen
PHENYLBUTAZONE
Phenylone Plus
Ponstan
Ponstel
PIROXICAM
Profen
Progesic
Relafen
Ro-Profen
Rufen
SULINDAC
Surgam
Synflex
Telectin DS
TIAPROFENIC ACID
TOLMETIN
Trendar
Voltaren
Voltaren SR
Voltarol
Voltarol Retard

ANTI-INFLAMMATORY DRUGS, STEROIDAL (Ophthalmic)

Ak-Dex
Ak-Pred
Ak-Tate
Baldex
BETAMETHASONE
Betnesol
Cortamed
Cortisol
Decadron
Dexair
DEXAMETHASONE
Dexotic
Econopred
Econopred Plus
Flarex
FLUOROMETHOLONE
Fluor-Op
FML Forte
FML Liquifilm
FML S.O.P.
HMS Liquifilm
HYDROCORTISONE
I-Methasone

I-Pred
Inflamase Forte
Inflamase-Mild
Life-Pred
Maxidex
MEDRYSONE
Ocu-Dex
Ocu-Pred
Ocu-Pred-A
Ocu-Pred Forte
Pred Forte
Pred Mild
Predair
Predair-A
Predair Forte
PREDNISOLONE
Ultra Pred

ANTISEBORRHEICS (Topical)

Buf-Bar
Capitrol
CHLOROXINE
DHS Zinc
Danex
Dan-Gard
Episel
Exsel
Glo-Sel
Head & Shoulders
Head & Shoulders
   Antidandruff Cream
   Shampoo Normal to Dry
   Formula
Head & Shoulders
   Antidandruff Cream
   Shampoo Normal to Oily
   Formula
Head & Shoulders
   Antidandruff Lotion
   Shampoo Normal to Dry
   Formula
Head & Shoulders
   Antidandruff Lotion
   Shampoo Normal to Oily
   Formula
Head & Shoulders
   Antidandruff Lotion
   Shampoo 2 in 1 Formula
Head & Shoulders Dry Scalp
   Conditioning Formula
   Lotion Shampoo
Head & Shoulders Dry Scalp
   Regular Formula Lotion
   Shampoo
Head & Shoulders Dry Scalp
   2 in 1 Formula Lotion
   Shampoo
Head & Shoulders Intensive
   Treatment Conditioning
   Formula Dandruff Lotion
   Shampoo
Head & Shoulders Intensive
   Treatment Regular
   Formula Dandruff Lotion
   Shampoo

Head & Shoulders Intensive
   Treatment 2 in 1 Formula
   Dandruff Lotion Shampoo
Meted Maximum Strength
   Anti-Dandruff Shampoo
   with Conditioners
PYRITHIONE
SALICYLIC ACID, SULFUR
   AND COAL TAR
Sebex-T Tar Shampoo
Sebulex Conditioning
   Suspension Shampoo
Sebulex Lotion Shampoo
Sebulon
Sebutone
SELENIUM SULFIDE
Selsun
Selsun Blue
Selsun Blue Regular Formula
SULFUR (scalp)
Vanseb-T
Vanseb Cream Dandruff
   Shampoo
Vanseb Lotion Dandruff
   Shampoo
Zincon
ZNP

APPETITE SUPPRESSANTS

Adipex-P
Adipost
Adphen
Anorex
Anoxine-AM
Appecon
Bacarate
BENZPHETAMINE
Bontril PDM
Bontril Slow Release
Dapex-37.5
Didrex
DIETHYLPROPION
Dital
Dyrexan-OD
Fastin
FENFLURAMINE
Ionamin
M-Orexic
Marlibar A
MAZINDOL
Mazanor
Melfiat-105 Unicelles
Metra
Nobesine
Obalan
Obe-Del
Obe-Mar
Obe-Nix
Obephen
Obermine
Obestin-30
Obeval
Obezine
Oby-Trim
Panrexin M
Panrexin MTP
Panshape

Parmine
Parzine
Phendiet
Phendimet
PHENDIMETRAZINE
PHENMETRAZINE
Phentercot
PHENTERMINE
Phenterxene
Phentra
Phentride
Phentrol
Phenzine
Plegine
Ponderal
Ponderal Pacaps
Pondimin
Pondimin Extentabs
Prelu-2
Preludin-Endurets
PT 105
Rexigen
Rexigen Forte
Sanorex
Slynn-LL
Span-RD
Statobex
T-Diet
Tega-Nil
Tenuate
Tenuate Dospan
Tepanil
Tepanil Ten-Tab
Teramin
Trimcaps
Trimstat
Trimtabs
Uni Trim
Wehless
Wehless Timecelles
Weightrol
Wescoid
Wilpowr
X-Trozine
X-Trozine LA
Zantryl

ASPIRIN

217
217 Strong
8-Hour Bayer Timed Release
A.S.A.
A.S.A. Enseals
Acetylsalicylic Acid
Alka-Seltzer Effervescent Pain
    Reliever & Antacid
Alka-Seltzer Plus
Alka-Seltzer Plus Maximum
    Strength Sinus Allergy
Alpha-Phed
Anacin
APAC Improved
APF Arthritic Pain Formula
Arthinol
Arthritis Pain Formula
Artria S.R.
Ascriptin
Ascriptin A/D
Aspergum
Astrin
Bayer

Bayer Timed-Release Arthritic
    Pain Formula
BC Cold Powder
Bexophene
Buffaprin
Bufferin
Buffinol
Cama Arthritis Reliever
Coricidin w/Codeine
Coryphen
Darvon Compound
Easprin
Ecotrin
Empirin
Entrophen
Equagesic
Excedrin
Halfprin
Lanorinal
Magnaprin
Magnaprin Arthritis Strength
Maprin
Maprin I-B
Measurin
Mepro Analgesic
Norgesic
Norwich Aspirin
Novasen
P-A-C Revised Formula
Presalin
Robaxisal
Rhinocaps
Riphen
Sal-Adult
Salatin
Saleto
Sal-Infant
Salocol
Supac
Supasa
Synalgos
Therapy Bayer
Triaphen
Ursinus Inlay
Viro-Med
Zorprin

BARBITURATES

Alurate
Amaphen
AMOBARBITAL
Amytal
Ancalixir
Anoquan
APROBARBITAL
Bancap
Barbita
Bucet
Busodium
BUTALBITAL
BUTABARBITAL
Butace
Butalan
Butisol
Dolmar
Endolor
Esgic
Ezol
Febridyne
Femcet
Fioricet
G-1

Gardenal
Gemonil
Isocet
Isopap
Lotusate Caplets
Luminal
Mebaral
Medigesic
MEPHOBARBITAL
METHARBITAL
Nembutal
Nova Rectal
Novopentobarb
Pacaps
PENTOBARBITAL
PHENOBARBITAL
Phrenilin
Repan
Rogesic
Sarisol No. 2
SECOBARBITAL
SECOBARBITAL AND
    AMOBARBITAL
Seconal
Sedapap
Semcet
Solfoton
TALBUTAL
Tencet
T.E.P.
Triad
Triaprin
Tuinal
Two-Dyne

BELLADONNA ALKALOIDS & BARBITURATES

Anaspaz PB
Antrocol
ATROPINE & PHENOBARBITAL
ATROPINE, HYOSCYAMINE,
    SCOPOLAMINE &
    BUTABARBITAL
ATROPINE, HYOSCYAMINE,
    SCOPOLAMINE &
    PHENOBARBITAL
Barbidonna
Barbidonna 2
Barophen
Belladenal
Belladenal-S
Belladenal Spacetabs
BELLADONNA & AMOBARBITAL
BELLADONNA &
    BUTABARBITAL
Bellalphen
Bellergal
Butibel
Chardonna-2
Donnapine
Donna-Sed
Donnatal
Donnatal Extentabs
Donphen
HYOSCYAMINE &
    PHENOBARBITAL
Hyosophen
Kinesed
Levsin with Phenobarbital
Levsinex with Phenobarbital
    Timecaps

Levsin-PB
Malatal
Pheno-Bella
Relaxadon
Spaslin
Spasmolin
Spasmophen
Spasquid
Susano

BENZODIAZEPINES

ALPRAZOLAM
Alzapam
Apo-Chlordiazepoxide
Apo-Diazepam
Apo-Flurazepam
Apo-Lorazepam
Apo-Oxazepam
Ativan
BROMAZEPAM
Centrax
CHLORDIAZEPOXIDE
CLONAZEPAM
CLORAZEPATE
Dalmane
Diazemuls
DIAZEPAM
Diazepam Intensol
Durapam
E-Pam
ESTAZOLAM
FLURAZEPAM
Gen-Xene
HALAZEPAM
KETAZOLAM
Klonopin
Lectopam
Libritabs
Librium
Lipoxide
Loftran
LORAZEPAM
Medilium
Meval
MIDAZOLAM
Mogadon
NITRAZEPAM
Novoclopate
Novodipam
Novoflupam
Novolorazem
Novopoxide
Novoxapam
Nu-Loraz
OXAZEPAM
Ox-Pam
Paxipam
PMS Diazepam
PMS Oxazepam
PRAZEPAM
ProSom
Razepam
Restoril
Rival
Rivotril
Serax
Sereen
Solium
Somnol
Som-Pam
TEMAZEPAM
Tranxene

Tranxene-SD
Tranxene T-Tab
Valium
Valrelease
Vasepam
Vivol
Xanax
Zapex
Zetran

BENZOYL PEROXIDE

Acetoxyl 2.5 Gel
Acetoxyl 5 Gel
Acetoxyl 10 Gel
Acetoxyl 20 Gel
Acne Aid 10 Cream
Acne-5 Lotion
Acne-10 Lotion
Acne-Mask
Acnomel B.P. 5 Lotion
Ben-Aqua 2½ Gel
Ben-Aqua 2½ Lotion
Ben-Aqua 5 Gel
Ben-Aqua 5 Lotion
Ben-Aqua 10 Gel
Ben-Aqua 10 Lotion
Ben-Aqua Masque 5
Benoxyl 5 Lotion
Benoxyl 10 Lotion
Benoxyl 20 Lotion
Benzac Ac 2½ Gel
Benzac Ac 5 Gel
Benzac Ac 10 Gel
Benzac W 2½ Gel
Benzac W 5 Gel
Benzac W 10 Gel
Benzagel 5 Acne Lotion
Benzagel 5 Acne Wash
Benzagel 5 Gel
Benzagel 10 Gel
Benzamycin
BenzaShave 5 Cream
BenzaShave 10 Cream
Brevoxyl 4 Gel
Buf-Oxal 10
Clear By Design 2.5 Gel
Clearasil BP Plus 5 Cream
Clearasil BP Plus 5 Lotion
Clearasil Maximum Strength
    Medicated Anti-Acne 10
    Tinted Cream
Clearasil Maximum Strength
    Medicated Anti-Acne 10
    Vanishing Cream
Clearasil Medicated Anti-Acne 10
    Vanishing Lotion
Cuticura Acne 5 Cream
Del-Aqua-5 Gel
Del-Aqua-10 Gel
Del-Ray
Dermoxyl 2.5 Gel
Dermoxyl 5 Gel
Dermoxyl 10 Gel
Dermoxyl 20 Gel
Dermoxyl Aqua
Desquam-E 2.5 Gel
Desquam-E 5 Gel
Desquam-E 10 Gel
Desquam-X 2.5 Gel
Desquam-X 5 Gel
Desquam-X 5 Wash
Desquam-X 10 Gel

Desquam-X 10 Wash
Dry and Clear 5 Lotion
Dry and Clear Double Strength
    10 Cream
Fostex 5 Gel
Fostex 10 Bar
Fostex 10 Cream
Fostex 10 Gel
Fostex 10 Wash
H₂Oxyl 2.5 Gel
H₂Oxyl 5 Gel
H₂Oxyl 10 Gel
H₂Oxyl 20 Gel
Loroxide 5 Lotion with Flesh-
    Tinted Base
Loroxide 5.5 Lotion
Neutrogena Acne Mask 5
Noxzema Clear-Ups Maximum
    Strength 10
Noxzema Clear-Ups On-the-Spot
    10 Lotion
Oxy 5 Tinted Lotion
Oxy 5 Vanishing Formula Lotion
Oxy 5 Vanishing Lotion
Oxy 10
Oxy 10 Daily Face Wash
Oxy 10 Tinted Lotion
Oxy 10 Vanishing Lotion
Oxyderm 5 Lotion
Oxyderm 10 Lotion
Oxyderm 20 Lotion
PanOxyl 5 Bar
PanOxyl 5 Gel
PanOxyl 10 Bar
PanOxyl 10 Gel
PanOxyl 15 Gel
PanOxyl 20 Gel
PanOxyl AQ 2½ Gel
PanOxyl AQ 5 Gel
Persa-Gel 5
Persa-Gel 10
Persa-Gel W 5
Persa-Gel W 10
pHisoAc BP 10
Propa P.H. 10 Acne Cover Stick
Propa P.H. 10 Liquid Acne Soap
Stri-Dex Maximum Strength
    Treatment 10 Cream
Theroxide 5 Lotion
Theroxide 10 Lotion
Theroxide 10 Wash
Topex 5 Lotion
Topex 10 Lotion
Vanoxide 5 Lotion
Xerac BP 5 Gel
Xerac BP 10 Gel
Zeroxin-5 Gel
Zeroxin-10 Gel

BETA-ADRENERGIC
BLOCKERS

ACEBUTOLOL
Apo-Metoprolol
Apo-Metoprolol (Type L)
Apo-Propranolol
Apo-Timol
ATENOLOL
Betaloc
Betaloc Durules
BETAXOLOL
Blocadren
CARTEOLOL

Cartrol
Corgard
Detensol
Inderal LA
Kerlone
LABETALOL
Levatol
Lopresor
Lopressor
Lopressor SR
METOPROLOL
Monitan
NADOLOL
Normodyne
Novometoprol
Novo-Pindol
Novopranol
Nu-Atenol
NuMetop
OXPRENOLOL
PENBUTOLOL
PINDOLOL
pms Propranolol
PROPRANOLOL
Sectral
Syn-Pindolol
Slow-Trasicor
Sotacor
SOTALOL
Tenormin
TIMOLOL
Toprol XL
Trandate
Trasicor
Visken

BETA-ADRENERGIC BLOCKING AGENTS & THIAZIDE DIURETICS

ATENOLOL &
 CHLORTHALIDONE
Co-Betaloc
Corzide
Inderide
Inderide LA
LABETALOL &
 HYDROCHLOROTHIAZIDE
Lopressor HCT
METOPROLOL &
 HYDROCHLOROTHIAZIDE
NADOLOL &
 BENDROFLUMETHIAZIDE
Normozide
PINDOLOL &
 HYDROCHLOROTHIAZIDE
PROPRANOLOL &
 HYDROCHLOROTHIAZIDE
Tenoretic
Timolide
TIMOLOL &
 HYDROCHLOROTHIAZIDE
Trandate HCT
Viskazide

BETAMETHASONE

Betnelan
Betnesol
Celestone
Celestone Phosphate
Celestone Soluspan
Lotrisone

Lotriderm
Selestoject

BRONCHODILATORS, ADRENERGIC

Adrenalin
Aerolone
ALBUTEROL
Alupent
Arm-a-Med Isoetharine
Arm-a-Med Metaproterenol
AsthmaHaler
AsthmaNefrin
Berotec
BITOLTEROL
Brethaire
Brethine
Bricanyl
Bronitin Mist
Bronkaid Mist
Bronkaid Mist Suspension
Bronkaid Mistometer
Bronkephrine
Bronkometer
Bronkosol
Dey-Dose Isoetharine
Dey-Dose Isoetharine S/F
Dey-Dose Isoproterenol
Dey-Dose Metaproterenol
Dey-Dose Racepinephrine
Dey-Lute Isoetharine
Dey-Lute Isoetharine S/F
Dey-Lute Metaproterenol
Dispos-a-Med Isoetharine
Dispos-a-Med Isoptroterenol
Ephed II
EPHEDRINE
EPINEPHRINE
EpiPen Auto-Injector
EpiPen Jr. Auto-Injector
ETHYLNOREPINEPHRINE
FENOTEROL
ISOETHARINE
ISOPROTERENOL
Isuprel
Isuprel Glossets
Isuprel Mistometer
Maxair
Medihaler-Epi
Medihaler-Iso
Metaprel
METAPROTERENOL
microNEFRIN
Norisodrine Aerotrol
Novosalmol
PIRBUTEROL
Primatene Mist
Primatene Mist Suspension
Pro-Air
PROCATEROL
Prometa
Proventil
Proventil Repetabs
Sus-Phrine
TERBUTALINE
Tornalate
Vapo-Iso
Vaponefrin
Ventolin
Ventolin Rotocaps

BRONCHODILATORS, XANTHINE

Accurbron
Aerolate
Aerophyllin
Aminophyllin
AMINOPHYLLINE
Apo-Oxtriphylline
Aquaphyllin
Asbron
Asmalix
Brondecon
Bronkodyl
Choledyl
Choledyl SA
Constant-T
Corophyllin
Dilor
Dilor-400
Duraphyl
Dyflex
DYPHILLINE
Elixicon
Elixomin
Elixophyllin
Elixophyllin SR
Lanophyllin
Lixolin
Lufyllin
Marax
Marax DF
Neothylline
Novotriphyl
OXTRIPHYLLINE
Palaron
Phyllocontin
PMS Theophylline
Primatene, P Formula
Protophylline
Pulmophylline
Quibron
Quibron Plus
Quibron-T
Quibron-T Dividose
Quibron-T/SR Dividose
Respbid
Slo-bid Gyrocaps
Slophyllin
Slo-Phyllin
Slo-Phyllin Gyrocaps
Solu-Phyllin
Somophyllin
Somophyllin-12
Somophyllin-CRT
Somophyllin-DF
Somophyllin-T
Sustaire
Synophylate
Tedral
T.E.H.
T.E.P.
Theobid Duracaps
Theobid Jr. Duracaps
Theochron
Theoclear
Theoclear L.A. Cenules
Theocot
Theo-Dur
Theo-Dur Sprinkle
Theolair
Theolair-Plus
Theolair-SR

Theomar
Theon
THEOPHYLLINE
Theophylline SR
Theo-Sav
Theospan SR
Theo-SR
Theostat
Theostat 80
Theo-Time
Theox
Theovent Long-acting
Thylline
Truphylline
Truxophyllin
Uniphyl

BUTALBITAL & ASPIRIN
(Also contains caffeine)

Axotal
B-A-C
Butalbital A-C
BUTALBITAL, ASPIRIN &
  CAFFEINE
Butalbital Compound
Butalgen
Farbital
Florex
Florgen PF
Fiorinal
Florital
Fortabs
Idenal
Isobutal
Isobutyl
Isolin
Isollyl (Improved)
Laniroif
Lanorinal
Marnal
Salipral
Tecnal
Vibutal

CAFFEINE

Amaphen
Anacin
Anoquan
A.P.C.
Aspirin Compound w/Codeine
Aspirin-Free Excedrin Caplets
Cafergot
Cafermine
Cafetrate
Caffedrine
Citrated Caffeine
Dexitac
Esgic
Excedrin Extra Strength
Fendol
Fiorinal
Korigesic
Lanorinal
Nodoz
Pacaps
P-A-C Compound
Propoxyphene Compound
Quick Pep
S-A-C
Salatin
Saleto-D
Salocol

Supac
Synalgos
Synalgos-DC
Tirend
Triaminicin with Codeine
Trigesic
Two-Dyne
Vanquish
Vivarin
Wigraine

CALCIUM CHANNEL
BLOCKERS

Adalat
AMLODIPINE
Apo-Nifed
Apo-Verap
Bepadin
BEPRIDIL
Calan
Calan SR
Cardene
Cardizem
Cardizem SR
Chase
Dilacor-XR
DILTIAZEM
Dyna Circ
FELODIPINE
Isoptin
Isoptin SR
ISRADIPINE
NICARDIPINE
NIFEDIPINE
Norvasc
Novo-Nifedin
Novo-Veramil
Nu-Diltiaz
Nu-Nifed
Nu-Verap
Plendil
Procardia
Syn-Diltiazem
Vascor
VERAPAMIL
Verelan

CALCIUM SUPPLEMENTS

BioCal
Calbarb 600
Calci-Chew
Calciday
Calcite
CALCIUM CARBONATE (also
  used as an antacid)
CALCIUM CITRATE
CALCIUM GLUBIONATE
CALCIUM GLUCONATE
CALCIUM GLYCEROPHOSPHATE
  & CALCIUM LACTATE
CALCIUM LACTATE
Calphosan
Caltrate
Citracal
DIBASIC CALCIUM PHOSPHATE
Gencalc
Mega-Cal
Neo-Calglucon
Nephro-Calci
Os-Cal
Oysco
Oyst-Cal

Oystercal
Posture
Rolaids-Calcium Rich
Super Calcium 1200
Titralac Extra Strength
TRIBASIC CALCIUM PHOSPHATE
Tums
Tums E-X

CHLORZOXAZONE &
ACETAMINOPHEN

Arlon Forte
Blanex
Cetazone
Chlorofon-F
Chlorzone Forte
Chlorzoxacet-F
Chlorzoxazone with APAP
Eze-DS
Flexaphen
Flextra
Lobac
Miflex
Mus-Lax
Panflex
Paracet Forte
Paraforte
Paragen-Forte
Parazone
Pargen Fortified
Polyflex
Pyregesic Forte
Rofon Forte
Saroflex
Spasgesic
Uni Para Plus

COAL TAR (Topical)

Alphosyl
Aquatar
Balnetar
Balnetar Therapeutic Tar Bath
Cutar Water Dispersible
  Emollient Tar
Denorex
Denorex Extra Strength
  Medicated Shampoo
Denorex Extra Strength
  Medicated Shampoo with
  Conditioners
Denorex Medicated Shampoo
Denorex Medicated Shampoo
  and Conditioner
Denorex Mountain Fresh Herbal
  Scent Medicated Shampoo
DHS Tar Gel Shampoo
DHS Tar Shampoo
Doak Oil
Doak Oil Forte
Doak Oil Forte Therapeutic Bath
  Treatment
Doak Oil Therapeutic Bath Treat-
  ment For All-Over Body Care
Doak Tar Lotion
Doak Tar Shampoo
Doctar
Doctar Hair & Scalp Shampoo
  and Conditioner
Estar
Fototar
Ionil-T Plus

LAVATAR
Liquor Carbonis Detergens
Medotar
Pentrax Extra-Strength
 Therapeutic Tar Shampoo
Pentrax Tar Shampoo
psoriGel
PsoriNail
Taraphilic
Tarbonis
Tar Doak
TARPASTE
Tarpaste Doak
T/Derm Tar Emollient
Tegrin Lotion for Psoriasis
Tegrin Medicated Cream
 Shampoo
Tegrin Medicated Shampoo
 Concentrated Gel
Tegrin Medicated Shampoo Extra
 Conditioning Formula
Tegrin Medicated Shampoo
 Herbal Formula
Tegrin Medicated Shampoo
 Original Formula
Tegrin Medicated Soap for
 Psoriasis
Tegrin Skin Cream for Psoriasis
Tersa-Tar Mild Therapeutic
 Shampoo with Protein and
 Conditioner
Tersa-Tar Soapless Tar Shampoo
Tersa-Tar Therapeutic Shampoo
T-Gel
T/Gel Therapeutic Conditioner
T/Gel Therapeutic Shampoo
Theraplex T Shampoo
Zetar
Zetar Emulsion
Zetar Medicated Antiseborrheic
 Shampoo

CONTRACEPTIVES, ORAL

Brevicon
Demulen
Enovid
Enovid-E
ETHYNODIOL DIACETATE &
 ETHINYL ESTRADIOL
ETHYNODIOL DIACETATE &
 MESTRANOL
Genora 1/35
Genora 1/50
Levlen
LEVONORGESTREL & ETHINYL
 ESTRADIOL
Loestrin
Lo-Ovral
Micronor
Minestrin
Min-Ovral
Modacon
Modicon
N.E.E. 1/35
Nelova
Norcept
Nordette
Norethin
NORETHINDRONE & ETHINYL
 ESTRADIOL

NORETHINDRONE &
 MESTRANOL
NORETHINDRONE ACETATE &
 ETHINYL ESTRADIOL
NORGESTREL & ETHINYL
 ESTRADIOL
Norlestrin
Norinyl
Nor-Q.D.
Norquest
NORTHYNODREL & MESTRANOL
Ortho
Ortho-Novum 0.5
Ortho-Novum 1/35
Ortho-Novum 1/50
Ortho-Novum 1/80
Ortho-Novum 2
Ortho-Novum 7/7/7
Ortho-Novum 10/11
Ovcon
Ovral
Ovrette
Ovulen
Program
Synphasic
Tri-Levlen
Tri-Norinyl
Triphasil

CONTRACEPTIVES, VAGINAL (Spermicides)

BENZALKONIUM CHLORIDE
Because
Conceptrol-Contraceptive Inserts
Conceptrol Gel
Delfen
Emko
Encare
Gynol II Extra Strength
Gynol II Original Formula
Intercept
Koromex Cream
Koromex Crystal Gel
Koromex Foam
Koromex Jelly
NONOXYNAL 9
OCTOXYNOL 9
Ortho-Creme
Ortho-Gynol
Pharmatex
Pre-Fil
Ramses Contraceptive Foam
Ramses Contraceptive Vaginal
 Jelly
Ramses Crystal Clear Gel
Semicid
Shur-Seal
Today
VCF

DEXAMETHASONE

Ak-Dex
Congespirin
Dalalone
Dalalone D.P.
Dalalone L.A.
Decadrol
Decadron
Decadron L.A.
Decadron Phosphate
Decadron Respihaler

Decaject
Decaject-L.A.
Deronil
Desasone L.A.
Dexacen
Dexacen L.A.
Dexasone
Dexone
Dexone LA
Hexadrol
Hexadrol Phosphate
Mymethasone
Oradexon
Solurex
Solurex LA

DEXTROMETHORPHAN

2/G-DM Cough
Actifed DM
Ambenyl-D Decongestant Cough
 Formula
Anatuss
Anti-Tuss DM Expectorant
Balminil DM
Bayaminicol
Baydec DM Drops
Bayer Cough Syrup for Children
Baytussin DM
Benylin-DM
Benylin Expectorant Cough
 Formula
Bromfed-AT
Bromfed-DM
Broncho-Grippol-DM
Brotane DX Cough
Carbinoxamine Compound
Carbodec DM Drops
Cerose-DM
Cheracol D Cough
Cheracol Plus
Chexit
Children's Nyquil Nighttime Cold
 Medicine
Co-Apap
Codimal DM
Codistan No. 1
Colrex Cough
Comtrex Daytime Caplets
Comtrex Multi-Symptom Cold
 Reliever
Comtrex Multi-Symptom Hot Flu
 Relief
Comtrex Multi-Symptom Non-
 Drowsy Caplets
Comtrex Nighttime
Conar
Conar-A
Conar Expectorant
Concentrin
Congespirin
Contac Jr. Children's Cold
 Medicine
Contac Severe Cold Formula
Contac Severe Cold Formula
 Night Strength
Coricidin Cough
CoTylenol Cold Medication
Cremacoat 1
Cremacoat 3 Throat Coating
 Cough Medicine
Cremacoat 4 Throat Coating
 Cough Medicine

Creo-Terpin
DayCare
DayQuil Liquicaps
DayQuil Non-Drowsy Cold/Flu
Delsym
DEXTROMETHORPHAN
HYDROBROMIDE AND TERPIN
HYDRATE
Dimacol
Dimetane-DX Cough
Dimetapp DM Cough and Cold
Dimetapp-DM
DM Cough
DM Syrup
Donatussin
Dondril
Dorcol Children's Cough
Dorcol DM
Dristan Cold and Flu
Efficol Cough Whip (Cough
Suppressant/Decongestant)
Efficol Cough Whip (Cough
Suppressant/Decongestant/
Antihistamine)
Efficol Cough Whip (Cough
Suppressant/Expectorant)
Extra Action Cough
Father John's Medicine Plus
Glycotuss-dM
Gulamid D.M. Liquid
Gulatuss-DM
Halls Mentho-Lyptus
Decongestant Cough Formula
Halotussin-DM Expectorant
Histalet-DM
Hold
Hold (Children's Formula)
Improved Sino-Tuss
Iotuss-DM
Ipsatol Cough Formula for
Children
Kiddy Koff
Koffex
Kolephrin/DM
Kolephrin GG/DM
Kolephrin NN Liquid
Kophane
Kophane Cough and Cold
Formula
Meda Syrup Forte
Medatussin
Medatussin Plus
Medi-Flu
Medi-Flu Caplets
Mediquell
Mediquell Decongestant Formula
Mytussin DM
Naldecon-DX
Naldecon-DX Adult Liquid
Naldecon-DX Children's Syrup
Naldecon-DX Pediatric Drops
Naldecon Senior DX
Neo-DM
Noratuss II Liquid
Novahistex DM
Novahistine Cough & Cold
Formula Liquid
Novahistine DMX Liquid
NyQuil Liquicaps
NyQuil Nighttime Colds Medicine
Nytime Cold Medicine Liquid
Omnicol
Ornade-DM 10

Ornade-DM 15
Ornade-DM 30
Orthoxicol Cough
PediaCare 1
PediaCare Children's Cold Relief
Night Rest Cough-Cold
Formula
PediaCare Children's Cough-Cold
Formula
Par Glycerol-DM
Pertussin AM
Pertussin CS
Pertussin PM
Phanadex
Phanatuss
Phenergan w/Dextromethorphan
Poly-Histine-DM
Prominicol Cough
Pseudo-Car DM
Quelidrine Cough
Queltuss
Remcol-C
Rhinosyn-DM
Rhinosyn-DMX Expectorant
Rhinosyn-X
Robidex
Robitussin-CF
Robitussin-DM
Robitussin Maximum Strength
Cough
Robitussin Night Relief
Robitussin Night Relief Colds
Formula Liquid
Robitussin-Pediatric
Rondec-DM
Rondec-DM Drops
Ru-Tuss Expectorant
Saleto-CF
Sedatuss
Silexin Cough
Snaplets-DM
Snaplets-Multi
St. Joseph for Children
Sucrets Cough Control
Sudafed Cough
Sudafed DM
Sudafed Severe Cold Formula
Syracol Liquid
Terphan
Terpin-Dex
TheraFlu/Flu, Cold & Cough
TheraFlu Nighttime Maximum
Strength
Tolu-Sed DM Cough
Triaminic-DM Cough Formula
Triaminic-DM Expectorant
Triaminic Nite Light
Triaminicol DM
Triaminicol Multi-Symptom Relief
Tricodene Forte
Tricodene NN
Tricodene Pediatric
Trimedine Liquid
Trind DM Liquid
Trocal
Tusquelin
Tussafed
Tussagesic
Tussar DM
Tuss-DM
Tussi-Organidin DM Liquid
Tusso-DM
Ty-Cold Cold Formula

Tylenol Cold and Flu
Tylenol Cold Medication
Tylenol Cold Medication,
Non-Drowsy
Tylenol Cold Night Time
Tylenol Cough
Unproco
Vicks Children's Cough
Vicks Formula 44 Cough Mixture
Vicks Formula 44D Decongestant
Cough Mixture
Vicks Formula 44M Multi-
symptom Cough Mixture
Viro-Med

DICYCLOMINE

A-Spas
Antispas
Bentyl
Bentylol
Byclomine
Dibent
Di-Cyclonex
Dilomine
Di-Spaz
Forulex
Lomine
Neoquess
Or-Tyl
Protylol
Spasmoban
Spasmoject
Viscerol

DIURETICS, THIAZIDE

Anhydron
Apo-Chlorthalidone
Apo-Hydro
Aquatensen
BENDROFLUMETHIAZIDE
BENZTHIAZIDE
CHLOROTHIAZIDE
CHLORTHALIDONE
CYCLOTHIAZIDE
Diucardin
Diuchlor H
Diulo
Diuril
Duretic
Enduron
Esidrix
Fluidil
HYDROCHLOROTHIAZIDE
HydroDIURIL
HYDROFLUMETHIAZIDE
Hydromox
Hygroton
Metahydrin
METHYCLOTHIAZIDE
METOLAZONE
Mykrox
Naqua
Naturetin
Neo-Codema
Novo-Hydrazide
Novo-Thalidone
Oretic
POLYTHIAZIDE
QUINETHAZONE
Renese
Saluron
Thalitone

TRICHLORMETHIAZIDE
Uridon
Urozide
Zaroxolyn

DOCUSATE SODIUM
Afko-Lube
Bilax
Bu-Lax
Colace
Colax
Correctol Extra Gentle
Dialose
Diocto
Dioeze
Diosuccin
Dio-Sul
Disonate
Di-Sosul
Doss
Doxidan
Doxinate
D-S-S
Duosol
Laxinate
Laxinate 100
Liqui-Doss
Modane Soft
Molatoc
Neolax
Peri-Colase
Pro-Sof
Pro-Sof Liquid Concentrate
Pro-Sof Plus
Regulax SS
Regulex
Regutol
Senokot-S
Stulex
Therevac Plus
Therevac-SB
Trilax

EPHEDRINE
Broncholate
Bronkotuss Expectorant
Ephed II
Histatuss Pediatric
KIE
Omni-Tuss
Quelidrine Cough
Rentamine
Rynatuss
Rynatuss Pediatric
T.E.P.

ERYTHROMYCINS
Akne-mycin
Apo-Erythro-S
A/T/S
Benzamycin
E-Base
E.E.S.
Emgel
E-Mycin
Eryc
Erycette
Ery-derm
Erygel
Erymax
EryPed

Ery-Sol
Ery-Tab
Erythro
Erythrocin
Erythrocot
Erythromid
ERYTHROMYCIN-BASE
ERYTHROMYCIN ESTOLATE
ERYTHROMYCIN
   ETHYLSUCCINATE
ERYTHROMYCIN GLUCEPTATE
ERYTHROMYCIN
   LACTOBIONATE
ERYTHROMYCIN STEARATE
Erythrozone
Ethril
ETS
Ilosone
Ilotycin
Kenmycin
My-E
Mythromycin
Novorythro
PCE Dispersatabs
Pediamycin
Robimycin
Ro-Mycin
Staticin
T-Stat
Wintrocin
Wyamycin E
Wyamycin S

ESTROGENS
Brevicon
C.E.S.
CHLOROTRIANISENE
CONJUGATED ESTROGENS
Deladiol-40
Delestrogen
Demulen
depGynogen
Depo Estradiol
Depogen
DES
DIETHYLSTILBESTROL
Dioval
Duragen
Dura-Estrin
E-Cypionate
ESTERIFIED ESTROGENS
Estinyl
Estrace
Estra-D
Estraderm
ESTRADIOL
Estradiol LA
Estra-L
Estratab
Estraval
Estro-Cyp
Estrofem
ESTROGEN
Estroject-2
Estroject-L.A.
ESTRONE
Estrone 5
Estrone Sulfate
Estrone-A
Estronol
ESTROPIPATE
Estrovis

ETHINYL ESTRADIOL
Etronol-LA
Feminone
Femogen Forte
Femogex
Foygen Aqueous
Gynogen
Honvol
Hormogen
Kestrin Aqueous
LAE 20
Loestrin
Lo-Ovral
Mannest
Menest
Modicon
Neo-Estrone
Norinyl
Norlestrin
Ogen
Ovcon
Ovral
Piperazine
Premarin
Progens
QUINESTROL
Stilphostrol
TACE
Tri-Norinyl
Unigen
Valergen
Wehgen

GUAIFENESIN
2/G-DM Cough
Adatuss D.C. Expectorant
Alamine Expectorant
Ambenyl-D Decongestant Cough
   Formula
Ami-Tex LA
Amonidrin
Anatuss
Anatuss with Codeine
Anti-Tuss
Anti-Tuss DM Expectorant
Balminil
Banex
Banex-LA
Bayaminic Expectorant
Bayhistine Expectorant
Baytussin AC
Baytussin DM
Benylin Expectorant Cough
   Formula
Breonesin
Brexin
Broncholate
Bronkotuss Expectorant
Cheracol
Cheracol D Cough
CoActifed Expectorant
Codegest-Expectorant
Codiclear DH
Codimal Expectorant
Codistan No. 1
Colrex Expectorant
Conar-A
Conar Expectorant
Concentrin
Conex
Conex w/Codeine Liquid
Congess JR

920

Congess SR
Coricidin Cough
Cremacoat 2
Cremacoat 3 Throat Coating
  Cough Medicine
C-Tussin Expectorant
DayCare
DayQuil Liquicaps
DayQuil Non-Drowsy Cold/Flu
Despec
Deproist Expectorant w/Codeine
Detussin Expectorant
Dilaudid Cough
Dimacol
Dimetane Expectorant
Dimetane Expectorant-C
Dimetane Expectorant-DC
Donatussin
Donatussin DC
Donatussin Drops
Dorcol Children's Cough
Dorcol DM
Dura-Vent
Efficol Cough Whip (Cough
  Suppressant/Expectorant)
Entex
Entex LA
Entex Liquid
Entex PSE
Entuss Expectorant
Entuss Pediatric Expectorant
Entuss-D
Extra Action Cough
Father John's Medicine Plus
Fedahist Expectorant
Fedahist Expectorant Pediatric
  Drops
Fendol
Gee-Gee
GG-CEN
Genatuss
Gentab LA
Glyate
Glycotuss
Glycotuss-dM
Glydeine Cough
Gualfed
Gualfed-PD
Guaipax
Guaitab
Guiamid D.M. Liquid
Guiatuss A.C.
Guiatuss-DM
Guiatussin w/Codeine Liquid
Guistrey Fortis
Gulatuss
Halotussin
Halotussin-DM Expectorant
Head & Chest
Histalet X
Humibid L.A.
Humibid Sprinkle
Hycotuss Expectorant
Hytuss
Hytuss-2X
Ipsatol Cough Formula for
  Children
Isoclor Expectorant
Kiddy Koff
Kolephrin GG/DM
Kwelcof Liquid
Lanatuss Expectorant
Malotuss

Meda Syrup Forte
Medatussin
Medatussin Plus
Myhistine Expectorant
Mytussin AC
Mytussin DAC
Mytussin DM
Naldecon
Naldecon-CX Adult Liquid
Naldecon-DX Adult Liquid
Naldecon-DX Children's Syrup
Naldecon-DX Pediatric Drops
Naldecon-EX
Naldecon Senior DX
Nolex LA
Noratuss II Liquid
Nortussin
Nortussin w/Codeine
Novahistex DH Expectorant
Novahistine DH Expectorant
Novahistine DMX Liquid
Novahistine Expectorant
Nucochem Expectorant
Nucochem Pediatric Expectorant
Nucofed Expectorant
Nucofed Pediatric Expectorant
Ornade Expectorant
Pertussin AM
Pertussin CS
Phanadex
Phanatuss
Phenhist Expectorant
Phenylfenesin L.A.
Polaramine Expectorant
Poly-Histine Expectorant Plain
Prominic Expectorant
Pseudo-Bid
Pseudo-Hist Expectorant
P-V-Tussin Tablets
Queltuss
Respaire-60 SR
Respaire-120 SR
Respinol-G
Respinol LA
Resyl
Rhinosyn-DMX Expectorant
Rhinosyn-X
Robafen
Robitussin
Robitussin with Codeine
Robitussin A-C
Robitussin-CF
Robitussin-DAC
Robitussin-DM
Robitussin-PE
Ru-Tuss Expectorant
Rymed
Rymed Liquid
Rymed-TR
Ryna-CX Liquid
Silexin Cough
Sinufed Timecelles
Snaplets-EX
Stamoist E
Stamoist LA
SRC Expectorant
Sudafed Cough
Sudafed Expectorant
T-Moist
Tolu-Sed Cough
Tolu-Sed DM Cough
Triaminic-DM Expectorant
Triaminic Expectorant

Triaminic Expectorant DH
Triaminic Expectorant w/Codeine
Trinex
Triphenyl Expectorant
Trocal
Tussanil DH Tablets
Tussar SF
Tussar-2
Tuss-DM
Tuss-LA
ULR-LA
Unproco
Utex-S.R.
Vicks Children's Cough
Vicks Formula 44D Decongestant
  Cough Mixture
Vicks Formula 44M Multi-
  symptom Cough Mixture
Viro-Med
Zephrex
Zephrex-LA

HYDROCORTISONE
  (Cortisol)

A-hydroCort
Cortef
Cortenema
Cortifoam
Hydrocortone
Hydrocortone Acetate
Hydrocortone Phosphate
Solu-Cortef

HYDROXYZINE

Anxanil
Apo-Hydroxyzine
Atarax
E-Vista
Hydroxacen
Hyzine
Marax
Multipax
Novohydroxyzin
Quiess
T.E.H. Tablets
Theozine
Vamate
Vistaject
Vistaquel
Vistaril
Vistazine

HYOSCYAMINE

Anaspaz
Anaspaz PB
Barbidonna
Barbidonna 2
Belladenal
Bellafoline
Donnatal
Donnatal Extentabs
Kinesed
Levsin
Levsinex
Levsinex Timecaps
Neoquess
Spasmolin
Spasquid
Spastolate

921

INSULIN

Humulin BR
Humulin L
Humulin N
Humulin R
Humulin U
Insulatard NPH
Insulatard NPH Human
Lente
Lente Iletin I
Lente Iletin II
Lente Insulin
Mixtard
Mixtard Human
Novolin 70/30
Novolin L
Novolin N
Novolin R
NPH
NPH Iletin I
NPH Iletin II
NPH Insulin
Protamine Zinc & Iletin
Protamine Zinc & Iletin I
Protamine Zinc & Iletin II
PZI
Regular
Regular (Concentrated) Iletin
Regular (Concentrated) Iletin II,
  U-500
Regular Iletin I
Regular Iletin II
Regular Insulin
Semilente
Semilente Iletin
Semilente Iletin I
Ultralente
Ultralente Iletin I
Velosulin
Velosulin Human

IRON SUPPLEMENTS

Apo-Ferrous Gluconate
Apo-Ferrous Sulfate
Femiron
Feosol
Feostat
Fergon
Fer-In-Sol
Fer-Iron
Fero-folic 500
Fero-Grad
Fero-Gradumet
Ferralet
Ferralyn
Ferra-TD
Ferrospace
FERROUS FUMARATE
FERROUS GLUCONATE
FERROUS SULFATE
Fertinic
Fumasorb
Fumerin
Geritol Tablets
Hemocyte
Hytinic
Iberet
Ircon
IRON POLYSACCHARIDE
Mol-Iron
Neo-Fer
Niferex

Niferex-150
Novoferrogluc
Novoferrosulfa
Novofumar
Nu-Iron
Nu-Iron 150
Palafer
Palmiron
PMS Ferrous Sulfate
Poly-Vi-Flor
Simiron
Slow Fe
Span-FF

MEPROBAMATE

Acabamate
Apo-Meprobamate
Equagesic
Equanil
Equanil Wyseals
Medi-Tran
Meprospan
Miltown
Neuramate
Novomepro
Novo-Mepro
Pax 400
Probate
Sedabamate
Trancot
Tranmep

METHYLPREDNISOLONE

A-methaPred
dep Medalone
Depo-Medrol
Depo-Pred-40
Depo-Pred-80
Depo-Predate
Depoject-40
Depoject-80
Duralone
Duralone-40
Duralone-80
Medralone-40
Medralone-80
Medrol
Meprolone
Rep-Pred
Solu-Medrol

MUSCLE RELAXANTS, SKELETAL

Carbacot
CARISOPRODOL
CHLORPHENESIN
CHLORZOXAZONE
Delaxin
Marbaxin
Maolate
METAXALONE
METHOCARBAMOL
Paraflex
Parafon Forte
Rela
Robamol
Robaxin
Robaxisal
Robomol
Skelaxin
Sodol

Soma
Soprodol
Soridol

NARCOTIC & ACETAMINOPHEN

Aceta with Codeine
Acetaco
ACETAMINOPHEN & CODEINE
Allay
Amacodone
Anexsia
Anodynos DHC
Anolor-DH5
APAP with Codeine
Atasol with Codeine
Bancap-HC
Capital with Codeine
Codalan
Codamin
Codaminophen
Co-gesic
Compal
Darvocet-N 100
Darvocet-N 50
Demerol-APAP
Dolacet
Dolene-AP 65
Doxapap
D-Rex
Duocet
Duradyne DHC
E-Lor
Empracet 30
Empracet 60
Emtec
Endocet
Exdol with Codeine
Genagesic
Hy-5
Hycomed
Hycopap
Hydrocet
HYDROCODONE & ACETAMINOPHEN
Hydrocodone with APAP
Hydrogesic
HY-PHEN
Lenoltec
Lorcet
Lorcet-HD
Lortab
Lortab 5
Lortab 7
Megagesic
MEPERIDINE & ACETAMINOPHEN
M-Gesic
Myapap with Codeine
Norcet
Novogesic
Oxycocet
OXYCODONE & ACETAMINOPHEN
PENTAZOCINE & ACETAMINOPHEN
Percocet
Percocet-Demi
Phenaphen with Codeine
Polygesic
Pro Pox with APAP
Propacet

Propain-HC
PROPOXYPHENE &
  ACETAMINOPHEN
Proval
Proxy 65
Pyregesic-C
Rogesic
Rounox with Codeine
Roxicet
Senefen III
Talacen
Tylaprin with Codeine
Tylenol with Codeine
Tylox
Ty-Pap with Codeine
Ty-Tabs
Ultragesic
Veganin
Vicodin
Wygesic
Zydone

NARCOTIC ANALGESICS
642
Actagen-C Cough
Actifed w/Codeine
Actifed w/Codeine Cough
Adatuss D.C.
Adatuss D.C. Expectorant
Alamine-C Liquid
Alamine Expectorant
Allerfrin w/Codeine
Ambay Cough
Ambenyl Cough
Ambophen Expectorant
Anamine HD
Anatuss with Codeine
Aspirin Compound w/Codeine
Astramorph
Astramorph-PF
Baycodan
Baycomine
Baycomine Pediatric
BayCotussend Liquid
Bayhistine DH
Bayhistine Expectorant
Baytussin AC
Benylin with Codeine
Biphetane DC Cough
Bromanate DC Cough
Bromphen DC w/Codeine Cough
Buprenex
BUPRENORPHINE
BUTORPHANOL
Calcidrine
Caldomine-DH Forte
Caldomine-DH Pediatric
Calmylin with Codeine
Cheracol
Chlorgest-HD
Citra Forte
CoActifed
CoActifed Expectorant
Codegest-Expectorant
Codamine
Codamine Pediatric
Codan
Codegest Expectorant
Codehist DH
CODEINE
CODEINE AND TERPIN
  HYDRATE

Codeine Sulfate
Codiclear DH
Codimal DH
Codimal PH
Colrex Compound
Conex w/Codeine Liquid
Cophene-S
Coricidin w/Codeine
Coristex-DH
Coristine-DH
C-Tussin Expectorant
Darvon
Darvon-N
De-Tuss
Demerol
Deproist Expectorant w/Codeine
Detussin Expectorant
Detussin Liquid
Dihistine DH
DIHYDROCODEINE
Dihydromorphinone
Dilaudid
Dilaudid Cough
Dilaudid-HP
Dimetane Expectorant-C
Dimetane Expectorant-DC
Dimetane-DC Cough
Dimetapp with Codeine
Dolene
Dolophine
Doloxene
Donatussin DC
Doraphen
Doxaphene
Dromoran
Duragesic
Duramorph
Efricon Expectorant Liquid
Empirin w/Codeine
Endal-HD
Endal-HD Plus
Entuss-D
Entuss Expectorant
Entuss Pediatric Expectorant
Epimorph
FENTANYL
Fortral
Glydeine Cough
Guiatuss A.C.
Gulatussin w/Codeine Liquid
Histafed C
Hycodan
Hycomine
Hycomine Compound
Hycomine Pediatric
Hycomine-S Pediatric
Hycotuss Expectorant
HYDROCODONE
HYDROCODONE AND
  HOMATROPINE
Hydromine
Hydromine Pediatric
HYDROMORPHONE
Hydropane
Hydrophen
Hystadyl E.C.
Iophen-C Liquid
Iotuss
Isoclor Expectorant
Kwelcof Liquid
Laudanum
Levo-Dromoran
Levorphan

LEVORPHANOL
Mallergan-VC w/Codeine
MEPERIDINE
METHADONE
Methadose
Midahist DH
MORPHINE
Morphitec
M.O.S.
M.O.S.-SR
MS Contin
MSIR
MST Continus
Mycotussin
Myhistine DH
Myhistine Expectorant
Myhydromine
Myhydromine Pediatric
Myphetane DC Cough
Mytussin AC
Mytussin DAC
NALBUPHINE
Naldecon-CX
Normatane DC
Nortussin w/Codeine
Novahistex C
Novahistex DH
Novahistex DH Expectorant
Novahistine DH
Novahistine DH Expectorant
Novahistine DH Liquid
Novahistine Expectorant
Novopropoxyn
Nubain
Nucochem
Nucochem Expectorant
Nucochem Pediatric Expectorant
Nucofed
Nucofed Expectorant
Nucofed Pediatric Expectorant
Numorphan
Omni-Tuss
OPIUM
Oramorph
Oramorph-SR
Oxycodan
OXYCODONE
OXYMORPHONE
P-V-Tussin
Pantopon
Par Glycerol C
Paveral
Pediacof Cough
Penntuss
PENTAZOCINE
Percodan
Pethidine
Phenameth VC
Phenergan w/Codeine
Phenergan VC with Codeine
Phenhist Expectorant
Pherazine VC w/Codeine
Physeptone
Poly-Histine w/Codeine
Poly-Histine-CS
Profene
Prometh VC w/Codeine
PROMETHAZINE AND CODEINE
Promist HD Liquid
Pro Pox
Propoxycon
PROPOXYPHENE
Prunicodeine

Pseudo-Hist Expectorant
Pseudodine C Cough
RMS Uniserts
Robidone
Robitussin with Codeine
Robitussin A-C
Robitussin-DAC
Roxanol
Roxanol SR
Roxicodone
Roxiprin
Ru-Tuss w/Hydrocodone Liquid
Ryna-C Liquid
Ryna-CX Liquid
Soma Compound w/Codeine
SRC Expectorant
Stadol
Stadol NS
Statex
Statuss Expectorant
Statuss Green
Supeudol
Synalgos-DC
Talwin
Talwin-NX
Temgesic
Terpin Hydrate w/Codeine
T-Koff
Tolu-Sed Cough
Triacin C Cough
Triaminic w/Codeine
Triaminic Expectorant w/Codeine
Triaminic Expectorant DH
Triaminicin w/Codeine
Tricodene #1
Trifed-C Cough
Tussaminic DH Forte
Tussaminic DH Pediatric
Tussanil DH
Tussar-2
Tussar SF
Tussi-Organidin
Tussi-Organidin Liquid
Tussigon
Tussionex
Tussirex w/Codeine Liquid
Vanex-HD

NARCOTIC & ASPIRIN

222
282
292
293
692
A.C.&C.
Anacin with Codeine
Ancasal
ASPIRIN & CODEINE
Azdone
Bexophrene
BUFFERED ASPIRIN & CODEINE
Coryphen with Codeine
Cotanal 65
Damason-P
Darvon Compound
Darvon with A.S.A.
Darvon-N with A.S.A.
Darvon-N Compound
Doraphen Compound 65
Doxaphene Compound
Drocade and Aspirin
DROCODE & ASPIRIN
Emcodeine

Empirin with Codeine
Endodan
HYDROCODONE & ASPIRIN
Lortab
Margesic A-C
Novopropoxyn Compound
Oxycodan
OXYCODONE & ASPIRIN
PENTAZOCINE & ASPIRIN
Percodan
Percodan-Demi
Pro Pox Plus
PROPOXYPHENE & ASPIRIN
Roxiprin
Synalgos-DC
Talwin Compound
Talwin Compound-50

NIACIN (Vitamin B-3, Nicotinic Acid)

Nia-Bid
Niac
Niacels
Niacin
Niacor
Nico-400
Nicobid
Nicolar
NICOTINAMIDE
Nicotinex
Nicotinyl alcohol
Papulex
Roniacol
Ronigen
Rycotin
Slo-Niacin
Span-Niacin
Tega-Span
Tri-B3
VITAMIN B-3
Numerous other multiple
    vitamin-mineral supplements.

NITRATES

Apo-ISDN
Cardilate
Cedocard-SR
Coradur
Coronex
Deponit
Dilatrate-SR
Duotrate
ERYTHRITYL TETRANITRATE
Glyceryl Trinitrate
ISMO
Iso-Bid
Isonate
Isorbid
Isordil
ISORBIDE MONONITRATE
ISOSORBIDE DINITRATE
Isotrate
Klavikordal
Naptrate
Niong
Nitro-Bid
Nitrocap
Nitrocap T.D.
Nitrocine
Nitrodisc
Nitro-Dur
Nitro-Dur II

Nitrogard-SR
NITROGLYCERIN (GLYCERYL
    TRINITRATE)
Nitroglyn
Nitrol
Nitrolin
Nitrolingual
Nitronet
Nitrong
Nitrong SR
Nitrospan
Nitrostat
Novosorbide
NTS
PENTAERYTHRITOL
    TETRANITRATE
Pentritol
Pentylan
Peritrate
Peritrate Forte
Peritrate SA
P.E.T.N.
Sorbitrate
Sorbitrate SA
Transderm-Nitro
Tridil

PAPAVERINE

Cerespan
Genabid
Pavabid
Pavabid Plateau Caps
Pavacap
Pavacen
Pavagen
Pavarine
Pavased
Pavatine
Pavatym
Paverolan

PHENOTHIAZINES

ACETOPHENAZINE
Apo-Fluphenazine
Apo-Perphenazine
Apo-Thioridazine
Apo-Trifluoperazine
Chlorpromanyl-20
Chlorpromanyl-40
CHLORPROMAZINE
Compazine
Compazine Spansule
Dartal
FLUPHENAZINE
Largactil
Largactil Liquid
Largactil Oral Drops
Levoprome
Majeptil
Mellaril
Mellaril Concentrate
Mellaril-S
MESORIDAZINE
METHOTRIMEPRAZINE
Modecate
Moditen Enanthate
Moditen HCl
Moditen HCl-H.P
Neuleptil
Novo-Chlorpromazine
Novo-Flurazine
Novo-Ridazine
Nozinan

Nozinan Liquid
Nozinan Oral Drops
PERICYAZINE
Permitil
Permitil Concentrate
PERPHENAZINE
Piportil L₄
PIPOTIAZINE
PMS Thioridazine
PROCHLORPERAZINE
Prolixin
Prolixin Concentrate
Prolixin Decanoate
Prolixin Enanthate
PROMAZINE
Prozine
Serentil
Serentil Concentrate
Solazine
Stelazine
Stelazine Concentrate
Stemetil
Stemetil Liquid
Suprazine
Terfluzine Concentrate
THIOPROPAZATE
THIOPROPERAZINE
THIORIDAZINE
Thorazine
Thorazine Concentrate
Thorazine Spansule
Thor-Prom
Tindal
TRIFLUOPERAZINE
TRIFLUPROMAZINE
Trilafon
Trilafon Concentrate
Vesprin

PHENYLEPHRINE

Alersule
Amaril D
Amaril D Spantab
Anamine HD
Anatuss
Atrohist Sprinkle
Banex
Banex Liquid
Bromophen T.D.
Cerose-DM
Citra Forte
Chlorgest-HD
Codimal DH
Codimal DM
Codimal PH
Colrex Compound
Colrex Cough
Coltab Children's
Comhist
Comhist LA
Conar
Conar Expectorant
Conar-A
Congespirin for Children Cold
    Tablets
Cophene-S
Cophene-X
Cophene-XP
Coristex-DH
Coristine-DH
Dallergy-D Syrup
Decohist

Decongestabs
Despec
Dihistine
Dimaphen S.A.
Dimetane Decongestant Caplets
Dimetane Expectorant
Dimetane Expectorant-C
Dimetane Expectorant-DC
Dimetapp Elixir
Dimetapp Oral Infant Drops
Dimetapp with Codeine
Dimetapp-DM
Donatussin
Donatussin DC
Donatussin Drops
Dondril
Dristan Cold
Efricon Expectorant Liquid
Endal-HD
Endal-HD Plus
Entex
Entex Liquid
Father John's Medicine Plus
Fendol
Guistrey Fortis
Histalet Forte
Histamic
Histatab
Histatan
Histatuss Pediatric
Hista-Vadrin
Histor-D
Hycomine
Hycomine Compound
Hycomine-S Pediatric
Improved Sino-Tuss
Mallergan-VC w/Codeine
Meda Syrup Forte
Myhistine
Naldecon
Naldecon Pediatric
Naldelate
Nalgest
Nasahist
Neo Citran Sinus Medicine
New-Decongest
New-Decongest Pediatric Syrup
Normatane
Novahistex C
Novahistex DH
Novahistex DH Expectorant
Novahistex DM
Novahistine
Novahistine DH
Novahistine DH Expectorant
Omnicol
P-V-Tussin
Par Decon
Pediacof Cough
Phenameth VC
Phenameth VC w/Codeine
Phenergan VC
Phenergan VC w/Codeine
Phentox Compound
Pherazine VC
Pherazine VC w/Codeine
Prometh VC Plain
Prometh VC w/Codeine
Promethazine VC
Quelidrine Cough
Respinol G
Respinol LA
Robitussin Night Relief

Robitussin Night Relief Colds
    Formula Liquid
R-Tannate
Ru-Tuss
Ru-Tuss w/Hydrocodone
Ru-Tuss Expectorant
Ru-Tuss w/Hydrocodone Liquid
Rymed
Rymed Liquid
Rynatan
Sinucon Pediatric Drops
Statuss Expectorant
Statuss Green
Tamine S.R.
T-Koff
Trimedine Liquid
Triotann
Tri-Phen-Chlor
Tri-Phen-Chlor T.D.
Tritann Pediatric
Tusquelin
Tussanil DH
Tussanil Plain
Tussirex w/Codeine
Tussirex w/Codeine Liquid
Vanex-HD
Vasominic T.D.
Veltap

PHENYLPROPANOLAMINE

Alamine
Alka-Seltzer Plus Maximum
    Strength Sinus Allergy
Allerest
Allerest 12 Hour
Allergy Relief Medicine
Amaril D
Ami-Tex LA
Anatuss
Anatuss with Codeine
A.R.M. Maximum Strength
    Caplets
BC Cold Powder
BC Cold Powder Non-Drowsy
    Formula
Banex
Banex Liquid
Banex-LA
Bayaminic Expectorant
Bayaminicol
Baycomine
Baycomine Pediatric
Bayer Cough Syrup
Bayer Cough Syrup for Children
Biphetane DC Cough Syrup
Bromanate DC Cough Syrup
Bromatap
Bromatapp
Bromophen T.D.
Bromphen DC w/Codeine Cough
Caldomine-DH Forte
Caldomine-DH Pediatric
Cheracol Plus
Chexit
Chlor-Rest
Chlor-Tripolon Decongestant
Codamine
Codamine Pediatric
Codegest Expectorant
Codimal Expectorant
Comtrex Multi-Symptom Cold
    Reliever

Condrin-LA
Conex
Conex D.A.
Conex w/Codeine Liquid
Congespirin for Children Liquid
    Cold Medicine
Contac Jr. Children's Cold
    Medicine
Contac 12-Hour
Contac Maximum Strength
    12-Hour
Cophene-S
Cophene-X
Cophene-XP
Coricidin Cough
Corsym
Decongestabs
Dehist
Demazin
Demazin Repetabs
Despec
Dilotab
Dimaphen S.A.
Dimetane Expectorant
Dimetane Expectorant-C
Dimetane Expectorant-DC
Dimetane-DC Cough
Dimetapp
Dimetapp with Codeine
Dimetapp Extentabs
Dimetapp Maximum Strength
    Liquigels
Dimetapp Oral Infant Drops
Dimetapp-DM
Dorcol DM
Drinophen
Drize
Dura-Vent
Dura-Vent/A
Effervescent Tylenol Cold
Efficol Cough Whip (Cough
    Suppressant/Decongestant)
Efficol Cough Whip (Cough
    Suppressant/Decongestant/
    Antihistamine)
Efficol Whip
Entex
Entex LA
Entex Liquid
Genamin
Genatap
Gencold
Genex
Gentab-LA
Guaipax
Halls Mentho-Lyptus
Halls Mentho-Lyptus
    Decongestant Cough Formula
Head & Chest
Histabid Duracaps
Histalet Forte
Histamic
Hista-Vadrin
Hold (Children's Formula)
Hycomine
Hycomine Pediatric
Hydromine
Hydromine Pediatric
Hydrophen
Ipsatol Cough Formula for
    Children
Kiddy Koff
Kolephrin/DM

Kolephrin NN Liquid
Kophane
Kophane Cough and Cold
    Formula
Lanatuss Expectorant
Medatussin Plus
Myhydromine
Myhydromine Pediatric
Myminic
Myphetane DC Cough
Myphetapp
Naldecon
Naldecon Pediatric
Naldecon-CX Adult Liquid
Naldecon-DX Adult Liquid
Naldecon-DX Children's Syrup
Naldecon-DX Pediatric Drops
Naldecon-EX
Naldelate
Naldelate Pediatric Syrup
Nalgest
Nasahist
New-Decongest
New-Decongest Pediatric Syrup
Nolamine
Nolex LA
Noraminic
Normatane
Normatane DC
Oragest S.R.
Oraminic Spancaps
Ornade
Ornade A.F.
Ornade-DM
Ornade-DM 10
Ornade-DM 15
Ornade-DM 30
Ornade Expectorant
Orthoxicol Cough
Panadyl
Par Decon
Pertussin AM
Phanadex
PhenAPAP No. 2
Phentox Compound
Phenylfenesin L.A.
Poly-Histine-CS
Poly-Histine-D
Poly-Histine-D Ped
Poly-Histine-DM
Prominic Expectorant
Prominicol Cough
Rentamine
Resaid S.R.
Rescaps-D S.R.
Respinol-G
Respinol LA
Rhinocaps
Rhinolar-EX
Rhinolar-EX 12
Robitussin-CF
Ru-Tuss II
Ru-Tuss w/Hydrocodone Liquid
Rymed
Rymed Liquid
Saleto-CF
Saleto-D
Sinucon Pediatric Drops
Snaplets-D
Snaplets-DM
Snaplets-EX
Snaplets-Multi

St. Joseph Cold Tablets for
    Children
Stamoist LA
Statuss Green
Syracol Liquid
Tamine S.R.
Tavist-D
T-Koff
Triaminic
Triaminic Allergy
Triaminic Chewables
Triaminic Cold
Triaminic Expectorant
Triaminic Expectorant DH
Triaminic Expectorant w/Codeine
Triaminic Oral Infant Drops
Triaminic TR
Triaminic-DM Cough Formula
Triaminic-DM Expectorant
Triaminicin w/Codeine
Triaminicol DM
Triaminicol Multi-Symptom Relief
Tricodene Forte
Tricodene NN
Tricodene NN Pediatric
    Medication
Tricodene Pediatric
Trind
Trind DM Liquid
Tri-Nefrin Extra Strength
Tripalgen Cold
Tri-Phen-Chlor
Tri-Phen-Chlor T.D.
Triphenyl
Triphenyl Expectorant
Triphenyl T.D.
Tusquelin
Tuss-Ade
Tuss Allergine Modified T.D.
Tuss-Ornade Liquid
Tuss-Ornade Spansules
Tussagesic
Tussaminic C Forte
Tussaminic C Pediatric
Tussaminic DH Forte
Tussaminic DH Pediatric
Tussanil DH Tablets
Tussogest
Tuss-Ornade Liquid
Tuss-Ornade Spansules
ULR-LA
Utex-S.R.
Vasominic T.D.
Veltap

POTASSIUM SUPPLEMENTS

Apo-K
Cena-K
K-10
Kallum Durules
Kaochlor
Kaochlor-Eff
Kaochlor S-F
Kaon
Kaon-Cl
Kaon-Cl 10
Kaon-Cl 20
Kato
Kay Ciel
Kay Ciel Elixir
Kaylixir

K+Care ET
KCL
K-Dur
K-G Elixir
K-Lease
K-Long
K-Lor
Klor-Con
Klor-Con/25
Klor-Con/EF
Klorvess
Klorvess 10% Liquid
Klotrix
K-Lyte
K-Lyte DS
K-Lyte/Cl
K-Lyte/Cl 50
K-Lyte/CL Powder
K-Norm
Kolyum
K-Tab
Micro-K
Micro-K 10
Micro-K LS
Neo-K
Novo-Lente-K
Potachlor 10%
Potachlor 20%
Potage
Potasalan
POTASSIUM ACETATE
POTASSIUM BICARBONATE
POTASSIUM BICARBONATE &
   POTASSIUM CHLORIDE
POTASSIUM BICARBONATE &
   POTASSIUM CITRATE
POTASSIUM CHLORIDE
POTASSIUM CHLORIDE,
   POTASSIUM BICARBONATE &
   POTASSIUM CITRATE
POTASSIUM GLUCONATE
POTASSIUM GLUCONATE &
   POTASSIUM CHLORIDE
POTASSIUM GLUCONATE &
   POTASSIUM CITRATE
POTASSIUM GLUCONATE,
   POTASSIUM CITRATE &
   AMMONIUM
Potassium-Rougier
Potassium-Sandoz
Potassium Triplex
Roychlor 10%
Roychlor 20%
Royonate
Rum-K
Slo-Pot 600
Slow-K
Ten K
Tri-K
TRIKATES
Twin-K
Twin-K-Cl

PREDNISOLONE

Articulose
Delta-Cortef
Hydeltrasol
Hydeltra-TBA
Key-Pred
Key-Pred-SP
Nor-Pred-TBA
Pediapred

Predaject
Predalone
Predate-50
Predate-S
Predate-TBA
Predcor 25
Predcor 50
Predicort-50
Prelone

PROGESTINS

Amen
Aygestin
Curretab
Cycrin
Depo-Provera
Duralutin
Femotrone
Gesterol
Gesterol L.A.
HYDROXYPROGESTERONE
Hylutin
Hyprogest
Hyproval P.A.
MEDROXYPROGESTERONE
Megace
MEGESTROL
Micronor
Nor-Q.D.
NORETHINDRONE
NORGESTREL
Norlutate
Norlutin
Norplant
Ovrette
Pro-Depo
Prodrox
Progestaject
PROGESTERONE
Progestilin
Provera

PSEUDOEPHEDRINE

Actacin
Actagen
Actagen-C Cough
Actifed
Actifed w/Codeine Cough
Actifed DM
Actifed 12-Hour
Afrinol Repetabs
Alamine-C Liquid
Alamine Expectorant
Allent
Allerest No-Drowsiness
Allerfrin Allergy Formula Sinutab
Allerfrin w/Codeine
AlleRid
Allerphed
Alpha-Phed
Ambenyl-D Decongestant Cough
Anamine
Anamine T.D.
Aprodrine
Atrofed
Formula
BayCotussend Liquid
Baydec DM Drops
Bayhistine DH
Bayhistine Expectorant
Benadryl Allergy/Sinus Headache
   Caplets

Benadryl Decongestant
Benylin Cold
Benylin Decongestant
Beta-Phed
Brexin
Brexin-L.A.
Bromfed
Bromfed-AT
Bromfed-DM
Bromphed-PD
Brompheril
Brotane DX Cough
Carbinoxamine Compound
Carbiset
Carbodec
Carbodec DM Drops
Carbodec TR
Cardec-S
Cenafed
Cenafed Plus
Cheracol Sinus
Children's NyQuil Nighttime Cold
   Medicine
Children's Sudafed Liquid
Chlorafed
Chlorafed H.S. Timecelles
Chlorafed Timecelles
Chlor-Trimeton Decongestant
Chlor-Trimetan Decongestant
   Repetabs
Chlor-Tripolon Decongestant
   Tablets
Chlor-Tripolon Decongestant
   Extra Strength
Chlor-Tripolon Decongestant
   Repetabs
CoActifed
CoActifed Expectorant
CoAdvil
CoAdvil Caplets
Co-Apap
Codehist DH
Codimal-LA
Coldrine
Comtrex Daytime Caplets
Comtrex Multi-Symptom Hot Flu
   Relief
Comtrex Multi-Symptom Non-
   Drowsy Caplets
Comtrex Nighttime
Concentrin
Congess JR
Congess SR
Congestac N.D. Caplets
Contac Maximum Strength Sinus
   Caplets
Contac Severe Cold Formula
Contac Severe Cold Formula
   Night Strength
Cophene No. 2
Co-Pyronil 2
CoTylenol Cold Medication
Cremacoat 3 Throat Coating
   Cough Medicine
Cremacoat 4 Throat Coating
   Cough Medicine
C-Tussin Expectorant
Dallergy-D
Dallergy Jr.
DayCare
DayQuil Liquicaps
DayQuil Non-Drowsy Cold/Flu
Decofed

927

Deconamine
Deconamine SR
Deproist Expectorant w/Codeine
De-Tuss
Detussin Expectorant
Detussin Liquid
Dexaphen SA
Dexophed
Dihistine DH
Dimacol
Dimetane-DX Cough
Disobrom
Disophrol
Disophrol Chronotabs
Dorcol Children's Cold Formula
Dorcol Children's Cough
Dorcol Children's Decongestant
Dristan Cold and Flu
Dristan Maximum Strength
  Caplets
Dristan Sinus Caplets
Drixoral
Drixoral Non-Drowsy Formula
Drixoral Plus
Drixoral Sinus
Drixtab
Duralex
Dura-Tap PD
Eltor-120
Endafed
Entuss-D
Entuss Pediatric Expectorant
Fedahist
Fedahist Decongestant
Fedahist Expectorant
Fedahist Expectorant Pediatric
  Drops
Fedahist Gyrocaps
Fedahist Timecaps
Genac
Genaphed
Guaifed
Guaifed-PD
Guaitab
Halofed
Halofed Adult Strength
Head & Chest
Histadyl E.C.
Histafed C
Histalet
Histalet-DM
Histalet X
Isoclor
Isoclor Expectorant
Isoclor Timesules
Klerist-D
Kronofed-A
Kronofed-A Jr.
Maxenal
Medi-Flu
Medi-Flu Caplets
Mediquell Decongestant Formula
Midahist DH
Mycotussin
Myfed
Myfedrine
Myfedrine Plus
Myhistine DH
Myhistine Expectorant
Mytussin DAC
Naldegesic
Napril
ND Clear T.D.

Neofed
Noratuss II Liquid
Novafed
Novafed A
Novahistex
Novahistine Cough & Cold
  Formula Liquid
Novahistine DH Liquid
Novahistine DMX Liquid
Novahistine Expectorant
Nucochem
Nucochem Expectorant
Nucochem Pediatric Expectorant
Nucofed
Nucofed Expectorant
Nucofed Pediatric Expectorant
NyQuil Liquicaps
NyQuil Nighttime Colds Medicine
Nytime Cold Medicine Liquid
Ornex Cold
Ornex No Drowsiness Caplets
Otrivin
PediaCare Children's Cough-Cold
  Formula
PediaCare Children's Cold Relief
  Night Rest Cough-Cold
  Formula
PediaCare Cold Formula
PediaCare Infants' Oral
  Decongestant Drops
Pertussin AM
Pertussin PM
Phenergan-D
Phenhist Expectorant
Polaramine Expectorant
Promist HD Liquid
Pseudo
Pseudo-Bid
Pseudo-Car DM
Pseudo-Chlor
Pseudodine C Cough
Pseudofrin
Pseudogest
Pseudogest Plus
Pseudo-Hist Expectorant
Respaire-60 SR
Respaire-120 SR
Resporal TR
Rhinosyn-DM
Rhinosyn-X
Rinade B.I.D.
Robidrine
Robitussin-DAC
Robitussin-PE
Rondec
Rondec Drops
Rondec-DM
Rondec-DM Drops
Ru-Tuss Expectorant
Rymed-TR
Ryna
Ryna-C Liquid
Ryna-CX Liquid
Seldane D
Sinarest No-Drowsiness
Sine-Aid
Sine-Aid Maximum Strength
Sine-Aid Maximum Strength
  Caplets
Sine-Off Maximum Strength No
  Drowsiness Formula Caplets
Sinufed Timecelles
Sinus Excedrin No Drowsiness

Sinus Excedrin No Drowsiness
  Caplets
SinuStat
Sinutab II Maximum Strength
Sinutab Maximum Strength
  Without Drowsiness
Sinutab Maximum Strength
  Without Drowsiness Caplets
Sinutab No Drowsiness
Sinutab No Drowsiness Extra
  Strength
SRC Expectorant
Stamoist E
Sudafed
Sudafed 12 Hour
Sudafed 60
Sudafed Cough
Sudafed DM
Sudafed Expectorant
Sudafed Plus
Sudafed Severe Cold Formula
  Caplets
Sudafed Sinus Maximum
  Strength
Sudafed Sinus Maximum
  Strength Caplets
Sudrin
Sufedrin
Super-Anahist
TheraFlu/Flu & Cold
TheraFlu/Flu, Cold & Cough
TheraFlu Nighttime Maximum
  Strength
T-Dry
T-Dry Junior
T-Moist
Triacin C Cough
Triaminic Nite Light
Trifed
Trifed-C Cough
Trinalin Repetabs
Trinex
Triofed
Tripodrine
Triposed
Tussafed
Tussar DM
Tussend
Tussend Expectorant
Tussend Liquid
Tuss-LA
Ty-Cold Cold Formula
Tylenol Allergy Sinus Gelcaps
Tylenol Cold Medication
Tylenol Cold Medication,
  Non-Drowsy
Tylenol Cold Night Time
Tylenol Cold and Flu
Tylenol Cough
Tylenol Sinus Maximum Strength
Tylenol Sinus Maximum Strength
  Caplets
Tylenol Sinus Maximum Strength
  Gelcaps
Tylenol Sinus Medication
Tylenol Sinus Medication Extra
  Strength
Ursinus Inlay
Vicks Formula 44D Decongestant
  Cough Mixture
Vicks Formula 44M Multi-
  symptom Cough Mixture
Viro-Med

Zephrex
Zephrex-LA

PSYLLIUM

Cillium
Effersyllium
Fiberall
Hydrocil
Hydrocil Instant
Karacil
Konsyl
Konsyl-D
Metamucil
Metamucil Instant Mix
Metamucil Instant Mix, Orange
  Flavor
Metamucil Orange Flavor
Metamucil Strawberry Flavor
Metamucil Sugar Free
Modane Bulk
Naturacil
Perdiem
Perdiem Plain
Pro-Lax
Prodiem
Prodiem Plain
Prompt
Reguloid Natural
Reguloid Orange
Serutan
Serutan Toasted Granules
Siblin
Syllact
V-Lax
Versabran

RADIO-PHARMACEUTICALS

Cyanocobalamin Co 57
Cyanocobalamin Co 60
Ferrous Citrate Fe 59
Gallium Citrate Ga 67
Indium In 111 Pentetate
Iodinated I 131 Albumin
Iodohippurate Sodium I 123
Iodohippurate Sodium I 131
Iothalamate Sodium I 125
Krypton KR 81m
Selenomethionine Se 75
Sodium Chromate Cr 51
Sodium Iodide I 123
Sodium Iodide I 131
Sodium Pertechnetate Tc 99m
Sodium Phosphate P 32
Technetium Tc 99m Albumin
  Aggregated
Technetium Tc 99m Disofenin
Technetium Tc 99m Gluceptate
Technetium Tc 99m Human
  Serum Albumin
Technetium Tc 99m Medronate
Technetium Tc 99m Oxidronate
Technetium Tc 99m Pentetate
Technetium Tc 99m
  Pyrophosphate
Technetium Tc 99m Succimer
Technetium Tc 99m Sulfur
  Colloid
Thallous Chloride Tl 201
Xenon Xe 127
Xenon Xe 133

RAUWOLFIA ALKALOIDS

ALSEROXYLON
Demi-Regroton
DESERPIDINE
Diupres
Diutensin-R
Enduronyl
Harmonyl
Hydromox R
Mallopress
Metatensin
Naquival
Novoreserpine
Oreticyl
Raudixin
Rauval
Rauverid
Rauwiloid
RAUWOLFIA SERPENTINA
Rauzide
Regroton
Renese-R
Reserfia
RESERPINE
Salutensin
Serpalan
Serpasil
Serpasil-Esidrix
Wolfina

RAUWOLFIA & THIAZIDE DIURETICS

Demi-Regroton
DESERPIDINE &
  HYDROCHLOROTHIAZIDE
DESERPIDINE &
  METHYCLOTHIAZIDE
Diupres
Diurese R
Diurigen with Reserpine
Diutensen-R
Dureticyl
Enduronyl
Enduronyl Forte
Hydromox-R
Hydropine
Hydropres
Hydrosine
Hydrotensin
Mallopres
Metatensin
Naquival
Oreticyl
Oreticyl Forte
RAUWOLFIA SERPENTINA &
  BENDROFLUMETHIAZIDE
Rauzide
Renese-R
RESERPINE & CHLOROTHIAZIDE
RESERPINE &
  CHLORTHALIDONE
RESERPINE &
  HYDROCHLOROTHIAZIDE
RESERPINE &
  HYDROFLUMETHIAZIDE
RESERPINE &
  METHYLCLOTHIAZIDE
RESERPINE & POLYTHIAZIDE
RESERPINE & QUINETHAZONE
RESERPINE &
  TRICHLORMETHIAZIDE
Salazide

Salutensin
Salutensin-Demi
Serpasil-Esidrix

SALICYLATES

Arthropan
CHOLINE MAGNESIUM
  SALICYLATES
Choline Magnesium Trisalicylate
CHOLINE SALICYLATE
Citra Forte
Disalcid
Doan's Pills
Fendol
Improved SinoTuss
Kolephrin NN Liquid
Magan
MAGNESIUM SALICYLATE
Mobidin
Mono-Gesic
Omnicol
Salflex
Salgesic
SALICYLAMIDE
SALSALATE
Salsitab
SODIUM SALICYLATE
Tricosal
Trilisate
Tussanil DH Tablets
Tussirex w/Codeine Liquid
Uracel
Uromide

SCOPOLAMINE (Hyoscine)

Barbidonna
Barbidonna 2
Buscopan
Donnatal
Donnatal Extentabs
Kinesed
Spasmolin
Spasquid
Transderm-Scop
Transderm-V

SULFAMETHOXAZOLE

Apo-Sulfamethoxazole
Apo-Sulfatrim
Azo Gantanol
Bactrim
Bactrim DS
Bethaprim
Cetamide
Cheragan w/TMP
Cotrim
Cotrim D.S.
Co-trimoxazole
Gantanol
Gantanol DS
Novotrimel
Protrin
Roubac
Septra
Septra DS
SMZ-TMP
Sulfamethoprim
Sulfamethoprim DS
Sulfaprim
Sulfaprim DS

Sulfatrim
Sulfatrim DS
Sulfoxaprim
Sulfoxaprim DS
Sulmeprim
Triazole
Triazole DS
Trimeth-Sulfa
Trisulfam
Uroplus DS
Uroplus SS

SULFISOXAZOLE

Apo-Sulfisoxazole
Azo-Gantrisin
Gantrisin
Lipo Gantrisin
Novosoxazole
Pediazole
Sulfafurazole

TESTOSTERONE & ESTRADIOL

Andrest
Andro-Estro
Andro/Fem
Androgyn L.A.
De-Comberol
Deladumone
Delatestadiol
depAndrogyn
Depo-Testadiol
Depotestogen
Ditate DS
Duo-Cyp
Duo-Gen L.A.
Duogex LA
Duoval PA
Duratestrin
Estrand
Estra-Testrin
Menoject-L.A.
Neo-Pause
Teev
T.E.-Ionate P.A.
Testadiate-Depo
Test-Estra-C
Test-Estro Cypionates
TESTOSTERONE CYPIONATE & ESTRADIOL CYPIONATE
TESTOSTERONE ENANTHATE & ESTRADIOL VALERATE
Testradiol
Testradiol L.A.
Valertest

TETRACYCLINES

Achromycin
Achromycin V
Apo-Doxy
Apo-Tetra
Declomycin
DEMECLOCYCLINE
Doryx
Doxy-Caps
Doxy-Tabs
DOXYCYCLINE
E.P. Mycin
METHACYCLINE
Minocin
MINOCYCLINE

Novotetra
OXYTETRACYCLINE
Panmycin
Robitet
Rondomycin
Sumycin
Terramycin
TETRACYCLINE
Tetracyn
Tija
Vibramycin
Vibratabs

TRIAMCINOLONE

Amcort
Aristocort Forte
Aristocort Intralesional
Aristospan
Articulose-L.A.
Azmacort
Cenocort A 40
Cenocort Forte
Cinalone 40
Cinonide 40
Dermacomb
Kanacort
Kenaject-40
Kenalog 10
Kenalog 40
Myco II
Myco-Triacet II
Mycobiotic II
Mycogen II
Mycolog II
Mykacet
Mykacet II
Mytrex
Tac-3
Triam A
Triam-Forte
Triamolone
Triamonide 40
Tri-Kort
Trilog
Trilone
Tristatin II
Tristoject
Some of these brands are avaiable as topical medicines (ointments, creams or lotions).
See ADRENOCORTICOIDS (Topical) in this section.

TRICYCLIC ANTIDEPRESSANTS

Adapin
AMITRYPTILINE
AMOXAPINE
Anafranil
Apo-Amitriptyline
Apo-Imipramine
Apo-Trimip
Asendin
Aventyl
CLOMIPRAMINE
DESIPRAMINE
DOXEPIN
Elavil
Emitrip
Endep
Enovil

IMIPRAMINE
Impril
Janimine
Levate
Norpramin
NORTRIPTYLINE
Novopramine
Novotriptyn
Pamelor
Pertofrane
PROTRIPTYLINE
Sinequan
Surmontil
Tipramine
Tofranil
Tofranil-PM
Triadapin
TRIMIPRAMINE
Triptil
Vivactil

VITAMIN B-12 (Cyanocobalamin)

Acti-B-12
Alphamin
Alpha Redisol
Anocobin
Bedoz
Berubigen
Betalin 12
Codroxomin
Cyanabin
CYANACOBALAMIN
Droxomin
HYDROXOCOBALAMIN
Kaybovite
Kaybovite-1000
Redisol
Rubion
Rubramin
Rubramin-PC
Numerous other multiple vitamin-mineral supplements.

VITAMIN C (Ascorbic Acid)

Ascorbicap
Cecon
Cemill
Cenolate
Cetane
Cevalin
Cevi-Bid
Ce-Vi-Sol
Cevita
C-Span
Flavorcee
Redoxon
Sunkist
Numerous other multiple vitamin-mineral supplements.

XYLOMETAZOLINE & OXYMETAZOLINE (Nasal)

4-Way Long Acting Nasal Spray
Afrin 12 Hour Nasal Spray
Afrin 12 Hour Nose Drops
Afrin Children's Strength 12 Hour Nose Drops

Afrin Children's Strength Nose
Drops
Afrin Menthol Nasal Spray
Afrin Nasal Spray
Afrin Nasal Spray Pump
Afrin Nose Drops
Allerest 12 Hour Nasal Spray
Chlorohist
Chlorohist-LA
Coricidin Nasal Mist
Dristan Long Lasting Menthol
Nasal Spray
Dristan Long Lasting Nasal
Pump Spray
Dristan Long Lasting Nasal
Spray
Dristan Long Lasting Nasal
Spray 12 Hour Metered Dose
Pump
Duramist Plus Up To 12 Hours
Decongestant Nasal Spray
Duration 12 Hour Nasal Spray
Pump

Nafrine Decongestant Nasal
Drops
Nafrine Decongestant Nasal
Spray
Nafrine Decongestant Pediatric
Nasal Spray/Drops
Neo-Synephrine 12 Hour Nasal
Spray
Neo-Synephrine 12 Hour Nasal
Spray Pump
Neo-Synephrine 12 Hour Nose
Drops
Neo-Synephrine 12 Hour Vapor
Nasal Spray
Neo-Synephrine II Long
Neo-Synephrine II Long Acting
Nasal Spray Adult Strength
Neo-Synephrine II Long Acting
Nose Drops Adult Strength
Nostril Nasal Decongestant Mild
Nostril Nasal Decongestant
Regular
Nostrilla 12 Hour Nasal
Decongestant

NTZ Long Acting Decongestant
Nose Drops
NTZ Long Acting Decongestant
Nose Spray
Otrivin
Otrivin Decongestant Nose
Drops
Otrivin Nasal Drops
Otrivin Nasal Spray
Otrivin Pediatric Decongestant
Nose Drops
Otrivin Pediatric Nasal Drops
Otrivin Pediatric Nasal Spray
Otrivin With M-D Pump
Sinarest 12 Hour Nasal Spray
Sinutab
Sinutab Sinus Spray
Vicks Sinex 12-Hour Formula
Decongestant Nasal Spray
Vicks Sinex 12-Hour Formula
Decongestant Ultra Fine Mist
Vicks Sinex Long-Acting 12 Hour
Nasal Spray

Additional Drug Interactions

The following lists of drugs and their interactions with other drugs are continuations of lists found in the alphabetized drug charts beginning on page 2. These lists are alphabetized by generic name or drug class name, shown in large capital letters. Only those lists too long for the drug charts are included in this section. For complete information about any generic drug, see the alphabetized chart.

GENERIC NAME OR DRUG CLASS	COMBINED EFFECT	GENERIC NAME OR DRUG CLASS	COMBINED EFFECT

ACETAMINOPHEN & SALICYLATES

GENERIC NAME OR DRUG CLASS	COMBINED EFFECT	GENERIC NAME OR DRUG CLASS	COMBINED EFFECT
Lisinopril	Decreased lisinopril effect.	Rifampin	Increased liver toxicity.
Methotrexate	Increased methotrexate effect.	Sotalol	Decreased antihypertensive effect of sotalol.
Non-steroidal anti-inflammatory drugs (NSAIDs)*	Risk of stomach bleeding and ulcers.	Spironolactone	Decreased spironolactone effect.
Para-aminosalicylic acid (PAS)	Possible salicylate toxicity.	Sulfinpyrazone	Decreased sulfinpyrazone effect.
Phenobarbital	Decreased effect of acetaminophen and salicylates because of quicker elimination.	Terazosin	Decreases effectiveness of terazosin. Causes sodium and fluid retention.
Phenytoin	Increased phenytoin effect.	Tetracyclines* (effervescent granules or tablets)	May slow tetracycline absorption. Space doses 2 hours apart.
Primidone	Increased liver toxicity.	Vancomycin	Hearing loss.
Probenecid	Decreased probenecid effect.	Verapamil	Increased risk of toxicity.
Propranolol	Decreased aspirin effect.	Vitamin C (large doses)	Possible aspirin toxicity.
Rauwolfia alkaloids*	Decreased aspirin effect.	Urinary alkalizers*	Increased risk of toxicity.
		Zidovudine	Increased toxicity of both.

AMILORIDE & HYDROCHLOROTHIAZIDE

GENERIC NAME OR DRUG CLASS	COMBINED EFFECT	GENERIC NAME OR DRUG CLASS	COMBINED EFFECT
Digitalis preparations*	Excessive potassium loss that causes dangerous heart rhythms.	Nicardipine	Dangerous blood pressure drop. Dosages may require adjustment.
Diuretics, thiazide*	Increased diuretic effect.	Nimodipine	Dangerous blood pressure drop.
Diuretics, other*	Increased effect of both drugs.	Nitrates*	Excessive blood pressure drop.
Indapamide	Increased diuretic effect.	Oxprenolol	Increased antihypertensive effect. Dosages may require adjustment.
Lisinopril	Increased antihypertensive effect. Dosage of each may require adjustment.	Probenecid	Decreased probenecid effect.
Lithium	Possible lithium toxicity.	Potassium supplements*	Increased potassium levels.
MAO inhibitors*	Increased hydrochlorothiazide effect.		

*See Glossary

GENERIC NAME OR DRUG CLASS	COMBINED EFFECT	GENERIC NAME OR DRUG CLASS	COMBINED EFFECT

AMILORIDE & HYDROCHLOROTHIAZIDE continued

Sodium bicarbonate	Decreased potassium levels.	Terazosin	Decreases effectiveness of terazosin.
Sotalol	Increased antihypertensive effect.	Zinc supplements	Increased need for zinc.

ANGIOTENSIN-CONVERTING ENZYME (ACE) INHIBITORS

Sotalol	Increased antihypertensive effects of both drugs. Dosages may require adjustment.	Terazosin	Decreases effectiveness of terazosin.
		Tiopronin	Increased risk of toxicity to kidneys.
Spironolactone	Possible excessive potassium in blood.	Triamterene	Possible excessive potassium in blood.

ANGIOTENSIN-CONVERTING ENZYME (ACE) INHIBITORS & HYDROCHLOROTHIAZIDE

Diuretics*	Decreased blood pressure.	Nitrates*	Excessive blood pressure drop.
Lisinopril	Increased antihypertensive effect. Dosage of each may require adjustment.	Non-steroidal anti-inflammatory drugs (NSAIDs)*	Decreased captopril effect.
Lithium	Increased effect of lithium.	Potassium supplements*	Excessive potassium in blood.
MAO inhibitors*	Increased hydrochlorothiazide effect.	Probenecid	Decreased probenecid effect.
Nicardipine	Blood pressure drop. Dosages may require adjustment.	Sotalol	Increased antihypertensive effects of both drugs. Dosages may require adjustment.
Nimodipine	Possible irregular heartbeat. May worsen congestive heart failure.	Spironolactone	Possible excessive potassium in blood.
		Triamterene	Possible excessive potassium in blood.

ANTICOAGULANTS (Oral)

Levamisole	Increased risk of bleeding.	Non-steroidal anti-inflammatory drugs (NSAIDs)*	Increased risk of bleeding.
Mineral oil	Decreased absorption of anticoagulant.	Omeprazole	Increased effect of anticoagulant.
Nicardipine	Possible increased effect of anticoagulant.	Phenytoin	Decreased phenytoin levels.
Nimodipine	Possible increased effect of anticoagulant.	Propafenone	May require adjustment of anticoagulant dosage.
Nizatidine	Increased effect of anticoagulant.	Rifampin	Decreased effect of anticoagulant.

*See Glossary

GENERIC NAME OR DRUG CLASS	COMBINED EFFECT	GENERIC NAME OR DRUG CLASS	COMBINED EFFECT
ANTICOAGULANTS (Oral) continued			
Sulfadoxine and pyrimethamine	Increased risk of toxicity.	**Vitamin E**	Increased risk of bleeding.
Suprofen	Increased risk of bleeding.	**Vitamin K**	Decreased effect of anticoagulant.
Testolactone	Increased effect of anticoagulant.	**Note: Any medicine**	Unpredictable absorption.

ANTIDIABETIC AGENTS

GENERIC NAME OR DRUG CLASS	COMBINED EFFECT	GENERIC NAME OR DRUG CLASS	COMBINED EFFECT
MAO inhibitors*	Increased blood-sugar lowering.	**Probenecid**	Increased blood-sugar lowering.
Nicotinic acid	Decreased blood-sugar lowering.	**Pyrazinamide**	Decreased blood-sugar lowering.
Non-steroidal anti-inflammatory drugs (NSAIDs)*	Increased blood-sugar lowering.	**Ranitidine**	Increased blood-sugar lowering.
Oxyphenbutazone	Increased blood-sugar lowering.	**Rifampin**	Decreased blood-sugar lowering.
Phenothiazines	Decreased blood-sugar lowering.	**Sulfa drugs***	Increased blood-sugar lowering.
Phenylbutazone	Increased blood-sugar lowering.	**Sulfadoxine and pyrimethamine**	Increased risk of toxicity.
Phenyramidol	Increased blood-sugar lowering.	**Sulfaphenazole**	Increased blood-sugar lowering.
Phenytoin	Decreased blood-sugar lowering.	**Thyroid hormones***	Decreased blood-sugar lowering.

ANTI-INFLAMMATORY DRUGS, NON-STEROIDAL (NSAIDs)

GENERIC NAME OR DRUG CLASS	COMBINED EFFECT	GENERIC NAME OR DRUG CLASS	COMBINED EFFECT
Minoxidil	Decreased minoxidil effect.	**Thyroid hormones***	Rapid heartbeat, blood pressure rise.
Probenecid	Increased pain relief.	**Tiopronin**	Increased risk of toxicity to kidneys.
Sotalol	Decreased antihypertensive effect of sotalol.	**Triamterene**	Reduced triamterene effect.
Terazosin	Decreases effectiveness of terazosin. Causes sodium and fluid retention.		

ASPIRIN

GENERIC NAME OR DRUG CLASS	COMBINED EFFECT	GENERIC NAME OR DRUG CLASS	COMBINED EFFECT
Ketoprofen	Increased risk of stomach ulcer.	**Minoxidil**	Decreased minoxidil effect.
Levamisole	Increased risk of bleeding.	**Non-steroidal anti-inflammatory drugs (NSAIDs)***	Risk of stomach bleeding and ulcers.
Methotrexate	Increased methotrexate effect.	**Oxprenolol**	Decreased antihypertensive effect of oxprenolol.

*See Glossary

GENERIC NAME OR DRUG CLASS	COMBINED EFFECT	GENERIC NAME OR DRUG CLASS	COMBINED EFFECT
ASPIRIN continued			
Para-aminosalicylic acid	Possible aspirin toxicity.	Spironolactone	Decreased spironolactone effect.
Penicillins*	Increased effect of both drugs.	Sulfinpyrazone	Decreased sulfin-pyrazone effect.
Phenobarbital	Decreased aspirin effect.	Terazosin	Decreases effectiveness of terazosin. Causes sodium and fluid retention.
Phenytoin	Increased phenytoin effect.		
Probenecid	Decreased probenecid effect.	Terfenadine	May conceal symptoms of aspirin overdose, such as ringing in ears.
Propranolol	Decreased aspirin effect.	Ticlopidine	Increased effect of both drugs.
Rauwolfia alkaloids*	Decreased aspirin effect.	Vitamin C (large doses)	Possible aspirin toxicity.
Salicylates, other*	Likely aspirin toxicity.	Valproic acid	May increase valproic acid effect.
Sotalol	Decreased antihypertensive effect of sotalol.		

ATROPINE, HYOSCYAMINE, METHENAMINE, METHYLENE BLUE, PHENYLSALICYLATE & BENZOIC ACID

GENERIC NAME OR DRUG CLASS	COMBINED EFFECT	GENERIC NAME OR DRUG CLASS	COMBINED EFFECT
MAO inhibitors*	Increased belladonna and atropine effect.	Phenytoin	Increased phenytoin effect.
Meperidine	Increased atropine and hyoscyamine effect.	Pilocarpine	Loss of pilocarpine effect in glaucoma treatment.
Methylphenidate	Increased atropine and hyoscyamine effect.	Potassium supplements*	Possible intestinal ulcers with oral potassium tablets.
Minoxidil	Decreased minoxidil effect.	Probenecid	Decreased probenecid effect.
Non-steroidal anti-inflammatory drugs (NSAIDs)*	Risk of stomach bleeding and ulcers.	Propranolol	Decreased salicylate effect.
Orphenadrine	Increased atropine and hyoscyamine effect.	Rauwolfia alkaloids*	Decreased salicylate effect.
Oxprenolol	Decreased antihypertensive effect of oxprenolol.	Salicylates, other*	Likely salicylate toxicity.
Para-aminosalicylic acid (PAS)	Possible salicylate toxicity.	Sedatives* or central nervous system (CNS) depressants*	Increased sedative effect of both drugs.
Penicillins*	Increased effect of both drugs.	Sodium bicarbonate	Decreased methenamine effect.
Phenobarbital	Decreased salicylate effect.	Spironolactone	Decreased spironolactone effect.
Phenothiazines*	Increased atropine and hyoscyamine effect.	Sulfa drugs*	Possible kidney damage.
		Sulfinpyrazone	Decreased sulfin-pyrazone effect.

*See Glossary

GENERIC NAME OR DRUG CLASS	COMBINED EFFECT	GENERIC NAME OR DRUG CLASS	COMBINED EFFECT

ATROPINE, HYOSCYAMINE, METHENAMINE, METHYLENE BLUE, PHENYLSALICYLATE & BENZOIC ACID continued

Terfenadine	May conceal symptoms of salicylate overdose, such as ringing in ears.	Vitamin C (1 to 4 grams per day)	Increased effect of methenamine, contributing to urine acidity; decreased atropine effect; possible salicylate toxicity.

BARBITURATES

Sertraline	Increased depressive effects of both drugs.	Tranquilizers*	Dangerous sedation. Avoid.
Sleep inducers*	Dangerous sedation. Avoid.	Valproic acid	Increased barbituate effect.
Sotalol	Increased barbiturate effect. Dangerous sedation.		

BELLADONNA ALKALOIDS & BARBITURATES

Contraceptives, oral*	Decreased contraceptive effect.	Narcotics*	Dangerous sedation. Avoid.
Cortisone drugs*	Increased internal eye pressure. Decreased cortisone effect.	Nitrates*	Increased internal eye pressure.
Digitoxin	Decreased digitoxin effect.	Nizatidine	Increased nizatidine effect.
Doxycycline	Decreased doxycycline effect.	Non-steroidal anti-inflammatory drugs (NSAIDs)*	Decreased anti-inflammatory effect.
Dronabinol	Increased effects of both drugs. Avoid.	Orphenadrine	Increased belladonna effect.
Furosemide	Possible orthostatic hypotension.	Pain relievers*	Dangerous sedation. Avoid.
Griseofulvin	Decreased griseofulvin effect.	Phenothiazines*	Increased belladonna effect. Danger of oversedation.
Haloperidol	Increased internal eye pressure.	Pilocarpine	Loss of pilocarpine effect in glaucoma treatment.
Indapamide	Increased indapamide effect.		
Ketoconazole	Decreased ketoconazole effect.	Potassium supplements*	Possible intestinal ulcers with oral potassium tablets.
MAO inhibitors*	Increased belladonna and barbiturate effect.	Quinidine	Increased belladonna effect.
Meperidine	Increased belladonna effect.	Sedatives* and central nervous system (CNS) depressants*	Dangerous sedation. Avoid.
Methylphenidate	Increased belladonna effect.		
Metronidazole	Decreased metronidazole effect.	Sleep inducers*	Dangerous sedation. Avoid.
Mind-altering drugs*	Dangerous sedation. Avoid.	Sotalol	Increased barbiturate effect. Dangerous sedation.

*See Glossary

GENERIC NAME OR DRUG CLASS	COMBINED EFFECT	GENERIC NAME OR DRUG CLASS	COMBINED EFFECT

BELLADONNA ALKALOIDS & BARBITURATES continued

GENERIC NAME OR DRUG CLASS	COMBINED EFFECT	GENERIC NAME OR DRUG CLASS	COMBINED EFFECT
Tranquilizers*	Dangerous sedation. Avoid.	Vitamin C	Decreased belladonna effect. Avoid large doses of vitamin C.
Valproic acid	Increased barbiturate effect.		

BETA-ADRENERGIC BLOCKERS

GENERIC NAME OR DRUG CLASS	COMBINED EFFECT	GENERIC NAME OR DRUG CLASS	COMBINED EFFECT
Encainide	Increased effect of toxicity on heart muscle.	Nitrates*	Possible excessive blood pressure drop.
Guanabenz	Additional blood pressure drop.	Non-steroidal anti-inflammatory drugs (NSAIDs)*	Decreased antihypertensive effect of beta-blocker.
Indomethacin	Decreased effect of beta-blocker.	Phenytoin	Decreased beta-blocker effect.
Insulin	Hypoglycemic effects may be prolonged.	Propafenone	Increased beta blocker effect.
Levobunolol eyedrops	Possible increased beta-blocker effect.	Quinidine	Slows heart excessively.
MAO Inhibitors*	High blood pressure following MAO discontinuation.	Reserpine	Increased reserpine effect. Excessive sedation and depression. Additional blood pressure drop.
Molindone	Increased tranquilizer effect.		
Narcotics*	Increased narcotic effect. Dangerous sedation.	Rifampin	Decreased beta-blocker effect.
		Symoathomimetics*	Decreases effect of both drugs.
Nicardipine	Possible irregular heartbeat and congestive heart failure.	Timolol eyedrops	Possible increased beta-blocker effect.
Nicotine	Increased beta blocker effect.	Tocainide	May worsen congestive heart failure.
Nimodipine	Possible irregular heartbeat. May worsen congestive heart failure.	Verapamil	Increased effects of both drugs.

BETA-ADRENERGIC BLOCKING AGENTS & THIAZIDE DIURETICS

GENERIC NAME OR DRUG CLASS	COMBINED EFFECT	GENERIC NAME OR DRUG CLASS	COMBINED EFFECT
Antihypertensives*	Increased antihypertensive effect.	Cortisone drugs*	Excessive potassium loss that causes dangerous heart rhythms.
Barbiturates*	Increased barbiturate effect. Dangerous sedation.	Diclofenac	Decreased antihypertensive effect.
Bumetanide	Increased diuretic effect.	Digitalis preparations*	Excessive potassium loss that causes dangerous heart rhythms. Can either increase or decrease heart rate. Improves irregular heartbeat.
Calcium channel blockers*	Increased antihypertensive effect. Dosages of both drugs may require adjustments.		
Cholestyramine	Decreased hydrochlorthiazide effect.	Diuretics, thiazide*	Increased effect of other thiazide diuretics.

*See Glossary

ADDITIONAL DRUG INTERACTIONS

GENERIC NAME OR DRUG CLASS	COMBINED EFFECT	GENERIC NAME OR DRUG CLASS	COMBINED EFFECT

BETA-ADRENERGIC BLOCKING AGENTS & THIAZIDE DIURETICS continued

GENERIC NAME OR DRUG CLASS	COMBINED EFFECT	GENERIC NAME OR DRUG CLASS	COMBINED EFFECT
Ethacrynic acid	Increased diuretic effect.	Nitrates*	Excessive blood pressure drop.
Furosemide	Increased diuretic effect.	Non-steroidal anti-inflammatory drugs (NSAIDs)*	Decreased anti-inflammatory effect.
Guanfacine	Increased effect of both drugs.	Phenytoin	Increased beta-adrenergic effect.
Hypoglycemics, oral*	Decreased ability to lower blood glucose.	Potassium supplements*	Decreased potassium effect.
Indapamide	Increased diuretic effect.	Probenecid	Decreased probenecid effect.
Insulin	Decreased ability to lower blood glucose.	Propafenone	Increased beta blocker effect.
Lisinopril	Increased antihypertensive effect. Dosage of each may require adjustment.	Quinidine	Slows heart excessively.
		Reserpine	Increased reserpine effect. Excessive sedation and depression.
MAO inhibitors*	Increased hydrochlorothiazide effect.	Sympathomimetics*	Decreased effectiveness of both.
Metolazone	Increased diuretic effect.	Theophylline, aminophylline	Decreased effectiveness of both.
Narcotics*	Increased narcotic effect. Dangerous sedation.	Tocainide	May worsen congestive heart failure.
Nicardipine	Possible irregular heartbeat and congestive heart failure.	Zinc supplements	Increased need for zinc.
Nicotine	Increased beta blocker effect.		

BETAMETHASONE

GENERIC NAME OR DRUG CLASS	COMBINED EFFECT	GENERIC NAME OR DRUG CLASS	COMBINED EFFECT
Ephedrine	Decreased betamethasone effect.	Insulin	Decreased insulin effect.
Estrogens*	Increased betamethasone effect.	Isoniazid	Decreased isoniazid effect.
Ethacrynic acid	Potassium depletion.	Oxyphenbutazone	Possible ulcers.
Furosemide	Potassium depletion.	Phenylbutazone	Possible ulcers.
Glutethimide	Decreased betamethasone effect.	Phenytoin	Decreased betamethasone effect.
Indapamide	Possible excessive potassium loss, causing dangerous heartbeat irregularity.	Potassium supplements*	Decreased potassium effect.
		Rifampin	Decreased betamethasone effect.
Indomethacin	Increased betamethasone effect.	Sympathomimetics*	Possible glaucoma.

BUTALBITAL & ASPIRIN (Also contains caffeine)

GENERIC NAME OR DRUG CLASS	COMBINED EFFECT	GENERIC NAME OR DRUG CLASS	COMBINED EFFECT
Cortisone drugs*	Increased cortisone effect. Risk of ulcer and stomach bleeding.	Digitoxin	Decreased digitoxin effect.

*See Glossary

GENERIC NAME OR DRUG CLASS	COMBINED EFFECT	GENERIC NAME OR DRUG CLASS	COMBINED EFFECT

BUTALBITAL & ASPIRIN (Also contains caffeine) continued

GENERIC NAME OR DRUG CLASS	COMBINED EFFECT	GENERIC NAME OR DRUG CLASS	COMBINED EFFECT
Doxycycline	Decreased doxycycline effect.	Pain relievers*	Dangerous sedation. Avoid.
Dronabinol	Increased effect of both drugs.	Rifampin	May decrease butalbital effect.
Furosemide	Possible aspirin toxicity.	Salicylates, others*	Likely aspirin toxicity.
Gold compounds*	Increased likelihood of kidney damage.	Sedatives*	Dangerous sedation. Avoid.
Griseofulvin	Decreased griseofulvin effect.	Sleep inducers*	Dangerous sedation. Avoid.
Indapamide	Increased indapamide effect.	Spironolactone	Decreased spironolactone effect.
Indomethacin	Risk of stomach bleeding and ulcers.	Sulfinpyrazone	Decreased sulfin-pyrazone effect.
MAO inhibitors*	Increased butalbital effect.	Terfenadine	May conceal symptoms of aspirin overdose, such as ringing in ears.
Methotrexate	Increased methotrexate effect.	Tranquilizers*	Dangerous sedation. Avoid.
Mind-altering drugs*	Dangerous sedation. Avoid.	Valproic acid	Increased butalbital effect.
Minoxidil	Decreased minoxidil effect.	Vitamin C (large doses)	Possible aspirin toxicity.
Narcotics*	Dangerous sedation. Avoid.	Zidovudine	Increased toxicity of both.
Non-steroidal anti-inflammatory drugs (NSAIDs)*	Risk of stomach bleeding and ulcers.		

BUTALBITAL, ASPIRIN & CODEINE (Also contains caffeine)

GENERIC NAME OR DRUG CLASS	COMBINED EFFECT	GENERIC NAME OR DRUG CLASS	COMBINED EFFECT
Antidepressants*	Decreased anti-depressant effect. Possible dangerous oversedation.	Digitoxin	Decreased digitoxin effect.
Antidiabetics, oral*	Increased butalbital effect. Low blood sugar.	Doxycycline	Decreased doxycycline effect.
Antihistamines*	Dangerous sedation. Avoid.	Dronabinol	Increased effect of drugs.
Aspirin, other	Likely aspirin toxicity.	Furosemide	Possible aspirin toxicity.
Beta-adrenergic blockers*	Decreased effect of beta-adrenergic blocker.	Gold compounds*	Increased likelihood of kidney damage.
Carteolol	Increased narcotic effect. Dangerous sedation.	Griseofulvin	Decreased griseofulvin effect.
Contraceptives, oral*	Decreased contra-ceptive effect.	Indapamide	Increased indapamide effect.
Cortisone drugs*	Increased cortisone effect. Risk of ulcer and stomach bleeding.	Indomethacin	Risk of stomach bleeding and ulcers.
		MAO inhibitors*	Increased butalbital effect.

*See Glossary

GENERIC NAME OR DRUG CLASS	COMBINED EFFECT	GENERIC NAME OR DRUG CLASS	COMBINED EFFECT

BUTALBITAL, ASPIRIN & CODEINE (Also contains caffeine) continued

GENERIC NAME OR DRUG CLASS	COMBINED EFFECT	GENERIC NAME OR DRUG CLASS	COMBINED EFFECT
Methotrexate	Increased methotrexate effect.	Propranolol	Decreased aspirin effect.
Mind-altering drugs*	Dangerous sedation. Avoid.	Rauwolfia alkaloids*	Decreased aspirin effect.
Minoxidil	Decreased minoxidil effect.	Salicylates, others*	Likely aspirin toxicity.
Narcotics*	Dangerous sedation. Avoid.	Sedatives*	Dangerous sedation. Avoid.
Nitrates*	Excessive blood pressure drop.	Sleep inducers*	Dangerous sedation. Avoid.
Non-steroidal anti-inflammatory drugs (NSAIDs)*	Risk of stomach bleeding and ulcers.	Sotalol	Increased narcotic effect. Dangerous sedation.
Pain relievers*	Dangerous sedation. Avoid.	Spironolactone	Decreased spironolactone effect.
Para-aminosalicylic acid	Possible aspirin toxicity.	Sulfinpyrazone	Decreased sulfinpyrazone effect.
Penicillins*	Increased effect of drugs.	Terfenadine	May conceal symptoms of aspirin overdose, such as ringing in ears.
Phenobarbital	Decreased aspirin effect.	Tranquilizers*	Dangerous sedation. Avoid.
Phenothiazines*	Increased phenothiazine effect.	Valproic acid	Increased phenobarbital effect.
Phenytoin	Increased phenytoin effect.	Vitamin C (large doses)	Possible aspirin toxicity.
Probenecid	Decreased probenecid effect.	Zidovudine	Increased toxicity of both.

CARBAMAZEPINE

GENERIC NAME OR DRUG CLASS	COMBINED EFFECT	GENERIC NAME OR DRUG CLASS	COMBINED EFFECT
MAO Inhibitors*	Dangerous over stimulation. Avoid.	Phenytoin	Decreased carbamazepine effect.
Mebendazole	Decreased effect of mebendazole.	Phenobarbital	Decreased carbamazepine effect.
Methyprylon	Increased sedative effect, perhaps to dangerous level. Avoid.	Primidone	Decreased carbamazepine effect.
Nabilone	Greater depression of central nervous system.	Propoxyphene (Darvon)	Increased toxicity of both. Avoid.
Nicardipine	May increase carbamazepine effect and toxicity.	Sertraline	Increased depressive effects of both drugs.
Nimodipine	May increase carbamazepine effect and toxicity.	Tiopronin	Increased risk of toxicity to bone marrow.
Nizatidine	Increased carbamazepine effect and toxicity.	Tranquilizers* (benzodiazepine)	Increased carbamazepine effect.
		Verapamil	Possible increased carbamazepine effect.

*See Glossary

CHLORDIAZEPOXIDE & AMITRIPTYLINE

GENERIC NAME OR DRUG CLASS	COMBINED EFFECT	GENERIC NAME OR DRUG CLASS	COMBINED EFFECT
Dronabinol	Increased effect of both drugs.	Narcotics*	Dangerous oversedation.
Erythromycin	Increased chlordiazepoxide effect.	Phenytoin	Decreased phenytoin effect.
Ethchlorvynol	Delirium.	Probenecid	Increased chlordiazepoxide effect.
Guanethidine	Decreased guanethidine effect.	Quinidine	Irregular heartbeat.
Ketoconazole	Increased chlordiazepoxide effect.	Sedatives*	Dangerous oversedation.
Levodopa	Possible decreased levodopa effect.	Sleep inducers*	Increased sedative effect of both drugs.
MAO inhibitors*	Convulsions, deep sedation, rage.	Sympathomimetics*	Increased sympathomimetic effect.
Methyldopa	Decreased methyldopa effect.	Thyroid hormones*	Irregular heartbeat.
Nabilone	Greater depression of central nervous system.	Tranquilizers*	Increased sedative effect of both drugs.

CHLORDIAZEPOXIDE & CLIDINIUM

GENERIC NAME OR DRUG CLASS	COMBINED EFFECT	GENERIC NAME OR DRUG CLASS	COMBINED EFFECT
MAO inhibitors*	Convulsions, deep sedation, rage.	Phenothiazines*	Increased clidinium effect.
Meperidine	Increased clidinium effect.	Pilocarpine	Loss of pilocarpine effect in glaucoma treatment.
Methylphenidate	Increased clidinium effect.	Potassium supplements*	Possible intestinal ulcers with oral potassium tablets.
Nabilone	Greater depression of central nervous system.		
Narcotics*	Increased sedative effect of both drugs.	Sedatives*	Increased sedative effect of both drugs.
Nitrates*	Increased internal-eye pressure.	Sleep inducers*	Increased sedative effect of both drugs.
Nizatidine	Increased nizatidine effect.	Tranquilizers*	Increased sedative effect of both drugs.
Orphenadrine	Increased clidinium effect.	Vitamin C	Decreased clidinium effect. Avoid large doses of vitamin C.

CLIDINIUM

GENERIC NAME OR DRUG CLASS	COMBINED EFFECT	GENERIC NAME OR DRUG CLASS	COMBINED EFFECT
Orphenadrine	Increased clidinium effect.	Tranquilizers*	Decreased clidinium effect.
Pilocarpine	Loss of pilocarpine effect in glaucoma treatment.	Vitamin C	Decreased clidinium effect. Avoid large doses of vitamin C.
Potassium supplements*	Possible intestinal ulcers with oral potassium tablets.		

*See Glossary

ADDITIONAL DRUG INTERACTIONS

GENERIC NAME OR DRUG CLASS	COMBINED EFFECT	GENERIC NAME OR DRUG CLASS	COMBINED EFFECT

CLONIDINE

Nimodipine	Dangerous blood pressure drop.	Sertraline	Increased depressive effects of both drugs.
Nitrates*	Possible excessive blood pressure drop.	Sotalol	Increased antihypertensive effect.
		Terazosin	Decreases effectiveness of terazosin.

CLONIDINE & CHLORTHALIDONE

Cholestyramine	Decreased chlorthalidone effect.	MAO inhibitors*	Increased chlorthalidone effect.
Cortisone drugs*	Excessive potassium loss that causes dangerous heart rhythms.	Nabilone	Greater depression of central nervous system.
Digitalis preparations*	Excessive potassium loss that causes dangerous heart rhythms.	Nicardipine	Blood pressure drop. Dosages may require adjustment.
		Nitrates*	Possible excessive blood pressure drop.
Diuretics*	Excessive blood pressure drop.	Potassium supplements*	Decreased potassium effect.
Fenfluramine	Possible increased clonidine effect.	Probenecid	Decreased probenecid effect.
Guanfacine	Blood pressure control impaired.	Sedatives* or central nervous system (CNS) depressants*	Increased sedative effect of both drugs.
Indapamide	Increased diuretic effect.	Sotalol	Decreased antihypertensive effect.
Lithium	Increased effect of lithium.	Terazosin	Decreases effectiveness of terazosin.

CONTRACEPTIVES, ORAL

Non-steroidal anti-inflammatory drugs (NSAIDs)*	Decreased contraceptive effect.	Terazosin	Decreases effectiveness of terazosin.
Phenothiazines*	Increased phenothiazine effect.	Tetracyclines*	Decreased contraceptive effect.
Rifampin	Decreased contraceptive effect.	Ursodiol	Decreased effect of ursodiol.
		Vitamin A	Vitamin A excess.
Sulfadoxine and pyrimethamine	Reduced reliability of the pill.	Vitamin C	Possible increased contraceptive effect.

CORTISONE

Indapamide	Possible excessive potassium loss, causing dangerous heartbeat irregularity.	Insulin	Decreased insulin effect.
		Isoniazid	Decreased isoniazid effect.
Indomethacin	Increased cortisone effect.		

*See Glossary

GENERIC NAME OR DRUG CLASS	COMBINED EFFECT	GENERIC NAME OR DRUG CLASS	COMBINED EFFECT

CORTISONE continued

GENERIC NAME OR DRUG CLASS	COMBINED EFFECT	GENERIC NAME OR DRUG CLASS	COMBINED EFFECT
Ketoprofen	Increased risk of stomach ulcer and bleeding.	Phenylbutazone	Possible ulcers.
		Potassium supplements*	Decreased potassium effect.
Mitotane	Decreased cortisone effect.	Rifampin	Decreased cortisone effect.
Non-steroidal anti-inflammatory drugs (NSAIDs)*	Increased risk of ulcers, increased cortisone effect.	Salicylates*	Decreased salicylate effect.
		Sodium bicarbonate	Sodium overload.
Oxyphenbutazone	Possible ulcers.	Sympathomimetics*	Possible glaucoma.
Phenobarbital	Decreased cortisone effect.	Theophylline	Possible increased theophylline effect.

DEXAMETHASONE

GENERIC NAME OR DRUG CLASS	COMBINED EFFECT	GENERIC NAME OR DRUG CLASS	COMBINED EFFECT
Estrogens*	Increased dexamethasone effect.	Non-steroidal anti-inflammatory drugs (NSAIDs)*	Increased risk of ulcers and dexamethasone effect.
Ethacrynic acid	Potassium depletion.	Oxyphenbutazone	Possible ulcers.
Furosemide	Potassium depletion.	Phenobarbital	Decreased dexamethasone effect.
Glutethimide	Decreased dexamethasone effect.		
Indapamide	Possible excessive potassium loss, causing dangerous heartbeat irregularity.	Phenylbutazone	Possible ulcers.
		Potassium supplements*	Decreased potassium effect.
		Rifampin	Decreased dexamethasone effect.
Indomethacin	Increased dexamethasone effect.	Salicylates*	Decreased salicylate effect.
Insulin	Decreased insulin effect.	Sympathomimetics*	Possible glaucoma.
Isoniazid	Decreased isoniazid effect.	Theophylline	Possible increased theophylline effect.
Mitotane	Decreased dexamethasone effect.		

DIGITALIS PREPARATIONS (Digitalis Glycosides)

GENERIC NAME OR DRUG CLASS	COMBINED EFFECT	GENERIC NAME OR DRUG CLASS	COMBINED EFFECT
Mineral Oil	Decreased digitalis effect.	Potassium supplements*	Overdosage of either drug may cause severe heartbeat irregularity.
Nicardipine	Increased digitalis effect. May need to reduce dose.	Propafenone	Increased digitalis absorption. May require decreased digitalis dosage.
Nizatidine	Increased digitalis effect.		
Oxyphenbutazone	Decreased digitalis effect.	PTU/Metronidazole	Decreased digitalis effect.
Phenobarbital	Decreased digitalis effect.	Quinidine	Increased digitalis effect.
Phenylbutazone	Decreased digitalis effect.	Rauwolfia alkaloids*	Increased digitalis effect.

*See Glossary

943

GENERIC NAME OR DRUG CLASS	COMBINED EFFECT	GENERIC NAME OR DRUG CLASS	COMBINED EFFECT

DIGITALIS PREPARATIONS (Digitalis Glycosides) continued

GENERIC NAME OR DRUG CLASS	COMBINED EFFECT	GENERIC NAME OR DRUG CLASS	COMBINED EFFECT
Rifampin	Possible decreased digitalis effect.	Tetracycline	May increase digitalis absorption.
Sotalol	Can either increase or decrease heart rate. Improves irregular heartbeat.	Thyroid hormones*	Digitalis toxicity.
		Ticlopidine	Slightly decreased digitalis effect (digoxin only).
Spironolactone	Increased digitalis effect. May require digitalis dosage reduction.	Trazodone	Possible increased digitalis toxicity.
Sulfasalazine	Decreased digitalis absorption.	Triamterene	Possible decreased digitalis effect.
Sympathmimetics*	Increased risk of heartbeat irregularities.	Verapamil	Increased digitalis effect.

DIURETICS, THIAZIDE

GENERIC NAME OR DRUG CLASS	COMBINED EFFECT	GENERIC NAME OR DRUG CLASS	COMBINED EFFECT
MAO inhibitors*	Increased antihypertensive effect.	Pentoxifylline	Increased antihypertensive effect.
Nicardipine	Blood pressure drop. Dosages may require adjustment.	Potassium supplements*	Decreased potassium effect.
		Probenecid	Decreased probenecid effect.
Nimodipine	Dangerous blood pressure drop.	Sotalol	Increased antihypertensive effect.
Nitrates*	Excessive blood pressure drop.	Terazosin	Decreases effectiveness of terazosin.
Opiates*	Dizziness or weakness when standing up after sitting or lying down.	Zinc supplements	Increased need for zinc.

ERGOTAMINE, BELLADONNA & PHENOBARBITAL

GENERIC NAME OR DRUG CLASS	COMBINED EFFECT	GENERIC NAME OR DRUG CLASS	COMBINED EFFECT
Digitoxin	Decreased digitoxin effect.	MAO inhibitors*	Increased belladonna and phenobarbital effect.
Doxycycline	Decreased doxycycline effect.	Meperidine	Increased belladonna effect.
Dronabinol	Increased effect of drugs.		
Ephedrine	Dangerous blood pressure rise.	Methylphenidate	Increased belladonna effect.
Epinephrine	Dangerous blood pressure rise.	Metoclopramide	May decrease metoclopramide effect.
Griseofulvin	Decreased griseofulvin effect.	Mind-altering drugs*	Dangerous sedation. Avoid.
Guanethidine	Decreased belladonna effect.	Narcotics*	Dangerous sedation. Avoid.
Haloperidol	Increased internal eye pressure.	Nitrates*	Increased internal eye pressure.
Indapamide	Increased indapamide effect.	Orphenadrine	Increased belladonna effect.

GENERIC NAME OR DRUG CLASS	COMBINED EFFECT	GENERIC NAME OR DRUG CLASS	COMBINED EFFECT

ERGOTAMINE, BELLADONNA & PHENOBARBITAL continued

GENERIC NAME OR DRUG CLASS	COMBINED EFFECT	GENERIC NAME OR DRUG CLASS	COMBINED EFFECT
Pain relievers*	Dangerous sedation. Avoid.	Sedatives*	Dangerous sedation. Avoid.
Phenothiazines*	Increased belladonna effect.	Sleep inducers*	Dangerous sedation. Avoid.
Pilocarpine	Loss of pilocarpine effect in glaucoma treatment.	Tranquilizers*	Dangerous sedation. Avoid.
Potassium supplements*	Possible intestinal ulcers with oral potassium tablets.	Troleandomycin	Increased adverse reactions of ergotamine.
Quinidine	Increased belladonna effect.	Valproic acid	Increased phenobarbital effect.
Reserpine	Decreased belladonna effect.	Vitamin C	Decreased belladonna effect. Avoid large doses of vitamin C.

ERGOTAMINE, CAFFEINE, BELLADONNA & PENTOBARBITAL

GENERIC NAME OR DRUG CLASS	COMBINED EFFECT	GENERIC NAME OR DRUG CLASS	COMBINED EFFECT
Anticonvulsants*	Changed seizure patterns.	Ephedrine	Dangerous blood pressure rise.
Antidepressants, tricyclics (TCA)*	Decreased antidepressant effect. Possible dangerous oversedation.	Epinephrine	Dangerous blood pressure rise.
Antidiabetics, oral*	Increased pentobarbital effect.	Estrogens*	Decreased estrogen effect.
Antihistamines*	Dangerous sedation. Avoid.	Griseofulvin	Possible decreased griseofulvin effect.
Aspirin	Decreased aspirin effect.	Guanethidine	Decreased belladonna effect.
Beta-adrenergic blockers*	Decreased effect of beta-adrenergic blocker.	Haloperidol	Increased internal eye pressure.
Cimetidine	Increased caffeine effect.	Indapamide	Increased indapamide effect.
Contraceptives, oral*	Decreased contraceptive effect.	Isoniazid	Increased caffeine effect.
Cortisone drugs*	Decreased cortisone effect. Increased internal eye pressure.	MAO inhibitors*	Increased belladonna effect, dangerous blood pressure rise.
Digitoxin	Decreased digitoxin effect.	Meperidine	Increased belladonna effect.
Disulfiram	Possible increased pentobarbital effect.	Methylphenidate	Increased belladonna effect.
Doxycycline	Decreased doxycycline effect.	Metoclopramide	May decrease metoclopramide effect.
Dronabinol	Increased effect of drugs.	Metronidazole	Possible decreased metronidazole effect.
		Mind-altering drugs*	Dangerous sedation. Avoid.

GENERIC NAME OR DRUG CLASS	COMBINED EFFECT	GENERIC NAME OR DRUG CLASS	COMBINED EFFECT

ERGOTAMINE, CAFFEINE, BELLADONNA & PENTOBARBITAL continued

GENERIC NAME OR DRUG CLASS	COMBINED EFFECT	GENERIC NAME OR DRUG CLASS	COMBINED EFFECT
Narcotics*	Dangerous sedation. Avoid.	Reserpine	Decreased belladonna effect.
Nitrates*	Increased internal eye pressure.	Rifampin	Possible decreased pentobarbital effect.
Non-steroidal anti-inflammatory drugs (NSAIDs)*	Decreased anti-inflammatory effect.	Sedatives*	Dangerous sedation. Avoid.
Orphenadrine	Increased belladonna effect.	Sleep inducers*	Dangerous sedation. Avoid.
Pain relievers*	Dangerous sedation. Avoid.	Sympathomimetics*	Overstimulation, blood pressure rise.
Phenothiazines*	Increased belladonna effect.	Thyroid hormones*	Increased thyroid effect.
Pilocarpine	Loss of pilocarpine effect in glaucoma treatment.	Tranquilizers*	Dangerous sedation. Avoid.
		Troleandomycin	Increased adverse reactions of ergotamine.
Potassium supplements*	Possible intestinal ulcers with oral potassium tablets.	Valproic acid	Increased pentobarbital effect.
Quinidine	Increased belladonna effect.	Vitamin C	Decreased belladonna effect. Avoid large doses of vitamin C.

ETHOTOIN

GENERIC NAME OR DRUG CLASS	COMBINED EFFECT	GENERIC NAME OR DRUG CLASS	COMBINED EFFECT
Phenylbutazone	Increased ethotoin effect.	Sedatives*	Increased sedative effect.
Propranolol	Increased propranolol effect.	Sulfa drugs*	Increased ethotoin effect.
Quinidine	Increased quinidine effect.	Theophylline	Reduced anticonvulsant effect.
		Valproic acid	Breakthrough seizures.

FLECAINIDE ACETATE

GENERIC NAME OR DRUG CLASS	COMBINED EFFECT	GENERIC NAME OR DRUG CLASS	COMBINED EFFECT
Propafenone	Increased effect of both drugs and increased risk of toxicity.	Verapamil	Possible decreased efficiency of heart-muscle contraction, leading to congestive heart failure.
Sodium bicarbonate	Possible increased flecainide acetate effect.		

GUANETHIDINE & HYDROCHLOROTHIAZIDE

GENERIC NAME OR DRUG CLASS	COMBINED EFFECT	GENERIC NAME OR DRUG CLASS	COMBINED EFFECT
Diuretics, thiazide*	Increased thiazide and guanethidine effect.	Indapamide	Possible increased effects of both drugs. When monitored carefully, combination may be beneficial in controlling hypertension.
Haloperidol	Decreased guanethidine effect.		
		Insulin	Increased insulin effect.

GENERIC NAME OR DRUG CLASS	COMBINED EFFECT	GENERIC NAME OR DRUG CLASS	COMBINED EFFECT

GUANETHIDINE & HYDROCHLOROTHIAZIDE continued

Lithium	Increased lithium effect.	Oxprenolol	Increased antihypertensive effect. Dosages of both drugs may require adjustments.
MAO inhibitors*	Increased hydrochlorothiazide effect.		
Minoxidil	Dosage adjustments may be necessary to keep blood pressure at proper level.	Phenothiazines*	Decreased guanethidine effect.
		Potassium supplements*	Decreased potassium effect.
Nicardipine	Blood pressure drop. Dosages may require adjustment.	Probenecid	Decreased probenecid effect.
Nimodipine	Dangerous blood pressure drop.	Sotalol	Increased antihypertensive effect.
Nitrates*	Excessive blood pressure drop.	Terazosin	Decreases effectiveness of terazosin.

GUANFACINE

Sympathomimetics*	May decrease antihypertensive effects of guanfacine.	Terazosin	Decreases effectiveness of terazosin.

HISTAMINE H₂ RECEPTOR ANTAGONISTS

Metronidazole	Increased effect and toxicity of metronidazole.	Propafenone	Increased effect of both drugs and increased risk of toxicity.
Moricizine	Increased concentration of H_2 receptor antagonist in the blood.	Propranolol	Possible increased propranolol effect.
Morphine	Increased effect and toxicity of morphine.	Quinidine	Increased quinidine effect.
Nicardipine	Possible increased effect and toxicity of nicardipine.	Tamoxifen	Decreased tamoxifen effect.
		Theophylline	Increased theophylline effect.
Nimodipine	Possible increased effect and toxicity of nimodipine.	Triazolam	Increased effect and toxicity of triazolam.
Phenytoin	Increased effect and toxicity of phenytoin.	Verapamil	Increased effect and toxicity of verapamil.
Procainamide	Increased effect and toxicity of procainamide.		

HYDRALAZINE & HYDROCHLOROTHIAZIDE

Diazoxide	Increased antihypertensive effect.	Diuretics, oral*	Increased effect of both drugs. When monitored carefully, combination may be beneficial in controlling hypertension.
Didanosine	Increased risk of peripheral neuropathy.		
Digitalis preparations*	Excessive potassium loss that causes dangerous heart rhythms.	Indapamide	Increased diuretic effect.

ADDITIONAL DRUG INTERACTIONS

GENERIC NAME OR DRUG CLASS	COMBINED EFFECT	GENERIC NAME OR DRUG CLASS	COMBINED EFFECT

HYDRALAZINE & HYDROCHLOROTHIAZIDE continued

Lithium	Increased effect of lithium.	Nitrates*	Excessive blood pressure drop.
MAO inhibitors*	Increased effect of drugs.	Potassium supplements*	Decreased potassium effect.
Nimodipine	Dangerous blood pressure drop.	Probenecid	Decreased probenecid effect.

HYDROCORTISONE (Cortisol)

Estrogens*	Increased hydro-cortisone effect.	Non-steroidal anti-inflammatory drugs (NSAIDs)*	Increased risk of ulcers and increased hydrocortisone effect.
Ethacrynic acid	Potassium depletion.	Oxyphenbutazone	Possible ulcers.
Furosemide	Potassium depletion.	Phenobarbital	Decreased hydro-cortisone effect.
Glutethimide	Decreased hydro-cortisone effect.	Phenylbutazone	Possible ulcers.
Indapamide	Possible excessive potassium loss, causing dangerous heartbeat irregularity.	Potassium supplements*	Decreased potassium effect.
		Rifampin	Decreased hydro-cortisone effect.
Indomethacin	Increased hydro-cortisone effect.	Salicylates*	Decreased salicylate effect.
Insulin	Decreased insulin effect.		
Isoniazid	Decreased isoniazid effect.	Sympathomimetics*	Possible glaucoma.
Mitotane	Decreased hydro-cortisone effect.	Theophylline	Possible increased theophylline effect.

KAOLIN, PECTIN, BELLADONNA & OPIUM

Ketoconazole	Decreased ketoconazole effect.	Pilocarpine	Loss of pilocarpine effect in glaucoma treatment.
Lincomycins*	Decreased absorption of lincomycin. Separate doses by at least 2 hours.	Potassium supplements*	Possible intestinal ulcers with oral potassium tablets.
MAO inhibitors*	Increased belladonna effect.	Sedatives*	Excessive sedation.
Meperidine	Increased belladonna effect.	Sleep inducers*	Increased effect of sleep inducers.
Methylphenidate	Increased belladonna effect.	Sotalol	Increased narcotic effect. Dangerous sedation.
Mind-altering drugs*	Increased sedative effect.	Tranquilizers*	Increased tranquilizer effect.
Narcotics, other*	Increased narcotic effect.	Vitamin C	Decreased belladonna effect. Avoid large doses of vitamin C.
Nitrates*	Increased internal-eye pressure.		
Orphenadrine	Increased belladonna effect.	All other oral medicines	Decreased absorption of other medicines. Separate doses by at least 2 hours.
Phenothiazines*	Increased sedative effect of paregoric.		

*See Glossary

GENERIC NAME OR DRUG CLASS	COMBINED EFFECT	GENERIC NAME OR DRUG CLASS	COMBINED EFFECT

LITHIUM

GENERIC NAME OR DRUG CLASS	COMBINED EFFECT	GENERIC NAME OR DRUG CLASS	COMBINED EFFECT
Nimodipine	Possible decreased lithium effect.	Phenytoin	Increased lithium effect.
Non-steroidal anti-inflammatory drugs (NSAIDs)*	Increased lithium toxicity.	Potassium iodide	Increased potassium iodide effect.
		Sodium bicarbonate	Decreased lithium effect.
Oxyphenbutazone	Increased lithium effect.	Tetracyclines*	Increased lithium effect.
Phenothiazines*	Decreased lithium effect.	Theophylline	Decreased lithium effect.
		Tiopronin	Increased risk of toxicity to kidneys.
Phenylbutazone	Increased lithium effect.	Verapamil	Decreased lithium effect.

MAPROTILINE

GENERIC NAME OR DRUG CLASS	COMBINED EFFECT	GENERIC NAME OR DRUG CLASS	COMBINED EFFECT
Fluoxetine	Increased depressant effects of both drugs.	Methyprylon	Increased sedative effect, perhaps to dangerous level. Avoid.
Guanabenz	Possible decreased clonidine effect.	Molindone	Increased tranquilizer effect.
Guanethidine	Decreased guanethidine effect.	Nabilone	Greater depression of central nervous system.
Guanfacine	May increase depressant effects of either drug.	Narcotics*	Dangerous oversedation.
Leucovorin	High alcohol content of leucovorin may cause adverse effects.	Phenothiazine	Possible increased antidepressant effect and toxicity.
Levodopa	May increase blood pressure.	Phenytoin	Decreased phenytoin effect.
Lithium	Possible decreased seizure threshold.	Procainamide	Possible irregular heartbeat.
MAO inhibitors*	Fever, delirium, convulsions.	Quinidine	Irregular heartbeat.
		Sedatives*	Dangerous oversedation.
Methyldopa	Decreased methyldopa effect.	Sertraline	Increased depressive effects of both drugs.
Methylphenidate	Possible increased antidepressant effect and toxicity.	Sympathomimetics*	Increased sympathomimetic effect.
		Thyroid hormones*	Irregular heartbeat.

MEPHENYTOIN

GENERIC NAME OR DRUG CLASS	COMBINED EFFECT	GENERIC NAME OR DRUG CLASS	COMBINED EFFECT
Propranolol	Increased propranolol effect.	Sulfa drugs*	Increased mephenytoin effect.
Quinidine	Increased quinidine effect.	Theophylline	Reduced anticonvulsant effect.
Sedatives*	Increased sedative effect.	Valproic acid	Breakthrough seizures.

*See Glossary

ADDITIONAL DRUG INTERACTIONS

GENERIC NAME OR DRUG CLASS	COMBINED EFFECT	GENERIC NAME OR DRUG CLASS	COMBINED EFFECT

MEPROBAMATE & ASPIRIN

GENERIC NAME OR DRUG CLASS	COMBINED EFFECT	GENERIC NAME OR DRUG CLASS	COMBINED EFFECT
MAO inhibitors*	Increased meprobamate effect.	Propranolol	Decreased aspirin effect.
Methotrexate	Increased methotrexate effect.	Rauwolfia alkaloids*	Decreased aspirin effect.
Minoxidil	Decreased minoxidil effect.	Salicylates, other*	Likely aspirin toxicity.
Narcotics*	Increased narcotic effect.	Sedatives*	Increased sedative effect.
Non-steroidal anti-inflammatory drugs (NSAIDs)*	Risk of stomach bleeding and ulcers.	Sleep inducers*	Increased effect of sleep inducer.
Oxprenolol	Decreased antihypertensive effect of oxprenolol.	Spironolactone	Decreased spironolactone effect.
		Sulfinpyrazone	Decreased sulfinpyrazone effect.
Para-aminosalicylic acid (PAS)	Possible aspirin toxicity.	Terfenadine	Possible excessive sedation. May conceal symptoms of aspirin overdose, such as ringing in ears.
Penicillins*	Increased effect of both drugs.		
Phenobarbital	Decreased aspirin effect.	Tranquilizers*	Increased tranquilizer effect.
Phenytoin	Increased phenytoin effect.	Vancomycin	Increased chance of hearing loss.
Probenecid	Decreased probenecid effect.	Vitamin C (large doses)	Possible aspirin toxicity.

METHYLDOPA

GENERIC NAME OR DRUG CLASS	COMBINED EFFECT	GENERIC NAME OR DRUG CLASS	COMBINED EFFECT
Nimodipine	Dangerous blood pressure drop.	Sotalol	Increased antihypertensive effect.
Phenoxybenzamine	Urinary retention.	Sympathomimetic drugs*	Increased risk of heart block and high blood pressure.
Pergolide	Decreased pergolide effect.		
Propranolol	Increased blood pressure (rarely).	Terazosin	Decreases effectiveness of terazosin.
Sertraline	Increased depressive effects of both drugs.	Tolbutamide	Increased tolbutamide effect.

METHYLDOPA & THIAZIDE DIURETICS

GENERIC NAME OR DRUG CLASS	COMBINED EFFECT	GENERIC NAME OR DRUG CLASS	COMBINED EFFECT
Cortisone drugs*	Excessive potassium loss that causes dangerous heart rhythms.	Diuretics, thiazide*	Increased effect of both drugs.
		Haloperidol	Increased sedation, possibly dementia.
Dapsone	Increased risk of adverse effect on blood cells.	Indapamide	Increased diuretic effect.
Didanosine	Increased risk of pancreatitis.	Levodopa	Increased effect of both drugs.
Digitalis preparations*	Excessive potassium loss that causes dangerous heart rhythms.	Lithium	Increased lithium effect.

*See Glossary

GENERIC NAME OR DRUG CLASS	COMBINED EFFECT	GENERIC NAME OR DRUG CLASS	COMBINED EFFECT

METHYLDOPA & THIAZIDE DIURETICS continued

GENERIC NAME OR DRUG CLASS	COMBINED EFFECT	GENERIC NAME OR DRUG CLASS	COMBINED EFFECT
MAO inhibitors*	Dangerous blood pressure changes.	Potassium supplements*	Decreased potassium effect.
Nabilone	Greater depression of central nervous system.	Propranolol	Increased blood pressure (rarely).
Nicardipine	Blood pressure drop. Dosages may require adjustment.	Sertraline	Increased depressive effects of both drugs.
Nimodipine	Dangerous blood pressure drop.	Sotalol	Increased antihypertensive effect.
Nitrates*	Excessive blood pressure drop.	Terazosin	Decreases effectiveness of terazosin.
Phenoxybenzanine	Urinary retention.	Tolbutamide	Increased tolbutamide effect.
		Zinc supplements	Increased need for zinc.

METHYLPREDNISOLONE

GENERIC NAME OR DRUG CLASS	COMBINED EFFECT	GENERIC NAME OR DRUG CLASS	COMBINED EFFECT
Digitalis preparations*	Dangerous potassium depletion. Possible digitalis toxicity.	Isoniazid	Decreased isoniazid effect.
Diuretics, thiazide*	Potassium depletion.	Mitotane	Decreased methylprednisolone effect.
Ephedrine	Decreased methylprednisolone effect.	Non-steroidal anti-inflammatory drugs (NSAIDs)*	Increased risk of ulcers and methylprednisolone effect.
Estrogens*	Increased methylprednisolone effect.	Oxyphenbutazone	Possible ulcers.
Ethacrynic acid	Potassium depletion.	Phenobarbital	Decreased methylprednisolone effect.
Furosemide	Potassium depletion.		
Glutethimide	Decreased methylprednisolone effect.	Phenylbutazone	Possible ulcers.
Indapamide	Possible excessive potassium loss, causing dangerous heartbeat irregularity.	Potassium supplements*	Decreased potassium effect.
		Rifampin	Decreased methylprednisolone effect.
Indomethacin	Increased methylprednisolone effect.	Salicylates*	Decreased salicylate effect.
Insulin	Decreased insulin effect.	Sympathomimetics*	Possible glaucoma.
		Theophylline	Possible increased theophylline effect.

MOLINDONE

GENERIC NAME OR DRUG CLASS	COMBINED EFFECT	GENERIC NAME OR DRUG CLASS	COMBINED EFFECT
Nabilone	Greater depression of central nervous system.	Sedatives*	Increased sedative effect.
Narcotics*	Increased narcotic effect.	Sertraline	Increased depressive effects of both drugs.
Pergolide	Decreased pergolide effect.	Sotalol	Increased tranquilizer effect.
Phenytoin	Increased phenytoin effect.	Tetracyclines*	May decrease absorption of both drugs.
Procarbazine	Increased sedation.	Tranquilizers, other*	Increased tranquilizer effect.
Quinidine	Impaired heart function. Dangerous mixture.		

*See Glossary

GENERIC NAME OR DRUG CLASS	COMBINED EFFECT	GENERIC NAME OR DRUG CLASS	COMBINED EFFECT

MONOAMINE OXIDASE (MAO) INHIBITORS

GENERIC NAME OR DRUG CLASS	COMBINED EFFECT	GENERIC NAME OR DRUG CLASS	COMBINED EFFECT
Ethinamate	Dangerous increased effects of ethinamate. Avoid combining.	Maprotiline	Dangerous blood pressure rise.
Fluoxetine	Increased depressant effects of both drugs.	Methyldopa	Sudden, severe blood pressure rise.
Furazolidine	Sudden, severe increase in blood pressure.	Methylphenidate	Increased blood pressure.
Guanadrel	High blood pressure.	Methyprylon	Increased sedative effect, perhaps to dangerous level. Avoid.
Guanethidine	Blood pressure rise to life-threatening level.	Nabilone	Greater depression of central nervous system.
Guanfacine	May increase depressant effects of either drug.	Narcotic analgesics	Severe high blood pressure.
Hypoglycemics, oral*	Increased hypoglycemic effect.	Phenothiazines*	Possible increased phenothiazine toxicity.
Indapamide	Increased indapamide effect.	Phenylpropanolamine	Increased blood pressure.
Insulin	Increased hypoglycemic effect.	Pseudoephedrine	Increased blood pressure.
Leucovorin	High alcohol content of leucovorin may cause adverse effects.	Sertraline	Increased depressive effects of both drugs.
Levodopa	Sudden, severe blood pressure rise.	Sympathomimetics*	Blood pressure rise to life-threatening level.
MAO inhibitors* (others, when taken together)	High fever, convulsions, death.	Tryptophan	Increased blood pressure.

NARCOTIC ANALGESICS

GENERIC NAME OR DRUG CLASS	COMBINED EFFECT	GENERIC NAME OR DRUG CLASS	COMBINED EFFECT
Naltrexone	Precipitates withdrawal symptoms. May lead to respiratory arrest, coma and death.	Phenytoin	Possible decreased narcotic effect.
		Rifampin	Possible decreased narcotic effect.
Narcotics, other*	Increased narcotic effect.	Sedatives*	Increased sedative effect.
Nicotine	Increased narcotic effect.	Selegiline	Severe toxicity characterized by breathing difficulties, seizures, coma.
Nitrates*	Excessive blood pressure drop.		
Non-steroidal anti-inflammatory drugs (NSAIDs)*	Increased narcotic effect.	Sertraline	Increased depressive effects of both drugs.
		Sleep inducers*	Increased sedative effect.
Pentazocine	Possibly precipitates withdrawal with chronic narcotic use.	Sotalol	Increased narcotic effect. Dangerous sedation.
Phenothiazines*	Increased sedative effect.	Tranquilizers*	Increased sedative effect.

*See Glossary

GENERIC NAME OR DRUG CLASS	COMBINED EFFECT	GENERIC NAME OR DRUG CLASS	COMBINED EFFECT
NARCOTIC & ASPIRIN			
Furosemide	Possible aspirin toxicity. May decrease furosemide effect.	Selegiline	Severe toxicity characterized by breathing difficulties, seizures, coma.
Gold compounds*	Increased likelihood of kidney damage.	Sleep inducers*	Increased sedative effect.
Indomethacin	Risk of stomach bleeding and ulcers.	Sotalol	Increased narcotic effect. Dangerous sedation.
Methotrexate	Increased methotrexate effect.	Spironolactone	Decreased spironolactone effect.
Minoxidil	Decreased minoxidil effect.	Sulfinpyrazone	Decreased sulfinpyrazone effect.
Narcotics, other*	Increased narcotic effect.	Terfenadine	Possible excessive sedation. May conceal symptoms of aspirin overdose, such as ringing in ears.
Nitrates*	Excessive blood pressure drop.		
Non-steroidal anti-inflammatory drugs (NSAIDs)*	Risk of stomach bleeding and ulcers.	Ticlopidine	Decreased effects of both drugs.
Propranolol	Decreased aspirin effect.	Tranquilizers*	Increased sedative effect.
Rauwolfia alkaloids*	Decreased aspirin effect.	Valproic acid	May increase valproic acid effect.
Salicylates, other*	Likely aspirin toxicity.	Vitamin C (large doses)	Possible aspirin toxicity.
Sedatives*	Increased sedative effect.		

GENERIC NAME OR DRUG CLASS	COMBINED EFFECT	GENERIC NAME OR DRUG CLASS	COMBINED EFFECT
NIMODIPINE			
Timolol eyedrops	May cause increased effect of nimodipine on heart function.	Tocainide	Increased likelihood of adverse reactions from either drug.
		Vitamin D (large doses)	Decreased nimodipine effect.

GENERIC NAME OR DRUG CLASS	COMBINED EFFECT	GENERIC NAME OR DRUG CLASS	COMBINED EFFECT
ORPHENADRINE, ASPIRIN & CAFFEINE			
Antidepressants, tricyclic (TCA)*	Increased sedation.	Griseofulvin	Decreased griseofulvin effect.
Antidiabetics, oral*	Low blood sugar.	Indomethacin	Risk of stomach bleeding and ulcers.
Aspirin, other	Likely aspirin toxicity.	Isoniazid	Increased caffeine effect.
Chlorpromazine	Hypoglycemia (low blood sugar).	Levodopa	Increased effect of levodopa. (Improves effectiveness in treating Parkinson's disease.)
Contraceptives, oral*	Increased caffeine effect.		
Cortisone drugs*	Increased cortisone effect. Risk of ulcers and stomach bleeding.	MAO inhibitors*	Dangerous blood pressure rise.
Furosemide	Possible aspirin toxicity.	Methotrexate	Increased methotrexate effect.
Gold compounds*	Increased likelihood of kidney damage.	Minoxidil	Decreased minoxidil effect.

*See Glossary

953

ADDITIONAL DRUG INTERACTIONS

GENERIC NAME OR DRUG CLASS	COMBINED EFFECT	GENERIC NAME OR DRUG CLASS	COMBINED EFFECT

ORPHENADRINE, ASPIRIN & CAFFEINE continued

GENERIC NAME OR DRUG CLASS	COMBINED EFFECT	GENERIC NAME OR DRUG CLASS	COMBINED EFFECT
Nitrates*	Increased internal-eye pressure.	Sedatives*	Decreased sedative effect.
Non-steroidal anti-inflammatory drugs (NSAIDs)*	Risk of stomach bleeding and ulcers.	Sleep inducers*	Decreased sedative effect.
Para-aminosalicylic acid (PAS)	Possible aspirin toxicity.	Spironolactone	Decreased spironolactone effect.
Penicillins*	Increased effect of drugs.	Sulfinpyrazone	Decreased sulfin-pyrazone effect.
Phenobarbital	Decreased aspirin effect.	Sympathomimetics*	Overstimulation.
Potassium supplements*	Increased possibility of intestinal ulcers with oral potassium tablets.	Terfenadine	May conceal symptoms of aspirin overdose, such as ringing in ears.
Probenecid	Decreased probenecid effect.	Thyroid hormones*	Increased thyroid effect.
Propoxyphene	Possible confusion, nervousness, tremors.	Tranquilizers*	Decreased tranquilizer effect.
Propranolol	Decreased aspirin effect.	Valproic acid	May increase valproic acid effect.
Rauwolfia alkaloids*	Decreased aspirin effect.	Vitamin C (large doses)	Possible aspirin toxicity.
Salicylates, other*	Likely aspirin toxicity.		

PANCREATIN, PEPSIN, BILE SALTS, HYOSCYAMINE, ATROPINE, SCOPOLAMINE & PHENOBARBITAL

GENERIC NAME OR DRUG CLASS	COMBINED EFFECT	GENERIC NAME OR DRUG CLASS	COMBINED EFFECT
Disopyramide	Increased atropine effect.	Non-steroidal anti-inflammatory drugs (NSAIDs)*	Decreased anti-inflammatory effects.
Dronabinol	Increased phenobarbital effect.	Orphenadrine	Increased atropine effect.
Griseofulvin	Decreased griseofulvin effect.	Phenothiazines*	Increased atropine effect.
Haloperidol	Increased internal-eye pressure.	Pilocarpine	Loss of pilocarpine effect in glaucoma treatment.
Indapamide	Increased indapamide effect.	Potassium supplements*	Possible intestinal ulcers with oral potassium tablets.
Ketoconazole	Decreased ketoconazole effect.		
MAO inhibitors*	Increased atropine effect.	Quinidine	Increased quinidine and scopolamine effect.
Meperidine	Increased atropine effect.	Sedatives*	Dangerous sedation. Avoid.
Methylphenidate	Increased atropine effect.	Sleep inducers*	Dangerous sedation. Avoid.
Mind-altering drugs*	Dangerous sedation. Avoid.	Tranquilizers*	Dangerous sedation. Avoid.
Narcotics*	Dangerous sedation. Avoid.	Valproic acid	Increased phenobarbital effect.
Nitrates*	Increased internal-eye pressure.	Vitamin C	Decreased atropine effect. Avoid large doses of vitamin C.
Nizatidine	Increased nizatidine effect.		

*See Glossary

GENERIC NAME OR DRUG CLASS	COMBINED EFFECT	GENERIC NAME OR DRUG CLASS	COMBINED EFFECT

PARAMETHASONE

GENERIC NAME OR DRUG CLASS	COMBINED EFFECT	GENERIC NAME OR DRUG CLASS	COMBINED EFFECT
Digitalis preparations*	Dangerous potassium depletion. Possible digitalis toxicity.	Isoniazid	Decreased isoniazid effect.
Diuretics, thiazide*	Potassium depletion.	Mitotane	Decreased paramethasone effect.
Ephedrine	Decreased paramethasone effect.	Non-steroidal anti-inflammatory drugs (NSAIDs)*	Increased risk of ulcers and paramethasone effect.
Estrogens*	Increased paramethasone effect.	Oxyphenbutazone	Possible ulcers.
Ethacrynic acid	Potassium depletion.	Phenobarbital	Decreased paramethasone effect.
Furosemide	Potassium depletion.	Phenylbutazone	Possible ulcers.
Glutethimide	Decreased paramethasone effect.	Potassium supplements*	Decreased potassium effect.
Indapamide	Possible excessive potassium loss, causing dangerous heartbeat irregularity.	Rifampin	Decreased paramethasone effect.
Indomethacin	Increased paramethasone effect.	Salicylates*	Decreased salicylate effect.
		Sympathomimetics*	Possible glaucoma.
Insulin	Decreased insulin effect.	Theophylline	Possible increased theophylline effect.

PERPHENAZINE & AMITRIPTYLINE

GENERIC NAME OR DRUG CLASS	COMBINED EFFECT	GENERIC NAME OR DRUG CLASS	COMBINED EFFECT
Guanabenz	Possible decreased guanabenz effect.	Nabilone	Greater depression of central nervous system.
Guanethidine	Decreased guanethidine effect.	Narcotics*	Increased narcotic effect and dangerous sedation.
Guanfacine	Possible decreased guanfacine effect.	Phenothiazines*	Possible increased antidepressant effect.
Levodopa	Decreased levodopa effect.	Procainamide	Possible irregular heartbeat.
Lithium	Possible decreased seizure threshold.	Procarbazine	Increased sedation.
MAO inhibitors*	Fever, delirium, convulsions.	Quinidine	Impaired heart function. Dangerous mixture.
Methyldopa	Possible decreased methyldopa effect.	Sedatives*	Dangerous oversedation.
Methylphenidate	Possible increased antidepressant effect.	Sympathomimetics*	Increased sympathomimetics effect.
Mind-altering drugs*	Increased effect of mind-altering drugs.	Thyroid hormones*	Irregular heartbeat.
		Tranquilizers, other*	Increased tranquilizer effect.

PHENOTHIAZINES

GENERIC NAME OR DRUG CLASS	COMBINED EFFECT	GENERIC NAME OR DRUG CLASS	COMBINED EFFECT
Narcotics*	Increased narcotic effect.	Sedatives*	Increased sedation.
Procarbazine	Increased sedation.	Tranquilizers* (other)	Increased tranquilizer effect.
Quinidine	Impaired heart function. Dangerous mixture.		

*See Glossary

PHENYTOIN

GENERIC NAME OR DRUG CLASS	COMBINED EFFECT	GENERIC NAME OR DRUG CLASS	COMBINED EFFECT
Leucovorin	May counteract the effect of phenytoin or any hydantoin anticonvulsant.	Para-aminosalicylic acid (PAS)	Increased phenytoin effect.
Loxapine	Decreased anticonvulsant effect of phenytoin or any hydantoin anticonvulsant.	Phenothiazines*	Increased phenytoin effect.
		Phenylbutazone	Increased phenytoin effect.
MAO inhibitors*	Increased polythiazide effect.	Potassium supplements*	Decreased potassium effect.
Methadone	Decreased methadone effect.	Probenecid	Decreased probenecid effect.
Methylphenidate	Increased phenytoin effect.	Propafenone	Increased effect of both drugs and increased risk of toxicity.
Molindone	Increased phenytoin effect.	Propranolol	Increased propranolol effect.
Nicardipine	Increased anticonvulsant effect.	Quinidine	Increased quinidine effect.
Nitrates*	Excessive blood pressure drop.	Sedatives*	Increased sedative effect.
Nizatidine	Increased effect and toxicity of phenytoin.	Sotalol	Decreased sotalol effect.
Omeprazole	Delayed excretion of phenytoin causing increased amount of phenytoin in blood.	Sulfa drugs*	Increased phenytoin effect.
		Theophylline	Reduced anticonvulsant effect.
Oxyphenbutazone	Increased phenytoin effect.	Trimethoprim	Increased phenytoin effect.
		Valproic acid	Unpredictable change in seizure control.

PRAZOSIN & POLYTHIAZIDE

GENERIC NAME OR DRUG CLASS	COMBINED EFFECT	GENERIC NAME OR DRUG CLASS	COMBINED EFFECT
Antidiabetics, other*	Increased blood sugar.	Diuretics, other*	Increased effect of other thiazide diuretics.
Antihypertensives*	Increased antihypertensive effect. Dosages may require adjustments.	Estrogen	Decreased prazosin effect.
Barbiturates*	Increased polythiazide effect.	Indapamide	Increased diuretic effect.
Carteolol	Increased antihypertensive effect.	Indomethacin	Decreased polythiazide effect.
Cholestyramine	Decreased polythiazide effect.	Lithium	Increased effect of lithium.
Chlorpromazine	Acute agitation.	MAO inhibitors*	Blood pressure drop. Increased polythiazide effect.
Cortisone drugs*	Excessive potassium loss that causes dangerous heart rhythms.	Nicardipine	Blood pressure drop. Dosages may require adjustment.
Digitalis preparations*	Excessive potassium loss that causes dangerous heart rhythms.	Nifedipine	Weakness and faintness when arising from bed or chair.

*See Glossary

GENERIC NAME OR DRUG CLASS	COMBINED EFFECT	GENERIC NAME OR DRUG CLASS	COMBINED EFFECT

PRAZOSIN & POLYTHIAZIDE continued

GENERIC NAME OR DRUG CLASS	COMBINED EFFECT	GENERIC NAME OR DRUG CLASS	COMBINED EFFECT
Nimodipine	Dangerous blood pressure drop.	Probenecid	Decreased probenecid effect.
Nitrates	Possible excessive blood pressure drop.	Sotalol	Decreased anti-hypertensive effect.
Non-steroidal anti-inflammatory drugs (NSAIDs)*	Decreased prazosin effect.	Sympathomimetics*	Decreased prazosin effect.
		Terazosin	Decreases effectiveness of terazosin.
Opiates*	Weakness and faintness when arising from bed or chair.	Verapamil	Weakness and faintness when arising from bed or chair.
Potassium	Decreased potassium effect.		

PREDNISOLONE

GENERIC NAME OR DRUG CLASS	COMBINED EFFECT	GENERIC NAME OR DRUG CLASS	COMBINED EFFECT
Digitalis preparations*	Dangerous potassium depletion. Possible digitalis toxicity.	Isoniazid	Decreased isoniazid effect.
		Mitotane	Decreased prednisolone effect.
Diuretics, thiazide*	Potassium depletion.	Non-steroidal anti-inflammatory drugs (NSAIDs)*	Increased risk of ulcers, increased prednisolone effect.
Ephedrine	Decreased prednisolone effect.		
Estrogens*	Increased prednisolone effect.	Oxyphenbutazone	Possible ulcers.
Ethacrynic acid	Potassium depletion.	Phenobarbital	Decreased prednisolone effect.
Furosemide	Potassium depletion.	Phenylbutazone	Possible ulcers.
Glutethimide	Decreased prednisolone effect.	Potassium supplements*	Decreased potassium effect.
Indapamide	Possible excessive potassium loss, causing dangerous heartbeat irregularity.	Rifampin	Decreased prednisolone effect.
		Salicylates*	Decreased salicylate effect.
Indomethacin	Increased prednisolone effect.	Sympathomimetics*	Possible glaucoma.
Insulin	Decreased insulin effect.	Theophylline	Possible increased theophylline effect.

PREDNISONE

GENERIC NAME OR DRUG CLASS	COMBINED EFFECT	GENERIC NAME OR DRUG CLASS	COMBINED EFFECT
Contraceptives, oral*	Increased prednisone effect.	Ethacrynic acid	Potassium depletion.
		Furosemide	Potassium depletion.
Digitalis preparations*	Dangerous potassium depletion. Possible digitalis toxicity.	Glutethimide	Decreased prednisone effect.
Diuretics, thiazide*	Potassium depletion.	Indapamide	Possible excessive potassium loss, causing dangerous heartbeat irregularity.
Ephedrine	Decreased prednisone effect.		
Estrogens*	Increased prednisone effect.	Indomethacin	Increased prednisone effect.

*See Glossary

ADDITIONAL DRUG INTERACTIONS

GENERIC NAME OR DRUG CLASS	COMBINED EFFECT	GENERIC NAME OR DRUG CLASS	COMBINED EFFECT

PREDNISONE continued

GENERIC NAME OR DRUG CLASS	COMBINED EFFECT	GENERIC NAME OR DRUG CLASS	COMBINED EFFECT
Insulin	Decreased insulin effect.	Phenylbutazone	Possible ulcers.
Isoniazid	Decreased isoniazid effect.	Potassium supplements*	Decreased potassium effect.
Mitotane	Decreased prednisone effect.	Rifampin	Decreased prednisone effect.
Non-steroidal anti-inflammatory drugs (NSAIDs)*	Increased risk of ulcers and prednisone effect.	Salicylates*	Decreased salicylate effect.
Oxyphenbutazone	Possible ulcers.	Sympathomimetics*	Possible glaucoma.
Phenobarbital	Decreased prednisone effect.	Theophylline	Possible increased theophylline effect.

PRIMIDONE

GENERIC NAME OR DRUG CLASS	COMBINED EFFECT	GENERIC NAME OR DRUG CLASS	COMBINED EFFECT
Nabilone	Greater depression of central nervous system.	Rifampin	Possible decreased primidone effect.
Narcotics*	Increased narcotic effect.	Sedatives*	Increased sedative effect.
Oxyphenbutazone	Decreased oxyphen-butazone effect.	Sertraline	Increased depressive effects of both drugs.
Phenylbutazone	Decreased phenyl-butazone effect.	Sleep inducers*	Increased effect of sleep inducer.
Phenytoin	Possible increased primidone toxicity.	Tranquilizers*	Increased tranquilizer effect.

PROBENECID & COLCHICINE

GENERIC NAME OR DRUG CLASS	COMBINED EFFECT	GENERIC NAME OR DRUG CLASS	COMBINED EFFECT
Para-aminosalicylic acid (PAS)	Increased effect of para-aminosalicylic acid.	Sleep inducers*	Oversedation.
Penicillins*	Enhanced penicillin effect.	Sulfa drugs*	Slows elimination. May cause harmful accumulation of sulfa.
Phenylbutazone	Decreased antigout effect of colchicine.	Thioguanine	More likelihood of toxicity of both drugs.
Pyrazinamide	Decreased probenecid effect.	Tranquilizers*	Oversedation.
Salicylates*	Decreased probenecid effect.	Vitamin B-12	Decreased absorption of vitamin B-12.
Sedatives*	Oversedation.	Zidovudine	Increased risk of zidovudine toxicity.

PROCARBAZINE

GENERIC NAME OR DRUG CLASS	COMBINED EFFECT	GENERIC NAME OR DRUG CLASS	COMBINED EFFECT
Guanethidine	Blood pressure rise to life-threatening level.	Leucovorin	High alcohol content of leucovorin may cause adverse effects.
Guanfacine	May increase depressant effects of either medicine.	Levamisole	Increased risk of bone marrow depression.
		Levodopa	Sudden, severe blood pressure rise.

*See Glossary

GENERIC NAME OR DRUG CLASS	COMBINED EFFECT	GENERIC NAME OR DRUG CLASS	COMBINED EFFECT
PROCARBAZINE continued			
MAO inhibitors, other*	High fever, convulsions, death.	**Phenothiazines***	Increased sedation.
Methyldopa	Severe high blood pressure.	**Rauwolfia alkaloids***	Very high blood pressure.
Methylphenidate	Excessive high blood pressure.	**Reserpine**	Increased blood pressure, excitation.
Methyprylon	May increase sedative effect to dangerous level. Avoid.	**Sertraline**	Increased depressive effects of both drugs.
Nabilone	Greater depression of central nervous system.	**Sympathomimetics***	Heartbeat abnormalities, severe high blood pressure.
Narcotics*	Increased sedation.	**Tiopronin**	Increased risk of toxicity to bone marrow.

RAUWOLFIA ALKALOIDS

GENERIC NAME OR DRUG CLASS	COMBINED EFFECT	GENERIC NAME OR DRUG CLASS	COMBINED EFFECT
Mind-altering drugs*	Excessive sedation.	**Pergolide**	Decreased pergolide effect.
Nabilone	Greater depression of central nervous system.	**Sertraline**	Increased depressive effects of both drugs.
Nicardipine	Blood pressure drop. Dosages may require adjustment.	**Sotalol**	Increased antihypertensive effect.
Nimodipine	Dangerous blood pressure drop.	**Terazosin**	Decreases effectiveness of terazosin.

RAUWOLFIA & THIAZIDE DIURETICS

GENERIC NAME OR DRUG CLASS	COMBINED EFFECT	GENERIC NAME OR DRUG CLASS	COMBINED EFFECT
Carteolol	Increased antihypertensive effect.	**MAO inhibitors***	Increased hydrochlorothiazide effect. Severe depression.
Cholestyramine	Decreased hydrocholorothiazide effect.	**Mind-altering drugs***	Excessive sedation.
Cortisone drugs*	Excessive potassium loss that causes dangerous heart rhythms.	**Nicardipine**	Blood pressure drop. Dosages may require adjustment.
Digitalis preparations*	Excessive potassium loss that causes dangerous heart rhythms.	**Nitrates***	Excessive blood pressure drop.
Diuretics, thiazide*	Increased effect of other thiazide diuretics.	**Oxprenolol**	Increased antihypertensive effect. Dosages of both drugs may require adjustments.
Dronabinol	Increased effect of both drugs. Avoid.		
Indapamide	Increased diuretic effect.	**Pergolide**	Decreased pergolide effect.
Levodopa	Decreased levodopa effect.	**Potassium supplements***	Decreased potassium effect.
Lisinopril	Increased antihypertensive effect. Dosage of each may require adjustment.	**Probenecid**	Decreased probenecid effect.
		Sotalol	Decreased antihypertensive effect.
Lithium	Increased effect of lithium.	**Terazosin**	Decreases effectiveness of terazosin.

*See Glossary

RESERPINE & HYDRALAZINE

GENERIC NAME OR DRUG CLASS	COMBINED EFFECT	GENERIC NAME OR DRUG CLASS	COMBINED EFFECT
Digitalis preparations*	Irregular heartbeat.	Mind-altering drugs*	Excessive sedation.
Diuretics, oral*	Increased effect of both drugs. When monitored carefully, combination may be beneficial in controlling hypertension.	Nicardipine	Blood pressure drop. Dosages may require adjustment.
		Nimodipine	Dangerous blood pressure drop.
Dronabinol	Increased effect of both drugs. Avoid.	Non-steroidal anti-inflammatory drugs (NSAIDs)*	Decreased hydralazine effect.
Levodopa	Decreased levodopa effect.	Pergolide	Decreased pergolide effect.
Lisinopril	Increased antihypertensive effect. Dosage of each may require adjustment.	Sotalol	Decreased antihypertensive effect.
MAO inhibitors*	Severe depression.	Terazosin	Decreases effectiveness of terazosin.

RESERPINE, HYDRALAZINE & HYDROCHLOROTHIAZIDE

GENERIC NAME OR DRUG CLASS	COMBINED EFFECT	GENERIC NAME OR DRUG CLASS	COMBINED EFFECT
Anticonvulsants*	Serious change in seizure pattern.	Diuretics, oral*	Increased effects of drugs. When monitored carefully, combination may be beneficial in controlling hypertension.
Antidepressants, tricyclic (TCA)*	Dangerous drop in blood pressure. Avoid combination unless under medical supervision.	Dronabinol	Increased effects of drugs.
Antihistamines*	Increased antihistamine effect.	Indapamide	Increased diuretic effect.
Antihypertensives, other*	Increased antihypertensive effect.	Levodopa	Decreased levodopa effect.
Aspirin	Decreased aspirin effect.	Lisinopril	Increased antihypertensive effect. Dosage of each may require adjustment.
Barbiturates*	Increased hydrochlorothiazide effect.		
Beta-adrenergic blockers*	Increased effect of rauwolfia alkaloids. Excessive sedation.	Lithium	Increased lithium effect.
		MAO inhibitors*	Increased effects of both drugs. Severe depression.
Carteolol	Increased antihypertensive effect.	Mind-altering drugs*	Excessive sedation.
Cholestyramine	Decreased hydrochlorothiazide effect.	Nicardipine	Blood pressure drop. Dosages may require adjustment.
Cortisone drugs*	Excessive potassium loss that causes dangerous heart rhythms.	Nimodipine	Dangerous blood pressure drop.
Diazoxide	Increased antihypertensive effect.	Nitrates*	Excessive blood pressure drop.
Digitalis preparations*	Excessive potassium loss that causes dangerous heart rhythms.		

*See Glossary

RESERPINE, HYDRALAZINE & HYDROCHLOROTHIAZIDE continued

GENERIC NAME OR DRUG CLASS	COMBINED EFFECT	GENERIC NAME OR DRUG CLASS	COMBINED EFFECT
Non-steroidal anti-inflammatory drugs (NSAIDs)*	Decreased hydralazine effect.	Potassium supplements*	Decreased potassium effect.
Oxprenolol	Increased antihypertensive effect. Dosages of drug may require adjustments.	Probenecid	Decreased probenecid effect.
		Sotalol	Decreased antihypertensive effect.
Pergolide	Decreased pergolide effect.	Terazosin	Decreases effectiveness of terazosin.

SALICYLATES

GENERIC NAME OR DRUG CLASS	COMBINED EFFECT	GENERIC NAME OR DRUG CLASS	COMBINED EFFECT
Penicillins*	Increased effect of both drugs.	Sulfinpyrazone	Decreased sulfinpyrazone effect.
Phenobarbital	Decreased salicylate effect.	Terazosin	Decreases effectiveness of terazosin. Causes sodium and fluid retention.
Phenytoin	Increased phenytoin effect.		
Probenecid	Decreased probenecid effect.	Urinary acidifiers*	Decreased excretion, increased salicylate effect.
Rauwolfia alkaloids*	Decreased salicylate effect.	Urinary alkalizers*	Increased excretion, decreased salicylate effect.
Salicylates, other*	Likely salicylate toxicity.		
Sotalol	Decreased antihypertensive effect of sotalol.	Valproic acid	Possible increased valproic acid toxicity.
Spironolactone	Decreased spironolactone effect.	Vitamin C (large doses)	Possible salicylate toxicity.
		Zidovudine	Increased zidovudine effect.

SCOPOLAMINE (Hyoscine)

GENERIC NAME OR DRUG CLASS	COMBINED EFFECT	GENERIC NAME OR DRUG CLASS	COMBINED EFFECT
Pilocarpine	Loss of pilocarpine effect in glaucoma treatment.	Sedatives* or central nervous system (CNS) depressants*	Increased sedative effect of both drugs.
Potassium supplements*	Possible intestinal ulcers with oral potassium tablets.	Sertraline	Increased depressive effects of both drugs.
Quinidine	Increased scopolamine effect.	Vitamin C	Decreased scopolamine effect. Avoid large doses of vitamin C.

SPIRONOLACTONE & HYDROCHLOROTHIAZIDE

GENERIC NAME OR DRUG CLASS	COMBINED EFFECT	GENERIC NAME OR DRUG CLASS	COMBINED EFFECT
Diuretics, other*	Increased effect of both drugs. Beneficial if needed and dose is correct.	Laxatives*	Reduced potassium levels.
		Lithium	Increased effect of lithium. Likely lithium toxicity.
Indapamide	Increased diuretic effect.		
Indomethacin	Decreased hydrochlorothiazide effect.	MAO inhibitors*	Increased hydrochlorothiazide effect.

*See Glossary

ADDITIONAL DRUG INTERACTIONS

SPIRONOLACTONE & HYDROCHLOROTHIAZIDE continued

GENERIC NAME OR DRUG CLASS	COMBINED EFFECT	GENERIC NAME OR DRUG CLASS	COMBINED EFFECT
Nicardipine	Blood pressure drop. Dosages may require adjustment.	Potassium iodide	May raise potassium level in blood to toxic levels.
Nimodipine	Dangerous blood pressure drop.	Probenecid	Decreased probenecid effect.
Nitrates*	Excessive blood pressure drop.	Salicylates*	May decrease spironolactone effect.
Opiates*	Weakness and faintness when arising from bed or chair.	Sodium bicarbonate	Reduces high potassium levels.
Potassium supplements*	Decreased potassium effect. Dangerous potassium retention, causing possible heartbeat irregularity.	Sotalol	Decreased anti-hypertensive effect.
		Terazosin	Decreases effectiveness of terazosin.
		Triamterene	Dangerous potassium retention.
		Zinc supplements	Increased need for zinc.

TESTOSTERONE & ESTRADIOL

GENERIC NAME OR DRUG CLASS	COMBINED EFFECT	GENERIC NAME OR DRUG CLASS	COMBINED EFFECT
Oxyphenbutazone	Decreased androgen and estrogen effect.	Rifampin	Decreased estrogen and testosterone effect.
Phenobarbital	Decreased androgen and estrogen effect.	Terazosin	Decreases effectiveness of terazosin.
Phenylbutazone	Decreased androgen and testosterone effect.	Thyroid hormones*	Decreased thyroid effect.
Primidone	Decreased estrogen and testosterone effect.	Ursodiol	Decreased effect of ursodiol.

THEOPHYLLINE, EPHEDRINE & BARBITURATES

GENERIC NAME OR DRUG CLASS	COMBINED EFFECT	GENERIC NAME OR DRUG CLASS	COMBINED EFFECT
Antihistamines*	Dangerous sedation. Avoid.	Cortisone drugs*	Decreased cortisone effect.
Antihypertensives*	Decreased antihypertensive effect.	Digitalis preparations*	Serious heart-rhythm disturbances.
Aspirin	Decreased aspirin effect.	Doxycycline	Decreased doxycycline effect.
Beta-adrenergic blockers*	Decreased effect of drugs.	Dronabinol	Increased effect of drugs. Avoid.
Carteolol	Increased barbiturate effect. Dangerous sedation.	Ephedrine	Increased effect of drugs.
Ciprofloxacin	Increased possibility of central nervous system poisoning, such as nausea, vomiting, restlessness, palpitations.	Epinephrine	Increased effect of drugs.
		Ergot preparations*	Serious blood pressure rise.
Clarithromycin	Increased concentration of theophylline.	Erythromycins*	Increased bronchodilator effect.
Contraceptives, oral*	Decreased contraceptive effect.	Finasteride	Decreased theophylline effect.

*See Glossary

GENERIC NAME OR DRUG CLASS	COMBINED EFFECT	GENERIC NAME OR DRUG CLASS	COMBINED EFFECT

THEOPHYLLINE, EPHEDRINE & BARBITURATES continued

GENERIC NAME OR DRUG CLASS	COMBINED EFFECT	GENERIC NAME OR DRUG CLASS	COMBINED EFFECT
Furosemide	Increased furosemide effect.	Non-steroidal anti-inflammatory drugs (NSAIDs)*	Decreased anti-inflammatory effect.
Griseofulvin	Decreased griseofulvin effect.	Probenecid	Decreased effect of drugs.
Guanethidine	Decreased effect of drugs.	Propranolol	Decreased broncho-dilator effect.
Indapamide	Increased indapamide effect.	Pseudoephedrine	Increased pseudo-ephedrine effect.
Lincomycins*	Increased broncho-dilator effect.	Rauwolfia alkaloids*	Rapid heartbeat.
Lithium	Decreased lithium effect.	Sotalol	Increased barbiturate effect. Dangerous sedation.
MAO inhibitors*	Increased ephedrine effect. Dangerous blood pressure rise.	Sulfinpyrazone	Decreased sulfin-pyrazone effect.
Mind-altering drugs*	Dangerous sedation. Avoid.	Terazosin	Decreased effect of terazosin.
Narcotics*	Dangerous sedation. Avoid.	Ticlopidine	Increased theophylline effect.
Nicardipine	May increase theophyl-line effect and toxicity.	Troleandomycin	Increased broncho-dilator effect.
Nicotine	Increased bronchodilator effect.	Valproic acid	Increased barbiturate effect.
Nitrates*	Possible decreased effect of drugs.		

THEOPHYLLINE, EPHEDRINE, GUAIFENESIN & BARBITURATES

GENERIC NAME OR DRUG CLASS	COMBINED EFFECT	GENERIC NAME OR DRUG CLASS	COMBINED EFFECT
Antidepressants, tricyclics (TCA)*	Decreased anti-depressant effect.	Cortisone drugs*	Increased cortisone effect.
Antidiabetics, oral*	Increased phenobarbital effect.	Digitalis preparations*	Serious heart-rhythm disturbances.
Antihistamines*	Dangerous sedation. Avoid.	Digitoxin	Decreased digitoxin effect.
Aspirin, other	Decreased aspirin effect.	Doxycycline	Decreased doxycycline effect.
Beta-adrenergic blockers*	Decreased effect of drugs.	Dronabinol	Increased effect of drugs.
Carteolol	Increased barbiturate effect. Dangerous sedation.	Ephedrine	Increased effect of drugs.
		Ergot preparations*	Serious blood pressure rise.
Clarithromycin	Increased concen-tration of theophylline.	Erythromycins*	Increased broncho-dilator effect.
Ciprofloxacin	Increased possibility of central nervous system poisoning, such as nausea, vomiting, rest-lessness, palpitations.	Finasteride	Decreased theophylline effect.
		Furosemide	Increased furosemide effect.
Contraceptives, oral*	Decreased contra-ceptive effect.	Griseofulvin	Decreased griseofulvin effect.

*See Glossary

963

GENERIC NAME OR DRUG CLASS	COMBINED EFFECT	GENERIC NAME OR DRUG CLASS	COMBINED EFFECT

THEOPHYLLINE, EPHEDRINE, GUAIFENESIN & BARBITURATES continued

GENERIC NAME OR DRUG CLASS	COMBINED EFFECT	GENERIC NAME OR DRUG CLASS	COMBINED EFFECT
Guanethidine	Decreased effect of drugs.	Pain relievers*	Dangerous sedation. Avoid.
Indapamide	Increased indapamide effect.	Probenecid	Decreased effect of drugs.
Lincomycins*	Increased broncho-dilator effect.	Propranolol	Decreased broncho-dilator effect.
Lithium	Decreased lithium effect.	Pseudoephedrine	Increased pseudo-ephedrine effect.
MAO inhibitors*	Increased pheno-barbital effect.	Rauwolfia alkaloids*	Rapid heartbeat.
Mind-altering drugs*	Dangerous sedation. Avoid.	Sedatives*	Dangerous sedation. Avoid.
Narcotics*	Dangerous sedation. Avoid.	Sleep inducers*	Dangerous sedation. Avoid.
Nicardipine	May increase theophylline effect and toxicity.	Sulfinpyrazone	Decreased sulfin-pyrazone effect.
Nicotine	Increased bronchodilator effect.	Terazosin	Decreased effect of terazosin.
Nitrates*	Possible decreased effect of drugs.	Ticlopidine	Increased theophylline effect.
Non-steroidal anti-inflammatory drugs (NSAIDs)*	Decreased anti-inflammatory effect.	Tranquilizers*	Dangerous sedation. Avoid.
		Troleandomycin	Increased broncho-dilator effect.
		Valproic acid	Increased phenobarbital effect.

THEOPHYLLINE, EPHEDRINE & HYDROXYZINE

GENERIC NAME OR DRUG CLASS	COMBINED EFFECT	GENERIC NAME OR DRUG CLASS	COMBINED EFFECT
Ciprofloxacin	May cause kidney dysfunction.	Guanethidine	Decreased effect of drugs.
Clarithromycin	Increased concen-tration of theophylline.	Lincomycins*	Increased broncho-dilator effect.
Digitalis preparations*	Serious heart-rhythm disturbances.	Lithium	Decreased lithium effect.
Dronabinol	Increased effect of drugs.	MAO inhibitors*	Increased ephedrine effect. Dangerous blood pressure rise.
Ephedrine	Increased effect of drugs.	Moricizine	Decreased antihistamine effect.
Epinephrine	Increased effect of drugs.	Nabilone	Greater depression of central nervous system.
Ergot preparations*	Serious blood pressure rise.	Nicardipine	May increase theophyl-line effect and toxicity.
Erythromycins*	Increased broncho-dilator effect.	Nicotine	Increased bronchodilator effect.
Finasteride	Decreased theophylline effect.	Nitrates*	Possible decreased effect of drugs.
Furosemide	Increased furosemide effect.		

*See Glossary

THEOPHYLLINE, EPHEDRINE & HYDROXYZINE continued

GENERIC NAME OR DRUG CLASS	COMBINED EFFECT	GENERIC NAME OR DRUG CLASS	COMBINED EFFECT
Pain relievers*	Increased effect of drugs.	Sulfinpyrazone	Decreased sulfinpyrazone effect.
Probenecid	Decreased effect of drugs.	Terazosin	Decreased effect of terazosin.
Propranolol	Decreased bronchodilator effect.	Ticlopidine	Increased theophylline effect.
Pseudoephedrine	Increased pseudoephedrine effect.	Tranquilizers*	Increased effect of drugs.
Rauwolfia alkaloids*	Rapid heartbeat.	Troleandomycin	Increased bronchodilator effect.
Sotalol	Decreased antihistamine effect.		

TRIAMCINOLONE

GENERIC NAME OR DRUG CLASS	COMBINED EFFECT	GENERIC NAME OR DRUG CLASS	COMBINED EFFECT
Furosemide	Potassium depletion.	Non-steroidal anti-inflammatory drugs (NSAIDs)*	Increased risk of ulcers and triamcinolone effect.
Glutethimide	Decreased triamcinolone effect.	Oxyphenbutazone	Possible ulcers.
Indapamide	Possible excessive potassium loss, causing dangerous heartbeat irregularity.	Phenobarbital	Decreased triamcinolone effect.
		Phenylbutazone	Possible ulcers.
Indomethacin	Increased triamcinolone effect.	Potassium supplements*	Decreased potassium effect.
Insulin	Decreased insulin effect.	Rifampin	Decreased triamcinolone effect.
Isoniazid	Decreased isoniazid effect.	Salicylates*	Decreased salicylate effect.
Mitotane	Decreased triamcinolone effect.	Sympathomimetics*	Possible glaucoma.
		Theophylline	Possible increased theophylline effect.

TRIAMTERENE & HYDROCHLOROTHIAZIDE

GENERIC NAME OR DRUG CLASS	COMBINED EFFECT	GENERIC NAME OR DRUG CLASS	COMBINED EFFECT
Indomethacin	Possible acute renal failure.	Nitrates*	Excessive blood pressure drop.
Lisinopril	Possible severe blood pressure drop with first dose.	Opiates*	Weakness and faintness when arising from bed or chair.
Lithium	Increased lithium effect.	Potassium supplements*	Possible excessive potassium retention. Decreased potassium effect.
MAO inhibitors*	Increased hydrochlorothiazide effect.		
Nicardipine	Dangerous blood pressure drop. Dosages may require adjustment.	Probenecid	Decreased probenecid effect.
		Spironolactone	Dangerous retention of potassium.
Nimodipine	Dangerous blood pressure drop.		

ADDITIONAL DRUG INTERACTIONS

TRICYCLIC ANTIDEPRESSANTS

GENERIC NAME OR DRUG CLASS	COMBINED EFFECT	GENERIC NAME OR DRUG CLASS	COMBINED EFFECT
Cimetidine	Possible increased tricyclic antidepressant effect and toxicity.	Methylphenidate	Possible increased tricyclic antidepressant effect and toxicity.
Clonidine	Possible decreased clonidine effect.	Methyprylon	Increased sedative effect, perhaps to dangerous level. Avoid.
Clozapine	Toxic effect on the central nervous system.		
Dextrothyroxine	Increased antidepressant effect. Irregular heartbeat.	Metyrosine	Increased sedative effect.
		Molindone	Increased molindone effect.
Disulfiram	Delirium.	Nabilone	Greater depression of central nervous system.
Ethchlorvynol	Delirium.		
Ethinamate	Dangerous increased effects of ethinamate. Avoid combining.	Narcotics*	Oversedation.
		Nicotine	Increased effect of antidepressant (imipramine).
Fluoxetine	Increased depressant effects of both drugs.		
Furazolidine	Sudden, severe increase in blood pressure.	Oral contraceptives	Increased depression.
		Phenothiazines*	Possible increased tricyclic antidepressant effect and toxicity.
Guanabenz	Decreased guanabenz effect.		
Guanethidine	Decreased guanethidine effect.	Phenytoin	Decreased phenytoin effect.
Leucovorin	High alcohol content of leucovorin may cause adverse effects.	Procainamide	Possible irregular heartbeat.
		Quinidine	Possible irregular heartbeat.
Levodopa	May increase blood pressure.	Sedatives*	Dangerous oversedation.
Lithium	Possible decreased seizure threshold.	Sertraline	Increased depressive effects of both drugs.
MAO inhibitors*	Fever, delirium, convulsions.	Sympathomimetics*	Increased sympathomimetic effect.
Methyldopa	Possible decreased methyldopa effect.	Thyroid hormones*	Irregular heartbeat.

TRIMEPRAZINE

GENERIC NAME OR DRUG CLASS	COMBINED EFFECT	GENERIC NAME OR DRUG CLASS	COMBINED EFFECT
Mind-altering drugs*	Increased effect of mind-altering drugs.	Sedatives*	Increased sedative effect.
Molindone	Increased sedative and antihistamine effect.	Sertraline	Increased depressive effects of both drugs.
Nabilone	Greater depression of central nervous system.	Sotalol	Increased antihistamine effect.
Narcotics*	Increased narcotic effect.	Tranquilizers*	Increased tranquilizer effect. Avoid.

*See Glossary

Glossary

The following medical terms are found in the drug charts. Where drug names are listed, the generic or drug class is first with brand names following in parentheses.

A

ACE Inhibitors/Angiotensin-Converting Enzyme (ACE) Inhibitors—A family of drugs used to treat hypertension and congestive heart failure. Inhibitors decrease the rate of conversion of Angiotensin I into Angiotensin II, which is the normal process for the angiotensin-converting enzyme. These drugs include benazepril captopril, enalapril, fosinopril, lisinopril and ramipril.

Acne Preparations—Creams, lotions and liquids applied to the skin to treat acne. These include alcohol and acetone; alcohol and sulfur; benzoyl peroxide; clindamycin; erythromycin; erythromycin and benzoyl peroxide; isotretinoin; meclocycline; resorcinol; resorcinol and sulfur; salicylic acid gel USP; salicylic acid lotion; salicylic acid ointment; salicylic acid pads; salicylic acid soap; salicylic acid and sulfur bar soap; salicylic acid and sulfur cleansing lotion; salicylic acid and sulfur cleansing suspension; salicylic acid and sulfur lotion; sulfurated lime; sulfur bar soap; sulfur cream; sulfur lotion; tetracycline, oral; tetracycline hydrochloride for topical solution; tretinoin.

Acute—Having a short and relatively severe course.

Addiction—Psychological or physiological dependence upon a drug.

Addictive drugs—Any drug that can lead to physiological dependence on the drug. These include alcohol, cocaine, marijuana, nicotine, opium, morphine, codeine, heroin (and other narcotics), and others.

Addison's Disease—Changes in the body caused by a deficiency of hormones manufactured by the adrenal gland. Usually fatal if untreated.

Adrenal Cortex—Center of the adrenal gland.

Adrenal Gland—Gland next to the kidney that produces cortisone and epinephrine (adrenalin).

Agranulocytosis—A symptom complex characterized by (1) a sharply decreased number of granulocytes (one of the types of white blood cells), (2) lesions of the throat and other mucous membranes, (3) lesions of the gastrointestinal tract, and (4) lesions of the skin. Sometimes also called granulocytopenia.

Alkalizers—These drugs neutralize acidic properties of the blood and urine by making them more alkaline (or basic). Systemic alkalizers include potassium citrate and citric acid, sodium bicarbonate, sodium citrate and citric acid, and tricitrates. Urinary alkalizers include potassium citrate, potassium citrate and citric acid, potassium citrate and sodium citrate, sodium citrate and citric acid.

Alkylating Agent—Chemical used to treat malignant diseases.

Allergy—Excessive sensitivity to a substance.

Amebiasis—Infection with amoebas, one-celled organisms. Causes diarrhea, fever and abdominal cramps.

Aminoglycosides—A family of antibiotics used for serious infections. Their usefulness is limited because of relative toxicity compared to some other antibiotics. These drugs include amikacin, gentamicin, kanamycin, neomycin, netilmicin, streptomycin, tobramycin.

Amphetamines—A family of drugs that stimulates the central nervous system, prescribed to treat attention-deficit disorders in children and also for narcolepsy. They are habit-forming, controlled under U.S. law, and are no longer prescribed as appetite suppressants. These drugs include amphetamine, dextro-amphetamine, methamphetamine. They may be ingredients of several combination drugs.

ANA Titers—A test to evaluate the immune system and to detect antinuclear antibodies (ANAs), substances which appear in the blood of some patients with autoimmune disease.

Analgesic—Agent that reduces pain without reducing consciousness.

Anaphylaxis—Severe allergic response to a substance. Symptoms are wheezing, itching, hives, nasal congestion, intense burning of hands and feet, collapse, loss of consciousness and cardiac arrest. Symptoms appear within a few seconds or minutes after exposure. Anaphylaxis is a severe medical emergency. Without appropriate treatment, it can cause death. Instructions for home treatment for anaphylaxis are on the front inside cover.

Androgens—Male hormones, including fluoxymesterone, methyltestosterone, testosterone.

Anemia—Not enough healthy red blood cells in the bloodstream or too little hemoglobin in the red blood cells. Anemia is caused by imbalance of blood loss and blood production.

Anemia, Aplastic—A form of anemia in which

the bone marrow is unable to manufacture adequate numbers of blood cells of all types—red cells, white cells, and platelets.

Anemia, Hemolytic—Anemia caused by a shortened lifespan of red blood cells. The body can't manufacture new cells fast enough to replace old cells.

Anemia, Iron-Deficiency—Anemia caused when iron necessary to manufacture red blood cells is not available.

Anemia, Pernicious—Anemia caused by a vitamin B-12 deficiency. Symptoms include weakness, fatigue, numbness and tingling of the hands or feet, and degeneration of the central nervous system.

Anemia, Sickle-Cell—Anemia caused by defective hemoglobin that deprives red blood cells of oxygen, making them sickle-shaped.

Anesthesias, General—Gases that are used in surgery to render patients unconscious and able to withstand the pain of surgical cutting and manipulation. They include enflurane, etomidate, fentanyl, halothane, isoflurane, ketamine, methohexital, methoxyflurane, nitrous oxide, propofol, thiamylal, thiopental, alfentanil, amobarbital, butabarbital, butorphanol, chloral hydrate, etomidate, fentanyl, tentanyl, hydroxyzine, ketamine, levorphanol, meperidine, midazolam, morphine parenteral, nalbuphine, oxymorphone, pentazocine, pentobarbital, phenobarbital, promethazine, propiomazine, scopolamine, secobarbital, sufentanil.

Anesthetic—Drug that eliminates the sensation of pain.

Angina (Angina Pectoris)—Chest pain with a sensation of suffocation and impending death. Caused by a temporary reduction in the amount of oxygen to the heart muscle through diseased coronary arteries.

Antacids—A large family of drugs prescribed to treat hyperacidity, peptic ulcer, esophageal reflux, and others. These drugs include aluminum carbonate, basic (Basaljel); aluminum hydroxide (Alagel, ALternaGEL, Alu-Cap, Alu-Tab, Amphojel, Dialume, Nephrox); dihydroxyaluminum aminoacetate (Robalate); dihydroxyaluminum sodium carbonate (Rolaids); alumina, magnesia and calcium carbonate (Camalox); alumina, magnesium carbonate and calcium carbonate (Duracid); simethicone, alumina, calcium carbonate and magnesia (Tempo); alumina and magnesia (Algenic Alka Improved, Aludrox, Alumid, Amphojel 500, Creamalin, Delcid, Diovol Ex, Gelamal, Gelusil, Gelusil Extra Strength, Kolantyl, Kudrox, Maalox, Maalox No. 1, Maalox No. 2, Maalox TC, Magmalin, Mintox, Mylanta 2 Plain, Neutralca-S, Rolox, Rulox, Rulox No. 1, Rulox No. 2, Univol, WinGel); alumina, magnesia and simethicone (Almacone, Almacone II, Alma-Mag Improved, Alma-Mag #4 Improved, Alumid Plus, Amphojel Plus, AntaGel, AntaGel-II, Di-Gel, Diovol, Gelusil, Gelusil-II, Gelusil-M, Maalox Plus, MiAcid, Mygel, Mygel II, Mylanta, Mylanta-II, Mylanta-2, Mylanta-2 Extra Strength, Newtrogel II, Silain-Gel, Simaal Gel, Simaal 2 Gel, Simeco); alumina and magnesium carbonate (Gaviscon, Liquimint, Magnagel, Remegel); alumina and magnesium trisilicate (Gaviscon, Gaviscon-2); dihydroxyaluminum aminoacetate, magnesia and alumina (Tralmag); magnesium trisilicate, alumina and magnesia (Magnatril); magnesium trisilicate, alumina and magnesium carbonate (Escot); simethicone, alumina, magnesium carbonate and magnesia (Amphojel Plus, Di-Gel); alumina, magnesium trisilicate and sodium bicarbonate (Gas-is-gon, Triconsil); calcium carbonate (Alka-Mints, Amitone, Chooz, Calcilac, Calglycine, Dicarbosil, Equilet, Gustalac, Pama No. 1, Titracin, Titralac, Tums, Tums E-X); calcium carbonate and magnesia (Bisodol, Calcitrel); calcium carbonate, magnesia and simethicone (Advanced Formula Di-Gel); calcium and magnesium carbonates (Marblen, Noralac, Spastosed); calcium and magnesium carbonates and magnesium oxide (Alkets); magaldrate (Lowsium, Riopan); magaldrate and simethicone (Riopan Plus, Lowsium); magnesium hydroxide (M.O.M., Phillips' Milk of Magnesia); magnesium oxide (Mag-Ox 400, Maox, Par-Mag, Uro-Mag); magnesium carbonate and sodium bicarbonate (Bisodol).

Antacids, Calcium Carbonate—These antacids include calcium carbonate and magnesium, calcium carbonate and simethicone, calcium carbonate and magnesium carbonates.

Antacids, Magnesium-Containing—These antacids include magnesium carbonate, magnesium hydroxide, magnesium oxide and magnesium trisilicate. All these medicines are designed to treat excess stomach acidity. In addition to being an effective antacid, magnesium can sometimes cause unpleasant side effects and drug interactions. Look for the presence of magnesium on non-prescription drugs.

Antiacne Topical Preparations—See Acne Preparations.

Antiadrenals—Medicines or drugs that prevent the effects of the hormones liberated by the adrenal glands.

Antianginals—A group of drugs used to treat *angina pectoris* (chest pain that comes and goes, caused by coronary artery disease). These drugs include acebutolol, amyl nitrite, atenolol, bepridril, carteolol, diltiazem, erythrityl tetranitrate, isosorbide dinitrate, labetalol, metoprolol, nadolol, nifedipine, nitroglycerin, oxprenolol, penbutolol, pentaerythritol, pindolol, propranolol, sotalol, timolol, verapamil.

Antianxiety—A group of drugs prescribed to treat anxiety. These drugs include alprazolam, bromazepam, buspirone, chlordiazepoxide, chlorpromazine, clomipramine, clorazepate, diazepam, halazepam, hydroxyzine, imipramine, ketazolam, lorazepam, meprobamate, oxazepam, prazepam, prochlorperazine, thioridazine, trifluoperazine.

Antiarrhythmics—A group of drugs used to treat heartbeat irregularities (arrhythmias). These drugs include acebutolol, amiodarone, atenolol, atropine, bretylium, deslanoside, digitalis, digitoxin, disopyramide, edrophonium, encainide, esmolol, flecainide, glycopyrrolate, hyoscyamine, lidocaine, methoxamine, metoprolol, mexiletine, moricizine, nadolol, oxprenolol, phenytoin, procainamide, propafenone, propranolol, quinidine, scopolamine, sotalol, timolol, tocainide, verapamil.

Antiasthmatics—Medicines used to treat asthma, which may be tablets, liquids or aerosols (to be inhaled to get directly to the bronchial tubes rather than through the bloodstream). These medicines include adrenocorticoids, glucocorticoid; albuterol; aminophylline; beclomethasone; bitolterol; corticotropin; cromolyn; dexamethasone; dyphylline; ephedrine; epinephrine; ethylnorepinephrine; fenoterol; flunisolide; isoetharine; isoproterenol; isoproterenol and phenylephrine; metaproterenol; oxtriphylline; oxtriphylline and guaifenesin; pirbuterol; racepinephrine; terbutaline; theophylline; theophylline and guaifenesin; triamcinolone.

Antibacterials (Antibiotics)—A group of drugs prescribed to treat infections. These drugs include aminocillin, amikacin, amoxicillin, amoxicillin and clavulanate, ampicillin, azlocillin, aztreonam, bacampicillin, carbenicillin, cefaclor, cefadroxil, cefamandole, cefazolin, cefonicid, cefoperazone, ceforanide, cefotaxime, cefotetan, cefoxitin, ceftazidime, ceftizoxime, ceftriaxone, cefuroxime, cephalexin, cephalothin, cephapirin, cephradine, chloramphenicol, cinoxacine, clindamycin, cloxacillin, cyclacillin, cycloserine, demeclocycline, dicloxacillin, doxycycline, erythromycin, erythromycin and sulfisoxazole, flucloxacillin, fusidic acid, gentamicin, imipenem and cilastatin, kanamycin, lincomycin, methacycline, methenamine,

methicillin, metronidazole, mezlocillin, minocycline, moxalactam, nafcillin, nalidixic acid, netilmicin, nitrofurantoin, norfloxacin, oxacillin, oxytetracycline, penicillin G, penicillin V, piperacillin, pivampicillin, rifampin, spectinomycin, streptomycin, sulfacytine, sulfadiazine and trimethoprim, sulfamethoxazole, sulfamethoxazole and trimethoprim, sulfisoxazole, tetracycline, ticarcillin, ticarcillin and clavulanate, tobramycin, trimethoprim, vancomycin.

Antibiotics—Chemicals that inhibit the growth of or kill germs. See Antibacterials.

Anticholinergics—Drugs that work against acetylcholine, a chemical found in many locations in the body, including connections between nerve cells and connections between muscle and nerve cells. Anticholinergic drugs include atropine, belladonna, clidinium, dicyclomine, glycopyrrolate, hyoscyamine, isopropamide, propantheline, scopolamine and tridihexethyl.

Anticoagulants—A family of drugs prescribed to slow the rate of blood-clotting. These drugs include acenocoumarol, anisindione, dicumarol, heparin, warfarin, dihydroergotamine and heparin.

Anticonvulsants—A group of drugs prescribed to treat or prevent seizures (convulsions). These drugs include these families: barbiturates, diones, hydantoins and succinamides. These are the names of the generic drugs in these families: amobarbital, carbamazepine, clonazepam, clorazepate, diazepam, divalproex, ethosuximide, ethotoin, lorazepam, magnesium sulfate, mephenytoin, mephobarbital, metharbital, methsuximide, metocurine, nitrazepam, paraldehyde, paramethadione, pentobarbital, phenobarbital, phensuximide, phenytoin, primidone, secobarbital, trimethadione, tubocurarine, valproic acid.

Antidepressants—A group of medicines prescribed to treat mental depression. These drugs include amitriptyline, amoxapine, clomipramine, desipramine, doxepin, imipramine, isocarboxazid, maprotiline, nortriptyline, phenelzine, protriptyline, tranylcypromine, trazodone, trimipramine.

Antidepressants, MAO (Monamine Oxidase Inhibitors)—A special group of drugs prescribed for mental depression. These are not as popular as in years past because of a relatively high incidence of adverse effects. These drugs include isocarboxazid (Marplan), phenelzine (Nardil), tranylcypromine (Parnate).

Antidepressants, Tricyclic (TCA)—A group of medicines with similar chemical structure and pharmacologic activity used to treat mental depression. These drugs include amitriptyline (Amitril, Apo-Amitriptyline, Elavil, Emitrip, Endep, Levate, Meravil, Novotriptyn); amoxapine (Asendin); clomipramine (Anafranil); desipramine (Pertofrane, Norpramin); doxepin (Adapin, Sinequan, triadapin); imipramine (Apo-Imipramine, Impril, Janimine, Novopramine, Tipramine, Tofranil, Tofranil-PM); nortriptyline (Aventyl, Pamelor); protriptyline (Triptil, Vivactil); trimipramine (Surmontil).

Antidiabetics—A group of drugs used in the treatment of *diabetes mellitus*. These medicines all reduce blood sugar. These drugs include acetohexamide, chlorpropamide, glipizide, glyburide, insulin, metformin, tolazamide, tolbutamide.

Antidiarrheal Preparations—Medicines that treat diarrhea symptoms. Most do not cure the cause. Oral medicines include aluminum hydroxide; charcoal, activated; kaolin and pectin; loperamide; polycarbophil; psyllium hydrophilic mucilloid. Systemic medicines include codeine; difenoxin and atropine; diphenoxylate and atropine; glucose and electrolytes; glycopyrrolate; kaolin, pectin, belladonna alkaloids and opium; kaolin, pectin and paregoric; opium tincture; paregoric.

Antidyskinetics—A group of drugs used for treatment of Parkinsonism (paralysis agitans) and drug-induced extrapyramidal reactions (see elsewhere in Glossary). These drugs include amantadine, benztropine, biperiden, bromocriptine, carbidopa and levodopa, diphenhydramine, ethopropazine, levodopa, levodopa and benserazide.

Antiemetics—A group of drugs used to treat nausea and vomiting. These drugs include buclizine, cyclizine, chlorpromazine, dimenhydrinate, diphenhydramine, diphenidol, domperidone, dronabinol, haloperidol, hydroxyzine, meclizine, metoclopramide, nabilone, perphenazine, prochlorperazine, promethazine, scopolamine, triflupromazine, trimethobenzamide.

Antifibronyltic Drugs—Drugs that are used to treat serious bleeding. These drugs include aminocaproic acid and tranexamic acid.

Antifungals—A group of drugs used to treat fungus infection. Those listed as systemic are taken orally or given by injection. Those listed as topical are applied directly to the skin and include liquids, powders, creams, ointments and liniments. Those listed as vaginal are used topically inside the vagina and sometimes on the vaginal lips. These drugs include Systemic—amphotericin B, miconazole, fluconazole, flucytosine, griseofulvin, ketoconazole, potassium iodide. Topical—carbol-fuchsin; ciclopirox; clioquinol; clotrimazole; econazole;

haloprogin; ketoconzaole; miconazole; nystatin; salicylic acid, sulfur and coal; tolnaftate. Vaginal—butoconazole, clotrimazole, gentian violet, miconazole, nystatin.

Antiglaucoma—Medicines used to treat glaucoma. Those listed as systemic are taken orally or given by injection. Those listed as ophthalmic are used as eye drops. These drugs include Systemic—acetazolamide, dichlorphenamide, glycerin, mannitol, methazolamide, timolol, urea. Ophthalmic—betaxolol, carbachol ophthalmic solution, demecarium, dipivefrin, echothiophate, epinephrine, epinephrine bitartrate, epinephryl borate, isoflurophate, levobunolol, physostigmine, pilocarpine, timolol.

Antigout Drugs—Drugs to treat the metabolic disease called gout. Gout causes recurrent attacks of joint pain caused by deposits of uric acid in the joints. Antigout drugs include allopurinol, carprofen, colchicine, fenoprofen, ibuprofen, indomethacin, ketoprofen, naproxen, phenylbutazone, piroxicam, probenecid, probenecid and colchicine, sulfinpyrazone, sulindac.

Anthelmintics—A family of drugs used to treat intestinal parasites. Names of these drugs include niclosamide, piperazine, pyrantel, pyrvinium, quinacrine, mebendazole, metronidazole, oxamniquine, praziquantel, thiabendazole.

Antihistamines—A family of drugs used to treat allergic conditions, such as hay fever, allergic conjunctivitis, itching, sneezing, runny nose, motion sickness, dizziness, sedation, insomnia and others. These drugs include azatadine (Optimine); brompheniramine (Bromamine, Brombay, Bromphen, Chlorphed, Dehist, Dimetane, Dimetane Extentabs, Dimetane-Ten, Histaject Modified, Nasahist B, ND-Stat Revised, Oraminic II, Veltane); carbinoxamine (Clistin); chlorpheniramine (Aller-Chlor, Allerid-O.D., Chlo-Amine, Chlor-100, Chlor-Mal, Chlor-Niramine, Chlorphen, Chlor-Pro, Chlorspan, Chlortab, Chlor-Trimeton, Chlor-Trimeton Repetabs, Chlor-Tripolon, Hal-Chlor, Histrey, Novopheniram, Phenetron, Phenetron Lanacaps, T.D. Alermine, Teldrin, Trymegen); clemastine (Tavist); cyproheptadine (Periactin); dexchlorpheniramine (Polaramine, Polaramine Repetabs); dimenhydrinate (Apo-Dimenhydrinate, Calm X, Dimentabs, Dinate, Dommanate, Dramamine, Dramilin, Dramocen, Dramoject, Dymenate, Gravol, Hydrate, Marmine, Motion-Aid, Nauseatol, Novodimenate, PMS-Dimenhydrinate, Reidamine, Travamine, Wehamine); diphenhydramine (Beldin, Benadryl, Benadryl Children's Allergy, Benadryl Complete Allergy, Bendylate, Benylin, Compoz, Diahist, Diphen, Diphenadril, Fenylhist, Fynex, Hydramine, Hydril, Insomnal,

Nervine Nighttime Sleep-Aid, Noradryl, Nordryl, Nytol with DPH, Robalyn, Sleep-Eze 3, Sominex Formula 2, Tusstate, Twilite, Valdrene); diphenylpyraline (Hispril); doxylamine (Unisom Nighttime Sleep-Aid); phenindamine (Nolahist); pyrilamine (Dormarex, Somnicaps, Sominex); terfenadine (Seldane); tripelennamine (PBZ, PBZ-SR); triprolidine (Actidil, Bayidyl).

Antihyperammonemias—Medications that decrease the amount of ammonia in the blood. The ones with this pharmacological property that are available in the United States are lactulose and sodium benzoate and sodium phenylacetate.

Antihypertensives—Drugs used to treat high blood pressure. These medicines can be used singly or in combination with other drugs. They work best if accompanied by a low-salt, low-fat diet plus an active exercise program. These drugs include acebutolol, alseroxylon, amiloride, amiloride and hydrochlorothiazide, atenolol, atenolol and chlorthalidone, bendroflumethiazide, benzthiazide, betaxolol, bumetanide, captopril, captopril and hydrochlorothiazide, carteolol, chlorothiazide, chlorthalidone, clonidine, clonidine and chlorthalidone, cyclothiazide, debrisoquine, deserpidine, deserpidine and hydrochlorothiazide, deserpidine and methyclothiazide, diazoxide, diltiazem, doxazosin, enalapril, enalapril and hydrochlorothiazide, ethacrynic acid, furosemide, guanabenz, guanadrel, guanethidine, guanethidine and hydrochlorothiazide, guanfacine, hydralazine, hydralazine and hydrochlorothiazide, hydrochlorothiazide, hydroflumethiazide, indapamide, labetalol, labetalol and hydrochlorothiazide, lisinopril, lisinopril and hydrochlorothiazide, mecamylamine, methyclothiazide, methyldopa, methyldopa and chlorothiazide, methyldopa and hydrochlorothiazide, metolazone, metoprolol, metoprolol and hydrochlorothiazide, minoxidil, nadolol, nadolol and bendroflumethiazide, nicardipine, nifedipine, nitroglycerin, nitroprusside, oxprenolol, pargyline, pargyline and methyclothiazide, penbutolol, pindolol, pindolol and hydrochlorothiazide, polythiazide, prazosin, prazosin and polythiazide, propranolol, propranolol and hydrochlorothiazide, quinethazone, rauwolfia serpentina, rauwolfia serpentina and bendroflumethazide, reserpine, reserpine and chlorothiazide, reserpine and chlorthalidone, reserpine and hydralazine, reserpine, hydralazine and hydrochlorothiazide, reserpine and hydrochlorothiazide, reserpine and hydroflumethiazide, reserpine and methyclothiazide, reserpine and polythiazide, reserpine and quinethazone, reserpine and trichlormethiazide, sotalol, spironolactone, spironolactone and hydrochlorothiazide, terazosin, timolol, timolol and hydrochlorothiazide, triamterene, triamterene and hydrochlorothiazide, trichlormethiazide, trimethaphan, verapamil.

Anti-Inflammatory Drugs, Non-Steroidal (NSAIDs)—A family of drugs not related to cortisone or other steroids that decrease inflammation wherever it occurs in the body. Used for treatment of pain, fever, arthritis, gout, menstrual cramps and vascular headaches. These drugs include aspirin; aspirin, alumina and magnesia tablets; buffered aspirin; bufexamac; choline salicylate; choline and magnesium salicylates; diflunisal; fenoprofen; ibuprofen; indomethacin; ketoprofen; magnesium salicylate; meclofenamate; naproxen; piroxicam; salsalate; sodium salicylate; sulindac; tolmetin.

Anti-Inflammatory, Steroidal—A family of drugs with similar pharmacologic characteristics of cortisone and cortisone-like drugs. They are used for many purposes to help the body deal with inflammation no matter what the cause. Steroidal drugs may be used orally or by injection (systemic), as local applications for the skin, eyes, ears, bronchial tubes (topical), and for others. These drugs include Nasal—beclomethasone, dexamethasone, flunisolide. Ophthalmic (eyes)—betamethasone, dexamethasone, fluorometholone, hydrocortisone, medrysone, prednisolone. Otic (ears)—betamethasone, desonide and acetic acid, dexamethasone, hydrocortisone, hydrocortisone and acetic acid, prednisolone. Systemic—betamethasone, corticotroprin, cortisone, dexamethasone, hydrocortisone, methylprednisolone, paramethasone, prednisolone, prednisone, triamcinolone. Topical—alclometasone; amcinonide; beclomethasone; betamethasone; clobetasol; clobetasone; clocortolone; desonide; desoximetasone; dexamethasone; diflorasone; diflucortolone; flumethasone; fluocinolone; fluocinonide; fluocinonide, procinonide and ciprocinonide; flurandrenolid; halcinonide; hydrocortisone; methylprednisolone; mometasone; triamcinolone.

Antimalarials (also called Antiprotozoals)—A group of drugs used to treat malaria. The choice depends on the precise type of malaria organism and its developmental state. These drugs include amphotericin B, chloroquine, dapsone, demeclocycline, doxycycline, hydroxychloroquine, iodoquinol, methacycline, mefloquine, metronidazole, minocycline, oxytetracycline, pentamidine, primaquine, pyrimethamine, quinacrine, quinidine, quinine, sulfadoxine and pyrimethamine, sulfamethoxazole, sulfamethoxazole and trimethoprim, sulfisoxazole, tetracycline.

Antimuscarines—Drugs that block the muscarinic action of acetylcholine and therefore decrease spasm of smooth muscles. They are prescribed for peptic ulcers, dysmenorrhea, dizziness, seasickness, bedwetting, slow heart rate, treatment of toxicity from pesticides made from organophosphates, and other medical problems. These drugs include anisotropine, atropine, belladonna, clidinium dicyclomine, glycopyrrolate, homatropine, hyoscyamine, hyoscyamine and scopolamine, isopropamide, mepenzolate, methantheline, methscopolamine, oxyphencyclimine, pirenzepine, propantheline, scopolamine, tridihexethyl.

Antimyasthenics—Medicines to treat myasthenia gravis, a muscle disorder (especially of the face and head) with increasing fatigue and weakness as muscles tire from use. These medicines include ambenonium, azathioprine, neostigmine, pyridostigmine.

Antineoplastics—Potent drugs used for malignant disease, they are listed here for completeness. Some of these are *not* described in this book. These drugs include Systemic— aminoglutethimide, amsacrine, antithyroid agents, asparaginase, azathioprine, bleomycin, busulfan, carboplatin, carmustine, chlorambucil, chloramphenicol, chlorotrianisene, chromic phosphate, cisplatin, colchicine, cyclophosphamide, cyclosporine, cyproterone, cytarabine, dacarbazine, dactinomycin, daunorubicin, deferoxamine, diethylstilbestrol, doxorubicin, dromostanolone, epirubicin, estradiol, estradiol valerate, estramustine, estrogens (conjugated and esterified), estrone, ethinyl estradiol, etoposide, floxuridine, flucytosine, fluorouracil, flutamide, fluoxymesterone, gold compounds, hexamethylmelamine, hydroxyprogesterone, hydroxyurea, interferon alfa-2a and alfa-2b (recombinant), ketoconazole, leuprolide, levamisole, levothyroxine, liothyronine, liotrix, lithium, lomustine, mechlorethamine, medroxyprogesterone, megestrol, melphalan, methyltestosterone, mercaptopurine, methotrexate, mitomycin, mitotane, mitoxantrone, nandrolone phenpropionate, penicillamine, plicamycin, procarbazine, sodium iodide I 131, sodium phosphate P 32, streptozocin, tamoxifen, teniposide, testolactone, testosterone, thioguanine, thiotepa, thyroglobulin, thyroid, thyrotropin, uracil mustard, vinblastine, vincristine, vindesine, zidovudine. Topical— fluorouracil, mechlorethamine.

Antiparkisonism Drugs—Drugs used to treat Parkinson's Disease. A disease of the central nervous system in older adults, it is characterized by gradual progressive muscle rigidity, tremors and clumsiness. These drugs include amantadine, benztropine, biperiden, bromocriptine, carbidopa and levodopa, diphenhydramine, ethopropazine, levodopa, levodopa and benserazide, orphenadrine, pergolide, procyclidine, seligiline, trihexyphenidyl.

Antipsychotic—A group of drugs used to treat the mental disease of psychosis, such as schizophrenia, manic-depressive illness, anxiety states, severe behavior problems and others. These drugs include acetophenazine, carbamazepine, chlorpromazine, chlorprothixene, fluphenazine, flupenthixol, fluspirilene, haloperidol, loxapine, mesoridazine, methotrimeprazine, molindone, pericyazine, perphenazine, pimozide, pipotiazine, prochlorperazine, promazine, thioproperazine, thioridazine, thiothixene, trifluoperazine, triflupromazine.

Antithyroid Drugs—These drugs decrease the amount of thyroid hormone produced by the thyroid gland.

Antitussive—A group of drugs used to suppress cough. These drugs include chlophedianol, codeine (oral), dextromethorphan, diphenhydramine syrup, hydrocodone, hydromorphone, methadone, morphine.

Antiulcer—A group of medicines used to treat peptic ulcer in the stomach, duodenum or the lower end of the esophagus. These drugs include antacids, anticholinergics, antispasmotics, cimetidine, doxepin, famotidine, omeprazole, ranitidine, sucralfate, trimipramine.

Antiurolithics—Medicines that prevent the formation of kidney stones.

Antiviral—A group of drugs to treat viral infection. These drugs include Ophthalmic (eye)—idoxuridine, trifluridine, vidarabine. Systemic—acyclovir, amantadine, ribavirin, zidovudine. Topical—acyclovir.

Appendicitis—Inflammation or infection of the appendix. Symptoms include loss of appetite, nausea, low-grade fever and tenderness in the lower right of the abdomen.

Appetite Suppressants—A group of drugs used to decrease the appetite as part of an overall treatment for obesity. These drugs include benzphetamine, diethylpropion, fenfluramine, mazindol, phendimetrazine, phenmetrazine, phentermine, phenylpropanolamine.

Artery—Blood vessel carrying blood away from the heart.

Asthma—Recurrent attacks of breathing difficulty due to spasms and contractions of the bronchial tubes.

Attentuated Virus Vaccines—Liquid products of killed germs used for injections to prevent certain diseases.

B

Bacteria—Microscopic organism. Some bacteria contribute to health; others (germs) cause disease.

Barbiturates—Powerful drugs used for sedation, to help induce sleep and sometimes to prevent seizures. Except for use in seizures (phenobarbital), barbiturates are being used less and less because there are better, less hazardous drugs that produce the same or better effects. These drugs include amobarbital, aprobarbital, butabarbital, mephobarbital, metharbital, pentobarbital, phenobarbital, secobarbital, secobarbital and amobarbital, talbutal.

Basal Area of Brain—Part of the brain that regulates muscle control and tone.

Beta Agonists—A group of drugs that act directly on cells in the body (beta-adrenergic receptors) to relieve spasm of the bronchial tubes and other organs consisting of smooth muscles. These drugs include albuterol, bitolerol, isoetharine, isoproterenol, methproterenol, terbutaline.

Beta Blockers (Beta-Adrenergic Blocking Agents)—A family of drugs with similar pharmacological actions with some variations. These drugs are prescribed for angina, heartbeat irregularities (arrhythmias), high blood pressure, hypertrophic subaortic stenosis, vascular headaches (as a preventative, not to treat once the pain begins), and others. Timolol is prescribed for treatment of open-angle glaucoma. These drugs include acebutolol (Monitan, Sectral); atenolol (Esmolol); labetalol (Normodyne, Trandate); metoprolol (Apo-Metoprolol, Betaloc, Betaloc Durules, Lopresor, Lopresor SR, Lopressor, Novometoprol); nadolol (Corgard); oxprenolol (Trasicor, Slow-Trasicor); pindolol (Visken); propranolol (Apo-Propranolol, Detensol, Inderal, Inderal LA, Novopranol, pms-Propranolol); sotalol (Sotacor); timolol (Blocadren).

Benzodiazepines—A family of drugs prescribed to treat anxiety, alcohol withdrawal, and sometimes for sedation. These drugs include alprazolam, bromazepam, chlordiazepoxide, clonazepam, clorazepate, diazepam, flurazepam, halazepam, ketazolam, lorazepam, midazolam, nitrazepam, oxazepam, prazepam, temazepam, triazolam.

Blood Count—Laboratory studies to count white blood cells, red blood cells, platelets and other elements of the blood.

Blood Dyscrasia-Causing Medicines—Drugs which cause unpredictable damaging effects to human bone marrow. These effects occur in a small minority of patients and are not dependent upon dosage. These medicines include the following (some of which are *not* described in this book): ACE inhibitors, anticonvulsants (dione, hydantoin, succinimide), antidepressants (tricyclic), antidiabetic agents (oral), anti-inflammatory analgesics, carbamazepine, chloramphenicol, dapsone, divalproex, ethosuximide, ethotoin, flecainide acetate, gold compounds, haloperidol, loxapine, maprotiline, mephenytoin, meth-suximide, mezlocillin, oxyphenbutazone, penicillins (some), penicillamine, phenothia-zines, phensuximide, phenytoin, primidone, procainamide, pyrimethamine (large doses), rifampin, sulfasalazine, thioxanthenes, tocainide, trimethoprim, valproic acid.

Blood Pressure, Diastolic—Pressure (usually recorded in millimeters of mercury) in the large arteries of the body when the heart muscle is relaxed and filling for the next contraction.

Blood Pressure, Systolic—Pressure (usually recorded in millimeters of mercury) in the large arteries of the body at the instant the heart muscle contracts.

Blood Sugar (Blood Glucose)—Necessary element in the blood to sustain life.

Bone Marrow Depressants—Medicines that affect the bone marrow to depress the normal function of forming blood cells. These medicines include the following (some of which are *not* described in this book): amophotericin B (systemic), anticancer drugs, anthithyroid drugs, azathioprine, busulfan, carboplatin, carmustine, chlorambucil, chloramphenicol, chromic phosphate, cisplatin, colchicine, cyclophosphamide, cytarabine, dacarbazine, dactinomycin, daunorubicin, doxorubicin, etoposide, floxuridine, flucytosine, fluorouracil, ganciclovir, hydroxyurea, ifos-famide, interferon, lomustine, mechlorethamine, melphalan, mercaptopurine, methotrexate, mitomycin, mitoxantrone, pentamidine, phenyl-butazone, plicamycin, procarbazine, rifampin, streptozocin, sulfa drugs, thioguanine, thiotepa, tocainide, trimethoprim, uracil mustard, vinblastine, vincristine, zidovudine.

Bone Marrow Depression—Many drugs taken for long periods of time in high doses can cause toxicity to the blood-producing capacity of human bone marrow.

Brain Depressants—Any drug that depresses brain function, such as tranquilizers, narcotics, alcohol, barbiturates.

Bronchodilators—A group of drugs used to dilate the bronchial tubes to treat such problems as asthma, emphysema, bronchitis, bronchiec-tasis, allergies and others. These drugs include albuterol, aminophylline, bitolterol, dyphilline, ephedrine, epinephrine, ethylnorepinephrine, fenoterol, ipratropium, isoetharine, isoproterenol, metaproterenol, oxtriphylline, oxtriphylline and guaifenesin, terbutaline, theophylline, theophylline and guaifenesin.

Bronchodilators, Xanthine Derivative—Drugs of similar chemical structure and pharmacological activity. They are prescribed to dilate bronchial tubes in disorders such as asthma, bronchitis, emphysema and other chronic lung diseases. These drugs include aminophylline, dyphylline, oxtriphylline, theophylline.

C

Calcium Channel Blockers—A group of drugs used to treat angina and heartbeat irregularities. These drugs include bepridril, diltiazem, felodipine, isradipine, nifedipine, nimodipine, quinapril, verapamil.

Calcium Supplements—Supplements used to increase calcium concentration in the blood in an attempt to make bones denser (as in osteoporosis). These supplements include calcium citrate, calcium glubionate, calcium gluconate, calcium glycerophosphate and calcium lactate, calcium lactate, dibasic calcium phosphate, tribasic calcium phosphate.

Carbonic Anhydrase Inhibitors—Drugs used to treat glaucoma, seizures and prevent high altitude sickness. They include acetazolamide, dichlorphenamide, methazolamid.

Cataract—Loss of transparency in the lens of the eye.

Cell—Unit of protoplasm, the essential living matter of all plants and animals.

Central Nervous System (CNS) Depressants—These drugs cause sedation or otherwise diminish brain activity and other parts of the nervous system. These drugs include alcohol, aminoglutethimide, anesthetics (general and injection-local), anticonvulsants, antidepressants (MAO inhibitors, TCA), antidyskinetics (except amantadine), antihistamines, apomorphine, baclofen, barbiturates, benzodiazepines, buclizine, carbamazepine, chlophedianol, chloral hydrate, chlorzoxazone, clonidine, cyclizine, difenoxin and atropine, diphenoxylate and atropine, disulfiram, dronabinol, ethchlorvynol, ethinamate, etomidate, fenfluramine, flavoxate, glutethimide, guanabenz, guanfacine, haloperidol, hydroxyzine, interferon, loxapine, magnesium sulfate (injection), maprotiline, meclizine, meprobamate, methyldopa, methyprylon, metoclopramide, metyrosine, mitotane, molindone, opioid (narcotic) analgesics, oxybutynin, paraldehyde, paregoric, pargyline, phenothiazines, pimozide, procarbazine, promethazine, propiomazine, rauwolfia alkaloids, scopolamine, skeletal muscle relaxants (centrally acting), thioxanthenes, trazodone, trimeprazine, trimethobenzamide.

Central Nervous System (CNS) Stimulants—Drugs that cause excitation, anxiety, nervousness or otherwise stimulate the brain and other parts of the central nervous system. These drugs include amantadine, amphetamines, anesthetics (local), appetite suppressants (except fenfluramine), bronchodilators (xanthine-derivative), caffeine, chlophedianol, cocaine, doxapram, methylphenidate, pemoline, sympathomimetics.

Cephalosporin—Antibiotic that kills many bacterial germs that penicillin and sulfa drugs can't destroy.

Cholinergic (Parasympathomimetic)—Chemical that facilitates passage of nerve impulses through the parasympathetic nervous system.

Cholinesterase Inhibitors—Drugs that prevent the action of cholinesterase (an enzyme that breaks down acetylcholine in the body).

Chronic—Long-term, continuing. Chronic illnesses may not be curable, but they can often be prevented from becoming worse. Symptoms usually can be alleviated or controlled.

Cirrhosis—Disease that scars and destroys liver tissue.

Citrates—Medicines taken orally to make urine more acid. Citrates include potassium citrate, potassium citrate and citric acid, potassium citrate and sodium citrate, sodium citrate and citric acid, tricitrates.

Coal Tar Preparations—Creams, ointments and lotions used on the skin for various skin ailments.

Cold Urticaria—Hives that appear in areas of the body exposed to the cold.

Colitis, Ulcerative—Chronic, recurring ulcers of the colon for unknown reasons.

Collagen—Support tissue of skin, tendon, bone, cartilage and connective tissue.

Colostomy—Surgical opening from the colon, the large intestine, to the outside of the body.

Congestive—Characterized by excess accumulation of blood. In congestive heart failure, congestion occurs in the lungs, liver, kidney and other parts of the body to cause shortness of breath, swelling of the ankles and feet, rapid heartbeat and other symptoms.

Constriction—Tightness or pressure.

Contraceptives, Oral (Birth Control Pills)—A group of hormones used to prevent ovulation, therefore preventing pregnancy. These hormones include ethynodiol diacetate and ethinyl estradiol, ethynodiol diacetate and mestranol, levonorgestrel and ethinyl estradiol, medroxyprogesterone, norethindrone tablets, norethindrone acetate and ethinyl estradiol, norethindrone and ethinyl estradiol, norethindrone and mestranol, norethynodrel and mestranol, norgestrel, norgestrel and ethinyl estradiol.

Contraceptives, Vaginal—Topical medications or devices applied inside the vagina to prevent pregnancy.

Convulsions—Violent, uncontrollable contractions of the voluntary muscles.

Corticosteroid (Adrenocorticosteroid)—Steroid hormones produced by the body's adrenal cortex or their synthetic equivalents.

Cortisone (Adrenocorticoids, Glucocorticoids) and Other Adrenal Steroids—Medicines that mimic the action of the steroid hormone cortisone, manufactured in the cortex of the adrenal gland. These drugs decrease the effects of inflammation within the body. They are available for injection, oral use, topical use for the skin and nose and inhalation for the bronchial tubes. These drugs include alclometasone; amcinonide; beclomethasone; benzyl benzoate; betamethasone; bismuth; clobetasol; clobetasone 17-butyrate; clocortolone; cortisone; desonide; desoximetasone; desoxycorticosterone; dexamethasone; diflorasone; diflucortolone; fludrocortisone; flumethasone; flunisolide; fluocinonide; fluocinonide, procinonide and ciprocinonide; fluorometholone; fluprednisolone, flurandrenolide; halcinonide; hydrocortisone; medrysone; methylprednisolone; mometasone; paramethasone; peruvian balsam; prednisolone; prednisone; triamcinolone; zinc oxide.

Cyclopegics—Eye drops that prevent the pupils from accommodating to varying degrees of light.

Cystitis—Inflammation of the urinary bladder.

D

Decongestants—Drugs used to open nasal passages by shrinking swollen lining membranes in the nose. These drugs include Cough-suppressing—phenylephrine and dextromethorphan, phenylpropanolamine and caramiphen, phenylpropanolamine and dextromethorphan, phenylpropanolamine and hydrocodone, pseudoephedrine and codeine, pseudoephedrine and dextromethorphan, pseudoephedrine and hydrocodone. Cough-suppressing and pain-relieving—phenylpropanolamine, dextromethorphan and acetaminophen. Cough-suppressing and sputum-thinning—phenylephrine, dextromethorphan and guaifenesin; phenylephrine, hydrocodone and guaifenesin; phenylpropanolamine, codeine and guaifenesin; phenylpropanolamine, dextromethorphan and guaifenesin;

pseudoephedrine, codeine and guaifenesin; pseudoephedrine, dextromethorphan and guaifenesin; pseudoephedrine, hydrocodone and guaifenesin; phenylephrine, dextromethorphan, guaifenesin and acetaminophen; pseudo-ephedrine, dextromethorphan, guaifenesin and acetaminophen. Sputum-thinning—ephedrine and guaifenesin; ephedrine and potassium iodide; phenylephrine, phenylpropanolamine and guaifenesin; phenylpropanolamine and guaifenesin; pseudoephedrine and guaifenesin. Nasal—ephedrine (oral), phenylpropanolamine, pseudoephedrine. Ophthalmic (eye)—naphazoline, oxymetazoline, phenylephrine. Topical—oxymetazoline, phenylephrine, xylometazoline.

Delirium—Temporary mental disturbance characterized by hallucinations, agitation and incoherence.

Diabetes—Metabolic disorder in which the body can't use carbohydrates efficiently. This leads to a dangerously high level of glucose (a carbohydrate) in the blood.

Dialysis—Procedure to filter waste products from the bloodstream of patients with kidney failure.

Digitalis Preparations (Digitalis Glycosides)—Important drugs to treat heart disease, such as congestive heart failure, heartbeat irregularities and cardiogenic shock. These drugs include deslanoside (Cedilanid); powdered digitalis (Crystodigin); digoxin (Lanoxin, Lanoxicaps).

Digoxin—One of the digitalis drugs used to treat heart disease. All digitalis products were originally derived from the foxglove plant.

Dilation—Enlargement.

Disulfiram Reaction—Disulfiram (Antabuse) is a drug to treat alcoholism. When alcohol in the bloodstream interacts with disulfiram, it causes a flushed face, severe headache, chest pains, shortness of breath, nausea, vomiting, sweating and weakness. Severe reactions may cause death. A disulfiram reaction is the interaction of any drug with alcohol or another drug to produce these symptoms.

Diuretics—Drugs that act on the kidneys to prevent reabsorption of electrolytes, especially chlorides. They are used to treat edema, high blood pressure, congestive heart failure, kidney and liver failure and others. These drugs include amiloride, amiloride and hydrochlorothiazide, bendroflumethiazide, benzthiazide, bumetanide, chlorothiazide, chlorthalidone, cyclothiazide, ethacrynic acid, furosemide, glycerin, hydrochlorothiazide, hydroflumethiazide, indapamide, mannitol, methyclothiazide, metolazone, polythiazide, quinethazone, spironolactone, sprionolactone and hydrochlorothiazide, triamterene, triamterene and hydrochlorothiazide, trichlormethiazide, urea.

Diuretics, Loop—Drugs that act on the kidneys to prevent reabsorption of electrolytes, especially chlorides. They are used to treat edema, high blood pressure, congestive heart failure, kidney and liver failure and others. These drugs include bumetanide, ethacrynic acid, furosemide.

Diuretics, Thiazide—Drugs that act on the kidneys to prevent reabsorption of electrolytes, especially chlorides. They are used to treat edema, high blood pressure, congestive heart failure, kidney and liver failure and others. These drugs include bendroflumethiazide (Naturetin); benzthiazide (Aquatag, Exna, Hydrex); chlorothiazide (Diuril); chlorthalidone (Apo-Chlorthalidone, Hygroton, Novothalidone, Thalitone, Uridon); cyclothiazide (Anhydron, Fluidil); hydrochlorothiazide (Apo-Hydro, Diuchlor H, Esidrix, Hydrochlorothiazide Intensol, HydroDIURIL, Mictrin, Natrimax, Neo-Codema, Novohydrazide, Oretic, Thiuretic, Urozide); hydroflumethiazide (Diucardin, Saluron); methyclothiazide (Aquatensen, Duretic, Enduron); metolazone (Diulo, Zaroxolyn); polythiazide (Renese); quinethazone (Aquamox, Hydromox); trichlormethiazide (Metahydrin, Naqua).

Diuretics, Potassium-Sparing—Drugs that act on the kidneys to prevent reabsorption of electrolytes, especially chlorides. They are used to treat edema, high blood pressure, congestive heart failure, kidney and liver failure and others. This particular group of diuretics does not allow the unwanted side effect of low potassium in the blood to occur. These drugs include amiloride, spironolactone, triamterene.

Duodenum—The first 12 inches of the small intestine.

E

ECG (or EKG)—Abbreviation for electrocardiogram or electrocardiograph. An ECG is a graphic tracing representing the electrical current produced by impulses passing through the heart muscle. This is a useful test in the diagnosis of heart disease, but used alone it usually can't make a complete diagnosis. An ECG is most useful in two areas: (1) demonstrating heart rhythm disturbances and (2) demonstrating changes when there is a myocardial infarction (heart attack). It will detect enlargement of either heart chamber, but will not establish a diagnosis of heart failure or disease of the heart valves.

Eczema—Disorder of the skin with redness, itching, blisters, weeping and abnormal pigmentation.

EEG—Electroencephalogram or electro-encephalograph. An EEG is a graphic recording of electrical activity generated spontaneously from nerve cells in the brain. This test is useful in the diagnosis of brain dysfunction, particularly in studying seizure disorders.

Electrolyte—Substance that can transmit electrical impulses when dissolved in body fluids.

Embolism—Sudden blockage of an artery by a clot or foreign material in the blood.

Emphysema—Disease in which the lung's air sacs lose elasticity and air accumulates in the lungs.

Endometriosis—Condition in which uterus tissue is found outside the uterus. Can cause pain, abnormal menstruation and infertility.

Enzyme—Protein chemical that can accelerate a chemical reaction in the body.

Epilepsy—Episodes of brain disturbance that cause convulsions and loss of consciousness.

Ergot Preparations—Medicines used to treat migraine and other types of throbbing headaches. Also used after delivery of babies to make the uterus clamp down and reduce excessive bleeding.

Erythromycins—A group of drugs with similar structure used to treat infections. These drugs include erythromycin (Eryc, Eryc Sprinkle, Erythromid, Novorythro, E-Mycin, Ery-Tab, Ilotycin, PCE Dispersatabs, Robimycin, RP-Mycin); erythromycin estolate (Ilosone, Novorythro); erythromycin ethylsuccinate (E.E.S., E-Mycin E, Pediamycin, Wyamycin E, EryPed); erythromycin gluceptate (Ilotycin); erythromycin lactobionate (Erythrocin); erythromycin stearate (ApoErythro-S).

Esophagitis—Inflammation of the lower part of the esophagus, the tube connecting the throat and the stomach.

Estrogens—Female hormones used to replenish the body's stores after the ovaries have been removed or become non-functional after menopause. Also used with progesterone in some birth control pills and for other purposes. These drugs include: Systemic—chlorotrianisene, diethylstilbestrol, estradiol, estrogens (conjugated and esterified), estrone, estropipate, ethinyl estradiol, quinestrol. Vaginal— dienestrol, estradiol, estrogens (conjugated), estrone, estropipate.

Eustachian Tube—Small passage from the middle ear to the sinuses and nasal passages.

Extrapyramidal Reactions—Drugs that may cause abnormal reactions in the power and coordination of posture and muscular movements. Movements are not under voluntary control. Some drugs associated with producing extrapyramidal reactions include antidepressants (tricyclic), droperidol, haloperidol, loxapine, methyldopa, metoclopramide, metyrosine, molindone, pemoline, phenothiazines, pimozide, rauwolfia alkaloids, thioxanthenes.

Extremity—Arm, leg, hand or foot.

F

Fecal Impaction—Condition in which feces become firmly wedged in the rectum.

Fibrocystic Breast Disease—Overgrowth of fibrous tissue in the breast, producing non-malignant cysts.

Fibroid Tumors—Non-malignant tumors of the muscular layer of the uterus.

Flu (Influenza)—A virus infection of the respiratory tract that lasts three to ten days. Symptoms include headache, fever, runny nose, cough, tiredness and muscle aches.

Fluoroquinolones—A class of drugs used to treat bacterial infections, such as urinary tract infections and some types of bronchitis. These drugs include ciprofloxacin, enoxacin, lomefloxacin, norfloxacin and ofloxacin.

Folliculitis—Inflammation of a follicle.

G

G6PD—Deficiency of glucose 6-phosphate, necessary for glucose metabolism.

Ganglionic Blockers—Medicines that block the passage of nerve impulses through a part of the nerve cell called a ganglion. Ganglionic blockers are used to treat urinary retention and other medical problems. Bethanechol is one of the best ganglionic blockers.

Gastritis—Inflammation of the stomach.

Gastrointestinal—Stomach and intestinal tract.

Gland—Organ that manufactures and excretes materials not required for its own metabolic needs.

Glaucoma—Eye disease in which increased pressure inside the eye damages the optic nerve, causes pain and changes vision.

Glucagon—Injectable drug that immediately elevates blood sugar by mobilizing glycogen from the liver.

Gold Compounds—Medicines which use gold as their base and are usually used to treat joint or arthritic disorders. These medicines include auranofin, aurothioglucose, gold sodium thiomalate.

H

H₂ Antagonists—Antihistamines that work against H₂ histamine. H₂ histamine may be liberated at any point in the body, but most often in the skin, bronchial tubes and gastrointestinal tract.

Hangover Effect—The same feelings as a "hangover" after too much alcohol consumption. Symptoms include headache, irritability and nausea.

Hemochromatosis—Disorder of iron metabolism in which excessive iron is deposited in and damages body tissues, particularly liver and pancreas.

Hemoglobin—Pigment that carries oxygen in red blood cells.

Hemolytics—Drugs that separate hemoglobin from the blood cells. These include acetohydroxamic acid, antidiabetic agents (oral), doxapram, furazolidone, methyldopa, nitrofurans, primaquine, procainamide, quinidine, quinine, sulfonamides (systemic), sulfones, vitamin K.

Hemorrhage—Heavy bleeding.

Hemorrheologic Agents—Medicines to help control bleeding.

Hemosiderosis—Increase of iron deposits in body tissues without tissue damage.

Hepatitis—Inflammation of liver cells, usually accompanied by jaundice.

Hepatotoxics—Medications that can possibly cause toxicity or decreased normal function of the liver. These drugs include the following (some of which are *not* described in this book): alcohol, amiodarone, anabolic steroids, androgens, antithyroid agents, asparaginase, azlocillin, carbamazepine, carmustine, dantrolene, daunorubicin, disulfiram, divalproex, erythromycins, estrogens, etretinate, gold compounds, halothane, isoniazid, ketoconazole (oral), mercaptopurine, methotrexate, methyldopa, mezlocillin, naltrexone, phenothiazines, phenytoin, piperacillin, plicamycin, rifampin, sulfonamides, testosterone, valproic acid.

Hiatal Hernia—Section of stomach that protrudes into the chest cavity.

Histamine—Chemical in body tissues that dilates the smallest blood vessels, constricts the smooth muscle surrounding the bronchial tubes and stimulates stomach secretions.

History—Past medical events in a patient's life.

Hives—Elevated patches on the skin that are redder or paler than surrounding skin and often itch severely.

Hormone—Chemical substance produced in the body to regulate other body functions.

Hypercalcemia—Too much calcium in the blood. This happens with some malignancies and in calcium overdose.

Hyperkalemia-Causing Medications—Medicines that cause too much potassium in the bloodstream. These include ACE inhibitors; anti-inflammatory analgesics, non-steroidal (NSAIAs); beta-adrenergic blocking agents;

cyclosporine; digitalis glycosides; diuretics (potassium-sparing); succinylcholine chloride; possibly any medicine that is combined with ptoassium.

Hypersensitivity—Serious reactions to many medications. The effects of hypersensitivity may be characterized by wheezing, shortness of breath, rapid heart rate, severe itching, faintness, unconsciousness and severe drop in blood pressure.

Hypertension—High blood pressure.

Hypervitaminosis—A condition due to an excess of one or more vitamins. Symptoms may include weakness, fatigue, loss of hair and changes in the skin.

Hypnotics—Drugs used to induce a sleeping state. See Barbiturates.

Hypocalcemia—Abnormally low level of calcium in the blood.

Hypoglycemia—Low blood sugar (blood glucose). A critically low blood-sugar level will interfere with normal brain function and can damage the brain permanently.

Hypoglycemics, Oral—Drugs that reduce blood sugar. These include insulin, acetohexamide, chlorpropamide, glipizide, glyburide, metformin, tolazamide, tolbutamide.

Hypokalemia-Causing Medications—Medicines that cause a depletion of potassium in the bloodstream. These include adrenocorticoids (systemic), alcohol, amphotericin B (systemic), carbonic anhydrase inhibitors, diuretics (loop and thiazide), insulin, laxatives (if dependent on), penicillins (some), salicylates, sodium bicarbonate, urea, vitamin D (overdose of).

Hypotension—Blood pressure decreased below normal. Symptoms may include weakness, lightheadedness, dizziness. Some medications that might cause hypotension include alcohol, alprostadil, amantadine, anesthetics (general), angiotensin-converting enzyme inhibitors (ACE inhibitors), antidepressants (MAO inhibitors, tricyclic), antihypertensives, benzodiazepines used as preanesthetics, beta-adrenergic blocking agents, bromocriptine, calcium channel-blocking agents, captopril, diuretics, edetate calcium disodium, edetate disodium, enalapril, encainide, haloperidol, hydralazine, levodopa, lidocaine (systemic), loxapine, maprotiline, molindone, nitrates, nitrites, opioid analgesics (including fentanil, fentanyl and sufentanil), pentamidine, phenothiazines, pimozide, prazosin, procainamide, quinidine, radiopaques (materials used in x-ray studies), thioxanthenes, tocainide, trazodone. If you take any of these medications, be sure to tell a dentist, anesthesiologist or anyone else who intends to give you an anesthetic to put you to sleep.

Hypothermia-Causing Medications—Medicines that can cause a significant lowering of body temperature. These drugs include alcohol, alpha-adrenergic blocking agents, barbiturates (large amounts), beta-adrenergic blocking agents, clonidine, insulin, lithium, magnesium sulfate, minoxidil, narcotic analgesics, vasodilators.

I

Ichthyosis—Skin disorder with dryness, scaling and roughness.

Ileitis—Inflammation of the ileum, the last section of the small intestine.

Ileostomy—Surgical opening from the ileum, the end of the small intestine, to the outside of the body.

Immunosuppressants—Powerful drugs that suppress the immune system. Immunosuppressants are used in patients who have had organ transplants or severe disease associated with the immune system. These drugs include the following (some of which are *not* described in this book): azathioprine, betamethasone, chlorambucil, corticotropin, cortisone, cyclophosphamide, cyclosporine, dexamethasone, hydrocortisone, mercaptopurine, methylprednisolone, muromonab, muromonab-CD3, paramethasone, prednisolone, prednisone, triamcinolone.

Impotence—Male's inability to achieve or sustain erection of the penis for sexual intercourse.

Insomnia—Sleeplessness.

Interaction—Change in the body's response to one drug when another is taken. Interaction may decrease the effect of one or both drugs, decrease the effect of one or both drugs, or cause toxicity.

Iron Supplements—Products that contain iron in a form that can be absorbed from the intestinal tract. Supplements include ferrous fumarate, ferrous gluconate, ferrous sulfate, iron dextran, iron-polysaccharide.

J

Jaundice—Symptoms of liver damage, bile obstruction or destruction of red blood cells. Symptoms include yellowed whites of the eyes, yellow skin, dark urine and light stool.

K

Keratosis—Growth that is an accumulation of cells from the outer skin layers.

Kidney Stones—Small, solid stones made from calcium, cholesterol, cysteine and other body chemicals.

L

Laxatives—Medicines prescribed to treat constipation. These medicines include bisacodyl;

bisacodyl and docusate; casanthranol; casanthranol and docusate; cascara sagrada; cascara sagrada and aloe; cascara sagrada and phenolphthalein; castor oil; danthron; danthron and docusate; danthron and poloxamer 188; dehydrocholic acid; dehydrocholic acid and docusate; docusate; docusate and phenolphthalein; docusate and mineral oil; docusate and phenolphthalein; docusate, carboxymethylcellulose and casanthranol glycerin; lactulose; magnesium citrate; magnesium hydroxide; magnesium hydroxide and mineral oil; magnesium oxide; magnesium sulfate; malt soup extract; malt soup extract and psyllium; methylcellulose; mineral oil; mineral oil and cascara sagrada; mineral oil and phenolphthalein; mineral oil, glycerin and phenolphthalein; phenolphthalein; poloxamer; polycarbophil; potassium bitartrate and sodium bicarbonate; psyllium; psyllium and senna; psyllium hydrophilic mucilloid; psyllium hydrophilic mucilloid and carboxymethylcellulose; psyllium hydrophilic mucilloid and sennosides; psyllium hydrophilic musilloid and senna; senna; senna and docusate; sennosides; sodium phosphate.

Lincomycins—A family of antibiotics used to treat certain infections. These antibiotics include erythromycin, erythromycin estolate, erythromycin ethylsuccinate, erythromycin glucaptate, erythromycin lactobionate, erythromycin stearate.

Low-Purine Diet—A diet that avoids high-purine foods, such as liver, sweetbreads, kidneys, sardines, oysters and others. If you need a low-purine diet, request instructions from your doctor.

Lupus—Serious disorder of connective tissue that primarily affects women. Varies in severity with skin eruptions, joint inflammation, low white blood cell count and damage to internal organs, especially the kidney.

Lymph Glands—Glands in the lymph vessels throughout the body that trap foreign and infectious matter and protect the bloodstream from infection.

M

MAO Inhibitors—Drugs that prevent the activity of the enzyme monoamine oxidase (MAO) in brain tissue, thus affecting mood. MAO inhibitors include antidepressants, the use of which is frequently restricted because of severe side effects. These side effects may be interactions with other drugs (such as ephedrine or amphetamine) or foods containing tyramine (such as cheese) and may produce a sudden increase in blood pressure. MAOs include isocarboxazid, pargyline, phenelzine, tranyclypromine.

Male Hormones—Chemical substances secreted by the testicles, ovaries and adrenal glands in humans. Some male hormones used by humans are derived synthetically. Male hormones include testosterone cypionate and estradiol cypionate, testosterone enanthate and estradiol valerate.

Manic-Depressive Illness—Psychosis with alternating cycles of excessive enthusiasm and depression.

Mast Cell—Connective tissue cell.

Menopause—The end of menstruation in the female, often accompanied by irritability, hot flashes, changes in the skin and bones and vaginal dryness.

Metabolism—Process of using nutrients and energy to build and break down wastes.

Migraine—Periodic headaches caused by constriction of arteries to the skull. Symptoms include severe pain, vision disturbances, nausea, vomiting and sensitivity to light.

Mind-Altering Drugs—Any drug that decreases alertness, perception, concentration, contact with reality or muscular coordination.

Mineral Supplements—Mineral substances added to the diet to treat or prevent mineral deficiencies. They include iron, copper, magnesium, calcium, etc.

Monoamine Oxidase (MAO) Inhibitors—See MAO Inhibitors.

Muscle Blockers—Same as muscle relaxants or skeletal muscle relaxants.

Muscle Relaxants—Medicines to lessen painful contractions and spasms of muscles. These include atracurium, carisoprodol, chlorphenesin, chlorzoxazone, cyclobenzaprine, metaxalone, methcarbamol, metocurine, orphenadrine citrate, pancuronium, succinylcholine, tubocurarine, vecuronium.

Myasthenia Gravis—Disease of the muscles characterized by fatigue and progressive paralysis. It is usually confined to muscles of the face, lips, tongue and neck.

Mydriatics—Eye drops that cause the pupils to dilate to a marked degree.

N

Narcotics—A group of habit-forming, addicting drugs used for treatment of pain, diarrhea, cough, acute pulmonary edema and others. They are all dervied from opium, a milky exudate in capsules of *Papaver somniferum*. Law requires licensed physicians to dispense by prescription. These drugs include alfentanil, buprenorphine, butorphanol, codeine, fentanyl, heroin, hydrocodone, hydromorphone, levorphanol, meperidine, methadone, morphine, nalbuphine, opium, oxycodone, oxymorphone, paregoric, pentazocine, propoxyphene, sufetanil.

Nephrotoxic Medications (Kidney-Poisoning)—Under some circumstances, these medicines can be toxic to the kidneys. These medicines include acyclovir; aminoglycosides; amphotericin B (given internally); analgesic combinations containing acetaminophen and aspirin or other salicylates (with chronic high-dose use); anti-inflammatory analgesics (non-steroidal); bacitracin (given internally); capreomycin; captopril; carmustine; cisplatin; cyclosporine; demeclocycline (nephrogenic diabetes insipidus); edetate calcium disodium (with high doses); edetate disodium (with high dose); enalapril; gold compounds; lithium; methotrexate (with high dose therapy); methoxyflurane; neomycin (oral); penicillamine; pentamidine; plicamycin; polymyxins (given internally); radiopaques (materials used for special x-ray examinations); rifampin; streptozocin; sulfonamides; tetracyclines (other, except doxycycline and minocycline); vancomycin (given internally).

Neuroleptic Malignant Syndrome—Ceaseless, involuntary, jerky movements of the tongue, facial muscles and hands.

Neuromuscular Blocking Agents—A group of drugs prescribed to relax skeletal muscles. They are all given by injection, and descriptions are not included in this book. These drugs include atracurium, edrohponium, gallamine, neostigmine, metocurine, pancuronium, pyridostigmine, succinylcholine, tubocurarine, vecuronium.

Neurotoxic Medications—Medicines that cause toxicity to the nerve tissues in the body. These drugs include anticonvulsants (hydantoin), carbamazepine, chloramphenicol (oral), cisplatin, cycloserine, disulfiram, isoniazid, lincomycins, lithium, metronidazole, mexiletine, nitrofurantoin, pemoline, pyridoxine (large amounts), quinacrine, quinine.

Nitrates—Medicines made from a chemical with a nitrogen base. Nitrates include erythrityl tetranitrate, isosorbide dinitrate, nitroglycerin, pentaerythritol tetranitrate.

Non-Steroidal Anti-Inflammatory Drugs (NSAIDs)—See Anti-Inflammatory Drugs, Non-Steroidal.

Nutritional Supplements—Substances used to treat and prevent deficiencies when the body is unable to absorb them by eating a well-balanced, nutritional diet. These supplements include Vitamins—ascorbic acid, ascorbic acid and sodium ascorbate, calcifediol, calcitriol, calcium pantothenate, cyanocobalamin, dihydrotachysterol, ergocalciferol, folate sodium, folic acid, hydroxocobalamin, niacin, niacinamide, pantothenic, pyridoxine, riboflavin, sodium ascorbate, thiamine, vitamin A, vitamin E. Minerals—calcium carbonate, calcium citrate, calcium glubionate, calcium gluconate, calcium lactate, calcium phosphate (dibasic and tribasic), sodium fluoride. Other—levocarnitine, omega-3 polyunsaturated fatty acids.

O

Opiates—Pain-killing medicines derived from opium that have a high index of addiction. Some of these include butorphanol, codeine, hydrocodone, hydromorphone, levorphanol, meperidine, methadone, morphine, nalbuphine, opium, oxycodone, oxymorphone, paregoric, pentazocine, propoxyphene.

Osteoporosis—Softening of bones caused by a loss of chemicals usually found in bone.

Ototoxic Medications—These medicines may possibly cause hearing damage. They include aminoglycosides, 4-aminoquinolines, anti-inflammatory analgesics (non-steroidal), bumetanide, capreomyucin, cisplatin, deferoxamine, erythromycins, ethacrynic acid, furosemide, minocycline, quinine, salicylates, vancomycin.

Ovary—Female sexual gland where eggs mature and ripen for fertilization.

P

Pain Relievers—Non-narcotic medicines to treat pain.

Palpitations—Rapid heartbeat noticeable to the patient.

Pancreatitis—Serious inflammation or infection of the pancreas that causes upper abdominal pain.

Parkinson's Disease or Parkinson's Syndrome—Disease of the central nervous system. Characteristics are a fixed, emotionless expression of the face, tremor, slower muscle movements, weakness, changed gait and a peculiar posture.

Pellagra—Disease caused by a deficiency of the water-soluble vitamin, thiamine (vitamin B-1). Symptoms include brain disturbance, diarrhea and skin inflammation.

Penicillin—Chemical substance (antibiotic) originally discovered as a product of mold, which can kill some bacterial germs.

Phenothiazines—Drugs used to treat mental, nervous and emotional conditions. These drugs include acetophenazine, chlorpromazine, fluphenazine, mesoridazine, perphenazine, prochlorperazine, promazine, thioridazine, trifluoperazine, triflupromazine.

Pheochromocytoma—A tumor of the adrenal gland which produces chemicals that cause high blood pressure, headache, nervousness and other symptoms.

Phlegm—Thick mucus secreted by glands in the respiratory tract.

Photophobia—Increased sensitivity to light as perceived by the human eye. Drugs that can cause photophobia include antidiabetic drugs*, atropine, belladonna, bromides, chloraquine, ciprofloxacin, chlordiazepoxide, clidinium, clomiphene, dicyclomine, digitalis drugs, doxepin, ethambutol, ethionamide, ethosuximide, etretinate, glycopyrrolate, hydroxychloroquine, hydroxyzine, hyoscyamine, mephenytoin, methenamine, methsuximide, monoamine oxidase (MAO) inhibitors, nalidixic acid, norfloxacin, oral contraceptives, orphenadrine, paramethadione, phenothiazines, propantheline, quinidine, quinine, scopolamine, sopropamide, tetracyclines, tridihexethyl, trimethadione.

Photosensitizing Medications—Medicines that can cause abnormally heightened skin reactions to the effects of sunlight. These medicines include acetohexamide, amiodarone, amitriptyline, amoxapine, anthralin, antidiabetic agents (oral), antihistamines, barbiturates, bendroflumethiazide, benzocaine, carbamazepine, chlordiazepoxide, chloroquine, chlorothiazide, chlorpromazine, chlorpropamide, chlortetracycline, chlorthalidone, clindamycin, coal tar, contraceptives (estrogen-containing, oral), cyproheptadine, demeclocycline, desipramine, diethylstilbestrol, diltiazem, diphenhydramine, diuretics (thiazide), doxepin, doxycycline, estrogens, ethionamide, etretinate, fluorouracil, fluphenazine, furosemide, griseofulvin, glyburide, gold preparations, hydrocholothiazide, hydroflumethiazide, imipramine, isotretinoin, ketoprofen, lincomycin, maprotiline, mesoridazine, methacycline, methotrexate, methoxsalen, nalidixic acid, naproxen, nortriptyline, oral contraceptives, oxyphenbutazone, oxytetracycline, perphenazine, phenobarbital, phenothiazines, phenylbutazone, phenytoin, piroxicam, prochlorperazine, promazine, promethazine, protriptyline, pyrazinamide, sulfonamides, sulindac, tetracyclines, thioridazine, thioxanthenes, tolazamide, tolbutamide, tranylcypromine, tretinoin, triamterene, trifluoperazine, trioxsalen, trimeprazine, trimipramine, triproldine.

Pinworms—Common intestinal parasite that causes rectal itching and irritation.

Pituitary Gland—Gland at the base of the brain that secretes hormones to stimulate growth and other glands to produce hormones.

Platelet—Disc-shaped element of the blood, smaller than red or white blood cells, necessary for blood clotting.

Polymixins—A family of antibiotics that kill bacteria.

Polyp—Growth on a mucous membrane.

Porphyria—Inherited metabolic disorder characterized by changes in the nervous system and kidney.

Post-Partum—Following delivery of a baby.

Potassium—Important chemical found in body cells.

Potassium Foods—Foods high in potassium content, including dried apricots and peaches, lentils, raisins, citrus and whole-grain cereals.

Potassium Supplements—Medicines needed by people who don't have enough potassium in their diets or by those who develop a deficiency due to illness or taking diuretics and other medicines. These supplements include chloride; potassium acetate; potassium bicarbonate; potassium bicarbonate and potassium chloride; potassium bicarbonate and potassium citrate; potassium chloride; potassium chloride, potassium bicarbonate and potassium citrate; potassium gluconate; potassium gluconate and potassium chloride; potassium gluconate and potassium citrate; potassium gluconate, potassium citrate and ammonium; trikates.

Prostate—Gland in the male that surrounds the neck of the bladder and the urethra.

Prothrombin—Blood substance essential in clotting.

Prothrombin Time—Laboratory study used to follow prothrombin activity and keep coagulation safe.

Psoriasis—Chronic, inherited skin disease. Symptoms are lesions with silvery scales on the edges.

Psychosis—Mental disorder characterized by deranged personality, loss of contact with reality and possible delusions, hallucinations or illusions.

Purine Foods—Foods that are metabolized into uric acid. Foods high in purines include anchovies, liver, brains, sweetbreads, sardines, kidney, oysters, gravy and meat extracts.

R

Rauwolfia Alkaloids—Drugs that belong to the family of antihypertensives (to lower blood pressure). Rauwolfia alkaloids are not used as extensively as in years past. They include alseroxylon, deserpidine, rauwolfia serpentina, reserpine.

RDA—Recommended daily allowance of a vitamin or mineral.

Rebound Effect—Return of a condition, often with increased severity, once the prescribed drug is withdrawn.

Renal—Pertaining to the kidney.

Retina—Innermost covering of the eyeball on which the image is formed.

Reye's Syndrome—Rare, sometimes fatal, disease of children that causes brain and liver damage.
Rickets—Bone disease caused by vitamin-D deficiency. Bones become bent and distorted during infancy or childhood.

S

Salicylates—Medicines to relieve pain and reduce fever. These include aspirin, aspirin and caffeine, buffered aspirin, choline salicylate, choline and magnesium salicylates, magnesium salicylate, salicylamide, salsalate, sodium salicylate.
Sedative—Drug that reduces excitement or anxiety.
Seizure—Brain disorder causing changes of consciousness or convulsions.
SGOT—Abbreviation for serum oxaloacetic transaminase. Measuring the level in the blood helps demonstrate liver disorders and diagnose recent heart damage.
SGPT—Abbreviation for a laboratory study measuring the blood level of serum glutamic-pyruvic transaminase. Deviations from a normal level may indicate liver disease.
Sick Sinus Syndrome—A complicated, serious heartbeat rhythm disturbance characterized by a slow heart rate alternating with a fast or slow heart rate with heart block.
Sinusitis—Inflammation or infection of the sinus cavities in the skull.
Skeletal Muscle Relaxants (Same as Skeletal Muscle Blockers)—A group of drugs prescribed to treat spasm of skeletal muscles. These drugs include carisoprodol, chlorphenesin, chlorzoxazone, cyclobenzaprine, diazepam, lorazepam, metaxalone, methocarbamol, orphenadrine, phenytoin.
Sleep Inducers—Night-time sedatives to aid in falling asleep. See Benzodiazepines.
Stimulants, Central Nervous System (CNS)—Drugs that stimulate the nerves of the brain and spinal cord. These drugs include amphetamine, caffeine, caffeine (citrated), caffeine and sodium benzoate, cocaine, dextroamphetamine, ephedrine (oral), methamphetamine, methylphenidate, pemoline.
Streptococcus—Bacteria that causes infections in the throat, respiratory system and skin. Improperly treated, can lead to disease in the heart, joints and kidneys.
Stroke—Sudden, severe attack. Usually sudden paralysis from injury to the brain or spinal cord caused by a blood clot or hemorrhage in the brain.
Stupor—Near unconsciousness.
Sublingual—Under the tongue. Some drugs are absorbed almost as quickly this way as by injection.

Sulfa Drugs—Shorthand for sulfonamide drugs, which are used to treat infections.
Sulfonamides—Sulfa drugs prescribed to treat infections. They include sulfacytine, sulfamethoxazole, sulfamethoxazole and trimethoprin, sulfasalazine, sulfisoxazole.
Sulfonureas—A family of drugs that lower blood sugar (hypoglycemic agents). Used in the treatment of some forms of diabetes.
Sympathomimetics—A large group of drugs that mimic the effects of stimulation of the *sympathetic* part of the autonomic nervous system. These drugs include adrenalin (epinephrine); appetite suppressants (such as benzphetamine, diethylpropion, fenfluramine, mazindol, phendimetrazine, phenmetrazine, phentermine, phenylpropanolamine); aramine; cocaine; dobutamine; ephedrine; epinephrine; mephentermine; methoxamine; norepinephrine; phenylephrine; phenylpropanolamine; metaraminol; isoproterenol.

T

Tardive Dyskinesia—Involuntary movements of the jaw, lips and tongue caused by an unpredictable drug reaction.
Tartrazine Dye—A dye used in foods and medicine preparations that may cause an allergic reaction in some people.
Tetracyclines—A group of medicines with similar chemical structure used to treat infections. These drugs include demeclocycline, doxycycline, methacycline, minocycline, oxytetracycline, tetracycline.
Thiazides—A group of chemicals that cause diuresis (loss of water through the kidney). Frequently used to treat high blood pressure and congestive heart failure. Thiazides include bendroflumethiazide, benzthiazide, chlorothiazide, cyclothiazide, hydrochlorothiazide, hydroflumethiazide, methyclothiazide, polythiazide, trichlormethiazide.
Thiothixines—See Thioxanthenes.
Thioxanthenes—Drugs used to treat emotional, mental and nervous conditions. These drugs include chlorprothixene, fluphenthixol, thiothixene.
Thrombocytopenias—Diseases characterized by inadequate numbers of blood platelets circulating in the bloodstream.
Thrombolytic Agents—Drugs that help to dissolve blood clots. They include alteplase, streptokinase, urokinase.
Thrombophlebitis—Inflammation of a vein caused by a blood clot in the vein.
Thyroid—Gland in the neck that manufactures and secretes several hormones.
Thyroid Hormones—Medications that mimic

the action of the thyroid hormone made in the thyroid gland. They include dextrothyroxine, levothyroxine, liothyronine, liotrix, thyroglobulin, thyroid.

Tic Douloureaux—Painful condition caused by inflammation of a nerve in the face.

Toxicity—Poisonous reaction to a drug that impairs body functions or damages cells.

Transdermal Patches—There are more and more medications in a form known as transdermal (stick-on) patches. If you are using this form, follow these instructions: Choose an area of skin without cuts, scars or hair, such as the upper arm, chest or behind the ear. Thoroughly clean the area where patch is to be applied. If patch gets wet and loose, cover with an additional piece of plastic. Apply a fresh patch if the first one falls off. Apply each dose to a different area of skin if possible.

Tranquilizer—Drug that calms a person without clouding consciousness.

Tremor—Involuntary trembling.

Trichomoniasis—Infestation of the vagina by *trichomonas*, an infectious organism. The infection causes itching, vaginal discharge and irritation.

Triglyceride—Fatty chemical manufactured from carbohydrates for storage in fat cells.

Tyramine—Normal chemical component of the body that helps sustain blood pressure. Can rise to fatal levels in combination with some drugs.

Tyramine is found in many foods:

Beverages—Alcohol beverages, especially Chianti or robust red wines, vermouth, ale, beer.

Breads—Homemade bread with a lot of yeast and breads or crackers containing cheese.

Fats—Sour cream.

Fruits—Bananas, red plums, avocados, figs, raisins.

Meats and meat substitutes—Aged game, liver, canned meats, salami, sausage, cheese, salted dried fish, pickled herring.

Vegetables—Italian broad beans, green-bean pods, eggplant.

Miscellaneous—Yeast concentrates or extracts, marmite, soup cubes, commercial gravy, soy sauce, any protein food that has been stored improperly or is spoiled.

U

Ulcer, Peptic—Open sore on the mucous membrane of the esophagus, stomach or duodenum caused by stomach acid.

Urethra—Hollow tube through which urine (and semen in men) is discharged.

Urethritis—Inflammation or infection of the urethra.

Urinary Acidifiers—Medications that cause urine to become acid. These include ascorbic acid, potassium phosphate, potassium and sodium phosphates.

Urinary Alkalizers—Medications that cause urine to become alkaline. These include potassium citrate, potassium citrate and citric acid, potassium citrate and sodium citrate, sodium bicarbonate, sodium citrate and citric acid, tricitrate.

Uterus—Also called womb. A hollow muscular organ in the female in which the embryo develops into a fetus.

V

Vascular—Pertaining to blood vessels.

Vascular Headache (Preventative)—Medicines prescribed to prevent the occurrence of or reduce the frequency and severity of vascular headache such as migraine. These drugs include atenolol; clonidine; ergotamine, belladonna alkaloids and phenobarbital; fenoprofen; ibuprofen; indomethacin; lithium; mefenamic acid; methysergide; metoprolol; nadolol; naproxen; pizotyline; propranolol; timolol.

Vascular Headache (Treatment)—Medicine prescribed to treat vascular headaches such as migraine. These drugs include dihydro-ergotamine; ergotamine; ergotamine and caffeine; ergotamine, caffeine, belladonna alkaloids and pentobarbital; fenoprofen; ibuprofen; indomethacin (capsules, oral suspension, rectal); isometheptene, dichloralphenazone and acetaminophen; naproxen.

Virus—Infectious organism that reproduces in the cells of the infected host.

Y

Yeast—A single-cell organism that can cause infections of the mouth, vagina, skin and parts of the gastrointestinal system.

GUIDE TO INDEX

Alphabetical entries in the index include three categories—generic names, brand names and drug-class names.

1. Generic names appear in capital letters, followed by their chart page number:
   ASPIRIN 108

2. Brand names appear in *italic,* followed by their generic ingredient and chart page number:
   Bayer - See ASPIRIN 108

   Some brand names contain two or more generic ingredients. These generic ingredients are listed in capital letters, following the brand name:
   Anacin - See
   ASPIRIN 108
   CAFFEINE 166

3. Drug-class names appear in regular type, capital and lower-case letters. All generic drug names in this book that fall into a drug class are listed after the class name:
   Anticonvulsant - See
   CARBAMAZEPINE 174
   DIVALPOREX 326
   PARALDEHYDE 650
   PRIMIDONE 716
   VALPROIC ACID (Dipropylacetic Acid) 880

INDEX

Afrin Nose Drops - See XYLOMETAZOLINE &
OXYMETAZOLINE (Nasal) 898
Afrinol Repetabs - See PSEUDOEPHEDRINE 736
Aftate for Athlete's Foot Aerosol Spray Liquid - See
ANTIFUNGALS (Topical) 84
Aftate for Athlete's Foot Aerosol Spray Powder -
See ANTIFUNGALS (Topical) 84
Aftate for Athlete's Foot Gel - See ANTIFUNGALS
(Topical) 84
Aftate for Athlete's Foot Sprinkle Powder - See
ANTIFUNGALS (Topical) 84
Aftate for Jock Itch Aerosol Spray Powder - See
ANTIFUNGALS (Topical) 84
Aftate for Jock Itch Gel - See ANTIFUNGALS
(Topical) 84
Aftate for Jock Itch Sprinkle Powder - See
ANTIFUNGALS (Topical) 84
Agoral - See
MINERAL OIL 562
PHENOLPHTHALEIN 676
A-hydroCort - See HYDROCORTISONE (Cortisol) 430
AK Homatropine - See CYCLOPEGIC, MYDRIATIC
(Ophthalmic) 266
Akarpine - See PILOCARPINE 690
Ak-Chlor Ophthalmic Solution - See
ANTIBACTERIALS (Ophthalmic) 64
Ak-Con - See DECONGESTANTS (Ophthalmic) 284
Ak-Dex - See
ANTI-INFLAMMATORY DRUGS, STEROIDAL
(Ophthalmic) 96
DEXAMETHASONE 290
Ak-Dilate - See PHENYLEPHRINE (Ophthalmic) 684
Akineton - See ANTIDYSKINETICS 80
Ak-Nefrin - See PHENYLEPHRINE (Ophthalmic) 684
Akne-mycin - See
ANTIBACTERIALS FOR ACNE (Topical) 72
ERYTHROMYCINS 354
Ak-Pentolate - See CYCLOPENTOLATE
(Ophthalmic) 268
Ak-Pred - See ANTI-INFLAMMATORY DRUGS,
STEROIDAL (Ophthalmic) 96
Ak-Sulf - See ANTIBACTERIALS (Ophthalmic) 64
Ak-Taine - See ANESTHETICS, LOCAL
(Ophthalmic) 50
Ak-Tate - See ANTI-INFLAMMATORY DRUGS,
STEROIDAL (Ophthalmic) 96
Ak-Zol - See CARBONIC ANHYDRASE
INHIBITORS 182
Ala-Cort - See ADRENOCORTICOIDS (Topical) 14
Alamag - See ANTACIDS 56
Alamine - See
ANTIHISTAMINES 92
PHENYLPROPANOLAMINE 686
Alamine Expectorant - See
GUAIFENESIN 408
NARCOTIC ANALGESICS 592
PSEUDOEPHEDRINE 736
Alamine-C Liquid - See
ANTIHISTAMINES 92
NARCOTIC ANALGESICS 592
PSEUDOEPHEDRINE 736

Ala-Scalp HP - See ADRENOCORTICOIDS
(Topical) 14
Alaxin - See POLOXAMER 188 694
Albalon - See DECONGESTANTS (Ophthalmic) 284
Alba-Temp 300 - See ACETAMINOPHEN 2
Albright's Solution - See CITRATES 220
ALBTEROL - See BRONCHODILATORS,
ADRENERGIC 150
Alcaine - See ANESTHETICS, LOCAL (Ophthalmic)
50
ALCLOMETASONE (Topical) - See
ADRENOCORTICOIDS (Topical) 14
ALCOHOL AND ACETONE - See ANTI-ACNE,
CLEANSING (Topical) 62
ALCOHOL AND SULFUR - See ANTI-ACNE,
CLEANSING (Topical) 62
Alcomicin - See ANTIBACTERIALS (Ophthalmic) 64
Aldactazide - See SPIRONOLACTONE &
HYDROCHLOROTHIAZIDE 798
Aldactone - See SPIRONOLACTONE 796
Aldoclor - See
METHYLDOPA 538
METHYLDOPA & THIAZIDE DIURETICS 540
Aldomet - See METHYLDOPA 538
Aldoril - See
METHYLDOPA 538
METHYLDOPA & THIAZIDE DIURETICS 540
Alersule - See
ANTIHISTAMINES 92
PHENYLEPHRINE 682
Algenic Alka - See ANTACIDS 56
Algenic Alka Improved - See ANTACIDS 56
Algicon - See ANTACIDS 56
Alka-Butazolidin - See ANTI-INFLAMMATORY
DRUGS, NON-STEROIDAL (NSAIDs) 94
Alkabutazone - See ANTI-INFLAMMATORY
DRUGS, NON-STEROIDAL (NSAIDs) 94
Alkalizer - See SODIUM BICARBONATE 790
Alka-Mints - See ANTACIDS 56
Alka-Phenylbutazone - See ANTI-INFLAMMATORY
DRUGS, NON-STEROIDAL (NSAIDs) 94
Alka-Seltzer Effervescent Pain Reliever & Antacid -
See ASPIRIN 108
Alka-Seltzer Plus - See ASPIRIN 108
Alka-Seltzer Plus Maximum Strength Sinus Allergy - See
ANTIHISTAMINES 92
ASPIRIN 108
PHENYLPROPANOLAMINE 686
Alkeran - See MELPHALAN (PAM, L-PAM,
Phenylalanine Mustard) 516
Alkets - See ANTACIDS 56
Allay - See NARCOTIC & ACETAMINOPHEN 590
Allent - See
ANTIHISTAMINES 92
PSEUDOEPHEDRINE 736
Alleract - See ANTIHISTAMINES 92
Aller-Chlor - See ANTIHISTAMINES 92
Allercort - See ADRENOCORTICOIDS (Topical) 14
Allerdryl - See ANTIHISTAMINES 92
Allerest - See
ANTIHISTAMINES 92

A-methaPred - See METHYLPREDNISOLONE 546
Amethopterin - See METHOTREXATE 532
AMFEBTAMONE - See BUPROPION 156
Amfetamine - See AMPHETAMINES 34
Amicar - See ANTIFIBRINOLYTIC AGENTS 82
Amidrin - See ISOMETHEPTENE,
    DICHLORALPHENAZONE &
    ACETAMINOPHEN 456
AMILORIDE 22
AMILORIDE & HYDROCHLOROTHIAZIDE 24
Aminobenzoate - See ANESTHETICS (Topical) 46
AMINOBENZOATE POTASSIUM 26
AMINOCAPROIC ACID - See ANTIFIBRINOLYTIC
    AGENTS 82
Aminofen - See ACETAMINOPHEN 2
Aminofen Max - See ACETAMINOPHEN 2
AMINOGLUTETHIMIDE 28
Aminophyllin - See BRONCHODILATORS,
    XANTHINE 152
AMINOPHYLLINE - See BRONCHODILATORS,
    XANTHINE 152
AMIODARONE 30
Ami-Tex LA - See
    GUAIFENESIN 408
    PHENYLPROPANOLAMINE 686
Amitone - See ANTACIDS 56
AMITRYPTILINE - See TRICYCLIC
    ANTIDEPRESSANTS 868
AMLODIPINE - See CALCIUM CHANNEL
    BLOCKERS 168
AMOBARBITAL - See BARBITURATES 122
Amogel PG - See KAOLIN, PECTIN,
    BELLADONNA & OPIUM 470
Amonidrin - See GUAIFENESIN 408
AMOXAPINE - See TRICYCLIC
    ANTIDEPRESSANTS 868
AMOXICILLIN 32
Amoxil - See AMOXICILLIN 32
AMPHETAMINE - See AMPHETAMINES 34
AMPHETAMINE SULFATE - See AMPHETAMINES
    34
AMPHETAMINES 34
Amphojel - See ANTACIDS 56
Amphojel 500 - See ANTACIDS 56
Amphojel Plus - See ANTACIDS 56
AMPHOTERACIN B - See ANTIFUNGALS (Topical)
    84
AMPICILLIN 36
Ampicin - See AMPICILLIN 36
Ampilean - See AMPICILLIN 36
Amyl Nitrite Inhalant - See AMYL NITRITE
    INHALANT 38
AMYL NITRITE INHALANT 38
Amytal - See BARBITURATES 122
Anabolin - See ANDROGENS 42
Anabolin LA 100 - See ANDROGENS 42
Anacin - See
    ASPIRIN 108
    CAFFEINE 166
Anacin with Codeine - See NARCOTIC & ASPIRIN
    594
Anacin-3 - See ACETAMINOPHEN 2

Anadrol - See ANDROGENS 42
Anafranil - See TRICYCLIC ANTIDEPRESSANTS
    868
Analgesic - See
    ACETAMINOPHEN 2
    ACETAMINOPHEN & SALICYLATES 4
    ASPIRIN 108
    BUTALBITAL & ASPIRIN (Also contains caffeine)
        162
    BUTALBITAL, ASPIRIN & CODEINE (Also
        contains caffeine) 164
    CARBAMAZEPINE 174
    CHLORZOXAZONE & ACETAMINOPHEN 212
    ERGOTAMINE, BELLADONNA &
        PHENOBARBITAL 348
    ERGOTAMINE & CAFFEINE 350
    ISOMETHEPTENE, DICHLORALPHENAZONE &
        ACETAMINOPHEN 456
    MEPROBAMATE & ASPIRIN 522
    NARCOTIC & ACETAMINOPHEN 590
    NARCOTIC & ASPIRIN 594
    ORPHENADRINE, ASPIRIN & CAFFEINE 632
    SALICYLATES 774
Analgesic (otic) - See ANALGESICS (Topical-Otic)
    40
Analgesic (topical) - See CAPSAICIN 172
Analgesic (urinary) - See
    ATROPINE, HYOSCYAMINE, METHENAMINE,
        METHYLENE BLUE, PHENYLSALICYLATE &
        BENZOIC ACID 112
    PHENAZOPYRIDINE 674
    SULFONAMIDES & PHENAZOPYRIDINE 814
ANALGESICS (Topical-Otic) 40
Anamine - See
    ANTIHISTAMINES 92
    PSEUDOEPHEDRINE 736
Anamine HD - See
    ANTIHISTAMINES 92
    NARCOTIC ANALGESICS 592
    PHENYLEPHRINE 682
Anamine T.D. - See
    ANTIHISTAMINES 92
    PSEUDOEPHEDRINE 736
Anapolon 50 - See ANDROGENS 42
Anaprox - See ANTI-INFLAMMATORY DRUGS,
    NON-STEROIDAL (NSAIDs) 94
Anaprox DS - See ANTI-INFLAMMATORY DRUGS,
    NON-STEROIDAL (NSAIDs) 94
Anaspaz - See HYOSCYAMINE 440
Anaspaz PB - See
    BELLADONNA ALKALOIDS & BARBITURATES
        128
    HYOSCYAMINE 440
Anatuss - See
    ACETAMINOPHEN 2
    ANTIHISTAMINES 92
    DEXTROMETHORPHAN 292
    GUAIFENESIN 408
    PHENYLEPHRINE 682
    PHENYLPROPANOLAMINE 686
Anatuss with Codeine - See
    ACETAMINOPHEN 2

INDEX

Apo-Keto-E - See ANTI-INFLAMMATORY DRUGS, NON-STEROIDAL (NSAIDs) 94

Apo-Lorazepam - See BENZODIAZEPINES 130

Apo-Meprobamate - See MEPROBAMATE 520

Apo-Methyldopa - See METHYLDOPA 538

Apo-Metoprolol (Type L) - See BETA-ADRENERGIC BLOCKERS 134

Apo-Metoprolol - See BETA-ADRENERGIC BLOCKERS 134

Apo-Metronidazole - See METRONIDAZOLE 554

Apo-Naproxen - See ANTI-INFLAMMATORY DRUGS, NON-STEROIDAL (NSAIDs) 94

Apo-Nifed - See CALCIUM CHANNEL BLOCKERS 168

Apo-Nitrofurantoin - See NITROFURANTOIN 616

Apo-Oxazepam - See BENZODIAZEPINES 130

Apo-Oxtriphylline - See BRONCHODILATORS, XANTHINE 152

Apo-Pen-VK - See PENICILLIN V 664

Apo-Perphenazine - See PHENOTHIAZINES 678

Apo-Piroxicam - See ANTI-INFLAMMATORY DRUGS, NON-STEROIDAL (NSAIDs) 94

Apo-Prednisone - See PREDNISONE 712

Apo-Primidone - See PRIMIDONE 716

Apo-Propranolol - See BETA-ADRENERGIC BLOCKERS 134

Apo-Quinidine - See QUINIDINE 752

Apo-Sulfamethoxazole - See SULFAMETHOXAZOLE 806

Apo-Sulfatrim - See SULFAMETHOXAZOLE 806 TRIMETHOPRIM 876

Apo-Sulfinpyrazone - See SULFINPYRAZONE 810

Apo-Sulfisoxazole - See SULFISOXAZOLE 812

Apo-Tetra - See TETRACYCLINES 828

Apo-Thioridazine - See PHENOTHIAZINES 678

Apo-Timol - See BETA-ADRENERGIC BLOCKERS 134

Apo-Timop - See ANTIGLAUCOMA, LONG-ACTING (Ophthalmic) 88

Apo-Tolbutamide - See ANTIDIABETIC AGENTS 78

Apo-Triazide - See TRIAMTERENE & HYDROCHLOROTHIAZIDE 864

Apo-Triazo - See TRIAZOLAM 866

Apo-Trifluoperazine - See PHENOTHIAZINES 678

Apo-Trihex - See ANTIDYSKINETICS 80

Apo-Trimip - See TRICYCLIC ANTIDEPRESSANTS 868

Apo-Verap - See CALCIUM CHANNEL BLOCKERS 168

Apo-Zidovudine - See ZIDOVUDINE (AZT, Azidothymidine) 900

Appecon - See APPETITE SUPPRESSANTS 106

Appetite suppressant - See APPETITE SUPPRESSANTS 106

APPETITE SUPPRESSANTS 106

Apresazide - See HYDRALAZINE & HYDROCHLOROTHIAZIDE 428

Apresoline - See HYDRALAZINE 426

Apresoline-Esidrix - See HYDRALAZINE & HYDROCHLOROTHIAZIDE 428

APROBARBITAL - See BARBITURATES 122

Aprodrine - See ANTIHISTAMINES 92

Aprozide - See HYDRALAZINE & HYDROCHLOROTHIAZIDE 428

Apsifen - See ANTI-INFLAMMATORY DRUGS, NON-STEROIDAL (NSAIDs) 94

Apsifen-F - See ANTI-INFLAMMATORY DRUGS, NON-STEROIDAL (NSAIDs) 94

Aquachloral - See CHLORAL HYDRATE 198

AquaMEPHYTON - See VITAMIN K 894

Aquaphyllin - See BRONCHODILATORS, XANTHINE 152

Aquasol A - See VITAMIN A 884

Aquasol E - See VITAMIN E 892

Aquatar - See COAL TAR (Topical) 242

Aquatensen - See DIURETICS, THIAZIDE 324

Aqueous Charcodote - See CHARCOAL, ACTIVATED 192

Aralen - See CHLOROQUINE 208

Aristocort - See ADRENOCORTICOIDS (Topical) 14

Aristocort A - See ADRENOCORTICOIDS (Topical) 14

Aristocort C - See ADRENOCORTICOIDS (Topical) 14

Aristocort D - See ADRENOCORTICOIDS (Topical) 14

Aristocort Forte - See TRIAMCINOLONE 860

Aristocort Intralesional - See TRIAMCINOLONE 860

Aristocort R - See ADRENOCORTICOIDS (Topical) 14

Aristospan - See TRIAMCINOLONE 860

Arlidin Forte - See NYLIDRIN 620

Arlon Forte - See CHLORZOXAZONE & ACETAMINOPHEN 212

A.R.M. Maximum Strength Caplets - See ANTIHISTAMINES 92 PHENYLPROPANOLAMINE 686

Arm & Hammer Pure Baking Soda - See SODIUM BICARBONATE 790

Arm-a-Med Isoetharine - See BRONCHODILATORS, ADRENERGIC 150

Arm-a-Med Metaproterenol - See BRONCHODILATORS, ADRENERGIC 150

Aromatic Cascara Fluidextract - See CASCARA 184

Artane - See ANTIDYSKINETICS 80

Artane Sequels - See ANTIDYSKINETICS 80

Arthinol - See ASPIRIN 108

Arthralgin - See ACETAMINOPHEN & SALICYLATES 4

Arthritis Pain Formula - See ASPIRIN 108

Arthropan - See SALICYLATES 774

Articulose - See PREDNISOLONE 710

Articulose-L.A. - See TRIAMCINOLONE 860

Artificial tears - See PROTECTANT (Ophthalmic) 734

Artria S.R. - See ASPIRIN 108

A.S.A. - See ASPIRIN 108

A.S.A. Enseals - See ASPIRIN 108

Asbron - See BRONCHODILATORS, XANTHINE 152

Asbron G - See THEOPHYLLINE & GUAIFENESIN 836

Asbron G Inlay Tablets - See THEOPHYLLINE & GUAIFENESIN 836

Azo-Sulfamethoxazole - See
 PHENAZOPYRIDINE 674
 SULFONAMIDES & PHENAZOPYRIDINE 814
Azo-Sulfisoxazole - See
 PHENAZOPYRIDINE 674
 SULFONAMIDES & PHENAZOPYRIDINE 814
Azo-Truxazole - See PHENAZOPYRIDINE 674
Azulfidine - See SULFASALAZINE 808
Azulfidine En-Tabs - See SULFASALAZINE 808

B

Baby Anbesol - See ANESTHETICS, DENTAL
 (Topical) 48
Baby Orajel - See ANESTHETICS, DENTAL
 (Topical) 48
B-A-C - See BUTALBITAL & ASPIRIN (Also
 contains caffeine) 162
B-A-C with Codeine - See BUTALBITAL, ASPIRIN
 & CODEINE (Also contains caffeine) 164
BACAMPICILLIN 118
Bacarate - See APPETITE SUPPRESSANTS 106
BACITRACIN - See ANTIBACTERIALS (Topical) 68
BACLOFEN 120
Bactine - See
 ADRENOCORTICOIDS (Topical) 14
 ANESTHETICS (Topical) 46
Bactine First Aid Antibiotic - See ANTIBACTERIALS
 (Topical) 68
Bactocill - See OXACILLIN 634
Bactrim - See
 SULFAMETHOXAZOLE 806
 TRIMETHOPRIM 876
Bactrim DS - See SULFAMETHOXAZOLE 806
Bactroban - See ANTIBACTERIALS (Topical) 68
Baldex - See ANTI-INFLAMMATORY DRUGS,
 STEROIDAL (Ophthalmic) 96
Balminil - See GUAIFENESIN 408
Balminil DM - See DEXTROMETHORPHAN 292
Balnetar - See COAL TAR (Topical) 242
Balnetar Therapeutic Tar Bath - See COAL TAR
 (Topical) 242
Bancap - See
 ACETAMINOPHEN 2
 BARBITURATES 122
Bancap-HC - See NARCOTIC &
 ACETAMINOPHEN 590
Banesin - See ACETAMINOPHEN 2
Banex - See
 GUAIFENESIN 408
 PHENYLEPHRINE 682
 PHENYLPROPANOLAMINE 686
Banex Liquid - See
 PHENYLEPHRINE 682
 PHENYLPROPANOLAMINE 686
Banex-LA - See
 GUAIFENESIN 408
 PHENYLPROPANOLAMINE 686
Barbidonna - See
 BELLADONNA ALKALOIDS & BARBITURATES
 128
 HYOSCYAMINE 440
 SCOPOLAMINE (Hyoscine) 776

Barbidonna 2 - See
 BELLADONNA ALKALOIDS & BARBITURATES
 128
 HYOSCYAMINE 440
 SCOPOLAMINE (Hyoscine) 776
Barbita - See BARBITURATES 122
Barbiturate - See THEOPHYLLINE, EPHEDRINE &
 BARBITURATES 830
BARBITURATES 122
Barc - See PEDICULISIDES (Topical) 656
Baridium - See PHENAZOPYRIDINE 674
Barophen - See BELLADONNA ALKALOIDS &
 BARBITURATES 128
Barriere-HC - See ADRENOCORTICOIDS (Topical) 14
Basaljel - See ANTACIDS 56
Bayaminic Expectorant - See
 GUAIFENESIN 408
 PHENYLPROPANOLAMINE 686
Bayaminicol - See
 ANTIHISTAMINES 92
 DEXTROMETHORPHAN 292
 PHENYLPROPANOLAMINE 686
Baycodan - See NARCOTIC ANALGESICS 592
Baycomine - See
 NARCOTIC ANALGESICS 592
 PHENYLPROPANOLAMINE 686
Baycomine Pediatric - See
 NARCOTIC ANALGESICS 592
 PHENYLPROPANOLAMINE 686
BayCotussend Liquid - See
 NARCOTIC ANALGESICS 592
 PSEUDOEPHEDRINE 736
Baydec DM Drops - See
 ANTIHISTAMINES 92
 DEXTROMETHORPHAN 292
 PSEUDOEPHEDRINE 736
Bayer - See ASPIRIN 108
Bayer Cough Syrup - See
 PHENYLPROPANOLAMINE 686
Bayer Cough Syrup for Children - See
 DEXTROMETHORPHAN 292
 PHENYLPROPANOLAMINE 686
Bayer Timed-Release Arthritic Pain Formula - See
 ASPIRIN 108
Bayhistine DH - See
 ANTIHISTAMINES 92
 NARCOTIC ANALGESICS 592
 PSEUDOEPHEDRINE 736
Bayhistine Expectorant - See
 GUAIFENESIN 408
 NARCOTIC ANALGESICS 592
 PSEUDOEPHEDRINE 736
Baytussin AC - See
 GUAIFENESIN 408
 NARCOTIC ANALGESICS 592
Baytussin DM - See
 DEXTROMETHORPHAN 292
 GUAIFENESIN 408
BC Cold Powder - See
 ANTIHISTAMINES 92
 ASPIRIN 108
 PHENYLPROPANOLAMINE 686

BC Cold Powder Non-Drowsy Formula - See
  PHENYLPROPANOLAMINE 686
Beben - See ADRENOCORTICOIDS (Topical) 14
Because - See CONTRACEPTIVES, VAGINAL
  (Spermicides) 252
BECLOMETHASONE 124
BECLOMETHASONE (Nasal) - See
  ADRENOCORTICOIDS (Nasal) 12
BECLOMETHASONE (Topical) - See
  ADRENOCORTICOIDS (Topical) 14
Beclovent - See BECLOMETHASONE 124
Beclovent Rotacaps - See BECLOMETHASONE
  124
Beconase - See ADRENOCORTICOIDS (Nasal) 12
Beconase AQ - See ADRENOCORTICOIDS (Nasal)
  12
Bedoz - See VITAMIN B-12 (Cyanocobalamin) 886
Beepen-VK - See PENICILLIN V 664
Beesix - See PYRIDOXINE (Vitamin B-6) 746
Beldin Cough - See ANTIHISTAMINES 92
Belix - See ANTIHISTAMINES 92
Belladenal - See
  BELLADONNA ALKALOIDS & BARBITURATES
    128
  HYOSCYAMINE 440
Belladenal-S - See BELLADONNA ALKALOIDS &
  BARBITURATES 128
Belladenal Spacetabs - See BELLADONNA
  ALKALOIDS & BARBITURATES 128
BELLADONNA 126
BELLADONNA & AMOBARBITAL - See
  BELLADONNA ALKALOIDS &
  BARBITURATES 128
BELLADONNA & BUTABARBITAL - See
  BELLADONNA ALKALOIDS &
  BARBITURATES 128
BELLADONNA ALKALOIDS & BARBITURATES
  128
Bellafoline - See HYOSCYAMINE 440
Bellalphen - See BELLADONNA ALKALOIDS &
  BARBITURATES 128
Bell/ans - See SODIUM BICARBONATE 790
Bellergal - See
  BELLADONNA ALKALOIDS & BARBITURATES
    128
  ERGOTAMINE, BELLADONNA &
    PHENOBARBITAL 348
Bellergal-S - See ERGOTAMINE, BELLADONNA &
  PHENOBARBITAL 348
Bellergal Spacetabs - See ERGOTAMINE,
  BELLADONNA & PHENOBARBITAL 348
Benacen - See PROBENECID 718
Bena-D - See ANTIHISTAMINES 92
Bena-D 50 - See ANTIHISTAMINES 92
Benadryl - See ANTIHISTAMINES 92
Benadryl Allergy/Sinus Headache Caplets - See
  ANTIHISTAMINES 92
  PSEUDOEPHEDRINE 736
Benadryl Complete Allergy - See ANTIHISTAMINES
  92
Benadryl Decongestant - See
  ANTIHISTAMINES 92

PSEUDOEPHEDRINE 736
Benahist 10 - See ANTIHISTAMINES 92
Benahist 50 - See ANTIHISTAMINES 92
Ben-Allergin-50 - See ANTIHISTAMINES 92
Benaphen - See ANTIHISTAMINES 92
Ben-Aqua 2 Gel - See BENZOYL PEROXIDE 132
Ben-Aqua 2 Lotion - See BENZOYL PEROXIDE
  132
Ben-Aqua 5 Gel - See BENZOYL PEROXIDE 132
Ben-Aqua 5 Lotion - See BENZOYL PEROXIDE
  132
Ben-Aqua 10 Gel - See BENZOYL PEROXIDE 132
Ben-Aqua 10 Lotion - See BENZOYL PEROXIDE
  132
Ben-Aqua Masque 5 - See BENZOYL PEROXIDE
  132
BENAZEPRIL - See ANGIOTENSIN-CONVERTING
  ENZYME (ACE) INHIBITORS 52
BENDROFLUMETHIAZIDE - See DIURETICS,
  THIAZIDE 324
Benemid - See PROBENECID 718
Benoject-10 - See ANTIHISTAMINES 92
Benoject-50 - See ANTIHISTAMINES 92
Benoxyl-5 Gel - See BENZOYL PEROXIDE 132
Benoxyl-5 Lotion - See BENZOYL PEROXIDE 132
Benoxyl-10 Gel - See BENZOYL PEROXIDE 132
Benoxyl-10 Lotion - See BENZOYL PEROXIDE 132
Benoxyl-20 Lotion - See BENZOYL PEROXIDE 132
Bensulfoid Cream - See ANTI-ACNE (Topical) 60
Bensylate - See ANTIDYSKINETICS 80
Bentyl - See DICYCLOMINE 300
Bentylol - See DICYCLOMINE 300
Benuryl - See PROBENECID 718
Benylin with Codeine - See
  ANTIHISTAMINES 92
  NARCOTIC ANALGESICS 592
Benylin Cold - See
  ANTIHISTAMINES 92
  PSEUDOEPHEDRINE 736
Benylin Cough - See ANTIHISTAMINES 92
Benylin Decongestant - See
  ANTIHISTAMINES 92
  PSEUDOEPHEDRINE 736
Benylin Expectorant Cough Formula - See
  DEXTROMETHORPHAN 292
  GUAIFENESIN 408
Benylin-DM - See ANTIHISTAMINES 92
Benzac Ac 2 Gel - See BENZOYL PEROXIDE 132
Benzac Ac 5 Gel - See BENZOYL PEROXIDE 132
Benzac Ac 10 Gel - See BENZOYL PEROXIDE 132
Benzac W 2 Gel - See BENZOYL PEROXIDE 132
Benzac W 5 Gel - See BENZOYL PEROXIDE 132
Benzac W 10 Gel - See BENZOYL PEROXIDE 132
Benzagel 5 Acne Lotion - See BENZOYL
  PEROXIDE 132
Benzagel 5 Acne Wash - See BENZOYL
  PEROXIDE 132
Benzagel 5 Gel - See BENZOYL PEROXIDE 132
Benzagel 10 Gel - See BENZOYL PEROXIDE 132
BENZALCONIUM CHLORIDE - See
  CONTRACEPTIVES, VAGINAL (Spermicides)
  252

Black-Draught Lax Senna - See SENNA 780
Blanex - See
  CHLORZOXAZONE & ACETAMINOPHEN 212
  ORPHENADRINE 630
Bleph-10 - See ANTIBACTERIALS (Ophthalmic) 64
Blue - See PEDICULISIDES (Topical) 656
Bonamine - See MECLIZINE 512
Bonine - See MECLIZINE 512
Bontril PDM - See APPETITE SUPPRESSANTS 106
Bontril Slow Release - See APPETITE
  SUPPRESSANTS 106
Bowel preparation - See KANAMYCIN 466
Bowel preparation adjunct - See NEOMYCIN
  (Topical) 600
Breonesin - See GUAIFENESIN 408
Brethaire - See BRONCHODILATORS,
  ADRENERGIC 150
Brethine - See BRONCHODILATORS,
  ADRENERGIC 150
Brevicon - See
  CONTRACEPTIVES, ORAL 250
  ESTROGENS 360
Brevoxyl 4 Gel - See BENZOYL PEROXIDE 132
Brexin - See
  ANTIHISTAMINES 92
  GUAIFENESIN 408
  PSEUDOEPHEDRINE 736
Brexin-L.A. - See
  ANTIHISTAMINES 92
  PSEUDOEPHEDRINE 736
Bricanyl - See BRONCHODILATORS,
  ADRENERGIC 150
Brokolixir - See THEOPHYLLINE, EPHEDRINE,
  GUAIFENESIN & BARBITURATES 832
Bromanate DC Cough - See
  ANTIHISTAMINES 92
  NARCOTIC ANALGESICS 592
Bromanate DC Cough Syrup - See
  PHENYLPROPANOLAMINE 686
Bromatap - See
  ANTIHISTAMINES 92
  PHENYLPROPANOLAMINE 686
Bromatapp - See
  ANTIHISTAMINES 92
  PHENYLPROPANOLAMINE 686
BROMAZEPAM - See BENZODIAZEPINES 130
Brombay - See ANTIHISTAMINES 92
Bromfed - See - See
  ANTIHISTAMINES 92
  PSEUDOEPHEDRINE 736
Bromfed-AT - See
  ANTIHISTAMINES 92
  DEXTROMETHORPHAN 292
  PSEUDOEPHEDRINE 736
Bromfed-DM - See
  ANTIHISTAMINES 92
  DEXTROMETHORPHAN 292
  PSEUDOEPHEDRINE 736
Bromfed-PD - See
  ANTIHISTAMINES 92
  PSEUDOEPHEDRINE 736
BROMOCRIPTINE 148

BROMODIPHENHYDRAMINE - See
  ANTIHISTAMINES 92
Bromophen T.D. - See
  ANTIHISTAMINES 92
  PHENYLEPHRINE 682
  PHENYLPROPANOLAMINE 686
Bromo-Seltzer - See ACETAMINOPHEN 2
Bromphem - See ANTIHISTAMINES 92
Bromphen DC - See ANTIHISTAMINES 92
Bromphen DC w/Codeine Cough - See
  NARCOTIC ANALGESICS 592
  PHENYLPROPANOLAMINE 686
BROMPHENIRAMINE - See ANTIHISTAMINES 92
Brompheril - See
  ANTIHISTAMINES 92
  PSEUDOEPHEDRINE 736
Bronchial - See THEOPHYLLINE & GUAIFENESIN 836
Broncho-Grippol-DM - See DEXTROMETHORPHAN
  292
Bronchodilator - See
  IPRATROPIUM 452
  ISOPROTERENOL & PHENYLEPHRINE 460
  THEOPHYLLINE & GUAIFENESIN 836
  THEOPHYLLINE, EPHEDRINE &
    BARBITURATES 830
Bronchodilator (xanthine) - See
  BRONCHODILATORS, XANTHINE 152
  OXTRIPHYLLINE & GUAIFENESIN 636
  THEOPHYLLINE, EPHEDRINE & HYDROXYZINE
    834
  THEOPHYLLINE, EPHEDRINE, GUAIFENESIN &
    BARBITURATES 832
BRONCHODILATORS, ADRENERGIC 150
BRONCHODILATORS, XANTHINE 152
Broncholate - See
  EPHEDRINE 340
  GUAIFENESIN 408
Brondecon - See
  BRONCHODILATORS, XANTHINE 152
  OXTRIPHYLLINE & GUAIFENESIN 636
Brondelate - See OXTRIPHYLLINE &
  GUAIFENESIN 636
Bronitin Mist - See BRONCHODILATORS,
  ADRENERGIC 150
Bronkaid Mist - See BRONCHODILATORS,
  ADRENERGIC 150
Bronkaid Mist Suspension - See
  BRONCHODILATORS, ADRENERGIC 150
Bronkaid Mistometer - See BRONCHODILATORS,
  ADRENERGIC 150
Bronkephrine - See BRONCHODILATORS,
  ADRENERGIC 150
Bronkodyl - See BRONCHODILATORS, XANTHINE
  152
Bronkometer - See BRONCHODILATORS,
  ADRENERGIC 150
Bronkosol - See BRONCHODILATORS,
  ADRENERGIC 150
Bronkotabs - See THEOPHYLLINE, EPHEDRINE,
  GUAIFENESIN & BARBITURATES 832
Bronkotuss Expectorant - See
  ANTIHISTAMINES 92

Cari-Tab - See VITAMINS & FLUORIDE 896
Carmol-HC - See ADRENOCORTICOIDS (Topical) 14
Carnitor - See LEVOCARNITINE 482
Caroid Laxative - See CASCARA 184
CARTEOLOL - See BETA-ADRENERGIC BLOCKERS 134
Carter's Little Pills - See BISACODYL 144
Cartrol - See BETA-ADRENERGIC BLOCKERS 134
CASCARA 184
Cascara Sagrada - See CASCARA 184
Castel Plus - See CARBOL-FUCHSIN (Topical) 180
Castellani Paint - See CARBOL-FUCHSIN (Topical) 180
CASTOR OIL 186
Catapres - See CLONIDINE 232
Catapres-TTS - See CLONIDINE 232
CCNU - See LOMUSTINE 492
Ceclor - See CEPHALOSPORINS 190
Cecon - See VITAMIN C (Ascorbic Acid) 888
Cedocard-SR - See NITRATES 614
CeeNU - See LOMUSTINE 492
CEFACHLOR - See CEPHALOSPORINS 190
CEFADROXIL - See CEPHALOSPORINS 190
Cefanex - See CEPHALOSPORINS 190
CEFIXIME - See CEPHALOSPORINS 190
CEFPODOXIME - See CEPHALOSPORINS 190
CEFPROZIL - See CEPHALOSPORINS 190
Ceftin - See CEPHALOSPORINS 190
CEFUROXIME - See CEPHALOSPORINS 190
Cefzil - See CEPHALOSPORINS 190
Celestoderm-V - See ADRENOCORTICOIDS (Topical) 14
Celestone Phosphate - See BETAMETHASONE 140
Celestone Soluspan - See BETAMETHASONE 140
Celestone - See BETAMETHASONE 140
Cellothyl - See METHYLCELLULOSE 536
CELLULOSE SODIUM PHOSPHATE 188
Celontin - See METHSUXIMIDE 534
Cemill - See VITAMIN C (Ascorbic Acid) 888
Cenafed - See PSEUDOEPHEDRINE 736
Cenafed Plus - See
    ANTIHISTAMINES 92
    PSEUDOEPHEDRINE 736
Cena-K - See POTASSIUM SUPPLEMENTS 704
Cenocort A 40 - See TRIAMCINOLONE 860
Cenocort Forte - See TRIAMCINOLONE 860
Cenolate - See VITAMIN C (Ascorbic Acid) 888
Central nervous system stimulant - See
    AMPHETAMINES 34
    PEMOLINE 658
Centrax - See BENZODIAZEPINES 130
CEPHALEXIN - See CEPHALOSPORINS 190
CEPHRADINE - See CEPHALOSPORINS 190
Ceporex - See CEPHALOSPORINS 190
Cerespan - See PAPAVERINE 646
Cerose-DM - See
    ANTIHISTAMINES 92
    DEXTROMETHORPHAN 292
    PHENYLEPHRINE 682
C.E.S. - See ESTROGENS 360

Cesamet - See NABILONE 580
Cetacort - See ADRENOCORTICOIDS (Topical) 14
Cetamide - See
    ANTIBACTERIALS (Ophthalmic) 64
    SULFAMETHOXAZOLE 806
Cetane - See VITAMIN C (Ascorbic Acid) 888
Cetazone - See CHLORZOXAZONE & ACETAMINOPHEN 212
Cevalin - See VITAMIN C (Ascorbic Acid) 888
Cevi-Bid - See VITAMIN C (Ascorbic Acid) 888
Ce-Vi-Sol - See VITAMIN C (Ascorbic Acid) 888
Cevita - See VITAMIN C (Ascorbic Acid) 888
Charcoaid - See CHARCOAL, ACTIVATED 192
CHARCOAL, ACTIVATED 192
Charcocaps - See CHARCOAL, ACTIVATED 192
Charcodote - See CHARCOAL, ACTIVATED 192
Chardonna-2 - See BELLADONNA ALKALOIDS & BARBITURATES 128
Chase - See CALCIUM CHANNEL BLOCKERS 168
Chelating agent - See PENICILLAMINE 660
Chenix - See CHENODIOL 194
CHENODIOL 194
Cheracol - See
    GUAIFENESIN 408
    NARCOTIC ANALGESICS 592
Cheracol D Cough - See
    DEXTROMETHORPHAN 292
    GUAIFENESIN 408
Cheracol Plus - See
    ANTIHISTAMINES 92
    DEXTROMETHORPHAN 292
    PHENYLPROPANOLAMINE 686
Cheracol Sinus - See
    ANTIHISTAMINES 92
    PSEUDOEPHEDRINE 736
Cheragan with TMP - See
    SULFAMETHOXAZOLE 806
    TRIMETHOPRIM 876
Cherapas - See RESERPINE, HYDRALAZINE & HYDROCHLOROTHIAZIDE 764
Chew-E - See VITAMIN E 892
Chexit - See
    ACETAMINOPHEN 2
    ANTIHISTAMINES 92
    DEXTROMETHORPHAN 292
    PHENYLPROPANOLAMINE 686
    TERPIN HYDRATE 822
Chibroxin - See ANTIBACTERIALS (Ophthalmic) 64
Children's Anacin 3 - See ACETAMINOPHEN 2
Children's Genapap - See ACETAMINOPHEN 2
Children's NyQuil Nighttime Cold Medicine - See
    ANTIHISTAMINES 92
    DEXTROMETHORPHAN 292
    PSEUDOEPHEDRINE 736
Children's Panadol - See ACETAMINOPHEN 2
Children's Sudafed Liquid - See
    PSEUDOEPHEDRINE 736
Children's Tylenol - See ACETAMINOPHEN 2
Children's Ty-Tab - See ACETAMINOPHEN 2
Chlo-Amine - See ANTIHISTAMINES 92
CHLOPHEDIANOL 196

BETHANECHOL 142
NEOSTIGMINE 602
PYRIDOSTIGMINE 744
Choloxin - See DEXTROTHYROXINE 296
Cholybar - See CHOLESTYRAMINE 214
Chooz - See ANTACIDS 56
Chronulac - See LACTULOSE 476
Cibalith-S - See LITHIUM 490
CICLOPIROX - See
 ANTIBACTERIALS, ANTIFUNGALS (Topical) 70
 ANTIFUNGALS (Topical) 84
Cillium - See PSYLLIUM 740
Ciloxam - See ANTIFUNGALS (Topical) 84
CIMETIDINE - See HISTAMINE H$_2$ RECEPTOR
 ANTAGONISTS 422
Cinalone 40 - See TRIAMCINOLONE 860
Cinchocaine - See ANESTHETICS (Topical) 46
Cinobac - See CINOXACIN 216
Cinonide 40 - See TRIAMCINOLONE 860
CINOXACIN 216
Cin-Quin - See QUINIDINE 752
Cipro - See CIPROFLOXACIN 218
CIPROFLOXACIN 218
Citra Forte - See
 ANTIHISTAMINES 92
 CITRATES 220
 NARCOTIC ANALGESICS 592
 PHENYLEPHRINE 682
 SALICYLATES 774
Citracal - See CALCIUM SUPPLEMENTS 170
Citrate of Magnesia - See MAGNESIUM CITRATE
 498
Citrated Caffeine - See CAFFEINE 166
CITRATES 220
Citrocarbonate - See SODIUM BICARBONATE 790
Citrocovorin Calcium - See LEUCOVORIN 478
Citrolith - See CITRATES 220
Citroma - See MAGNESIUM CITRATE 498
Citro-Mag - See MAGNESIUM CITRATE 498
Citro-Nesia - See MAGNESIUM CITRATE 498
Citrovorum Factor - See LEUCOVORIN 478
Citrucel - See METHYLCELLULOSE 536
Claripex - See CLOFIBRATE 228
CLARITHROMYCIN 222
Claritin - See ANTIHISTAMINES 92
Clavulin - See AMOXICILLIN 32
Cleansing agent - See ANTI-ACNE, CLEANSING
 (Topical) 62
Clear Away - See ANTI-ACNE (Topical) 60
Clear by Design 2.5 Gel - See BENZOYL
 PEROXIDE 132
Clear by Design Medicated Cleansing Pads - See
 ANTI-ACNE (Topical) 60
Clear Eyes - See DECONGESTANTS (Ophthalmic)
 284
Clearasil Adult Care Medicated Blemish - See
 ANTI-ACNE Cream (Topical) 58
Clearasil Adult Care Medicated Blemish Stick - See
 ANTI-ACNE (Topical) 60
Clearasil BP Plus 5 Cream - See BENZOYL
 PEROXIDE 132

Clearasil BP Plus 5 Lotion - See BENZOYL
 PEROXIDE 132
*Clearasil Clearstick Maximum Strength Topical
 Solution* - See ANTI-ACNE (Topical) 60
*Clearasil Clearstick Regular Strength Topical
 Solution* - See ANTI-ACNE (Topical) 60
Clearasil Double Textured Pads Maximum Strength
 - See ANTI-ACNE (Topical) 60
Clearasil Double Textured Pads Regular Strength -
 See ANTI-ACNE (Topical) 60
*Clearasil Maximum Strength Medicated Anti-Acne
 10 Tinted Cream* - See BENZOYL PEROXIDE
 132
*Clearasil Maximum Strength Medicated Anti-Acne
 10 Vanishing Cream* - See BENZOYL
 PEROXIDE 132
Clearasil Medicated Anti-Acne 10 Vanishing Lotion
 - See BENZOYL PEROXIDE 132
Clearasil Medicated Deep Cleanser Topical Solution
 - See ANTI-ACNE (Topical) 60
CLEMASTINE FUMARATE - See ANTIHISTAMINES
 92
Cleocin - See CLINDAMYCIN 226
Cleocin T - See
 ANTIBACTERIALS (Topical) 68
 ANTIBACTERIALS FOR ACNE (Topical) 72
C-Lexin - See CEPHALOSPORINS 190
CLIDINIUM 224
CLINDAMYCIN 226
CLINDAMYCIN - See ANTIBACTERIALS (Topical)
 68
CLINDAMYCIN (topical) - See ANTIBACTERIALS
 FOR ACNE (Topical) 72
Clindex - See CHLORDIAZEPOXIDE & CLIDINIUM
 206
Clinoril - See ANTI-INFLAMMATORY DRUGS,
 NON-STEROIDAL (NSAIDs) 94
Clinoxide - See CHLORDIAZEPOXIDE &
 CLIDINIUM 206
CLIOQUINOL - See ANTIBACTERIALS,
 ANTIFUNGALS (Topical) 70
CLIOQUINOL & HYDROCORTISONE - See
 ANTIBACTERIALS, ANTIFUNGALS (Topical)
 70
Clipoxide - See
 CHLORDIAZEPOXIDE & CLIDINIUM 206
 CLIDINIUM 224
Clistin - See ANTIHISTAMINES 92
CLOBETASOL (Topical) - See
 ADRENOCORTICOIDS (Topical) 14
CLOBETASONE (Topical) - See
 ADRENOCORTICOIDS (Topical) 14
CLOCORTOLONE (Topical) - See
 ADRENOCORTICOIDS (Topical) 14
Cloderm - See ADRENOCORTICOIDS (Topical) 14
CLOFIBRATE 228
Clomid - See CLOMIPHENE 230
CLOMIPHENE 230
CLOMIPRAMINE - See TRICYCLIC
 ANTIDEPRESSANTS 868
CLONAZEPAM - See BENZODIAZEPINES 130

Colrex Expectorant - See GUAIFENESIN 408
Coltab Children's - See
  ANTIHISTAMINES 92
  PHENYLEPHRINE 682
Coly-Mycin S - See ANTIBACTERIALS (Otic) 66
Combipres - See CLONIDINE &
  CHLORTHALIDONE 234
Comfort - See DECONGESTANTS (Ophthalmic)
  284
Comhist - See
  ANTIHISTAMINES 92
  PHENYLEPHRINE 682
Comhist LA - See
  ANTIHISTAMINES 92
  PHENYLEPHRINE 682
Compal - See NARCOTIC & ACETAMINOPHEN
  590
Compazine - See PHENOTHIAZINES 678
Compazine Spansule - See PHENOTHIAZINES 678
Compound W Gel - See ANTI-ACNE (Topical) 60
Compound W Liquid - See ANTI-ACNE (Topical)
  60
Compoz - See ANTIHISTAMINES 92
Comtrex - See ACETAMINOPHEN 2
Comtrex Daytime Caplets - See
  ACETAMINOPHEN 2
  DEXTROMETHORPHAN 292
  PSEUDOEPHEDRINE 736
Comtrex Multi-Symptom Cold Reliever - See
  ACETAMINOPHEN 2
  ANTIHISTAMINES 92
  DEXTROMETHORPHAN 292
  PHENYLPROPANOLAMINE 686
Comtrex Multi-Symptom Hot Flu Relief - See
  ACETAMINOPHEN 2
  ANTIHISTAMINES 92
  DEXTROMETHORPHAN 292
  PSEUDOEPHEDRINE 736
Comtrex Multi-Symptom Non-Drowsy Caplets - See
  ACETAMINOPHEN 2
  DEXTROMETHORPHAN 292
  PSEUDOEPHEDRINE 736
Comtrex Nighttime - See
  ACETAMINOPHEN 2
  ANTIHISTAMINES 92
  DEXTROMETHORPHAN 292
  PSEUDOEPHEDRINE 736
Conacetol - See ACETAMINOPHEN 2
Conar - See
  DEXTROMETHORPHAN 292
  PHENYLEPHRINE 682
Conar Expectorant - See
  DEXTROMETHORPHAN 292
  GUAIFENESIN 408
  PHENYLEPHRINE 682
Conar-A - See
  ACETAMINOPHEN 2
  DEXTROMETHORPHAN 292
  GUAIFENESIN 408
  PHENYLEPHRINE 682
Conceptrol Gel - See CONTRACEPTIVES,
  VAGINAL (Spermicides) 252

Conceptrol-Contraceptive Inserts - See
  CONTRACEPTIVES, VAGINAL (Spermicides)
  252
Concentrin - See
  DEXTROMETHORPHAN 292
  GUAIFENESIN 408
  PSEUDOEPHEDRINE 736
Condrin-LA - See
  ANTIHISTAMINES 92
  PHENYLPROPANOLAMINE 686
Conex - See
  GUAIFENESIN 408
  PHENYLPROPANOLAMINE 686
Conex w/Codeine Liquid - See
  GUAIFENESIN 408
  NARCOTIC ANALGESICS 592
  PHENYLPROPANOLAMINE 686
Conex D.A. - See PHENYLPROPANOLAMINE 686
Congespirin - See
  ACETAMINOPHEN 2
  DEXAMETHASONE 290
  DEXTROMETHORPHAN 292
Congespirin for Children Cold Tablets - See
  ACETAMINOPHEN 2
  PHENYLEPHRINE 682
Congespirin for Children Liquid Cold Medicine -
  See
  ACETAMINOPHEN 2
  PHENYLPROPANOLAMINE 686
Congess JR - See
  GUAIFENESIN 408
  PSEUDOEPHEDRINE 736
Congess SR - See
  GUAIFENESIN 408
  PSEUDOEPHEDRINE 736
Congestac N.D. Caplets - See
  PSEUDOEPHEDRINE 736
Conjec-B - See ANTIHISTAMINES 92
CONJUGATED ESTROGENS - See ESTROGENS
  360
Constant-T - See BRONCHODILATORS,
  XANTHINE 152
Constilac - See LACTULOSE 476
Contac 12-Hour - See
  ANTIHISTAMINES 92
  PHENYLPROPANOLAMINE 686
Contac Jr. Children's Cold Medicine - See
  ACETAMINOPHEN 2
  DEXTROMETHORPHAN 292
  PHENYLPROPANOLAMINE 686
Contac Maximum Strength 12-Hour - See
  PHENYLPROPANOLAMINE 686
Contac Maximum Strength Sinus Caplets - See
  ACETAMINOPHEN 2
  PSEUDOEPHEDRINE 736
Contac Severe Cold Formula - See
  ACETAMINOPHEN 2
  ANTIHISTAMINES 92
  DEXTROMETHORPHAN 292
  PSEUDOEPHEDRINE 736
Contac Severe Cold Formula Night Strength - See
  ACETAMINOPHEN 2

Corzide - See BETA-ADRENERGIC BLOCKING
AGENTS & THIAZIDE DIURETICS 136
Cotanal 65 - See NARCOTIC & ASPIRIN 594
Cotazym - See PANCRELIPASE 642
Cotazym E.C.S. - See PANCRELIPASE 642
Cotazym-65B - See PANCRELIPASE 642
Cotazym-S - See PANCRELIPASE 642
Cotrim - See
  SULFAMETHOXAZOLE 806
  TRIMETHOPRIM 876
Cotrim D.S. - See SULFAMETHOXAZOLE 806
Co-trimoxazole - See SULFAMETHOXAZOLE 806
Co-Tylenol - See ACETAMINOPHEN 2
CoTylenol Cold Medication - See
  ACETAMINOPHEN 2
  ANTIHISTAMINES 92
  DEXTROMETHORPHAN 292
  PSEUDOEPHEDRINE 736
Cough suppressant - See
  CHLOPHEDIANOL 196
  DEXTROMETHORPHAN 292
Cough/cold preparation - See
  GUAIFENESIN 408
  OXTRIPHYLLINE & GUAIFENESIN 636
  THEOPHYLLINE, EPHEDRINE, GUAIFENESIN &
    BARBITURATES 832
Coumadin - See ANTICOAGULANTS (Oral) 74
Covangesic - See ACETAMINOPHEN 2
Creamalin - See ANTACIDS 56
Cremacoat 1 - See DEXTROMETHORPHAN 292
Cremacoat 2 - See GUAIFENESIN 408
Cremacoat 3 Throat Coating Cough Medicine - See
  DEXTROMETHORPHAN 292
  GUAIFENESIN 408
  PSEUDOEPHEDRINE 736
Cremacoat 4 Throat Coating Cough Medicine - See
  ANTIHISTAMINES 92
  DEXTROMETHORPHAN 292
  PSEUDOEPHEDRINE 736
Creon - See PANCRELIPASE 642
Creo-Terpin - See DEXTROMETHORPHAN 292
CROMOLYN 256
Cruex Aerosol Powder - See ANTIFUNGALS
  (Topical) 84
Cruex Antifungal Cream - See ANTIFUNGALS
  (Topical) 84
Cruex Antifungal Powder - See ANTIFUNGALS
  (Topical) 84
Cruex Antifungal Spray Powder - See
  ANTIFUNGALS (Topical) 84
Cruex Cream - See ANTIFUNGALS (Topical) 84
Cruex Powder - See ANTIFUNGALS (Topical) 84
Crystapen - See PENICILLIN G 662
Crysticillin - See PENICILLIN G 662
Crystodigin - See DIGITALIS PREPARATIONS
  (Digitalis Glycosides) 306
C-Span - See VITAMIN C (Ascorbic Acid) 888
C-Tussin Expectorant - See
  GUAIFENESIN 408
  NARCOTIC ANALGESICS 592
  PSEUDOEPHEDRINE 736

Cultivate - See ADRENOCORTICOIDS (Topical) 14
Cuplex Gel - See ANTI-ACNE (Topical) 60
Cuprimine - See PENICILLAMINE 660
Curretab - See PROGESTINS 728
Cutar Water Dispersible Emollient Tar - See COAL
  TAR (Topical) 242
Cuticura Acne 5 Cream - See BENZOYL
  PEROXIDE 132
Cuticura Ointment - See ANTI-ACNE (Topical) 60
Cyanabin - See VITAMIN B-12 (Cyanocobalamin)
  886
CYANACOBALAMIN - See VITAMIN B-12
  (Cyanocobalamin) 886
Cyanocobalamin Co 57 - See RADIO-
  PHARMACEUTICALS 756
Cyanocobalamin Co 60 - See RADIO-
  PHARMACEUTICALS 756
Cyantin - See NITROFURANTOIN 616
CYCLACILLIN 258
CYCLANDELATE 260
Cyclapen-W - See CYCLACILLIN 258
CYCLIZINE 262
CYCLOBENZAPRINE 264
Cyclocort - See ADRENOCORTICOIDS (Topical) 14
Cyclogyl - See CYCLOPENTOLATE (Ophthalmic) 268
Cyclokapron - See ANTIFIBRINOLYTIC AGENTS 82
Cyclomen - See DANAZOL 276
CYCLOMETHYCAINE - See ANESTHETICS
  (Topical) 46
Cyclopegic, mydriatic - See
  CYCLOPEGIC, MYDRIATIC (Ophthalmic) 266
  CYCLOPENTOLATE (Ophthalmic) 268
CYCLOPEGIC, MYDRIATIC (Ophthalmic) 266
CYCLOPENTOLATE (Ophthalmic) 268
CYCLOPHOSPHAMIDE 270
CYCLOSERINE 272
Cyclospasmol - See CYCLANDELATE 260
CYCLOSPORINE 274
CYCLOTHIAZIDE - See DIURETICS, THIAZIDE 324
Cycrin - See PROGESTINS 728
Cylert - See PEMOLINE 658
Cylert Chewable - See PEMOLINE 658
CYPROHEPTADINE - See ANTIHISTAMINES 92
Cyraso-400 - See CYCLANDELATE 260
Cytadren - See AMINOGLUTETHIMIDE 28
Cytomel - See THYROID HORMONES 846
Cytotec - See MISOPROSTOL 568
Cytotoxic (topical) - See PODOPHYLLUM (Topical)
  692
Cytoxan - See CYCLOPHOSPHAMIDE 270

D

Dacodyl - See BISACODYL 144
Dalacin - See ANTIBACTERIALS FOR ACNE
  (Topical) 72
Dalalone - See DEXAMETHASONE 290
Dalalone D.P. - See DEXAMETHASONE 290
Dalalone L.A. - See DEXAMETHASONE 290
Dallergy Jr. - See
  ANTIHISTAMINES 92
  PSEUDOEPHEDRINE 736

INDEX

Delatestryl - See ANDROGENS 42
Delaxin - See MUSCLE RELAXANTS, SKELETAL 578
Delcid - See ANTACIDS 56
Delestrogen - See ESTROGENS 360
Delfen - See CONTRACEPTIVES, VAGINAL (Spermicides) 252
Del-Ray - See BENZOYL PEROXIDE 132
Delsym - See DEXTROMETHORPHAN 292
Delta-Cortef - See PREDNISOLONE 710
Deltalin - See VITAMIN D 890
Deltamine - See METHENAMINE 528
Deltasone - See PREDNISONE 712
Demazin - See
  ANTIHISTAMINES 92
  PHENYLPROPANOLAMINE 686
Demazin Repetabs - See
  ANTIHISTAMINES 92
  PHENYLPROPANOLAMINE 686
DEMECARIUM - See ANTIGLAUCOMA, LONG-ACTING (Ophthalmic) 88
DEMECLOCYCLINE - See TETRACYCLINES 828
Demerol - See NARCOTIC ANALGESICS 592
Demerol-APAP - See NARCOTIC & ACETAMINOPHEN 590
Demi-Regroton - See
  RAUWOLFIA & THIAZIDE DIURETICS 760
  RAUWOLFIA ALKALOIDS 758
Demser - See METYROSINE 558
Demulen - See
  CONTRACEPTIVES, ORAL 250
  ESTROGENS 360
Denorex - See COAL TAR (Topical) 242
Denorex Extra Strength Medicated Shampoo - See COAL TAR (Topical) 242
Denorex Extra Strength Medicated Shampoo with Conditioners - See COAL TAR (Topical) 242
Denorex Medicated Shampoo - See COAL TAR (Topical) 242
Denorex Medicated Shampoo and Conditioner - See COAL TAR (Topical) 242
Denorex Mountain Fresh Herbal Scent Medicated Shampoo - See COAL TAR (Topical) 242
Denta-Fl - See SODIUM FLUORIDE 792
Dep Andro - See ANDROGENS 42
dep Medalone - See METHYLPREDNISOLONE 546
Depa - See VALPROIC ACID (Dipropylacetic Acid) 880
Depakene - See VALPROIC ACID (Dipropylacetic Acid) 880
Depakote - See DIVALPROEX 326
depAndrogyn - See TESTOSTERONE & ESTRADIOL 826
Depen - See PENICILLAMINE 660
depGynogen - See ESTROGENS 360
Depo Estradiol - See ESTROGENS 360
Depogen - See ESTROGENS 360
Depoject-40 - See METHYLPREDNISOLONE 546
Depoject-80 - See METHYLPREDNISOLONE 546
Depo-Medrol - See METHYLPREDNISOLONE 546
Deponit - See NITRATES 614

Depo-Pred-40 - See METHYLPREDNISOLONE 546
Depo-Pred-80 - See METHYLPREDNISOLONE 546
Depo-Predate - See METHYLPREDNISOLONE 546
Depo-Provera - See PROGESTINS 728
Depotest - See ANDROGENS 42
Depo-Testadiol - See TESTOSTERONE & ESTRADIOL 826
Depotestogen - See TESTOSTERONE & ESTRADIOL 826
Depo-Testosterone - See ANDROGENS 42
Deproist Expectorant w/Codeine - See
  GUAIFENESIN 408
  NARCOTIC ANALGESICS 592
  PSEUDOEPHEDRINE 736
Derbac - See PEDICULISIDES (Topical) 656
Derma & Soft Creme - See ANTI-ACNE (Topical) 60
Dermabet - See ADRENOCORTICOIDS (Topical) 14
Dermacomb - See
  ANTIBACTERIALS, ANTIFUNGALS (Topical) 70
  NYSTATIN 622
  TRIAMCINOLONE 860
Dermacort - See ADRENOCORTICOIDS (Topical) 14
DermiCort - See ADRENOCORTICOIDS (Topical) 14
Dermolate - See HYDROCORTISONE Rectal) 432
Dermovate - See ADRENOCORTICOIDS (Topical) 14
Dermovate Scalp Application - See ADRENOCORTICOIDS (Topical) 14
Dermoxyl 2.5 Gel - See BENZOYL PEROXIDE 132
Dermoxyl 5 Gel - See BENZOYL PEROXIDE 132
Dermoxyl 10 Gel - See BENZOYL PEROXIDE 132
Dermoxyl 20 Gel - See BENZOYL PEROXIDE 132
Dermoxyl Aqua - See BENZOYL PEROXIDE 132
Dermtex HC - See ADRENOCORTICOIDS (Topical) 14
Deronil - See DEXAMETHASONE 290
DES - See ESTROGENS 360
Desasone L.A. - See DEXAMETHASONE 290
Desenex Aerosol Powder - See ANTIFUNGALS (Topical) 84
Desenex Antifungal Cream - See ANTIFUNGALS (Topical) 84
Desenex Antifungal Liquid - See ANTIFUNGALS (Topical) 84
Desenex Antifungal Ointment - See ANTIFUNGALS (Topical) 84
Desenex Antifungal Powder - See ANTIFUNGALS (Topical) 84
Desenex Antifungal Penetrating Foam - See ANTIFUNGALS (Topical) 84
Desenex Antifungal Spray Powder - See ANTIFUNGALS (Topical) 84
Desenex Ointment - See ANTIFUNGALS (Topical) 84
Desenex Powder - See ANTIFUNGALS (Topical) 84
Desenex Solution - See ANTIFUNGALS (Topical) 84
DESERPIDINE - See RAUWOLFIA ALKALOIDS 758

Diasporal Cream - See ANTI-ACNE (Topical) 60
Diazemuls - See BENZODIAZEPINES 130
DIAZEPAM - See BENZODIAZEPINES 130
Diazepam Intensol - See BENZODIAZEPINES 130
DIBASIC CALCIUM PHOSPHATE - See CALCIUM
    SUPPLEMENTS 170
DIBASIC POTASSIUM & SODIUM PHOSPHATES -
    See POTASSIUM & SODIUM PHOSPHATES 702
Dibent - See DICYCLOMINE 300
DIBUCAINE - See
    ANESTHETICS (Rectal) 44
    ANESTHETICS (Topical) 46
Dicarbosil - See ANTACIDS 56
DICHLORPHENAMIDE - See CARBONIC
    ANHYDRASE INHIBITORS 182
DICLOFENAC - See ANTI-INFLAMMATORY
    DRUGS, NON-STEROIDAL (NSAIDs) 94
DICLOXACILLIN 298
DICUMAROL - See ANTICOAGULANTS (Oral) 74
DICYCLOMINE 300
Di-Cyclonex - See DICYCLOMINE 300
DIDANOSINE 302
Didrex - See APPETITE SUPPRESSANTS 106
Didronel - See ETIDRONATE 372
Dietary replacement - See CALCIUM
    SUPPLEMENTS 170
DIETHYLPROPION - See APPETITE
    SUPPRESSANTS 106
DIETHYLSTILBESTROL (DES) - See ESTROGENS
    360
DIFENOXIN & ATROPINE 304
DIFLORASONE (Topical) - See
    ADRENOCORTICOIDS (Topical) 14
DIFLUCORTOLONE (Topical) - See
    ADRENOCORTICOIDS (Topical) 14
DIFLUNISAL - See ANTI-INFLAMMATORY
    DRUGS, NON-STEROIDAL (NSAIDs) 94
Difulcan - See FLUCONAZOLE 384
Di-Gel - See
    ANTACIDS 56
    SIMETHICONE 786
Digestant - See PANCREATIN, PEPSIN, BILE
    SALTS, HYOSCYAMINE, ATROPINE,
    SCOPOLAMINE & PHENOBARBITAL 640
DIGITALIS - See DIGITALIS PREPARATIONS
    (Digitalis Glycosides) 306
Digitalis Preparations - See DIGITALIS
    PREPARATIONS (Digitalis Glycosides) 306
DIGITALIS PREPARATIONS (Digitalis Glycosides)
    306
DIGITOXIN - See DIGITALIS PREPARATIONS
    (Digitalis Glycosides) 306
DIGOXIN - See DIGITALIS PREPARATIONS
    (Digitalis Glycosides) 306
Dihistine - See
    ANTIHISTAMINES 92
    PHENYLEPHRINE 682
Dihistine DH - See
    ANTIHISTAMINES 92
    NARCOTIC ANALGESICS 592
    PSEUDOEPHEDRINE 736

Dihydrex - See ANTIHISTAMINES 92
DIHYDROCODEINE - See NARCOTIC
    ANALGESICS 592
Dihydromorphinone - See NARCOTIC
    ANALGESICS 592
DIHYDROTACHYSTEROL - See VITAMIN D 890
Dihydrotesterone inhibitor - See FINASTERIDE 378
DIHYDROXYALUMINUM AMINOACETATE - See
    ANTACIDS 56
DIHYDROXYALUMINUM AMINOACETATE,
    MAGNESIA, AND ALUMINA - See ANTACIDS
    56
DIHYDROXYALUMINUM SODIUM CARBONATE -
    See ANTACIDS 56
Dilantin - See PHENYTOIN 688
Dilantin-30-Pediatric - See PHENYTOIN 688
Dilantin-125 - See PHENYTOIN 688
Dilantin Infatabs - See PHENYTOIN 688
Dilantin Kapseals - See PHENYTOIN 688
Dilatair - See PHENYLEPHRINE (Ophthalmic) 684
Dilatrate-SR - See NITRATES 614
Dilaudid - See NARCOTIC ANALGESICS 592
Dilaudid Cough - See
    GUAIFENESIN 408
    NARCOTIC ANALGESICS 592
Dilaudid-HP - See NARCOTIC ANALGESICS 592
Dilodohydroxyquin - See IODOQUINOL 448
Dilomine - See DICYCLOMINE 300
Dilor - See BRONCHODILATORS, XANTHINE 152
Dilor-400 - See BRONCHODILATORS, XANTHINE
    152
Dilotab - See
    ACETAMINOPHEN 2
    PHENYLPROPANOLAMINE 686
DILTIAZEM - See CALCIUM CHANNEL
    BLOCKERS 168
Dimacol - See
    DEXTROMETHORPHAN 292
    GUAIFENESIN 408
    PSEUDOEPHEDRINE 736
Dimaphen S.A. - See
    ANTIHISTAMINES 92
    PHENYLEPHRINE 682
    PHENYLPROPANOLAMINE 686
Dimelor - See ANTIDIABETIC AGENTS 78
DIMENHYDRINATE - See ANTIHISTAMINES 92
Dimentabs - See ANTIHISTAMINES 92
Dimetane - See ANTIHISTAMINES 92
Dimetane Decongestant - See ANTIHISTAMINES 92
Decongestant Caplets - See PHENYLEPHRINE 682
Dimetane Expectorant - See
    ANTIHISTAMINES 92
    GUAIFENESIN 408
    PHENYLEPHRINE 682
    PHENYLPROPANOLAMINE 686
Dimetane Expectorant-C - See
    ANTIHISTAMINES 92
    GUAIFENESIN 408
    NARCOTIC ANALGESICS 592
    PHENYLEPHRINE 682
    PHENYLPROPANOLAMINE 686

INDEX

EpiPen Auto-Injector - See BRONCHODILATORS, ADRENERGIC 150
EpiPen Jr. Auto-Injector - See BRONCHODILATORS, ADRENERGIC 150
Episel - See ANTISEBORRHEICS (Topical) 100
Epistatin -See HMG-CoA REDUCTASE INHIBITORS 424
Epitol - See CARBAMAZEPINE 174
Epitrate - See ANTIGLAUCOMA, SHORT-ACTING (Ophthalmic) 90
Epival - See DIVALPROEX 326
Eppy/N - See ANTIGLAUCOMA, SHORT-ACTING (Ophthalmic) 90
Eprolin - See VITAMIN E 892
Epromate-M - See MEPROBAMATE & ASPIRIN 522
Epsikapron - See ANTIFIBRINOLYTIC AGENTS 82
Epsilan-M - See VITAMIN E 892
Epsom Salts - See MAGNESIUM SULFATE 500
Eptastatin - See HMG-CoA REDUCTASE INHIBITORS 424
Equagesic - See
  ASPIRIN 108
  MEPROBAMATE & ASPIRIN 522
  MEPROBAMATE 520
Equalactin - See POLYCARBOPHIL CALCIUM 696
Equanil - See MEPROBAMATE 520
Equanil Wyseals - See MEPROBAMATE 520
Equazine-M - See MEPROBAMATE & ASPIRIN 522
Equilet - See ANTACIDS 56
Ercaf - See ERGOTAMINE & CAFFEINE 350
Ercatabs - See ERGOTAMINE & CAFFEINE 350
Ergamisol - See LEVAMISOLE 480
Ergo-Caff - See ERGOTAMINE & CAFFEINE 350
ERGOCALCIFEROL - See VITAMIN D 890
ERGOLOID MESYLATES 342
Ergomar - See ERGOTAMINE 346
Ergometrine - See ERGONOVINE 344
ERGONOVINE 344
Ergostat - See ERGOTAMINE 346
Ergot preparation - See
  ERGONOVINE 344
  ERGOLOID MESYLATES 342
  METHYLERGONOVINE 542
ERGOTAMINE 346
ERGOTAMINE, BELLADONNA & PHENOBARBITAL 348
ERGOTAMINE & CAFFEINE 350
ERGOTAMINE, CAFFEINE, BELLADONNA & PENTOBARBITAL 352
Ergotrate - See ERGONOVINE 344
Ergotrate Maleate - See ERGONOVINE 344
Eridium - See PHENAZOPYRIDINE 674
Eryc - See ERYTHROMYCINS 354
Erycette - See
  ANTIBACTERIALS FOR ACNE (Topical) 72
  ERYTHROMYCINS 354
EryDerm - See ANTIBACTERIALS FOR ACNE (Topical) 72
Ery-derm - See ERYTHROMYCINS 354
Erygel - See
  ANTIBACTERIALS FOR ACNE (Topical) 72

ERYTHROMYCINS 354
Erymax - See
  ANTIBACTERIALS FOR ACNE (Topical) 72
  ERYTHROMYCINS 354
EryPed - See ERYTHROMYCINS 354
Ery-Sol - See
  ANTIBACTERIALS FOR ACNE (Topical) 72
  ERYTHROMYCINS 354
Ery-Tab - See ERYTHROMYCINS 354
ERYTHRITYL TETRANITRATE - See NITRATES 614
Erythro - See ERYTHROMYCINS 354
Erythrocin - See ERYTHROMYCINS 354
Erythrocot - See ERYTHROMYCINS 354
Erythromid - See ERYTHROMYCINS 354
ERYTHROMYCIN (Ophthalmic) - See ANTIBACTERIALS (Ophthalmic) 64
ERYTHROMYCIN (Topical) - See ANTIBACTERIALS FOR ACNE (Topical) 72
ERYTHROMYCIN & SULFISOXAZOLE 356
ERYTHROMYCIN ESTOLATE - See ERYTHROMYCINS 354
ERYTHROMYCIN ETHYLSUCCINATE - See ERYTHROMYCINS 354
ERYTHROMYCIN GLUCEPTATE - See ERYTHROMYCINS 354
ERYTHROMYCIN LACTOBIONATE - See ERYTHROMYCINS 354
ERYTHROMYCIN STEARATE - See ERYTHROMYCINS 354
ERYTHROMYCIN-BASE - See ERYTHROMYCINS 354
ERYTHROMYCINS 354
Erythrozone - See ERYTHROMYCINS 354
Escot - See ANTACIDS 56
Eserine - See ANTIGLAUCOMA, SHORT-ACTING (Ophthalmic) 90
Esgic - See
  ACETAMINOPHEN 2
  BARBITURATES 122
  CAFFEINE 166
Esidrix - See DIURETICS, THIAZIDE 324
Esimil - See GUANETHIDINE & HYDROCHLOROTHIAZIDE 416
Eskalith - See LITHIUM 490
Eskalith CR - See LITHIUM 490
Espotabs - See PHENOLPHTHALEIN 676
Estar - See COAL TAR (Topical) 242
ESTAZOLAM - See BENZODIAZEPINES 130
ESTERIFIED ESTROGENS - See ESTROGENS 360
Estinyl - See ESTROGENS 360
Estivin II - See DECONGESTANTS (Ophthalmic) 284
Estrace - See ESTROGENS 360
Estra-D - See ESTROGENS 360
Estraderm - See ESTROGENS 360
ESTRADIOL - See ESTROGENS 360
Estradiol L.A. - See ESTROGENS 360
Estra-L - See ESTROGENS 360
ESTRAMUSTINE 358
Estrand - See TESTOSTERONE & ESTRADIOL 826
Estratab - See ESTROGENS 360
Estra-Testrin - See TESTOSTERONE & ESTRADIOL 826

INDEX

Feldene - See ANTI-INFLAMMATORY DRUGS,
    NON-STEROIDAL (NSAIDs) 94
FELODIPINE - See CALCIUM CHANNEL
    BLOCKERS 168
Female sex hormone - See CONTRACEPTIVES,
    ORAL 250
Female sex hormone (estrogen) - See
    ESTROGENS 360
Female sex hormone (progestin) - See
    LEVONORGESTREL 486
    PROGESTINS 728
FemCare - See ANTIFUNGALS (Vaginal) 86
Femcet - See
    ACETAMINOPHEN 2
    BARBITURATES 122
Feminone - See ESTROGENS 360
Femiron - See IRON SUPPLEMENTS 454
Femogen Forte - See ESTROGENS 360
Femogex - See ESTROGENS 360
Femotrone - See PROGESTINS 728
Femstat - See ANTIFUNGALS (Vaginal) 86
Fendol - See
    ACETAMINOPHEN 2
    CAFFEINE 166
    GUAIFENESIN 408
    PHENYLEPHRINE 682
    SALICYLATES 774
FENFLURAMINE - See APPETITE
    SUPPRESSANTS 106
Fenicol Ophthalmic Ointment - See
    ANTIBACTERIALS (Ophthalmic) 64
FENOPROFEN - See ANTI-INFLAMMATORY
    DRUGS, NON-STEROIDAL (NSAIDs) 94
Fenopron - See ANTI-INFLAMMATORY DRUGS,
    NON-STEROIDAL (NSAIDs) 94
FENOTEROL - See BRONCHODILATORS,
    ADRENERGIC 150
FENTANYL - See NARCOTIC ANALGESICS 592
Fenylhist - See ANTIHISTAMINES 92
Feosol - See IRON SUPPLEMENTS 454
Feostat - See IRON SUPPLEMENTS 454
Fergon - See IRON SUPPLEMENTS 454
Fer-In-Sol - See IRON SUPPLEMENTS 454
Fer-Iron - See IRON SUPPLEMENTS 454
Fero-folic-500 - See IRON SUPPLEMENTS 454
Fero-Grad - See IRON SUPPLEMENTS 454
Fero-Gradumet - See IRON SUPPLEMENTS 454
Ferospace - See IRON SUPPLEMENTS 454
Ferralet - See IRON SUPPLEMENTS 454
Ferralyn - See IRON SUPPLEMENTS 454
Ferra-TD - See IRON SUPPLEMENTS 454
Ferrous Citrate Fe 59 - See RADIO-
    PHARMACEUTICALS 756
FERROUS FUMARATE - See IRON
    SUPPLEMENTS 454
FERROUS GLUCONATE - See IRON
    SUPPLEMENTS 454
FERROUS SULFATE - See IRON SUPPLEMENTS 454
Fertinic - See IRON SUPPLEMENTS 454
Festal II - See PANCRELIPASE 642

Feverall Sprinkle Caps - See ACETAMINOPHEN 2
Fever-reducer - See
    ACETAMINOPHEN 2
    ACETAMINOPHEN & SALICYLATES 4
    CHLORZOXAZONE & ACETAMINOPHEN 212
    NARCOTIC & ACETAMINOPHEN 590
Fevernol Children's Strength - See
    ACETAMINOPHEN 2
Fevernol Junior Strength - See ACETAMINOPHEN 2
Fiberall - See PSYLLIUM 740
FiberCon - See POLYCARBOPHIL CALCIUM 696
FINASTERIDE 378
Fiomor with Codeine - See BUTALBITAL, ASPIRIN
    & CODEINE (Also contains caffeine) 164
Fiorgen with Codeine - See BUTALBITAL, ASPIRIN
    & CODEINE (Also contains caffeine) 164
Fioricet - See
    ACETAMINOPHEN 2
    BARBITURATES 122
Fiorinal with Codeine - See BUTALBITAL, ASPIRIN
    & CODEINE (Also contains caffeine) 164
Fivent - See CROMOLYN 256
Flagyl - See METRONIDAZOLE 554
Flagyl I.V. - See METRONIDAZOLE 554
Flagyl I.V. RTU - See METRONIDAZOLE 554
Flamazine - See
    ANTIBACTERIALS (Topical) 68
    ANTIFUNGALS (Topical) 84
Flarex - See ANTI-INFLAMMATORY DRUGS,
    STEROIDAL (Ophthalmic) 96
Flavorcee - See VITAMIN C (Ascorbic Acid) 888
FLAVOXATE 380
FLECAINIDE ACETATE 382
Fleet Bisacodyl - See BISACODYL 144
Fleet Bisacodyl Prep - See BISACODYL 144
Fleet Enema - See SODIUM PHOSPHATE 794
Fleet Enema Mineral Oil - See MINERAL OIL 562
Fleet Flavored Castor Oil - See CASTOR OIL 186
Fleet Phospho-Soda - See SODIUM PHOSPHATE
    794
Fleet Relief - See ANESTHETICS (Rectal) 44
Fletcher's Castoria - See SENNA 780
Flexagin - See ORPHENADRINE 630
Flexain - See ORPHENADRINE 630
Flexaphen - See CHLORZOXAZONE &
    ACETAMINOPHEN 212
Flexeril - See CYCLOBENZAPRINE 264
Flexoject - See ORPHENADRINE 630
Flexon - See ORPHENADRINE 630
Flextra - See CHLORZOXAZONE &
    ACETAMINOPHEN 212
Flint SSD - See ANTIBACTERIALS, ANTIFUNGALS
    (Topical) 70
FLOCTAFENINE - See ANTI-INFLAMMATORY
    DRUGS, NON-STEROIDAL (NSAIDs) 94
Florene E - See ADRENOCORTICOIDS (Topical) 14
Florex - See BUTALBITAL & ASPIRIN (Also
    contains caffeine) 162
Florgen PF - See BUTALBITAL & ASPIRIN (Also
    contains caffeine) 162

INDEX

G

G-1 Capsules - See
BARBITURATES 122
CAFFEINE 166
GALLBLADDER X-RAY TEST DRUGS
(Cholecystographic Agents) 396
Gallium Citrate Ga 67 - See RADIO-
PHARMACEUTICALS 756
Gantanol - See SULFAMETHOXAZOLE 806
Gantanol DS - See SULFAMETHOXAZOLE 806
Gantrisin - See
ANTIBACTERIALS (Ophthalmic) 64
SULFISOXAZOLE 812
Garamycin - See
ANTIBACTERIALS (Ophthalmic) 64
ANTIBACTERIALS (Otic) 66
ANTIBACTERIALS (Topical) 68
Gardenal - See BARBITURATES 122
Gas-is-gon - See ANTACIDS 56
Gastrocrom - See CROMOLYN 256
Gastrolyte - See DEXTROSE & ELECTROLYTES
294
Gaviscon - See ANTACIDS 56
Gaviscon Extra Strength Relief Formula - See
ANTACIDS 56
Gaviscon-2 - See ANTACIDS 56
GBH - See PEDICULISIDES (Topical) 656
Gee-Gee - See GUAIFENESIN 408
Gelamal - See ANTACIDS 56
Gelpirin - See ACETAMINOPHEN & SALICYLATES 4
Gelusil - See
ANTACIDS 56
SIMETHICONE 786
Gelusil Extra Strength - See ANTACIDS 56
Gelusil-II - See ANTACIDS 56
Gelusil-M - See ANTACIDS 56
GEMFIBROZIL 398
Gemnisyn - See ACETAMINOPHEN &
SALICYLATES 4
Gemonil - See BARBITURATES 122
Genabid - See PAPAVERINE 646
Genac - See
ANTIHISTAMINES 92
PSEUDOEPHEDRINE 736
Genagesic - See NARCOTIC & ACETAMINOPHEN
590
Genalac - See ANTACIDS 56
Genallerate - See ANTIHISTAMINES 92
Genamin - See
ANTIHISTAMINES 92
PHENYLPROPANOLAMINE 686
Genapap - See ACETAMINOPHEN 2
Genapap Extra Strength - See ACETAMINOPHEN 2
Genapax - See ANTIFUNGALS (Vaginal) 86
Genaphed - See PSEUDOEPHEDRINE 736
Genaspore Cream - See ANTIFUNGALS (Topical)
84
Genatap - See
ANTIHISTAMINES 92
PHENYLPROPANOLAMINE 686
Genatuss - See GUAIFENESIN 408
Gencalc - See CALCIUM SUPPLEMENTS 170

Gencold - See
ANTIHISTAMINES 92
PHENYLPROPANOLAMINE 686
Genebs - See ACETAMINOPHEN 2
Genebs Extra Strength - See ACETAMINOPHEN 2
Generiac - See LACTULOSE 476
Genex - See
ACETAMINOPHEN 2
PHENYLPROPANOLAMINE 686
Genoptic - See
ANTIBACTERIALS (Ophthalmic) 64
ANTIBACTERIALS (Otic) 66
Genora 1/35 - See CONTRACEPTIVES, ORAL 250
Genora 1/50 - See CONTRACEPTIVES, ORAL 250
Genpril - See ANTI-INFLAMMATORY DRUGS,
NON-STEROIDAL (NSAIDs) 94
Gentab LA - See
ANTIHISTAMINES 92
GUAIFENESIN 408
PHENYLPROPANOLAMINE 686
Gentacidin - See ANTIBACTERIALS (Ophthalmic)
64
Gentafair - See ANTIBACTERIALS (Ophthalmic) 64
Gentak - See ANTIBACTERIALS (Ophthalmic) 64
Gentamar - See ANTIBACTERIALS (Topical) 68
GENTAMICIN - See
ANTIBACTERIALS (Otic) 66
ANTIBACTERIALS (Topical) 68
GENTAMICIN (Ophthalmic) - See
ANTIBACTERIALS (Ophthalmic) 64
Gentian Violet - See ANTIFUNGALS (Vaginal) 86
Gentle Nature - See SENNOSIDES A & B 782
Gentrasul - See ANTIBACTERIALS (Ophthalmic) 64
Gen-Xene - See BENZODIAZEPINES 130
Geocillin - See CARBENICILLIN 176
Geopen - See CARBENICILLIN 176
Geopen Oral - See CARBENICILLIN 176
Geridium - See PHENAZOPYRIDINE 674
Geritol Tablets - See IRON SUPPLEMENTS 454
Gesterol - See PROGESTINS 728
Gesterol L.A. - See PROGESTINS 728
GG-CEN - See GUAIFENESIN 408
Glaucon - See ANTIGLAUCOMA, SHORT-ACTING
(Ophthalmic) 90
GLIPIZIDE - See ANTIDIABETIC AGENTS 78
Glo-Sel - See ANTISEBORRHEICS (Topical) 100
GLUCAGON 400
Glucagon for Injection - See GLUCAGON 400
Glucamide - See ANTIDIABETIC AGENTS 78
Glucotrol - See ANTIDIABETIC AGENTS 78
Gly-Cort - See ADRENOCORTICOIDS (Topical) 14
Glyate - See GUAIFENESIN 408
GLYBURIDE - See ANTIDIABETIC AGENTS 78
Glycate - See ANTACIDS 56
Glyceryl T - See THEOPHYLLINE & GUAIFENESIN
836
Glyceryl Trinitrate - See NITRATES 614
GLYCOPYRROLATE 402
Glycotuss - See GUAIFENESIN 408
Glycotuss-dM - See
DEXTROMETHORPHAN 292
GUAIFENESIN 408

Hydropine - See RAUWOLFIA & THIAZIDE DIURETICS 760

Hydropres - See RAUWOLFIA & THIAZIDE DIURETICS 760

Hydrosalic - See ANTI-ACNE (Topical) 60

Hydrosine - See RAUWOLFIA & THIAZIDE DIURETICS 760

Hydrotensin - See RAUWOLFIA & THIAZIDE DIURETICS 760

Hydro-Tex - See ADRENOCORTICOIDS (Topical) 14

Hydroxacen - See HYDROXYZINE 438

HYDROXOCOBALAMIN - See VITAMIN B-12 (Cyanocobalamin) 886

HYDROXYCHLOROQUINE 434

HYDROXYPROGESTERONE - See PROGESTINS 728

HYDROXYPROPYL CELLULOSE - See PROTECTANT (Ophthalmic) 734

HYDROXYPROPYL METHYL-CELLULOSE - See PROTECTANT (Ophthalmic) 734

HYDROXYUREA 436

HYDROXYZINE 438

HYDROXYZINE - See ANTIHISTAMINES 92

Hygroton - See DIURETICS, THIAZIDE 324

Hylorel - See GUANADREL 412

Hylutin - See PROGESTINS 728

HYOSCYAMINE 440

HYOSCYAMINE & PHENOBARBITAL - See BELLADONNA ALKALOIDS & BARBITURATES 128

Hyosophen - See BELLADONNA ALKALOIDS & BARBITURATES 128

HY-PHEN - See NARCOTIC & ACETAMINOPHEN 590

Hypnotic - See CHLORAL HYDRATE 198

Hypnotic (barbiturate) - See BARBITURATES 122

Hyprogest - See PROGESTINS 728

Hyproval P.A. - See PROGESTINS 728

Hyrexin-50 - See ANTIHISTAMINES 92

Hystadyl E.C. - See NARCOTIC ANALGESICS 592

Hytakerol - See VITAMIN D 890

Hytinic - See IRON SUPPLEMENTS 454

Hytone - See ADRENOCORTICOIDS (Topical) 14

Hytrin - See TERAZOSIN 818

Hytuss - See GUAIFENESIN 408

Hytuss-2X - See GUAIFENESIN 408

Hyzine - See HYDROXYZINE 438

I

Iberet - See IRON SUPPLEMENTS 454

Ibren - See ANTI-INFLAMMATORY DRUGS, NON-STEROIDAL (NSAIDs) 94

Ibumed - See ANTI-INFLAMMATORY DRUGS, NON-STEROIDAL (NSAIDs) 94

Ibuprin - See ANTI-INFLAMMATORY DRUGS, NON-STEROIDAL (NSAIDs) 94

Ibupro-600 - See ANTI-INFLAMMATORY DRUGS, NON-STEROIDAL (NSAIDs) 94

IBUPROFEN - See ANTI-INFLAMMATORY DRUGS, NON-STEROIDAL (NSAIDs) 94

Ibutex - See ANTI-INFLAMMATORY DRUGS, NON-STEROIDAL (NSAIDs) 94

I-Chlor Ophthalmic Solution - See ANTIBACTERIALS (Ophthalmic) 64

I.D.A - See ISOMETHEPTENE, DICHLORALPHENAZONE & ACETAMINOPHEN 456

Idarac - See ANTI-INFLAMMATORY DRUGS, NON-STEROIDAL (NSAIDs) 94

Idenal - See BUTALBITAL & ASPIRIN (Also contains caffeine) 162

IDOXURIDINE DROPS & OINTMENT - See ANTIVIRALS (Ophthalmic) 104

Ifen - See ANTI-INFLAMMATORY DRUGS, NON-STEROIDAL (NSAIDs) 94

I-Homatropine - See CYCLOPEGIC, MYDRIATIC (Ophthalmic) 266

Ilosone - See ERYTHROMYCINS 354

Ilotycin - See
ANTIBACTERIALS (Ophthalmic) 64
ERYTHROMYCINS 354

Ilozyme - See PANCRELIPASE 642

Imbrilon - See ANTI-INFLAMMATORY DRUGS, NON-STEROIDAL (NSAIDs) 94

I-Methasone - See ANTI-INFLAMMATORY DRUGS, STEROIDAL (Ophthalmic) 96

IMIPRAMINE - See TRICYCLIC ANTIDEPRESSANTS 868

Immunosuppressant - See
AZATHIOPRINE 116
BUSULFAN 160
CHLORAMBUCIL 200
CYCLOPHOSPHAMIDE 270
CYCLOSPORINE 274
MERCAPTOPURINE 524

Imodium - See LOPERAMIDE 494

Imodium A-D - See LOPERAMIDE 494

Impril - See TRICYCLIC ANTIDEPRESSANTS 868

Improved Sino-Tuss - See
ACETAMINOPHEN 2
ANTIHISTAMINES 92
DEXTROMETHORPHAN 292
PHENYLEPHRINE 682
SALICYLATES 774

Imuran - See AZATHIOPRINE 116

I-Naphline - See DECONGESTANTS (Ophthalmic) 284

Indameth - See ANTI-INFLAMMATORY DRUGS, NON-STEROIDAL (NSAIDs) 94

INDAPAMIDE 442

Inderal LA - See BETA-ADRENERGIC BLOCKERS 134

Inderide - See BETA-ADRENERGIC BLOCKING AGENTS & THIAZIDE DIURETICS 136

Inderide LA - See BETA-ADRENERGIC BLOCKING AGENTS & THIAZIDE DIURETICS 136

Indium In 111 Pentetate - See RADIO-PHARMACEUTICALS 756

Indocid - See ANTI-INFLAMMATORY DRUGS, NON-STEROIDAL (NSAIDs) 94

Indocid SR - See ANTI-INFLAMMATORY DRUGS, NON-STEROIDAL (NSAIDs) 94

BARBITURATES 122
ISOPROTERENOL - See BRONCHODILATORS, ADRENERGIC 150
ISOPROTERENOL & PHENYLEPHRINE 460
Isoptin - See CALCIUM CHANNEL BLOCKERS 168
Isoptin SR - See CALCIUM CHANNEL BLOCKERS 168
Isopto - See CYCLOPEGIC, MYDRIATIC (Ophthalmic) 266
Isopto Alkaline - See PROTECTANT (Ophthalmic) 734
Isopto Atropine - See CYCLOPEGIC, MYDRIATIC (Ophthalmic) 266
Isopto Carbachol - See ANTIGLAUCOMA, SHORT-ACTING (Ophthalmic) 90
Isopto Carpine - See PILOCARPINE 690
Isopto Cetamide - See ANTIBACTERIALS (Ophthalmic) 64
Isopto Eserine - See ANTIGLAUCOMA, SHORT-ACTING (Ophthalmic) 90
Isopto Fenicol - See ANTIBACTERIALS (Ophthalmic) 64
Isopto Frin - See PHENYLEPHRINE (Ophthalmic) 684
Isopto Homatropine - See CYCLOPEGIC, MYDRIATIC (Ophthalmic) 266
Isopto Hyoscine - See CYCLOPEGIC, MYDRIATIC (Ophthalmic) 266
Isopto Plain - See PROTECTANT (Ophthalmic) 734
Isopto Tears - See PROTECTANT (Ophthalmic) 734
Isorbid - See NITRATES 614
ISORBIDE MONONITRATE - See NITRATES 614
Isordil - See NITRATES 614
ISOSORBIDE DINITRATE - See NITRATES 614
Isotamine - See ISONIAZID 458
Isotrate - See NITRATES 614
ISOTRETINOIN 462
ISOXSUPRINE 464
ISRADIPINE - See CALCIUM CHANNEL BLOCKERS 168
I-Sulfacet - See ANTIBACTERIALS (Ophthalmic) 64
Isuprel - See BRONCHODILATORS, ADRENERGIC 150
Isuprel Glossets - See BRONCHODILATORS, ADRENERGIC 150
Isuprel Mistometer - See BRONCHODILATORS, ADRENERGIC 150
I-Tropine - See CYCLOPEGIC, MYDRIATIC (Ophthalmic) 266

J

Janimine - See TRICYCLIC ANTIDEPRESSANTS 868
Jumex - See SELEGILINE 778
Jumexal - See SELEGILINE 778
Just Tears - See PROTECTANT (Ophthalmic) 734

K

K + Care ET - See POTASSIUM SUPPLEMENTS 704
K-10 - See POTASSIUM SUPPLEMENTS 704

K-Lease - See POTASSIUM SUPPLEMENTS 704
Kabolin - See ANDROGENS 42
Kainaire - See ANESTHETICS, LOCAL (Ophthalmic) 50
Kallum Durules - See POTASSIUM SUPPLEMENTS 704
Kanacort - See TRIAMCINOLONE 860
KANAMYCIN 466
Kantrex - See KANAMYCIN 466
Kaochlor - See POTASSIUM SUPPLEMENTS 704
Kaochlor S-F - See POTASSIUM SUPPLEMENTS 704
Kaochlor-Eff - See POTASSIUM SUPPLEMENTS 704
Kao-Con - See KAOLIN & PECTIN 468
Kaodene with Paregoric - See KAOLIN, PECTIN, BELLADONNA & OPIUM 470
Kaodonna-PG - See KAOLIN, PECTIN, BELLADONNA & OPIUM 470
Kaolin - See KAOLIN & PECTIN 468
KAOLIN & PECTIN 468
KAOLIN, PECTIN & PAREGORIC 472
KAOLIN, PECTIN, BELLADONNA & OPIUM 470
Kaon - See POTASSIUM SUPPLEMENTS 704
Kaon-Cl - See POTASSIUM SUPPLEMENTS 704
Kaon-Cl 10 - See POTASSIUM SUPPLEMENTS 704
Kaon-Cl 20 - See POTASSIUM SUPPLEMENTS 704
Kaopectate - See
  ATTAPULGITE 114
  KAOLIN & PECTIN 468
Kapectolin - See KAOLIN & PECTIN 468
Kapectolin with Paregoric - See KAOLIN, PECTIN & PAREGORIC 472
Kapectolin PG - See KAOLIN, PECTIN, BELLADONNA & OPIUM 470
Karacil - See PSYLLIUM 740
Karidium - See SODIUM FLUORIDE 792
Kasof - See DOCUSATE POTASSIUM 330
Kato - See POTASSIUM SUPPLEMENTS 704
Kay Ciel - See POTASSIUM SUPPLEMENTS 704
Kay Ciel Elixir - See POTASSIUM SUPPLEMENTS 704
Kaybovite - See VITAMIN B-12 (Cyanocobalamin) 886
Kaybovite-1000 - See VITAMIN B-12 (Cyanocobalamin) 886
Kaylixir - See POTASSIUM SUPPLEMENTS 704
Kaypectol - See KAOLIN & PECTIN 468
K-C - See KAOLIN & PECTIN 468
KCL - See POTASSIUM SUPPLEMENTS 704
K-Dur - See POTASSIUM SUPPLEMENTS 704
Keflet - See CEPHALOSPORINS 190
Keflex - See CEPHALOSPORINS 190
Keftab - See CEPHALOSPORINS 190
Kellogg's Castor Oil - See CASTOR OIL 186
Kemadrin - See ANTIDYSKINETICS 80
Kenac - See ADRENOCORTICOIDS (Topical) 14
Kenaject-40 - See TRIAMCINOLONE 860
Kenalog - See ADRENOCORTICOIDS (Topical) 14
Kenalog 10 - See TRIAMCINOLONE 860

INDEX

L

LABETALOL - See BETA-ADRENERGIC
  BLOCKERS 134
LABETALOL & HYDROCHLOROTHIAZIDE - See
  BETA-ADRENERGIC BLOCKING AGENTS &
  THIAZIDE DIURETICS 136
Labor inhibitor - See RITODRINE 772
Lacril (ophthalmic) - See PROTECTANT
  (Ophthalmic) 734
Lacrisert - See PROTECTANT (Ophthalmic) 734
Lacticare-HC - See ADRENOCORTICOIDS (Topical)
  14
Lactisol - See ANTI-ACNE (Topical) 60
LACTULOSE 476
L.A.E. 20 - See ESTROGENS 360
Lanacort - See ADRENOCORTICOIDS (Topical) 14
Lanacort 10 - See ADRENOCORTICOIDS (Topical)
  14
Lanatuss Expectorant - See
  ANTIHISTAMINES 92
  CITRATES 220
  GUAIFENESIN 408
  PHENYLPROPANOLAMINE 686
Laniazid - See ISONIAZID 458
Lanirolf - See BUTALBITAL & ASPIRIN (Also
  contains caffeine) 162
Lanophyllin - See BRONCHODILATORS,
  XANTHINE 152
Lanophyllin-GG - See THEOPHYLLINE &
  GUAIFENESIN 836
Lanorinal - See
  ASPIRIN 108
  BUTALBITAL & ASPIRIN (Also contains caffeine)
  162
  CAFFEINE 166
Lanoxicaps - See DIGITALIS PREPARATIONS
  (Digitalis Glycosides) 306
Lanoxin - See DIGITALIS PREPARATIONS (Digitalis
  Glycosides) 306
Lansoyl - See MINERAL OIL 562
Lanvis - See THIOGUANINE 842
Largactil - See PHENOTHIAZINES 678
Largactil Liquid - See PHENOTHIAZINES 678
Largactil Oral Drops - See PHENOTHIAZINES 678
Lariam - See MEFLOQUINE 514
Larodopa - See LEVODOPA 484
Lasan - See ANTHRALIN (Topical) 58
Lasan HP - See ANTHRALIN (Topical) 58
Lasan Pomade - See ANTHRALIN (Topical) 58
Lasan Unguent - See ANTHRALIN (Topical) 58
Lasix - See DIURETICS, LOOP 322
Lasix Special - See DIURETICS, LOOP 322
Laudanum - See
  NARCOTIC ANALGESICS 592
  PAREGORIC 654
LAVATAR - See COAL TAR (Topical) 242
Laxative (bulk-forming) - See
  MALT SOUP EXTRACT 502
  METHYLCELLULOSE 536
  POLYCARBOPHIL CALCIUM 696
  PSYLLIUM 740
Laxative (emollient) - See POLOXAMER 188 694

Laxative (hyperosmotic) - See
  LACTULOSE 476
  MAGNESIUM CITRATE 498
  MAGNESIUM SULFATE 500
  SODIUM PHOSPHATE 794
Laxative (lubricant) - See MINERAL OIL 562
Laxative (stimulant) - See
  BISACODYL 144
  CASCARA 184
  CASTOR OIL 186
  DANTHRON AND DOCUSATE 278
  DEHYDROCHOLIC ACID 286
  PHENOLPHTHALEIN 676
  SENNA 780
  SENNOSIDES A & B 782
Laxative (stool softener) - See
  DOCUSATE CALCIUM 328
  DOCUSATE POTASSIUM 330
  DOCUSATE SODIUM 332
Laxinate - See DOCUSATE SODIUM 332
Laxinate 100 - See DOCUSATE SODIUM 332
Laxit - See BISACODYL 144
LazerSporin-C - See ANTIBACTERIALS (Otic) 66
L-Carnitine - See LEVOCARNITINE 482
Lectopam - See BENZODIAZEPINES 130
Ledercillin VK - See PENICILLIN V 664
Lemoderm - See ADRENOCORTICOIDS (Topical)
  14
Lenoltec - See NARCOTIC & ACETAMINOPHEN
  590
Lente - See INSULIN 444
Lente Iletin I - See INSULIN 444
Lente Iletin II - See INSULIN 444
Lente Insulin - See INSULIN 444
Leponex - See CLOZAPINE 240
LEUCOVORIN 478
Leukeran - See CHLORAMBUCIL 200
LEVAMISOLE 480
Levate - See TRICYCLIC ANTIDEPRESSANTS 868
Levatol - See BETA-ADRENERGIC BLOCKERS 134
Levlen - See CONTRACEPTIVES, ORAL 250
LEVOBUNOLOL - See ANTIGLAUCOMA, SHORT-
  ACTING (Ophthalmic) 90
LEVOCARNITINE 482
LEVODOPA 484
Levo-Dromoran - See NARCOTIC ANALGESICS
  592
LEVONORGESTREL 486
LEVONORGESTREL & ETHINYL ESTRADIOL - See
  CONTRACEPTIVES, ORAL 250
Levoprome - See PHENOTHIAZINES 678
Levorphan - See NARCOTIC ANALGESICS 592
LEVORPHANOL - See NARCOTIC ANALGESICS
  592
Levothroid - See THYROID HORMONES 846
Levoxine - See THYROID HORMONES 846
Levsin - See HYOSCYAMINE 440
Levsin with Phenobarbital - See BELLADONNA
  ALKALOIDS & BARBITURATES 128
Levsin-PB - See BELLADONNA ALKALOIDS &
  BARBITURATES 128
Levsinex - See HYOSCYAMINE 440

MELPHALAN (PAM, L-PAM, Phenylalanine
  Mustard) 516
MEPHENYTOIN 518
MEPHOBARBITAL - See BARBITURATES 122
Mephyton - See VITAMIN K 894
Mepro Analgesic - See
  ASPIRIN 108
  MEPROBAMATE & ASPIRIN 522
METAXALONE - See MUSCLE RELAXANTS,
  SKELETAL 578
  RAUWOLFIA & THIAZIDE DIURETICS 760
  RAUWOLFIA ALKALOIDS 758
MEPROBAMATE 520
MEPROBAMATE & ASPIRIN 522
Meprogese - See MEPROBAMATE & ASPIRIN 522
Meprogesic - See MEPROBAMATE & ASPIRIN 522
Meprogesic Q - See MEPROBAMATE & ASPIRIN
  522
Meprolone - See METHYLPREDNISOLONE 546
Meprospan - See MEPROBAMATE 520
MERCAPTOPURINE 524
Mercurochrome II - See ANESTHETICS (Topical)
  46
MESALAMINE (Rectal) 526
Mesalazine - See MESALAMINE (Rectal) 526
Mesantoin - See MEPHENYTOIN 518
MESORIDAZINE - See PHENOTHIAZINES 678
Mestinon - See PYRIDOSTIGMINE 744
Mestinon Timespans - See PYRIDOSTIGMINE 744
Metaderm - See ADRENOCORTICOIDS (Topical)
  14
Metahydrin - See DIURETICS, THIAZIDE 324
Metamucil - See PSYLLIUM 740
Metamucil Instant Mix - See PSYLLIUM 740
Metamucil Instant Mix, Orange Flavor - See
  PSYLLIUM 740
Metamucil Orange Flavor - See PSYLLIUM 740
Metamucil Strawberry Flavor - See PSYLLIUM 740
Metamucil Sugar Free - See PSYLLIUM 740
Metandren - See ANDROGENS 42
Metaprel - See BRONCHODILATORS,
  ADRENERGIC 150
METAPROTERENOL - See BRONCHODILATORS,
  ADRENERGIC 150
Metatensin - See
  RAUWOLFIA ALKALOIDS 758
  RAUWOLFIA ALKALOIDS & THIAZIDE
  DIURETICS 760
*Meted Maximum Strength Anti-Dandruff Shampoo
  with Conditioners* - See
  ANTI-ACNE (Topical) 60
  ANTISEBORRHEICS (Topical) 100
METHACYCLINE - See TETRACYCLINES 828
METHADONE - See NARCOTIC ANALGESICS 592
Methadose - See NARCOTIC ANALGESICS 592
METHAMPHETAMINE - See AMPHETAMINES 34
Methandine - See METHENAMINE 528
METHARBITAL - See BARBITURATES 122
METHAZOLAMIDE - See CARBONIC ANHYDRASE
  INHIBITORS 182
METHENAMINE 528
Methendelate - See METHENAMINE 528

Methergine - See METHYLERGONOVINE 542
METHICILLIN 530
METHIMAZOLE - See ANTITHYROID DRUGS 102
METHOCARBAMOL - See MUSCLE RELAXANTS,
  SKELETAL 578
METHOTREXATE 532
METHOTRIMEPRAZINE - See PHENOTHIAZINES
  678
METHOXSALEN - See PSORALENS 738
Methoxsalen Lotion (Topical) - See PSORALENS
  738
METHSUXIMIDE 534
METHYCLOTHIAZIDE - See DIURETICS, THIAZIDE
  324
METHYLCELLULOSE 536
METHYLDOPA 538
METHYLDOPA & CHLOROTHIAZIDE - See
  METHYLDOPA & THIAZIDE DIURETICS 540
METHYLDOPA & HYDROCHLOROTHIAZIDE - See
  METHYLDOPA & THIAZIDE DIURETICS 540
METHYLDOPA & THIAZIDE DIURETICS 540
Methylergometrine - See METHYLERGONOVINE
  542
METHYLERGONOVINE 542
METHYLPHENIDATE 544
METHYLPREDNISOLONE 546
METHYLPREDNISOLONE (Topical) - See
  ADRENOCORTICOIDS (Topical) 14
METHYLTESTOSTERONE - See ANDROGENS 42
METHYPRYLON 548
METHYSERGIDE 550
Meticorten - See PREDNISONE 712
METIPRANOLOL - See ANTIGLAUCOMA, SHORT-
  ACTING (Ophthalmic) 90
Metizol - See METRONIDAZOLE 554
METOCLOPRAMIDE 552
METOLAZONE - See DIURETICS, THIAZIDE 324
METOPROLOL - See BETA-ADRENERGIC
  BLOCKERS 134
METOPROLOL & HYDROCHLOROTHIAZIDE - See
  BETA-ADRENERGIC BLOCKING AGENTS &
  THIAZIDE DIURETICS 136
Metopirone - See METYRAPONE 556
Metosyn - See ADRENOCORTICOIDS (Topical) 14
Metosyn FAPG - See ADRENOCORTICOIDS
  (Topical) 14
Metra - See APPETITE SUPPRESSANTS 106
Metric 21 - See METRONIDAZOLE 554
Metro I.V. - See METRONIDAZOLE 554
MetroGel - See METRONIDAZOLE 554
MetroGel-Vaginal - See METRONIDAZOLE 554
Metronid - See METRONIDAZOLE 554
METRONIDAZOLE 554
Metryl - See METRONIDAZOLE 554
Metryl IV - See METRONIDAZOLE 554
METYRAPONE 556
METYROSINE 558
Mevacor - See HMG-CoA REDUCTASE
  INHIBITORS 424
Meval - See BENZODIAZEPINES 130
Mevinolin - See HMG-CoA REDUCTASE
  INHIBITORS 424

INDEX

Monistat-Derm - See ANTIFUNGALS (Topical) 84
Monitan - See BETA-ADRENERGIC BLOCKERS
134
MONOBASIC POTASSIUM & SODIUM
PHOSPHATES - See POTASSIUM & SODIUM
PHOSPHATES 702
Mono-Gesic - See SALICYLATES 774
Monopril - See ANGIOTENSIN-CONVERTING
ENZYME (ACE) INHIBITORS 52
M-Orexic - See APPETITE SUPPRESSANTS 106
MORICIZINE 576
MORPHINE - See NARCOTIC ANALGESICS 592
Morphitec - See NARCOTIC ANALGESICS 592
M.O.S. - See NARCOTIC ANALGESICS 592
M.O.S.-SR - See NARCOTIC ANALGESICS 592
Motion-Aid - See ANTIHISTAMINES 92
Motofen - See DIFENOXIN & ATROPINE 304
Motrin - See ANTI-INFLAMMATORY DRUGS, NON-
STEROIDAL (NSAIDs) 94
Motrin-IB - See ANTI-INFLAMMATORY DRUGS,
NON-STEROIDAL (NSAIDs) 94
Motrin-IB Caplets - See ANTI-INFLAMMATORY
DRUGS, NON-STEROIDAL (NSAIDs) 94
Movergan - See SELEGILINE 778
MS Contin - See NARCOTIC ANALGESICS 592
MSIR - See NARCOTIC ANALGESICS 592
MST Continus - See NARCOTIC ANALGESICS 592
Mucolysin - See TIOPRONIN 852
Mudrane GG - See THEOPHYLLINE, EPHEDRINE,
GUAIFENESIN & BARBITURATES 832
Mudrane GG2 - See THEOPHYLLINE &
GUAIFENESIN 836
Multipax - See HYDROXYZINE 438
MULTIPLE VITAMINS & FLUORIDE - See
VITAMINS & FLUORIDE 896
Mulvidren-F - See VITAMINS & FLUORIDE 896
MUPIROCIN - See ANTIBACTERIALS (Topical) 68
Murine - See DECONGESTANTS (Ophthalmic) 284
Muro's Opcon - See DECONGESTANTS
(Ophthalmic) 284
Muscle relaxant - See
CHLORZOXAZONE & ACETAMINOPHEN 212
CYCLOBENZAPRINE 264
DANTROLENE 280
MUSCLE RELAXANTS, SKELETAL 578
ORPHENADRINE 630
ORPHENADRINE, ASPIRIN & CAFFEINE 632
Muscle relaxant in multiple sclerosis - See
BACLOFEN 120
MUSCLE RELAXANTS, SKELETAL 578
Mus-Lax - See CHLORZOXAZONE &
ACETAMINOPHEN 212
Mustargen - See MECHLORETHAMINE (Topical)
510
My Cort - See ADRENOCORTICOIDS (Topical) 14
Myapap with Codeine - See NARCOTIC &
ACETAMINOPHEN 590
Myapap Elixir - See ACETAMINOPHEN 2
Mycelex - See
ANTIFUNGALS (Topical) 84
CLOTRIMAZOLE (Oral-Local) 236

Mycelex Troches - See ANTIFUNGALS (Topical)
84
Mycelex-G - See ANTIFUNGALS (Vaginal) 86
Mycifradin - See
NEOMYCIN (Oral) 598
NEOMYCIN (Topical) 600
Myciguent - See ANTIBACTERIALS (Topical) 68
Mycitracin - See
ANTIBACTERIALS (Ophthalmic) 64
ANTIBACTERIALS (Topical) 68
Myclo - See ANTIFUNGALS (Vaginal) 86
Myclo Cream - See ANTIFUNGALS (Topical) 84
Myclo Solution - See ANTIFUNGALS (Topical) 84
Myclo Spray - See ANTIFUNGALS (Topical) 84
Myco II - See
NYSTATIN 622
TRIAMCINOLONE 860
Myco-Triacet II - See
NYSTATIN 622
TRIAMCINOLONE 860
Mycobiotic - See ANTIBACTERIALS,
ANTIFUNGALS (Topical) 70
Mycobiotic II - See
NYSTATIN 622
TRIAMCINOLONE 860
Mycogen - See ANTIBACTERIALS, ANTIFUNGALS
(Topical) 70
Mycogen II - See
NYSTATIN 622
TRIAMCINOLONE 860
Mycostatin - See
ANTIFUNGALS (Topical) 84
ANTIFUNGALS (Vaginal) 86
NYSTATIN 622
Mycotussin - See
NARCOTIC ANALGESICS 592
PSEUDOEPHEDRINE 736
Mydfrin - See PHENYLEPHRINE (Ophthalmic) 684
Mydriatic - See PHENYLEPHRINE (Ophthalmic)
684
My-E - See ERYTHROMYCINS 354
Myfed - See
ANTIHISTAMINES 92
PSEUDOEPHEDRINE 736
Myfedrine - See PSEUDOEPHEDRINE 736
Myfedrine Plus - See
ANTIHISTAMINES 92
PSEUDOEPHEDRINE 736
Mygel - See
ANTACIDS 56
SIMETHICONE 786
Mygel II - See ANTACIDS 56
Myhistine - See PHENYLEPHRINE 682
Myhistine DH - See
ANTIHISTAMINES 92
NARCOTIC ANALGESICS 592
PSEUDOEPHEDRINE 736
Myhistine Expectorant - See
GUAIFENESIN 408
NARCOTIC ANALGESICS 592
PSEUDOEPHEDRINE 736

INDEX

Niloric - See ERGOLOID MESYLATES 342
Nilstat - See
  ANTIFUNGALS (Topical) 84
  ANTIFUNGALS (Vaginal) 86
  NYSTATIN 622
NIMODIPINE 612
Nimotop - See NIMODIPINE 612
Niong - See NITRATES 614
NITRATES 614
NITRAZEPAM - See BENZODIAZEPINES 130
Nitrex - See NITROFURANTOIN 616
Nitro-Bid - See NITRATES 614
Nitrocap - See NITRATES 614
Nitrocap T.D. - See NITRATES 614
Nitrocine - See NITRATES 614
Nitrodisc - See NITRATES 614
Nitro-Dur - See NITRATES 614
Nitro-Dur II - See NITRATES 614
Nitrofan - See NITROFURANTOIN 616
Nitrofor - See NITROFURANTOIN 616
Nitrofuracot - See NITROFURANTOIN 616
NITROFURANTOIN 616
Nitrogard-SR - See NITRATES 614
NITROGLYCERIN (GLYCERYL TRINITRATE) - See
  NITRATES 614
Nitroglyn - See NITRATES 614
Nitrol - See NITRATES 614
Nitrolin - See NITRATES 614
Nitrolingual - See NITRATES 614
Nitronet - See NITRATES 614
Nitrong - See NITRATES 614
Nitrong SR - See NITRATES 614
Nitrospan - See NITRATES 614
Nitrostat - See NITRATES 614
Nix Cream Rinse - See PEDICULISIDES (Topical)
  656
NIZATIDINE - See HISTAMINE H$_2$ RECEPTOR
  ANTAGONISTS 422
Nizoral - See KETOCONAZOLE 474
Nizoral Shampoo - See ANTIFUNGALS (Topical) 84
Nobesine - See APPETITE SUPPRESSANTS 106
Noctec - See CHLORAL HYDRATE 198
Nodoz - See CAFFEINE 166
Nolahist - See ANTIHISTAMINES 92
Nolamine - See
  ANTIHISTAMINES 92
  PHENYLPROPANOLAMINE 686
Nolex LA - See
  GUAIFENESIN 408
  PHENYLPROPANOLAMINE 686
Noludar - See METHYPRYLON 548
Nolvadex - See TAMOXIFEN 816
Nolvadex-D - See TAMOXIFEN 816
NONOXYNAL 9 - See CONTRACEPTIVES,
  VAGINAL (Spermicides) 252
Non-steroidal anti-inflammatory (salicylates) - See
  ACETAMINOPHEN & SALICYLATES 4
Noradex - See ORPHENADRINE 630
Noradryl - See ANTIHISTAMINES 92
Norafed - See ANTIHISTAMINES 92
Noralac - See ANTACIDS 56
Noraminic - See

ANTIHISTAMINES 92
PHENYLPROPANOLAMINE 686
Noratuss II Liquid - See
  DEXTROMETHORPHAN 292
  GUAIFENESIN 408
  PSEUDOEPHEDRINE 736
Norcept - See CONTRACEPTIVES, ORAL 250
Norcet - See NARCOTIC & ACETAMINOPHEN 590
Nordette - See CONTRACEPTIVES, ORAL 250
Nordryl - See ANTIHISTAMINES 92
Nordryl Cough - See ANTIHISTAMINES 92
Norethin - See CONTRACEPTIVES, ORAL 250
NORETHINDRONE - See PROGESTINS 728
NORETHINDRONE & ETHINYL ESTRADIOL - See
  CONTRACEPTIVES, ORAL 250
NORETHINDRONE & MESTRANOL - See
  CONTRACEPTIVES, ORAL 250
NORETHINDRONE ACETATE & ETHINYL
  ESTRADIOL - See CONTRACEPTIVES, ORAL
  250
Norflex - See ORPHENADRINE 630
NORFLOXACIN 618
Norgesic - See
  ASPIRIN 108
  ORPHENADRINE, ASPIRIN & CAFFEINE 632
Norgesic Forte - See ORPHENADRINE, ASPIRIN &
  CAFFEINE 632
NORGESTREL - See PROGESTINS 728
NORGESTREL & ETHINYL ESTRADIOL - See
  CONTRACEPTIVES, ORAL 250
Norinyl - See ESTROGENS 360
Norisodrine Aerotrol - See BRONCHODILATORS,
  ADRENERGIC 150
Norlestrin - See
  CONTRACEPTIVES, ORAL 250
  ESTROGENS 360
Norlinyl - See CONTRACEPTIVES, ORAL 250
Norlutate - See PROGESTINS 728
Norlutin - See PROGESTINS 728
Normatane - See
  ANTIHISTAMINES 92
  PHENYLEPHRINE 682
  PHENYLPROPANOLAMINE 686
Normatane DC - See
  ANTIHISTAMINES 92
  NARCOTIC ANALGESICS 592
  PHENYLPROPANOLAMINE 686
Nor-Mil - See DIPHENOXYLATE & ATROPINE 314
Normodyne - See BETA-ADRENERGIC BLOCKERS
  134
Normozide - See BETA-ADRENERGIC BLOCKING
  AGENTS & & THIAZIDE DIURETICS 136
Noroxin - See NORFLOXACIN 618
Norpace - See DISOPYRAMIDE 318
Norpace CR - See DISOPYRAMIDE 318
Norphadrine - See ORPHENADRINE, ASPIRIN &
  CAFFEINE 632
Norphadrine Forte - See ORPHENADRINE,
  ASPIRIN & CAFFEINE 632
Norplant - See
  LEVONORGESTREL 486
  PROGESTINS 728

Novolorazem - See BENZODIAZEPINES 130
Novomedopa - See
  METHYLDOPA 538
  METHYLDOPA & THIAZIDE DIURETICS 540
Novomepro - See MEPROBAMATE 520
Novo-Mepro - See MEPROBAMATE 520
Novomethacin - See ANTI-INFLAMMATORY
  DRUGS, NON-STEROIDAL (NSAIDs) 94
Novometoprol - See BETA-ADRENERGIC
  BLOCKERS 134
Novonaprox - See ANTI-INFLAMMATORY DRUGS,
  NON-STEROIDAL (NSAIDs) 94
Novonidazol - See METRONIDAZOLE 554
Novo-Nifedin - See CALCIUM CHANNEL
  BLOCKERS 168
Novopen-G - See PENICILLIN G 662
Novopentobarb - See BARBITURATES 122
Novopen-VK - See PENICILLIN V 664
Novoperidol - See HALOPERIDOL 420
Novopheniram - See ANTIHISTAMINES 92
Novo-Pindol - See BETA-ADRENERGIC
  BLOCKERS 134
Novopirocam - See ANTI-INFLAMMATORY
  DRUGS, NON-STEROIDAL (NSAIDs) 94
Novopoxide - See BENZODIAZEPINES 130
Novopramine - See TRICYCLIC
  ANTIDEPRESSANTS 868
Novopranol - See BETA-ADRENERGIC BLOCKERS
  134
Novoprofen - See ANTI-INFLAMMATORY DRUGS,
  NON-STEROIDAL (NSAIDs) 94
Novopropamide - See ANTIDIABETIC AGENTS 78
Novopropoxyn - See NARCOTIC ANALGESICS
  592
Novopropoxyn Compound - See NARCOTIC &
  ASPIRIN 594
Novopurol - See ALLOPURINOL 16
Novopyrazone - See SULFINPYRAZONE 810
Novoquinidin - See QUINIDINE 752
NovoQuinine - See QUININE 754
Novoreserpine - See RAUWOLFIA ALKALOIDS
  758
Novo-Ridazine - See PHENOTHIAZINES 678
Novorythro - See ERYTHROMYCINS 354
Novosalmol - See BRONCHODILATORS,
  ADRENERGIC 150
Novosemide - See DIURETICS, LOOP 322
Novosorbide - See NITRATES 614
Novosoxazole - See SULFISOXAZOLE 812
Novospiroton - See SPIRONOLACTONE 796
Novospirozine - See SPIRONOLACTONE &
  HYDROCHLOROTHIAZIDE 798
Novo-Sundac - See ANTI-INFLAMMATORY
  DRUGS, NON-STEROIDAL (NSAIDs) 94
Novotetra - See TETRACYCLINES 828
Novo-Thalidone - See DIURETICS, THIAZIDE 324
Novotriamzide - See TRIAMTERENE &
  HYDROCHLOROTHIAZIDE 864
Novotrimel - See
  SULFAMETHOXAZOLE 806
  TRIMETHOPRIM 876
Novotriolam - See TRIAZOLAM 866

Novotriphyl - See BRONCHODILATORS,
  XANTHINE 152
Novotriptyn - See TRICYCLIC ANTIDEPRESSANTS
  868
Novo-Veramil - See CALCIUM CHANNEL
  BLOCKERS 168
Novoxapam - See BENZODIAZEPINES 130
Noxzema Anti-Acne Gel - See ANTI-ACNE (Topical)
  60
Noxzema Anti-Acne Pads Maximum Strength - See
  ANTI-ACNE (Topical) 60
Noxzema Anti-Acne Pads Regular Strength - See
  ANTI-ACNE (Topical) 60
Noxzema Clear-Ups Maximum Strength 10 - See
  BENZOYL PEROXIDE 132
Noxzema Clear-Ups On-the-Spot 10 Lotion - See
  BENZOYL PEROXIDE 132
Nozinan - See PHENOTHIAZINES 678
Nozinan Liquid - See PHENOTHIAZINES 678
Nozinan Oral Drops - See PHENOTHIAZINES 678
NP-27 Cream - See ANTIFUNGALS (Topical) 84
NP-27 Powder - See ANTIFUNGALS (Topical) 84
NP-27 Solution - See ANTIFUNGALS (Topical) 84
NP-27 Spray Powder - See ANTIFUNGALS
  (Topical) 84
NPH - See INSULIN 444
NPH Iletin I - See INSULIN 444
NPH Iletin II - See INSULIN 444
NPH Insulin - See INSULIN 444
NTS - See NITRATES 614
NTZ Long Acting Decongestant Nose Drops - See
  XYLOMETAZOLINE & OXYMETAZOLINE
  (Nasal) 898
NTZ Long Acting Decongestant Nose Spray - See
  XYLOMETAZOLINE & OXYMETAZOLINE
  (Nasal) 898
Nu-Atenol - See BETA-ADRENERGIC BLOCKERS
  134
Nubain - See NARCOTIC ANALGESICS 592
Nu-Cephalex - See CEPHALOSPORINS 190
Nucochem - See
  NARCOTIC ANALGESICS 592
  PSEUDOEPHEDRINE 736
NucoChem Expectorant - See
  GUAIFENESIN 408
  NARCOTIC ANALGESICS 592
  PSEUDOEPHEDRINE 736
NucoChem Pediatric Exptectorant - See
  GUAIFENESIN 408
  NARCOTIC ANALGESICS 592
  PSEUDOEPHEDRINE 736
Nucofed - See
  NARCOTIC ANALGESICS 592
  PSEUDOEPHEDRINE 736
Nucofed Expectorant - See
  GUAIFENESIN 408
  NARCOTIC ANALGESICS 592
  PSEUDOEPHEDRINE 736
Nucofed Pediatric Expectorant - See
  GUAIFENESIN 408
  NARCOTIC ANALGESICS 592
  PSEUDOEPHEDRINE 736

Nu-Diltiaz - See CALCIUM CHANNEL BLOCKERS 168

Nu-Indo - See ANTI-INFLAMMATORY DRUGS, NON-STEROIDAL (NSAIDs) 94

Nu-Iron - See IRON SUPPLEMENTS 454

Nu-Iron 150 - See IRON SUPPLEMENTS 454

Nujol - See MINERAL OIL 562

Nu-Loraz - See BENZODIAZEPINES 130

Nu-Medopa - See METHYLDOPA 538

NuMetop - See BETA-ADRENERGIC BLOCKERS 134

Numorphan - See NARCOTIC ANALGESICS 592

Nu-Nifed - See CALCIUM CHANNEL BLOCKERS 168

Nupercainal - See ANESTHETICS (Rectal) 44

Nupercainal Cream - See ANESTHETICS (Topical) 46

Nupercainal Ointment - See ANESTHETICS (Topical) 46

Nu-Pirox - See ANTI-INFLAMMATORY DRUGS, NON-STEROIDAL (NSAIDs) 94

Nuprin - See ANTI-INFLAMMATORY DRUGS, NON-STEROIDAL (NSAIDs) 94

Nuprin Caplets - See ANTI-INFLAMMATORY DRUGS, NON-STEROIDAL (NSAIDs) 94

Nutracort - See ADRENOCORTICOIDS (Topical) 14

Nutritional supplement - See
BETA CAROTENE 138
LEVOCARNITINE 482

Nu-Verap - See CALCIUM CHANNEL BLOCKERS 168

Nyaderm - See
ANTIFUNGALS (Topical) 84
ANTIFUNGALS (Vaginal) 86
NYSTATIN 622

Nydrazid - See ISONIAZID 458

NYLIDRIN 620

NyQuil Liquicaps - See
ACETAMINOPHEN 2
ANTIHISTAMINES 92
DEXTROMETHORPHAN 292
PSEUDOEPHEDRINE 736

NyQuil Nighttime Colds Medicine - See
ACETAMINOPHEN 2
ANTIHISTAMINES 92
DEXTROMETHORPHAN 292
PSEUDOEPHEDRINE 736

Nystaform - See NYSTATIN 622

NYSTATIN 622

NYSTATIN - See
ANTIFUNGALS (Topical) 84
ANTIFUNGALS (Vaginal) 86

Nystex - See
ANTIFUNGALS (Topical) 84
NYSTATIN 622

Nytilax - See SENNOSIDES A & B 782

Nytime Cold Medicine Liquid - See
ACETAMINOPHEN 2
ANTIHISTAMINES 92
DEXTROMETHORPHAN 292
PSEUDOEPHEDRINE 736

Nytol with DPH - See ANTIHISTAMINES 92

O

Obalan - See APPETITE SUPPRESSANTS 106

Obe-Del - See APPETITE SUPPRESSANTS 106

Obe-Mar - See APPETITE SUPPRESSANTS 106

Obe-Nix - See APPETITE SUPPRESSANTS 106

Obephen - See APPETITE SUPPRESSANTS 106

Obermine - See APPETITE SUPPRESSANTS 106

Obestin-30 - See APPETITE SUPPRESSANTS 106

Obeval - See APPETITE SUPPRESSANTS 106

Obezine - See APPETITE SUPPRESSANTS 106

Oby-Trim - See APPETITE SUPPRESSANTS 106

Occlusal Topical Solution - See ANTI-ACNE (Topical) 60

Occlusal-HP Topical Solution - See ANTI-ACNE (Topical) 60

OCTOXYNOL 9 - See CONTRACEPTIVES, VAGINAL (Spermicides) 252

Ocu-Caine - See ANESTHETICS, LOCAL (Ophthalmic) 50

Ocu-Carpine - See PILOCARPINE 690

Ocu-Chlor Ophthalmic Ointment - See ANTIBACTERIALS (Ophthalmic) 64

Ocu-Chlor Ophthalmic Solution - See ANTIBACTERIALS (Ophthalmic) 64

Ocu-Dex - See ANTI-INFLAMMATORY DRUGS, STEROIDAL (Ophthalmic) 96

Ocugestrin - See PHENYLEPHRINE (Ophthalmic) 684

Ocu-Mycin - See ANTIBACTERIALS (Ophthalmic) 64

Ocu-Pentolate - See CYCLOPENTOLATE (Ophthalmic) 268

Ocu-Phrin - See PHENYLEPHRINE (Ophthalmic) 684

Ocu-Pred - See ANTI-INFLAMMATORY DRUGS, STEROIDAL (Ophthalmic) 96

Ocu-Pred Forte - See ANTI-INFLAMMATORY DRUGS, STEROIDAL (Ophthalmic) 96

Ocu-Pred-A - See ANTI-INFLAMMATORY DRUGS, STEROIDAL (Ophthalmic) 96

Ocusert Pilo - See PILOCARPINE 690

Ocu-Sul-10 - See ANTIBACTERIALS (Ophthalmic) 64

Ocu-Sul-15 - See ANTIBACTERIALS (Ophthalmic) 64

Ocu-Sul-30 - See ANTIBACTERIALS (Ophthalmic) 64

Ocusulf-10 - See ANTIBACTERIALS (Ophthalmic) 64

Ocu-Tropine - See CYCLOPEGIC, MYDRIATIC (Ophthalmic) 266

Ocu-Zoline - See DECONGESTANTS (Ophthalmic) 284

Off-Ezy - See ANTI-ACNE (Topical) 60

Off-Ezy Topical Solution Corn & Callus Remover Kit - See ANTI-ACNE (Topical) 60

Off-Ezy Topical Solution Wart Removal Kit - See ANTI-ACNE (Topical) 60

O-Flex - See ORPHENADRINE 630

OFLOXACIN 624

Ogen - See ESTROGENS 360

OLSALAZINE 626

OMEPRAZOLE 628
Omnicol - See
  ACETAMINOPHEN 2
  ANTIHISTAMINES 92
  DEXTROMETHORPHAN 292
  PHENYLEPHRINE 682
  SALICYLATES 774
Omnipen - See AMPICILLIN 36
Omnipen-N - See AMPICILLIN 36
Omni-Tuss - See
  ANTIHISTAMINES 92
  EPHEDRINE 340
  NARCOTIC ANALGESICS 592
o,p'-DDD - See MITOTANE 570
Opcon - See DECONGESTANTS (Ophthalmic) 284
Ophthacet - See ANTIBACTERIALS (Ophthalmic)
  64
Ophthaine - See ANESTHETICS, LOCAL
  (Ophthalmic) 50
Ophthetic - See ANESTHETICS, LOCAL
  (Ophthalmic) 50
Ophthochlor Ophthalmic Solution - See
  ANTIBACTERIALS (Ophthalmic) 64
Ophtho-chloram Ophthalmic Solution - See
  ANTIBACTERIALS (Ophthalmic) 64
OPIUM - See NARCOTIC ANALGESICS 592
Opium Tincture - See PAREGORIC 654
Opticrom - See CROMOLYN 256
Optimine - See ANTIHISTAMINES 92
Optipranolol - See ANTIGLAUCOMA, SHORT-
  ACTING (Ophthalmic) 90
Orabase with Benzocaine - See ANESTHETICS,
  DENTAL (Topical) 48
Oracit - See CITRATES 220
Oradexon - See DEXAMETHASONE 290
Oragest S.R. - See
  ANTIHISTAMINES 92
  PHENYLPROPANOLAMINE 686
Oragrafin Calcium - See GALLBLADDER X-RAY
  TEST DRUGS (Cholecystographic Agents) 396
Oragrafin Sodium - See GALLBLADDER X-RAY
  TEST DRUGS (Cholecystographic Agents) 396
Orajel - See ANESTHETICS, DENTAL (Topical) 48
Oramide - See ANTIDIABETIC AGENTS 78
Oraminic II - See ANTIHISTAMINES 92
Oraminic Spancaps - See
  ANTIHISTAMINES 92
  PHENYLPROPANOLAMINE 686
Oramorph - See NARCOTIC ANALGESICS 592
Oramorph-SR - See NARCOTIC ANALGESICS 592
Orap - See ANTIDYSKINETICS 80
Oraphen-PD - See ACETAMINOPHEN 2
Orasone - See PREDNISONE 712
Ora-Testryl - See ANDROGENS 42
Orazinc - See ZINC SUPPLEMENTS 902
Orbenin - See CLOXACILLIN 238
Oretic - See DIURETICS, THIAZIDE 324
Oreticyl - See
  RAUWOLFIA ALKALOIDS 758
  RAUWOLFIA & THIAZIDE DIURETICS 760
Oreticyl Forte - See RAUWOLFIA & THIAZIDE
  DIURETICS 760

Oreton - See ANDROGENS 42
Orflagen - See ORPHENADRINE 630
Orfro - See ORPHENADRINE 630
Organic-1 - See IODINATED GLYCEROL 446
Organidin - See IODINATED GLYCEROL 446
Orinase - See ANTIDIABETIC AGENTS 78
Ornade - See PHENYLPROPANOLAMINE 686
Ornade A.F. - See PHENYLPROPANOLAMINE 686
Ornade Expectorant - See
  ANTIHISTAMINES 92
  GUAIFENESIN 408
  PHENYLPROPANOLAMINE 686
Ornade Spansules - See ANTIHISTAMINES 92
Ornade-DM - See PHENYLPROPANOLAMINE 686
Ornade-DM 10 - See
  ANTIHISTAMINES 92
  DEXTROMETHORPHAN 292
  PHENYLPROPANOLAMINE 686
Ornade-DM 15 - See
  ANTIHISTAMINES 92
  DEXTROMETHORPHAN 292
  PHENYLPROPANOLAMINE 686
Ornade-DM 30 - See
  ANTIHISTAMINES 92
  DEXTROMETHORPHAN 292
  PHENYLPROPANOLAMINE 686
Ornex Cold - See PSEUDOEPHEDRINE 736
Ornex No Drowsiness Caplets - See
  ACETAMINOPHEN 2
  PSEUDOEPHEDRINE 736
ORPHENADRINE 630
ORPHENADRINE, ASPIRIN & CAFFEINE 632
Orphenagesic - See ORPHENADRINE, ASPIRIN &
  CAFFEINE 632
Orphenagesic Forte - See ORPHENADRINE,
  ASPIRIN & CAFFEINE 632
Orphenate - See ORPHENADRINE 630
Ortega Otic-M - See ANTIBACTERIALS (Otic) 66
Ortho - See CONTRACEPTIVES, ORAL 250
Ortho-Creme - See CONTRACEPTIVES, VAGINAL
  (Spermicides) 252
Ortho-Cyclen 21 - See ESTROGENS 360
Ortho-Cyclen 28 - See ESTROGENS 360
Ortho-Gynol - See CONTRACEPTIVES, VAGINAL
  (Spermicides) 252
Ortho-Novum 0.5 - See CONTRACEPTIVES, ORAL
  250
Ortho-Novum 1/35 - See CONTRACEPTIVES,
  ORAL 250
Ortho-Novum 1/50 - See CONTRACEPTIVES,
  ORAL 250
Ortho-Novum 1/80 - See CONTRACEPTIVES,
  ORAL 250
Ortho-Novum 2 - See CONTRACEPTIVES, ORAL 250
Ortho-Novum 7/7/7 - See CONTRACEPTIVES,
  ORAL 250
Ortho-Novum 10/11 - See CONTRACEPTIVES,
  ORAL 250
Orthoxicol Cough - See
  ANTIHISTAMINES 92
  DEXTROMETHORPHAN 292
  PHENYLPROPANOLAMINE 686

INDEX

Oxyderm 20 Lotion - See BENZOYL PEROXIDE 132

Oxydess II - See AMPHETAMINES 34

OXYMETHOLONE - See ANDROGENS 42

OXYMORPHONE - See NARCOTIC ANALGESICS 592

OXYTETRACYCLINE - See TETRACYCLINES 828

Oysco - See CALCIUM SUPPLEMENTS 170

Oyst-Cal - See CALCIUM SUPPLEMENTS 170

Oystercal - See CALCIUM SUPPLEMENTS 170

P

P&S - See ANTI-ACNE (Topical) 60

P-A-C Compound - See CAFFEINE 166

P-A-C Revised Formula - See ASPIRIN 108

Pacaps - See
  ACETAMINOPHEN 2
  BARBITURATES 122
  CAFFEINE 166

Palafer - See IRON SUPPLEMENTS 454

Palaron - See BRONCHODILATORS, XANTHINE 152

Palmiron - See IRON SUPPLEMENTS 454

Pama No. 1 - See ANTACIDS 56

Pamelor - See TRICYCLIC ANTIDEPRESSANTS 868

Pamprin-IB - See ANTI-INFLAMMATORY DRUGS, NON-STEROIDAL (NSAIDs) 94

Panadol - See ACETAMINOPHEN 2

Panadol Junior Strength - See ACETAMINOPHEN 2

Panadyl - See
  ANTIHISTAMINES 92
  PHENYLPROPANOLAMINE 686

Pancoate - See PANCRELIPASE 642

Pancrease - See PANCRELIPASE 642

Pancrease MT4 - See PANCRELIPASE 642

Pancrease MT10 - See PANCRELIPASE 642

Pancrease MT16 - See PANCRELIPASE 642

PANCREATIN, PEPSIN, BILE SALTS, HYOSCYAMINE, ATROPINE, SCOPOLAMINE & PHENOBARBITAL 640

PANCRELIPASE 642

Panectyl - See TRIMEPRAZINE 872

Panex - See ACETAMINOPHEN 2

Panex 500 - See ACETAMINOPHEN 2

Panflex - See CHLORZOXAZONE & ACETAMINOPHEN 212

Panmycin - See TETRACYCLINES 828

PanOxyl 5 Bar - See BENZOYL PEROXIDE 132

PanOxyl 5 Gel - See BENZOYL PEROXIDE 132

PanOxyl 10 Bar - See BENZOYL PEROXIDE 132

PanOxyl 15 Gel - See BENZOYL PEROXIDE 132

PanOxyl 20 Gel - See BENZOYL PEROXIDE 132

PanOxyl AQ 2 Gel - See BENZOYL PEROXIDE 132

PanOxyl AQ 5 Gel - See BENZOYL PEROXIDE 132

Panrexin M - See APPETITE SUPPRESSANTS 106

Panrexin MTP - See APPETITE SUPPRESSANTS 106

Panshape - See APPETITE SUPPRESSANTS 106

Pantapon - See NARCOTIC ANALGESICS 592

PANTOTHENIC ACID (Vitamin B-5) 652

Panwarfin - See ANTICOAGULANTS (Oral) 74

PAPAVERINE 646

Paplex - See ANTI-ACNE (Topical) 60

Paplex Ultra - See ANTI-ACNE (Topical) 60

Papulex - See NIACIN (Vitamin B-3, Nicotinic Acid) 604

Par Glycerol - See IODINATED GLYCEROL 446

Par Glycerol C - See
  IODINATED GLYCEROL 446
  NARCOTIC ANALGESICS 592

Par Glycerol-DM - See
  DEXTROMETHORPHAN 292
  IODINATED GLYCEROL 446

PARA-AMINOSALICYLIC ACID (Aminosalicylate Sodium) 648

Paracet Forte - See CHLORZOXAZONE & ACETAMINOPHEN 212

Paracetamol - See ACETAMINOPHEN 2

Paradione - See ANTICONVULSANTS, DIONE-TYPE 76

Paraflex - See MUSCLE RELAXANTS, SKELETAL 578

Parafon Forte - See
  ACETAMINOPHEN 2
  MUSCLE RELAXANTS, SKELETAL 578

Parafon Forte DSC - See MUSCLE RELAXANTS, SKELETAL 578

Paraforte - See CHLORZOXAZONE & ACETAMINOPHEN 212

Paragen-Forte - See CHLORZOXAZONE & ACETAMINOPHEN 212

Paral - See PARALDEHYDE 650

PARALDEHYDE 650

PARAMETHADIONE - See ANTICONVULSANTS, DIONE-TYPE 76

PARAMETHASONE 652

Parazone - See CHLORZOXAZONE & ACETAMINOPHEN 212

Parbenem - See PROBENECID 718

Par Decon - See
  ANTIHISTAMINES 92
  PHENYLEPHRINE 682
  PHENYLPROPANOLAMINE 686

PAREGORIC 654

Parepectolin - See
  KAOLIN & PECTIN 468
  KAOLIN, PECTIN & PAREGORIC 472

Pargen Fortified - See CHLORZOXAZONE & ACETAMINOPHEN 212

PARGYLINE - See MONOAMINE OXIDASE (MAO) INHIBITORS 574

Pariodel - See BROMOCRIPTINE 148

Par-Mag - See ANTACIDS 56

Parmine - See APPETITE SUPPRESSANTS 106

Parnate - See MONOAMINE OXIDASE (MAO) INHIBITORS 574

Parsidol - See ANTIDYSKINETICS 80

Parsitan - See ANTIDYSKINETICS 80

Parviscon - See ANTACIDS 56

Parzine - See APPETITE SUPPRESSANTS 106

Propa pH 10 Liquid Acne Soap - See BENZOYL
PEROXIDE 132
Propa pH Medicated Acne Cream Maximum
Strength - See ANTI-ACNE (Topical) 60
Propa pH Medicated Cleansing Pads Maximum
Strength - See ANTI-ACNE (Topical) 60
Propa pH Medicated Cleansing Pads Sensitive Skin
- See ANTI-ACNE (Topical) 60
Propa pH Perfectly Clear Skin Cleanser Topical
Solution Normal/Combination Skin - See ANTI-
ACNE (Topical) 60
Propa pH Perfectly Clear Skin Cleanser Topical
Solution Oily Skin - See ANTI-ACNE (Topical)
60
Propa pH Perfectly Clear Skin Cleanser Topical
Solution Sensitive Skin Formula - See ANTI-
ACNE (Topical) 60
Propacet - See NARCOTIC & ACETAMINOPHEN
590
Propaderm - See ADRENOCORTICOIDS (Topical)
14
PROPAFENONE 730
Propain-HC - See NARCOTIC &
ACETAMINOPHEN 590
Propanthel - See PROPANTHELINE 732
PROPANTHELINE 732
PROPARACAINE - See ANESTHETICS, LOCAL
(Ophthalmic) 50
Propine - See ANTIGLAUCOMA, SHORT-ACTING
(Ophthalmic) 90
Propoxycon - See NARCOTIC ANALGESICS 592
PROPOXYPHENE - See NARCOTIC ANALGESICS
592
PROPOXYPHENE & ACETAMINOPHEN - See
NARCOTIC & ACETAMINOPHEN 590
PROPOXYPHENE & ASPIRIN - See NARCOTIC &
ASPIRIN 594
Propoxyphene Compound - See CAFFEINE 166
PROPRANOLOL - See BETA-ADRENERGIC
BLOCKERS 134
PROPRANOLOL & HYDROCHLOROTHIAZIDE -
See BETA-ADRENERGIC BLOCKING AGENTS
& THIAZIDE DIURETICS 136
Propyl-Thyracil - See ANTITHYROID DRUGS 102
PROPYLTHIOURACIL - See ANTITHYROID
DRUGS 102
Proscar - See FINASTERIDE 378
Prosed - See ATROPINE, HYOSCYAMINE,
METHENAMINE, METHYLENE BLUE,
PHENYLSALICYLATE & BENZOIC ACID 112
Pro-Sof - See DOCUSATE SODIUM 332
Pro-Sof Liquid Concentrate - See DOCUSATE
SODIUM 332
Pro-Sof Plus - See DOCUSATE SODIUM 332
Prostaphlin - See OXACILLIN 634
PROSTEP - See NICOTINE (Skin Patch) 608
Prostigmin - See NEOSTIGMINE 602
Prostin E2 - See DINOPROSTONE (Vaginal) 310
Protamine Zinc & Iletin - See INSULIN 444
Protamine Zinc & Iletin I - See INSULIN 444
Protamine Zinc & Iletin II - See INSULIN 444

Protectant (ophthalmic) - See PROTECTANT
(Ophthalmic) 734
PROTECTANT (Ophthalmic) 734
Protophylline - See BRONCHODILATORS,
XANTHINE 152
Protostat - See METRONIDAZOLE 554
Protrin - See
SULFAMETHOXAZOLE 806
TRIMETHOPRIM 876
PROTRIPTYLINE - See TRICYCLIC
ANTIDEPRESSANTS 868
Protylol - See DICYCLOMINE 300
Proval - See NARCOTIC & ACETAMINOPHEN 590
Proventil - See BRONCHODILATORS,
ADRENERGIC 150
Proventil Repetabs - See BRONCHODILATORS,
ADRENERGIC 150
Provera - See PROGESTINS 728
Prov-U-Sep - See METHENAMINE 528
Proxy 65 - See NARCOTIC & ACETAMINOPHEN
590
Prozac - See FLUOXETINE 388
Prozine - See PHENOTHIAZINES 678
Prunicodeine - See
NARCOTIC ANALGESICS 592
TERPIN HYDRATE 822
Pseudo - See PSEUDOEPHEDRINE 736
Pseudo-Bid - See
GUAIFENESIN 408
PSEUDOEPHEDRINE 736
Pseudo-Car DM - See
ANTIHISTAMINES 92
DEXTROMETHORPHAN 292
PSEUDOEPHEDRINE 736
Pseudo-Chlor - See
ANTIHISTAMINES 92
PSEUDOEPHEDRINE 736
Pseudodine C Cough - See
ANTIHISTAMINES 92
NARCOTIC ANALGESICS 592
PSEUDOEPHEDRINE 736
PSEUDOEPHEDRINE 736
Pseudofrin - See PSEUDOEPHEDRINE 736
Pseudogest - See PSEUDOEPHEDRINE 736
Pseudogest Plus - See
ANTIHISTAMINES 92
Pseudo-Hist Expectorant - See
GUAIFENESIN 408
NARCOTIC ANALGESICS 592
PSEUDOEPHEDRINE 736
PSORALENS 738
Psorcon - See ADRENOCORTICOIDS (Topical) 14
psoriGel - See COAL TAR (Topical) 242
PsoriNail - See COAL TAR (Topical) 242
PSYLLIUM 740
PT 105 - See APPETITE SUPPRESSANTS 106
Pulmophylline - See BRONCHODILATORS,
XANTHINE 152
Purge - See CASTOR OIL 186
Purinethol - See MERCAPTOPURINE 524
Purinol - See ALLOPURINOL 16

INDEX

Razepam - See BENZODIAZEPINES 130
Reclomide - See METOCLOPRAMIDE 552
Rectocort - See HYDROCORTISONE Rectal) 432
Rederm - See ADRENOCORTICOIDS (Topical) 14
Redisol - See VITAMIN B-12 (Cyanocobalamin) 886
Redoxon - See VITAMIN C (Ascorbic Acid) 888
Reese's Pinworm Medicine - See PYRANTEL 742
Reglan - See METOCLOPRAMIDE 552
Regonol - See PYRIDOSTIGMINE 744
Regroton - See RAUWOLFIA ALKALOIDS 758
Regular - See INSULIN 444
Regular (Concentrated) Iletin - See INSULIN 444
Regular (Concentrated) Iletin II, U-500 - See
    INSULIN 444
Regular Iletin I - See INSULIN 444
Regular Iletin II - See INSULIN 444
Regular Insulin - See INSULIN 444
Regulax SS - See DOCUSATE SODIUM 332
Regulex - See DOCUSATE SODIUM 332
Regulex-D Doss - See DANTHRON AND
    DOCUSATE 278
Reguloid Natural - See PSYLLIUM 740
Reguloid Orange - See PSYLLIUM 740
Regutol - See DOCUSATE SODIUM 332
Rehydralyte - See DEXTROSE & ELECTROLYTES 294
Reidamine - See ANTIHISTAMINES 92
Rela - See MUSCLE RELAXANTS, SKELETAL 578
Relafen - See ANTI-INFLAMMATORY DRUGS,
    NON-STEROIDAL (NSAIDs) 94
Relaxadon - See BELLADONNA ALKALOIDS &
    BARBITURATES 128
Relief - See PHENYLEPHRINE (Ophthalmic) 684
Remcol-C - See
    ACETAMINOPHEN 2
    ANTIHISTAMINES 92
    DEXTROMETHORPHAN 292
Renalgin - See METHENAMINE 528
Renese - See DIURETICS, THIAZIDE 324
Renese-R - See
    RAUWOLFIA ALKALOIDS 758
    RAUWOLFIA & THIAZIDE DIURETICS 760
Renoquid - See SULFACYTINE 802
Rentamine - See
    ANTIHISTAMINES 92
    EPHEDRINE 340
    PHENYLPROPANOLAMINE 686
Repan - See
    ACETAMINOPHEN 2
    BARBITURATES 122
Repigmenting agent (psoralen) - See PSORALENS
    738
Rep-Pred - See METHYLPREDNISOLONE 546
Resaid S.R. - See
    ANTIHISTAMINES 92
    PHENYLPROPANOLAMINE 686
Rescaps-D S.R. - See PHENYLPROPANOLAMINE
    686
Reserfia - See RAUWOLFIA ALKALOIDS 758
RESERPINE - See RAUWOLFIA ALKALOIDS 758
RESERPINE & CHLOROTHIAZIDE - See
    RAUWOLFIA & THIAZIDE DIURETICS 760

RESERPINE & CHLORTHALIDONE - See
    RAUWOLFIA & THIAZIDE DIURETICS 760
RESERPINE & HYDRALAZINE 762
RESERPINE & HYDROCHLOROTHIAZIDE - See
    RAUWOLFIA & THIAZIDE DIURETICS 760
RESERPINE & HYDROFLUMETHIAZIDE - See
    RAUWOLFIA & THIAZIDE DIURETICS 760
RESERPINE & METHYLCLOTHIAZIDE - See
    RAUWOLFIA & THIAZIDE DIURETICS 760
RESERPINE & POLYTHIAZIDE - See RAUWOLFIA
    & THIAZIDE DIURETICS 760
RESERPINE & QUINETHAZONE - See
    RAUWOLFIA & THIAZIDE DIURETICS 760
RESERPINE & TRICHLORMETHIAZIDE - See
    RAUWOLFIA & THIAZIDE DIURETICS 760
RESERPINE, HYDRALAZINE &
    HYDROCHLOROTHIAZIDE 764
Resol - See DEXTROSE & ELECTROLYTES 294
RESORCINOL - See ANTI-ACNE (Topical) 60
RESORCINOL & SULFUR - See ANTI-ACNE
    (Topical) 60
Respaire-60 SR - See
    GUAIFENESIN 408
    PSEUDOEPHEDRINE 736
Respaire-120 SR - See
    GUAIFENESIN 408
    PSEUDOEPHEDRINE 736
Respbid - See BRONCHODILATORS, XANTHINE
    152
Respinol G - See PHENYLEPHRINE 682
Respinol LA - See
    GUAIFENESIN 408
    PHENYLEPHRINE 682
    PHENYLPROPANOLAMINE 686
Respinol-G - See
    GUAIFENESIN 408
    PHENYLPROPANOLAMINE 686
Resporal TR - See
    ANTIHISTAMINES 92
    PSEUDOEPHEDRINE 736
Restoril - See BENZODIAZEPINES 130
Resyl - See GUAIFENESIN 408
Retin-A Cream - See TRETINOIN (Topical) 858
Retin-A Cream Regimen Kit - See TRETINOIN
    (Topical) 858
Retin-A Gel - See TRETINOIN (Topical) 858
Retin-A Gel Regimen Kit - See TRETINOIN
    (Topical) 858
Retin-A Solution - See TRETINOIN (Topical) 858
Retinoic Acid - See TRETINOIN (Topical) 858
Retrovir - See ZIDOVUDINE (AZT, Azidothymidine)
    900
Rexigen - See APPETITE SUPPRESSANTS 106
Rexigen Forte - See APPETITE SUPPRESSANTS
    106
Rezamid Lotion - See ANTI-ACNE (Topical) 60
Rheaban - See ATTAPULGITE 114
Rheumatrex - See METHOTREXATE 532
Rhinalar - See ADRENOCORTICOIDS (Nasal) 12
Rhinocaps - See
    ACETAMINOPHEN 2

BARBITURATES 122
NARCOTIC & ACETAMINOPHEN 590
Rolaids - See ANTACIDS 56
Rolaids Calcium Rich - See
ANTACIDS 56
CALCIUM SUPPLEMENTS 170
Rolaids Sodium Free - See ANTACIDS 56
Ro-Mycin - See ERYTHROMYCINS 354
Rondec - See
ANTIHISTAMINES 92
PSEUDOEPHEDRINE 736
Rondec Drops - See
ANTIHISTAMINES 92
PSEUDOEPHEDRINE 736
Rondec-DM - See
ANTIHISTAMINES 92
DEXTROMETHORPHAN 292
PSEUDOEPHEDRINE 736
Rondec-DM Drops - See
ANTIHISTAMINES 92
DEXTROMETHORPHAN 292
PSEUDOEPHEDRINE 736
Rondec-TR - See
ANTIHISTAMINES 92
PSEUDOEPHEDRINE 736
Rondomycin - See TETRACYCLINES 828
Roniacol - See NIACIN (Vitamin B-3, Nicotinic Acid)
604
Ronigen - See NIACIN (Vitamin B-3, Nicotinic Acid)
604
Ro-Profen - See ANTI-INFLAMMATORY DRUGS,
NON-STEROIDAL (NSAIDs) 94
Roubac - See
SULFAMETHOXAZOLE 806
TRIMETHOPRIM 876
Rounox - See ACETAMINOPHEN 2
Rounox with Codeine - See NARCOTIC &
ACETAMINOPHEN 590
Rowasa - See MESALAMINE (Rectal) 526
Roxanol - See NARCOTIC ANALGESICS 592
Roxanol SR - See NARCOTIC ANALGESICS 592
Roxicet - See NARCOTIC & ACETAMINOPHEN 590
Roxicodone - See NARCOTIC ANALGESICS 592
Roxiprin - See
NARCOTIC & ASPIRIN 594
NARCOTIC ANALGESICS 592
Roychlor 10% - See POTASSIUM SUPPLEMENTS
704
Roychlor 20% - See POTASSIUM SUPPLEMENTS
704
Royonate - See POTASSIUM SUPPLEMENTS 704
R-Tannate - See
ANTIHISTAMINES 92
PHENYLEPHRINE 682
Rubion - See VITAMIN B-12 (Cyanocobalamin) 886
Rubramin - See VITAMIN B-12 (Cyanocobalamin) 886
Rubramin-PC - See VITAMIN B-12
(Cyanocobalamin) 886
Rufen - See ANTI-INFLAMMATORY DRUGS, NON-
STEROIDAL (NSAIDs) 94
Rulox - See ANTACIDS 56
Rulox No. 1 - See ANTACIDS 56

Rulox No. 2 - See ANTACIDS 56
Rum-K - See POTASSIUM SUPPLEMENTS 704
Ru-Tuss - See
ANTIHISTAMINES 92
PHENYLEPHRINE 682
Ru-Tuss II - See
ANTIHISTAMINES 92
PHENYLPROPANOLAMINE 686
Ru-Tuss Expectorant - See
DEXTROMETHORPHAN 292
GUAIFENESIN 408
PHENYLEPHRINE 682
PSEUDOEPHEDRINE 736
Ru-Tuss w/Hydrocodone - See PHENYLEPHRINE
682
Ru-Tuss w/Hydrocodone Liquid - See
ANTIHISTAMINES 92
NARCOTIC ANALGESICS 592
PHENYLEPHRINE 682
PHENYLPROPANOLAMINE 686
Ru-Vert-M - See MECLIZINE 512
Rycotin - See NIACIN (Vitamin B-3, Nicotinic Acid)
604
Rymed - See
GUAIFENESIN 408
PHENYLEPHRINE 682
PHENYLPROPANOLAMINE 686
Rymed Liquid - See
GUAIFENESIN 408
PHENYLEPHRINE 682
PHENYLPROPANOLAMINE 686
Rymed-TR - See
GUAIFENESIN 408
PSEUDOEPHEDRINE 736
Ryna - See
ANTIHISTAMINES 92
PSEUDOEPHEDRINE 736
Ryna-C Liquid - See
ANTIHISTAMINES 92
NARCOTIC ANALGESICS 592
PSEUDOEPHEDRINE 736
Ryna-CX Liquid - See
GUAIFENESIN 408
NARCOTIC ANALGESICS 592
PSEUDOEPHEDRINE 736
Rynacrom - See CROMOLYN 256
Rynatan - See
ANTIHISTAMINES 92
PHENYLEPHRINE 682
Rynatuss - See
ANTIHISTAMINES 92
EPHEDRINE 340
Rynatuss Pediatric - See
ANTIHISTAMINES 92
EPHEDRINE 340
Rythmodan - See DISOPYRAMIDE 318
Rythmodan-LA - See DISOPYRAMIDE 318

S
S-A-C - See
ACETAMINOPHEN & SALICYLATES 4
CAFFEINE 166

Salac - See ANTI-ACNE (Topical) 60
Salacid - See ANTI-ACNE (Topical) 60
Sal-Acid Plaster - See ANTI-ACNE (Topical) 60
Salactic Film Topical Solution - See ANTI-ACNE
  (Topical) 60
Sal-Adult - See ASPIRIN 108
Salatin - See
  ACETAMINOPHEN & SALICYLATES 4
  ASPIRIN 108
  CAFFEINE 166
Salazide - See RAUWOLFIA & THIAZIDE
  DIURETICS 760
Salazopyrin - See SULFASALAZINE 808
Salazosulfapyridine - See SULFASALAZINE 808
Sal-Clens Plus Shampoo - See ANTI-ACNE
  (Topical) 60
Sal-Clens Shampoo - See ANTI-ACNE (Topical) 60
Saleto - See
  ACETAMINOPHEN & SALICYLATES 4
  ASPIRIN 108
Saleto-CF - See
  ACETAMINOPHEN 2
  DEXTROMETHORPHAN 292
  PHENYLPROPANOLAMINE 686
Saleto-D - See
  ACETAMINOPHEN 2
  CAFFEINE 166
  PHENYLPROPANOLAMINE 686
Salflex - See SALICYLATES 774
Salgesic - See SALICYLATES 774
Sal Hepatica - See SODIUM PHOSPHATE 794
SALICYLAMIDE - See SALICYLATES 774
SALICYLATES 774
Salicylazosulfapyridine - See SULFASALAZINE 808
SALICYLIC ACID - See ANTI-ACNE (Topical) 60
SALICYLIC ACID & SULFUR - See ANTI-ACNE
  (Topical) 60
SALICYLIC ACID, SULFUR AND COAL TAR - See
  ANTISEBORRHEICS (Topical) 100
Saligel - See ANTI-ACNE (Topical) 60
Sal-Infant - See ASPIRIN 108
Salipral - See BUTALBITAL & ASPIRIN (Also
  contains caffeine) 162
Salocol - See
  ACETAMINOPHEN & SALICYLATES 4
  ASPIRIN 108
  CAFFEINE 166
Salofalk - See MESALAMINE (Rectal) 526
Salonil - See ANTI-ACNE (Topical) 60
Salphenyl - See ACETAMINOPHEN &
  SALICYLATES 4
Sal-Plant Gel Topical Solution - See ANTI-ACNE
  (Topical) 60
SALONATE - See SALICYLATES 774
Salsitab - See SALICYLATES 774
Saluron - See DIURETICS, THIAZIDE 324
Salutensin - See
  RAUWOLFIA ALKALOIDS 758
  RAUWOLFIA & THIAZIDE DIURETICS 760
Salutensin-Demi - See RAUWOLFIA & THIAZIDE
  DIURETICS 760

Sandimmune - See CYCLOSPORINE 274
Sanorex - See APPETITE SUPPRESSANTS 106
Sansert - See METHYSERGIDE 550
Sarisol No. 2 - See BARBITURATES 122
Sarna HC - See ADRENOCORTICOIDS (Topical) 14
Sarodant - See NITROFURANTOIN 616
Saroflex - See CHLORZOXAZONE &
  ACETAMINOPHEN 212
S.A.S. - See SULFASALAZINE 808
S.A.S. Enteric - See SULFASALAZINE 808
Sastid - See ANTI-ACNE (Topical) 60
Sastid (AL) Scrub - See ANTI-ACNE (Topical) 60
Sastid Plain - See ANTI-ACNE (Topical) 60
Sastid Plain Shampoo and Acne Wash - See ANTI-
  ACNE (Topical) 60
Sastid Soap - See ANTI-ACNE (Topical) 60
Satric - See METRONIDAZOLE 554
Scabene - See PEDICULISIDES (Topical) 656
Scabicide - See PEDICULISIDES (Topical) 656
SCOPOLAMINE - See CYCLOPEGIC, MYDRIATIC
  (Ophthalmic) 266
SCOPOLAMINE (Hyoscine) 776
Seba-Nil - See ANTI-ACNE, CLEANSING (Topical)
  62
Sebasorb Liquid - See ANTI-ACNE (Topical) 60
Sebex - See ANTI-ACNE (Topical) 60
Sebex-T Tar Shampoo - See ANTISEBORRHEICS
  (Topical) 100
Sebulex Antiseborrheic Treatment and Conditioning
  Shampoo - See ANTI-ACNE (Topical) 60
Sebulex Antiseborrheic Treatment Shampoo - See
  ANTI-ACNE (Topical) 60
Sebulex Conditioning Shampoo - See ANTI-ACNE
  (Topical) 60
Sebulex Conditioning Suspension Shampoo - See
  ANTISEBORRHEICS (Topical) 100
Sebulex Cream Medicated Shampoo - See ANTI-
  ACNE (Topical) 60
Sebulex Lotion Shampoo - See
  ANTISEBORRHEICS (Topical) 100
Sebulex Medicated Dandruff Shampoo with
  Conditioners - See ANTI-ACNE (Topical) 60
Sebulex Medicated Shampoo - See ANTI-ACNE
  (Topical) 60
Sebulex Regular Medicated Dandruff Shampoo -
  See ANTI-ACNE (Topical) 60
Sebulex Shampoo - See ANTI-ACNE (Topical) 60
Sebulon - See ANTISEBORRHEICS (Topical) 100
SECOBARBITAL - See BARBITURATES 122
SECOBARBITAL AND AMOBARBITAL - See
  BARBITURATES 122
Seconal - See BARBITURATES 122
Sectral - See BETA-ADRENERGIC BLOCKERS 134
Sedabamate - See MEPROBAMATE 520
Sedapap-10 - See
  ACETAMINOPHEN 2
  BARBITURATES 122
Sedative - See
  BARBITURATES 122
  BUTALBITAL & ASPIRIN (Also contains caffeine)
  162

INDEX

1057

ERGOTAMINE, CAFFEINE, BELLADONNA &
PENTOBARBITAL 352
ISOMETHEPTENE, DICHLORALPHENAZONE &
ACETAMINOPHEN 456
PANCREATIN, PEPSIN, BILE SALTS,
HYOSCYAMINE, ATROPINE, SCOPOLAMINE
& PHENOBARBITAL 640
THEOPHYLLINE, EPHEDRINE &
BARBITURATES 830
THEOPHYLLINE, EPHEDRINE, GUAIFENESIN &
BARBITURATES 832
Sedative (hypnotic) - See
ETHINAMATE 364
METHYPRYLON 548
TRIAZOLAM 866
Sedatuss - See DEXTROMETHORPHAN 292
Seldane - See TERFENADINE 820
Seldane D
ANTIHISTAMINES 92
PSEUDOEPHEDRINE 736
TERFENADINE 820
SELEGILINE 778
SELENIUM - See ANTISEBORRHEICS (Topical)
100
Selenomethionine Se 75 - See RADIO-
PHARMACEUTICALS 756
Selestoject - See BETAMETHASONE 140
Selsun - See ANTISEBORRHEICS (Topical) 100
Selsun Blue - See ANTISEBORRHEICS (Topical)
100
Selsun Blue Regular Formula - See
ANTISEBORRHEICS (Topical) 100
Semcet - See
ACETAMINOPHEN 2
BARBITURATES 122
Semicid - See CONTRACEPTIVES, VAGINAL
(Spermicides) 252
Semilente - See INSULIN 444
Semilente Iletin - See INSULIN 444
Semilente Iletin I - See INSULIN 444
Senefen III - See NARCOTIC & ACETAMINOPHEN
590
Senexon - See SENNA 780
SENNA 780
SENNOSIDES A & B 782
Senokot - See SENNA 780
Senokot-S - See DOCUSATE SODIUM 332
Senolax - See SENNA 780
Sential - See ADRENOCORTICOIDS (Topical) 14
Septra - See
SULFAMETHOXAZOLE 806
TRIMETHOPRIM 876
Septra DS - See SULFAMETHOXAZOLE 806
Ser-A-Gen - See RESERPINE, HYDRALAZINE &
HYDROCHLOROTHIAZIDE 764
Seralazide - See RESERPINE, HYDRALAZINE &
HYDROCHLOROTHIAZIDE 764
Ser-Ap-Es - See
HYDRALAZINE 426
RESERPINE, HYDRALAZINE &
HYDROCHLOROTHIAZIDE 764
Serax - See BENZODIAZEPINES 130

Sereen - See BENZODIAZEPINES 130
Serentil - See PHENOTHIAZINES 678
Serentil Concentrate - See PHENOTHIAZINES 678
Seromycin - See CYCLOSERINE 272
Serophene - See CLOMIPHENE 230
Serpalan - See RAUWOLFIA ALKALOIDS 758
Serpasil - See RAUWOLFIA ALKALOIDS 758
Serpasil-Apresoline - See RESERPINE &
HYDRALAZINE 762
Serpasil-Esidrix - See
RAUWOLFIA ALKALOIDS 758
RAUWOLFIA & THIAZIDE DIURETICS 760
Serpazide - See RESERPINE, HYDRALAZINE &
HYDROCHLOROTHIAZIDE 764
Sertan - See PRIMIDONE 716
SERTRALINE 784
Serutan - See PSYLLIUM 740
Serutan Toasted Granules - See PSYLLIUM 740
Shur-Seal - See CONTRACEPTIVES, VAGINAL
(Spermicides) 252
Siblin - See PSYLLIUM 740
Silain - See SIMETHICONE 786
Silain-Gel - See ANTACIDS 56
Sildimac - See ANTIBACTERIALS, ANTIFUNGALS
(Topical) 70
Silexin Cough - See
DEXTROMETHORPHAN 292
GUAIFENESIN 408
Silphen - See ANTIHISTAMINES 92
Silvadene - See ANTIBACTERIALS, ANTIFUNGALS
(Topical) 70
SILVER SULFADIAZINE - See ANTIBACTERIALS,
ANTIFUNGALS (Topical) 70
Simaal 2 Gel - See ANTACIDS 56
Simaal Gel - See ANTACIDS 56
SIMETHICONE 786
SIMETHICONE, ALUMINA, CALCIUM
CARBONATE, AND MAGNESIA - See
ANTACIDS 56
SIMETHICONE, ALUMINA, MAGNESIUM
CARBONATE, AND MAGNESIA - See
ANTACIDS 56
Simron - See IRON SUPPLEMENTS 454
SIMVASTATIN - See HMG-CoA REDUCTASE
INHIBITORS 424
Sinarest - See ACETAMINOPHEN 2
Sinarest 12 Hour Nasal Spray - See
XYLOMETAZOLINE & OXYMETAZOLINE
(Nasal) 898
Sinarest No Drowsiness - See
ACETAMINOPHEN 2
PSEUDOEPHEDRINE 736
Sincomen - See SPIRONOLACTONE 796
Sine-Aid - See
ACETAMINOPHEN 2
PSEUDOEPHEDRINE 736
Sine-Aid Maximum Strength - See
ACETAMINOPHEN 2
PSEUDOEPHEDRINE 736
Sine-Aid Maximum Strength Caplets - See
ACETAMINOPHEN 2
PSEUDOEPHEDRINE 736

Sofarin - See ANTICOAGULANTS (Oral) 74
Solatene - See BETA CAROTENE 138
Solazine - See PHENOTHIAZINES 678
Solfoton - See BARBITURATES 122
Solium - See BENZODIAZEPINES 130
Solu-Cortef - See HYDROCORTISONE (Cortisol) 430
Solu-Flur - See SODIUM FLUORIDE 792
Solu-Medrol - See METHYLPREDNISOLONE 546
Solu-Phyllin - See BRONCHODILATORS, XANTHINE 152
Solurex - See DEXAMETHASONE 290
Solurex LA - See DEXAMETHASONE 290
Soma - See MUSCLE RELAXANTS, SKELETAL 578
Soma Compound w/Codeine - See NARCOTIC ANALGESICS 592
Sominex Liquid - See ANTIHISTAMINES 92
Somnol - See BENZODIAZEPINES 130
Somophyllin - See BRONCHODILATORS, XANTHINE 152
Somophyllin-12 - See BRONCHODILATORS, XANTHINE 152
Somophyllin-CRT - See BRONCHODILATORS, XANTHINE 152
Somophyllin-DF - See BRONCHODILATORS, XANTHINE 152
Somophyllin-T - See BRONCHODILATORS, XANTHINE 152
Som-Pam - See BENZODIAZEPINES 130
Sopamycetin - See ANTIBACTERIALS (Otic) 66
Sopamycetin Ophthalmic Ointment - See ANTIBACTERIALS (Ophthalmic) 64
Sopamycetin Ophthalmic Solution - See ANTIBACTERIALS (Ophthalmic) 64
Soprodol - See MUSCLE RELAXANTS, SKELETAL 578
Sorbitrate - See NITRATES 614
Sorbitrate SA - See NITRATES 614
Soridol - See MUSCLE RELAXANTS, SKELETAL 578
Sotacor - See BETA-ADRENERGIC BLOCKERS 134
SOTALOL - See BETA-ADRENERGIC BLOCKERS 134
Spancap - See AMPHETAMINES 34
Span-FF - See IRON SUPPLEMENTS 454
Span-Niacin - See NIACIN (Vitamin B-3, Nicotinic Acid) 604
Span-RD - See APPETITE SUPPRESSANTS 106
Spasgesic - See CHLORZOXAZONE & ACETAMINOPHEN 212
Spaslin - See BELLADONNA ALKALOIDS & BARBITURATES 128
Spasmoban - See DICYCLOMINE 300
Spasmoject - See DICYCLOMINE 300
Spasmolin - See
  BELLADONNA ALKALOIDS & BARBITURATES 128
  HYOSCYAMINE 440
  SCOPOLAMINE (Hyoscine) 776

Spasmophen - See BELLADONNA ALKALOIDS & BARBITURATES 128
Spasquid - See
  BELLADONNA ALKALOIDS & BARBITURATES 128
  HYOSCYAMINE 440
  SCOPOLAMINE (Hyoscine) 776
Spastolate - See HYOSCYAMINE 440
Spastosed - See ANTACIDS 56
Spec T - See ANESTHETICS, DENTAL (Topical) 48
Spectazole - See ANTIFUNGALS (Topical) 84
Spectrobid - See BACAMPICILLIN 118
Spectro-Chlor Ophthalmic Ointment - See ANTIBACTERIALS (Ophthalmic) 64
Spectro-Chlor Ophthalmic Solution - See ANTIBACTERIALS (Ophthalmic) 64
Spectro-Genta - See ANTIBACTERIALS (Ophthalmic) 64
Spectro-Homatropine - See CYCLOPEGIC, MYDRIATIC (Ophthalmic) 266
Spectro-Pentolate - See CYCLOPENTOLATE (Ophthalmic) 268
Spectro-Sulf - See ANTIBACTERIALS (Ophthalmic) 64
SPIRONOLACTONE 796
SPIRONOLACTONE & HYDROCHLOROTHIAZIDE 798
Spirozide - See SPIRONOLACTONE & HYDROCHLOROTHIAZIDE 798
SRC Expectorant - See
  GUAIFENESIN 408
  NARCOTIC ANALGESICS 592
  PSEUDOEPHEDRINE 736
SSKI - See POTASSIUM IODIDE 698
S-T Cort - See ADRENOCORTICOIDS (Topical) 14
St. Joseph Antidiarrheal - See ATTAPULGITE 114
St. Joseph Aspirin Free - See ACETAMINOPHEN 2
St. Joseph Cold Tablets for Children - See
  ACETAMINOPHEN 2
  PHENYLPROPANOLAMINE 686
St. Joseph for Children - See
  DEXTROMETHORPHAN 292
Stadol - See NARCOTIC ANALGESICS 592
Stadol NS - See NARCOTIC ANALGESICS 592
Stamoist E - See
  GUAIFENESIN 408
  PSEUDOEPHEDRINE 736
Stamoist LA - See
  GUAIFENESIN 408
  PHENYLPROPANOLAMINE 686
STANOZOLOL - See ANDROGENS 42
Staphcillin - See METHICILLIN 530
Statex - See NARCOTIC ANALGESICS 592
Staticin - See
  ANTIBACTERIALS FOR ACNE (Topical) 72
  ERYTHROMYCINS 354
Statobex - See APPETITE SUPPRESSANTS 106
Statuss Expectorant - See
  NARCOTIC ANALGESICS 592
  PHENYLEPHRINE 682

INDEX

SULFISOXAZOLE & PHENAZOPYRIDINE - See
SULFONAMIDES & PHENAZOPYRIDINE 814
Sulfonamide - See SULFONAMIDES &
PHENAZOPYRIDINE 814
SULFONAMIDES (Ophthalmic) - See
ANTIBACTERIALS (Ophthalmic) 64
SULFONAMIDES & PHENAZOPYRIDINE 814
Sulfone - See DAPSONE 282
Sulfonurea - See ANTIDIABETIC AGENTS 78
Sulforcin - See ANTI-ACNE (Topical) 60
Sulfoxaprim - See
SULFAMETHOXAZOLE 806
TRIMETHOPRIM 876
Sulfoxaprim DS - See SULFAMETHOXAZOLE 806
SULFUR (Scalp) - See ANTISEBORRHEICS
(Topical) 100
SULFUR (Topical) - See ANTI-ACNE (Topical) 60
SULFURATED LIME - See ANTI-ACNE,
CLEANSING (Topical) 62
SULINDAC - See ANTI-INFLAMMATORY DRUGS,
NON-STEROIDAL (NSAIDs) 94
Sulmeprim - See
SULFAMETHOXAZOLE 806
TRIMETHOPRIM 876
Sulpho-Lac - See ANTI-ACNE (Topical) 60
Sulsal Soap - See ANTI-ACNE (Topical) 60
Sulten-10 - See ANTIBACTERIALS (Ophthalmic) 64
Summit - See ACETAMINOPHEN 2
Sumycin - See TETRACYCLINES 828
Sunkist - See VITAMIN C (Ascorbic Acid) 888
Supac - See
ACETAMINOPHEN & SALICYLATES 4
ASPIRIN 108
CAFFEINE 166
Supasa - See ASPIRIN 108
Super-Anahist - See
ACETAMINOPHEN 2
PSEUDOEPHEDRINE 736
Super Calcium 1200 - See CALCIUM
SUPPLEMENTS 170
SuperChar - See CHARCOAL, ACTIVATED 192
Supeudol - See NARCOTIC ANALGESICS 592
Suppap - See ACETAMINOPHEN 2
Suprax - See CEPHALOSPORINS 190
Suprazine - See PHENOTHIAZINES 678
Surfak - See DOCUSATE CALCIUM 328
Surgam - See ANTI-INFLAMMATORY DRUGS,
NON-STEROIDAL (NSAIDs) 94
Surmontil - See TRICYCLIC ANTIDEPRESSANTS
868
Susano - See BELLADONNA ALKALOIDS &
BARBITURATES 128
Sus-Phrine - See BRONCHODILATORS,
ADRENERGIC 150
Sust-A - See VITAMIN A 884
Sustaire - See BRONCHODILATORS, XANTHINE
152
Sutilan - See TIOPRONIN 852
Syllact - See PSYLLIUM 740
Symadine - See AMANTADINE 18
Symmetrel - See AMANTADINE 18

Sympathomimetic - See
BRONCHODILATORS, ADRENERGIC 150
EPHEDRINE 340
ISOPROTERENOL & PHENYLEPHRINE 460
METHYLPHENIDATE 544
PHENYLEPHRINE 682
PHENYLPROPANOLAMINE 686
PSEUDOEPHEDRINE 736
THEOPHYLLINE, EPHEDRINE &
BARBITURATES 830
THEOPHYLLINE, EPHEDRINE & HYDROXYZINE
834
THEOPHYLLINE, EPHEDRINE, GUAIFENESIN &
BARBITURATES 832
XYLOMETAZOLINE & OXYMETAZOLINE (Nasal)
898
Synacort - See ADRENOCORTICOIDS (Topical) 14
Synalar - See ADRENOCORTICOIDS (Topical) 14
Synalgos - See
ASPIRIN 108
CAFFEINE 166
Synalgos-DC - See
CAFFEINE 166
NARCOTIC & ASPIRIN 594
NARCOTIC ANALGESICS 592
Synamol - See ADRENOCORTICOIDS (Topical) 14
Synandone - See ADRENOCORTICOIDS (Topical)
14
Synarel - See NAFARELIN 582
Syn-Captopril - See ANGIOTENSIN-CONVERTING
ENZYME (ACE) INHIBITORS 52
Syncophylate-GG - See THEOPHYLLINE &
GUAIFENESIN 836
Syn-Diltiazem - See CALCIUM CHANNEL
BLOCKERS 168
Synemol - See ADRENOCORTICOIDS (Topical) 14
Synflex - See ANTI-INFLAMMATORY DRUGS,
NON-STEROIDAL (NSAIDs) 94
Synkayvite - See VITAMIN K 894
Synophylate - See BRONCHODILATORS,
XANTHINE 152
Synphasic - See CONTRACEPTIVES, ORAL 250
Syn-Pindolol - See BETA-ADRENERGIC
BLOCKERS 134
Synthroid - See THYROID HORMONES 846
Synvinolin - See HMG-CoA REDUCTASE
INHIBITORS 424
Syracol Liquid - See
DEXTROMETHORPHAN 292
PHENYLPROPANOLAMINE 686

T

Tac-3 - See TRIAMCINOLONE 860
TACE - See ESTROGENS 360
Tagamet - See HISTAMINE H$_2$ RECEPTOR
ANTAGONISTS 422
Talacen - See NARCOTIC & ACETAMINOPHEN
590
TALBUTAL - See BARBITURATES 122
Talwin - See NARCOTIC ANALGESICS 592
Talwin Compound - See NARCOTIC & ASPIRIN 594

INDEX

INDEX

Triamonide 40 - See TRIAMCINOLONE 860
TRIAMTERENE 862
TRIAMTERENE & HYDROCHLOROTHIAZIDE 864
Trianide - See ADRENOCORTICOIDS (Topical) 14
Triaphen - See ASPIRIN 108
Triaprin - See
  ACETAMINOPHEN 2
  BARBITURATES 122
Triasox - See THIABENDAZOLE 838
Triavil - See PERPHENAZINE & AMITRIPTYLINE
  672
TRIAZOLAM 866
Triazole - See
  SULFAMETHOXAZOLE 806
  TRIMETHOPRIM 876
Triazole DS - See SULFAMETHOXAZOLE 806
Tri-B3 - See NIACIN (Vitamin B-3, Nicotinic Acid)
  604
TRIBASIC CALCIUM PHOSPHATE - See CALCIUM
  SUPPLEMENTS 170
Tribavirin - See RIBAVIRIN 766
TRICHLORMETHIAZIDE - See DIURETICS,
  THIAZIDE 324
TRICITRATES - See CITRATES 220
Tricodene –1 - See
  NARCOTIC ANALGESICS 592
  TERPIN HYDRATE 822
Tricodene Forte - See
  ANTIHISTAMINES 92
  DEXTROMETHORPHAN 292
  PHENYLPROPANOLAMINE 686
Tricodene NN - See
  ANTIHISTAMINES 92
  DEXAMETHASONE 290
  PHENYLPROPANOLAMINE 686
Tricodene NN Cough and Cold Medication - See
  CITRATES 220
  TERPIN HYDRATE 822
Tricodene Pediatric - See
  DEXTROMETHORPHAN 292
  PHENYLPROPANOLAMINE 686
Triconsil - See ANTACIDS 56
Tricosal - See SALICYLATES 774
TRICYCLIC ANTIDEPRESSANTS 868
Tridesilon Solution - See ANTIBACTERIALS (Otic)
  66
Tridil - See NITRATES 614
Tridione - See ANTICONVULSANTS, DIONE-TYPE
  76
Trifed - See
  ANTIHISTAMINES 92
  PSEUDOEPHEDRINE 736
Trifed-C Cough - See
  ANTIHISTAMINES 92
  NARCOTIC ANALGESICS 592
  PSEUDOEPHEDRINE 736
TRIFLUOPERAZINE - See PHENOTHIAZINES 678
Trifluorothymidine - See ANTIVIRALS (Ophthalmic)
  104
TRIFLUPROMAZINE - See PHENOTHIAZINES 678
TRIFLURIDINE - See ANTIVIRALS (Ophthalmic)
  104

Trigesic - See
  ACETAMINOPHEN & SALICYLATES 4
  CAFFEINE 166
Trihexane - See ANTIDYSKINETICS 80
Trihexy - See ANTIDYSKINETICS 80
TRIHEXYPHENIDYL - See ANTIDYSKINETICS 80
Tri-Hydroserpine - See RESERPINE,
  HYDRALAZINE & HYDROCHLOROTHIAZIDE
  764
Tri-K - See POTASSIUM SUPPLEMENTS 704
Trikacide - See METRONIDAZOLE 554
TRIKATES - See POTASSIUM SUPPLEMENTS 704
Tri-Kort - See TRIAMCINOLONE 860
Trilafon - See PHENOTHIAZINES 678
Trilafon Concentrate - See PHENOTHIAZINES 678
Trilax - See
  DEHYDROCHOLIC ACID 286
  DOCUSATE SODIUM 332
  PHENOLPHTHALEIN 676
Tri-Levlen - See CONTRACEPTIVES, ORAL 250
Trilisate - See SALICYLATES 774
Trilog - See TRIAMCINOLONE 860
Trilombrin - See PYRANTEL 742
Trilone - See TRIAMCINOLONE 860
Trimcaps - See APPETITE SUPPRESSANTS 106
Trimedine Liquid - See
  ANTIHISTAMINES 92
  DEXTROMETHORPHAN 292
  PHENYLEPHRINE 682
TRIMEPRAZINE 872
Trimeth-Sulfa - See
  SULFAMETHOXAZOLE 806
  TRIMETHOPRIM 876
TRIMETHADIONE - See ANTICONVULSANTS,
  DIONE-TYPE 76
TRIMETHOBENZAMIDE 874
TRIMETHOPRIM 876
TRIMIPRAMINE - See TRICYCLIC
  ANTIDEPRESSANTS 868
Trimox - See AMOXICILLIN 32
Trimpex - See TRIMETHOPRIM 876
Trimstat - See APPETITE SUPPRESSANTS 106
Trimtabs - See APPETITE SUPPRESSANTS 106
Trinalin Repetabs - See
  ANTIHISTAMINES 92
  PSEUDOEPHEDRINE 736
Trind - See
  ANTIHISTAMINES 92
  PHENYLPROPANOLAMINE 686
Trind DM Liquid - See
  ANTIHISTAMINES 92
  DEXTROMETHORPHAN 292
  PHENYLPROPANOLAMINE 686
Tri-Nefrin Extra Strength - See
  ANTIHISTAMINES 92
  PHENYLPROPANOLAMINE 686
Trinex - See
  ANTIHISTAMINES 92
  GUAIFENESIN 408
  PSEUDOEPHEDRINE 736
Tri-Norinyl - See
  CONTRACEPTIVES, ORAL 250

ESTROGENS 360
TRILOSTANE 870
Triofed - See
  ANTIHISTAMINES 92
  PSEUDOEPHEDRINE 736
Triotann - See
  ANTIHISTAMINES 92
  PHENYLEPHRINE 682
TRIOXSALEN - See PSORALENS 738
Tri-Pain - See ACETAMINOPHEN & SALICYLATES 4
Tripalgen Cold - See
  ANTIHISTAMINES 92
  PHENYLPROPANOLAMINE 686
TRIPELENNAMINE - See ANTIHISTAMINES 92
Triphasil - See CONTRACEPTIVES, ORAL 250
Tri-Phen-Chlor - See
  ANTIHISTAMINES 92
  PHENYLEPHRINE 682
  PHENYLPROPANOLAMINE 686
Tri-Phen-Chlor T.D. - See
  ANTIHISTAMINES 92
  PHENYLEPHRINE 682
  PHENYLPROPANOLAMINE 686
Triphenyl - See
  ANTIHISTAMINES 92
  PHENYLPROPANOLAMINE 686
Triphenyl Expectorant - See
  GUAIFENESIN 408
  PHENYLPROPANOLAMINE 686
Triphenyl T.D. - See
  ANTIHISTAMINES 92
  PHENYLPROPANOLAMINE 686
Triple X - See PEDICULISIDES (Topical) 656
Tripodrine - See
  ANTIHISTAMINES 92
  PSEUDOEPHEDRINE 736
Triposed - See
  ANTIHISTAMINES 92
  PSEUDOEPHEDRINE 736
TRIPROLIDINE - See ANTIHISTAMINES 92
Triptil - See TRICYCLIC ANTIDEPRESSANTS 868
Trip-Tone - See ANTIHISTAMINES 92
Trisatin - See NYSTATIN 622
Trisoralen - See PSORALENS 738
Tristatin - See ANTIBACTERIALS, ANTIFUNGALS
  (Topical) 70
Tristatin II - See TRIAMCINOLONE 860
Tristoject - See TRIAMCINOLONE 860
Trisulfam - See
  SULFAMETHOXAZOLE 806
  TRIMETHOPRIM 876
Tritann Pediatric - See
  ANTIHISTAMINES 92
  PHENYLEPHRINE 682
Tri-Vi-Flor - See VITAMINS & FLUORIDE 896
Trocal - See
  DEXTROMETHORPHAN 292
  GUAIFENESIN 408
Tronolane - See ANESTHETICS (Rectal) 44

Tronothane - See
  ANESTHETICS (Rectal) 44
  ANESTHETICS (Topical) 46
Truphylline - See BRONCHODILATORS,
  XANTHINE 152
Truxophyllin - See BRONCHODILATORS,
  XANTHINE 152
Trymegen - See ANTIHISTAMINES 92
Trymex - See ADRENOCORTICOIDS (Topical) 14
T-Stat - See
  ANTIBACTERIALS FOR ACNE (Topical) 72
  ERYTHROMYCINS 354
Tubasal - See PARA-AMINOSALICYLIC ACID
  (Aminosalicylate Sodium) 648
Tubizid - See ISONIAZID 458
Tuinal - See BARBITURATES 122
Tums - See
  ANTACIDS 56
  CALCIUM SUPPLEMENTS 170
Tums E-X - See
  ANTACIDS 56
  CALCIUM SUPPLEMENTS 170
Tums Liquid Extra Strength - See ANTACIDS 56
Tums Liquid Extra Strength with Simethicone - See
  ANTACIDS 56
Tusquelin - See
  ANTIHISTAMINES 92
  DEXTROMETHORPHAN 292
  PHENYLEPHRINE 682
  PHENYLPROPANOLAMINE 686
Tuss Allergine Modified T.D. - See
  PHENYLPROPANOLAMINE 686
Tuss-Ade - See PHENYLPROPANOLAMINE 686
Tussafed - See
  ANTIHISTAMINES 92
  DEXTROMETHORPHAN 292
  PSEUDOEPHEDRINE 736
Tussagesic - See
  ACETAMINOPHEN 2
  ANTIHISTAMINES 92
  DEXTROMETHORPHAN 292
  PHENYLPROPANOLAMINE 686
  TERPIN HYDRATE 822
Tussaminic C Forte - See
  PHENYLPROPANOLAMINE 686
Tussaminic C Pediatric - See
  PHENYLPROPANOLAMINE 686
Tussaminic DH Forte - See
  ANTIHISTAMINES 92
  NARCOTIC ANALGESICS 592
  PHENYLPROPANOLAMINE 686
Tussaminic DH Pediatric - See
  ANTIHISTAMINES 92
  NARCOTIC ANALGESICS 592
  PHENYLPROPANOLAMINE 686
Tussanil DH Tablets - See
  ANTIHISTAMINES 92
  GUAIFENESIN 408
  NARCOTIC ANALGESICS 592

INDEX

INDEX

Valisone - See ADRENOCORTICOIDS (Topical) 14
Valisone Scalp Lotion - See ADRENOCORTICOIDS (Topical) 14
Valium - See BENZODIAZEPINES 130
Valmid - See ETHINAMATE 364
Valnac - See ADRENOCORTICOIDS (Topical) 14
Valorin - See ACETAMINOPHEN 2
Valorin Extra - See ACETAMINOPHEN 2
VALPROIC ACID (Dipropylacetic Acid) 880
Valrelease - See BENZODIAZEPINES 130
Vamate - See HYDROXYZINE 438
Vancenase - See ADRENOCORTICOIDS (Nasal) 12
Vancenase AQ - See ADRENOCORTICOIDS (Nasal) 12
Vanceril - See BECLOMETHASONE 124
Vancocin - See VANCOMYCIN 882
VANCOMYCIN 882
Vanex-HD - See
  ANTIHISTAMINES 92
  NARCOTIC ANALGESICS 592
  PHENYLEPHRINE 682
Vanoxide 5 Lotion - See BENZOYL PEROXIDE 132
Vanquin - See PYRVINIUM 748
Vanquish - See
  ACETAMINOPHEN & SALICYLATES 4
  CAFFEINE 166
Vanseb - See ANTI-ACNE (Topical) 60
Vanseb Cream Dandruff Shampoo - See ANTISEBORRHEICS (Topical) 100
Vanseb Lotion Dandruff Shampoo - See ANTISEBORRHEICS (Topical) 100
Vanseb-T - See ANTISEBORRHEICS (Topical) 100
Vapo-Iso - See BRONCHODILATORS, ADRENERGIC 150
Vaponefrin - See BRONCHODILATORS, ADRENERGIC 150
Vascor - See CALCIUM CHANNEL BLOCKERS 168
Vascular headache suppressant - See ISOMETHEPTENE, DICHLORALPHENAZONE & ACETAMINOPHEN 456
Vasepam - See BENZODIAZEPINES 130
Vaseretic - See ANGIOTENSIN-CONVERTING ENZYME (ACE) INHIBITORS & HYDROCHLOROTHIZIDE 54
VasoClear - See DECONGESTANTS (Ophthalmic) 284
Vasocon - See DECONGESTANTS (Ophthalmic) 284
Vasoconstrictor - See
  ERGOTAMINE 346
  ERGOTAMINE, BELLADONNA & PHENOBARBITAL 348
  ERGOTAMINE & CAFFEINE 350
  ERGOTAMINE, CAFFEINE, BELLADONNA & PENTOBARBITAL 352
  METHYSERGIDE 550
  ORPHENADRINE, ASPIRIN & CAFFEINE 632
Vasodilan - See ISOXSUPRINE 464
Vasodilator - See
  CYCLANDELATE 260
  ISOXSUPRINE 464

NIACIN (Vitamin B-3, Nicotinic Acid) 604
NYLIDRIN 620
PAPAVERINE 646
Vasominic T.D. - See
  ANTIHISTAMINES 92
  PHENYLEPHRINE 682
  PHENYLPROPANOLAMINE 686
Vasoprine - See ISOXSUPRINE 464
Vasotec - See ANGIOTENSIN-CONVERTING ENZYME (ACE) INHIBITORS 52
Vaxoconstrictor - See CAFFEINE 166
VCF - See CONTRACEPTIVES, VAGINAL (Spermicides) 252
V-Cillin K - See PENICILLIN V 664
VC-K - See PENICILLIN V 664
Veetids - See PENICILLIN V 664
Veganin - See NARCOTIC & ACETAMINOPHEN 590
Velosef - See CEPHALOSPORINS 190
Velosulin - See INSULIN 444
Velosulin Human - See INSULIN 444
Veltane - See ANTIHISTAMINES 92
Veltap - See
  ANTIHISTAMINES 92
  PHENYLEPHRINE 682
  PHENYLPROPANOLAMINE 686
Ventolin - See BRONCHODILATORS, ADRENERGIC 150
Ventolin Rotocaps - See BRONCHODILATORS, ADRENERGIC 150
VePesid - See ETOPOSIDE 374
VERAPAMIL - See CALCIUM CHANNEL BLOCKERS 168
Verazinc - See ZINC SUPPLEMENTS 902
Verelan - See CALCIUM CHANNEL BLOCKERS 168
Vermox - See MEBENDAZOLE 506
Versabran - See PSYLLIUM 740
Verukan Topical Solution - See ANTI-ACNE (Topical) 60
Verukan-HP Topical Solution - See ANTI-ACNE (Topical) 60
Vesprin - See PHENOTHIAZINES 678
Vibramycin - See TETRACYCLINES 828
Vibratabs - See TETRACYCLINES 828
Vibutal - See BUTALBITAL & ASPIRIN (Also contains caffeine) 162
Vicks Children's Cough - See
  DEXTROMETHORPHAN 292
  GUAIFENESIN 408
Vicks Formula 44 Cough Mixture - See
  ANTIHISTAMINES 92
  DEXTROMETHORPHAN 292
Vicks Formula 44D Decongestant Cough Mixture - See
  DEXTROMETHORPHAN 292
  GUAIFENESIN 408
  PSEUDOEPHEDRINE 736
Vicks Formula 44M Multi-symptom Cough Mixture - See
  ACETAMINOPHEN 2
  DEXTROMETHORPHAN 292

Wolfina - See RAUWOLFIA ALKALOIDS 758
Wyamycin E - See ERYTHROMYCINS 354
Wyamycin S - See ERYTHROMYCINS 354
Wycillin - See PENICILLIN G 662
Wygesic - See NARCOTIC & ACETAMINOPHEN
  590
Wymox - See AMOXICILLIN 32
Wytensin - See GUANABENZ 410

X

Xanax - See BENZODIAZEPINES 130
Xenon Xe 127 - See RADIO-PHARMACEUTICALS
  756
Xenon Xe 133 - See RADIO-PHARMACEUTICALS
  756
Xerac 5 Lotion - See ANTI-ACNE, CLEANSING
  (Topical) 62
Xerac BP 5 Gel - See BENZOYL PEROXIDE 132
Xerac BP 10 Gel - See BENZOYL PEROXIDE 132
X-Prep Liquid - See SENNA 780
Xseb - See ANTI-ACNE (Topical) 60
X-Trozine - See APPETITE SUPPRESSANTS 106
X-Trozine LA - See APPETITE SUPPRESSANTS
  106
Xylocaine - See
  ANESTHETICS (Topical) 46
  ANESTHETICS, DENTAL (Topical) 48
Xylocaine Viscous - See ANESTHETICS, DENTAL
  (Topical) 48
XYLOMETAZOLINE & OXYMETAZOLINE (Nasal)
  898

Y

Yodoxin - See IODOQUINOL 448
Yutopar - See RITODRINE 772

Z

Zantac - See HISTAMINE H$_2$ RECEPTOR
  ANTAGONISTS 422
Zantryl - See APPETITE SUPPRESSANTS 106
Zapex - See BENZODIAZEPINES 130
Zarontin - See ETHOSUXIMIDE 368
Zaroxolyn - See DIURETICS, THIAZIDE 324
Zeasorb-AF Powder - See ANTIFUNGALS (Topical)
  84
Zephrex - See
  GUAIFENESIN 408

PSEUDOEPHEDRINE 736
Zephrex-LA - See
  GUAIFENESIN 408
  PSEUDOEPHEDRINE 736
Zeroxin-5 Gel - See BENZOYL PEROXIDE 132
Zeroxin-10 Gel - See BENZOYL PEROXIDE 132
Zestoretic - See ANGIOTENSIN-CONVERTING
  ENZYME (ACE) INHIBITORS &
  HYDROCHLOROTHIZIDE 54
Zestril - See ANGIOTENSIN-CONVERTING
  ENZYME (ACE) INHIBITORS 52
Zetar - See COAL TAR (Topical) 242
Zetar Emulsion - See COAL TAR (Topical) 242
Zetar Medicated Antiseborrheic Shampoo - See
  COAL TAR (Topical) 242
Zetran - See BENZODIAZEPINES 130
ZIDOVUDINE (AZT, Azidothymidine) 900
ZINC CHLORIDE - See ZINC SUPPLEMENTS 902
ZINC GLUCONATE - See ZINC SUPPLEMENTS
  902
ZINC SULFATE - See ZINC SUPPLEMENTS 902
ZINC SUPPLEMENTS 902
Zinc-220 - See ZINC SUPPLEMENTS 902
Zincate - See ZINC SUPPLEMENTS 902
Zincaps-220 - See ZINC SUPPLEMENTS 902
Zincon - See ANTISEBORRHEICS (Topical) 100
ZNP - See ANTISEBORRHEICS (Topical) 100
Zocor - See HMG-CoA REDUCTASE INHIBITORS
  424
Zoloft - See SERTRALINE 784
Zorprin - See ASPIRIN 108
Zostrix - See
  ANESTHETICS (Topical) 46
  CAPSAICIN 172
Zostrix-HP - See
  ANESTHETICS (Topical) 46
  CAPSAICIN 172
Zovirax - See ACYLOVIR (Oral & Topical) 10
Zovirax Ointment - See ACYLOVIR (Oral & Topical)
  10
Zurinol - See ALLOPURINOL 16
Zydone - See NARCOTIC & ACETAMINOPHEN
  590
Zyloprim - See ALLOPURINOL 16
Zymase - See PANCRELIPASE 642
Zymenol - See MINERAL OIL 562

An invaluable medical information library from one of America's most trusted family physicians, Dr. H. Winter Griffith.

Complete Guide to Symptoms, Illness & Surgery, 2nd Edition
Featuring hundreds of signs and symptoms, this guide helps you diagnose, understand, and seek treatment for a wide variety of illnesses and disorders.

Complete Guide to Symptoms, Illness & Surgery for People Over 50
The most comprehensive medical reference available for older Americans.

Complete Guide to Prescription & Non-Prescription Drugs, 1994 Edition
The latest edition of the bestselling reference, offering easy-to-understand, dependable information on thousands of brand-name and generic drugs.

Complete Guide to Pediatric Symptoms, Illness & Medications
A comprehensive guide to diagnosing and treating childhood illnesses and disorders.

Complete Guide to Sports Injuries
An essential reference for recognizing and caring for sports-related injuries.

These books are available at your bookstore or wherever books are sold,
or for your convenience, we'll send them directly to you.
Just call 1-800-631-8571 (press 1 for inquiries and orders)
or fill out the coupon below and send it to:
The Putnam Publishing Group
390 Murray Hill Parkway, Dept. B — East Rutherford, NJ 07073

		Price	
		U.S.	Canada
_____Complete Guide to Symptoms, Illness & Surgery	399-51709-X	$15.95	$20.95
_____Complete Guide to Symptoms, Illness & Surgery for People Over 50	399-51749-9	18.95	24.95
_____Complete Guide to Prescription & Non-Prescription Drugs, 1994 Edition	399-51835-5	15.95	20.95
_____Complete Guide to Pediatric Symptoms, Illness & Medications	895-86816-4	14.95	19.50
_____Complete Guide to Sports Injuries	399-51712-X	14.95	19.50

Subtotal	$_____
Postage & handling	$_____
Sales tax (CA, NJ, NY, PA)	$_____
Total amount due	$_____

Payable in U.S. funds (no cash orders accepted). $15.00 minimum on credit card orders.
*Postage & handling: $2.50 for 1 book, 75¢ for each additional book up to a maximum of $6.25.

Enclosed is my   □check □money order
Please charge my   □Visa □MasterCard □American Express
Card #_____ Expiration date_____
Signature as on charge card_____
Name_____
Address_____
City_____ State_____ Zip_____
Please allow six weeks for delivery. Prices subject to change without notice.

Source key #44

EMERGENCY GUIDE FOR OVERDOSE VICTIMS

This section lists *basic* steps in recognizing and treating immediate effects of drug overdose.

Study the information before you need it. If possible, take a course in first aid and learn external cardiac massage and mouth-to-mouth breathing techniques, called *cardiopulmonary resuscitation* (CPR).

For quick reference, list emergency telephone numbers in the spaces provided on the inside front cover for fire department paramedics, ambulance, poison-control center and your doctor. These numbers, except for doctor, are usually listed on the inside cover of your telephone directory.

IF VICTIM IS UNCONSCIOUS, NOT BREATHING:

1. Yell for help. Don't leave victim.

2. Begin mouth-to-mouth breathing immediately.

3. If there is no heartbeat, give external cardiac massage.

4. Have someone call 0 (operator) or 911 (emergency) for an ambulance or medical help.

5. Don't stop CPR until help arrives.

6. Don't try to make victim vomit.

7. If vomiting occurs, save vomit to take to emergency room for analysis.

8. Take medicine or empty bottles with you to emergency room.

IF VICTIM IS UNCONSCIOUS AND BREATHING:

1. Dial 0 (operator) or 911 (emergency) for an ambulance or medical help.

2. If you can't get help immediately, take victim to the nearest emergency room.

3. Don't try to make victim vomit.

4. If vomiting occurs, save vomit to take to emergency room for analysis.

5. Watch victim carefully on the way to the emergency room. If heart or breathing stops, use cardiac massage and mouth-to-mouth breathing (CPR).

6. Take medicine or empty bottles with you to emergency room.